Contact Lenses

This third edition is dedicated to the memory of
Fred 'Budge' Wilmot, original coordinator of
the first edition in its formative days at The City
University, London. Without his enthusiasm
and persistence *Contact Lenses* would not have
come into being.

Janet Stone
Tony Phillips

Contact Lenses
A Textbook for Practitioner and Student
Third Edition

Edited by

Anthony J. Phillips MPhil, FBOA HD, FBCO, FAAO, DCLP
Contact Lens Practitioner and Optometrist, Contact Lens Department,
Flinders Medical Centre, Adelaide, South Australia

Janet Stone FBOA HD, FBCO, FAAO, DCLP
Contact Lens Practitioner, Shrewsbury.
Formerly Senior Lecturer, The London Refraction Hospital

Butterworths
London Boston Singapore Sydney Toronto Wellington

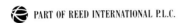 PART OF REED INTERNATIONAL P.L.C.

First published 1972
Reprinted 1976
Second edition (2 vols) 1980, 1981
Combined second edition 1984
Third edition 1989

© **Butterworth & Co. (Publishers) Ltd, 1989**

British Library Cataloguing in Publication Data

Contact lenses – 3rd ed.
  1. Contact lenses
  I. Phillips, A. J. (Anthony John), *1942–*
  II. Stone, Janet, *1935–*
617.7′523

  ISBN 0-407-93275-5

Library of Congress Cataloguing in Publication Data

Contact lenses: a textbook for practitioner and
  student / edited by Anthony J. Phillips and
  Janet Stone. -- 3rd ed.
    p.   cm.
  Bibliography: p.
  Includes index.
  ISBN 0-407-93275-5 :
  1. Contact lenses. I. Phillips, Anthony John.
  II. Stone, Janet.
RE977.C6C59   1989
617.7′523--dc19   89-803
                         CIP

Photoset by Butterworths Litho Preparation Department
Printed and bound in Great Britain by Butler and Tanner,
Frome, Somerset

Preface to the third edition

This third edition of *Contact Lenses*, to be published at the conclusion of 100 years of contact lens practice, incorporates all the latest thinking and knowledge in the contact lens field. It also includes the terminology agreed in 1986 by the International Standards Organisation.

Since the publication of the second edition the advances of gas permeable hard lenses and extended wear lenses have made a major impact. In addition the specialized uses of contact lenses in keratoconus, aphakia, post-keratoplasty, paediatrics, and as prosthetic devices, have become increasingly important. Knowledge of the technical, physiological and pathological aspects has also increased and a much wider and more profound understanding of the whole field has been achieved. Several new contributors have joined the team involved in the preparation of the book, each of these being an acknowledged expert in his or her specific area.

The editors would like to express their thanks to all the co-authors for the work they have put in, not only into their own chapters but often for advice and comments on other chapters where they may also have had a special interest. In addition, we would like to thank the many contact lens prescription laboratories and solution manufacturers who have provided information and photographs and apologize to readers for any omissions.

We would also like to acknowledge the generous financial support provided by the laboratories in sponsoring the colour plate sections. These vital sections are produced at considerable expense and their sponsorship assists in reducing the overall cost of the book.

Finally we must acknowledge the logistical help of certain individuals: Professor Douglas Coster, Head of the Eye Department at Flinders Medical Centre, Adelaide, for providing the facilities of the Eye Department and many of the colour plates; Jennifer Taylor, Librarian, the British College of Optometrists; Eva Lefty for the enormous volume of typing and correspondence; and all of the many individuals who provided information and help.

Janet Stone,
Shrewsbury

Tony Phillips,
Adelaide

Preface to the second edition

The writing of a scientific textbook has one particular frustration. This is, of course, the fact that by the time it has passed through the various stages of production, the proofs read and the final corrections made, over a year will have passed since the manuscript was submitted to the publisher. During this time, scientific progress will have continued to advance at a phenomenal pace. Thus, whilst the manuscript may be completely up to date at the time of submission to the publisher, it is, of unfortunate necessity, that much out of date by the time it reaches the reader. For example, in the twelve months between submission of manuscript and publication of the first edition, hydrophilic lenses came to the forefront of contact lens development.

The second edition has been largely re-written to incorporate not only current knowledge on hydrophilic lenses but several new topics not dealt with in the first edition. This has been done to provide both a greater compass of this rapidly increasing science and also to cover more completely the examination syllabuses in contact lenses as laid down by the British Optical Association, now the British College of Ophthalmic Opticians (optometrists).

The editors would like to welcome the several new contributors to the book and to take the opportunity of thanking all the contributors for the work they have put in, not only into their own chapters but often for advice and comments on other chapters where they may also have had a special interest. In addition, we would like to thank the many prescription laboratories and solution manufacturers who have provided information and photographs as well as Mr W. S. Hodges of the British Standards Institution. Tony Phillips would also like to record his appreciation to four members of his staff – Linda Cholerton, Anne Collison, Julie Perrin and Pamela Bates – who dealt with much of the enormous volume of correspondence and the typing of illegible manuscripts at the Loughborough end of the editorial link. In particular, he would like to thank his wife, Susan, for her forebearance.

We would also like to acknowledge the great help of Miss J. M. Taylor, BA, ALA, Librarian and Museum Curator of the British Optical Association, in providing many of the references to other works used by various contributors. Without the availability of this service to the profession the production of a text of this nature, much of it written by people in practice without the facilities of a university library available to them, would be extremely difficult, if not impossible.

Finally, we would like to acknowledge the assistance of the British Optical Association without whose backing the book would not have come into being.

Janet Stone and Tony Phillips
London and Loughborough

Acknowledgements

The Publishers are most grateful to the following for their generous sponsorship of the colour plates contained in this book:

Abatron

Alcon Laboratories, Australia

Allergan Pharmaceuticals Pty Ltd, Australia

Bausch & Lomb UK Ltd

CIBA Vision, UK

CooperVision Ltd

David Thomas (Contact Lenses) Ltd

G. N. L. Contact Lenses, Australia

Hydron Europe Ltd

Madden & Layman Ltd

Pilkington Visioncare

Contributors

Christine L. K. Astin, BSc, FBCO, DCLP
Principal Optometrist, Contact Lens and Prosthesis
Department, Moorfields Eye Hospital, London, UK

Kerry W. Atkinson, FBCO, DCLP
Contact Lens Practitioner and Academic Associate
and Clinical Associate in Contact Lens Practice,
Department of Optometry, University of Auckland,
New Zealand

David Campbell-Burns, FBCO, FAAO, FBIM, ARPS
Contact Lens Practitioner, Crowborough,
Sussex, UK

John T. de Carle, FBCO, FAAO, DCLP
Contact Lens Practitioner, London, and Past
President, British Contact Lens Association,
London, UK

Bill A. Douthwaite, MSc, PhD, FBCO, DCLP
Lecturer in Optometry, Department of Optometry,
University of Bradford, Bradford, UK

Morley W. Ford, FBCO, FAAO, DCLP
Contact Lens Practitioner, North Shields, Tyne and
Wear, UK

John L. Francis, FBOA HD, DOrth
Formerly Senior Lecturer, The London Refraction
Hospital, London, UK

Andrew Gasson, FBCO, FAAO, DCLP
Contact Lens Practitioner, London, UK

Brien A. Holden, LOSc, PhD, FAAO
Associate Professor and Director, Cornea and
Contact Lens Research Unit, School of Optometry,
University of New South Wales, Kensington, NSW,
Australia

Graham A. Hopkins, BPharm, PhD, MRPharmS
Ophthalmic Products Manager, Smith & Nephew
Pharmaceuticals, Romford, UK

Donald F. C. Loran, MSc, FBCO, DCLP, AMCT
Clinical Director and Senior Lecturer, Department of
Optometry and Vision Sciences, University of
Manchester Institute of Science and Technology,
Manchester, UK

Charles W. McMonnies, MSc, FAAO
Contact Lens Practitioner and Senior Research
Consultant, Cornea and Contact Lens Research Unit,
School of Optometry, University of New South
Wales, Kensington, NSW, Australia

Anthony J. Phillips, MPhil, FBOA HD, FBCO, FAAO,
DCLP
Contact Lens Practitioner and Optometrist, Contact
Lens Department, Flinders Medical Centre,
Adelaide, South Australia

Michael J. A. Port, MSc, FBCO, DCLP, FAAO
Lecturer, Department of Optometry and Visual
Science, The City University, London, UK

Edmund J. D. Proctor, BSc, FBCO, FAAO, DCLP
Optometrist/Contact Lens Practitioner,
Kidderminster, Worcestershire, UK

Kenneth W. Pullum, BSc, FBCO, DCLP
Contact Lens Practitioner, Hertford, UK; Senior
Optometrist, Contact Lens and Prosthesis
Department, Moorfields Eye Hospital, London, UK,
and Oxford Eye Hospital, Oxford, UK

Roy H. Rengstorff, BSc, OD, MSc, PhD, FAAO
Contact Lens Practitioner, Maryland, USA; Adjunct
Faculty, Pennsylvania College of Optometry,
Philadelphia, USA

Gordon L. Ruskell, MS, PhD, DSc, FBCO
Professor of Ocular Anatomy, Department of
Optometry and Visual Science, The City University,
London, UK

Anthony G. Sabell, MSc, FBCO, DCLP
Ophthalmic Practitioner to the University of
Birmingham Health Service and Contact Lens
Practitioner to Birmingham Children's Hospital,
Birmingham, UK

Michael Sheridan, MSc, FBOA HD, FBCO, DCLP
Senior Lecturer in Optometry, Department of
Optometry, University of Bradford, Bradford, UK

Lynne Speedwell, BSc, FBCO, DCLP
Senior Optometrist, Contact Lens and Prosthesis
Department, Moorfields Eye Hospital and Great
Ormond Street Hospital for Sick Children,
London, UK

John H. Stewart-Jones, MPhil, SRN, OND, RNT
Senior Lecturer, Department of Optometry and
Visual Science, The City University, London, UK

Janet Stone, FBOA HD, FBCO, FAAO, DCLP
Contact Lens Practitioner, Shrewsbury,
Shropshire, UK

Helen Swarbrick, MSc
Senior Research Optometrist, Cornea and Contact
Lens Research Unit, School of Optometry, University
of New South Wales, Kensington, NSW, Australia

Brian J. Tighe, PhD, CChem, FRSC
Reader in Polymer Science, Department of Applied
Chemistry, The University of Aston,
Birmingham, UK

Rita Watts, FBCO
Optometrist, Leicestershire, UK; Formerly Lecturer,
Department of Optometry and Visual Science, The
City University, London, UK

David Westerhout, FBCO, FAAO, CLCert(SMC)
Contact Lens Practitioner, Harare, Zimbabwe;
Visiting Professor, The College of Optometry,
University of Houston, Texas, USA

E. Geoffrey Woodward, PhD, FBCO, DCLP
Professor of Optometry and Visual Science and
Head, Department of Optometry and Visual Science,
The City University, London, UK

Contents

Glossary of terms

Pharmaceutical terminology

British Pharmacopoeia terminology is used throughout the book with the exception of thiomersalate which is referred to by its American term of thimerosal since this is in wide international use and the BP term may cause confusion.

Contact lens terminology

Previous editions of the book have adopted British Standard terminology (BS 5562:1978 and BS 3521:1979). Because of the relatively small size of the eye-care professions and the ongoing interchange of journals, books and lectures it became increasingly apparent that confusion would result from the differing terminology used in different countries. To avoid this problem the International Standards Organisation published ISO 8320-1986 which has proposed a universal terminology which it is hoped will eventually be used in all countries. This standard has now been adopted as the British Standard BS 3521: Part 3: 1988 and it is expected that other countries will also adopt the new International Standard as their own Standards come up for revision. For these reasons the new ISO Standard terminology is used throughout this Third Edition. A brief summary of the most commonly used terms are set out below but both students and practitioners are urged to obtain and study the full Standard.

Extracts from BS 3521: Part 3 : 1988 are reproduced below with the permission of the British Standards Institute, complete copies of the Standard can be obtained by post from BSI Sales, Linford Wood, Milton Keynes, MK14 6LE.

Obsolete terms

Former British terms			Former American terms
Back central optic radius (BCOR)	=		Base curve (BC)
		or	Central posterior curve radius (PCCR)
Back central optic diameter (BCOD)	=		Posterior optic zone diameter (POZD) or optic zone (OZ)
Back peripheral optic radius (BPOR)	=		Peripheral curve radius (PCR)
Overall size (OS)	=		Lens diameter (LD)
		or	Total diameter (TD)

Summary of new terms relating to contact lens manufacture and materials

Reference in Standard

2.4.1	Water content	The proportion by mass of water retained within a lens under specified conditions
2.4.2	Wettability	A property of the contact lens surface as defined by the contact angle and measured under specified conditions
2.4.3	Oxygen permeability, *Dk*	The rate of oxygen flow under specified conditions through the unit area of contact lens material of unit thickness when subjected to unit pressure difference:

$$Dk = \frac{\text{amount of oxygen} \times \text{thickness}}{\text{area} \times \text{time} \times \text{pressure difference}}$$

2.4.4	Oxygen transmissibility, *Dk/t*	The value for oxygen permeability divided by the thickness of the measured sample under specified conditions
2.4.5	Oxygen transmission rate	The amount of oxygen, per unit of time, which diffuses through a contact lens under specified conditions, when subjected to unit pressure difference
2.4.8	Hard lens; rigid lens	Contact lens which, in its final form and under normal conditions, retains its form without support
2.4.9	Gas permeable hard (rigid) lens	Hard lens which allows passage through the material of all, or a substantial part, of the oxygen required for corneal metabolism
2.4.10	Soft lens	Contact lens which, in its final form, requires support to maintain its form
2.4.11	Hydrogel lens	Soft lens containing water
2.4.12	Hydrophilic lens	Lens which requires a quantity of water to obtain its functional form and properties

Summary of terms relating to corneal and soft lenses

2.1.14	Optic zone	Zone of a contact lens that has a prescribed optical effect
2.1.15	Central optic zone	Central region of a contact lens that has a prescribed optical effect where there is a peripheral optic zone or zones.
2.1.16	Peripheral zone	Region of specified dimensions surrounding the optic zone. *Notes*: (1) These zones are numbered first, second, third etc., beginning with the zone immediately surrounding the central optic zone. (2) The term may be qualified, for example 'back peripheral zone', or 'front peripheral zone'.

2.1.18	Optic zone diameter	Diameter of a specified optic zone, measured to the surrounding junction. If the latter is not circular, the major and minor diameters define the size *Note*: The term may be qualified, for example 'back central optic zone diameter'.
2.1.19	Back optic zone radius, r_o	Radius of curvature of the back optic zone
2.1.20	Back peripheral radius, $r, r_2 \ldots$	Radius of curvature of a back peripheral zone *Note*: These zones are numbered first, second, third etc., beginning with the zone immediately surrounding the central optic zone
2.1.24	Transition	Junction modified to smooth the change between adjacent curvatures
2.1.25	Blending	Process of forming a transition
2.1.27	Front vertex power, F_v	Reciprocal of the focal length, in metres, of the optic zone(s) of the lens, measured in air, or calculated for the lens, from the front vertex of the lens
2.1.28	Back vertex power, F_v'	Reciprocal of the focal length, in metres, of the optic zone(s) of the lens, measured in air, or calculated for the lens, from the back vertex of the lens
2.1.29	Total diameter, θ_T	Maximum external dimension(s) of the finished lens or shell
2.1.30	Lenticular lens	Lens having a front optic zone made smaller than the total diameter
2.1.31	Carrier	That part of a lenticular lens surrounding the front optic zone
2.1.35	Geometrical centre thickness, t_c	Thickness of the lens or shell at its geometrical centre
2.1.37	Carrier junction thickness, t_{suffix}	Thickness of the lens measured normal to the back surface at the junction of the front optic and carrier
2.1.39	Radial edge thickness	Thickness of the lens measured normal to the front surface at a specified point near the edge
2.1.45	Axial edge lift, l_a	Distance between a point on the back surface of a lens at a specified diameter and the continuation of the back central optic zone, measured parallel to the lens axis
2.1.46	Radial edge lift, l_r	Distance between a point on the back surface of a lens at a specified diameter and the continuation of the back central optic zone, measured along a radius of curvature of the latter
2.1.10	Aspheric lens	Lens with at least one surface (front and/or back) having a form generated by the rotation of a curve of continuously varying radius about the lens axis
2.1.11	Toric lens	Lens with front or back central optic zone of toroidal form
2.1.12	Bi-toric lens	Lens having both front and back central optic zones of toroidal form
2.1.13	Peripheral toric lens	Lens with one or more peripheral front or back zones of toroidal form

The most commonly used terms are represented diagramatically in the tri-curve lens below.

Abbreviation	Symbol	Term	Former abbreviations
BOZR	r_o	back optic zone radius	BCOR, BC, PCCR
BOZD	θ_o	back optic zone diameter	BCOD, POZD, OZ
BPR	r_1, r_2	back peripheral radius	BPOR, PCR
BPZD	θ_1, θ_2	back peripheral zone diameter	BPOD, PCD
TD	θ_T	total diameter	OS, OD, TD
t_o	t_c	geometrical centre thickness	t_c

Note: The above terms apply to single vision lenses. The terms back central optic zone radius (BCOZR) and back central optic zone diameter (BCOZD) are now applicable to concentric bifocal lenses, where the addition is on the back surface or FCOZR and FCOZD where the addition is on the front surface.

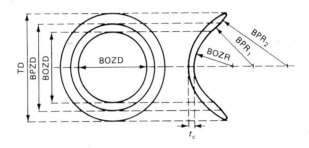

Summary of new terms relating to scleral lenses and shells

Reference in Standard

2.2.1	Scleral zone	That zone of a scleral lens (or shell) designed to lie in front of the sclera
2.2.2	Scleral shell	Contact shell with a scleral zone
2.2.3	Impression lens	Scleral lens the back scleral surface of which has been produced by moulding from a cast of the eye
2.2.7	Preformed scleral lens	Scleral lens, not an impression lens, the back surface of which is of a predetermined form
2.2.8	Primary optic diameter	Longest optic diameter of a lens in which the junction of the back optic and back central scleral surfaces is not circular
2.2.9	Primary optic plane	Plane perpendicular to the lens axis and containing the primary optic diameter
2.2.10	Primary sagitta	Distance along the lens axis from the back optic surface to the primary optic plane
2.2.11	Back scleral size	Maximum internal dimension of the back scleral surface before the sharp edge has been rounded
2.2.12	Scleral thickness	Thickness of the scleral zone measured normal to the front scleral surface at any specified point
2.2.13	Scleral chord	In a specified meridian, the distance from the optic–scleral junction to the junction of the back scleral surface with edge
2.2.14	Displacement of optic	Half the difference between the (two) maximum and minimum scleral chords

Abbreviation	Term
LA	lens axis
BOZR	back optic zone radius
PS	primary sagitta
POD	primary optic diameter
POP	primary optic plane
SC	scleral chord
BSR	back scleral radius
BSS	back scleral size
TD	total diameter
d	displacement

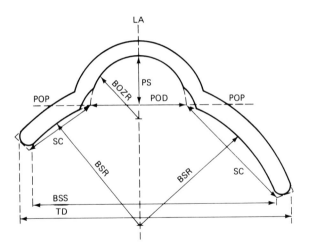

Chapter 1

The history of contact lenses

A. G. Sabell

A study of the history of contact lenses is necessary if only to appreciate how fruitful of ideas were our predecessors. The greatest achievement for which most of us can hope is to revive a previously described idea which may have been abandoned because of some missing component of technical knowledge or prowess, and to pursue this to success within the framework of present-day technology. It is hoped, therefore, that readers will not pass over this chapter as having little relevance to modern contact lens practice, for it is upon the foundations of the past that we operate today. Likewise, the contributions which we may make help to cement the structure upon which our successors will continue to build.

Look, therefore, very carefully at what has gone before and think deeply on these past efforts, their successes and their failures, for few ideas are completely new and the dividing line between success and failure may be very fine and may well depend, not on one's own efforts, but on the availability of supporting technology.

This history in its original form was compiled between 1975 and 1977 and at that time it seemed difficult, if not inappropriate, to include too recent events. For that reason, the subject of hydrogel lenses, a development of the previous decade was treated in a very cursory manner. The reader was referred to the later chapters of the book in which current thinking and practice were to be presented. Now, some 10 years later we may legitimately examine some of the trends of the 1970s.

It would be appropriate to say that the introduction of the hydrophilic gel contact lens by Professor Wichterle and his colleagues heralded a period in which the polymer chemist was and perhaps still is at the spearhead of contact lens progress. We have moved into the era of 'materials' rather than design as a means

of satisfying an increasing proportion of those who elect, for one reason or another, to wear their optical correction in direct proximity to their corneas.

General developments in the contact lens field

Optical principles

Several well-defined periods of development are recognizable from a survey of the broader aspects of contact lens history. The first of these hinges on theorizing about the optics of neutralization of the corneal surface in water. Experimental work of this period does little more than illustrate something of the optical theory which underlies the use of the contact lens as a vision aid. This period begins with our earliest known reference, by Leonardo da Vinci, and the reader is referred to the detailed papers by Ferrero (1952) and by Hofstetter and Graham (1953) for a fuller description of this work. A useful general paper on Leonardo is that by Gasson (1976). The actual work by Leonardo da Vinci, claimed by some authors to pertain to the history of contact lenses, appears to consist of the construction of a large transparent globe intended to form a model of the human eye. This globe being filled with water, into which the observer immersed his face, resulted in the optical neutralization of the observer's corneas. Other than the fact that the corneal surface is neutralized it is difficult to see precisely what relevance this has to the history of the contact lens.

The work of René Descartes (1637; *Figure 1.1*) has been well described by Enoch (1956) and does perhaps begin, if somewhat remotely, to have some bearing on the contact lens. The elongated water-filled tube used by Descartes to

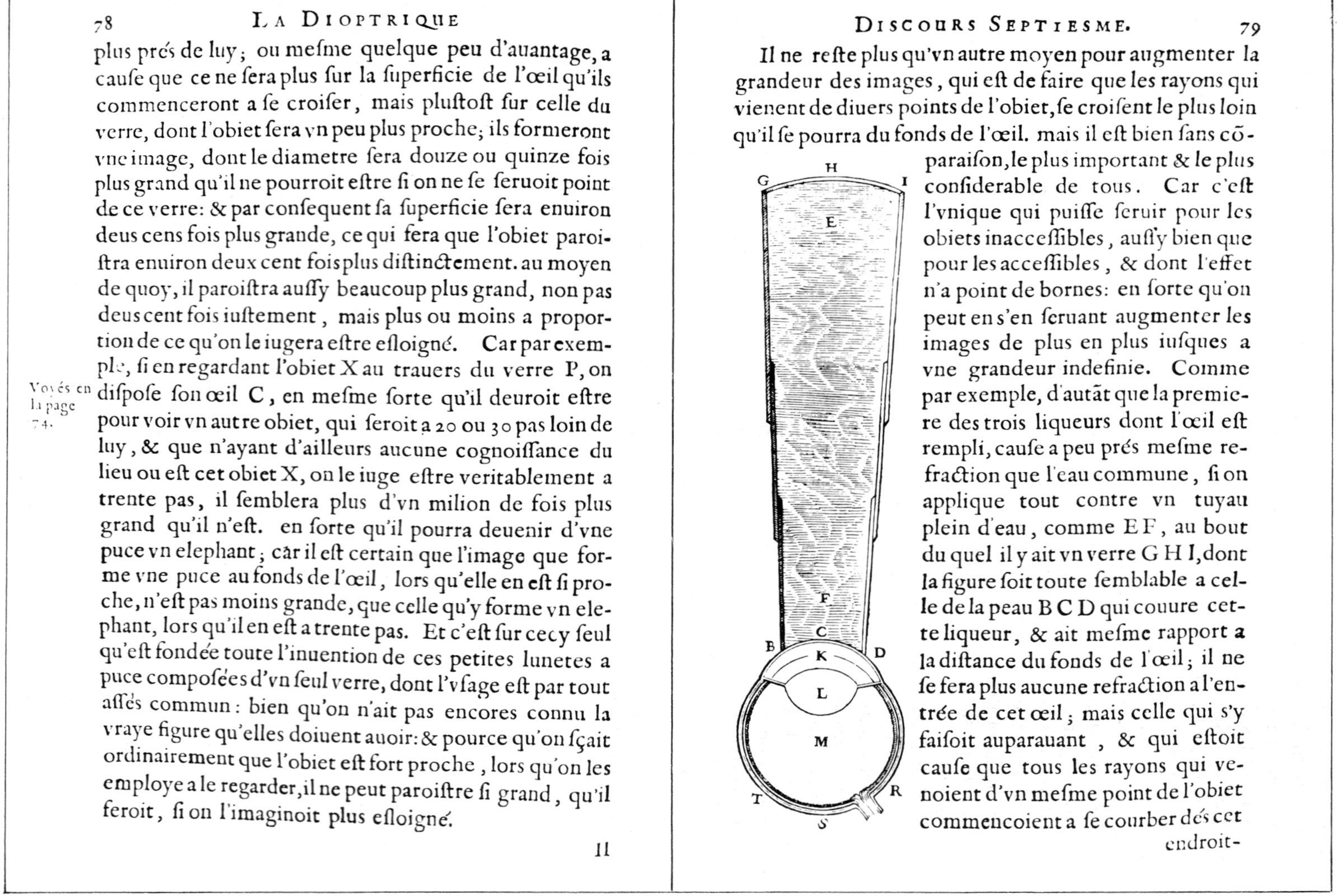

LA DIOPTRIQUE

78

plus prés de luy; ou mefme quelque peu d'auantage, a caufe que ce ne fera plus fur la fuperficie de l'œil qu'ils commenceront a fe croifer, mais pluftoft fur celle du verre, dont l'obiet fera vn peu plus proche; ils formeront vne image, dont le diametre fera douze ou quinze fois plus grand qu'il ne pourroit eftre fi on ne fe feruoit point de ce verre: & par confequent fa fuperficie fera enuiron deus cens fois plus grande, ce qui fera que l'obiet paroiftra enuiron deux cent fois plus diftinctement. au moyen de quoy, il paroiftra auffy beaucoup plus grand, non pas deus cent fois iuftement, mais plus ou moins a proportion de ce qu'on le iugera eftre efloigné. Car par exemple, fi en regardant l'obiet X au trauers du verre P, on difpofe fon œil C, en mefme forte qu'il deuroit eftre pour voir vn autre obiet, qui feroit a 20 ou 30 pas loin de luy, & que n'ayant d'ailleurs aucune cognoiffance du lieu ou eft cet obiet X, on le iuge eftre veritablement a trente pas, il femblera plus d'vn milion de fois plus grand qu'il n'eft. en forte qu'il pourra deuenir d'vne puce vn elephant; car il eft certain que l'image que forme vne puce au fonds de l'œil, lors qu'elle en eft fi pro-che, n'eft pas moins grande, que celle qu'y forme vn ele-phant, lors qu'il en eft a trente pas. Et c'eft fur cecy feul qu'eft fondée toute l'inuention de ces petites lunetes a puce compofées d'vn feul verre, dont l'vfage eft par tout affés commun : bien qu'on n'ait pas encores connu la vraye figure qu'elles doiuent auoir: & pource qu'on fçait ordinairement que l'obiet eft fort proche, lors qu'on les employe a le regarder, il ne peut paroiftre fi grand, qu'il feroit, fi on l'imaginoit plus efloigné.

Voyés en la page 74.

II

DISCOURS SEPTIESME.

79

Il ne refte plus qu'vn autre moyen pour augmenter la grandeur des images, qui eft de faire que les rayons qui vienent de diuers points de l'obiet, fe croifent le plus loin qu'il fe pourra du fonds de l'œil. mais il eft bien fans cõ-paraifon, le plus important & le plus confiderable de tous. Car c'eft l'vnique qui puiffe feruir pour les obiets inacceffibles, auffy bien que pour les acceffibles, & dont l'effet n'a point de bornes: en forte qu'on peut ens'en feruant augmenter les images de plus en plus iufques a vne grandeur indefinie. Comme par exemple, d'autãt que la premie-re des trois liqueurs dont l'œil eft rempli, caufe a peu prés mefme re-fraction que l'eau commune, fi on applique tout contre vn tuyau plein d'eau, comme EF, au bout du quel il y ait vn verre GHI, dont la figure foit toute femblable a cel-le de la peau BCD qui couure cet-te liqueur, & ait mefme rapport a la diftance du fonds de l'œil, il ne fe fera plus aucune refraction a l'en-trée de cet œil; mais celle qui s'y faifoit auparauant, & qui eftoit caufe que tous les rayons qui ve-noient d'vn mefme point de l'obiet commencoient a fe courber dés cet endroit-

Figure 1.1 Pages from the seventh discourse of René Descartes (1637) showing his contact appliance

enlarge the size of the retinal image would certainly have been impossible to wear as an appliance for the correction of vision. Duke-Elder (1970) also cites the experiments of Philip de la Hire around 1685 as having relevance to the history of contact lenses.

The contribution of Thomas Young (1801) provided the immediate stimulus leading to the first optical correction of astigmatism by Airy (1827) and in turn triggered the now famous speculation by Sir John F. W. Herschel (1845) (*Figure 1.2*). Herschel's far-seeing comments link the early period associated with optical theories with the beginnings of the clinical struggle. To this man, therefore, should go the honour of envisaging the more important of the present-day areas of clinical application of the contact lens. The reason for some confusion over the dates of Herschel's publications, whether 1827 or 1845, have been discussed by Bennett (1961). Although undoubtedly of great optical significance, the work of this period contributes nothing to the subsequent struggle to achieve toleration of a corrective appliance which must be worn on the eye of a visually handicapped individual. It might well be claimed that the earlier work had greater relevance to the development of the hydrodiascope by Lohnstein (1896) and Siegrist (1916).

Early practical trials

The second phase, that of practical clinical development, began with the work of Fick (1888), an English translation of which was made by May in the same year. This publication was preceded by two loosely related occurrences. The first was an idea put forward in 1886 by Galezowsky that a gelatin disc might be applied to the cornea immediately following cataract extraction. This disc was to be impregnated with cocaine and sublimate of mercury which would provide corneal anaesthesia to relieve postoperative pain and an antiseptic cover to prevent infection. This suggestion has been quoted by Mann (1938) although she gives no specific reference to the publication. Despite the horrifying implications of such a procedure, we may see in the proposal not only the first use of a soft and hydrophilic contact appliance but also the forerunner of the hydrophilic lens as a dispenser of ophthalmic medication. The second event preceding Fick's publication was, of

course, the frequently described work by the firm of F.Ad. Müller Sohne at Wiesbaden for Dr Theodore Saemisch's patient. This consisted of the supplying of a protective contact device and does not appear to have been intended primarily as a visual aid. This contribution has been described by many authors amongst whom Nissel (1965) published a description of the origins of the firm of Müller and Sons of Wiesbaden. He quotes extensively from the work by Müller (1920) and also that of Müller and Müller (1910), both documents of great interest to the contact lens historian.

There also appeared in 1889 the inaugural thesis of August Müller of Gladbach, presented at the University of Kiel for his degree of Doctorate in Medicine and entitled 'Spectacle lenses and corneal lenses' (*Figure 1.3*). This work incorporates the first known use of the expression 'corneal lens'. August Müller's interests lay in the correction of high myopia, while Fick had been eager to produce usable vision for keratoconus patients. Pearson (1978) has published a detailed review of Müller's contact lens contribution.

Almost simultaneously Eugene Kalt in Paris was investigating contact lenses which were undoubtedly of corneal lens form, as 'orthopaedic appliances' in the treatment of keratoconus. This we may regard as laying down the groundwork which has led to the consideration of the contact lens as a means of myopia control and to its use in orthokeratology.

To return to the paper by Fick (1888), this is undoubtedly worthy of being read and re-read by all contact lens practitioners because it contains some astonishingly accurate observations and one wonders, in the light of some of Fick's observations, why the subsequent development of contact lenses took place so slowly. For example, in addition to recommending the use of contact lenses for keratoconus, Fick suggested their potential usefulness in aphakia, as prosthetic/cosmetic lenses and also postulated the use of pinhole contact lenses. He clearly foresaw the future high cosmetic demand for the wearing of contact lenses. Fick is, of course, best remembered for his description of what, much later, became called Sattler's veil or, less commonly, Fick's phenomenon. He recognized that an adaptational process occurred enabling the wearer to become more tolerant, due to the regular usage of the contact

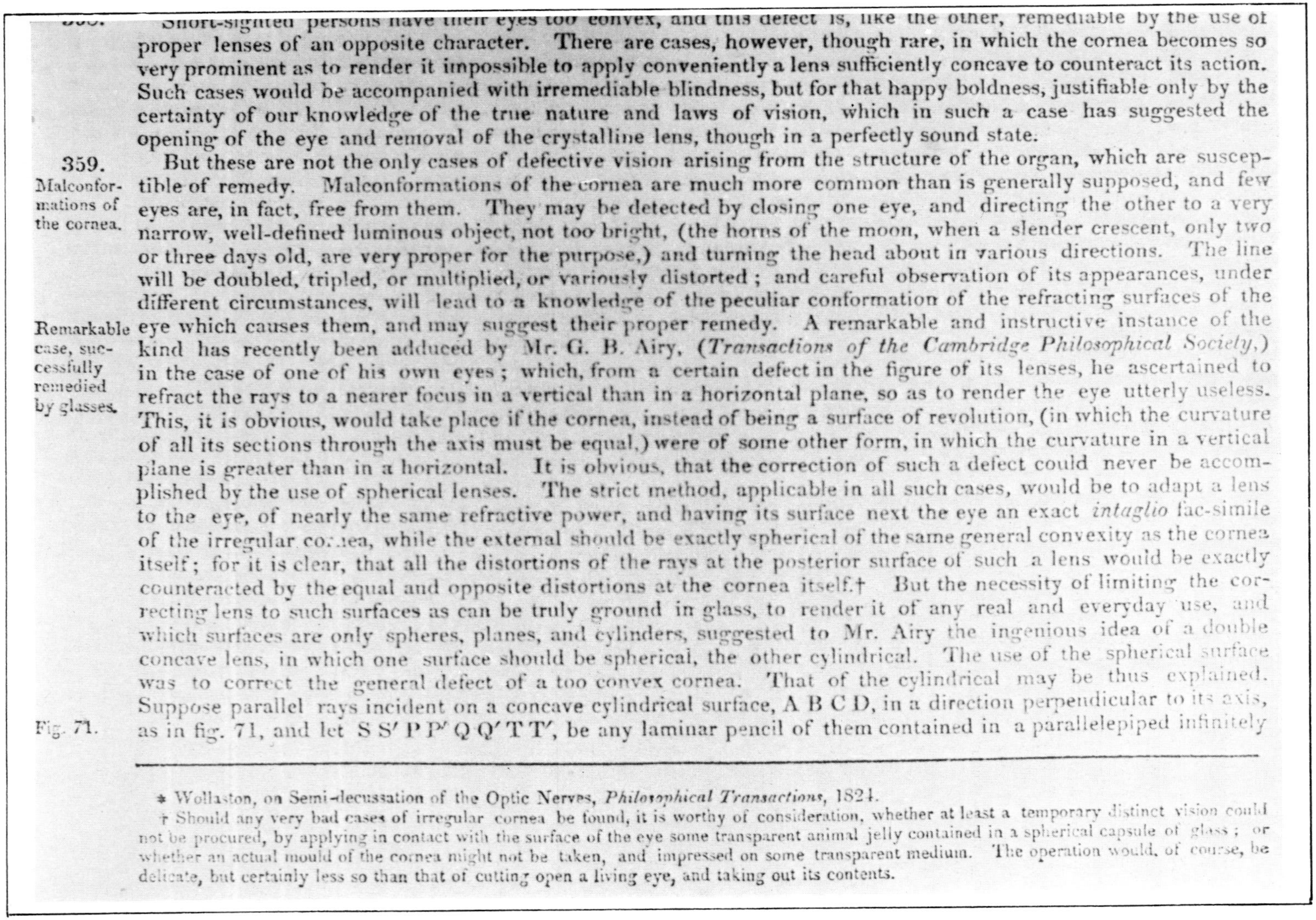

Short-sighted persons have their eyes too convex, and this defect is, like the other, remediable by the use of proper lenses of an opposite character. There are cases, however, though rare, in which the cornea becomes so very prominent as to render it impossible to apply conveniently a lens sufficiently concave to counteract its action. Such cases would be accompanied with irremediable blindness, but for that happy boldness, justifiable only by the certainty of our knowledge of the true nature and laws of vision, which in such a case has suggested the opening of the eye and removal of the crystalline lens, though in a perfectly sound state.

359.

Malconformations of the cornea.

But these are not the only cases of defective vision arising from the structure of the organ, which are susceptible of remedy. Malconformations of the cornea are much more common than is generally supposed, and few eyes are, in fact, free from them. They may be detected by closing one eye, and directing the other to a very narrow, well-defined luminous object, not too bright, (the horns of the moon, when a slender crescent, only two or three days old, are very proper for the purpose,) and turning the head about in various directions. The line will be doubled, tripled, or multiplied, or variously distorted ; and careful observation of its appearances, under different circumstances, will lead to a knowledge of the peculiar conformation of the refracting surfaces of the cornea.

Remarkable case, successfully remedied by glasses.

A remarkable and instructive instance of the kind has recently been adduced by Mr. G. B. Airy, (*Transactions of the Cambridge Philosophical Society*,) in the case of one of his own eyes ; which, from a certain defect in the figure of its lenses, he ascertained to refract the rays to a nearer focus in a vertical than in a horizontal plane, so as to render the eye utterly useless. This, it is obvious, would take place if the cornea, instead of being a surface of revolution, (in which the curvature of all its sections through the axis must be equal,) were of some other form, in which the curvature in a vertical plane is greater than in a horizontal. It is obvious, that the correction of such a defect could never be accomplished by the use of spherical lenses. The strict method, applicable in all such cases, would be to adapt a lens to the eye, of nearly the same refractive power, and having its surface next the eye an exact *intaglio* fac-simile of the irregular cornea, while the external should be exactly spherical of the same general convexity as the cornea itself; for it is clear, that all the distortions of the rays at the posterior surface of such a lens would be exactly counteracted by the equal and opposite distortions at the cornea itself.† But the necessity of limiting the correcting lens to such surfaces as can be truly ground in glass, to render it of any real and everyday use, and which surfaces are only spheres, planes, and cylinders, suggested to Mr. Airy the ingenious idea of a double concave lens, in which one surface should be spherical, the other cylindrical. The use of the spherical surface was to correct the general defect of a too convex cornea. That of the cylindrical may be thus explained.

Fig. 71.

Suppose parallel rays incident on a concave cylindrical surface, A B C D, in a direction perpendicular to its axis, as in fig. 71, and let S S' P P' Q Q' T T', be any laminar pencil of them contained in a parallelepiped infinitely

---

* Wollaston, on Semi-decussation of the Optic Nerves, *Philosophical Transactions*, 1824.

† Should any very bad cases of irregular cornea be found, it is worthy of consideration, whether at least a temporary distinct vision could not be procured, by applying in contact with the surface of the eye some transparent animal jelly contained in a spherical capsule of glass ; or whether an actual mould of the cornea might not be taken, and impressed on some transparent medium. The operation would, of course, be delicate, but certainly less so than that of cutting open a living eye, and taking out its contents.

Figure 1.2 The footnote in Sir John Herschel's dissertation on light (1845) which constituted the beginning of modern thinking on contact lenses

lens, and even recognized that air trapped behind the contact lens on insertion retarded the onset of visual clouding. Fick was aware that the cause of this clouding lay in the epithelium.

Thus, by 1890 the foundations had been laid for: correction of visual errors, protection of the exposed cornea, remoulding of corneal shape, neutralization of corneal irregularity and the use of the contact lens as an applicator of ophthalmic drugs. Within this period also, the successes and failures of ocular toleration had been recognized and the pattern of events set which were to last until about 1930. This second period of development was therefore characterized by a lack of ability to ensure both good toleration and good vision by the majority of contact lens patients. The underlying reasons for such lack of success are to be found in the limited understanding of detailed topography, of the physiology of the anterior segment of the eye and of its responses to the contact lens. Although Fick had, in 1888, made a succession of very relevant observations, it appears that before many years were to pass he would have lost much of his interest in the contact lens. In his textbook *Diseases of the Eye and Ophthalmoscopy* (1896), he devoted only eight lines to the use of contact lenses. August Müller (1889) had described his

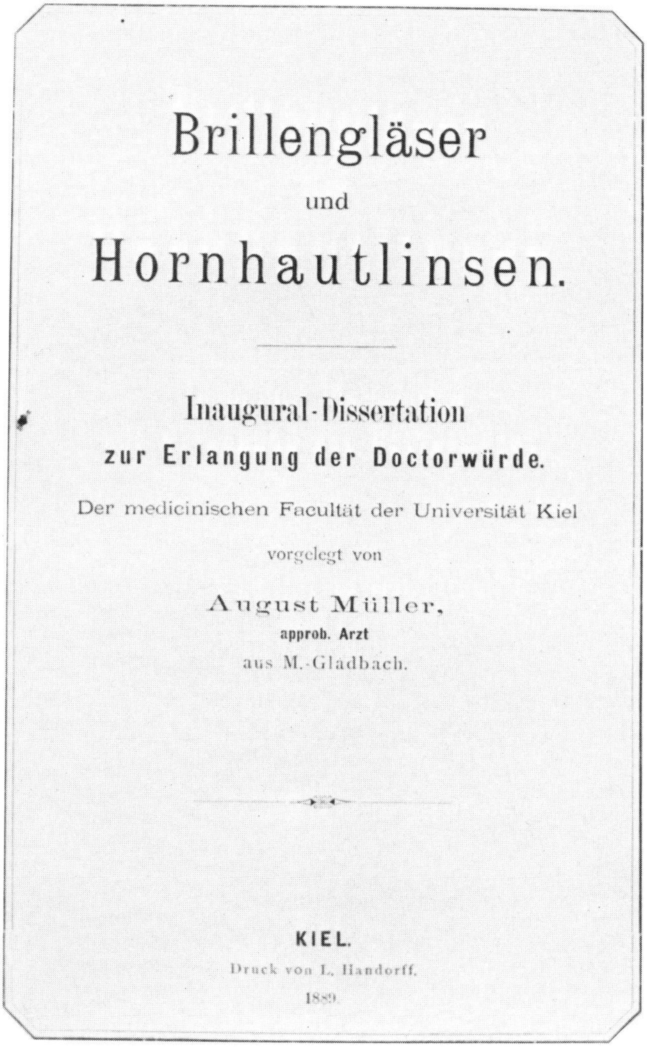

Brillengläser

und

Hornhautlinsen.

Inaugural-Dissertation

zur Erlangung der Doctorwürde.

Der medicinischen Facultät der Universität Kiel

vorgelegt von

August Müller,

approb. Arzt

aus M.-Gladbach.

KIEL.

Druck von L. Handorff.

1889.

Figure 1.3 Title page of August Müller's doctoral thesis (1889) using, for the first time, the term 'corneal lenses'

own disappointing tolerance of contact lenses. He believed that the discomfort arose from pressure of the scleral zone of the lens on the conjunctiva. He also described the difficulty found in applying his contact lenses without air bubbles and his avoidance of this problem by inserting the lenses under water. From our understanding of the osmotic principles involved, this factor alone would account for a very limited toleration because corneal oedema would develop within about 15 minutes. Indeed, the physical discomfort which must have resulted from the marked hypotonicity of the liquid behind the contact lens probably accounts for Müller's use of cocaine eye drops prior to inserting his lenses. It would seem, therefore, quite apart from any defects in physical fit of Müller's lenses, that he was doomed to failure by such physiological factors.

It should be noted that Fick (1888) had pronounced on the subject of suitable fluids for inserting contact lenses and had settled on 2% grape sugar solution, which he claimed was capable of giving 8–10 hours wear by his rabbits before corneal clouding developed. It seems likely, had a slit lamp been available at this time, even of the level of sophistication of that used by Sattler (1938), that he would have observed the corneal clouding at an earlier stage. Fick stressed the need for sterilization of his dextrose solution by boiling prior to use and also pronounced on the need for careful disinfection of the lenses themselves. Dor (1892) of Paris recommended the use of physiological saline solution as an insertion medium for contact lenses and this seems to have remained a popular choice up to the early 1940s. Perusal of Fick's 1888 paper shows that he had experimented with 'salt solutions, with various organic additions' and had discarded these in favour of his 2% dextrose. Personal experiences of various contact lens solutions around 1946 with full clearance sealed lenses convinced the author that sodium chloride solutions of various concentrations between 0.5 and 1.5% were usually rejected by patients who complained of smarting sensation and redness of the eyes.

It seems, therefore, that from about 1895 until around 1930 an impasse was reached in terms of patient usage of contact lenses. Over this period the choice lay between the blown glass lenses produced by the firm of Müller's of Wiesbaden and the ground glass contact lenses such as those made by Carl Zeiss of Jena. The former were inferior in consistency of optical quality, but superior to the latter in comfort and duration of wearing. The author has described the optical and physical characteristics of several Müller and Zeiss lenses of this period (Sabell, 1980a). This lack of progress in achievement of longer wearing times with good vision did not prevent the development of ideas for utilization of contact appliances requiring only short-term application. Thus, the use of the contact splint to retain a corneal graft in position during healing has been attributed by Mann (1938) to de Weckers in 1900. Ideas progressed on the use of contact lenses in keratoconus and the classic form of the ground Zeiss lens began to emerge. Possibly the development by Koeppe (1918) of contact lenses for gonioscopy and for slit lamp microscopy of the fundus best illustrate the exploitation of short wearing time potential of contact lenses.

Preformed fitting sets

During the 1920–30 period, the trial fitting set as we know it today began to emerge, although Fick had in fact established the principles of preformed fitting on his rabbits around 1887 saying 'after many trials I abandoned the use of the casts and satisfied myself with obtaining glass vesicles, 21, 20, and 19 mm in diameter . . . From a large number of such small glass shells I selected the best-fitting one for each individual rabbit'. The Zeiss preformed development of the 1920–30 period began with Dr W. Stock's four lens set and developed to the massive afocal lens sets devised by Professor Leopold Heine (1929). It would seem then, although many attempts had been made from way back in the 1880s to produce good impressions of the eye surface, a lack of achievement in this quarter had allowed the preformed lens method to be developed to a reasonable level of sophistication by 1930.

Ophthalmic impressions

It was, therefore, the development of successful methods of making eye impressions to produce accurate casts of the eye surface which opened up the next phase in contact lens development. From this point, around 1930, considerably more information on ocular topography began to accumulate, although one should note that

Fick, in 1888, from his plaster of Paris impressions of the eyes of human cadavers had described the aspherical character of the scleral contours with considerable accuracy. In his paper of 1937, Obrig, while conscious of the potential of impression lenses, still appeared to favour the Zeiss preformed lens. He commented on the improved knowledge of ocular topography which by this time had indicated the need for larger back optic diameters. This he felt had made the use of the Zeiss lens preferable to the less consistent Müller lenses. Such views were in contrast to the opinions expressed 5 years earlier by Sitchevska. Obrig did, however, have certain reservations, commenting for instance 'raised corneal portions on Zeiss lenses are to be avoided wherever possible'. In the light of modern contact lens procedures, as recommended by the makers of one of the proprietary brands of hydrophilic contact lenses, it is interesting to read Obrig's (1937) recorded thoughts regarding the afocal lens system of Heine: 'Heine's method of fitting contact lenses has one decided disadvantage. It requires the investment of from $1,000 to $3,500 in trial lenses. This fact alone would prevent many ophthalmologists from working with these interesting and practical devices.' It is interesting to note that in recent years we have moved once more towards the use of large lens banks, particularly in the hospital eye service.

Obrig (1938a) reported rapid strides in the use of moulded contact lenses. By this time he considered the moulded lens to be 'the ideal conception of the perfect contact lens'. He clearly recognized that much intolerance was due to limbal pressure, especially at the nasal and temporal positions. This had been confirmed by the measurement of eye casts and he realized the inaccuracy of trying to assess corneal diameter by direct measurement of the eye itself. In some cases the cast dimensions of the cornea were 3 mm larger than those given by the measurement of visible horizontal iris diameter. From the measurement of a large number of impression casts, Obrig produced his famous table showing average corneal dimensions, which set the pattern of full corneal clearance fitting during the following decade.

Curiously, although Obrig referred to clouding of the contact lens fluid by accumulation of mucus and sebaceous secretions inside the optic zone, he makes little reference to Sattler's veil, other than the mention in passing of 'transient corneal opacities' which may or may not be a part of that phenomenon. He was certainly aware of corneal clouding, because this was mentioned in his case summaries. The occurrence of limbal pressure from contact lenses was made more easily recognizable by Obrig's discovery (1938b) of the value of blue light with fluorescein solution in the fitting of contact lenses. Prior to this, the method of checking corneal clearance had been by the use of the slit lamp, a technique requiring considerable expertise with this instrument.

This improvement in understanding of ocular topography and of corneal physiology, together with the gradual refinement of methods of fitting and observation constitute the main elements in contact lens progress prior to World War II. The pendulum was swinging from progress in the preformed field as depicted by the development of Zeiss fitting sets, to exploitation of the possibilities offered by the impression lens. Treissman and Plaice (1946) compared the advantages and disadvantages of impression and preformed lenses, and it should be remembered that their concept of the latter at that time was based on the Zeiss contact lens of the pre-war period and the Dixey plastics lens of very similar design which was developed in the UK during the early war years.

Ocular topography and physiology

The 1930s, then, was a period in which the comfort of contact lenses was improved by the realization that sustained corneal pressure from the lens was undesirable. From this stemmed the large optic zone giving, initially, enhanced comfort to the wearer. This full clearance method of fitting scleral lenses was initiated by Obrig in the USA and became widely accepted in that country and also in the UK in the first half of the 1940s. The technique has been thoroughly discussed by Dickinson and Hall (1946), especially in relation to the Dixey preformed lenses of that period. Unfortunately, the advantages gained in comfort by a wide corneal clearance are rapidly eroded by concomitant disadvantages. First, the cosmetic appearance of this type of contact lens leaves something to be desired. Secondly, the full clearance optic must remain fluid filled if visual performance is to be unimpaired. This calls for a glove-like seal by the scleral zone of the lens because loose channels offer the possibility of air seepage and the resultant growth of an air bubble behind the optic zone. This zone, in this type of lens, was often fitted steeper than the cornea with a positive liquid lens which encouraged the location of any such air bubble in front of the pupil. The third and major adverse effect of the full clearance optic was the revealing of all the implications of Sattler's veil. It may seem curious that epithelial oedema induced by the wearing of contact lenses, which had been observed as early as 1888, should have attracted little detailed attention until the investigation by Sattler around 1936. A possible explanation may lie in the physical discomfort induced by the ground spherical contact lenses which would often force removal of the lens long before the visual phenomena associated with Sattler's veil became pronounced. If a lens is wearable only for one hour, there is insufficient time for Sattler's veil to become objectionable (provided of course that an isotonic or slightly hypertonic solution is used to start with). The Müller lenses, on the other hand, appear to have been relatively untroubled by Sattler's veil for two possible reasons. First, the very hit-and-miss methods of selection of these lenses and the characteristic aspherical shapes of their scleral zones no doubt allowed loose channels for the relatively free passage of fresh tears to carry off the waste products of corneal metabolism. Secondly, such channels would be highly likely

to allow seepage of air which would accumulate in the optic zone and help retard the onset of veiling. We should consider the method in use at this time for detecting loose channels beneath the scleral zone. This was the application of a small quantity of 2% fluorescein solution to the upper edge of the lens and the observation in white light (blue or ultraviolet light not being introduced until later) of the amber liquid tracking behind the scleral zone. But it must be remembered that the Müller blown lenses (*Figure 1.4*) were commonly made with white scleral zones akin to artificial eyes and such observations on these lenses would have been difficult.

As seen previously, such an accumulation of air behind the optic zone is likely to affect vision adversely unless of course that portion of the lens has been fitted with such a relationship to the cornea as to ensure that the air remains in the limbal region at all times. Such fine control of the fit of the optic zone was certainly not possible with the blown Müller lenses. But what if the inherent optical quality of the lens itself was poor, as were many of these blown lenses? Might not the presence of air go relatively unnoticed along with the general mediocre visual performance? Moreover, if the patient had a markedly irregular or hazy cornea and, thus, very low spectacle visual acuity, even a poor optical quality contact lens might effect considerable improvement, and a little disturbance such as that resulting from the presence of

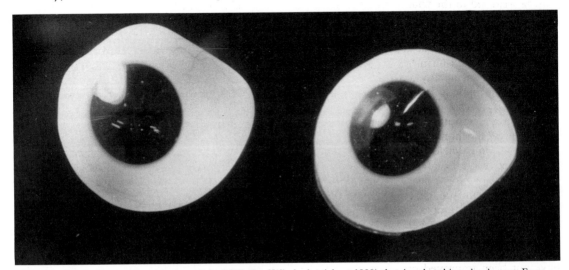

Figure 1.4 Blown glass contact lenses made by Müller's of Wiesbaden (about 1900) showing the white scleral zones. From the museum, Department of Vision Sciences, University of Aston

an air bubble might be regarded as of very secondary importance.

With the enhanced comfort offered by the full clearance optic it was hoped that longer wearing times might be possible. However, the new limiting factor of Sattler's veil was now revealed and indeed remained as the major cause of reduced contact lens toleration until the late 1940s. In a totally sealed lens, Sattler's veil would commence after some 2 hours of wear, visible to the wearer more readily indoors, as a faint blue haze resembling tobacco smoke. This haze became gradually more noticeable but without any gross reduction in visual acuity in the early stages. Shortly after onset, the classic rainbow rings resembling glaucoma haloes would become apparent. Few patients were able to pursue contact lens wear for more than about 30 minutes after the onset of these symptoms because the developing corneal oedema brought gradual onset of photophobia, blepharospasm, and an unpleasant sensation of heat to the eyes.

Contact lens solutions

The observation that tonicity and pH of solution may have some bearing on the onset time of Sattler's veil, led to considerable time being wasted during the late 1930s and early 1940s in the search for the ideal contact lens solution. Obrig and Salvatori (1957) describe vividly the wide range of possibilities which were explored. Changes noted in pH of the contact lens liquid during wear led to the trial of buffered solutions such as those formulated by Gifford and Smith (1933), Gifford (1935) and by Feldman (1937). This, in turn, led to the adoption by contact lens practitioners of the term 'buffer solution', used incorrectly to mean any suitable fluid used to form the liquid lens behind an unfenestrated contact lens, a term now rarely heard. It seems likely that this adoption of the term arose out of the supposed mechanical cushioning effect of the reservoir of liquid held behind the contact lens.

However, not all workers were led astray by the apparent comfort of wide corneal clearance, and the search for the 'elixir' of an ideal contact lens solution. Two notable exceptions in the 1930s were A. Mueller-Welt and Joseph Dallos, the latter laying down physiological principles for the fitting of scleral contact lenses which have not been improved on since. Working on the assumption that the natural body fluid offers the best chance of success, Dallos in the 1930s set out to conserve the tear reservoir and to allow for its interchange by fresh tears. This process is discussed more fully later.

Acrylic contact lenses

Several other developments at this time were to stimulate interest in contact lenses and to herald in the current era of widespread contact lens usage. First, the gradual introduction of plastics materials to largely, but not yet completely, replace glass. Several plastics scleral lenses which predate the introduction of polymethyl methacrylate (PMMA) have been described by the author (Sabell, 1980b). Early attempts with plastics in the USA failed principally through unsuitability of available materials. The compromise introduced by Feinbloom (1937) of a plastics scleral zone holding a glass optic zone presents us with the 'half-way house'. Among the earliest users of PMMA as a material for scleral contact lenses in Eastern Europe was Györrfy in Budapest, following the move of Dallos to London shortly before World War II. Dr Györrfy in 1939 began to investigate the use of plastics to overcome some of the technical difficulties associated with the manufacture of glass lenses of the Dallos type. Györrfy (1950) described the therapeutic use of plastics scleral lenses in Hungary. His later paper (1968) described in considerable detail the Hungarian methods for production of both scleral and corneal lenses in PMMA. Dr Istvan Györrfy has also a considerable interest in the history of contact lenses and has published several excellent papers on this aspect (Györrfy, 1980, 1981). The final introduction of the all acrylic moulded lenses in the USA by Obrig Laboratories and of acrylic lathe-turned preformed lenses by the firm of C. W. Dixey in the UK, led not only to easier lens modification, but also opened the way to the development of successful corneal lenses. A second development at this time, also attributed to Obrig (1943), was the modification of existing cold dental alginates to produce the first specifically ophthalmic impression material.

A third step forward, perhaps at the time appearing to be of relatively minor significance, was the discovery by Obrig, referred to earlier, of the value of cobalt blue light for viewing fluorescein solution behind the contact lens.

Solutions of fluorescein had been used in ophthalmology since first introduced by Straub in 1888, for the investigation of corneal lesions. In the fitting of scleral leneses, while white tungsten light was adequate for detecting the presence of the amber concentrated fluorescein solution tracking through loose channels beneath the scleral zone, the interpretation of varying depths of dilute fluorescein within the optic zone was not possible with this illumination. Corneal clearance had been determined by viewing the lens *in situ* by slit lamp microscopy. It was during such an inspection that Obrig (1938b) fortuitously discovered the value of the cobalt blue filter and thus provided a more ready means of detecting limbal pressure in his scleral lenses. This method of observation must have contributed greatly to the comfort of many patients. The enormous value of this discovery, leading as it did in later years to considerable improvements in the activating light source, is undeniable. It is hard to envisage the handicap to the development of corneal lenses had this simple step not been taken.

By 1948, therefore, the way lay open to the attainment of all day tolerance for the contact lens wearer. The principles of tear interchange in scleral lenses derived from Dallos' minimum clearance principles, over the next 5 years allowed the widespread achievement of long tolerance for many scleral lens wearers.

It should be emphasized that, for most contact lens practitioners, there occurred, in the late 1940s, a great boost to morale as the work of Dallos (1946) and of Bier (1945, 1948) in developing the fenestrated method of fitting scleral lenses began to be widely applied. The difference in duration of wear between the unfenestrated scleral lens as fitted by most practitioners of the time and that of the minimum clearance fenestrated contact lens had to be seen to be believed. Lenses of full corneal clearance rarely allowed longer wearing time than 3 hours without removal to allow the subsidence of Sattler's veil. Scleral lenses, unfenestrated, but with a suitable minimum clearance optic and a suitably loose scleral fitting, might, by accident or design, allow 8–10 hours to be achieved without removal. However, more frequently the figure for this type of lens would be around 4–6 hours. Overnight as it seemed, patients could be transformed into all-day-long wearers of contact lenses for the

very first time. Norman Bier (1982, personal communication) states that his work on fenestration of scleral lenses began in 1944; his original patent application was made on 25th January 1945. The work by Dallos is more difficult to date precisely because it stems from his minimum clearance fitting with narrow upper scleral zones of the mid-1930s, leading to the more conventionally shaped scleral lens having a loose fitting scleral zone used in the late 1930s. This led, from the discovery of improved toleration when a large circular hole was cut in the upper limbal region of the lens, to conventional methods of interpalpebral fenestration and also to the slotted scleral lens developed later by Trodd at Moorfields Eye Hospital (*see* Chapter 18). A photograph of these original Dallos lenses has been published by the author (Sabell, 1980d). The development, as with all others, revealed several minor problems not previously of great consequence; annoying clicking sounds produced in some lenses by the fenestration and frothing, often accompanied by 'dimple veil' causing visual inconvenience to the patient (*see* Chapters 17, 18 and 19).

Corneal lenses

The introduction of acrylic materials around 1938 allowed, from 1948 onwards, the development of corneal lenses, eventually capable of giving all day wear. The gradual refinement of lens design of these two forms of contact lenses has allowed them to cater for nearly all potential users. The progressive development in design of contact lenses is discussed later. One more radical innovation remains to be mentioned. The announcement in the *New Scientist* on 18th January, 1962, that O. Wichterle and D. Lim in Prague had developed contact lenses made of a new 'hydrocolloid' material, did not give rise to any great elation here in the UK. The short report announced that the Czechs had, with the new soft lenses, been able to achieve wearing times of up to 8 hours in 10% of patients fitted. By this time, the bi-curve hard corneal lenses of the late 1950s had been even further improved by multi-curve designs similar to those in wide use today. Some 75% of patients were able to achieve 12–16 hours of continuous daily wear with such lenses. The prospect, therefore, of 8 hours tolerance from the hydrophilic lens did not raise much enthusiasm (Wichterle, Lim and

Dreifus, 1961). The hidden potential in the Czechoslovakian lens lay in the ability, by employing mass production methods, to provide 'off the peg' contact lenses which might be fitted in a matter of minutes. If the lifespan of these new contact lenses was only a few weeks, why worry, the mass production methods would soon bring down the manufacturing costs so low that we would all have disposable 'throw away and get replacement' type contact lenses.

Developments within the soft lens field and the subsequent rigid lenses will be discussed later in this chapter.

The development of eye impression procedures

The concept of reproducing a cast or model of the eye surface as a means of manufacturing contact lenses is a natural one. Indeed, Herschel (1845), had said '. . . or whether an actual mould of the cornea might not be taken, and impressed on some transparent medium'. It is natural that Fick should have explored this possibility and he refers in the 1888 paper to his plaster of Paris eye impressions of rabbits and also of human cadavers. With respect to the rabbits, Fick described his technique in the following terms: 'In one of these animals, I drew the lids and nictitating membrane from the eyeball and filled the resulting sac with plaster of Paris of fluid consistence.' No mention is made of the use of a shell and because the plaster would set to a completely rigid state, such an appliance would seem unnecessary.

August Müller (1889) also makes mention of living eye impressions taken in plaster of Paris, and regarded it as a potentially suitable technique. From the present viewpoint, the setting characteristics of plaster of Paris make it obvious to most that it is an unsuitable material for reproducing accurately the shape of a living and potentially mobile organ which can be distorted by pressure or indeed from its own movement. This factor apart, the absorbent qualities of the drying plaster must create marked disturbance of the epithelial surface and its mucin coating. Additionally, these very early workers would have had only cocaine eye drops available as a local anaesthetic, a drug which, because of local cellular toxicity, is now regarded as unsuitable for eye impressions even

in conjunction with the greatly improved modern impression materials. From around 1890, although various attempts at refining the technique were made, little progress was achieved until after 1930.

Among the methods which had been tried were those of von Csapody (1929). He tried plaster of Paris on animal eyes but was unable to prevent it adhering and damaging the eye on removal. After trying other materials such as cocoa butter, whale fat and the paraffins, he settled for paraffin wax adjusted to a setting temperature around 40°C. This he poured in molten state into a glass cylinder which rested on the eye surface and which served to hold the eyelids apart. As the wax began to set, von Csapody poured on top a layer of iced liquid paraffin to render the paraffin wax sufficiently rigid to avoid distortion while being removed. After removal, a plaster of Paris positive cast was made as a stage towards making a lead die which was then electroplated with copper or nickel, according to Mann (1938). Von Csapody is also credited (Much, 1931) with attempting to make eye impressions in a material called Dentakoll.

In 1928, Joseph Dallos, approaching final qualification as a physician, joined the staff of the No.1 Eye Clinic at the Royal Hungarian Peter Pázmány University at Budapest (*Figure 1.5*). Dallos quickly developed an interest in the use of contact lenses for correction of visual defects, but was frustrated by the limited choice afforded between the ground Zeiss lenses and blown Müller lenses of the time. Around 1931, Dr Alphons Poller of Zurich had described a material derived from seaweed which was intended for preparation of surface impressions to make anatomical models. Shortly afterwards, in turning his thoughts towards eye impressions, Dallos' attention was drawn to Poller's Negocoll. His first trial with this material was made on a cadaver, the skin of the face, nose and eyelids being reproduced. Between the partially closed eyelids, a section of the corneal surface was reproduced with a smooth polished texture. Dallos prepared a positive cast of this impression in the wax-like substance Hominit (*Figure 1.6*) and the smooth appearance of the visible corneal segment convinced him that Negocoll would be a suitable medium for ophthalmic impressions (J. Dallos, 1977, personal communication). Dallos went on to evolve a

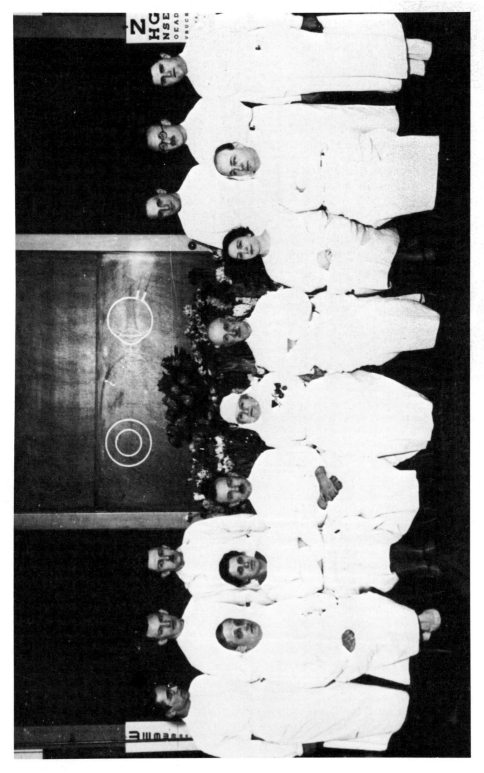

Figure 1.5 The staff of the No.1 Eye Clinic at the Royal Hungarian Peter Pázmány University, Budapest (about 1930). Dr Joseph Dallos is standing, second from the right. Professor Le Grosz is seated, front row, third from the right

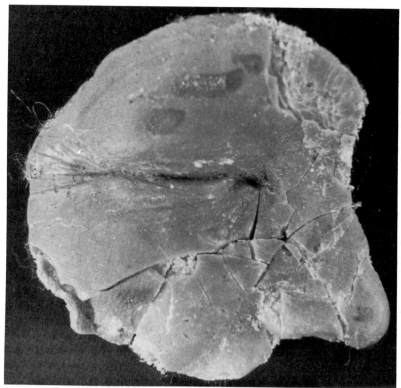

Figure 1.6 The original Hominit cast made from the first impression made by Dallos using the new material 'Poller's Negocoll' (about 1932). The right eyelids and nasal profile of the cadaver are clearly visible. (From the museum, Department of Vision Sciences, University of Aston)

satisfactory impression routine by using Müller contact lenses as impression trays. Some early Dallos impression casts were illustrated by the author (Sabell, 1980c). Although he was the originator of the modern impression technique, Dallos was never completely satisfied with the results achieved. After a few years he accumulated a large enough collection of glass shells made from his earlier impressions to enable him to avoid, with most patients, the necessity of taking further impressions. Gradually this set of 'type shells' grew until it contained several thousand shells from which a very near fit could be selected for almost any eye. As Dallos has demonstrated, it is not the initial selection or the initial impression which provides the finished lens, but the careful tailoring of this preliminary form to the precise requirements of the individual eye. To this modification procedure Dallos gave the title 'haptics', which he described in 1936, as 'a new branch of prosthetics'.

Despite the apparent sound footing on which Dallos had placed Negocoll eye impressions, a few workers still attempted to use wax by various methods. Such a technique was described by Prister (1933) who devised an instrument in which a thin sheet of dental modelling wax could be suspended for application to the eye surface. The application of hot wet packs of cotton wool was used to soften the wax sheet and mould it to the shape of the eye. After this had been achieved, cold swabs were applied before the wax impression and its carrier were removed. Prister recommended making two plaster models from each wax impression, the cornea of one being varnished so that keratometry on the varnished cast could be compared with direct keratometry of the patient's cornea. This, he suggested, would act as an index of distortion resulting from the impression procedure.

A modification of this method using dental wax was, in fact, still being recommended by

Feinbloom (1937) and also by Town as late as 1940. In Town's method, thin sheets of dental modelling wax approximately 0.7 mm thick were employed to make a shell by moulding over a hemishere of the same radius of curvature as a preformed contact lens of approximately correct fit. Town, while agreeing that the Negocoll method resulted in the best impression of the cornea and limbus, nevertheless believed that as good an approximation of the somewhat variable shape of the scleral zone was to be obtained by the wax shell method. Having moulded his wax shell, he removed the central zone and substituted a small glass optic segment of 12 mm diameter. He then cut the external dimensions of the wax shell to an approximate size between 20 × 22 mm and 24 × 26 mm. This he placed on the anaesthetized eye for a period of 15 minutes. The eye was then sprayed with iced water to ensure rigidity of the wax model during removal.

Stevens (1936) described a method of eye impressions using Negocoll. In contrast to Dallos' use of a Müller lens as an impression tray, she reverted to the use of aluminium tubes used in the same manner as von Csapody's glass cylinders. These metal tubes, about 1 inch (2.5 cm) in length, were squeezed to form an oval section corresponding more nearly to the palpebral aperture. The technique resulted in a good impression of the cornea and limbus but the area of sclera reproduced was minimal and to this end it was an unsatisfactory method for the contact lens practitioner. In all fairness it should be added that the procedure was employed for making corneal models as part of an investigation into keratoconus and was not primarily intended as a basis for contact lens fitting.

Obrig (1937) described a technique for eye impressions essentially similar to that of Dallos, using Müller contact lenses as trays to hold Negocoll. He regarded the use of a speculum, recommended by Stevens, as unnecessary and undesirable and believed that the lens would achieve its natural centration if the lids were allowed to resume their normal position. Obrig did, however, recommend irrigation of the Negocoll impression with cold water to aid setting before attempting to remove it from the eyes. He attributed the idea of specially designed shells or trays for eye impressions to Dr Harry Eggers who suggested the attachment of a

fixed handle to a Müller-type contact lens. Obrig at this time was himself employing a funnel-shaped blown glass shell, some 22 mm in diameter and 7 mm deep, having a handle about 25 mm long. He recommended plugging the hollow blown handle with cotton wool to aid retention of the Negocoll. These shells were marked with coloured spots or lines, red for right and light blue for left, which also served to indicate the position of the nasal canthus on the otherwise round shell. A problem was encountered when too much Negocoll was inserted with the shell. This tended to flow out beneath the lids extending away from the shell and encouraged the Negocoll to adhere to the eye surface so that it pulled away from the impression tray during removal. These early glass trays had no perforations to encourage the material to key on.

It is interesting to note that the early Zeiss moulded lenses introduced about 1936, which Obrig (1937) envisaged ordering from his casts, were stated to be oval in shape with dimensions of only 20 × 19 mm. Another curiosity of the time is a recommendation that right and left markers on the finished lenses be placed at the nasal side of the scleral zone to aid correct positioning of the lenses. These markers were recommended to consist of coloured lines and one cannot help thinking that such marks would not be very acceptable cosmetically. Obrig mentioned, incidentally, that delivery time of the moulded glass lenses from Jena was some 2 months, rather longer than the time taken for them to supply their ground preformed lenses.

Obrig's (1938b) paper described a new design of impression tray and recognized the need to have a range of different sizes to cater for variations in eye size, palpebral aperture, lid tension etc. Obrig's choice of material was still Negocoll, but his impression trays, although still of blown glass, were now oval in a range of sizes from 22 × 24 mm to 24 × 26 mm, the bowl being much nearer in shape to that of the Müller contact lens. He reported having performed well over 400 impressions and had obviously resolved many of the points of difficulty encountered by earlier workers. He did, however, remark on the necessity in several instances to take up to three impressions of each eye in order to achieve a successful result. The time scale for these impressions is interesting when the various techniques are compared. Obrig (1938a) for instance, allowed his shell of Negocoll to remain on the eye for about 5 minutes before removal was attempted. The actual removal time averaged 2–3 minutes, but he reported one case in which he required 9 minutes to achieve successful removal. Against such problems should be judged therefore, the slightly earlier decision by Dallos to abandon the impression method in favour of using 'type shells'. Although the 'type shell' approach may appear potentially lengthy and tedious, it should not be judged against the very easy and successful impressions made possible by modern materials and by the accumulated experience of the subsequent years, but against the less reliable methods of that time.

It is clear that, with the use of such non-perforated shells, excess Negocoll would be forced outwards into the fornices and it does appear that large particles had to be sought for and extracted following the removal of the impression itself. This problem has been largely eliminated with modern impression materials and perforated trays (see Chapter 18). Although attention was paid to the improvement of impression techniques by various workers, for example, Chisholm (1940) in developing methods and ideas for fixation and positioning of the eye, it is probably in the field of improved impression materials that most progress has been made. Maisler (1939) described the adaptation to ophthalmic use of 'a reversible hydrocolloid gel' introduced some months earlier by a San Francisco dental surgeon. This material — Kerr's hydrocolloid — was manufactured by the Detroit Dental Manufacturing Company, and was packaged in collapsible toothpaste-type tubes. The tube was immersed in hot water and kneaded to soften the consistency of the material. The hydrocolloid was employed on the eye between 104°F and 100°F (40°C and 38°C). After removal, dental plaster or stone was used to make the positive eye cast. Maisler found that the blown glass impression trays as recommended by Obrig (1938a) were too fragile and described his own trays made in silver which could be made sufficiently thin to be malleable and therefore adjusted in contour to suit the individual eye. Maisler's shells were described as having perforations 'to obtain a better fixation between the gel and the moulding shell'. This may well be the origin of this design feature which is almost universally applied today. Maisler

claimed a very fast setting time for Kerr's hydrocolloid — 'it is possible to obtain a hard gel within a minute's time by flushing the highly conductable silver shell with iced water from an undine'. He postulated the idea of a double-walled silver shell with inlet and outlet so that iced water could pass through the tray itself instead of being run over the patient's face and lids.

The introduction of cold-water mixed impression materials provided a considerable improvement in this method of fitting contact lenses. Obrig (1943) introduced the first cold alginate impression material intended specifically for ophthalmic work. This was Ophthalmic Moldite, a material available until comparatively recently and therefore used by practitioners over nearly 30 years. Obrig had received the first supplies of this new material in the summer of 1942 and had made a considerable number of impressions before the publication of his paper. By this time, he was employing acrylic impression trays in place of his earlier blown glass ones. These new shells also had hollow tubular handles but had perforations around the bowl and he would appear, therefore, to have adopted this feature of the Maisler shells. From experience with Ophthalmic Moldite, it would not appear to be a very suitable material for use with an unperforated shell after the manner in which Negocoll had been employed. On the other hand, Moldite did not seem so likely to leave large particles behind in the fornices. Essentially the routine described by Obrig (1943) is the classic 'insertion method' as used earlier with Negocoll and as still preferred by some practitioners to this day.

Obrig's 1943 paper, however, was not the first to describe the use of a cold alginate impression material. Boshoff, earlier that year, had described his experience using the dental alginate Zelex (Figure 1.7), manufactured in London by the Amalgamated Dental Manufacturing Company. Curiously, Boshoff recommended that after anaesthetization, 'the soft paste is now ladled into the conjunctival sac while the lids are retracted and lifted slightly off the eyeball'. After this, he filled 'a large contact glass with the paste' and applied this also to the eye. He made the point that if the eye moves, the paste and contact lens move with it. This principle of the natural centration of a handle-less shell had been advocated by Obrig (1937) who had,

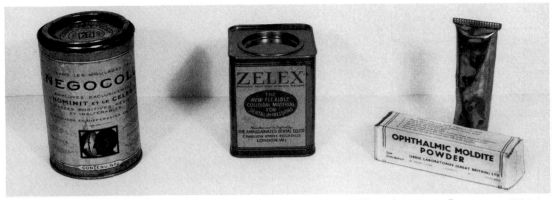

Figure 1.7 The principal eye impression materials in use between 1933 and 1950. (From the museum, Department of Vision Sciences, University of Aston)

according to Dallos (1977, personal communication), seen the handle-less Müller trays used in Budapest in 1935. This was obviously to form the basis for the so-called 'concentric moulding' technique described later by Jessen and Wesley (1949). The contact lens used seems to have employed no perforations to aid adhesion of the Zelex, and Boshoff applied a rubber suction holder to the 'contact glass' to facilitate removal of the impression. He claimed that one advantage of Zelex lay in the shorter preparation time — some 3–6 minutes as compared to that of Negocoll. Obrig, in describing Ophthalmic Moldite, also claimed a 5-minute time from the mixing to the gelling points.

Sugar (1943) referred to recent improvements in dental impression materials and related these to developments in eye impressions. He surveyed the advantages and disadvantages already discussed and introduced another dental alginate, 'Coe-Loid powder', manufactured by Coe Laboratories of Chicago. This material was mixed at room temperature using water in which was dissolved a chemical retarder. Sugar was apparently using perforated impression trays as described by Obrig (1943). Setting time with Coe-Loid varied from 5 minutes at 65°F (18°C) to 2.5 minutes at 80°F (27°C) in very much the same way as currently used alginate materials. Like Moldite, immersion in a fixing solution after removal from the eye was deemed necessary.

By the end of World War II (i.e. 1945), therefore, cold setting impression materials were firmly established. Dental Zelex was commonly employed in the UK until about 1947 when Obrig Laboratories opened a London branch

and Moldite became readily available. Along with the arrival of Obrig Laboratories, came an impression technique new to the UK. This was the so-called 'injection method' still widely used.

Steele (1948) drew attention to the development by American optometrists of the technique of taking eye impressions without using any form of anaesthetization. The need for this variation in procedure was brought about by the drugs laws in the USA which necessitated the presence of a physician to instil the local anaesthetic drops. (The same legal restriction also led to the development by US optometrists of the technique of scleral tonometry.) It would seem logical that the injection method was developed so that the patient's eye could remain stationary while the impression material was being applied and avoid unseen contact between the cornea and the impression shell. The author was a subject for a demonstration of this non-anaesthetic method by one of Obrig's staff shortly after the opening of the London branch. It was certainly not a painful process but would have been unsuitable for use on the more apprehensive type of patient because good relaxation is an essential feature of first class impressions.

Shortly after this time, Jessen and Wesley (1949) published their account of what was claimed to be a new method of taking eye impressions, which they called 'concentric molding'. The technique hinged on the use of a contact lens-like impression tray with no handle. A description was given of the design for such an impression tray, no perforations being mentioned and the description of the procedure suggests that none was employed. The inside of the tray was 'scored or grooved' for good adhesion of the Moldite. The photograph of trays for concentric moulding published in Wesley and Jessen's later book (1953) shows a pair of impression trays each having four large perforations through the scleral zone. This would support the contention that Ophthalmic Moldite did not adhere well to an unperforated tray. The theory behind the concentric method was that, provided the impression tray has the same dimensions and proportions as that required in the finished lens, it will centre itself accurately with its optic zone corresponding to the patient's cornea. Therefore, the positioning of the eye by means of visual fixation of the contralateral eye will be unnecessary. The patient may either look straight ahead or may, in fact, close both eyes while the impression material gels.

Over more recent years the method of using trays without handles has been developed to a very high level of efficiency by F. A. B. Hodd and provides, in certain circumstances, a technique superior to the use of trays with fixed handles. It is interesting to speculate that this technique has evolved from what was undoubtedly the very first method to give a successful impression. It is possible with the correct application of this type of impression tray, to reach the point where little or no modification to the scleral zone of the resultant shell is required.

Returning to the subject of impression materials, the introduction in the UK around 1950 of a specifically prepared Ophthalmic Zelex packaged into single-dose plastic tubes is worthy of note. Ophthalmic Moldite had always been available in multiple dose metal foil packages, so that the introduction of the correctly measured amount of Ophthalmic Zelex supplied in a tube which could be used as a measure for the correct volume of water, did offer a great attraction at first. However, it should be noted that materials packaged in such small quantities appear to suffer loss of their setting characteristics more rapidly than when packaged in greater bulk.

In more recent years there has been a reversion to dental alginates as shown by the current popularity of materials such as Tissutex and Kromopan. Storey (1972) has also published some observations on the possible use of polysulphide rubber impression materials and the use of silicone rubber impression materials

has become popular with some practitioners (A. Silk, 1982, personal communication).

In retrospect, therefore, rapid progress in understanding ocular topography and the principles of 'haptics' followed close on the successful eye impressions first achieved by Dallos around 1932. Although much time and effort has been expended on preformed lens designs by many workers over three-quarters of a century of contact lens history, the good eye impression still remains an unrivalled basis for the fitting of scleral contact lenses. As a final observation on eye impressions, the reader's attention is drawn to the work of Dallos (1964) in attempting to apply the technique of precise corneal impressions to the fitting of acrylic corneal lenses. One of these Dallos corneal casts has been illustrated (Sabell, 1980b). It is appropriate to conclude this section on the development of eye impressions by quoting Obrig and Salvatori (1957): 'The original work of Dallos in discovering and proving the use of Negocoll as a practical, satisfactory medium for making accurate molds of the living human eye has done more than anything else to make modern contact lenses a reality.'

Development in contact lens design and materials

The gradual progress in contact lens design is, to a great extent, the product of developing knowledge of ocular topography and of ocular physiology. A starting point may be taken as the words of Herschel (1845) '. . . spherical capsules of glass'. No simpler concept could be expressed than this and it would seem to represent the commencement of contact lens design.

Fick (1888) had begun by describing the contact lens as 'a thin glass shell bounded by concentric and parallel spherical segments'. Graham (1959) contends that this description can only be interpreted as 'the simple form characteristic of corneal lenses'. Fick, in fact, goes on to describe his initial experiment using large rabbits and, from his plaster casts of these animals' eyes, he concluded that 'the radius of curvature of the cornea did not differ materially from that of the sclera, and the eyeball of the rabbit is pretty nearly a sphere'. After having a number of shells blown over the rabbit casts, Fick 'abandoned the use of the casts and satisfied myself with obtaining glass vesicles 21,

20 and 19 mm in diameter and with having a segment separated from these, the base of which was distant but a few millimetres from the equator of the sphere'. From these stock sizes he selected the best fit for each individual rabbit. Thus, Fick was the first to use a preformed lens approach.

The author has some doubts, therefore, over Graham's contention that Fick's description of a contact lens was necessarily that of a corneal lens. It seems equally feasible that such a description fits his scleral lenses for rabbits. It is some four pages later, after discussing the effects of contact lens wear on the eyes of rabbits, that Fick turns his attention to the human eye. He concluded, from his plaster casts of the eyes of a cadaver, that 'the cast of a human eye shows very plainly that the cornea is the segment of a sphere of smaller radius of curvature than the rest of the globe'. He then described having a glass sphere made and then 'a portion of this small glass globe was heated and a protrusion blown out'. Fick himself wore this first human lens for 2 hours and described his observations. Later, other subjects repeated these wearing trials. It would seem, therefore, that his first human lenses were of scleral form and that single segment types were, in fact, scleral lenses for rabbits and not corneal lenses for human eyes. Indeed, Fick's first paper on the subject was published before any of his patients were actually wearing a contact lens and was concerned with the results of his preliminary experiments and with speculation as to useful fields of application for the appliance. The lenses which he subsequently requested Professor Abbe to make for him are described as having an optic radius of curvature of 8 mm with a diameter of 14 mm and a scleral band of 3 mm width having a radius of curvature of 15 mm. This made a total diameter of just under 20 mm — decidedly a scleral contact lens.

What is certainly interesting and has a bearing on contact lens design, is that Fick recognized the following features, many of which were not utilized until many decades later:

(1) From the cast of the human eye 'the radius of curvature of the conjunctiva increases steadily from before, backwards as we would naturally expect when we consider that only in the immediate neighbourhood of the cornea does the conjunctiva lie directly on the globe, while further back it is separated from this by a constantly thickening layer of tendons, connective tissue, fat and muscles'.

(2) 'Concerning the clouding of the cornea, it was easily demonstrated that it was produced solely by the liquid. For if a glass be applied without filling it with liquid, the cornea will remain clear.'

Thus, Fick recognized the factor which has provided the limitation to usefulness of scleral lenses with spherical scleral zones. He had observed the crucial feature on which the fenestrated scleral lens was to be based many decades later as a means of solving the very phenomenon of corneal clouding with which his name was to be associated. Fick is usually, and rightly credited with an interest in correcting the sight of keratoconus patients. Such patients may have central corneal opacification for which he described the treatment of iridectomy, often followed at that time by corneal tattooing. He described the potential usefulness of a pinhole contact lens, saying 'a contact lens which has been rendered opaque except opposite the artificial pupil'. This device he suggested as an alternative to corneal tattooing which too often resulted in severe infection of the eye.

Several authors have attributed the suggestion of contact lenses for aphakia to later writers, but Fick in 1888 wrote 'at the same time the high degree of hypermetropia in aphakia could be diminished by increased curvature of the glass cornea'. Fick described also the potential use of the cosmetic (prosthetic) contact shell 'by the use of a contact lens upon which the iris and a black pupil is painted'. In retrospect, therefore, Eugen Fick showed an astonishing insight into the future of the contact lens field.

Scleral lenses

If we follow, first, the development of the scleral contact lens, practitioners were, for the next few decades, confined either to the blown lens such as that made at Wiesbaden, or to the solid ground lens being made primarily by Carl Zeiss of Jena. We may gain some concept of the former type by reference to the writings of Sitchevska (1932). In this paper, which compared the design of the two forms of contact lens, she drew attention to the empirical fitting procedure necessary for the Müller lenses. The necessity to try very large numbers of lenses was tedious both to the patient and the practitioner and, if subsequently the lens should break or become roughened, the whole process had to be repeated. Sitchevska reported several cases fitted with Müller contact lenses around 1929 to 1931. The numbers of lenses tried in during the fitting sessions were as follows: '100 trials to select lenses for a pair of eyes, 20 tried for one eye, 45 for one eye and 20–30 for the other, 35 lenses tried for one eye'. Clearly as with the Zeiss–Heine system, a very large fitting bank of Müller lenses was necessary.

The problems in selecting a suitably fitting Müller lens become very apparent. Nevertheless, toleration was often surprisingly good, Sitchevska quoting 8–10 hours, 12–14 hours, 6–9 hours, 10–12 hours, 4–5 hours, 8–9 hours, and 6–8 hours in successive patients. In contrast, a number of these patients had already tried wearing the ground Zeiss lenses with typical wearing times recorded as 'could not wear, 1–2 hours or half to one hour'. The chances of good visual correction, however, were much higher when using the Zeiss lens.

To what can we attribute the greater toleration of the Müller lenses? Sitchevska quoted a weight of 0.5 g for the Zeiss and a little more for the Müller lens, so weight seems not to provide the answer. She described the classic design of the Zeiss lens 'the glass until recently was standardized to four precise corneal curvatures, the radii of which are 6.5, 7.1, 8.1 and 9 mm. The diameter of the corneal segment is 12 mm and the height of the corneal segment or its depth varies with the various radii — 3.0, 4.0, 4.5 and 5.0 mm respectively'. Therein lies the reason for the choice of such a curious range of back optic zone radii. If we remember that up to this time no method had been devised for obtaining detailed impressions of the cornea, and what dimensions had been obtained were the result of optically measuring the visible iris diameter, the reasons for regarding a back optic zone diameter of 12 mm as satisfactory, become apparent.

Duke-Elder (1961) quotes the average corneal diameter from the findings of many different workers as 11.7 mm horizontally by 10.6 mm vertically and slightly less in females. From these figures, an optic zone diameter of 12 mm seems more than adequate. It was not until 1938 when Obrig first published his table of corneal dimensions as determined from the measurements of several hundred eye casts resulting from Negocoll impressions, that the inadequacy of back optic zone diameter of the Zeiss lens became completely apparent. The reader should remember that the means of determining lack of corneal touch at this time lay in slit lamp examination of the contact lens on the eye. The slit lamps of this period had nowhere near reached the present level of sophistication and ease of use. Moreover, the assessment of clearance at the limbal region would have been more uncertain with the slit lamp than would apical clearance. Fluorescein solution, long used for the detection of corneal lesions, had been recommended as an aid to detection of loose channels under the scleral zone of contact lenses. Von der Heydt and Gradle (1930) had recommended the slit lamp in conjunction with fluorescein for these observations. The examination, however, was made with white tungsten light so the fluorescence of the dye was only poorly activated. It was not until 1938 that Obrig drew attention to the value of using cobalt blue light for this work. Thus, it is not surprising that the significance of the small back optic zone diameter of the Zeiss contact lens was not recognized earlier.

In contrast to the Zeiss lens, with its scleral zone about 4.5 mm wide, Sitchevska described the Müller lens as having a scleral band nasally of 4–5 mm, superiorly and inferiorly of 7–8 mm and temporally of 10–12 mm and comments on its 'gradual transition from the corneal into the scleral part'. Here then were reasons for the greater acceptability of the blown Müller lens. Obrig and Salvatori (1957) cite both Sommer (1927) and Gill (1928) as attributing the greater comfort of the Müller lens in part to its natural fire polish as a consequence of the techniques of its manufacture. Having examined the quality of finish on Zeiss lenses of the period, the author does not accept this factor as being sufficient to account for the marked discrepancy. We must look to the design of the back surfaces to account for the better toleration and to the greater likelihood of loose channels in the Müller lens allowing tear interchange. One should remember that in those days of restricted tolerance, high ametropes often managed to use the Müller contact lenses throughout the day, by wearing monocularly and alternating between right and left lenses.

The development of design in the Zeiss ground lens is in itself an interesting study. Mann (1938) states that the Zeiss ground lens was first produced in 1911. The first vestiges of a preformed fitting set approach were seen around 1920 with the introduction of the four lens set already referred to. Dr W. Stock, its originator, was himself a sufferer from keratoconus and intended this four lens set primarily for the investigation of that condition. Dallos (1936) credits Professor Hans Hartinger with the idea of blending the sharp junction between optic and scleral zones of the Zeiss lens and Zeiss trade literature of around 1933 offers the option of a totally blended transition. Over the course of the 1920s, an increasing range of back scleral radii was added to the original 12 mm standard radius. First, a choice of three radii 11.0 mm, 12.0 mm and later 13.0 mm. Later, the 0.5-mm steps and ultimately, according to Dallos (1936), a full range in 0.25-mm steps from 10.0 mm to 14.0 mm were available.

Around this time was also being evolved the 'afocal lens approach' of Professor Leopold Heine. This offered a choice of a large range of afocal Zeiss lenses of varying back optic zone radii with which a wide range of ametropia could be corrected purely by means of the liquid lens. The ultimate range of back optic zone radii extended from 5.0 mm to 11.0 mm and eventually these could be procured in steps of 0.1 mm. Towards 1930 it had become the practice to grind some optical power on to the Zeiss prescription lens so that a total correction could be achieved partly from the liquid lens and partly from the optical power of the contact lens. However, such optical power was limited to the order of ±7.00 D. It was not until 1933 that Dallos made the suggestion that if the front optic diameter be restricted to some 8 mm, much higher optical values would become possible and a great saving effected in thickness and weight. Despite this technical progress, Dallos (1936), remarking that the University of Kiel Eye Clinic had a set of over 300 different Zeiss lenses, voiced the opinion that these were able to satisfy only a very small percentage of those who needed to be fitted with contact lenses. Dallos went on to survey the developing topographic knowledge of the eye which was accruing from successful eye impressions, noting the changes in scleral curvature from one meridian to another and naturally concluding that a lens

construction based on segments of a sphere, could not possibly result in the uniform contact necessary to achieve a high level of comfort.

Another of the major contributions by Dallos to contact lens technology in the early 1930s was the development of glass moulding as a means of producing the initial contact shell. It became necessary to perfect a series of stages by which the Negocoll impression and its resultant Hominit positive could be transposed via plaster of Paris into a brass die suitable for the glass moulding procedure. This process has been described in some detail and illustrated by the author (Sabell, 1980d). Moreover, it was important that such shells should be capable of being optically ground and polished in the central zone in order to form the clinically important link between the wearable but optically imperfect Müller lens and the optically good but less well tolerated Zeiss lens. The attempts at optically grinding the Müller lenses by Erggelet and von Hippel, reported by Sitchevska (1932), had all ended in complete failure. That this process is not intrinsically impossible was later demonstrated by Dallos, although for normal scleral lens manufacture it would not appear to be a sound production method. From this point on, therefore, a third method of manufacturing contact lenses had begun, a method which was to dominate the field until well into the 1950s. It was a method equally applicable to the new acrylic materials which were to be introduced some 10 years later.

Dallos' earlier attempts at glass moulding were made in the bacteriology laboratory of the No.1 Eye Clinic, Budapest, and were begun using sections of cleaned photographic plates. The earliest attempts (*Figure 1.8*) were made with equipment no more elaborate than a standard laboratory tripod with bunsen burner to heat the glass plate. The metal die, which is an essential feature in the process of moulding a glass contact lens, was held by means of forceps, or some other suitable attachment, in the hand of the technician. When the glass had reached a suitable temperature as judged by its colour the metal die was quickly thrust through the softened glass plate and the source of heat removed. On removal of the heat, the glass solidifies so rapidly that unlike moulding acrylic materials it is not strictly necessary that the die should be held in a mechanically rigid clamp. Later, presses as developed by Dallos and his

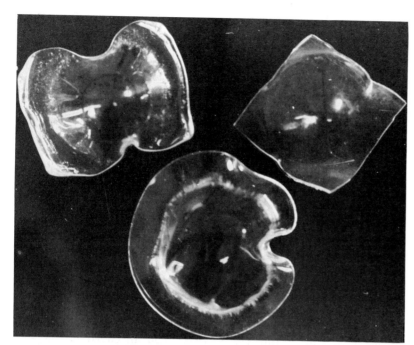

Figure 1.8 The results of initial experiments at moulding sheet glass made by Dallos in Budapest (about 1932). (From the museum, Department of Vision Sciences, University of Aston)

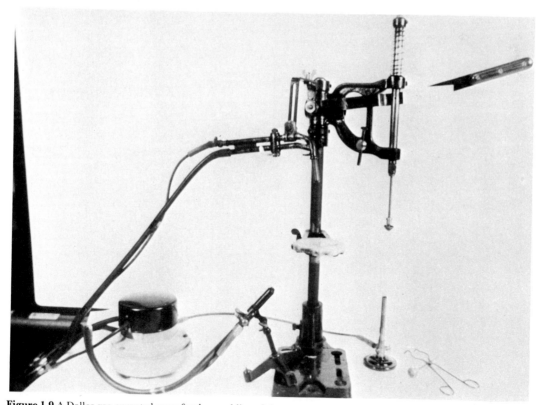

Figure 1.9 A Dallos gas-operated press for the moulding of glass contact shells (about 1942). Two gas jets heat the glass blank from above and below simultaneously, while the bunsen burner heats the brass die in readiness for the moulding process. (From the museum, Department of Vision Sciences, University of Aston)

team became rather more sophisticated and an example of one produced in the early 1940s is shown in *Figure 1.9*.

It was from this time on that Dallos established what he referred to as 'haptics, a new branch of prosthetics'. It was this establishment of rules for the modification of casts and shells leading systematically to the achievement of a well balanced contact lens, that placed Dallos at the forefront of contact lens practitioners of the inter-war years. Dallos himself said in 1936 'one does not now select at random among the ready made shells or bowls and trust a patient's judgement as to the best one to use; but with the same precision with which the dioptric requirements are prescribed one forms the shells for the individual patient'.

It is interesting, however, that by 1938, Dallos, although still thoroughly disenchanted with the Zeiss lens, was also showing signs of moving away from eye impressions. With respect to the Zeiss lens he said '. . . the scleral periphery of these spherical glass bowls will reach the conjunctiva and touch it, but only over certain circumscribed areas. These areas are always at the edge of this ring-shaped scleral part, either on the peripheral margin, or on the limbus inside, so that even if the glass does rest on the scleral conjunctiva it never fits with its surface, but rather with sharp edges'. We were later to see, using this same reasoning, the introduction by Forknall (1948) of the 'offset scleral lens'. Although Dallos did not for one instant accept that a uniform scleral fit could be achieved by using even the very narrow scleral zone of the 20 mm Zeiss lens, he had become sceptical of the necessity of taking eye impressions for each individual patient. Dallos (1938) went on to say: 'you start every case with an approximately fitting shell. If you have got a set consisting of 30 pairs of differently shaped forms, you will very probably find a type that will not differ or differs only slightly from the eye to be fitted. If you have not got this set, then you had better take a mould from the eye.' A case of 100 pairs of brass dies to accompany the type shell set has been illustrated by the author (Sabell, 1980d). We see therefore that by 1938 Dallos, by now working in London at the Cavendish Square 'centre' (Rugg-Gunn, 1938), had firmly established his technique of fitting from 'type shells' in preference to making new impressions for each patient.

There followed the development of this unique approach to the fitting of scleral contact lenses, a method which comparatively few practitioners have learned and fewer still have mastered. It was an achievement which for years to come, set Dallos far ahead of his contemporaries in the achievement of long toleration combined with good visual results. The natural outcome of these complexities in scleral lens fitting was to encourage rather than to discourage an interest in the potentialities of the spherical preformed lens.

Impetus was given to the preformed lens following the introduction of acrylic materials. In the USA this development occurred predominantly in the field of the moulded impression lenses pioneered by Obrig, although Feinbloom (1937) had, some years earlier, introduced a contact lens with a plastic scleral zone and a glass optic. In England, by contrast, the early moves were made in the preformed field. C. W. Dixey and Co. made their first experiments which led to their 'flexible contact lenses' in 1938. Although these were at first plastic replicas of the Zeiss lens, their manufacturing process was unique and marks the introduction of the fourth major lens-making process. According to Ridley (1946), Dixey's were the first to use a precision lathe for cutting contact lenses from solid blocks of ICI Transpex material. This lathe-cutting process allowed much greater variability in dimensions than was readily obtainable from the glass-grinding methods of Zeiss. The Dixey lenses were of the same order of thickness as the Zeiss lens but could readily be made thinner (down to 0.3 mm) without becoming excessively fragile. Thus, a saving of about 60% on the weight of the glass Zeiss lens could be achieved. Dallos consistently condemned this flexibility which resulted from very thin acrylic lenses, which he saw as an obstacle to achieving the precision of corneal fit which he required (J. Dallos, personal communication).

The image of this almost infinite variety of sizes and shapes offered by the 'Dixey flexible contact lens' encouraged an increase in the number of contact lens practitioners, especially in the non-medical sphere. Names like Frank Dickinson and Keith Clifford Hall began to be closely associated with the fitting of this form of lens. Their textbook in 1946 contained considerable information on the development from the

Zeiss to the Dixey forms of contact lens. In the medical sphere, Ridley (1946) came out with enthusiasm on the side of the Dixey lens. He presented an analysis of results of 200 consecutive patients and said 'it is believed that this series justifies a revival of interest in the spherical or regular types of lens'. Ridley believed that 80% of contact lens patients were suitable for fitting by this method and that the lens could be prescribed by an ophthalmologist in the same way that prescriptions for spectacles were handed out.

Dallos' message of the direct involvement of the contact lens practitioner in the achievement of a personally tailored contact lens seemed unattractive to seekers after an easier road. It should be remembered that in the UK, for the period between the introduction of the Dixey lens, until about 1947, the only plastics contact lenses available were of preformed design. Patients for whom impressions were necessary still had to be supplied with glass lenses. This factor swung preference somewhat artificially towards the preformed lens approach.

This interest in preformed lenses was further accentuated by the introduction, between 1945 and the end of 1948, of a number of apparently new ideas. From America came a new concept by Feinbloom who had pioneered the early transition from glass to plastics. Feinbloom (1945) discarded the concept that the weight of a scleral lens was best supported over as broad an area as possible. He felt that a minimal tangential touch would not only evoke less sensation but would enable a better balance on the toroidally shaped sclera, and he introduced the 'Feincone lens'. At this time, no toric preformed scleral lenses were in regular production and the only alternative lay in the impression. It has been suggested in the section on development of impression techniques that this limitation of choice in the USA may have placed the optometrist in an embarrassing situation vis-à-vis the drugs laws. Thus, any preformed lens able to make further inroads into the 20% or so of patients for whom impressions seemed the only answer must have been welcomed. The 'Feincone lens' offered a preview of the apparent simplicity of fitting which was to reappear in the corneal lens sphere in later years as a result of similar tangential designs. Certainly reduction of the sharp corneoscleral junction and making the conic scleral zone

approximately tangential to the globe, resulted in an initially favourable sensory response. It was, however, in the American tradition set by Obrig, a full clearance lens and therefore did nothing to reduce the effects of Sattler's veil. Watson (1947) commented on its prominent appearance and, introducing his 'Kelvin lens', he described his attempts at improving cosmetically on this American design. A fitting set of these Kelvin conic lenses has been described and illustrated (Sabell, 1980b). Curiously, a second conical design was announced in the same issue of The Optician, by Cohen (1947), whose design was also manifestly based on Feinbloom's lens. These designs were reviewed by McKellen (1949).

By far the best known design in the UK said to be based on the Feincone lens was the 'wide angle lens' of Nissel, introduced in 1947. This and the other two conical designs mentioned had one aim in common, to reduce the vast numbers of permutations introduced by the Dixey system. In theory, it was possible to order well over 3000 different Dixey lenses without repeating oneself, and this did not include variations in optical power. By standardizing the diameter of the optic zone and relating the apical cone angle of its transition region to a fixed relationship with the back optic zone radius, a considerable reduction in permutations was achieved by the wide angle design. For specific detail of the construction of wide angle lenses and of typical fitting sets the reader is referred to Chapter 17 on preformed fitting techniques.

This post-war period saw the introduction of two other concepts worthy of note. The first, by Bier and Cole (1948), was introduced as a small set of preformed fitting shells intended to supplement the fitting sets of Dixey lenses then in use. Once again, the rationale was one of simplification of the processes of scleral lens fitting to reduce the number of fitting lenses needed by the less experienced practitioner. This was the 'transcurve lens' and its originators claimed cosmetic superiority by virtue of a larger total diameter than that of the Dixey-type preformed lens. The most significant contribution associated with the transcurve lens was the introduction of the separate corneal measuring caps now referred to as FLOMS (fenestrated lenses for optic measurement). In the author's opinion, these provide one of the most useful aids for teaching students the fundamental principles of the optic fit. Again, the design features of these measuring lenses are dealt with in Chapter 17.

The second of these post-war concepts was the 'offset lens' of Forknall (1948), designed with an aspherical scleral zone to obtain a more even pressure on the sclera. This also aided simplification of fitting by the elimination of the necessity to adjust scleral zone radius when total diameter was changed. As McKellen (1963) later pointed out, this design was neglected by most contact lens practitioners and the concept achieved wider prominence only after its re-introduction by Ruben within the sphere of corneal lenses around 1966. The use of 'offset scleral lenses' is also dealt with under Preformed fitting in Chapter 17.

One should not end this account of aspheric scleral lens development without reference to the lenses of A. Mueller-Welt. Starting with experience of making and fitting artificial eyes, Mueller-Welt established the ability to grind optical surfaces on blown lenses and later, using acrylic materials, expressed a preference for polymerization in making the initial shell rather than cutting or grinding. Mueller-Welt (1950) described the design of his lenses as having a capillary tear layer over the cornea and retaining an air cushion beneath the scleral zone. This part of the lens may incorporate several areas of differing curvature, seeking to take account of the anatomy of the insertions of the four recti muscles. Thus, with these two designs we can see the preformed advocates attempting to reproduce, in mathematical terms, the natural asphericity achieved by the practitioners using the impression or 'type-shell' approach to fitting.

The design of scleral lenses and the principles on which their fitting is based has therefore changed little over the last 40 years. One or two more recent developments are worthy of note, such as the methods of Marriott (1967, 1970) for the manufacture of impression shells and also the scleral lens design developed by Lewis (1970) both of which are particularly useful in hospital eye service contact lens work.

Glass and acrylic corneal lenses

For some time after 1948, corneal lenses were believed by many to have originated with those devised by Tuohy and by Woehlk. These lenses have been described by Bier (1957) and it is interesting to note that, while the name of Tuohy is much more widely known as a corneal lens pioneer, the lenses being used at that time by Woehlk more nearly conform in size to those corneal lenses in use today.

However, Obrig and Salvatori (1957) and Graham (1959) have put forward evidence of the attempted use of corneal lenses from as early as 1888. According to Graham, one of the first to draw attention to earlier usage of corneal lenses was Emerich Rakoss, who published a paper entitled 'How new is the corneal lens?' in May 1950. Both authors refer to the lenses by Kalt of Paris as being of corneal lens design. Obrig and several other authors have described M. Kalt as an optician. This seems unlikely in view of his participation in meetings of the Société Française d'Ophtalmologie, as reported (in the discussion following a paper) by Chevallereau (1893). It would seem likely that this was Eugene Kalt of Paris whose photograph is published by Duke-Elder (1969). In addition, Graham presents reasons for supposing that Fick's early lenses were also of corneal design and this point has already been discussed.

There can be little doubt, however, that August Müller of Kiel University was the first to use the name corneal lenses — 'Hornhautlinsen' — although it is doubtful whether this is an accurate description of the type of lens which he employed because it is described as having a scleral radius of 12.0 mm.

Experimental corneal lenses were made by Carl Zeiss and were described by von Rohr and Stock (1912). Erggelet also used such lenses experimentally and Obrig and Salvatori (1957) published a letter from Dr Hans Hartinger confirming this. The purpose of these lenses was to induce artificial ametropia for subjective testing of various designs of spectacle lens.

Some years later, H. J. M. Weve used glass corneal lenses to aid observation of the retina during detachment surgery. This lens was referred to by Mann (1938), and Obrig and Salvatori (1957) again published a letter from Weve on their use. These authors also quoted Zeiss records as showing a number of companies and institutions to whom glass corneal-type contact lenses were supplied in the 1935/36 period.

It is safe to assume that, while these early

glass corneal lenses may have been of value for experimental work or as aids to eye surgery, they were unsuccessful as routine corrective appliances for ametropia. Obrig and Salvatori (1957) quote from a letter by Dr L. L. Forchheiner saying that these lenses could not be worn satisfactorily owing to their weight. Graham (1959) published a comparison of dimensions between a Zeiss-made 1932 glass corneal lens of thickness 0.6 mm and a 1948 variety acrylic lens of thickness 0.3 mm. Because, apart from thickness, these lenses were of similar dimensions and allowing for the specific gravity of the two materials, it would appear that the glass lens would be at least four times the weight of the plastics one. One must also bear in mind the surface characteristics of the two materials. Glass wets more readily and has a more slippery surface when on the eye. This factor has been quoted to account for a preference for glass artificial eyes by patients who have changed over to wearing an acrylic prosthesis. Because successful performance and comfort of a corneal lens depends on the ability of the upper lid to raise the lens on the cornea after each blink, it seems unlikely that glass would offer a suitable material for a corneal lens. Thus, the key factor necessary for successful development of corneal lenses was the development of polymethyl methacrylate around 1936 and its introduction as a contact lens material around 1938 by Obrig in the USA and by C. W. Dixey and Company in England. Indeed, it may well be claimed that Dixey's development of the first precision lathes for cutting contact lenses also played indirectly a major part in the success of this type of lens.

By 1952, the Tuohy lens had become well known and yet was still a poor competitor with the scleral lenses of that period. This may be judged by reference to the American Army Report which is quoted extensively by Obrig and Salvatori (1957). It was not until the introduction of the single curve 'Microlens' in 1954 that corneal lenses appeared to offer an effective alternative to scleral lenses. This lens (Dickinson, 1954), devised jointly by W. P. Soehnges in Germany, Frank Dickinson in England and John C. Neil in the USA, proved a considerable improvement on the larger Tuohy lenses. Reference to *Table 1.1* will make clear the design differences.

For comparison of fit, the reader should

Table 1.1 Comparison of parameters of the Tuohy and 'Microlens' corneal lenses

Parameters	Tuohy lens	'Microlens'
Total diameter (mm)	11–12	9.5
Centre thickness (mm)	0.25–0.35	0.20 (afocal)
BOZD (mm)	8.0–9.0	9.5
Back surface peripheral curve	One	None
Width of peripheral curve (mm)	1.5	Nil
Relationship of peripheral curve to BOZR (mm)	0.3–0.6 flatter	Identical

consider only the zone of constant curvature. Thus, we are effectively comparing a 'Microlens' of total diameter 9.5 mm fitted 0.3–0.6 mm flatter than the corneal keratometer reading, with a Tuohy lens effectively of 8.5 mm diameter fitted about 0.35 mm flatter than the keratometer reading. The central bearing zone was therefore similar in size in both cases. The Tuohy lens being considerably larger, the resultant fluorescein band of edge clearance was broader. This, in turn, limited the application of this larger lens for the fitting of astigmatic eyes and Bier (1957) considered 2.00 D of corneal astigmatism to represent the limit of usefulness for the Tuohy lens. By contrast, the 'Microlens' allowed fitting of up to 4.00 D of corneal toricity. Both designs, giving a hard apical pressure zone, tended to result in apical corneal erosions. With this factor in mind, the smaller and thinner microlens had obvious advantages and its designers specified that centre thickness should be calculated on the basis of an afocal lens of centre thickness 0.2 mm. This is a realistic standard which could still be usefully followed by many of today's corneal lens manufacturers.

About this time, an interesting, if unproductive, design of corneal lens was introduced by de Carle (1953) which was designated the 'corneal flange lens'. This was a peripheral bearing lens having minimal central clearance and a fairly large fenestration. It was an interesting attempt to apply scleral lens principles to the fitting of corneal lenses. As such it was unsuccessful through inability to control air bubble movement.

Concern over corneal apical erosion and corneal curvature changes resulting from long periods of microlens wear led to the establishment by Bier (1956a,b) of a new principle of fitting. His 'contour lens' of similar size and thickness to the 'microlens' could, by virtue of its smaller back optic zone diameter (BOZD), be fitted nearly in alignment with the central zone of the cornea, thereby minimizing to a considerable degree the central erosion problem. Edge clearance was still maintained by a peripheral curve some 1.25 mm wide. Bier postulated that flatter corneas were likely to require a greater peripheral curve flattening relative to back optic zone radius (BOZR) than steeper corneas. He therefore recommended fitting sets in which the degree of peripheral flattening ranged from 0.3 mm at the 7.3 mm BOZR region to 0.7 mm at the 8.5 mm end of the range. This system does make for some complications in using such a set and from about 1960 it became more common to employ fitting sets with a standard peripheral flattening throughout the full lens range. It is interesting to note that with later trends to establish fitting sets having a constant edge lift, we may be moving back towards the principle established loosely by Bier in 1956. With his introduction of the contour lens, Bier also laid down the principles of apical clearance fitting, producing a slightly modified design of lens for this purpose. This mode of fit, however, was not popular and did not gain acceptance until later design changes allowed its full exploitation.

Two main changes in design paved the way to apical clearance fitted corneal lenses. The first of these was the addition of a flat edge bevel or narrow peripheral curve of some 12 mm radius. This feature was introduced into the UK by de Carle, with the Sphercon corneal lenses which were modifications of a slightly earlier American design of the same name. The popularity of these lenses developed in the UK over the early 1960s and established firmly the multi-curve principle.

The second feature, also seen in the Sphercon range of lenses, which helped to establish successful apical clearance fitting, was the reduction of total diameter. This resulted from the manufacturing of fitting sets of standard lenses around 9.20 mm and smaller lenses of 8.70 mm.

The trend towards narrower intermediate and peripheral zones in tri-curve, tetra-curve and penta-curve corneal lenses at the this time led, via various degrees of blending of transitions, to the manufacturing of various continuous back surface designs. Thus, the late 1960s were characterized by the establishment of a series of aspheric corneal lenses ranging from the tangential conic periphery designs of Thomas (1968) and Stek (1969) through the continuous offset bi-curve principle (Ruben, 1966; Nissel, 1967), to the lathe-cut continuous aspheric lens of Nissel (1968). Over this period, and before the wider acceptance of the small ultrathin PMMA lenses, fenestration was frequently employed with corneal lenses to minimize central corneal oedema. This was particularly required with steeply fitted lenses such as the conic design of Thomas (1968). With such lenses the 'cupping glass effect' of negative hydrostatic pressure which occurred in the absence of fenestration, readily produced such central oedema. Unfortunately, the fenestration of such lenses seemed, not infrequently, to encourage so-called 'dimple veil' (*see* Chapter 19 and *Plate 22*). Occasionally the urge to fenestrate corneal lenses seems to have got out of hand (*Figure 1.10*). Despite the apparently enhanced tear exchange, this particular patient had developed extensive superior corneal neovascularization. We have thus reached the present-day period with a wide range of corneal lens design including toric and multifocal lenses available for selection by practitioners in order to fit successfully the vast majority of prospective patients.

A discussion of hard corneal lenses should not end without reference to the 'Apex lens' of

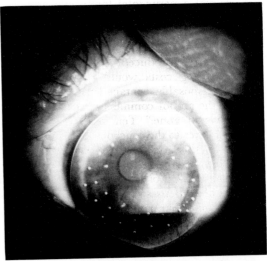

Figure 1.10 A multifenestrated PMMA corneal lens made in the USA around 1970. A laser beam was used to produce the 40 fenestrations simultaneously

Fraser and Gordon (1967). This, like the scleral design of Lewis (1970) was a lens designed specifically for the hospital service. The name 'Apex' — said to be derived from 'aphakic experiment' — not perhaps the most tactful of designations, nevertheless clearly defines its area of application. It is a large corneal/perilimbal design which in an aphakic prescription is necessarily fairly thick and heavy. It is a design likely to be tolerated well only by corneas which have suffered a fair depletion of sensibility as is commonly the case following cataract surgery. The great advantage of this design which has been discussed by Ruben (1967) lies, for aphakics, in the great stability of vision resulting from the limbal locating characteristics.

'Soft' lenses and rigid gas permeable corneal lenses

Dreifus (1978) has reviewed the early work leading to the announcement of hydrophilic plastics for medical applications and has described the investigations using experimental animals to assess toxicity to the intraocular tissues and to determine the effect of the early hydrogel (soft) lenses on corneal metabolism. He describes some of the initial resistance by clinicians to the use of this new and revolutionary form of contact lens, some of the early clinical experiences using these Geltakt lenses, the original experimental forms, and the later Czechoslovakian commercially distributed Spofalenses. As stated in the first section of this chapter, the early Czechoslovakian hydrophilic lenses were introduced in the belief that manufacturing costs would be so low as to provide disposable contact lenses. In the last edition, the author commented 'Where has this happy vision gone?' Ten years later we are slightly nearer to the concept of throw away soft lenses, yet this goal is still recognized as most desirable. Morris (1980), in reviewing soft lens progress, speaks of the need for prepacked supplies of soft lenses so that perhaps one year's supply of, say, four pairs can be dispensed at one time. Whether such a system would be open to abuse is of course a debatable point but at least it would by-pass some of the present day unsatisfactory cleaning facilities which plague some patients, especially those using extended wear systems.

The centenary year of Fick's publication, 1988, saw the introduction by Messrs Johnson & Johnson of the first disposable extended wear soft lens system. The running costs of this 'Acuvue' lens are, however, appreciably higher than those of conventional extended wear soft lenses and in this respect we are still a long way from the original Czech dream of a cheap, disposable, visual correction.

The second hope was that, being a very flexible material, a single back surface curve, steeper than the human cornea would suffice and such a lens could be pressed into place and would conform to all corneal contours. The original lenses therefore had an aspherical rear surface derived from the centrifugal force employed in their spin-casting mode of fabrication. Visual instability rapidly forced the multiplication of back surface curves and led to lens design studies such as that of Larke and Sabell (1971). From around 1967, the availability of buttons of the dehydrated HEMA material allowed development of lathe-cutting techniques and the application of conventional back surface designs as had been employed in various hard corneal and perilimbal lenses. One of the earliest enthusiasts for the new soft lenses in the UK was Robert Turner who from December 1963 held a series of meetings to introduce this new concept to practitioners. His report in the *Ophthalmic Optician* (Turner, 1964a) appears to be among the earliest in British journals. Despite this early enthusiasm, by July 1964 doubts were already being raised over the available procedures for sterilizing these lenses. By November of that year Turner (1964b) commented 'disadvantages in the use of hydrophilic gel contact lenses have led to experiments with silicone'. A further statement in this paper is interesting in the light of subsequent developments: '. . . it is not possible to maintain stability in a hydrophilic gel when we have a combination of only 25 per cent of plastic macromolecular structure, and 75 per cent of water.' In discussing the observable 'Sattler's veil' in some patients using the hydrogel lenses of the period, Turner makes the prophetic statement: 'The soft plastics are such a new and revolutionary development it must be expected that we shall have to face many greater problems than this before we are fully satisfied and completely happy with the results.' This paper also discusses difficulties of soft lens measurement and problems arising from both heat and chemical systems of disinfection. It sounds strange to us today to read '. . . that daily wear lenses should be sterilised at least once every two weeks, if not once each week'.

Over the last two decades we have seen the worldwide explosion in contact lens-related research into corneal physiology. This has run concurrently with the great interest, often commercially inspired, in the development of new contact lens materials. The great obsession of the 1970s has been the importance of oxygen to the corneal well being, the importance of which was questioned by Dallos (1980).While practitioners were well aware of the necessity to ensure good tear exchange behind both scleral and PMMA corneal lenses, it appeared to be the advent of the hydrogel lens which turned thoughts towards the possibility of diffusion of oxygen through the lens material itself. The early belief that the original low water content hydrogel lenses were oxygen permeable was dispelled by research of workers such as Hill and Fatt (1964). Nevertheless, investigations into corneal uptake of oxygen following occlusion by various forms of contact lens stimulated the development, first of high water content materials such as Permalens and Sauflon, and, more latterly, of the ultrathin soft lens in lower water content material in the hope of increasing the lifespan of the contact lens.

Towards the end of the 1970s a growing disillusionment on the part of many practitioners with flexible forms of contact lens has led to the current popularity of the rigid gas permeable (RGP) corneal lens. The advent of RGP materials has offered some relief from limited correction of corneal astigmatism by flexible lenses. We can say in looking back that the 1970s was the decade of the soft lens but that, although they are still widely employed, many practitioners have become disillusioned with this form of correction. The reasons were many. Transmitted corneal astigmatism, despite valiant attempts by lens manufacturers to produce satisfactory toric soft lenses, still constitutes, in the private sector at least, a great nuisance. With soft lenses, the added complexity and cost of maintenance systems still proves a great disadvantage. The inability to effectively remove some forms of deposit remains a source of frustration. The red eye syndrome, whether the result of anoxia, entrapped debris or toxic

response to chemical antiseptics used in lens care is still with us to a noticeable degree.

Purification of hydrogel material to eliminate intrinsic toxicity together with much time and thought spent on lens design, have eliminated many of the early problems associated with hydrogel lenses. We now have a bewildering array of proprietary brands of soft contact lenses from a multiplicity of makers and suppliers. This is matched by a large array of care systems, each claiming superiority over its competitors. Prescription restrictions of the early years have been overcome and it is now possible to obtain very high optical powers as well as astigmatic corrections and even bifocal forms of soft lens. This is not to say that these more specialized types are free of their own mechanical problems. It is still true to say that the simplest designs of both corneal and soft lenses are the ones giving least problems in toleration.

To reach this stage of development with soft lenses has demanded huge research expenditure. This has been further increased by demands made by government departments both in the UK and in the USA and other countries in order to safeguard the public from various potential hazards, both real and imaginary. The rules and regulations of both the DHSS (in the UK) and the Food and Drugs Administration (in the USA) now apply both to soft lenses and to care products for both hard (rigid) and soft contact lenses. The outcome of these events has been the almost total elimination of what the author has heard disparagingly referred to as 'the cottage industry' of contact lens manufacturing of former years. Since the early 1960s, contact lens manufacturing has been increasingly taken over by large multinational organizations often associated directly or indirectly with the pharmaceutical industry on which the contact lens practitioner had become dependent for all contact lens support systems. We see regular 'take-overs' and financial manoeuvrings within the present-day contact lens industry which have tended to destroy that close personal working relationship which, in earlier days, existed between the practitioner and his supply house.

In the last edition, the author expressed the opinion that the greatest potential for soft lenses lay in their use for medically indicated conditions, especially those lenses intended for extended wear. It is now difficult to imagine how a hospital eye service would cope with the contact lens needs of, for example, the aphakic elderly if it were not for the ready availability of extended wear soft lenses. Equally, the paediatric field has become very dependent on this form of correction. Not that these are trouble free by any stretch of the imagination. The deposition and cleaning difficulties already mentioned, together with the microbial risks associated with soft lens wear, continue to call forth a steady stream of publications in the professional journals. Nevertheless, within the hospital sector the soft lens has become indispensible. Both for visual and therapeutic needs, it has taken its place alongside rigid lenses of both corneal and scleral forms. While corneal lenses play an important role for hospital patients, it is within this area that the scleral lens has retained a vital place. For this reason it is disturbing that, almost worldwide, the undergraduate teaching curriculum has largely eliminated practical scleral lens experience. Teaching of this is of course time consuming and, if absent from undergraduate programmes, it seems vital that adequate provision be made for postgraduate work in this area if the future of this lens form is to be safeguarded.

The apparent insolubility of the various soft lens problems already outlined makes understandable the trend over more recent years of reversion to rigid lenses. A return to well-tried PMMA? Certainly not! Such a move would imply retreat. Besides which the polymer chemists by now had the bit between their teeth and were forging ahead with apparently unlimited variations of the so-called oxygen permeable rigid copolymers. The 1980s can therefore truly be labelled as the decade of the RGP contact lens. There have even been attempts in Australia and the UK to produce scleral lenses in RGP materials (*see* Chapters 17 and 18), although with the necessary thickness of a scleral lens it is difficult to imagine how much oxygen could permeate through. Both lathe-turning and moulding have been attempted as methods of manufacture.

Little change seems to have taken place in corneal lens designs for use with the new RGP materials, which did, however, allow a return to the fitting of larger corneal lenses. With PMMA, the trend over the 1970s had been towards very small and ultrathin lenses in an attempt to minimize corneal oedema and corneal warping.

The small lenses sometimes gave rise to complaints of edge flare, especially in patients who had previously worn larger corneal lenses. The increased visual stability afforded by the larger RGP lenses was therefore welcomed by practitioner and patient alike.

Unhappily the new materials, apart from being more susceptible to mechanical damage than PMMA, have also shown themselves much more prone to surface deposits although not so badly as the hydrogels. RGP lenses are therefore more demanding of specialized care systems than their impermeable predecessors. An interesting comment was made to the author recently by a fellow examiner in the professional examinations to the effect that he found today's graduates tended to think exclusively in terms of either hydrogel or RGP lenses and already to regard PMMA as 'something from the Ark'. In contrast, the older practitioner, having cut his teeth on PMMA corneal lenses, tends to have an increasing respect for the characteristics of that material. It does seem astonishing that the first of the plastics to be widely adopted for contact lens use, albeit not having been devised for that purpose, should have turned out to be such a success. One so frequently hears these older practitioners say that where possible they still prefer to employ PMMA for corneal lenses. Can this be a parallel to the expressed preference right until the end of his life, by Joseph Dallos, for glass rather than PMMA, for the construction of scleral lenses? It would appear that where PMMA corneal lenses are tolerated by the patient they have given excellent long-term service and we are seeing today increasing numbers still happily wearing such lenses for upwards of 30 years. It is, for the sake of perspective, worth remembering that, prior to the coming of the hydrogel lens and the RGP lens, experienced contact lens practitioners were claiming between 70 and 80% success rate using PMMA. The mere availability of alternative forms and materials encourages switching from PMMA in the hope of a quick solution to an immediate problem. Such a decision is not necessarily in the best long-term interests of the patient.

The currently used materials and the design of contact lenses made from these materials will be dealt with in greater technical detail in later chapters of this book.

Epilogue

The history of any subject is, to a considerable extent, a story of human endeavour. In the field of contact lenses, two names stand out above all others. A. Eugen Fick made so many significant observations and predictions in his paper of 1888 that one is left with the feeling that all subsequent work has been tying up the loose ends which he indicated. Fick seems to have provided so many of the clues necessary to assist later workers.

The second of these great names is that of Joseph Dallos, for what other worker in the field of ophthalmology has devoted an entire working life to the furtherance of contact lenses? The work of Dallos from 1928, began to dominate the contact lens field, making a series of practical contributions which carried the contact lens from the status of an interesting novelty to that of a routinely applied correction. Indeed, when one looks at the maintenance routine which today's patient has to apply daily to hydrophilic contact lenses, one wonders whether Dallos had not reached the optimum point by 1936, when he said: 'its care is simple. In the evening after it is removed it is washed in water, dried with a clean cloth and put away in a padded box'. When one considers the present-day dependence of the contact lens wearer and, indeed, of the contact lens practitioner on technologists in many spheres, which in turn usually ends in inconvenience to both patient and practitioner, one may look back with nostalgia to the period during which contact lenses were truly regarded as 'solutionless lenses'.

We find, therefore, from the study of past events, that a recurrent pattern emerges. Initial concepts often represent over-simplification and the uncovering of problems leads to increasing complexity in design, materials and procedures in order to solve these problems. This increasing complexity may eventually reach proportions which become self-restrictive and which therefore call for attempts at re-simplification, at the same time retaining those features proven to be useful during the phase of increasing complexity. The overall trend is towards greater intricacy but conscious effort should be made to limit unnecessary technical complication. This is also true of contact lens economics; the most widespread application and usage of contact lenses will be aided by striving for simplicity of maintenance and handling procedures because, in the end, each appliance must be used by a lay person with very limited supervision. Development work aimed at reducing both supply and manufacturing costs of contact lenses is also important if maximum use is to be achieved. To these ends, the processes of re-simplification become important.

Some contact lens personalities

The last few years since the preparation of the previous edition of this book has included the deaths of several notables of the contact lens world.

On 27th June 1979 died Joseph Dallos whose early work formed the pivot between the previous 40 years of strictly limited progress in the contact lens field and the next 40 of rapid progress and expansion leading us to the present-day situation. Obituary notices were published in the *Journal of the British Contact Lens Association* by George Nissel (1979), erstwhile brother-in-law of the deceased, and also by M. Ruben (1979) in the *British Medical Journal*, followed 3 weeks later by two letters of appreciation by professional colleagues. The author (Sabell, 1979) also published a review of the work of Joseph Dallos in September of that year.

The death of George Nissel referred to above, occurred unexpectedly in Switzerland on 12th September 1982. An obituary notice written by Mr S. L. Sasieni (1982) appeared soon after, which outlines Nissel's career as a foremost contact lens manufacturer. A most comprehensive review of his life and work was given as the George Nissel Memorial Lecture by Ruben (1983).

A second well-liked personality from the contact lens manufacturing sphere to have died was Peter Madden. His sudden death at the early age of 59 years, took place on 25th November 1983 and left a sad and noticeable gap in the ranks of the contact lens fraternity of the UK.

A fourth well-known contact lens figure has also more recently passed on. This was Geoff McKellen who died on 25th January 1985 at the age of 81 years. G. D. McKellen was one of the few remaining practitioners who can claim to have had contact lens experience prior to World War II. It is appropriate that the North

Midland Optical Society should have instituted a McKellen Memorial Lecture, the first of which was given on 8th October 1986 by Mr Norman Bier.

No attempt has been made in this chapter to deal with the history of contact lens instrumentation. Neither has any detailed consideration been possible of development of knowledge relating corneal physiology and pathology to the use of contact lenses. One day, perhaps, a detailed history of contact lens manufacturing will be written, but such items must wait for the future and it is time for the reader to turn to a consideration of present-day knowledge and techniques.

Acknowledgements

I am indebted to the following persons for guidance and assistance in the preparation of this chapter.

Dr Joseph Dallos for many hours spent in discussion and for the most generous donation of many items of great historic interest to the Museum of the Department of Ophthalmic Optics, now the Department of Vision Sciences, at Aston University. Mr George Nissel for most useful advice and suggestions as well as to Mr Norman Bier. The University of Kiel Library for the loan of August Müller's dissertation 'Brillengläser und hornhautlinsen'. The University of Durham Library for the loan of Volume 4 of *Encyclopaedia Metropolitana* (1845). Mr Richard Hildred of the Birmingham and Midland Eye Hospital for photographic assistance. Mrs Ursula Bridgewater and Mrs Juliet Townsend for various translations, and last but by no means least to Mrs Margaret Jones of the University of Birmingham Health Centre for typing during the revision of this chapter.

References

AIRY, G. B. (1827). On a peculiar defect in the eye, and a mode of correcting it. *Trans. Camb. Phil. Soc.* **2**, 267–271

BENNETT, A. G. (1961). Contact lenses: origin. *Optician* **141**(3663), 644

BIER, N. (1945). Application For British Patent No.592055, 25th January 1945. Published in *Contact Lens Theory and Practice*, 2nd edn. London: Butterworths

BIER, N. (1948). The practice of ventilated contact lenses. *Optician* **116**, 497–501

BIER, N. (1956a). A study of the cornea. *Am. J. Optom.* **33**, 291–304

BIER, N. (1956b). The contour lens — a new form of corneal lens. *Optician* **132**(3422), 397–399

BIER, N. (1957). *Contact Lens Routine and Practice*, 2nd edn. London: Butterworths

BIER, N. and COLE, P. J. (1948). The 'transcurve' contact lens fitting shell. *Optician* **115**(2987), 605–606

BOSHOFF, P. H. (1943). Use of Zelex in making impressions of the eye for molded contact glasses. *Archs Ophthal.* **29**, 282–284

DE CARLE, J. (1953). Corneal flange contact lenses. *Optician* **125**(3248), 616–620

CHEVALLEREAU, M. A. (1893). Traitement du kératocone. *Bull. Mém. Soc. fr. Ophtal.* **11**, 385–392

CHISHOLM, J. F. (1940). Corneal molding for contact lenses. *Archs Ophthal.* **24**, 552–553

COHEN, L. B. (1947). The new 'Lewcone' contact lens. *Optician* **114**, 226–227

VON CSAPODY, I. (1929). Abgusse der lebenden augapfeloberfläche für verordnung von kontaktgläsern. *Klin. Mbl. Augenheilk.* **82**, 818–822

DALLOS, J. (1933). 'Ueber haftgläser und kontaktschalen. *Klin. Mbl. Augenheilk.* **91**, 640–659

DALLOS, J. (1936). Contact glasses, the 'invisible' spectacles. *Archs Ophthal.* **15**, 617–623

DALLOS, J. (1938). The individual fitting of contact glasses. *Trans. Ophthal. Soc. UK* **57**, 509–520

DALLOS, J. (1946). Sattler's veil. *Br. J. Ophthal.* **30**, 607–613

DALLOS, J. (1964). Individually fitted corneal lenses made to corneal moulds. *Br. J. Ophthal.* **48**, 510–512

DALLOS, J. (1980). The myth of oxygen permeability. *J. Br. Contact Lens Ass.* **3**(1), 28–29

DESCARTES, R. (1637). *Discours de la Methode*, Discours No. 7, *La Dioptrique* p.79

DICKINSON, F. (1954). Report on a new corneal lens. *Optician* **128**(3303), 3–6

DICKINSON, F. and HALL, K. G. C. (1946). *An Introduction to the Prescribing and Fitting of Contact lenses*. London: Hammond and Hammond

DOR, H. (1892). Sur les verres de contact. *Revue Gén. Ophtal.* **11**, 493–497

DREIFUS, M. (1978). The development of PHEMA for contact lens wear. In *Soft Contact Lenses*, edited by M. Ruben, pp. 7–16. London: Baillière Tindall

DUKE-ELDER, S. (1961). *The Anatomy of the Visual System, System of Ophthalmology*, Vol.2, p.93. London: Kimpton

DUKE-ELDER, S. (1969). *Diseases of the Lens and Vitreous: Glaucoma and Hypotony, System of Ophthalmology*, Vol.11, p.260. London: Kimpton

DUKE-ELDER, S. (1970). *Ophthalmic Optics and Refraction, System of Ophthamology*, Vol.5, p.713. London: Kimpton

ENOCH, J. M. (1956). Descartes' contact lens. *Am. J. Optom.* **33**, 77–85

FEINBLOOM, W. (1937). A plastic contact lens. *Am. J. Optom.* **14**, 41–49

FEINBLOOM, W. (1945). The tangent cone contact lens series. *Optom. Wkly* **36**, 1159–1161

FELDMAN, J. B. (1937). pH and buffers in relation to ophthalmology. *Archs Ophthal.* **17**, 797–810

FERRERO, N. (1952). Leonardo da Vinci: of the eye. *Am. J. Ophthal.* **35**, 507–521

FICK, A. E. (1888). A contact lens. (Translation by C. H. May.) *Archs Ophthal.* **19**, 215–226

FICK, A. E. (1896). *Diseases of the Eye and Ophthalmoscopy.* Translation by A. B. Hale (1902). p.261. Manchester: King

FORKNALL, A. J. (1948). Offset contact lenses. *Optician* **116**(3006), 419–421

FRASER, J. P. and GORDON, S. P. (1967). The 'apex' lens for uniocular aphakia. *Ophthal. Optician* **7**, 1190–1194, 1247–1253

GASSON, W. (1976). Leonardo da Vinci — ophthalmic scientist. *Ophthal. Optician* **16**, 393–541

GIFFORD, S. R. (1935). 'Reaction of buffer solution and ophthalmic drugs. *Archs Ophthal.* **13**, 78–82

GIFFORD, S. R. and SMITH, R. D. (1933). Effect of reaction on ophthalmic solutions. *Archs Ophthal.* **9**, 227–233

GILL, R. R. (1928). Korrektion des keratokonus durch kontakgläser. *Klin. Mbl. Augenheilk.* **80**, 100

GRAHAM, R. (1959). The evolution of corneal contact lenses. *Am. J. Optom.* **36**, 55–72

GYÖRRFY, I. (1950). Therapeutic contact lenses from plastic. *Br. J. Ophthal.* **34**, 115–118

GYÖRRFY, I. (1968). The manufacture of haptic and corneal lenses in Budapest. *Contact Lens* **2**(1), 9–15

GYÖRRFY, I. (1980). Geschichte der Sklerallinsen aus PMMA. *Contactologia* **2**, 143–149

GYÖRRFY, I. (1981). Zur Geschichte der Korneallinsen aus PMMA. *Contactologia* **3**, 106–109

HEINE, L. (1929). Die korrektur saemtlichr ametropien durch geschliffene kontaktschalen. *Ber. 13' Congr. Ophthal. Amst.* **1**, 232–234

HERSCHEL, J. F. W. (1845). 'Light' Section XII 'Of the structure of the eye, and of vision'. *Encyclopaedia Metropolitana* **4**, 396–404

VON DER HEYDT, R. and GRADLE, H. (1930). Concerning contact glasses. *Am. J. Ophthal.* **13**, 867–868

HILL, R. M. and FATT, I. (1964). Oxygen measurements under a contact lens. *Am. J. Optom.* **41**, 382–387

HOFSTETTER, H. W. and GRAHAM, R. (1953). Leonardo and contact lenses. *Am. J. Optom.* **30**, 41–44

JESSEN, G. N. and WESLEY, N. K. (1949). Concentric molding. *Optom. Wkly* **40**, 753

KOEPPE, L. (1918). Die mikroskopie des lebenden augenhintergrundes mit starken vergrösserungen im fokalen lichte der Gullstrandschen Nernstspaltlampe. *Albrecht v. Graefes Arch. Ophthal.* **95**, 282–306

LARKE, J. R. and SABELL, A. G. (1971). Some basic design concepts of hydrophilic gel contact lenses. *Br. J. physiol. Optics* **26**, 49–60

LEWIS, E. M. T. (1970). A haptic lens design. *Ophthal. Optician* **10**, 56–59, 86

LOHNSTEIN, T. (1896). Zur gläserbehandlung des unregelmässigen hornhaut-astigmatismus. *Klin. Mbl. Augenheilk.* **34**, 405–423

McKELLEN, G. D. (1949). Conical contact lenses. *Br. J. Ophthal.* **33**, 120–127

McKELLEN, G. D. (1963). The 'offset' haptic lens. *Optician* **14**(3479), 105–107

MAISLER, S. (1939). Casts of the human eye for contact lenses. *Archs Ophthal.* **21**, 359–361

MANN, I. (1938). The history of contact lenses. *Trans. Ophthal. Soc. UK* **58**, 109–136

MARRIOTT, P. J. (1967). The construction of impression haptic lenses. *Contact Lens* **1**(3), 8–14

MARRIOTT, P. J. (1970). The use of acrylic laminates in fitting impression haptic lenses. *Br. J. physiol. Optics* **25**, 29–43

MORRIS, J. (1980). Contact lenses in the eighties. *Contact Lens J.* **9**(2), 3–5

MUCH, V. (1931) Der gegenwärtige stand des haftglasproblems, sowie die möglichkeiten und grenzen der haftglastherapie. *Acta ophthal.* **9**, 247–274

MUELLER-WELT, A. (1950). The Mueller-Welt fluidless contact lens. *Optom Wkly* **41**, 831–834

MÜLLER, A. (1889). Brillengläser und hornhautlinsen. *Inaugural Dissertation*, University of Kiel, p.20

MÜLLER, F. A. and MÜLLER, A. C. (1910). *Das Kunstliche auge*, pp. 68–75. Wiesbaden: J. F. Bergmann

MÜLLER, F. E. (1920). Ueber die korrektion des keratokonus und anderer brechungsanomalien des auges mit müllerschen kontaktschalen. *Inaugural Dissertation*, University of Marburg

NISSEL, G. (1965). The Müllers of Wiesbaden. *Optician* **150**(3897), 591–594

NISSEL, G. (1967). Off-set corneal contact lenses. *Ophthal. Optician* **6**, 857–860

NISSEL, G. (1968). Aspheric contact lenses. *Ophthal. Optician* **7**, 1007–1010

NISSEL, G. (1979). Obituary. *J. Br. Contact Lens Ass.* **2**(3), 21

OBRIG, T. E. (1937). Fitting of contact lenses for persons with ametropia. *Archs Ophthal.* **17**, 1089–1120

OBRIG, T. E. (1938a). Molded contact lenses. *Archs Ophthal.* **19**, 735–758

OBRIG, T. E. (1938b). A cobalt blue filter for observation of the fit of contact lenses. *Archs Ophthal.* **20**, 657–658

OBRIG, T. E. (1943). A new ophthalmic impression material. *Archs Ophthal.* **30**, 626–630

OBRIG, T. E. and SALVATORI, P. L. (1957). *Contact Lenses*. 3rd edn. pp.340–345. New York: Obrig Laboratories

PEARSON, R. M. (1978). August Müller's inaugural dissertation. *J. Br. Contact Lens Ass.* **1**(2), 33–36

PRISTER, B. (1933). I vetri adesivi ed il calco del segmento anteriore del bulbo. *Boll. Oculist.* **12**, 149–160

RAKOSS, E. (1950). How new is the corneal lens? *Ophthal. Dispenser*, May 1950, cited by Graham, R. (1959)

RIDLEY, F. (1946). Recent developments in the manufacture, fitting and prescription of contact lenses of regular shape. *Proc. R. Soc. Med.* **39**, 842–848

VON ROHR, M. and STOCK, W. (1912). Ueber eine methode zur subjektiven prüfung von brillenwirkungen. *Albrecht v. Graefes Arch. Ophthal.* **83**, 189–205

RUBEN, M. (1966). The use of conoidal curves in corneal contact lenses. *Br. J. Ophthal.* **50**, 642–645

RUBEN, M. (1967). The apex lens. *Contact Lens* **1**(4), 14–28

RUBEN, M. (1979). J. Dallos, M.D. *Br. Med. J.* **2**(6183), 217

RUBEN, M. (1983). The era of the master lens makers. *J. Br. Contact Lens Ass.* **7**(2), 98–102

RUGG-GUNN, A. (1938). The contact lens centre: its purpose and policy. *Br. Med. J.* **2**(1770), 278–279

SABELL, A. G. (1979). Joseph Dallos, an appreciation. *Contact Lens J.* **8**(5), 16–18

SABELL, A. G. (1980a). An ophthalmic museum. *Contact Lens J.* **9**(2), 15–19

SABELL, A. G. (1980b). An ophthalmic museum. *Contact Lens J.* **9**(6), 3–18

SABELL, A. G. (1980c). An ophthalmic museum. *Contact Lens J.* **9**(3), 16–22

SABELL, A. G. (1980d). An ophthalmic museum. *Contact Lens J.* **9**(4), 10–18

SASIENI, L. S. (1982). Mr George Nissel. *Ophthal. Optician* **22**(20), 695

SATTLER, C. H. (1938). Erfahrungen mit haftgläsern. *Klin. Mbl. Augenheilk.* **100**, 172–177

SIEGRIST, A. (1916). Die behandlung des keratokonus. *Klin. Mbl. Augenheilk.* **56**, 400–421

SITCHEVSKA, O. (1932). Contact glasses in keratoconus and in ametropia. *Am. J. Ophthal.* **15**, 1028–1038

SOMMER, F. (1927). Ueber kontaktgläser zue korrektion des keratokonus. *Inaugural Dissertation*, University of Freiburg

STEELE, E. (1948). American modifications of the contact lens moulding technique. *Optician* **115**(2968), 87

STEK, A. W. (1969). The Percon contact lens — design and fitting techniques. *Contact Lens* **2**(2), 12–14

STEVENS, C. L. (1936). A method for making casts of the human cornea. *Am. J. Ophthal.* **19**, 593–595

STOCK, W. (1920). Ueber korrektion des keratokonus durch verbesserte geschliffene kontaktgläser. *Ber. 42 Versamml. dt. ophthal. Ges.*

STOREY, J. K. (1972). The possible use of polysulphide rubber impression material in contact lens work. *Ophthal Optician* **12**, 1017–1018

STRAUB (1888). Paper published in *Centralblatt f. Augenheilk.* (Title, vol. and page unknown) cited in Benson, A. H. (1902). A note on the value of the fluorescein test. *Ophthal. Review* **21**, 121–130

SUGAR, H. S. (1943). A new material for anterior-segment impressions. *Am. J. Ophthal.* **26**, 1210–1212

THOMAS, P. (1968). The prescribing and fitting of conoid contact lenses. *Contacto* **12**(1), 66–69

TOWN, A. E. (1940). Impression technic for contact glasses. *Archs Ophthal.* **23**, 822–824

TREISSMAN, H. and PLAICE, E. A. (1946). *Principles of the Contact Lens.* pp.64–65. London: Kimpton

TURNER, R. (1964a). Hydrophilic contact lenses. *Ophthal. Optician* **4**(7,8), 343–346, 404–406

TURNER, R. (1964b). An appraisal of the problems of hydrophilic contact lenses. *Ophthal. Optician* **4**(22), 1151–1159

WATSON, R. K. (1947). The 'Kelvin' contact lens. *Optician* **114**(2948), 228–230

WESLEY, N. K. and JESSEN, G. N. (1953). *Contact Lens Practice.* p.86. Chicago: Professional Press

WICHTERLE, O., LIM, D. and DREIFUS, M. (1961). A contribution to the problem of contact lenses. *Cesk. Oftal.* **17**, 70–75

YOUNG, T. (1801). On the mechanism of the eye. *Phil. Trans. R. Soc.* **16**, 23–88

Chapter 2

Anatomy and physiology of the cornea and related structures

G.L. Ruskell

So much new information on the structure and function of the cornea has been produced recently that it becomes a considerable task to keep up to date. For a variety of reasons, the contact lens practitioner probably has more need to be aware of new information on these subjects than anyone else engaged in eye care, and in this chapter an attempt is made to refer to all recent significant advances in knowledge and to emphasize those items which are of most interest to the clinician. Indeed, a large part of recent work has been triggered by the desire to know of the structural and functional changes that may be produced by placing a lens in contact with the eye.

The epithelium (epithelium anterius corneae)

The outermost of the five layers of the cornea consists of stratified epithelium mounted on a fine basement membrane with anchoring filaments extending into the underlying collagen layer (Gipson, Spurr-Michaud and Tisdale, 1987). Next to the membrane are the basal cells, which are columnar and possess an approximately spherical nucleus which is displaced towards the anterior pole or the head of the cell. Two or three rows of smaller interlocked wing or umbrella cells are mounted on the basal cells. Their nuclei differ from those of the basal cells in being smaller, more oval in section and in having their long axes orientated in the plane of the cornea. The wing cells become thinner with increased displacement from the basal cells and they are in turn capped by two or three layers of surface squamous cells (*Figure 2.1*).

The epithelium is of regular thickness (about 70 μm in the fixed adult eye) and it is continuous with that of the conjunctiva where it thickens and becomes folded. Generation of new cells by mitosis occurs mainly in the basal cell layer but also to a limited extent in the second layer (Machemer, 1966). Epithelial mitosis appears to display a circadian distribution in rats, being most common at 7 a.m. and least common at 7 p.m. (Cardoso *et al.*, 1968). Basal cells make room for new ones by migrating to the next layer and they subsequently move up to the surface of the cornea, becoming squamosed and sloughed away by the action of the eyelids.

Autoradiographic studies of epithelial cell nuclei labelled with tritiated thymidine indicate that the life cycle of cells lasts between 3.5 and 7 days in a variety of young animals (Hanna and O'Brien, 1960; Süchting, Machemer and Welz, 1966). By arresting the division of cells at metaphase with colchicine, Bertanlanffy and Lau (1962) determined that 14.5% of epithelial cells are renewed daily in rats. Assuming that surface cells desquamate at the same rate, then the epithelium would be totally regenerated in a period of 7 days. The life cycle of corneal epithelial cells in man was estimated, from the results of isotope studies of enucleated eyes, to take about 7 days (Hanna, Bicknell and O'Brien, 1961).

Adrenaline (epinephrine) and sympathectomy were each found to decrease the mitotic rate in rats (Friedenwald and Buschke, 1944a). This interesting phenomenon has not been explained satisfactorily. If, as seems probable, this decrease is related to innervation and not simply to circulating adrenaline, then it may not occur in man because, unlike rats, adrenergic terminals are not present (Ehinger, 1964, 1971) or are rare in the human cornea (Toivanen *et al.*, 1987).

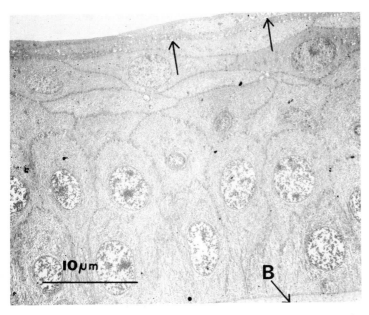

Figure 2.1 Electron micrograph of epithelium taken from close to the centre of the cornea. The cell borders are pronounced because of the presence of numerous desmosomes which have a high electron density. Relatively wide intercellular spacings (arrows) occur between the desmosomes of the flat surface epithelial cells; this feature is a preliminary stage in desquamation. B, Bowman's layer or anterior limiting layer. Lead citrate, monkey

In contrast to the surface cells of skin, those of the cornea are unkeratinized and they retain their organelles — which suggests that metabolic processes are still functioning. Superficially, the cells present a smooth regular surface as seen through an optical microscope but, as Jakus (1964) has shown with the electron microscope, the shallowest of furrows exist between adjacent surface cells which, she suggests, offer a favourable surface for the adherence of tears. However, the most prominent irregularity is caused by the microvilli and microplicae (*Figure 2.2*), which range up to 0.75 μm in height in man (Ehlers, 1965a; Payrau *et al.*, 1967). Pedler (1962) described surface processes or microvilli in kitten corneae and he considered them to be remaining components of desmosomes previously attached to desquamated cells, a view supported by observations on the epithelium of perilimbal conjunctiva in monkeys (Macintosh, 1968). *Figure 2.3* illustrates the commencement of surface cell sloughing; protrusions of cytoplasm and the consequent development of microvilli occur as a result of desmosome resistance to sloughing.

If the eye has been bandaged, or if pressure is exerted through the lids, the epithelium wrinkles (Bron, 1968). This gives rise to a quickly fading mosaic, which is made visible with fluorescein staining.

The space between epithelial cells is uniformly very narrow. The apposed cell membranes are remarkable for their steep, short and fairly regular undulations (*see Figure 2.1*). These occur at all cell interfaces except between apposed basal cells. The cell membrane is modified by the frequent occurrence of attachment zones or desmosomes, which appear as electron-dense plaques, and each one is paired by a similar modification of the apposed cell membrane (*see Figures 2.1, 2.2 and 2.3*). A fine fibrillar substance occupies part of the intercellular space between the plaques. The interlocking of cells, together with the abundant desmosomes, might offer an explanation for the commonly occurring clean detachment of the full thickness of epithelium as opposed to an irregular excavation of the cells following trauma. However, basal cells also possess numerous desmosomes linking them to the basement membrane, and consequently one

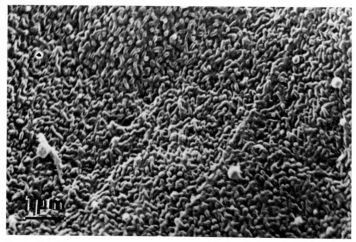

Figure 2.2 Scanning electron micrograph of the surface of the cornea showing microvilli and microplicae with a line marking the borders of adjacent epithelial cells, monkey

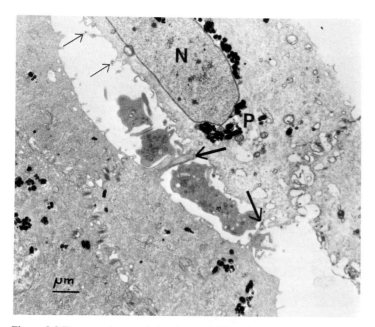

Figure 2.3 Electron micrograph showing partial detachment of surface cells from the perilimbal epithelium prior to sloughing. Cytoplasmic extrusions opposite desmosomes (thick arrows) mark the persisting attachment zones. Desmosomes have broken away from the attached cells and are suspended from microvilli of the detaching cell (thin arrows). N, nucleus; P, pigment granules. Lead citrate, monkey

might expect the basement membrane to detach with the epithelium; but experimental lesions of rabbit corneal epithelium revealed that basement membranes were commonly left in place (Khodadoust *et al.*, 1968). Less frequent gap junctions contribute to the binding of epithelial cells at all levels and the intercellular space between the superficial cells is closed by a tight junction girdle, probably providing a barrier to most molecules.

Another type of epithelial cell, the dendritic or polygonal cell, has been described (Sugiura,

1965). These cells are small in man with a limited perikaryon and numerous long thin processes and they are mostly between basal cells (Segawa, 1964). They are normal residents of the epithelium, present at birth and decreasing in number with distance from the limbus (Chandler, Cummings and Gillette, 1985). They are probably the equivalent of skin Langerhan cells and are thus derived from bone marrow with a lifespan of weeks. Corneal dendritic cells presumably migrate from the conjunctival epithelium which receives them from the blood stream. These cells have aroused considerable interest recently because they bear HLA-DR antigens and may provide the first signal in host sensitization to a corneal graft leading to rejection (Rodrigues et al., 1981; Braude and Chandler, 1983; Treseler, Foulkes and Sanfilippo, 1984).

The nerve fibre terminals of the epithelium are described on pages 47 and 52, together with other nerve fibres of the cornea.

Epithelial damage

In the context of this book, it is appropriate to consider at some length the reactions of corneal epithelium to damage. The smallest corneal wounds — such as a pinprick — are covered in about 3 hours by the neighbouring basal cells, which send out pseudopodia to cover the excavated area (Friedenwald and Buschke, 1944a). Normal mitosis is inhibited and plays no part in healing. Although these observations were made on rats, a similar time course probably obtains in man: a small lesion observed by fluorescein staining one day and absent on the next is a common clinical observation. If a somewhat larger area of the cornea is denuded, cells from all layers of the surrounding epithelium migrate and flatten to cover the wound. In this event, mitosis is again at first inhibited; but after a few hours, it recommences and takes an active part in repair. In experiments on rabbits, Mann (1944) found that an area 2–3 mm in diameter will become covered within 24 hours, and in 3 days the area will have a normal appearance as determined by fluorescein staining. The time course of repair is independent of the cause of the lesion except in the case of thermal burns, when it is delayed, and the time course applies whether or not the underlying tissues are affected. Other experiments on rabbits have shown that the establish-

ment of a tight adhesion of newly regenerated epithelium takes only a few days if the basement membrane is largely intact, but initially the new epithelium is very susceptible to damage (Khodadoust et al., 1968). The results of this study serve to emphasize the need to discontinue wearing contact lenses for a few days after incurring significant epithelial damage. On theoretical grounds at least, the concept that continued wearing of lenses will afford protection to the regenerating epithelium is questionable. If the lesion lies close to the limbus, conjunctival cells will take part in the migration, as may be ascertained by the movement into the cornea of pigment cells from the limbus in rabbits; and the same process was confirmed in man by observations on Negro patients (Mann, 1944). Such migration may represent an acceleration of a normal slow centripetal movement of epithelial cells (Buck, 1985). After massive or total denudation of the corneae of rabbits, it was found that 50% coverage occurs after 24 hours, 75% after 48 hours (Langham, 1960), and total coverage takes from 4 to 12 days (Mann, 1944; Heydenreich, 1958; Khodadoust et al., 1968). On completion of coverage of the cornea, the epithelium is one or two cells thick (Khodadoust et al., 1968), and after 2 weeks it is two to three cells thick (Heydenreich, 1958), but several weeks pass before the epithelium is of normal thickness. Langham found that normal thickness may be attained in one region of a previously completely denuded cornea while another remains uncovered.

Three hours following epithelial abrasions in rabbits, polymorphonuclear leucocytes appeared in the basal lamina and at the edge of the abrasion. Epithelial cells bordering the abrasion were flattened and they developed surface ruffles and filopodia at their free edges (Pfister, 1975). The ruffles and the long, fine filopodia extended to form attachments to the basal lamina giving the impression of a capacity to draw the cells forward into the area of the defect. Epithelial cells bordering a defect appear to increase their water content and surface area, facilitating the production of cell extensions (Cintron, Kublin and Covington, 1982).

One might expect that epithelial repair slows with age, and Marré (1967) found that this was so in rabbits; but the difference in rate of repair in 4- to 6-month-old and 4- to 6-year-old animals was very slight.

There is evidence to suggest that chemotactic substances liberated from the epithelium are responsible for initiating the early stages of healing both in the epithelium and in the stroma (Weimar, 1960). Immediately after deep corneal wounding in rats, a period of proteolytic activity gives rise to the invasion of the cornea by polymorphonuclear leucocytes and to phagocytic activity by the stromal cells. The epithelium appears to be the source of the proteolytic enzymes which trigger these early responses to injury.

Anaesthetics — being protoplasmic poisons — necessarily alter cellular metabolism, and Freidenwald and Buschke (1944b) showed that, if these or other agents such as adrenergic drugs are applied locally in experimental animals, mitosis is inhibited. Gunderson and Liebman (1944) found that the epithelial healing process in guinea-pigs was delayed by anaesthetics. Healing was retarded by inhibition of both mitosis and migration. This effect varied with concentration and tonicity but not with pH. If local anaesthetics are applied excessively, epithelial and possibly stromal opacification is caused, accompanied by the eruption of cells and bleb formation. The whole cornea will stain in this condition. Certain synthetic anaesthetics have a less toxic effect on the epithelium than cocaine (Gunderson and Liebman, 1944; Boozan and Cohen, 1953; Rycroft, 1964), but with prolonged use they are all capable of producing serious corneal damage (Epstein and Paton, 1968).

The epithelium in contact lens wearers is subject to the development of microcysts at basal cell level that are often visible only with the most careful inspection (*Plate 61*). All 45 subjects taking part in a controlled study developed microcysts during 6 months of continuous wear of soft contact lenses (Humphreys, Larke and Parrish, 1980). The subjects were symptomless and the cysts disappeared 10 weeks or so after lens wear was discontinued. A variety of other cellular changes may occur (Bergmanson and Chu, 1982).

Imprinting of the corneal epithelium by corneal contact lenses has been reported by Dixon (1964) and others in a small proportion of patients. Imprinting usually takes the form of a

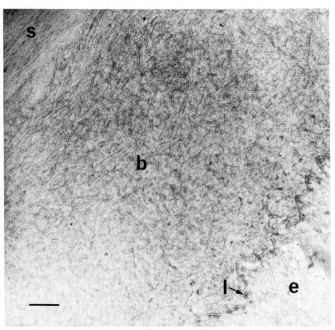

Figure 2.4 Electron micrograph of Bowman's layer (b). Note the random orientation of the collagen fibres. Bowman's layer merges with the stroma (s) in which the fibrils are regularly orientated. The basement membrane of the epithelium (e) is not smooth; the densities opposite the membrane are hemidesmosomes (the arrow indicates one). Marker = 1 µm, human

raised crescent inferiorly. It has been argued by Cochet that the softness or fragility of the epithelium is variable, and he observed a marked fragility in 5% of patients seeking to wear contact lenses (Guilbert, 1963). Fragility was determined by fitting an engraved spherical cone to the Goldmann applanation tonometer and assessing the extent of imprinting of the epithelium when applied to the cornea. Apparently, in France fragility testing is widely used in determining the suitability of patients for wearing contact lenses.

Imprinting in rabbit corneal epithelium was accompanied by the loss of a wing cell layer and increased mitosis (Greenberg and Hill, 1973) indicating a faster turnover of cells, but this has been questioned and a reduced turnover claimed (Hamano *et al.*, 1983).

Bowman's layer
(lamina limitans anterior)

Beneath the fine basement membrane of the epithelium is a layer of uniform thickness of about 12 μm which, histologically, appears homogeneous. Recently, with the aid of electron microscopy, a very fine unorientated fibrillar meshwork has been resolved, the elements of which resemble the collagen fibrils of the stroma, suggesting a common origin for the two layers (*Figure 2.4*). Microscopic inspection reveals that the anterior limiting layer terminates abruptly at the limbus, but short, fine extensions to the conjunctiva have been described by a number of authors. Over the whole of its area, the layer is penetrated by fine unmyelinated nerve fibres which pass from the stroma to the epithelial cells; the nerve fibres lose their Schwann cell sheaths as they leave the stroma.

The frequency of epithelial damage without involvement of this layer is evidence of its relative toughness; but if it does become damaged, fibrous scar tissue is laid down, resulting in a permanent opacity — although some reduction of the initial scar area usually occurs. To ascribe a stronger tendency for this layer to retain scar tissue compared with the underlying stroma is questionable in view of their similar structural elements. Significant mechanical damage to Bowman's layer by a contact lens, however grossly mishandled, is an unlikely occurrence.

The stroma
(substantia propria cornea)

The stroma constitutes 90% of the corneal thickness and gives the cornea its strength. It is remarkable for its regular structure and the absence of blood vessels, which are the two basic features on which corneal transparency rests. The stroma consists of about 200 layers or lamellae of collagen fibrils. The fibrils, which are buried in a mucoid matrix, have a periodicity which is characteristic of collagen. Despite several earlier light microscopic descriptions of elastic fibres in the stroma, they have not been observed with the electron microscope except in areas immediately adjacent to the trabecular meshwork. The fibril diameters are of a regular size at any given depth in the stroma but they vary between an average of 19 nm in the anterior layers and 34 nm in the posterior layers in man (Jakus, 1961).

A majority of the lamellae have a similar thickness (1.5–2.5 μm) and they lie parallel to each other (*Figure 2.5*), but the fibrillar orienta-

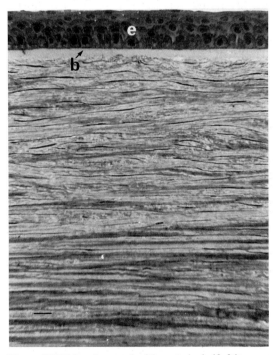

Figure 2.5 Light micrograph of the anterior half of the cornea in transverse section. The difference in density of the lamellae of the stroma is partly attributable to a difference in fibril orientation. The slight irregularity of the lamellae underlying Bowman's layer (b) is a normal feature. e, epithelium. Marker = 20 μm, human

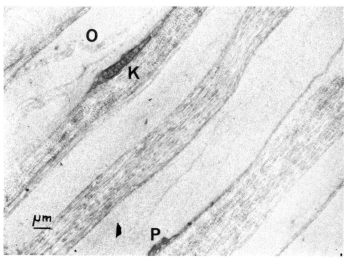

Figure 2.6 Electron micrograph of the lamellae of the stroma. Alternate lamellae are of similar fibril orientation but have different thicknesses. Thin, oblique fibril bundles (O) connect alternate lamellae in places. A dense keratocyte (K) is sectioned transversely through its nucleus and lies in a lamellar interface. The narrow intercellular space between adjacent keratocyte cell processes (P) is also shown. Phosphotungstic acid, monkey

tion of adjacent lamellae is angled (Jakus, 1964). A randomness of lamellar orientation is widely accepted but there is evidence that corneal collagen is predominantly orientated diagonally upward and outward (Schute, 1974). The lamellae probably extend uninterrupted across the cornea without lateral changes in direction, and they are continuous with lamellae of the sclera. Their widths are difficult to assess, but some appear to be in excess of 1 mm. A few lamellae are extremely thin, as may be seen with the electron microscope. Although an impression of separateness of adjacent lamellae prevails when viewing the ultrastructure of the stroma, here and there, thin, slightly oblique branches connect one lamella with another (*Figure 2.6*). This general arrangement explains the ease with which the stroma may be slit along its thickness, as in preparation for lamellar corneal grafting. Towards the periphery of the cornea, some lamellae lie approximately concentric with the limbus (Kokott, 1938; Polack, 1961); these are responsible, in part, for the peripheral thickening of the cornea.

At the corneoscleral margin, the stromal lamellae undulate, branch and probably interweave. The fibrils of single lamellae remain parallel to each other but their diameters vary ten-fold or more (*Figure 2.7*), and some variation

in diameter is present throughout the sclera. At the deep surface of this region, the canal of Schlemm and the corneoscleral meshwork are located; a description of their structure and relationships is beyond the scope of this chapter.

The main cellular element of the stroma is the keratocyte (corneal fibrocyte, corpuscle or fixed cell), which is a flattened, dendritic cell disposed in the interface between adjacent lamellae (*see Figure 2.6*). In a single interface, the cell bodies are well spaced across the cornea; but their thin, lengthy processes are so extensive that many come into contact with processes from neighbouring cells, giving the appearance of a delicate wide-mesh network (*Figure 2.8*). This is repeated at each lamellar interface. The nuclei of these cells are flat, approximately oval discs embedded in a sparse perikaryon. More than one nucleus may be present.

There is good evidence that the fibrocytes of the cornea are exceptional in displaying a phagocytic function. Klintworth (1969) has reviewed and extended the literature in which phagocytosis of a wide variety of foreign particulate substances by these cells has been described. Polymorphonuclear leucocytes and mast cells are present in the periphery of the stroma. Autoradiographic studies of thymidine-labelled nuclei reveals little or no evidence of

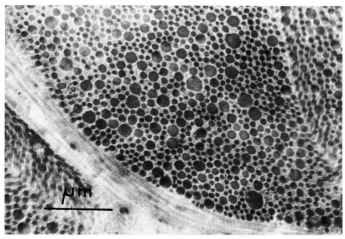

Figure 2.7 Electron micrograph of a transverse section through collagen fibrils of the scleral spur. The difference between adjacent collagen fibril diameters is marked. Lead citrate, monkey

DNA synthesis among the keratocytes, which indicates that they seldom divide (Hanna and O'Brien, 1961; Machemer, 1966).

Descemet's layer (lamina limitans posterior)

Descemet's layer is a product of the endothelium and is thinner than Bowman's layer in the young, but it thickens continuously throughout life, rapidly during gestation and the first postnatal year when it is about 5 μm thick, then slowly, increasing by approximately 1.3 μm each decade (Murphy, Alvarado and Juster, 1984); corneal stroma thickness, by comparison, is unchanged. It appears devoid of internal structure under the light microscope but electron microscopy reveals a fine regular organization anteriorly. In tangential sections, it has a two-dimensional lace network appearance with a repeating hexagonal unit with seven dense nodes marking the angles; these are connected by fine filaments of equal length. The networks are stacked in depth in register as revealed by transverse sections; dark bands are discernible perpendicular to the plane of the cornea consisting of columns of dark granules, which are the nodes of the tangential section network (Jakus, 1964). In contrast, the posterior part of this layer has the same fine granular appearance in whichever plane it is sectioned and it shows no signs of a patterned organization. The granular layer is thinner at birth, becoming thicker than the fibrillar layer with age.

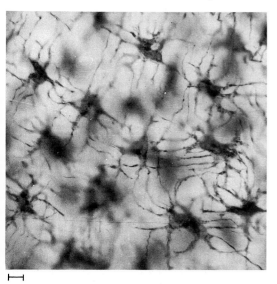

Figure 2.8 Stromal keratocytes. The full thickness of the cornea is viewed from the front and focused at a superficial stromal level. The keratocytes in focus probably all lie at a single lamellar interface. Marker = 20 μm

The endothelium (endothelium camerae anterioris)

This deepest layer of the cornea lacks the thin basement membrane usually associated with endothelia. The endothelium consists of a single thin layer of predominantly hexagonal cells which present a smooth surface to the anterior chamber. Seen in tangential sections, the cell borders are ill defined because of the oblique cell interfaces and the interdigitation of broad processes of adjacent cells. The nucleus may have an oval or a kidney shape and the cytoplasm often appears granular. The cells are well stocked with organelles, especially mitochondria, and the endoplasmic reticulum is prominent. Near the posterior border of this layer, the intercellular space is reduced to form a tight junction of 10 nm width which presumably restricts the movement of substances in and out of the cornea between the endothelial cells (Iwamoto and Smelser, 1965). A few mitotic patterns occur in very young but not adult animals (Sallmann, Caravaggio and Grimes, 1961) and cell division probably ceases before birth in man (Murphy, Alvarado and Juster, 1984). Cells increase in size during growth of the eye and probably spread to cover damaged areas when injured.

The endothelial mosaic is not quite regular because some variation in size (and in number of facets) or polymegathism occurs; this increases with age and is exaggerated as a consequence of wearing hard or rigid contact lenses. Lens-induced increments in polymegathism develop quickly and progress slowly and the irregular mosaic pattern, readily seen by specular microscopy (*see Figures 6.11* and *6.12*), persists at least as long as the contact lenses continue to be worn (Stocker and Schoessler, 1985). Polymegathism may indicate a loss of endothelial functional capacity (Rao *et al.*, 1979) and perhaps explains the *corneal exhaustion phenomenon* when hard contact lenses cannot be tolerated after many years (Stocker and Schoessler, 1985).

The conjunctival sac and the epithelial surface

The conjunctiva is a mucous membrane which lines the posterior surface of each eyelid, reflecting sharply at the fornix to line the anterior eyeball where it becomes continuous with the corneal epithelium. The opposite faces of the conjunctiva are presumably in contact, apart from a very thin liquid film. Estimates of the depth of the sac vary, and the measurements of the sac superiorly and inferiorly presented in

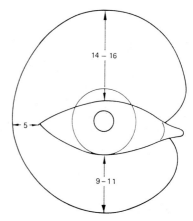

Figure 2.9 Approximate contours of the fornix and the dimensions of the unextended conjunctival sac in millimetres when the eye is open. (Based on the data of Whitnall (after Baker) and Ehlers, 1965b)

Figure 2.9 are those of Ehlers (1965b). The circumference of the sac has a mean value of about 9.5 cm, and Ehlers showed that the circumference varies with the width of the palpebral fissure. The conjunctiva covering the eyeball (bulbar), and especially that of the fornix, is thrown into numerous horizontal folds and consequently the sac is potentially larger than is shown in *Figure 2.9*. Ehlers found that the sac may be distended inferiorly to 14–16 mm and superiorly to 25–30 mm, which is more than enough to lodge a displaced contact lens.

The following description of the histology of the conjunctiva is largely restricted to the epithelium. The form of the conjunctival epithelium varies considerably with position. At the limbus, and again at the lid margin, the epithelium is stratified, unkeratinized and several cells thick. In these positions, the cellular arrangement is quite similar to that of the cornea except that the flat-surfaced epithelium varies in thickness because of the undulations of the basement membrane and because — at least in the limbal conjunctiva — the intercellular spaces are larger. Goblet cells are occasionally present in the limbal epithelium, but these become gradually more numerous through the bulbar conjunctiva increasing to a maximum at the fornix and plica semilunaris. The epithelium of the bulbar conjunctiva becomes thinner with increasing distance from the limbus until at the fornix it is only two cells thick. Surface

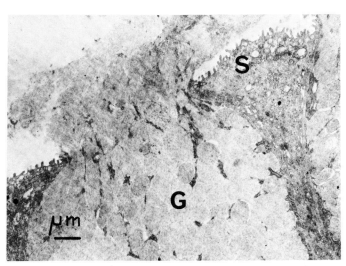

Figure 2.10 Electron micrograph of the apex of a conjunctival goblet cell. Nearly all the cytoplasm consists of secretion granules (G). At the goblet cell borders apposed cell processes are discernible. The conjunctival surface is indicated by the microvilli of adjacent supporting cells (S). The material extruding from the apex of the cell includes secretion granules and other organelles of which granular endoplasmic reticulum can be recognized. Lead citrate, monkey

squamous cells are present at the limbus but not at the fornix. The intercellular spaces are greatest at the fornix except towards the surface, where the bulky goblet cells lie in close apposition to the adjacent, tall, narrow supporting cells (*Figure 2.10*). The concentration of goblet cells continues into the orbital portion of the palpebral conjunctiva, reducing in frequency opposite the tarsal plate where the epithelium consists of two layers of flattened cells in the upper eyelid and three or four layers in the lower eyelid (Wolff, 1948). The medial half of the conjunctiva is richer in goblet cells especially at the plica and caruncle (Kessing, 1968).

No information is available regarding the turnover rate of cells in the conjunctival epithelium except at the limbus, where tritiated thymidine-labelled basal cells are sloughed away after 132–154 hours in rats — which according to Süchting, Machemer and Welz (1966), is rather slower than in the corneal epithelium. It is likely that the turnover rate of cells is much reduced in the glandular parts of the conjunctiva. The goblet cells, which are apocrine glands, probably survive total evacuation of their secretion granules and become recharged, as appears to be the case in goblet cells of the gut (Freeman, 1962).

Many of the superficial cells of the conjunctival epithelium have vesicular inclusions capable of discharging their mucoprotein content onto the surface of the epithelium. The long branched mucoprotein chains remain attached to the cell membrane on the surface and provide an anchor for the mucous layer secreted by the goblet cells, according to Dilly (1985). Whether or not this novel and well-supported theory can be extended to the corneal surface remains to be shown. Vesicles increase in number in contact lens wearers (Greiner *et al.*, 1980). Some cells also appear to have the capacity to remove substances from the surface of the conjunctiva by ingestion through pinocytotic vesicles which then discharge into the intercellular spaces; substances subsequently pass to the subepithelium for removal by the vascular system (Steuhl and Rohen, 1983).

A slight circumscribed elevation of the bulbar conjunctiva, called a pinguecula, may occur opposite the palpebral aperture close to the limbus on one or both sides. Pingueculae are yellow with a fatty appearance due to their content of connective tissue subjected to elastoid degeneration. Pingueculae are uncommon in young eyes but occur frequently in elderly people, especially among those exposed to high levels of ultraviolet radiation and it is therefore more common in countries close to the extremes of latitude. Among other age changes is a reduction in the number of epithelial cells including goblet cells (Gornig and Pommer, 1971).

The blood vessels of the bulbar conjunctiva tend towards a radial arrangement. Arterioles pass from the anterior ciliary arteries before they penetrate the sclera and others pass round the fornix from arterioles of the palpebral conjunctiva. At the limbus, capillaries are again radially disposed mainly between the palisades (radial thickenings of epithelium) and form fine vascular loops at the margin of the cornea. Venules pass back, converge and anastomose frequently and many of the larger venules lie adjacent to the arterioles. The sclera overlaps the cornea anteriorly about the vertical meridian so that transparency loss is gradual across the transition. Consequently, the limbal vessels may give the impression of penetrating the cornea. Many of the conjunctival capillaries are closed in the normal eye but irritation of the cornea or conjunctiva will increase the number and size of blood-bearing vessels.

Small lymphatic vessels are present in the conjunctiva including fine lymphatic capillaries that extend to the corneoscleral border. They drain into larger subconjunctival vessels.

The conjunctiva is served by sensory nerves that branch from certain divisions of the ophthalmic nerve and the infraorbital nerve. Most of them probably terminate in the subepithelial tissues but some pass into the epithelium and lie on the basement membrane or between basal cells. A few terminals penetrate closer to the surface. Although special forms of terminal, including encapsulated endings, have been reported in the conjunctiva in the past, it now appears that practically all sensory fibres form free nerve endings. Sympathetic nerves are also present in the conjunctiva and parasympathetic terminals of pterygopalatine ganglion origin were described recently in monkeys (Macintosh, 1974); both are probably exclusively vasomotor.

Conjunctival injection is commonly present when contact lenses are worn and rarely, in persistent cases, may lead to corneal vascularization (McMonnies, 1984). Modest routine changes in the upper tarsal conjunctival epithelium are unsurprising and occur, no doubt, as a

result of mechanical effects of the lens. Cell borders are more prominent and microvilli tend to clump at the centre of the surface cells (Richard and Allensmith, 1981). Normal topography of the conjunctiva is occasionally disturbed by the development of giant papillary conjunctivitis producing discomfort and lens intolerance (see Chapter 19 and Plate 71).

Eyelids

The skin of the eyelids is very thin. The epidermis consists of only six or seven layers of epithelial cells beneath the keratinized surface layer. At the lid margin, the epithelium thickens and becomes moist and the keratinized layer terminates in front of the orifices of the tarsal glands. Here the epithelium is continuous with that of the marginal conjunctiva where the epithelium is the thickest in the eyelid. The dermis contains small sweat glands. The hairs of the skin are extremely fine and short and, where the skin is regularly folded upon itself in the palpebral furrows, the hairs barely extend beyond their follicles. Sebaceous glands associated with the hairs are commensurately small.

Nearly a third of the thickness of the eyelid is made up of the striated orbicularis oculi muscle, which is bordered anteriorly and posteriorly by loose non-adipose connective tissue. The orbicularis is a thin muscle surrounding the palpebral aperture and extending well beyond the orbital margin on to the face. Structurally and functionally, the muscle is divisible into orbital and palpebral portions. Most of the orbital portion lies beyond the orbital margin and its border describes a horizontal ellipse approximately. It is continuous with the palpebral portion, which itself is clearly divisible into preseptal (lying in front of the orbital septum) and pretarsal parts, the latter terminating near the palpebral margins. Jones (1961) described the orbicularis muscle with considerable precision. He showed that the fascicles of the pretarsal muscle are broadest in the central region of the eyelid, tapering laterally to terminate just beyond the outer canthus. In contrast, the fascicles of the preseptal muscle maintain a regular width, terminating laterally in the raphe, where fibres of the upper and lower eyelids meet. A weak lateral palpebral ligament joins the posterior face of the raphe to the lateral orbital margin at the orbital tubercle. The upper fascicles of the orbital division are continuous with the lower ones laterally. The palpebral furrows or sulci mark the transition from pretarsal to preseptal portions. The divisions of the orbicularis oculi taper and fuse medially and they are anchored to the orbital margin by the strong medial palpebral ligament. Jones distinguished separate ligaments of the three portions of the muscle, and each of them possessed a deep and a superficial ligament or head. According to Jones, the deep heads of the inferior and superior preseptal muscles terminate in the fascial sheet bridging the lacrimal fossa laterally (the lacrimal diaphragm). This structural arrangement — which has been questioned by Brienen and Snell (1967) — figures prominently in a postulated mechanism of lacrimal liquid drainage. The whole of the orbicularis is innervated by the facial nerve.

Behind the orbicularis oculi lies the tarsal plate, which may be regarded as the skeleton of the eyelid. It consists of a very dense plate of fibrous tissue that has a base close to the lid margin. In the upper lid, it extends to the level of the superior palpebral furrow and its upper boundary describes an arc from the medial to the lateral canthus. In the lower lid the plate is only a third as deep.

If pressure is applied inwards and downwards along the superior palpebral furrow, using the fingers or a glass rod, and the lid margin is pulled upwards, the upper lid may be everted. This position is maintained without assistance by the strength of the tarsal plate, provided that the eyes are directed downwards. This manoeuvre is used to permit inspection of the palpebral conjunctiva. When the eyes look upwards, the lid reverts to its normal position. Foreign bodies are frequently lodged in the conjunctiva between the base of the upper tarsal plate and the lid margin where the subtarsal sulcus is formed.

Eversion of the lid reveals the tarsal (meibomian) glands, which are buried within the tarsal plate. The glands run nearly the full length of the tarsus and, in fact, beyond the tarsus at the lid margin, and they are arranged approximately parallel. There are about 25 in the upper eyelid and about 20 in the lower eyelid. The openings of the gland ducts are disposed in a single row along the lid margin, behind the lashes. The glands are sebaceous and holocrine,

the ruptured pyknotic cells forming the oily secretion. Overflow of tears is prevented by a coating of tarsal gland secretion along the lid margins, and this is extended in a thin film across the precorneal tear layer (see Tears, p. 62).

Tarsal glands quite commonly become infected, forming a chalazion or internal stye. Although not painful itself, the chalazion frequently produces a small, hard, discrete elevation of the inner surface of the eyelid, and irritation of the cornea may ensue. Irregularity of the tarsal conjunctiva of whatever cause potentially presents a problem for the contact lens wearer. Hodd, in a personal communication, considers that in numerous cases of lens intolerance a chalazion is the culprit.

The palpebral conjunctiva lines the posterior face of the eyelids. It is firmly attached to the tarsal plate by a thin fibrous subepithelial layer that is rich in capillaries and venules. There is good evidence that the vessels nourish the cornea when the lids are closed. Some small lymphatic vessels are also present in this layer, and they communicate with other lymphatics of the eyelids at the upper and lower margins of the tarsal plate. The epithelium is described above (pp. 42, 43).

The levator palpebrae superioris is a striated muscle with the function of elevating the upper eyelid. It therefore opposes the action of the orbicularis oculi. The levator passes above the superior rectus muscle within the orbit and it has a broad tendonous insertion in the lid. Part of the insertion terminates at the upper border of the tarsus, and the remainder passes in front of the tarsus between the fascicles of the orbicularis to the skin. The levator is innervated by the oculomotor nerve.

A thin layer of smooth muscle — the superior tarsal muscle of Müller — contributes to the elevation of the eyelid. It is a short muscle connecting the inferior fascial sheath of the levator with the upper margin of the tarsus. The superior tarsal muscle is innervated by sympathetic nerve fibres, and it has a weak action compared to that of the levator. This is suggested by the difference in the sizes of the two muscles and by the observation that sympathectomy produces a modest depression of the upper lid compared with the marked ptosis after oculomotor neurectomy. The specific role of the superior tarsal muscle in effecting elevation of the lid is uncertain. An inferior tarsal muscle is found in the lower lid with attachments to the fascial sheaths of the inferior rectus and inferior oblique muscles and to the inferior tarsus. No counterpart to the levator palpebrae superioris is present in the lower lid. The limited capacity to depress the lid is therefore produced by contraction of the inferior rectus muscle and the inferior tarsal muscle.

Structure of the eyelid margins

The line of tarsal gland orifices at the margins of the lids marks the sharp transition from unkeratinized epithelium of the conjunctiva posteriorly to the keratinized epithelium of the skin. Two or three irregular rows of cilia, or eyelashes, emerge from the skin in front of the tarsal gland orifices. The lashes are thick and strong, and those of the upper eyelid are longer and more numerous. The lash follicles are disposed between the terminations of the pretarsal portion of the orbicularis muscle and the lid margin and they lack arrectores pilorum. Lashes are replaced two or three times a year and regrow quickly after epilation. They are normally curved outwards, but in rare instances they may grow inwards (trichiasis) to touch the cornea and give rise to pain (*Plate 7*).

Paired sebaceous glands (of Zeis) open into the lash follicles, and their oily secretion moistens the lashes. Sweat glands (of Moll) are also present in small numbers in the lid margins. Unlike sweat glands elsewhere, they are un-coiled and possess a wide lumen. Although they sometimes open into lash follicles, they usually exhibit the common feature of sweat glands of opening directly on to the skin.

Small bundles of striped muscle fibres (of Riolan) are present immediately beneath the skin of the lid margins. Most of these lie anterior to the tarsal gland ducts but a few are present posterior to the ducts. In general, they run approximately parallel to the lid margins but some fibres pass obliquely between the ducts. It has been postulated that these fibres control the lumina of the ducts. However, this appears unlikely other than as an occurrence incidental to their function of maintaining the lid margins in apposition to the eye during lid closure.

The eyelid sometimes catches the edge of a corneal contact lens. This problem is caused by the lens periphery standing off from the cornea, but an unusual configuration of the posterior margin of the eyelid might be a predisposing factor. However, Shanks (1965) employed a moulding technique to examine this feature in a small group and found little variation between individuals.

Lid movements

In waking hours, the upper eyelid is very active as a result of reflex blinking. A basic rhythm of blinking occurs at a frequency of 12 blinks a minute according to King and Michels (1957), or rather more than this according to others. Alterations of the rate of blinking are produced by many factors such as anxiety, noise or a stuffy atmosphere — but, interestingly, not by a dry atmosphere. A blink is completed in less than one-third of a second. During this period, the eye makes a rapid upwards and inwards movement and returns. Ginsborg (1952) found this movement to be between 20 and 100 minutes of arc nasally and between 40 and 70 superiorly when the eyes were initially in the primary position; but the direction and extent varies with the initial position of the eyes. In secondary positions of gaze, there is a tendency for the eye to move towards the primary position during blinking (Ginsborg and Maurice, 1959). This small displacement is insufficient to account for the movement of a contact lens relative to the eye during a blink; clearly it is the traction of the eyelid that causes the lens movement. The blink rate is reduced when contact lenses are worn, the more so with hard lenses (Brown *et al.*, 1973).

If closure of one eye is prevented by holding the lid when a person attempts to shut both eyes, a movement upwards and outwards is usually seen. This displacement is known as Bell's phenomenon, and it is most strikingly displayed in some cases of facial paralysis (Bell's palsy). The movement is far greater than that induced by blinking as measured by Ginsborg.

Closure in blinking is produced by relaxation of the levator followed by contraction of the palpebral portion of the orbicularis oculi. The whole orbicularis and frequently the accessory muscles contract when the eyes are squeezed shut. This may occur reflexly (optical blinking or menace reflex) together with a backward movement of the head when, for example, the eyes are exposed to a dazzling light, or when a tonometer or contact lens approaches the eye. All contact lens practitioners, however considerate their manner, must have faced the problem of a patient's prolonged blepharospasm prior to the initial insertion of a contact lens.

Gordon (1951) held that in downward gaze, as in reading, the orbicularis muscle plays no active part and that relaxation of the levator is alone responsible for the partial closure of the palpebral aperture. In upward gaze, contraction of both the levator and the frontalis muscle occurs.

Corneal innervation

The cornea is served by 70–80 small sensory nerves. They issue from ciliary nerves which branch from the ophthalmic division of the trigeminal nerve. They enter the sclera from the uvea at the level of the ciliary body and pass anteriorly to enter the cornea radially and predominantly in the middle corneal layers. Other nerves from the same source enter the cornea superficially. They enter the conjunctival epithelium from the subepithelial tissue at the limbus and pass directly into the corneal epithelium at basal cell level (Lim and Ruskell, 1978). A minority of the nerve fibres entering the cornea possess a myelin sheath but this is lost at the limbus or within 0.5 mm of entering the cornea. Occasionally, myelin persists a little further and, exceptionally, even to the centre of the cornea; such fibres are, of course, opaque and they present a striking picture when viewed through a biomicroscope. The perineurium and the fibres and cells of the endoneurium also terminate at the limbus. Only the nerve fibre bundles advance into the cornea. Each bundle consists of several axons enclosed by a Schwann cell sheath (Matsuda, 1968).

Initially, the fibre bundles of each nerve are grouped together; these separate and spread, overlapping and running together with branches from neighbouring nerves producing the plexiform arrangement seen in full thickness preparations of the cornea under low magnification with methylene blue stain (Zander and Weddell, 1951a; Oppenheimer, Palmer and Weddell, 1958) or with a stain for acetylcholinesterase (*Figure 2.11*). The plexus is particularly dense beneath Bowman's layer.

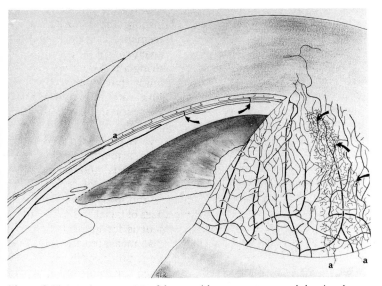

Figure 2.11 Anterior structures of the eye with a segment removed showing the nerves of the cornea topographically and in section. The finer and denser arborization of epithelial fibres is shown on the right superimposed on part of the stromal fibre arborization. Most of the epithelial fibres issue from the stromal supply, having penetrated Bowman's layer at points indicated by arrows, but peripherally at a the epithelial supply is augmented by fibres entering the epithelium directly from the limbus. The drawing is based on the nerve pattern seen in rabbit corneae. In man, the arrangement is similar except that epithelial fibres are often longer and straighter

Axons separate and some divide at intervals and form fine terminal branches, some of which may lose their Schwann cell investment; the terminal axons follow a lengthy and tortuous course between the stromal fibrils. They bear numerous small bead-like varicosities, with a final, often larger one marking the end of the axon.

Fibres from single nerve bundles at the limbus may be distributed to as much as two-thirds of the area of the cornea. Consequently, there is a considerable overlapping by nerve fibres from different nerve bundles. Measurements of receptive fields of the cornea of the cat recorded from ciliary nerves are consistent with the anatomical arrangement of nerve fibre bundles and, indeed, overlapping of receptive fields of single nerve fibres has been demonstrated (Belmonte and Giraldez, 1981). This arrangement explains why sensitivity persists in all areas of the cornea subsequent to large, full-penetration, perilimbal incisions as undertaken in the surgical treatment of cataract and glaucoma (Schirmer and Mellor, 1961). It also explains inability to localize stimuli on the cornea.

The epithelium receives a prolific supply of terminal nerve fibres which pass perpendicularly from the plexus of the anterior stroma and penetrate Bowman's layer. The small nerve fibre bundles lose their Schwann cell investment before entering the epithelium whereupon the fine naked axons disperse and turn sharply to lie nearly parallel to Bowman's layer. They arborize dichotomously as they pass between the basal cells. Varicosities similar to those present in the stroma occur in the epithelium. Such axons may run a course, often with little weaving, up to a length of 2 mm with fine beaded branches issuing from them directed through successive layers of epithelial cells nearly to the surface of the cornea (Schimmelpfennig, 1982; Tervo et al., 1985). Matsuda observed epithelial nerve terminal beads of two types in rabbits and man; one contained mitochondria and the other contained both mitochondria and vesicles. Beads without vesicles probably serve a sensory function, and those with vesicles are probably motor, he suggested. But sympathetic motor fibres are rarely present in primate eyes (Ehinger, 1971) and there is no reliable evidence for the presence of parasympathetic fibres. Moreover, morphological subclasses of beads are not obvious in human

material and it is reasonable to assume that, in contrast to some animals, only sensory fibres are present in substantial numbers in the primate cornea. Variety in their chemistry suggests that sensory fibres may form functionally distinct subgroups; some contain the neuropeptide substance P (Tervo et al., 1981; Stone, Laties and Brecha, 1982), which is recognized as a neurotransmitter in the central nervous system, and others, of unknown chemical identity, do not (Lehtosalo, 1984). Calcitonin gene-related protein (CGRP), another neuropeptide identified in the cornea, may coexist with substance P in the same terminal (Stone et al., 1986). Various functions of corneal nerves are mentioned in these pages but none can yet be attributed to a specific nerve fibre form.

If the sensory nerves of the cornea are destroyed by ophthalmic nerve or trigeminal ganglion lesions, changes in the structure and properties of the cornea occur and a neuroparalytic keratitis often develops (see Chapter 21). This has led to the concept of a trophic function of corneal nerves, parallel to that of cutaneous nerves, responsible for the maintenance of tissue integrity (Beuerman and Schimmelpfennig, 1980). The mechanism of the trophic function is not understood, but it may be dependent on antidromic stimulation of sensory nerves.

Sensitivity of the cornea and conjunctiva

Common experience and the earliest measurements of surface sensitivity indicate that the sensitivity of the cornea is probably unsurpassed by that of any other part of the body. The measurement of threshold sensitivity has been practised throughout this century, but it is probably true to state that progress has only recently been made in calibrating the stimulus with accuracy. Notwithstanding, the technique of aesthesiometry remains blunted by uncertainties, and the data it provides — whether absolute or relative — can only be accepted with caution in so far as they apply to the cornea and conjunctiva. The stimulus employed was classically a fine hair or a series of hairs of different lengths and weights applied to the surface of the cornea, but, more recently, a nylon monofilament has been used. The force exerted is measured in weight per unit area of contact; the area of contact is assumed to remain constant and the weight or pressure is varied. The method of varying the unsupported length of monofilament between the holder and the point of contact is usually employed in corneal aesthesiometers. Pressure on the instrument is increased until the monofilament bends and the force required to achieve this end-point for any length of monofilament is precalibrated. The length of monofilament is decreased until a threshold response is elicited. The shorter the length of monofilament the greater the pressure required to bend it. An electronic aesthesiometer making use of an induction coil to produce preset forces of the stimulus body placed in contact with the cornea before measurements are taken is now available (Draeger, 1984). Threshold and differential responses may be measured electrophysiologically in experimental animals.

The sensitivity of the cornea varies from a maximum apically to a minimum at the periphery with a considerable drop in sensitivity at the limbal conjunctiva. Sensitivity reduces further to a minimum at the fornix, then increases again at the lid margins (Boberg-Ans, 1955; Cochet and Bonnet, 1960; Schirmer and Mellor, 1961). Using a nylon monofilament the average central threshold stimulus is 12–15 mg/mm^2 and the peripheral corneal threshold is highest at 12 o'clock where the cornea is normally partially covered by the eyelid (Draeger, 1984; Millodot, 1984). A summary of threshold values is given in *Figure 2.12*. According to Cochet, in a personal communication, Sédan observed an annular zone of raised sensitivity (lower threshold) about 4 mm from the centre of the cornea in 30% of cases and Draeger (1984) claimed to find the increase regularly with his instrument.

Sensitivity varies with age. In a study of 150 patients whose ages ranged between 10 and 90 years, Boberg-Ans (1956) found a peak sensitivity in young patients three times that of his oldest patients, a slightly greater difference than that found by Millodot (1977). Most of the sensitivity reduction occurs between the ages of 50 and 65 years (Jalavisto, Orma and Tawast, 1951) or even later (Sédan, Farnarier and Ferrand, 1958). Sensitivity is usually approximately the same in both eyes, and there is no reliable evidence to indicate a difference in sensitivity between the sexes but it is worth noting Millodot and Lamont's (1974) observations that the average sensitivity in nine women

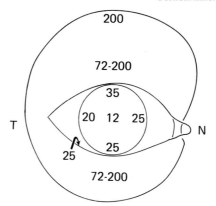

Figure 2.12 Touch thresholds (in mg/mm^2) representing a synthesis of published results. Absolute values vary according to the technique used and those shown are considered the most likely to be obtained with careful use of a hand-held 0.12 mm nylon suture Cochet–Bonnet aesthesiometer. Lower thresholds would be obtained using a 0.08 mm instrument with mechanical control of application and microscopic viewing. The arrow indicates the marginal conjunctiva where it lies in contact with the eye

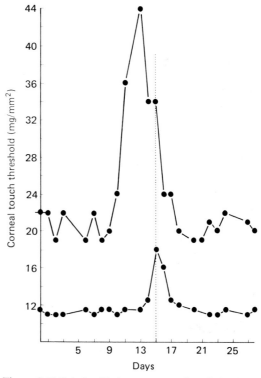

Figure 2.13 Relationship between corneal touch threshold and number of days of the menstrual cycle in women. Days are numbered from the assumed occurrence of ovulation and the dotted line represents onset of menstruation. (From Millodot, M., 1974, *Br. J. Ophthal.*, Vol. 58, pp. 752–756, by kind permission of the author and publishers)

was approximately halved during the premenstruum and at the onset of menstruation (*Figure 2.13*). Moreover, women may exhibit a transient reduction of sensitivity in the later weeks of pregnancy (Millodot, 1977; Riss and Riss, 1981). Corneae display a diurnal variation in sensitivity with about a third greater sensitivity as the day progresses from morning to evening (Millodot, 1972). Perhaps the most striking variation is that displayed between people of different iris colour. Millodot (1975b) found that blue-eyed people have a greater sensitivity than those with dark-brown irises (*Figure 2.14*). Non-white people with dark-brown irises have less sensitive corneae than Caucasians with similar iris colour. On average, non-white people have four times less sensitive corneae than blue-eyed people and half as sensitive corneae as brown-eyed Caucasians.

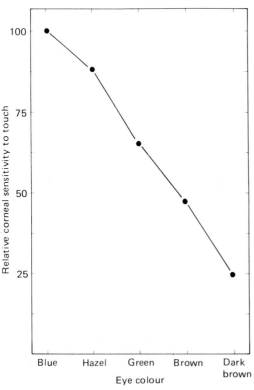

Figure 2.14 Relative corneal sensitivity to touch as a function of the colour of the iris (112 subjects). The dark-brown group consists of non-white subjects. The sensitivity is the reciprocal of the touch threshold measured in mg/mm^2 and the group with greatest sensitivity has been assigned 100. (From Millodot, M., 1975b, by kind permission of the author and publishers)

Depression of corneal sensitivity as a consequence of limbal transection for cataract extraction is surprisingly slight. The threshold value adjacent to the incision is raised to little more than twice the normal (Schirmer and Mellor, 1961); but recovery of sensitivity was found to be negligible over a period of 2 years. The survival of nerve fibres entering the cornea across half its circumference is adequate to maintain a high degree of sensitivity over the whole of the cornea. One might expect some recovery of sensitivity subsequent to a limbal incision if one is free to extend Zander and Weddell's (1951b) observations on rabbits to man. They found that normal innervation was recovered in favourable cases 9 months after keratotomy of up to one-third of the corneal circumference, but the speed of regeneration of corneal nerve fibres is related to age, being more rapid in the young (Rexed and Rexed, 1951).

The opportunities to study reinnervation of corneal grafts in man are obviously rare and the limited information available so far suggests that epithelial reinnervation may reach normal levels, whereas stromal reinnervation is sparse (Tervo *et al.*, 1985). Recovery of sensitivity in the graft area after several years is practically nil in some cases and slow and fractional in others (Ruben and Colebrook, 1979; Lyne, 1982; Draeger, 1984). Similarly, the cornea close to the keratotomy wound associated with cataract extraction recovers little of its lost sensitivity (Draeger, 1984).

All diseases affecting the cornea tend to reduce sensitivity and a summary of the conditions so far studied by aesthesiometry is available (Millodot, 1984). Contrary to common belief, keratoconus provides an example of reduced sensitivity (Millodot and Owens, 1983; Bleshoy, 1986). The reduction is largely confined to the central cornea but with little or no correlation with cone steepness. The general polyneuropathy of diabetes is expressed in the cornea by a reduced sensitivity (O'Leary and Millodot, 1981). Low sensitivity is also associated with the inherited condition of albinism (Millodot, 1978).

The effects of contact lenses on corneal sensitivity

Corneal sensitivity is reduced as a result of wearing hard contact lenses. Sensitivity testing, in the past, produced some extraordinarily discrepant results with claims that sensitivity reduces to a fraction of the normal level with the use of hard contact lenses or, contrariwise, that lenses are commonly innocent of any effect when fitted properly. Freehand aesthesiometry and possibly bias must take the blame for the confusion. When the aesthesiometer is attached to a biomicroscope, providing stability, improved control of application speed and adequate visibility, sensitivity reduction of relatively modest proportions is recorded as a routine response to contact lens wear. Millodot's (1975a,b) results are typical of more recent studies using the Cochet–Bonnet nylon aesthesiometer under controlled conditions. Touch threshold value was approximately doubled on average in 11 young subjects after wearing hard contact lenses for 8 hours (*Figure 2.15*). Sensitiv-

ity reduction was proportionately similar for the central and peripheral cornea and full recovery occurred 2 hours after removal of the lenses.

Lower eyelid margin sensitivity is substantially reduced by wearing hard contact lenses (Lowther and Hill, 1968).

Sensitivity reduction is chronic and slowly progressive and after some years of daily hard contact lens wear corneal sensitivity no longer returns to a normal level upon removal of the lenses. *Figure 2.16* shows a considerable reduction in sensitivity after 5–8 years wear reducing further after 15–21 years with a three-fold rise or more in threshold, yet the wearers displayed no symptoms and corneal oedema was insignificant. Some of the long-term wearers in the group abandoned their lenses and normal levels of sensitivity returned after 1–3 months confirming that contact lens wear was responsible for the reduction (Millodot, 1978).

Soft contact lenses also depress corneal sensitivity but the amount is relatively small. In the earliest studies, Larke and Sabell (1971) found none while Knoll and Williams (1970) observed a loss that was not statistically significant. However, when sensitivity was measured subsequent to the removal of soft contact lenses, a small but significant increase

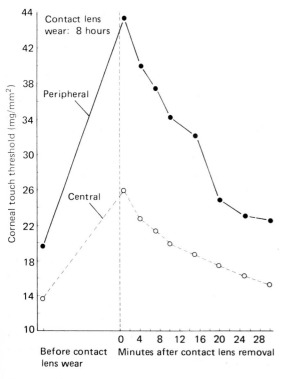

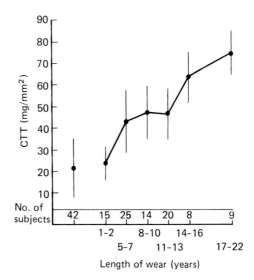

Figure 2.15 The effect of hard contact lenses on corneal touch threshold averaged from the eyes of 11 subjects. Thresholds before lens insertion and at frequent intervals after 8 hours wear are plotted. Threshold at the centre of the cornea is about half that at the periphery. Recovery of sensitivity after contact lens removal is comparable in both positions. (After Millodot, 1975a)

Figure 2.16 Chronic sensitivity reduction in hard contact lens wearers using a daily wear routine. The corneal touch threshold (CTT) was measured early in the day before insertion of lenses. Vertical lines represent ±s.d. (From Millodot, M., 1984, by kind permission of the author and publishers)

was found (Millodot, 1974). Evidently sensitivity had been reduced. This loss was probably obscured in earlier studies by the diurnal increment of sensitivity as the day progresses.

The long-term effect of soft contact lenses on sensitivity is unknown but the results of short-term prospective studies imply that reduction of sensitivity is again chronic and progressive. Extended wear lenses appear to hasten the process as sensitivity was more than halved after 20 weeks (Larke and Hirji, 1979); the reduction was slightly less when a lens cleaning solution was used at 8-week intervals. The rate of sensitivity loss evidently also depends upon the nature of the lens material and the frequency of lens removal (*Figure 2.17*).

Oxygen deprivation appears to be the major cause of corneal sensitivity loss and, presumably, mechanical assault is responsible for eyelid margin effects. The cornea in sleep is deprived of atmospheric oxygen and after sleep sensitivity is found to be depressed. When deprivation is extended by taping the lids, sensitivity reduction is much increased (Millodot and O'Leary, 1980). When atmospheric gases are controlled by using goggles, sensitivity reduction is highly correlated with time of exposure to reduced oxygen levels.

Schirmer (1963) has suggested that in determining the suitability of patients before prescribing contact lenses corneal sensitivity should

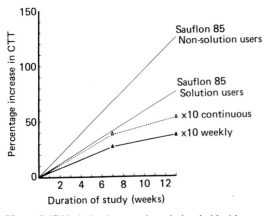

Figure 2.17 Variation in corneal touch threshold with two types of high water content soft lenses worn differently. The Sauflon data were taken from the 20-week study of Larke and Hirji (1979) referred to in the text. ×10 is assumed to be an abbreviation for another type of extended wear lens worn continuously (--△--) or removed weekly (—▲—). (From Millodot, M., 1984, by kind permission of the author and publishers)

be taken into account; but in particular, he values the degree of tolerance of a sustained stimulus as a better criterion. High tolerance and low sensitivity, as Schirmer suggests, would appear to be suitable features for successful contact lens wear on the evidence of his data using his instrument. But others take a different view (for example, Cochet and Bonnet, 1960), and the general value of these criteria has yet to be demonstrated. At the present time, there appears to be little reason to promote the routine use of aesthesiometry in contact lens practice: and it must be remembered that the technique is not without hazard.

Sensibility of the cornea and conjunctiva

One associates the sensations of pain and irritation with the cornea, possibly to the exclusion of any others. Von Frey and his co-workers proposed and maintained this view over several decades against the evidence of other groups who claimed that the cornea exhibits several sensibilities. The problem is of broad interest in that von Frey postulated the well-known correlation between specific forms of cutaneous sensory end-organs with particular functions. Free nerve endings mediate pain sensitivity, according to this hypothesis and, as we have seen, the cornea is populated exclusively by them. The qualitative evaluation of sensitivity is of limited practical importance to the contact lens practitioner, but he is dealing with a structure which is at the centre of an engaging physiological dispute and he may be interested in a brief account of the views of the opponents of von Frey's conception of cutaneous sensitivity.

Lele and Weddell (1956) claimed that the sensibilities of touch, cold, warmth and pain may be experienced if the cornea is suitably stimulated. Strughold (1953) himself, although a principal proponent of the von Frey concept, appeared to concede the possibility of touch sensibility as distinct from irritation. Nafe and Wagoner (1937) claimed that either touch or pain sensations may be elicited from the cornea according to the intensity of the stimulus. Based on the understanding that pain impulses conducted by the trigeminal nerve — and therefore including those initiated in the cornea — are chiefly presented at the caudal end of the nucleus of the spinal trigeminal tract in the lower brainstem, Sjöqvist (1938) incised the tract at this level in cases of trigeminal neuralgia. This procedure effectively reduces the sensibility of pain while sufficient tactile sensibility is retained to avoid the possibly blinding consequences associated with total anaesthesia which results from the alternative operation of trigeminal neurectomy (Rowbotham, 1939; Grant, Groff and Lewy, 1940). Patients treated by this procedure experience no discomfort if the cornea is moderately stimulated, and they recognize the predominating sensation as touch.

One is, perhaps, at liberty to conclude from this evidence that the sensation of touch is fully differentiated from pain, but it is noteworthy that in cats the representation of pain sensation is spread throughout the nucleus of the spinal trigeminal tract (Eisenman, Landgren and Novin, 1963; Kerr, 1963). The separate representation of pain in the trigeminal nerve nucleus is inconsistent with the 'gate control' theory of Melzack and Wall (1965). They argue that pain is experienced as a consequence of increased strength of any form of stimulation sufficient to release the central inhibition set up by activity of cells of the substantia gelatinosa. On this basis, Sjöqvist's incision may be considered to so reduce total sensory input that the threshold for pain is not reached or the gate is not opened.

Perhaps the most controversial aspect of corneal sensibility is that of temperature. Von Frey concluded, from experiments in which he stimulated the cornea with cooled and heated rods, that temperature sensations were absent. He also noted the absence of Ruffini endings and Krause end-bulbs. In the adjacent conjunctiva, Strughold and Karbe (1925) found many warm and cold spots. Employing intravital staining of nerves and the low magnification level of the biomicroscope, they concluded that warm spots related to Ruffini endings and cold spots to Krause end-bulbs. These observations supported their view that warmth and cold sensibilities are not experienced from the cornea. Subsequent studies by Weddell and Zander (1950) and Oppenheimer, Palmer and Weddell (1958) unequivocally reject this correlation in the conjunctiva. Complex nerve endings are rare and irregularly occurring, and in some species they are altogether absent. They therefore cannot be considered to relate to the function of temperature reception. This leads to the conclusion that morphologically unspecial-ized nerve endings are related to a variety of sensibilities, and that absence of all but free nerve endings in the cornea does not preclude the reception of stimuli giving rise to sensations other than pain.

Nafe and Wagoner (1937) concluded from their experiments that both warm and cold sensations are absent from the cornea. Lele and Weddell (1956), in challenging the validity of these experiments, pointed out that these investigators were searching to establish that vascular receptors are responsible for the sensations of warmth and cold and that it was in their interest to find a negative response to these stimuli in the avascular cornea. Kenshalo (1960) showed that thermal changes may be recognized by the cornea, but he claimed that the quality of the sensation is irritation rather than warmth. The temperature difference required for threshold sensitivity was found to be much in excess of that necessary in the conjunctiva, lips and skin. However, the detectable temperature changes in Lele and Weddell's subjects, employing short-duration warm and cold air jets, indicated an accurate discrimination: a cold jet was never confused with a warm jet. Although the elicited sensations were equated approximately with those of warmth and cold, these workers recognized them to be somewhat singular in quality.

Corneal transparency

The most obvious and simple explanation for the transparency of the cornea is that its components all have the same refractive index; but a number of easily observed factors discount this. For instance, an anatomist might doubt the validity of this explanation because he is able to discern the structure of the cornea in unstained sections using phase contrast microscopy which is dependent on refractive index differences. Similarly, cellular detail is discernible in the living eye with a biomicroscope. The birefringence of the cornea is evident from the interference figures it displays when examined with polarized light, and this property has been examined in detail (Naylor, 1953; Stanworth and Naylor, 1953).

Cogan and Kinsey (1942b), accepting a difference in refractive index of the stromal components, proposed that refraction at their surfaces is minimized as a consequence of a limited liquid component, and one may point to the phenomenon of scleral transparency *in situ* in the dehydrated state in support of this. But this concept is at variance with the facts that the liquid component is of the order of 80% by weight and collagen fibrils constitute only 18% of the volume of the stroma.

Caspersson and Engström (1946) postulated that the fibrils of the stroma are positioned parallel to the surface of the cornea in rows which are perpendicular to it. Light rays would be refracted to and fro along a row of fibrils and finally emerge undeviated. The gaps between fibrils were considered to be 'plugged' by the mucoid ground substance of graduated refractive index with a peak equal and adjacent to that of the fibril, thereby avoiding reflection at interfaces. This scheme is untenable for a number of reasons — one of which is that it accounts only for light rays of normal incidence.

No satisfactory hypothesis explaining the transparency of the cornea as a whole has appeared, but Maurice (1957, 1962a) has offered an explanation of the transparency of the stroma. His hypothesis is precisely stated and does not invoke extravagant assumptions. It embraces light of all incidences and satisfactorily explains how transparency is lost in various circumstances. Maurice proposed that the stromal fibrils, which were found to have a refractive index of about 1.55 in the dry state, are so arranged to behave as a series of diffraction gratings permitting transmission through the liquid ground substance (refractive index 1.34). We have already seen that the fibrils in adjacent regions of the stroma are of remarkably regular diameter and that they are probably regularly spaced so that, neglecting the curvature of the cornea, in any plane a reasonable facsimile of a diffraction grating exists. It is of interest to note that the fibrils of the opaque sclera do not show these properties. A diffraction grating eliminates scattered light by destructive interference and permits the transmission of light energy maxima at angles θ to a normally incident beam, the angles depending on the physical characteristics of the grating and the light. Accordingly, $\sin \theta = m\lambda/d$, where m is any integer and d is the space between grating elements. The fibrils are the grating elements which, it is suggested, are

disposed in an hexagonal lattice as shown in *Figure 2.18*. Only the first of the energy maxima applies because the grating or fibril interval is shorter than the wavelength of light of $\lambda/d > 1$, and the equation is only satisfied when m is zero and consequently θ is 0°. In this manner the transmission of normally incident light through the stroma, without deviation or significant scattering, is explained. As shown in *Figure 2.18*, a light beam of other than normal incidence is covered by the hypothesis simply by considering an oblique lattice plane. Other planes can be drawn, and together they explain the transmission of light through the cornea at different incidences. The lattice theory has been questioned — for example, Smith (1969) argued that Maurice's calculations of refractive index differences were incorrect — but the theory has gained wide acceptance as a reasonable explanation of transparency of the stroma.

The slight irregularities of collagen fibril separation as seen with the electron microscope were regarded by Maurice as preparation artefacts. Others have taken them into account such as Hart and Farrell (1969) who computed the probability distribution function for the relative position of fibrils from electron micrographs. They found that the mathematical summation of the phases of light waves scattered by the partially ordered array gave magnitude and wavelength dependence of the scattered light in good agreement with that found experimentally. Benedek (1971) presented proof that the scattering of light is produced only by fluctuations in the index of refraction of wavelengths larger than one-half the wavelength of light in the medium. Since the index fluctuations are far shorter than this value, transparency of the stroma is explained without the need for a perfect lattice of collagen fibrils. It has the added advantage of explaining the transparency of Bowman's layer.

When the cornea is oedematous its transparency is reduced and this may be explained in terms of the lattice theory in that the regularity of the fibrillar spacing is disturbed by the excess liquid and the efficiency of fibrils as grating elements is reduced. Local pressure on the cornea reduces transparency in the compressed region, again as a result of fibril disarray, but normal transparency returns immediately the pressure is withdrawn, allowing the forces maintaining the regular fibrillar spacing to

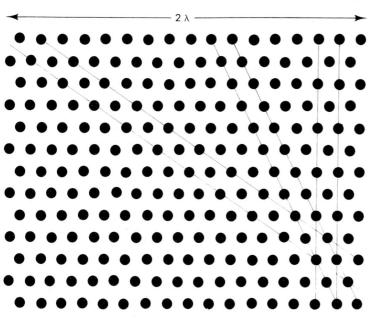

Figure 2.18 Lattice arrangement of the fibrils of the corneal stroma. If lines were drawn joining the adjacent fibrils, they would describe a lattice. The parallel lines pass through rows of fibrils and represent light wave fronts. The rows of fibrils may act as diffraction gratings (Maurice, 1957) and hence, wave fronts of widely differing orientations may traverse the stroma

operate once more. The haze and haloes around bright lights which often become very noticeable when contact lenses are worn are the result of corneal swelling, and again this may be explained in terms of the lattice theory. Alternatively, transparency loss with oedema may be explained by the formation of spaces within the stroma free of collagen fibrils and larger than the critical size of half the wavelength of light.

If our understanding of the transparency of the stroma were satisfactory, we would still be left without an explanation of transparency of other layers of the cornea. They have a different structure from that of the stroma and yet a biomicroscope reveals that the epithelium scatters less light than does the stroma. This problem awaits solution.

A most interesting study by Bernhard, Miller and Møller (1965) showed that many insects have a surface corneal nipple array which has the property of increasing light transmission. The minute nipples are shorter than the wavelength of light, as is their separation, so that they become visible only by means of electron microscopy. They are approximately cone shaped with adjacent bases in contact, and

they cover the whole surface of each ommatidium. This transmission phenomenon applies only to visible wavelengths. As noted earlier, microvillus-like structures are present on the surface of the human cornea but their irregularity does not allow comparison with the insect nipple array — but Bernhard's studies serve to emphasize that there is still much to be learned about light transmission through cellular structures.

The maintenance of corneal transparency is clearly dependent on the forces which limit its hydration. These forces are very susceptible to disturbances such as that produced by an inserted contact lens. Corneal hydration undoubtedly follows the insertion of a contact lens; some lenses are worse offenders than others and some persons are more affected than others. The dehydrating forces are discussed in the following section.

Maintenance of corneal transparency

The cornea functions in a liquid environment and yet it has the capacity to maintain a steady solid/liquid ratio of about 1:4. If this ratio is increased by liquid uptake, the cornea loses its transparency. As the excised or damaged cornea is remarkably hygroscopic (the excised cornea in water increases to about four times its normal thickness), we may conclude that the transparent, living cornea, as a significant part of its workload, has to pump out water.

The integrity of its surface layers is essential for maintenance of corneal transparency, indicating that the pump operates through them. It is widely accepted that the endothelium carries the major burden in this active process, and much recent evidence supports this view. The pumping function could explain the high oxygen consumption by the endothelium per unit volume compared with that of the epithelium (Freeman, 1972). In experiments on rabbits, Maurice (1972) showed that the endothelium has the capacity to pump out water up to 12 times its own thickness in an hour. But both epithelium and endothelium have been shown to act as inert partial barriers to ion and liquid influx under experimental conditions such as hypothermia or anoxia, when the pump cannot be working, and therefore one may consider the pump to complement the action of the structural barriers in effecting the deturgescence of the cornea. The barrier characteristics of the limiting layers are different in that the epithelium is far more impermeable to organic ions than is the endothelium, while the endothelium is more resistant than the epithelium to diffusion of water (Maurice, 1951; Donn, Miller and Mallett, 1963).

The pump probably operates by expelling ions from the stroma to the fluids bathing the cornea, setting up an osmotic flow of water from the cornea. It is therefore an active process and if corneal metabolism is inhibited the pump cannot operate and the cornea swells and loses transparency due to the uptake of water. A 'metabolic pump' is therefore actively transporting substances across the surface layers. Active transport describes the movement of a substance across a biological membrane against an electrochemical gradient, requiring the use of energy. The potential gradient results from the inequality of distribution of electrolytes on the two sides of the membrane.

The precise nature of the pump is not known but there is little doubt that more than one type of ion is involved. Hodson and Miller (1976) demonstrated active transport of HCO_3^- from endothelium to aqueous activated by the enzyme carbonic anhydrase located adjacent to the posterior membrane of the endothelium. The enzyme converts carbon dioxide to bicarbonate which is then pumped into the aqueous. They showed that the endothelial pump was partly inhibited when carbon dioxide and bicarbonate were removed from the cornea. The presence of Na^+ and HCO_3^- was found to be necessary for the full activity of the pump in maintaining the cornea dehydrated (Hodson, 1977) indicating that the transport of bicarbonate was linked to that of sodium. Other ions have been implicated in the endothelial pump.

The importance of metabolic forces in this process is established by experiments in which transparency loss and thickening occurs when the temperature is reduced to a level sufficient to inhibit metabolism followed by recovery when the temperature is raised (Davson, 1955; Harris and Nordquist, 1955; Mishima, 1968). Deprivation of oxygen or the application of metabolic inhibitors such as ouabain also produce reversible swelling and opacification of the cornea (Trenberth and Mishima, 1968).

Recovery of normal thickness at body temperature after cooling of the excised cornea, whether or not the epithelium is present, vividly demonstrates that deturgescence is substantially the responsibility of the endothelium (Harris and Nordquist, 1955). A punctate lesion of the corneal endothelium causes a well-circumscribed region of stromal opacification opposite the lesion, suggesting that liquid intake is confined to the traumatized zone by the vigorous activity of the adjacent endothelium (Langham, 1960). Removal of the epithelium in vivo does lead to some hydration of the cornea but to a lesser extent than when the endothelium is removed (Maurice and Giardini, 1951). Corneal swelling in rabbits caused by removing the epithelium is reversed first at the periphery as cells from the conjunctiva slowly migrate across the cornea, while the remaining denuded area stays swollen. This situation is maintained even after 72 hours when 90% of the cornea is covered (Langham, 1960). The contribution of the epithelium to corneal deturgescence is unlikely to be attributable to its inert barrier characteristics alone, and Klyce and Crosson (1985) have shown that Cl^- is actively transported by the epithelium to the tear film. The duties of the epithelium in deturgescence of the cornea, however small, obviously warrants the attention of the contact lens practitioner.

At the corneoscleral junction there is a potential liquid leak into the cornea, but Maurice (1962b) calculated that the endothelium has more than sufficient pumping power to deal with the influx of water from this region.

In summary, it has been shown that the surface layers of the cornea act as inert, partial barriers to water influx and that, superimposed on this, a metabolic pump opposes the swelling pressure of the cornea. The nature of the pump is uncertain, but it is vigorous — particularly across the endothelium — and it probably consumes a large proportion of the cellular energy of the cornea.

Metabolic processes

The following description of the metabolic processes in the cornea is confined to a consideration of glucose metabolism. De Roetth (1950) has shown that carbohydrate metabolism predominates in the cornea as indicated by a respiratory quotient of unity, and glucose is the principal monosaccharide of this process. Much of the energy released in the metabolism of glucose is used in the phosphorylation of ADP (adenosine disphosphate) to ATP (adenosine triphosphate), and energy is stored in this form. The efficiency of a metabolic pathway may therefore be measured in terms of the number of ATP molecules produced. The processes of greatest importance in the metabolism of glucose are, first, the glycolytic pathway followed by the tricarboxylic or citric acid cycle and, second, the oxidation of glucose directly by the pentose phosphate pathway or hexose monophosphate shunt. These will be considered in turn and then related specifically to corneal metabolism.

Glycolysis

In this complex glycolytic process, enzymes called dehydrogenases act as catalysts for each stage in the process and finally split the glucose molecule into two molecules of pyruvic acid. In the third of the four stages of the glycolytic process, liberated energy is used to form two molecules of ATP from ADP and inorganic phosphate.

Under anaerobic conditions, pyruvic acid is converted to lactic acid without significant liberation or uptake of energy. Under aerobic conditions, glucose metabolism does not stop at this point but continues until the final products are carbon dioxide and water. This further breakdown is brought about by the citric acid cycle. During the cycle, carbon dioxide and hydrogen atoms are released. The hydrogen atoms, at length, become oxidized to form water and the combined cycle and oxidative processes synthesize a further 36 ATP molecules (*Figure 2.19*).

Hexose monophosphate shunt

Although the glycolytic pathway just described is the principal pathway for the oxidation of glucose, others are available. Of these, the hexose monophosphate shunt is the most important. In this process, glucose 6-phosphate takes part in a cyclic mechanism which, rather than producing ATP for general metabolic functions, has the main purposes of providing reducing power in the form of NADPH (reduced nicotinamide adenine dinucleotide phosphate) which can be used for biosynthesis and to produce the ribose 5-phosphate necessary for the synthesis of nucleotides and nucleic acids. Due to the rapid production of epithelial cells, the cornea has a substantial requirement for these molecules.

Carbohydrate metabolism in the cornea

Glycolysis is predominantly exhibited in the epithelium. The high level of enzyme and pyridine nucleotide concentration and the rate of oxygen consumption indicate that the endothelium also has a high glycolytic activity, but the relative inaccessibility of this layer has limited studies upon it. In contrast, the stroma shows very little metabolic activity. Tissues exhibiting aerobic glycolysis accumulate lactate because the glycolytic pathway is more efficient than the aerobic mechanisms which cause the combustion of pyruvate to carbon dioxide and water (Langham, 1954).

Anaerobic glycolysis alone, with its low energy yield, is evidently inadequate to maintain the cornea in its normal state as, in the absence of oxygen, the cornea swells and loses its transparency (Heald and Langham, 1956, and many others).

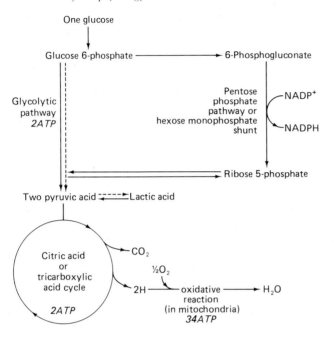

Figure 2.19 Outline of glucose metabolism in the cornea. Free oxygen does not take a direct part in the citric acid cycle, but its presence is essential and the cycle cannot operate in anaerobic conditions. Note the reversible connections between the pentose phosphate and glycolytic pathways. The broken lines indicate glycolysis in anaerobic conditions

Kinoshita and his colleagues have demonstrated that the hexose monophosphate shunt is unusually active in the cornea (Kinoshita and Masurat, 1959; Kinoshita, 1962). They estimated that, in the bovine corneal epithelium, about 65% of the glucose is metabolized by way of the glycolytic pathway followed by the citric acid cycle and 35% by means of the hexose monophosphate shunt. Kuhlman and Resnick (1959) estimated that, in the total cornea of rabbits, up to 70% of glucose is oxidized to carbon dioxide via the shunt mechanism. There is evidence that the metabolism of the corneal layers is interrelated. For example, it is found that lactic acid, which is produced in all layers of the cornea, cannot be utilized in the absence of the epithelium (Hermann and Hickman, 1948).

Sources of metabolites

The avascularity of the cornea promotes enquiry into the possible routes of metabolite supply. There are clearly three possibilities: from the perilimbal blood vessels, from the aqueous humour, and from the tear liquid. A common method of investigation is to alter the availability of metabolites from one of these possible sources and note if the cornea shows any alteration.

There is little reason to doubt that the perilimbal blood vessels provide metabolites for the cornea — at least, for the peripheral cornea; but that this route is of limited importance is indicated by experiments and observations where blood flow has been interrupted. Gunderson (1939) noted that corneal transparency was unaltered in his patients following complete peritomy of the cornea. Scarification of the conjunctiva in cases of perilimbal melanomas, and experimental thermocoagulation of the perilimbal tissues in rabbits, fails to interfere with corneal transparency. Diffusion of radioactive substances from the limbus into the cornea following subconjunctival or systemic injection has been observed. These substances are found to be in greater concentration peripherally than centrally (Maurice, 1951; Pratt-Johnson, 1959). Maurice (1962b) found that large molecules are the most likely to diffuse to the central cornea, and the conditions for this occurrence are least favourable for oxygen and glucose.

The question of the relative importance of tear liquid and aqueous humour as sources of glucose for the cornea appears to be settled in favour of the aqueous, but it is still uncertain whether or not the tear liquid route is of any practical importance. Bock and Maumenee (1953) inserted thin polythene sheets between stromal lamellae in rabbits and observed a thickening of the overlying stroma with complete degeneration of the epithelium in the central zone after 2 days. The deep underlying stroma and the endothelium were normal during this period and the epithelium maintained its integrity when the polythene sheet was trephined with several 2-mm holes. The conclusion was reached that the epithelium and stroma are dependent on the aqueous humour for metabolites. But these results are not altogether consistent with more recent studies. For example, water-impermeable polypropylene sheets inserted between stromal lamellae in cats were tolerated for more than a year without pathological changes, deep or superficial to the sheet (Pollack, 1962). In similar experiments, Knowles (1961) reported an absence of pathological changes for periods of up to 10 weeks in rabbits. Clearly, the deeper layers may flourish when isolated from the anterior layers and hence the aqueous must be a source of metabolites for the cornea. It is unlikely that much glucose moves in the other direction, from the tears to the cornea, as the concentration of 2.6 mg/100 ml in tears in man (Giardini and Roberts, 1950) is far too little to be of much significance in the nourishment of the cornea (Maurice, 1962b). Glucose concentration is more than 10 times as great in the aqueous (Reim et al., 1967). A reduction in epithelial glycogen and ATP as well as glucose was demonstrated following the insertion of intralamellar membrane barriers (Turss, Friend and Dohlman, 1970) and these changes could not be prevented by tarsorrhaphy or the topical application of glucose.

Thoft and Friend (1972) observed a passive diffusion of a labelled amino acid through the endothelium. The rapid turnover of epithelial cells demands a considerable utilization of amino acids in the synthesis of protein and, as expected, the concentration was high, but it was actively accumulated by the epithelium only after it had appeared in the stroma, suggesting that none was taken up from the tears despite their rich amino acid content (Balik, 1958). It appears that epithelium has a very low permeability to amino acids and glucose.

The utilization of atmospheric oxygen by the cornea through the tear film has been demonstrated in a number of ways. In man, symptoms of corneal irritation together with the haze and haloes known as Sattler's veil (Finkelstein, 1952) were experienced when the cornea was deprived of atmospheric oxygen (Smelser, 1952; Smelser and Ozanics, 1952). These symptoms were induced 2.5 hours after pumping nitrogen saturated with water vapour into tight-fitting goggles. The introduction of oxygen relieved the symptoms. Langham (1952) exposed the eyes of rabbits to a pure oxygen atmosphere for 3–3.5 hours and found that the lactic acid concentration in the cornea was reduced by a third. Using a nitrogen atmosphere for the same period of time, lactic acid concentration was increased by a third. These observations indicated an increase in aerobic glycolysis in the first case and a decrease in the second, again establishing that atmospheric oxygen is utilized by the cornea. Hill and Fatt (1964) measured the rate of oxygen uptake by the corneal epithelium in man by using oxygen electrodes embedded in a tight-fitting scleral lens with an oxygen-filled reservoir between the lens and cornea. They observed a rapid reduction in the oxygen tension in the reservoir as a result of oxygen uptake by the cornea. A rate of oxygen uptake of $4.8\,\mu l/cm^2$ per h was calculated from their results. However, Farris, Takahashi and Donn (1967), using the same technique, interpreted their data differently to arrive at a figure of $1.4\,\mu l/cm^2$ per h.

Langham (1952) concluded that the rabbit cornea also utilizes aqueous oxygen. The lactic acid concentration decreased from a value of unity to 0.7, 3–3.5 hours after introducing an oxygen bubble into the anterior chamber; the concentration was increased to 1.26 if nitrogen was used in place of oxygen. But whether provision of oxygen to the endothelium is the responsibility of the tear film or the aqueous is open to debate. Barr and his co-workers found an oxygen gradient reducing from the front surface of the cornea to the anterior chamber in rabbits and concluded that atmospheric oxygen normally diffuses through the full thickness of the cornea to the anterior chamber (Barr and

Roetman, 1974; Barr, Hennessey and Murphy, 1977). On the other hand, Fatt and Bieber (1968) and Fatt, Freeman and Lin (1974) concur with Langham on the basis of calculated oxygen distribution profiles through the cornea knowing the partial oxygen pressures at the two surfaces, stromal consumption, diffusion coefficients and solubility. The profile (*Figure 2.20*) displays a trough at the stromal aspect of the endothelium indicating that the endothelial layer receives oxygen from the aqueous. However, the crucial datum at the deep surface is difficult to determine and is supported by a single measurement.

Although equivalent data in man are limited, Fatt and Bieber believe that the oxygen distribution profiles in rabbits '. . . represent, at least qualitatively, the situation in the human cornea'. When the lids were closed long enough for equilibrium levels to be reached, the partial oxygen pressure at the epithelium reduced from 155 mmHg to the same level (55 mmHg) obtaining at the endothelial surface (*Figure 2.20*), with a trough within the stroma. Under these circumstances, it appears, first, that the vessels

of the palpebral conjunctiva must provide the epithelium with oxygen because if contact between these surfaces is prevented the partial oxygen pressure falls to zero. Earlier, Langham (1952) reached the same conclusion. Secondly, the altered profile suggests that aqueous oxygen is being used now by deeper structures of the cornea. This interpretation is based on the assumption that aqueous oxygen level is maintained, whereas Barr and Silver (1973) claim that it reduces as oxygen levels at the anterior surface of the cornea are reduced. Similar studies of the carbon dioxide partial pressures indicated that corneal and aqueous carbon dioxide passed out to the tears when the lids were open, but when they were closed some passed to the aqueous from the cornea.

The effects of contact lenses on corneal metabolism

A contact lens presents a barrier between the cornea and the atmosphere, and from the foregoing it follows that the most likely interference with corneal metabolism that a contact lens

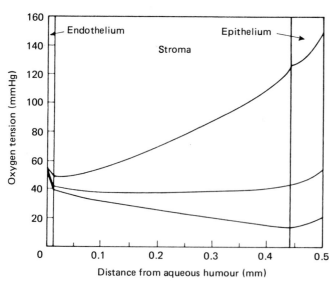

Figure 2.20 Summary of oxygen tension profiles for various conditions based on measurements made under each condition at the epithelial surface and under the normal condition at the endothelial surface in rabbits. The curves joining the surface points were calculated. The upper and middle curves represent the eye open and closed conditions respectively. The lowest curve represents the profile with a soft contact lens of low permeability on the eye. (Modified from Fatt, Freeman and Lin, 1974)

might cause is deprivation of oxygen with a consequent reduction in aerobic glycolysis. Oxygen uptake by the tears in front of the lens would continue, but transference of oxygen to the film behind the lens may be prevented. Normally, this situation is avoided with hard corneal lenses because they move and produce tear circulation, permitting some degree of oxygen and carbon dioxide exchange between the cornea and atmosphere.

Soft lenses also move on the eye but the circulation of tears behind the lens is less although they have the advantage of transmitting oxygen in amounts varying with the nature and thickness of the material (Fatt and St Helen, 1971; Refojo and Leong, 1979; Holden and Mertz, 1984). Tear exchange is least with scleral lenses; in the case of fenestrated lenses Ruben (1967) calculated the rate of tear exchange to be half that obtained with hard corneal lenses.

Presumably, the cornea can comfortably tolerate a reduction of the partial oxygen pressure at the epithelial surface from 155 to 55 mmHg, for this occurs when the lids are closed for some length of time and there is evidence that the cornea can tolerate levels as low as 11–19 mmHg (Polse and Mandell, 1970). Farris, Takahashi and Donn (1967), using the oxygen electrode method, observed a transient increase in oxygen uptake by the corneal epithelium measured a few seconds after comfortably fitted corneal lenses had been worn for a period of 8 hours. But even after only 2 minutes wear, a large increase in oxygen uptake occurred (Hill and Leighton, 1968). The increased uptake of oxygen was about the same whether soft hydrophilic or hard methacrylate lenses were worn (Hill, 1967). The increase was due to the replenishment of the supply of dissolved oxygen normally present when an unlimited supply is available from the atmosphere. The level of oxygen deprivation induced by wearing corneal lenses was found to be slightly greater than that caused by lid closure for 5 minutes (Farris, Takahashi and Donn, 1967). Following the argument of Fatt and his colleagues, aqueous oxygen utility extends deeper than the endothelium when the level of tear liquid oxygen is depressed by the presence of a contact lens.

Interference with normal corneal metabolism will produce a thickening and a reduction of transparency of the cornea. The thickening which is observed with corneal lens wear varies between individuals. Most people show a measurable thickening and it seems likely that when none is reported the thickening is simply too little to permit detection. Increases in

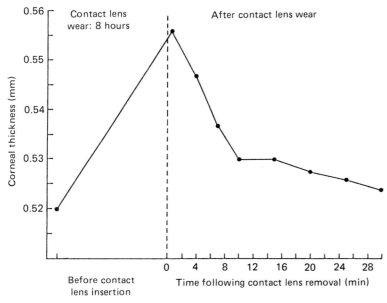

Figure 2.21 Relationship between central corneal thickness and the wearing of hard contact lenses for 8 hours. Each point represents the mean of 11 subjects. (After Millodot, 1975a)

thickness average between 4% (Honda, Sakaue and Kyoko, 1968; Farris, Kubota and Mishima, 1971) and about 7 or 8% (*Figure 2.21*) (Manchester, 1970; Millodot, 1975a). Increases of 20% have been recorded. The increase usually takes more than one hour after insertion of a lens to reach a maximum thickness (El Hage *et al.*, 1974) and within 2 hours of removing the lens normal thickness is recovered. Epithelial swelling contributes to the thickening (Farris, Kubota and Mishima, 1971) and increased curvature has been recorded (Miller, 1969). Early claims that soft lenses in general do not cause swelling of the cornea have not been confirmed (El Hage *et al.*, 1974) and the amount of swelling incurred may compare with that associated with hard lenses (Bailey and Carney, 1973; Polse, Sarver and Harris, 1975). Oxygen transmission characteristics and mean thickness of the material used are the major factors in determining the amount of swelling which varies from practically nothing up to 5% or exceptionally 8% according to lens type (Holden and Mertz, 1984). Vertical striae are quite commonly present while soft lenses are worn but corneal curvature does not appear to be altered. Much has been written favouring the concept that oedema reduces as the eyes adapt to contact lenses but specific data are often lacking. Some recovery from oedema seems likely but it is probably slow (Farris, Kubota and Mishima, 1971) and possibly incomplete. Evidence of sustained oedema may be found with greater facility. In this context it is worth noting that corneal thickening with soft daily wear lenses is, at most, little more than the 4% or so incurred normally during sleep. If a lens is not worn the cornea gradually thins over a period of 1 or 2 hours (Mandell and Fatt, 1965; Gerstman, 1972).

When lenses are worn continuously, lens- and sleep-induced effects are compounded and swelling is consequently greater than with daily wear. Holden and Mertz (1984) measured a thickening of 7–15% on awakening after a single day/night cycle of wear, varying according to soft lens type and reducing to 1–6% during the course of the day. Corneal thickness increases during the first week of continuous wear and, although a subsequent reduction has been reported (Schoessler and Barr, 1980), this may be deceptive (Holden *et al.*, 1985) and a stable chronic swelling is more likely.

Alterations in glycolysis have been measured after fitting contact lenses to experimental animals. The corneae of guinea-pigs fitted with scleral lenses became thicker and less transparent and the lactic acid content increased rapidly (Smelser and Chen, 1955). An increased lactic acid content would be expected as a result of reduced aerobic glycolysis, and Hirano's (1959) observation of depleted glycogen content in rabbit corneae fitted with corneal lenses indicates an increased consumption of glycogen by means of the less productive anaerobic glycolytic cycle in an endeavour to compensate. Morley and McCulloch (1961) also observed an increased lactic acid content in both the stroma and epithelium of rabbits fitted with contact lenses and, in addition, they observed a slight decrease of oxidized pyridine nucleotides and a decrease in the percentage of protein in the epithelium. These results suggest that both aerobic glycolysis and protein synthesis were reduced.

The loss of transparency associated with induced thickening is so slight that it cannot be measured objectively.

Tears

The basic secretion of tears is largely derived from the lacrimal gland, with small additional contributions from the accessory lacrimal glands, the mucous conjunctival glands and the sebaceous tarsal (meibomian) glands. A conjunctival gland or goblet cell is shown in *Figure 2.10* in the process of releasing mucin granules into the tear film. The lacrimal gland has usually been classified as a serous gland, but recent evidence shows that it is in fact a seromucous gland in man and monkeys (Ruskell, 1969, 1975; Allen, Wright and Reid, 1972). The watery secretion is explained by the greater activity of the serous cells. It has been proposed that the lacrimal gland does not take part in the basic secretion of tears because the eye remains moist if the lacrimal gland is congenitally absent, or when the gland is removed or its motor nerve supply is interrupted. It may be true that the eye usually remains sufficiently moist for comfort in these circumstances with retention of an optically adequate corneal surface, but denervation or removal of the gland nonetheless produces a radical reduction in the basic secretion of tears (Golding-Wood, 1964; Ruskell, 1969).

Superimposed on the basic secretion are the phasic increments in secretion induced reflexly by mechanical or chemical irritation and by psychogenic factors. To distinguish between the two, the words 'lacrimation', to describe reflex tears, and 'weeping', for psychogenic tears, have been suggested.

The precorneal film

Wolff (1948) considered the precorneal film to consist of a triple-layered structure with a central watery phase made up of the serous secretion of the lacrimal gland and constituting the bulk of the film; a thin superficial oily layer was thought to issue from the tarsal glands and a deep layer of mucoproteins from the conjunctival glands.

The presence of a thin superficial oily layer is suggested by the coloured interference fringes which may be observed with a biomicroscope. Further evidence of the surface film and of its origin is provided by Mishima and Maurice (1961), who demonstrated in rabbits that tear film evaporation increases at least 10-fold in the absence of tarsal gland secretion. This amount of increased evaporation is approximately that expected of water in the absence of a surface lipid film. Despite this apparently straightforward evidence for tarsal gland function, when secretion, expressed from human tarsal glands, was spread over a saline solution no significant reduction in evaporation was observed (Brown and Dervichian, 1969). Although the experimental conditions of this study are not beyond criticism, the results are at least sufficient to re-open discussion of the matter.

The superficial lipid layer contributes to the stability of the tear film by lowering the surface tension at the air/tear film interface.

Lacrimal secretion is substantially serous but a small mucus content is present and hence the watery phase of the tear film has mucus dispersed within it, probably augmented by goblet cell mucus. Mucins from the conjunctival goblet cells are adsorbed by the epithelium producing a wettable hydrophilic surface providing further stability for the tear film (Holly and Lemp, 1971; Holly, 1973). Most superficial cells of the conjunctiva contain a number of vesicular inclusions thought to discharge their content onto the surface (Greiner et al., 1980), and Dilly (1985) showed that upon opening onto the surface, vesicles presented branched mucoprotein chains providing an anchor for the mucous layer of the tear film. The surface coating so produced is presumably equivalent to the glycocalyx of other surface cells and it is reasonable to suppose that similar provision is made for the cornea but a vesicular method of production has not yet been demonstrated.

The precorneal film is of nearly uniform thickness of between 6 and 9 μm (Ehlers, 1965a; Mishima, 1965). Ehlers observed that it reduces by about 20% 5 seconds after blinking and by nearly 50% after 30 seconds. There is little flow across the cornea between blinks. The limited flow and the uniform thickness are the consequences of the 'framing' function of the eyelids which is eliminated if the eyelids are withdrawn from the eyeball, causing a spotty drying of the precorneal film.

Apposition of the eyelid margins during blinking permits replenishment of lipid from the tarsal glands which is then spread across the surface of the reconstructed film as the eyelids part. Similarly, mucus is spread over the corneal and conjunctival epithelium by the massaging action of the eyelids. It should be added that the spreading of the tear film is facilitated by the movement of the eyelids across the cornea. In the presence of a contact lens, the interfacial tension at three surfaces has to be considered. The desirable establishment of low interfacial tension at the two surfaces of the contact lens is partly related to the nature and to the condition of the lens.

Function of tears

Tear liquid is essential for the maintenance of the normal optical properties of the cornea; without it, corneal metabolic processes are impaired, as noted earlier, with consequent loss of transparency. Further, the excellent refracting surface which the smooth tear film provides would be lost and an irregularly refracting, dessicated epithelial surface would be substituted. Tear liquid is the lubricant for eyelid movement over the cornea and the medium for flushing away foreign matter which potentially endangers the optical integrity of the cornea.

Tears have antibacterial properties. Lysozyme, the enzyme originally described by Fleming (1922) in tear liquid, is selectively bacteriolytic by destruction of the cell wall providing a degree of protection against certain Gram-positive bacteria lodged in the conjunctival sac. Claims for the presence of a non-lysozyme antibacterial factor (NLAF) in tears with far greater activity than lysozyme have been criticized. It is argued that inappropriate analytical methods were used giving grossly misleading results. However, the presence of some NLAF activity is broadly agreed. Lactoferrin, present in abundance in tears (Kijlstra, Jerissen and Koning, 1983), has non-specific bactericidal properties (Arnold, Cole and McGhee, 1977) and moreover may have an anti-inflammatory function (Veerhuis and Kijlstra, 1982). Among the antibody proteins, IgA and IgG are prominent in tears but other immunoglobulins are present.

Tear drainage

Much of the tear liquid lies in strips (the rivus lacrimalis) along the lid margins and against the cornea, presenting a concave cylindrical free surface. Medially, the strips terminate in the so-called lacrimal lake which is often described as a reservoir of tear liquid bathing the caruncle and bounded by the inner canthus and the free edge of the plica semilunaris. This delimitation is obviously changed as the eye moves from the primary position. But, as Wolff (1948) pointed out, under normal circumstances the inner canthus is moist but does not contain a pool of fluid. The punctum lacrimale of each papilla is turned in towards the cornea and interrupts the marginal tear strip.

Drainage of tears is initiated by the movement of tear liquid from the marginal tear strips through the punctum and into the canaliculus by capillary attraction. This is facilitated by the continuous movement of liquid nasally which is effected by lid closure; closure occurs first at the outer canthus and then, progressively, to the inner canthus. If a very small spot of dye is applied to a marginal tear strip, blinking will cause the dye to spread towards the punctum. It will neither move to the fornix nor to the outer canthus (Ehlers, 1965a).

The canaliculi are embedded in the orbicularis muscle so that on contraction of the muscle the canaliculi are closed and shortened and the tear liquid is driven into the lacrimal sac. Regurgitation is prevented by the simultaneous closure of the ampulla of each canaliculus. The

muscular activity amounts to a milking action rather than a peristalsis. The preseptal portion of the orbicularis muscle is claimed to have a deep insertion from each lid to the lacrimal diaphragm which is the lateral fascial wall of the lacrimal sac, with the consequence that contraction causes a lateral movement of the lacrimal diaphragm. It follows that the sac becomes dilated, and it is thought to produce a reduction of the pressure in the sac which produces a siphoning of tear liquid. This postulated mechanism (Jones, 1961), which constitutes a lacrimal pump, would appear to demand closure of the 'valve' of Hasner which occludes the nasal exits of the nasolacrimal duct (ostium lacrimalis), in order to create an effective vacuum for siphoning. This probably does not occur, and pressure measurements within the sac reveal no change during eyelid movement (Wright and Maurice, personal communication). Further, the existence of the necessary structures for operating the lacrimal pump, postulated by Jones, has been questioned (Brienen and Snell, 1967). Hence, it appears that an elaborate pumping mechanism may not be present and that gravitation alone may account for the movement of the tears out of the lacrimal sac.

Tear output

The daily output of tears is usually considered to be rather less than 1 g. This figure is based on the data of Schirmer (1903), but it has been questioned because of the probable inaccuracy of his measuring technique. Tests developed recently, that measure the rate of dilution of a stain applied to the marginal tear strip, probably introduce less error, but results are not consistent. Originally, Nover and Jaeger (1952) calculated the surprisingly high average rate of 14 g of tear secretion daily, but Kirschner's (1964) results were similar to those of Schirmer. However, Norn (1965) subsequently reported a daily tear output of 15–30 g measured from 186 eyes. The instillation of a stain (rose bengal and/or fluorescein) will obviously tend to elevate the recorded figure for basic tear secretion both by its own bulk and by its irritant effect. But the method neither involves the aspiration of tears nor neglects to account for tears escaping through the puncta, and these are important shortcomings of other tests, some of which also share the error invoked by corneal irritation. Hence, it may be tentatively concluded that the lacrimal secretion normally produced is well in excess of 1 g as suggested by Schirmer but rather less than the 15–30 g measured by Norn.

In a study of a large number of full-term infants, Penbharkkul and Karelitz (1962) encountered shedding of tears as early as 5.5 hours of age and as late as 84 days. The onset of lacrimation occurred during the first 4 weeks in a majority of infants, and in most it occurred first with crying associated with hunger and pain. Sjögren (1955) used nasal irritants to determine the onset of reflex lacrimation in infants and found that it occurred in all but 13% during the first few weeks of life.

With advancing years, basic tear secretion decreases gradually: the difference between the sexes is negligible (Norn, 1965) except in early adult life, when females have a higher rate of secretion (Henderson and Prough, 1950; de Roetth, 1953). Sex differences concerning psychogenic tears or weeping are clearly a separate matter.

Schirmer's popular tear secretion test is unsatisfactory as a precise quantitative test for tear secretion but it is of considerable value in comparing the production of tears between eyes of a pair and between eyes of different persons. The test should find a place in routine contact lens practice, according to some authorities (for example, Halberg, 1967), as an aid in determining the suitability of a patient for contact lens wear. It is argued that patients with a low rate of tear secretion are more likely than others to be intolerant of lenses. If this is too indulgent a view, it is at least reasonable that practitioners should be aware of the problems of limited or reduced lacrimal gland secretion. Lacrimal hypersecretion, induced by contact lenses, has been held responsible for corneal oedema on rather insubstantial grounds and the idea has been refuted (Uniacke and Hill, 1970; Farris, Kubota and Mishima, 1971).

In Schirmer's test, filter paper strips (Whatman's No.1 are satisfactory), 5 mm in width are folded 5 mm from one end. This short end is trimmed at the corners and inserted into the inferior conjunctival sac, displaced laterally to avoid contact with the cornea (*see Figure 11.8a* and *b*, Chapters 8, 11 and 21). Anaesthesia is not used. After 5 minutes, the exposed length of moistened filter paper is measured to the fold. A 15 mm length is moistened, on average, in a 5-minute period. Standardized sterile strips are available if preferred (Schirmer tear test — CooperVision and Sno Strips — Smith & Nephew). The test should not be undertaken immediately after any procedure that may induce hypersecretion of tears.

Neural control of tears

Irritation of the cornea, conjunctiva, nasal mucosa and of any area served by the trigeminal nerve causes reflex lacrimation. The trigeminal nerve is responsible for the sensory input of the reflex pathway and if it is blocked, or surface anaesthesia applied, reflex lacrimation is abolished. The paths of the central nervous system associated with psychogenic weeping are unknown, and a knowledge of the link between the trigeminal nerve and the facial nerve in the reflex lacrimation pathway is lacking.

Both parasympathetic nerve fibres (from the pterygopalatine or sphenopalatine ganglion) and sympathetic nerve fibres (from the superior cervical ganglion) have been thought to be responsible for motor control of lacrimal gland secretion; but in recent experiments on cats and monkeys, only parasympathetic fibres could be shown to exercise this control (Botelho, Hisada and Fuenmayor, 1966; Ruskell, 1969). There is no clear evidence of motor control of the tarsal and conjunctival glands.

References

ALLEN, M., WRIGHT, P. and REID, L. (1972). The human lacrimal gland. A histochemical and organ culture study of the secretory cells. *Archs Ophthal.* **88**, 493–497

ARNOLD, R. R., COLE, M. F. and McGHEE, J. R. (1977). A bactericidal effect for human lactoferrin. *Science* **197**, 263–265

BAILEY, I. L. and CARNEY, L. G. (1973). Corneal changes from hydrophilic contact lenses. *Am. J. Optom.* **50**, 299–304

BALIK, J. (1958). The amino acid content of tears. *Sborn. Lék.* **60**, 332–336, as cited in *Ophthal. Lit.* **12**, No.4847 (1958)

BARR, R. E. and ROETMAN, E. L. (1974). Oxygen radients in the anterior chamber of anesthetized rabbits. *Invest. Ophthal.* **13**, 386–389

BARR, R. E. and SILVER, I. A. (1973) Effects of corneal environment on oxygen tension in the anterior chambers of rabbits. *Invest. Ophthal.* **12**, 140–144

BARR, R. E., HENNESSEY, M. and MURPHY, V. G. (1977). Diffusion of oxygen at the endothelial surface of the rabbit cornea. *J. Physiol.* **270**, 1–8

BELMONTE, C. and GIRALDEZ, F. (1981). Responses of cat corneal sensory receptors to mechanical and thermal stimulation. *J. Physiol.* **321**, 355–368

BENEDEK, G. B. (1971). Theory of transparency of the eye. *Appl. Optics* **10**, 459–472

BERGMANSON, J. P. G. and CHU, L. W. F. (1982). Corneal response to rigid contact lens wear. *Br. J. Ophthal.* **66**, 667–675

BERNHARD, C. G., MILLER, W. H. and MØLLER, A. R. (1965). The insect corneal nipple array. *Acta physiol. scand.* **63**, Suppl. 243

BERTANLANFFY, F. D. and LAU, C. (1962). Mitotic rate and renewal time of the corneal epithelium in the rat. *Archs Ophthal.* **68**, 546–551

BEUERMAN, R. W. and SCHIMMELPFENNIG. B. (1980). Sensory denervation of the rabbit cornea affects epithelial properties. *Expl Neurol.* **69**, 196–201

BLESHOY, H. (1986). Corneal sensitivity in keratoconus. *Trans. Br. Contact Lens Ass.* 9–12

BOCK, R. H. and MAUMENEE, A. E. (1953). Corneal fluid metabolism: experiments and observations. *Archs Ophthal.* **50**, 282–285

BOBERG-ANS, J. (1955). Experience in clinical examination of corneal sensitivity. *Br. J. Ophthal.* **39**, 705–726

BOBERG-ANS, J. (1956). On the corneal sensitivity. *Acta ophthal.* **35**, 149–162

BOOZAN, C. W. and COHEN, I. J. (1953). Ophthaine; new topical anesthetic for eye. *Am. J. Ophthal.* **36**, 1619–1621

BOTELHO, S. Y., HISADA, M. and FUENMAYOR, N. (1966). Functional innervation of the lacrimal gland in the cat. *Archs Ophthal.* **76**, 581–588

BRAUDE, L. S. and CHANDLER, J. W. (1983). Corneal allograft rejection. The role of the major histocompatibility complex. *Survey Ophthal.* **27**, 290–305

BRIENEN, J. A. and SNELL, C. A. R. D. (1967). A new examination of the orbicularis oculi. *Ophthalmologica* **154**, 104–113

BRON, A. J. (1968). Anterior corneal mosaic. *Br. J. Ophthal.* **52**, 659–669

BROWN, M., CHINN, S., FATT, I. and HARRIS, M. G. (1973). The effect of soft and hard contact lenses on blinkrate, amplitude and length. *J. Am. optom. Ass.* **44**, 254–257

BROWN, S. I. and DERVICHIAN, D. G. (1969). The oils of the meibomian glands. *Archs Ophthal.* **82**, 537–540

BUCK, R. C. (1985). Measurement of centripetal migration of normal corneal epithelial cells in the mouse. *Invest. Ophthal. Vis. Sci.* **26**, 1296–1298

CARDOSO, S. S., FERREIRA, A. L., CAMARGO, A. C. M. and BÖHN, G. (1968). The effect of partial hepatectomy upon circadian distribution of mitosis in the cornea of rats. *Experientia* **24**, 569–570

CASPERSSON, T. and ENGSTRÖM, A. (1946). Hornhinne-vävnadens transparens. *Nord. Med.* **30**, 1279–1282, cited by D. M. Maurice (1957)

CHANDLER, J. W., CUMMINGS, M. and GILLETTE, T. E. (1985). Presence of Langerhans cells in the central corneas of normal human infants. *Invest. Ophthal. Vis. Sci.* **26**, 113–115

CINTRON, C., KUBLIN, C. L. and COVINGTON, H. (1982).

Quantitative studies of corneal epithelial wound healing in rabbits. *Curr. Eye Res.* **1**, 507–516

COCHET, P. and BONNET, R. (1960). L'esthésia cornéenne. Sa measure clinique ses variations physiologiques et pathologiques. *Clin. Ophthal.* **4**, 1–27

COGAN, D. G. and KINSEY, V. E. (1942). The cornea. V: Physiological aspects. *Archs Ophthal.* **28**, 661–669

DAVSON, H. (1955). The hydration of the cornea. *Biochem. J.* **59**, 24–28

DILLY, P. N. (1985). Contribution of the epithelium to the stability of the tear film. *Trans. Ophthal. Soc. UK* **104**, 381–389

DONN, A., MILLER, S. and MALLETT, N. (1963). Water permeability of the living cornea. *Archs Ophthal.* **70**, 515–521

DRAEGER, J. (1984). *Corneal Sensitivity: Measurement and Clinical Importance.* Vienna: Springer Verlag

EHINGER, B. (1964). Adrenergic nerves to the eye and its adnexa in rabbit and guinea-pig. *Acta Univ. Lund.* (2), No.20.

EHINGER, B. (1971). A comparative study of the adrenergic nerves to the anterior eye segment of some primates. *Z. Zellforsch. mikroskop. Anat.* **116**, 157–177

EHLERS, N. (1965a). The precorneal film. Biomicroscopical, histological and chemical investigations. *Acta ophthal.* Suppl. 81

EHLERS, N. (1965b). On the size of the conjunctival sac. *Acta ophthal.* **43**, 205–210

EISENMAN, J., LANDGREN, S. and NOVIN, P. (1963). Functional organization in the main sensory trigeminal nucleus and in the rostral subdivision of the nucleus of the spinal trigeminal tract in the cat. *Acta physiol. scand.* **59**, Suppl. 214

EL HAGE, S. G., HUGHES, C. C., SCHLAUER, K. R. and JARELL, R. L. (1974). Evaluation of corneal thickness induced by hard and flexible contact lens wear. *Am. J. Optom.* **51**, 24–33

EPSTEIN, D. L. and PATON, D. (1968). Keratitis from misuse of corneal anaesthetics. *N. Engl. J. Med.* **279**, 396–399. Annotated in *Lancet*, 16 Nov. (1968)

FARRIS, R. L., TAKAHASHI, G. H. and DONN, A. (1967). Corneal oxygen flux in contact lens wearers. In *Corneal and Scleral Contact Lenses*, edited by L. J. Girard, pp.413–425. St Louis: Mosby

FARRIS, R. L., KUBOTA, Z. and MISHIMA, S. (1971). Epithelial decompensation with corneal contact lens wear. *Archs Ophthal.* **85**, 651–660

FATT, I. and BIEBER, M. T. (1968). The steady-state distribution of oxygen and carbon dioxide in the *in vivo* cornea. 1: The open eye in air and the closed eye. *Expl Eye Res.* **7**, 103–112

FATT, I. and ST HELEN, R. (1971). Oxygen tension under an oxygen-permeable contact lens. *Am. J. Optom.* **48**, 545–555

FATT, I., FREEMAN, R. D. and LIN, D. (1974). Oxygen tension distributions in the cornea: a re-examination. *Expl Eye Res.* **18**, 357–365

FINKELSTEIN, I. S. (1952). The biophysics of corneal scatter and diffraction of light induced by contact lenses. *Am. J. Optom.* **29**, 231–259

FLEMING, A. (1922). On a remarkable bacteriolytic element

found in tissues and secretions. *Proc. R. Soc. Lond.* **B 93**, 306–317

FREEMAN, J. A. (1962). Fine structure of the goblet cell mucous secretory process. *Anat. Rec.* **144**, 341–357

FREEMAN, R. D. (1972). Oxygen consumption by the component layers of the cornea. *J. Physiol.* **225**, 15–32

FRIEDENWALD, J. S. and BUSCHKE, W. (1944a). The effect of excitement of epinephrine and of sympathectomy on the mitotic activity of corneal epithelium in rats. *Am. J. Physiol.* **141**, 689–694

FRIEDENWALD, J. S. and BUSCHKE, W. (1944b). Mitotic and wound-healing activities of the corneal epithelium. *Archs Ophthal.* **32**, 410–413

GERSTMAN, D. R. (1972). The biomicroscope and Vickers image-splitting eyepiece applied to the diurnal variation in human central corneal thickness. *J. Microsc.* **96**, 385–388

GIARDINI, A. and ROBERTS, J. R. E. (1950). Concentration of glucose and total chloride in tears. *Br. J. Ophthal.* **34**, 737–743

GINSBORG, B. L. (1952). Rotation of the eyes during involuntary blinking. *Nature* **169**, 412–413

GINSBORG, B. L. and MAURICE, D. M. (1959). Involuntary movements of the eye during fixation and blinking. *Br. J. Ophthal.* **43**, 435–437

GIPSON, I. K., SPURR-MICHAUD, S. J. and TISDALE, A. S. (1987). Anchoring fibrils form a complex network in human and rabbit corneas. *Invest. Ophthal. Vis. Sci.* **28**, 212–220

GOLDING-WOOD, P. H. (1964). The ocular effects of autonomic surgery. *Proc. R. Soc. Med.* **57**, 494–497

GORDON, G. (1951). Observations upon the movement of the eyelids. *Br. J. Ophthal.* **35**, 339–351

GORNIG, H. and POMMER, G. (1971). Alternsveranderungen des Konjunktivalepithels. *Z. Altensforsch.* **23**, 391–395

GRANT, F. C., GROFF, R. A. and LEWY, F. H. (1940). Section of descending spinal root of fifth cranial nerve. *Archs Neurol. Psychiat.* **43**, 498–509

GREENBERG, M. H. and HILL, R. M. (1973). The physiology of contact lens imprints. *Am. J. Optom.* **50**, 699–702

GREINER, J. V., KENYON, K. R., HENRIQUEZ, A. S., KORB, D. R., WEIDMAN, T. A. and ALLANSMITH, M. R. (1980). Mucus secretory vesicles in conjunctival epithelial cells of wearers of contact lenses. *Archs Ophthal.* **98**, 1843–1846

GUILBERT, J. (1963). Contact lens fitting in France. *J. Am. Optom. Ass.* **34**, 1403–1405

GUNDERSON, T. (1939). Vascular obliteration for various types of keratitis. Its significance regarding nutrition of corneal epithelium. *Archs Ophthal.* **21**, 76–107

GUNDERSON, T. and LIEBMAN, S. D. (1944). Effect of local anaesthetics on regeneration of corneal epithelium. *Archs Ophthal.* **31**, 29–33

HALBERG, G. P. (1967). Lacrimal function and contact lenses. In *XXth International Congress of Ophthalmology, Munich, 1966. Contact Lens Symposium*, pp.149–154. Basel: Karger

HAMANO, H. (1960). Topical and systemic influences of wearing contact lenses. *Contacto* **4**, 41–48

HAMANO, H., HORI, M., HAMANO, T., KAWABE, H., MIKAMI, M., MITSUNAGA, S. and HAMANO, T. (1983). Effects of contact lens wear on mitosis of corneal epithelium and lactate

content in aqueous humor of rabbit. *Jap. J. Ophthal.* **27**, 451–458

HANNA, C. and O'BRIEN, J. E. (1960). Cell production and migration in the epithelial layer of the cornea. *Archs Ophthal.* **64**, 536–539

HANNA, C. and O'BRIEN, J. E. (1961). Thymidine-tritium labelling of the cellular elements of the corneal stroma. *Archs Ophthal.* **66**, 362–365

HANNA, C., BICKNELL, D. S. and O'BRIEN, J. E. (1961). Cell turnover in the adult human eye. *Archs Ophthal.* **65**, 695–698

HARRIS, J. E. and NORDQUIST, L. T. (1955). The hydration of the cornea. 1: The transport of water from the cornea. *Am. J. Ophthal.* **40**, 100–110

HART, R. W. and FARRELL, R. A. (1969). Light scattering in the cornea. *J. opt. Soc. Am.* **59**, 766–774

HEALD, K. and LANGHAM, M. E. (1956). Permeability of the cornea and blood-aqueous barrier to oxygen. *Br. J. Ophthal.* **40**, 705–720

HENDERSON, J. W. and PROUGH, W. L. (1950). Influence of age and sex on flow of tears. *Archs Ophthal.* **43**, 224–231

HERRMANN, H. and HICKMAN, F. H. (1948). The adhesion of epithelium to stroma in the cornea. *Bull. Johns Hopkins Hosp.* **82**, 182–207

HEYDENREICH, A. (1958). *Die Hornhautregeneration.* Marhold: Halle

HILL, R. M. (1967). Effects of hydrophilic plastic lenses on corneal respiration. *J. Am optom. Ass.* **38**, 181–184

HILL, R. M. and FATT, I. (1964). Oxygen measurements under a contact lens. *Am. J. Optom.* **41**, 382–387

HILL, R. M. and LEIGHTON, A. J. (1968). Effects of contact lens apertures on corneal respiration under dynamic conditions. *Am. J. Optom.* **45**, 65–79

HIRANO, J. (1959). Histochemical studies on the corneal changes induced by corneal contact lenses. *Jap. J. Ophthal.* **3**, 1–8

HODSON, S. (1977). Endothelial pump of cornea (editorial). *Invest. Ophthal. Vis. Sci.* **16**, 589–591

HODSON, S. and MILLER, F. (1976). The bicarbonate ion pump in the endothelium which regulates the hydration of rabbit cornea. *J. Physiol.* **263**, 563–577

HOLDEN, B. A. and MERTZ, G. W. (1984). Critical oxygen levels to avoid corneal edema for daily and extended wear contact lenses. *Invest. Ophthal. Vis. Sci.*, **25**, 1161–1167

HOLDEN, B. A., SWEENEY, D. F., EFRON, N., VANNAS, A. and NILSSON, K. T. (1985). Effects of long-term extended contact lens wear on the human cornea. *Invest. Ophthal. Vis. Sci.* **26**, 1489–1501

HOLLY, F. J. (1973). Formation and rupture of the tear film. *Expl Eye Res.* **15**, 515–525

HOLLY, F. J. and LEMP, M. A. (1971). Wettability and wetting of corneal epithelium. *Expl Eye Res.* **11**, 239–250

HONDA, Y., SAKAUE, E. and KYOKO, O. (1968). Studies on the thickness of the cornea wearing contact lenses. (In Japanese). *J. Jap. Contact Lens Soc.* **10**, 133–141. In *Fol. ophthal. Jap.* **19**, No.11

HUMPHREYS, J. A., LARKE, J. R. and PARRISH, S. T. (1980). Microepithelial cysts observed in extended contact lens wearing subjects. *Br. J. Ophthal.* **64**, 888–889

IWAMOTO, T. and SMELSER, G. K. (1965). Electron microscopy of the human corneal endothelium with reference to transport mechanisms. *Invest. Ophthal.* **4**, 270–284

JAKUS, M. A. (1961). The fine structure of the human cornea. In *The Structure of the Eye*, edited by G. K. Smelser. New York: Academic Press

JAKUS, M. A. (1964). *Ocular Fine Structure. Selected Electron Micrographs*. Retina Foundation, Inst. Biol. Med. Sci. Monographs & Conferences, Vol. 1. London: Churchill

JALAVISTO, E., ORMA, E. and TAWAST, M. (1951). Ageing and relation between stimulus intensity and duration in corneal sensibility. *Acta physiol. scand.* **23**, 224–233

JONES, L. T. (1961). An anatomical approach to problems of the eyelids and lacrimal apparatus. *Archs Ophthal.* **66**, 111–124

KENSHALO, D. R. (1960). Comparison of thermal sensitivity of the forehead, lip, conjunctiva and cornea. *J. appl. Physiol.* **15**, 987–991

KERR, F. W. L. (1963). The divisional organization of afferent fibres of the trigeminal nerve. *Brain* **86**, 721–732

KESSING, S. V. (1968). Mucous gland system of the conjunctiva. *Acta ophthal.* Suppl. 85, 36–59

KHODADOUST, A. A., SILVERSTEIN, A. M., KENYON, K. R. and DOWLING, J. E. (1968). Adhesions of regenerating corneal epithelium: The role of basement membrane. *Am. J. Ophthal.* **65**, 339–348

KIJLSTRA, H., JEURISSEN, S. H. M. and KONING, K. M. (1983). Lactoferrin levels in normal human tears. *Br. J. Ophthal.* **67**, 199–202

KING, D. C. and MICHELS, K. M. (1957). Muscular tension and the human blink rate. *J. exp. Psychol.* **53**, 113–116

KINOSHITA, J. H. (1962). Some aspects of the carbohydrate metabolism of the cornea. *Invest Ophthal.* **1**, 178–186

KINOSHITA, J. H. and MASURAT, T. (1959). Aerobic pathways of glucose metabolism in bovine corneal epithelium. *Am. J. Ophthal.* **48**, 47–52

KIRCHNER, C. (1964). Untersuchungen über das Ausmass der Tränensekretion beim Menschen. *Klin. Mbl. Augenheilk.* **144**, 412–417

KLINTWORTH, G. K. (1969). Experimental studies on the phagocytic capability of the corneal fibroblast. *Am. J. Path.* **55**, 283–294

KLYCE, S. D. and CROSSON, C. E. (1985). Transport processes across the rabbit corneal epithelium — a review. *Curr. Eye Res.* **4**, 323–332

KNOLL, H. A. and WILLIAMS, J. (1970). Effects of hydrophilic contact lenses on corneal sensitivity. *Am. J. Optom.* **47**, 561–563

KNOWLES, W. F. (1961). Effect of intra-lamellar plastic membranes on corneal physiology. *Am. J. Ophthal.* **51**, 274–284

KOKOTT, W. (1938). Über mechanisch funktionelle Strukturen des Auges. *Graefes Arch. klin. exp. Ophthal.* **138**, 424–485

KUHLMAN, R. E. and RESNICK, R. A. (1959). The oxidation of C-14-labelled glucose and lactate by the rabbit cornea. *Archs Biochem. Biophys.* **8**, 29–36

LANGHAM, M. E. (1952). Utilization of oxygen by the component layers of the living cornea. *J. Physiol.* **117**, 461–470

LANGHAM, M. E. (1954). Glycolysis in the cornea of the rabbit. *J. Physiol.* **126**, 396–403

LANGHAM, M. E. (1960). Corneal metabolism and its influence on corneal hydration in the excised eye and in the living animal. In *The Transparency of the Cornea*, edited by Sir Stewart Duke-Elder and E. S. Perkins. Oxford: Blackwell

LARKE, J. R. and HIRJI, N. K. (1979). Some clinically observed phenomena in extended contact lens wear. *Br. J. Ophthal.* **63**, 475–477

LARKE, J. R. and SABELL, A. G. (1971). A comparative study of the ocular responses to two forms of contact lenses. *Optician* **162**(4187), 8–12 and (4188), 10–17

LEHTOSALO, J. I. (1984). Substance P-like immunoreactive trigeminal ganglion cells supplying the cornea. *Histochemistry* **80**, 273–276

LELE, P. P. and WEDDELL, G. (1956). The relationship between neurohistology and corneal sensibility. *Brain* **79**, 119–154

LIM, C. H. and RUSKELL, G. L. (1978). Corneal nerve access in monkeys. *Albrecht v. Graefes Arch. Ophthal.* **208**, 15–23

LOWTHER, G. E. and HILL, R. M. (1968). Sensitivity threshold of the lower lid margin in the course of adaptation to contact lenses. *Am. J. Optom.* **45**, 587–594

LYNE, A. (1982). Corneal sensitivity after surgery. *Trans. Ophthal. Soc. UK* **102**, 302–305

MACHEMER, R. (1966). Autoradiographische Untersuchungen des Regenerationzonen der Hornhaut. *Graefes Arch. klin. exp. Ophthal.* **170**, 286–297

MACINTOSH, S. R. (1968). The ultrastructure of conjunctival epithelium in monkeys. Student special study, The City University, London

MACINTOSH, S. R. (1974). The innervation of the conjunctiva in monkeys. An electron microscopic and nerve degeneration study. *Graefes Arch. klin. exp. Ophthal.* **192**, 105–116

McMONNIES, C. W. (1984). Risk factors in the etiology of contact lens induced corneal vascularization. *Int. Contact Lens Clin.* **11**, 286–213

MANCHESTER, P. T. (1970). Hydration of the cornea. *Trans. Am. ophthal. Soc.* **68**, 425–461

MANDELL, R. B. and FATT, I. (1965). Thinning of the human cornea on awakening. *Nature* **208**, 292–293

MANN, I. (1944). A study of epithelial regeneration in the living eye. *Br. J. Ophthal.* **28**, 26–40

MARRÉ, M. (1967). Zur Altersabhängigkeit der Heilung von Hornhautepitheldefekten. *Graefes Arch. klin. exp. Ophthal.* **173**, 250–255

MATSUDA, H. (1968). Electron microscopic study of the corneal nerve with special reference to its endings. *Jap. J. Ophthal.* **12**, 163–173

MAURICE, D. M. (1951). The permeability to sodium ions of the living rabbit's cornea. *J. Physiol.* **122**, 367–391

MAURICE, D. M. (1957). The structure and transparency of the cornea. *J. Physiol.* **136**, 263–286

MAURICE, D. M. (1962a). Clinical physiology of the cornea. *Int. ophthal. Clin.* **2**, 561–572

MAURICE, D. M. (1962b). The cornea and sclera. In *The Eye*, edited by H. Davson, Vol. 1, pp.289–368. New York and

London: Academic Press

MAURICE, D. M. (1972). The location of the fluid pump in the cornea. *J. Physiol.* **221**, 43–54

MAURICE, D. M. and GIARDINI, A. (1951). Swelling of the cornea *in vivo* after the destruction of its limiting layers. *Br. J. Ophthal.* **35**, 791–797

MELZACK, R. and WALL, P. D. (1965). Pain mechanisms: a new theory. *Science* **150**, 971–979

MILLER, D. (1969). Contact lens-induced corneal curvature and thickness change. *Archs Ophthal.* **80**, 430–432

MILLODOT, M. (1972). Diurnal variation of corneal sensitivity. *Br. J. Ophthal.* **56**, 844–847

MILLODOT, M. (1974). Effect of soft lenses on corneal sensitivity. *Acta ophthal.* **52**, 603–608

MILLODOT, M. (1975a). Effect of hard contact lenses on corneal sensitivity and thickness. *Acta ophthal.* **53**, 576–584

MILLODOT, M. (1975b). Do blue-eyed people have more sensitive corneas than brown-eyed people? *Nature* **255**, 151–152

MILLODOT, M. (1976). Effect of the length of wear of contact lenses on corneal sensitivity. *Acta ophthal.* **54**, 721–730

MILLODOT, M. (1977). The influence of pregnancy on the sensitivity of the cornea. *Br. J. Ophthal.* **61**, 646–649

MILLODOT, M. (1978). Corneal sensitivity in albinos. *Archs Ophthal.* **96**, 1225

MILLODOT, M. (1984). A review of research on the sensitivity of the cornea. *Ophthal. physiol. Optics* **4**, 305–318

MILLODOT, M. and LAMONT, A. (1974). Influence of menstruation on corneal sensitivity. *Br. J. Ophthal.* **58**, 752–756

MILLODOT, M. and O'LEARY, D. J. (1980). Effect of oxygen deprivation on corneal sensitivity. *Acta ophthal.* **58**, 434–439

MILLODOT, M. and OWENS, H. (1983). Sensitivity and fragility in keratoconus. *Acta ophthal.* **61**, 908–917

MISHIMA, S. (1965). Some physiological aspects of the precorneal tear film. *Archs Ophthal.* **73**, 233–241

MISHIMA, S. (1968). Corneal thickness. *Survey Ophthal.* **13**, 57–96

MISHIMA, S. and HAYAKAWA, M. (1972). The function of the corneal endothelium in relation to corneal dehydration and nutrition. *Israel J. med. Sci.* **8**, 1507–1518

MISHIMA, S. and MAURICE, D. M. (1961). The oily layer of the tear film and evaporation from the corneal surface. *Expl Eye Res.* **1**, 39–45

MORLEY, N. and McCULLOCH, C. (1961). Corneal lactate and pyridine nucleotides (PNS) with contact lenses. *Archs Ophthal.* **66**, 379–382

MURPHY, C., ALVARADO, J. and JUSTER, R. (1984). Prenatal and postnatal growth of the human Descemet's membrane. *Invest. Ophthal. Vis. Sci.* **25**, 1402–1415

NAFE, J. and WAGONER, K. (1937). Insensitivity of cornea to heat and pain derived from high temperatures. *Am. J. Psychol.* **49**, 631–635

NAYLOR, E. J. (1953). Polarised light studies of corneal structure. *Br. J. Ophthal.* **38**, 77–84

NORN, M. S. (1965). Tear secretion in normal eyes estimated by a new method. The lacrimal streak dilution test. *Acta ophthal.* **43**, 567–573

NOVER, A. and JAEGER, W. (1952). Kolorimetrische Methode zur Messung der Tränensekretion (Fluoreszein-Verdünnungstest). *Klin. Mbl. Augenheilk.* **121**, 419–425

O'LEARY, D. J. and MILLODOT, M. (1981). Abnormal epithelial fragility in diabetes and contact lens wear. *Acta ophthal.* **59**, 827–833

OPPENHEIMER, D. R., PALMER, E. and WEDDELL, G. (1958). Nerve endings in the conjunctiva. *J. Anat.* **92**, 321–352

PAYRAU, P., POULIQUEN, Y., FAURE, J.-P. and OFFRET, G. (1967). *La Transparence de la Cornée. Les Mécanismes de ses Altérations*, p.49. Paris: Masson

PEDLER, C. (1962). The fine structure of the corneal epithelium. *Expl Eye Res.* **1**, 286–289

PENBHARKKUL, S. and KARELITZ, S. (1962). Lacrimation in the neonatal and early infancy period of premature and full-term infants. *J. Pediat.* **61**, 859–863

PFISTER, R. R. (1975). The healing of corneal epithelial abrasions in the rabbit: a scanning electron microscope study. *Invest. Ophthal.* **14**, 648–661

PHILPOT, F. J. (1955). Factors affecting the hydration of the rabbit cornea. *J. Physiol.* **128**, 504–510

POLACK, F. M. (1961). Morphology of the cornea. 1: Study with silver stains. *Am. J. Ophthal.* **51**, 179–184

POLLACK, I. P. (1962). Corneal hydration studied in stromal segments separated by intralamellar discs. *Invest. Ophthal.* **1**, 661–665

POLSE, K. A. and MANDELL. R. B. (1970). Critical oxygen tension at the corneal surface. *Archs Ophthal.* **84**, 505–508

POLSE, K. A., SARVER, M. D. and HARRIS, M. G. (1975). Corneal edema and vertical striae accompanying the wearing of hydrogel lenses. *Am. J. Optom.* **52**, 185–191

PRATT-JOHNSON, J. A. (1959). Studies on the anatomy and pathology of the peripheral cornea. *Am. J. Ophthal.* **47**, 478–488

RAO, G. N., SHAW, E. L., ARTHUR, E. J. and AQUAVELLA, J. V. (1979). Endothelial cell morphology and corneal deturgescence. *Ann. Ophthal.* **11**, 885–899

REFOJO, M. F. and LEONG, F. L. (1979). Water-dissolved oxygen permeability coefficients of hydrogel contact lenses and boundary layer effects. *J. Membrane Sci.* **4**, 415–420

REIM, M., LAX, F., LICHTE, H. and TURSS, R. (1967). Steady state levels of glucose in the different layers of the cornea, aqueous humor, blood and tears *in vivo*. *Ophthalmologica* **154**, 39–50

REXED, B. and REXED, V. (1951). Degeneration and regeneration of corneal nerves. *Br. J. Ophthal.* **35**, 38–49

RICHARD, P. R. and ALLANSMITH, M. R. (1981). Giant papillary conjunctivitis. *Int. ophthal. Clin.* **21**, 65–82

RISS, B. and RISS, P. (1981). Corneal sensitivity in pregnancy. *Ophthalmologica* **183**, 57–62

RODRIGUES, M. M., ROWDEN, G., HACKETT, J. and BAKOS, I. (1981). Langerhans cells in the normal conjunctiva and peripheral cornea of selected species. *Invest. Ophthal. Vis. Sci.* **21**, 759–765

DE ROETTH, A., JR (1950). Respiration of the cornea. *Archs Ophthal.* **44**, 666–676

DE ROETTH, A., SR (1953). Lacrimation in normal eyes. *Archs Ophthal.* **49**, 185–189

ROWBOTHAM, G. (1939). Observations on effects of trigeminal denervation. *Brain* **62**, 364–380

RUBEN, M. (1967). Corneal changes in contact lens wear. *Trans. ophthal. Soc. UK* **87**, 27–43

RUBEN, M. and COLEBROOK, E. (1979). Keratoplasty sensitivity. *Br. J. Ophthal.* **63**, 265–267

RUSKELL, G. L. (1969). Changes in nerve terminals and acini of the lacrimal gland and changes in secretion induced by autonomic denervation. *Z. Zellforsch. mikroscop. Anat.* **94**, 261–281

RUSKELL, G. L. (1975). Nerve terminals and epithelial cell variety in the human lacrimal gland. *Cell Tiss. Res.* **158**, 121–136

RYCROFT, P. V. (1964). Ophthaine (proparacaine hydrochloride): local anaesthetic for ophthalmic surgery. *Br. J. Ophthal.* **48**, 102–104

SALLMANN, C., CARAVAGGIO, L. L. and GRIMES, P. (1961). Studies on corneal epithelium of the rabbit. 1: Cell division and growth. *Am. J. Ophthal.* **51**, 83–94

SCHIMMELPFENNIG, B. (1982). Nerve structures in human central corneal epithelium. *Graefes Arch. klin. exp. Ophthal.* **218**, 14–20

SCHIRMER, O. (1903). Studien zur Physiologie und Pathologie der Träanenabsonderung und Thränenabfur. *Graefes Arch. klin. exp. Ophthal.* **56**, 197–291

SCHIRMER, K. E. (1963). Corneal sensitivity and contact lenses. *Br. J. Ophthal.* **47**, 493–495

SCHIRMER, K. E. and MELLOR, L. D. (1961). Corneal sensitivity after cataract extraction. *Archs Ophthal.* **65**, 433–436

SCHOESSLER, J. P. and BARR, J. T. (1980). Corneal thickness changes with extended contact lens wear. *Am. J. Optom. physiol. Optics* **57**, 729–733

SCHUTE, C. C. D. (1974). Haidinger's brushes and predominant orientation of collagen in corneal stroma. *Nature* **250**, 163–164

SEDAN, J., FARNARIER, G. and FERRAND, G. (1958). Contribution a l'étude de la keraesthésie. *Ann. Oculist* **191**, 736–751

SEGAWA, K. (1964). Electron microscopic studies on the human corneal epithelium: dendritic cells. *Archs Ophthal.* **72**, 650–659

SHANKS, K. R. (1965). The shape of the margin of the upper eyelid, related to corneal lenses. *Br. J. physiol. Optics* **22**, 71–83

SJÖGREN, H. (1955). The lacrimal secretion in newborn, premature and fully developed children. *Acta ophthal.* **33**, 557–560

SJÖQVIST, O. (1938). Studies on pain conduction in the trigeminal nerve. *Acta psychiat. neurol. Suppl.* 17, 1–139

SMELSER, G. K. (1952). Relation of factors involved in maintenance of optical properties of cornea to contact-lens wear. *Archs Ophthal.* **47**, 328–343

SMELSER, G. K. and CHEN, D. K. (1955). Physiological changes in cornea induced by contact lenses. *Archs Opthal.* **53**, 676–679

SMELSER, G. K. and OZANICS, O. (1952). Importance of atmospheric oxygen for maintenance of the optical properties of the human cornea. *Science* **115**, 140

SMITH, J. W. (1969). The transparency of the corneal stroma. *Vision Res.* **9**, 393–396

STANWORTH, A. and NAYLOR, E. S. (1953). Polarised light studies of the cornea. I. The isolated cornea. *J. exp. Biol.* **30**, 160–163

STEUHL, P. and ROHEN, J. W. (1983). Absorption of horse-radish peroxide by the conjunctival epithelium of monkeys and rabbits. *Albrecht v. Graefes Arch. Ophthal.* **220**, 13–18

STOCKER, E. G. and SCHOESSLER, J. P. (1985). Corneal endothelial polymegathism induced by PMMA contact lens wear. *Invest. Ophthal. Vis. Sci.* **26**, 857–863

STONE, R. A., LATIES, A. M. and BRECHA, N. C. (1982). Substance P-like immunoreactive nerves in the anterior segment of the rabbit, cat and monkey eye. *Neuroscience* **7**, 2459–2468

STONE, R. A., KUWAYAMA, X., TERENGHI, G. and POLAK, J. M. (1986). Calcitonin gene-related peptide: occurrence in corneal sensory nerves. *Expl Eye Res.* **43**, 279–284

STRUGHOLD, H. (1953). The sensitivity of cornea and conjunctiva of the human eye and the use of contact lenses. *Am. J. Optom.* **30**, 625–630

STRUGHOLD, H. and KARBE, M. (1925). Die Topographie des Kältesinnes auf Cornea und Conjunctiva, ein Beitrag zur Frage nach den spezifischen Empgängern desselben. *Z. Biol.* **83**, 189–212

SÜCHTING, P., MACHEMER, R. and WELZ, S. (1966). Die Lebenszeit der Epithelzelle der Rattencornea und conjunctiva. *Graefes Arch. klin. exp. Ophthal.* **170**, 297–310

SUGIURA, B. (1965). The polygonal cell system of the corneal epithelium. In *Die Struktur des Auges. II. Symposium*, edited by J. Rohen, Eighth International Congress of Anatomists, Wiesbaden, pp.463–479. Stuttgart: Schattauer

TERVO, K., TERVO, T., ERÄNKÖ, L., ERÄNKÖ, O. and CUELLO, C. (1981). Immunoreactivity for substance P in the Gasserian ganglion, ophthalmic nerve and anterior segment of the rabbit eye. *Histochem. J.* **13**, 435–443

TERVO, T., VANNAS, A., TERVO, K. and HOLDEN, B. A. (1985). Histochemical evidence of limited reinnervation of human corneal grafts. *Acta ophthal.* **63**, 207–214

THOFT, R. A. and FRIEND, J. (1972). Corneal amino acid supply and distribution. *Invest. Ophthal.* **11**, 723–727

TOIVANEN, M., TERVO, T., PARTANEN, M., VANNAS, A. and HERVONEN, A. (1987). Histochemical demonstration of adrenergic nerves in the stroma of human cornea. *Invest. Ophthal. Vis. Sci.* **28**, 398–400

TRENBERTH, S. M. and MISHIMA, S. (1968). The effect of ouabain on the rabbit corneal endothelium. *Invest. Ophthal.* **7**, 44–52

TRESELER, P. S., FOULKS, G. N. and SANFILIPPO, F. (1984). The expression of HLA antigens by cells in the human cornea. *Am. J. Ophthal.* **98**, 763–712

TURSS, R., FRIEND, J. and DOHLMAN, C. H. (1970). Effect of a corneal barrier on the nutrition of the epithelium. *Expl Eye Res.* **9**, 254–259

UNIACKE, N. P. and HILL, R. M. (1970). Osmotic pressure of the tears during adaptation to contact lenses. *J. Am. optom.*

Ass. **41**, 932–936

VEERHUIS, R. and KIJLSTRA, A. (1982). Inhibition of hemolytic complement activity by lactoferrin in tears. *Expl Eye Res.* **34**, 257–265

WEDDELL, G. and ZANDER, E. (1950). A critical evaluation of methods used to demonstrate tissue neural elements, illustrated by reference to the cornea. *J. Anat.* **84**, 168–195

WEIMAR, V. (1960). Healing processes in the cornea. In *The Transparency of the Cornea*, edited by Sir Stewart Duke-Elder and E. S. Perkins, pp.111–124. Oxford: Blackwell

WOLFF, E. (1948). *The Anatomy of the Eye and Orbit*, 3rd edn. p. 166. London: Lewis

ZANDER, E. and WEDDELL, G. (1951a). Observations on the innervation of the cornea. *J. Anat.* **85**, 68–99

ZANDER, E. and WEDDELL, G. (1951b). Reaction of corneal nerve fibres to injury. *Br. J. Ophthal.* **35**, 61–88

Chapter 3

Contact lens materials

B. J. Tighe

It is perhaps not immediately obvious that the use of polymers for contact lenses in recent years represents an example of the biomedical application of synthetic materials. It is, nevertheless, quite true for just as the use of quite similar materials in joint replacement, heart valves, membrane oxygenators and haemodialysis membranes presents specific problems associated with, for example, their biocompatibility, strength and permeability so, in contact lens usage, the question of the material design to give a balance of properties appropriate to the environment in which the material will ultimately be used is of prime importance. The situation is obviously less critical in the case of lenses intended for daily wear only, than it is in the case of extended or 'continuous' wear lenses. In both cases, however, very similar properties to those mentioned above in connection with other biomedical applications are involved.

The contact lens, of course, does have certain unique features which tend to set it apart from other areas of biomedicine. The design and fitting of the lens can play an overriding part in governing the patient's response to a given material, although this is to a large extent offset by the relative ease of insertion and removal of the device. Thus, it is much easier in this than most other fields to compare the response of reasonably large numbers of patients to different materials under conditions in which variables related to design and fitting have been isolated. For this reason, the research carried out in recent years into the use of hydrogel polymers in contact lenses has provided information on a wide range of materials of this type which is currently assisting work on their use in other biomedical applications.

The historical aspect of the development of contact lens materials is quite interesting and is covered in detail in Chapter 1. Glass was used

exclusively for some years and it was conventional for lenses to be individually ground. When polymethyl methacrylate began to replace glass in the 1940s it was because of its toughness, optical properties and physiological inactivity coupled with ease of processing by existing turning techniques. It was not, therefore, in any sense a purpose-designed polymer and yet, as will be seen, it possesses a combination of properties that are difficult to surpass in a thermoplastic or conventional elastomeric polymer. There have been many attempts to find alternative materials but it was not until the class of polymers known as hydrogels appeared on the scene that any serious competitor emerged. In order to appreciate the reasons for this, it is necessary to review briefly some of the general characteristics of 'polymers', which is a general term for a group of materials that includes plastics (both thermoplastics and thermosetting), fibres, rubbers (or more correctly elastomers) and hydrogels.

Classification of contact lens materials

We can all readily appreciate the differences in behaviour between gases, liquids and solids. It is helpful to consider the difference in molecular make-up of these three groups before dealing with polymers as a particular class of solid materials.

In gases, we are dealing with a collection of individual small molecules well separated from each other and moving rapidly and randomly in the space that encloses them. The resistance that a gas offers to anything moving through it is, therefore, negligible. When we move to liquids we are talking about a 'condensed' phase and although the molecules are still small individual entities, the resistance to motion within them is greater. (Think, for example, of the difference in ease of movement in the air and in a swimming pool.) Motion in a liquid can be likened to placing a hand into a large bag of ball-bearings or marbles. There is some resistance, but the hand can move by displacing the ball-bearings if the force that it exerts is greater than the force of attraction between the individual ball-bearings.

In the case of solid materials the individual molecules are packed more efficiently. Alternatively, it could be said that the forces of attraction between them have increased. In the absence of reasonably strong deforming forces, the material retains its shape whereas a liquid, of course, will take the shape of the vessel into which it is poured — being deformed simply by the force of gravity. There are within this group of solid materials all sorts of different behaviours ranging from that of toffee or thick treacle to that of metals. Toffee and treacle are in some aspects liquid-like in their behaviour and in some respects resemble solids.

If solids, then, are materials in which the constituent molecules are well packed together we have to consider in more detail the way in which the molecules are packed or associated or bonded together since this will play a large part in determining the strength of the material in question. Metals, ceramics or glasses, and polymers represent three different types of solid material in which the constituent atoms or molecules are in some way linked together. The ways in which they are linked together are quite different and so we get different types of behaviour in passing from one class to another.

The unique properties that polymers have arise from the ability of certain atoms to bond together to form stable covalent bonds. Foremost among the atoms that can do this is carbon (C) which can link together with four other atoms either of its own kind or alternatively atoms of, for example, hydrogen (H), oxygen (O), nitrogen (N), sulphur (S) or chlorine (Cl). It is because of this unique property of carbon that most of the polymers that we are concerned with fall within the realm of what is called organic chemistry or the chemistry of carbon compounds. These polymers may be purely natural (such as cellulose), modified natural polymers (such as cellulose acetate) or completely synthetic (such as polymethyl methacrylate).

The single characteristic that unites these and other polymers is the fact that, as the name (polymer) suggests, they are composed of many units linked together in long chains. Thus, if we can imagine a molecule of oxygen and a molecule of water enlarged to the size of a tennis ball (the molecular size of water and oxygen is very similar) a molecule of polymethyl methacrylate on the same scale would be of similar cross-sectional diameter but anything up to 200 feet in length. It is the gigantic length of polymers (sometimes called macromolecules) in relation to their cross-sectional diameter that gives them their unique properties.

Most of the polymers that we shall be concerned with are synthetic and prepared from monomers by the process of polymerization. In this way, the simplest polymer, polyethylene, is obtained by polymerization of ethylene monomer.

$$
\begin{array}{c}
\text{H}\ \ \text{H} \\
|\ \ \ | \\
\text{C}=\text{C} \\
|\ \ \ | \\
\text{H}\ \ \text{H}
\end{array}
\longrightarrow
\begin{array}{c}
\text{H}\ \ \text{H}\ \ \text{H}\ \ \text{H}\ \ \text{H}\ \ \text{H} \\
|\ \ \ |\ \ \ |\ \ \ |\ \ \ |\ \ \ | \\
\sim\text{C}-\text{C}-\text{C}-\text{C}-\text{C}-\text{C}\sim \\
|\ \ \ |\ \ \ |\ \ \ |\ \ \ |\ \ \ | \\
\text{H}\ \ \text{H}\ \ \text{H}\ \ \text{H}\ \ \text{H}\ \ \text{H}
\end{array}
$$

This is more usually represented by a general equation showing the conversion of n ethylene units to a polyethylene chain that is n units long, i.e.:

$$ n\,\text{CH}_2=\text{CH}_2 \longrightarrow -(\text{CH}_2-\text{CH}_2)_n- $$

In a commercial polymer n might have a value of several thousand.

The polymerization of methyl methacrylate can be shown in a similar manner.

$$
n\,\text{CH}_2=
\begin{array}{c}
\text{CH}_3 \\
| \\
\text{C} \\
| \\
\text{C}=\text{O} \\
| \\
\text{O} \\
| \\
\text{CH}_3
\end{array}
\longrightarrow
-\!\!\left(\text{CH}_2-
\begin{array}{c}
\text{CH}_3 \\
| \\
\text{C} \\
| \\
\text{C}=\text{O} \\
| \\
\text{O} \\
| \\
\text{CH}_3
\end{array}
\right)_{\!n}\!\!-
$$

The structure enclosed within the bracket is known as the 'repeating unit' and it is conventional when writing the name of the polymer to indicate precisely what this is. Thus, we should write poly(ethylene) or poly(methyl methacrylate) but since these are well known commercial polymers the brackets are often omitted. The same is true of polystyrene (a) and polyvinyl chloride (b):

$$-(CH_2-CH)_n- \atop | \atop C_6H_5 \qquad\qquad -(CH_2-CH)_n- \atop | \atop Cl$$

(a)   (b)

To indicate that a polymer contains more than one type of repeating unit obtained by polymerizing together two different monomers the term 'copolymer' is used. Thus, by copolymerizing styrene and methyl methacrylate a styrene–methyl methacrylate copolymer is obtained. This would more correctly be described as poly(methyl methacrylate–costyrene). Although the term 'copolymer' is a general one and can be used to describe polymers obtained from mixtures of more than two monomers, the term 'terpolymer' is frequently used for the specific case of a polymer produced by the polymerization of three monomers. The more common usage, however, is that involving the term 'copolymer' to describe a polymer obtained from at least (but not necessarily exactly) two different monomers.

Perhaps the best way of visualizing the way in which polymer molecules arrange themselves is by taking several pieces of string to represent individual molecules. The most usual arrangement will be a random one in which the pieces of string are loosely entangled (in a heap or ball rather than being extended). It is the interaction and entanglement of the individual molecules in this way that gives polymers their characteristic physical properties. By changing the chemical nature of the polymer chain and their arrangement together we can change the physical properties and thus obtain either flexible, elastomeric behaviour or, at the other extreme, hard glassy behaviour.

These variations arise from differences in mobility of the constituent polymer chains. Thus, at very low temperatures all polymers are hard and glassy. As the temperature is raised, however, the thermal energy of the system increases and eventually the individual polymer chains will possess enough energy to begin to undergo rotation. If we think of the tangled string as a plate of spaghetti at this point, the rotational energy that it achieves would be enough to give it the mobility of a plate of worms. In terms of physical properties this corresponds to a change from glassy behaviour to rubbery or leathery behaviour. For this reason the temperature at which this occurs is known as the 'glass–rubber transition temperature' (T_g). The actual temperature at which the transition occurs will depend on the chemical nature of the polymer. Thus, for natural rubber it is below 0°C and for polymethyl methacrylate it is above 100°C. For this reason at room temperature natural rubber is readily deformed whereas polymethyl methacrylate is glassy.

There are several additional subtleties involved in the design of polymers that have the ability to undergo the large deformation with instantaneous recovery which is characteristic of ideal elastomeric behaviour. Despite this, the principle of intramolecular mobility and the glass transition temperature is the fundamental factor and provides an adequate basis for understanding the difference between 'hard' and 'soft' lens materials.

There is another important way in which a hard glassy thermoplastic material such as polymethyl methacrylate or polyvinyl chloride can be converted into a flexible material and that is by the incorporation of a 'plasticizer'. This is a mobile component, often an organic liquid having a high boiling point, that will act as an 'internal lubricant'. Its presence separates the polymer chains, and allows them to move more freely. Its function is to lower the temperature at which the transition from glassy to flexible behaviour takes place.

Thus, polyvinyl chloride in its unmodified state is a rigid glassy material and will be familiar as the clear corrugated roofing material used on car ports and similar domestic extensions. When a plasticizer is incorporated the material is converted into the flexible material used, for example, as 'vinyl' seat coverings in cars and general domestic applications. In these cases, pigments and various processing aids will also have been added in order to enable the polymer to be produced in a variety of colours and textures.

An almost identical principle is involved in the formation of so-called 'hydrogel' polymers. The structure of polymethyl methacrylate can be made more hydrophilic by the incorporation of hydroxyl groups. The simplest structure that can be made in this way is poly(2-hydroxyethyl methacrylate) which is obtained by polymerizing 2-hydroxyethyl methacrylate monomer:

$$n\,CH_2{=}\underset{\underset{\underset{\underset{OH}{|}}{CH_2}}{\underset{|}{CH_2}}}{\overset{\overset{\overset{CH_3}{|}}{C}}{\underset{|}{C}}}{\overset{|}{\underset{|}{\underset{O}{\|}}}} \longrightarrow {+}CH_2{-}\underset{\underset{\underset{\underset{OH}{|}}{CH_2}}{\underset{|}{CH_2}}}{\overset{\overset{\overset{CH_3}{|}}{C}}{\underset{|}{C}}}{\overset{|}{\underset{|}{\underset{O}{\|}}}}{}_n$$

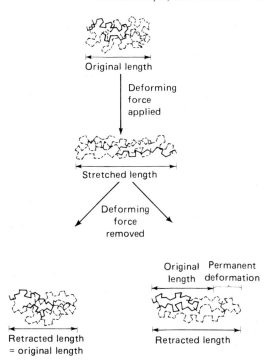

Original length

Deforming force applied

Stretched length

Deforming force removed

Original length   Permanent deformation

Retracted length
= original length

Retracted length

Good elastic recovery   Poor elastic recovery

Figure 3.1 Diagrammatic representation of the deformation of entangled polymer chains illustrating both good and poor elastic recovery

The monomer and polymer are often referred to as HEMA and PHEMA*, respectively.

In the dry state polymethyl methacrylate and poly(2-hydroxyethyl methacrylate) have very similar characteristics — both are hard glassy polymers as their structures would indicate. Whereas polymethyl methacrylate is relatively unaffected by water, however (it absorbs approximately 0.5% of its own weight), the more hydrophilic poly(2-hydroxyethyl methacrylate) swells to form an elastic hydrogel. The water acts as a plasticizer in the manner previously described. It behaves as an 'internal lubricant' and allows the chains to move more freely with respect to each other, and as a result the glass transition temperature of the hydrogel is well below room temperature whereas that of the dehydrated polymer is about 100°C.

It is necessary to describe one more molecular feature that is required in elastic polymers (both hydrogels and synthetic elastomers), i.e. the 'cross-link'. So far polymer chains have been considered to be individual molecular species unattached to each other. In some cases, however, it is necessary to link individual chains to their neighbours at intervals along each polymer backbone. In this way, a polymer 'network' is formed and the frequency at which these linkages occur is called the 'cross-link density'. The necessity for doing this can be best understood by considering *Figure 3.1* which illustrates good and bad elastic behaviour. To obtain good elastic behaviour the chains must be mobile enough to change their positions when a deforming force is applied but they also need some restraining links to ensure that they

are able to return to their original positions. The incorporation of an excessively large number of cross-links will of course restrict deformability and destroy elastic behaviour. For good elastic behaviour, the upper limit of cross-link density is in the region of one cross-link per 100 backbone atoms. The theoretical basis of elastic behaviour in polymers is of course much more complex than this but the simplified picture given above enables the behaviour exhibited by the types of polymer that are important in contact lens usage to be understood.

The nature of polymeric materials

It is convenient to consider the polymers that have been used or suggested for use as contact lens materials under four headings: (1) thermoplastics; (2) synthetic elastomers; (3) hybrid rigid 'gas permeable' copolymers (RGP materials); and (4) hydrogels. Each group has its own characteristic advantages and disadvantages

*In clinical practice the term 'HEMA' is used for simplicity but actually refers to 'PHEMA'.

which may be best illustrated by taking a typical member of each group and making a comparative list of appropriate properties.

The thermoplastics

The thermoplastics are the group of polymers that are capable of being shaped or moulded under the application of heat and pressure but which at room temperature are fairly rigid, possibly showing some flexibility, but certainly not elastic. Foremost among this group is polymethyl methacrylate which, since its introduction in the 1940s, has been the most widely used contact lens material. It is apparent that several of its advantageous properties are shared by other thermoplastics. Among these properties are optical clarity, processability, toughness and ease of sterilization. On the other hand, the rigidity and virtual impermeability to oxygen must certainly count as disadvantages, and prevent the material from being considered for anything other than daily wear. The rigidity and impermeability to oxygen are obviously interrelated because although rigidity is a prime factor in producing discomfort it does permit the lens to be fitted in such a manner as to promote the flow of tear fluid behind the lens, thus compensating for the absence of oxygen transmission through the lens itself. This does mean, however, that attempts to reduce the rigidity of the lens material to any marked extent have the consequence of requiring a greater permeability of the lens to oxygen. It is largely to improve on the behaviour of polymethyl methacrylate in these two areas that other polymers have been suggested as replacements.

At first sight the task of finding an improved material would not seem too difficult since almost all thermoplastics are less rigid and more oxygen permeable than polymethyl methacrylate. Materials patented for contact lens use range from simple structures such as polyethylene (Studies Inc., 1969) and polyvinyl chloride (Rosen, 1969) to complex copolymers of tetrafluoroethylene with perfluoro-2-methylene-4-methyl-1,3-dioxolane or with hexafluoroacetone and ethylene (Dupont, 1971). None of these materials has, however, achieved any success largely because of inadequate surface properties, a point which will be elaborated in due course. More promising results were obtained with both poly(4-methyl

pent-1-ene), a form of which is known commercially as TPX (Kamath, 1970):

$$-(CH_2-CH)_{\overline{n}}$$
$$|$$
$$CH_2$$
$$|$$
$$CH$$
$$CH_3 \quad CH_3$$

and with cellulose esters such as cellulose acetate butyrate.

The structures of cellulose such as cellulose acetate, cellulose acetate butyrate or cellulose acetate propionate are quite different from those of the carbon-backbone polymers previously considered. Cellulose itself consists of a series of rings or cyclic structures linked together by oxygen atoms:

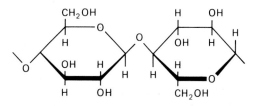

The hydroxyl groups in the polymer can be partially or completely reacted. If all three hydroxyl groups in each ring are acetylated the resultant polymer is the well known cellulose triacetate, which will be familiar as the textile fibre Tricel.

Two variations now become apparent. In the first place, some of the hydroxyl groups may be left unreacted (the average number of hydroxyl groups per ring that have been reacted is referred to as the 'degree of substitution'). Secondly, propionyl (CH_3CH_2CO-) or butyryl ($CH_3CH_2CH_2CO-$) groups may be used wholly or partially in place of acetyl groups. Cellulose acetate butyrate therefore describes the case in which we have some acetyl, some butyryl and usually some free hydroxyl groups. This highlights one of the problems with this material in that, unlike polymethyl methacrylate and other polymers previously discussed, it does not have a fixed composition. For this reason, supplies from different sources can have somewhat different properties. In general, higher concentrations of free hydroxyl groups will result in a greater tendency to take up water and will produce rather more hydrophilic surfaces. On the other hand, increasing the relative concentrations of butyryl groups produces rather greater flexibility and a slight increase in oxygen permeability.

Poly(4-methyl pent-1-ene) and cellulose acetate butyrate resemble each other in many ways. Both polymers are less rigid and less brittle than polymethyl methacrylate — they can conveniently be described as tougher. It is debatable, however, as to whether the greater flexibility is of any substantial advantage in relation to comfort. Poly(4-methyl pent-1-ene) is unique in having a glass transition temperature between room temperature and the temperature of the eye ($T_g \simeq 29°C$). In principle this should mean that the polymer is more resistant to deformation and damage during handling at room temperature, but when placed in the eye its flexibility and therefore comfort should increase. In practice, however, the increase in flexibility makes virtually no difference to comfort. This will be clarified when the effect of rigidity modulus on lens comfort and visual performance is discussed (pp. 83–85). The most relevant point is that the flexibility associated with these two polymers is very much less than that associated with elastomers and hydrogels.

The oxygen permeability of both cellulose acetate butyrate and poly(4-methyl pent-1-ene) is appreciably (of the order of 100 times) greater than that of polymethyl methacrylate. This is not as advantageous as it may seem at first sight, however, since even in the case of poly(4-methyl pent-1-ene) which is by far the more permeable of the two, a lens of minimal centre thickness prevents normal functioning of the cornea during the closed eye condition. This point will be discussed in more detail in the general context of oxygen permeability requirements (p. 92).

In certain other respects, cellulose acetate butyrate has some advantages over poly(4-methyl pent-1-ene). Although it has a variable composition this does mean that it is possible to produce a grade of polymer that will be adequately wettable and able to sustain a film of tear fluid. On the other hand, poly(4-methyl pent-1-ene) lenses have to undergo surface treatment to enable them to do this. In addition, cellulose acetate butyrate is somewhat easier to process.

On balance there is little advantage over polymethyl methacrylate in the case of either poly(4-methyl pent-1-ene) or cellulose acetate butyrate. Neither polymer is sufficiently flexible to produce substantially greater comfort and neither polymer has a sufficiently high oxygen permeability to make them obvious candidates for rigid extended wear lenses. In neither case is lens fabrication as straightforward as with PMMA and, despite the fact that CAB suffers from poor dimensional stability, its better processability and lack of need for surface treatment have enabled it to obtain a small share of the market. One potential advantage of this group (thermoplastics) is the fact that they can be used to make lenses by melt pressing. This type of hard lens fabrication process has, however, never been widely used. Some of the problems associated with surface treatment of flexible thermoplastics and results of a clinical trial with poly(4-methyl pent-1-ene) have been presented in more detail elsewhere (Larke, Pedley and Tighe, 1973; Larke et al., 1973; Ng, Pedley and Tighe, 1976).

The synthetic elastomers

The synthetic elastomers are the group of polymers which are not only flexible but show rubber-like behaviour, i.e. they are capable of being compressed or stretched and when the deforming force is removed they instantaneously return to their original shape. They consist of polymer chains that possess high mobility and which are cross-linked at intervals along the polymer backbones. Their properties are in many ways intermediate between those of thermoplastics and hydrogels. Thus, they possess to a degree the toughness associated with the former group of materials and the softness of the latter. In this sense they are ideal candidates for contact lens usage. Unfortunately, however, they possess one inherent disadvantage. The molecular features required for true elastic behaviour invariably produce polymers with hydrophobic surfaces. All polymers in this group require some form of surface treatment, therefore, to render them sufficiently hydrophilic for use as contact lenses. In general, it has been the absence of a suitably permanent treatment that has prevented their use on a wide scale.

In addition to natural rubber itself many synthetic elastomers have been patented in connection with contact lens manufacture (Dow Corning, 1971). These include ethylene propylene terpolymer (EPT) which may be simply represented as

$$\underset{\displaystyle (CH_2-CH_2-CH_2-CH)_n}{\overset{\displaystyle CH_3 \atop |}{}}$$

cis-polybutadiene

$$\underset{CH=CH}{-(CH_2 \qquad CH_2)_n}$$

and *cis*-polyisoprene

$$-(CH_2 \qquad CH_2)_n \atop CH=C \atop | \atop CH_3$$

which is synthetic natural rubber.

Although these polymers have oxygen permeabilities more than 100 times greater than that of polymethyl methacrylate, the most significant member of this group has an oxygen permeability which is over 1000 times greater than that of polymethyl methacrylate. For this reason this polymer, silicone rubber or poly(dimethyl siloxane), has received considerable attention as a potential contact lens material.

$$-(O-Si)_n \atop \overset{\displaystyle CH_3 \atop |}{\underset{| \atop CH_3}{}}$$

The high oxygen permeability arises from the backbone of alternate silicone and oxygen atoms which has not only great freedom of rotation but a much higher solubility for oxygen than polymers with all-carbon backbones.

Surface-treated silicone rubber lenses were developed in the mid-1960s (Becker, 1966; Dow Corning, 1967) and found clinically to have little effect on corneal respiration (Hill and Schloessler, 1967; Burns, Roberts and Rich, 1971). Despite the apparent attraction of a soft yet tough, highly oxygen permeable material, problems have been encountered in its clinical use (Bitonte and Keates, 1972). Not the least of these is the fact that surface treatments tend to be non-permanent and to cause some reduction in the optical qualities of the lens surface. Despite this it is to be anticipated that an adequate surface-treatment technique will be developed in the course of time. Lenses made of current materials (p. 429, Chapter 11) are used very little. In conclusion it is appropriate to note that because of the nature of the materials, elastomer lenses are normally produced by some form of compression moulding technique.

The hybrid rigid gas permeable materials

The third group (hybrid rigid gas permeable materials) combine to a degree the ease of preparation of PMMA and the oxygen permeability of silicone rubber. The history and underlying chemistry of this group of materials is more fully described in a subsequent section.

The hydrogels

The fourth group, hydrogels, is also potentially the largest in terms of structural variety. These are hydrophilic polymers which are plasticized by the water that they absorb and can be conveniently described as soft, elastic, water-containing gels. The first of these to achieve commercial significance, PHEMA, was developed by Wichterle and his co-workers in Czechoslovakia as a general purpose surgical material (Wichterle and Lim, 1960, 1961, 1965). PHEMA is in many ways typical of other hydrogels and unfortunately the terms have been used synonymously on many occasions. The range of properties obtainable with hydrogels is, however, extremely wide and with this class of material it is possible to 'purpose-design' or 'tailor-make' polymers for contact lens use.

Before turning to a fuller consideration of the nature and properties of hydrogels and RGP materials, however, it is necessary to discuss those material properties that are important in the design and function of contact lenses together with the various ways in which the lenses themselves are fabricated. Chapters 10 and 11 should also be consulted for discussions on material characteristics in relation to the fitting requirements for particular types of eye and refractive error.

Routes to lens manufacture

As a prelude to reviewing the property requirements of lens materials it is appropriate to outline the routes by which monomers are converted into polymers in lens form. As will become apparent the use of some routes makes demands on the properties of hydrogel in its dehydrated state. The four types of formation considered (lathe-cut lenses, spin-cast lenses, static cast polymerization lenses, and melt pressed lenses) are used to widely differing extents. The order in which they are dealt with probably represents order of decreasing usage. Because of factors such as production costs and interest in disposable lenses, the less labour intensive techniques, particularly static polymerization, will undoubtedly find more widespread use.

Lathe-cut lenses

The monomers are bulk polymerized in polyolefin moulds using conventional free radical techniques. Polymer rods 10–15 mm in diameter with lengths of 20 cm upwards are prepared and sliced into buttons 5–10 mm thick for the lathe-cutting operation. Alternatively the polymerization may be carried out in individual button-shaped moulds.

Conversion of the button to lens form involves first mounting the button in the lathe to cut and polish the back curve, then reversing the button and mounting onto a brass stub by means of a pitch adhesive in order that the front surface and edge of the lens may be cut and polished. The polish consists typically of alumina dispersed in a hydrocarbon or silicone oil fluid.

Removal of the lens from the mounting stub and cleaning all traces of adhesive and polish involves the use of solvents (such as chlorinated hydrocarbons) and surfactants. This process, which is undoubtedly the most widely used in lens manufacture, places demands on those mechanical properties of the lens that govern susceptibility to high speed cutting and polishing. In particular the generation of heat in these operations places a lower limit on the glass transition temperature of the polymers. The technique is equally useful for PMMA, hydrogels and RGPs.

Spin-cast lenses

This process was developed by Wichterle and is described in his patents. A mixture of liquid monomer, cross-linking agent, initiator and optionally a diluent such as ethylene glycol, is introduced into a concave mould. The mould is rotated about its central axis (i.e. spun) during the polymerization and the centrifugal force results in the direct formation of a lens form. The mould may be fabricated from glass or polymers such as polypropylene and nylon. The quality of the mould surface has a direct influence on that of the front surface of the lens. The technology involved in this form of lens production has been extended and developed by Bausch & Lomb Inc. in the USA, who are now its foremost users in the production of soft lenses.

Static cast polymerization lenses

This technique also involves the direct conversion of monomer mixture into lens form. In principle a two part mould fabricated from a flexible polymer such as polypropylene or nylon is filled with monomer mixture which subsequently polymerizes. The mould is opened yielding the finished lens, ready for hydration.

In practice a great deal of design skill is needed in overcoming the problems associated with filling and closing the mould, and with contraction during polymerization but especially in obtaining good and reproducible edge quality. The lenses are inspected and checked following hydration and it is common for appreciable numbers to be rejected at this stage. Because of the fact that the unit production cost is potentially very low this technique and variants of it are of great current interest. Although principally used in hydrogel manufacture, its successful extension to RGP production is to be anticipated.

Melt pressed lenses

Although techniques of this type are used commercially for the production of poly(methyl methacrylate) and silicone rubber lenses, their use in hydrogel and RGP lens manufacture does not appear to have gone beyond the patent literature and pilot scale work. The monomers are polymerized to give a linear polymer which is isolated and converted to sheet, powder or granules, depending upon the type of mould to be used. The next stage involves use of conventional compression or injection moulding techniques, sometimes with a subsequent cross-linking stage which may involve irradiation. The moulded lens may require edging and local polishing to remove moulding flash, prior to hydration. The major problems in melt processing techniques lie in achieving a balance of flow and cross-linking in these highly functionalized polymers together with good mould release without the addition of conventional processing aids.

Each of the foregoing techniques has its own particular requirements in terms of monomer and polymer properties. In contrast to the behaviour of the lens in the eye, which makes demands on the behaviour of the hydrated polymer, manufacturing techniques frequently make behavioural demands of the polymer in its completely dehydrated state.

Properties of contact lens materials

The following properties are among the most important in affecting the performance of materials as contact lenses.

(1) Density.
(2) Refractive index.
(3) Optical transmittance.
(4) Dimensional stability with respect to: time, temperature, pH and tonicity.
(5) Surface properties.
(6) Water content.
(7) Mechanical properties, including tensile strength, tear strength and rigidity modulus.
(8) Permeability to oxygen, carbon dioxide etc.
(9) Ocular compatibility.
(10) Toxicity and chemical stability.
(11) Method and ease of sterilization.

The relative importance of the various properties will depend on whether the lens is intended for daily wear or extended wear. In addition, some properties such as refractive index and density vary by relatively small amounts within the range of polymers that are otherwise suitable for contact lens use. Consequently, the potential value of a material as a lens material is not greatly affected by its density or refractive index.

Similarly, the dimensional stability of a material with respect to changes in temperature is less important than the reversibility of any changes that occur. This aspect of lens behaviour will usually be most important during heat sterilization procedures, if these are employed. To a lesser extent, some dimensional changes with changing pH and tonicity can be tolerated provided that such changes are reversible and small over the range of pH and tonicity encountered on the eye. Dimensional stability with respect to time is extremely important since instability will result in irreversible flattening or distortion of the lens. Dimensional instability in PMMA is invariably the result of strain induced during lens manufacture. With CAB and RGP materials, however, water uptake results in a degree of plasticization of the matrix and this causes dimensional instability, particularly flattening.

One of the problems associated with the measurement of mechanical properties of lens materials is that no single property measurement reflects accurately the 'in use' situation. Thus, 'tensile strength' indicates the resistance of the material to deformation under tension, 'tear strength' the resistance of the material to tear propagation from a notch or imperfection and 'rigidity modulus' the resistance to deformation under compression. The first two give some indication of the behaviour of a material during handling whilst the third indicates the extent to which the eyelid will deform it. Thus, a 'hard' or rigid material would have a high rigidity modulus whereas a 'soft' material would have a much lower value. Whilst a low rigidity modulus is associated with greater comfort, in extreme cases poor visual stability is encountered, thus setting a lower limit to this property.

Attempts have been made to define the properties of the 'ideal contact lens' (Kamath, 1969) but in view of the divergence of clinical preference in relation to the wide range of lenses presently available such an approach is unlikely to succeed. It is possible, however, to define acceptable ranges of certain situations (i.e. daily wear, extended wear, hard lenses, soft lenses). It is useful in doing this to compare the properties of a member of each of the three classes of 'pure' (i.e. excluding 'hybrid' RGP) material previously discussed. It is also useful to include for comparison the properties of the cornea although collection of the relevant information

Table 3.1 Properties of representative contact lens materials (all reported at 25°C unless otherwise stated)

	Polymethyl methacrylate (thermoplastics)	Silicone rubber (elastomers)	PHEMA (hydrogels)	Cornea
Density (g/cm^3)	1.18	1.10	1.16	1.03
Refractive index	1.49	1.43	1.43	1.37
Dimensional stability with respect to: Time Temperature pH Toxicity	Generally good unless strain induced during processing	Generally good	Generally good	
Surface wettability				
Critical surface tension (dyn/cm)	39	25	≈50	≈30
Equilibrium water contact angle (°)	65–70	≈96	≈20	≈47
Water content (%)	≈0.5	≈0	≈39	≈8
Tensile strength (dyn/cm^2)	≈50 × 10^7	≈10 × 10^7	≈0.5 × 10^7	≈5 × 10^7
Rigidity modulus (dyn/cm^2)	≈1 × 10^{10}	≈8 × 10^7	≈5 × 10^7	≈10 × 10^7
Tear strength (g/mm)	Strong but brittle	≈2000	≈10	≈1500
Oxygen permeability (0.1 mm thick sample)				
P_g (ml(STP) mm)/(cm^2 s cmHg)	≈1 × 10^{-10}	≈5000 × 10^{-10}	—	—
P_d (ml(STP) mm)/(cm^2 s cmHg)	≈1 × 10^{-10}	≈1500 × 10^{-10}	75 × 10^{-10}	≈300 × 10^{-10}

in this case is not easy (Kamath, 1969; Anderton, 1973; Tighe, 1976).

A comparison of various properties of polymethyl methacrylate, poly(dimethyl siloxane) or silicone rubber, PHEMA hydrogel and the cornea is presented in *Table 3.1*. In the light of these figures and the preceding discussion it will be apparent that relatively few properties are absolutely critical in determining whether or not a material is suitable for contact lens use. From the point of view of lens description, rigidity modulus and surface wettability will be sufficient to define the material (in the commonly used terms) as hard hydrophobic, soft hydrophobic or soft hydrophilic (corresponding to each of the three classes). In addition, the oxygen permeability will indicate whether the material is suitable for daily wear only or may be investigated as an extended wear candidate. Most of the other properties are either relatively unimportant or affect only convenience of use and ease of handling (tensile and tear strengths for example). In either case, absolute limits cannot be put on their magnitude although in the case of both tear and tensile strengths it should be as high as possible.

If an alternative approach is taken, that of considering the contact lens as an extension of the cornea, a similar conclusion is reached. Thus, the lens must allow the cornea to respire normally, it must resist the deforming force of the eyelid and it must permit a continuous tear film to be maintained on the lens. These factors can be discussed in terms of mechanical properties, surface properties and oxygen permeability. Some attempt must therefore be made to put quantitative limits on these very important properties.

The underlying problem that has bedevilled the field of contact lens materials has been the lack of adequate standardization. Whereas legislation and common scientific practice have made it possible to compare most pharmaceutical products, one with another, no such situation exists with contact lenses. Given the relative explosion in the number and types of material that have become available in the last 15 years, this is a serious problem. Even the activities of the Food and Drugs Administration (FDA) in the USA have failed to produce a satisfactory and generally observed basis for the assessment and comparison of different lens materials of the same type with respect to an adequate range of properties. The following section outlines the type of information that can be obtained, and its relevance to contact lens performance. An agreed international basis for the determination and reporting of such properties is urgently needed.

Mechanical properties

It is generally believed that variations in mechanical properties of what are essentially polymers whose properties lie in a tough to glassy regime (the RGPs) will be less critical in relation to clinical performance than is the case with soft elastic hydrogels. This does not mean to say that the mechanical properties of RGPs are unimportant in this respect, but they are more obviously related to problems associated with manufacturing and durability. Perhaps for this reason, less attention has been given to determination of mechanical properties of hard contact lens materials, than has been given to, say, permeability or wettability. It is important, however, to recognize the important clinical consequences of dimensional instability of some RGPs and the fact that this instability has its roots in the underlying mechanical properties of the materials. For this reason determination, with reasonable accuracy, of some fundamental mechanical properties of materials in the form of contact lenses is a desirable aim. This is in fact a major problem, for although many test procedures, techniques and materials' characteristics are known in the field of mechanical properties they are not designed for small curved samples of changing cross-section. To provide a basis for discussion, the types of information obtained in conventional mechanical testing must first be outlined.

In general, mechanical property testing involves the application of some form of deforming force to a sample and a concurrent study of the way that the sample responds. The results are often expressed in the form of strength or modulus. The strength of a material is usually defined in terms of the force per unit area required to cause failure when the material is subjected to a particular type of test procedure (e.g. tensile, shear, impact, tear). The modulus, on the other hand, is defined as the true stress (i.e. force per unit area) required to produce a true unit strain (i.e. deformation) in the direction of the force (e.g. tensile modulus, rigidity modulus). The most common types of mechanical property tests are described below

but first it is necessary to comment on the units used in quoting the results.

Several different units of stress are used (e.g. tsi, ton weight per square inch; psi, pound weight per square inch; kg or kgf/mm^2, kilogram weight per square millimetre, and dyn/cm^2, dynes per square centimetre). The SI unit of stress is N/m^2 (newtons per square metre), but this is an extremely small quantity and MN/m^2 (mega-newtons per square metre, equal to 10^6 N/m^2) is a more useful unit. The units are related in the following way:

$$1\,\text{dyn/cm}^2 = 0.1\,\text{N/m}^2 = 10^{-7}\,\text{MN/m}^2$$
$$= 1.45 \times 10^{-5}\,\text{psi}$$
$$= 6.46 \times 10^{-9}\,\text{tsi} = 1.02 \times 10^{-8}\,\text{kg/mm}^2$$

Some of the ways in which this information is obtained are outlined below.

Examination of materials under tension

A polymer specimen is stretched if a tensile stress is applied to it. The tensile test is normally carried out with a tensometer (which measures the extension produced as the load is applied). A stress–strain curve produced in this way provides wide-ranging mechanical data of the material under test:

(1) How strong it is, i.e. the ultimate tensile strength of the material.
(2) How much it can be deformed before fracture, i.e. the elongation at break of the material.
(3) How stiff it is, i.e. the tensile modulus (Young's modulus) of the material.
(4) How tough it is, which can be determined from the area under the whole stress–strain curve.

In addition, the profile of the stress–strain curve provides valuable guidance as to the mechanism of failure of the specimen.

The relationships, with appropriate units, are shown below.

Units

$$\text{Tensile strength} = \frac{\text{Load at break (N)}}{\text{Cross-sectional area (m}^2)} \qquad \text{N/m}^2$$

$$\text{Tensile modulus} = \frac{\text{Stress (N/m}^2)}{\text{Strain}} \qquad \text{N/m}^2$$

Percentage elongation at break

$$= \frac{\text{Extension at break (m)}}{\text{Original length (m)}} \times 100\% \qquad \%$$

Examination of materials under compression: rigidity modulus

The type of test selected for a given polymeric material should relate to the stresses it will experience in service. Simulating the actual service conditions of the polymer in experimental tests may provide many difficulties since no single commercially available technique can provide all the experimental conditions for testing polymers in different applications. The nearer the experimental conditions are to the service conditions, the more potentially significant will be the results obtained. One of the more useful and significant tests for soft lens materials is the time-dependent deformation and recovery of the materials under successive periods of load application and removal. Unlike ideally elastic materials, most polymers are viscoelastic (i.e. they deform time dependently when a load is applied to them and recover time dependently when the load is removed) and this may result in a progressive deformation of the materials.

Instruments for the study of deformational properties under compression are fundamentally similar. Typically, the instrument allows the indentation of any test sample (e.g. in the form of a thin film or coating) by a small sphere under a small constant load, to be measured as a function of time. The recovery of the specimen after the load has been removed can also be measured as a function of time. Both the indentation and recovery curves are recorded automatically and the time scales of each can be set separately. Because wide variation of both magnitude of load and indenter diameter or form is possible, a wide range of material properties can be monitored with this technique. The non-destructive nature of the method coupled with its ability to handle small specimen sizes make it particularly suitable for the examination of contact lens materials. As a consequence, values of the rigidity modulus for a wide range of types of material are known and some general comments on the relationship with clinical performance can be made.

The value of the rigidity modulus indicates the force (stress) necessary to compress (strain) the material by a given amount. It is therefore a bulk property and has units of 'force per unit area' such as lb/in^2 or dyn/cm^2. Although this gives a good indication of the flexibility of the material, it bears no relationship to properties that are measured in tension, such as tensile strength and tear strength. Some indication of the way in which the rigidity modulus is related to comfort and visual performance is given in *Figure 3.2*. The two latter parameters are expressed in arbitrary units since a general rather than precise relationship is intended.

It is apparent from the figure that there are two regions (A and C) in which the visual performance has markedly deteriorated. Region C corresponds to the very low rigidity modulus associated with some hydrogels, often of high

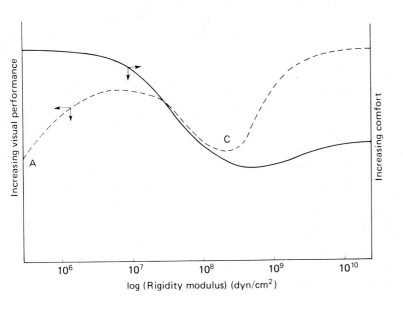

Figure 3.2 The general relationship between the rigidity modulus of a contact lens material and the comfort (—) and visual performance (---) of the lens

water content. In this case, the poor visual performance is due to the inability of the material to adequately resist the deforming force of the eyelid. Region A corresponds to flexible thermoplastics that have poor elastic recovery and poor dimensional stability. Plasticized polyvinyl chloride of the type encountered in vinyl seat coverings is an example of polymers showing this behaviour. Here the material is insufficiently rigid for the lens to be fitted as a conventional hard lens but insufficiently flexible and elastic to be accommodated to the corneal profile in the way that conventional 'soft' lenses are.

This illustrates the difficulty in achieving a balance between comfort, visual performance and flexibility and in particular the problems associated with a 'semi-rigid' lens which would of course otherwise have many attractive features. In practical terms, materials in regions C and A are unsuitable for contact lens usage. Although the exact limits are difficult to define, it is apparent from clinical studies that poly(4-methyl pent-1-ene) or TPX is approaching the point where reduced rigidity (in comparison with polymethyl methacrylate) results in some loss in visual performance when conventional fitting techniques are used (Larke, Pedley and Tighe, 1973; Larke et al., 1973; Ng, Pedley and Tighe, 1976).

Rigidity modulus and related measurements have been made on a wide range of contact lens materials using a microindentation apparatus (Ng, 1974; Tighe, 1976). This technique enables samples of similar thickness to that of contact lenses (0.1–0.4 mm) to be studied. Rigidity modulus measurements are made by measuring the deformation produced in the sample by a spherical indenter to which a series of loads is applied. *Figure 3.3* illustrates the relationship between log load and log indentation for a spherical indenter of 0.16 mm radius. Materials of decreasing rigidity are found on moving from left to right and it is relevant to note that the cornea corresponds to line *g* in this figure. From this figure it is also easy to appreciate that under a load (say, 1 g) that causes moderate deformation of elastomers, hydrogels and the cornea (*f–h*), the effect on the group of thermoplastics (*a–e*) is negligible. Thus, although we can detect manually the difference in flexibility or rigidity between, say, polymethyl methacrylate and a 'semi-rigid' plastic such as poly(4-methyl pent-

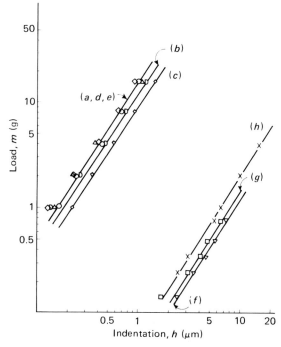

Figure 3.3 Microindentation studies. The correlation of a log(load) with log(indentation) for various materials: (*a*) △ PMMA; (*b*) **D** polystyrene; (*c*) ◇ poly(4-methyl pent-1-ene); (*d*) ○ dehydrated PHEMA; (*e*) ◇ dehydrated HEMA–styrene (90:10); (*f*) ▽ PHEMA hydrogel; (*g*) □ HEMA–styrene (90:10) hydrogel; (*h*) × EPT

1-ene), the cornea is unable to detect any difference.

This point is illustrated more clearly when the microindentation technique is used with a flattened indenter and load calibrated to produce a pressure similar to that exerted by the eyelid ($\approx 2.6 \times 10^4 \, \text{dyn/cm}^2$). Using this procedure the deformation and recovery of polymer samples of contact lens thickness under eyelid load can be studied. No detectable deformation is produced in any of the thermoplastic polymers previously discussed. It must be remembered, however, that this is compression of a supported material and not 'flattening' of an unsupported lens which does begin to occur with less rigid polymers.

Indentation studies of this type under eyelid load correlate well with clinical studies. Although the ideal elastic behaviour exhibited (*Figure 3.4*) by synthetic elastomers under these low loads is preferable, appreciable deviations from this situation still produce acceptable

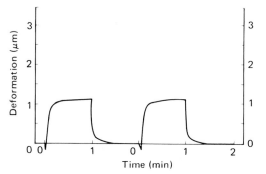

Figure 3.4 Deformation properties of ethylene–propylene terpolymer under eyelid pressure

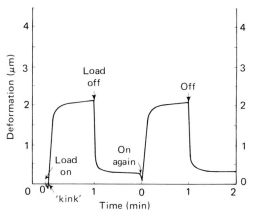

Figure 3.5 Deformation properties of PHEMA under eyelid pressure

clinical behaviour. Thus, materials whose behaviour is more time dependent (i.e. less than instantaneous deformation and recovery) produce acceptable visual stability levels in lenses provided that the overall deformation is not more than about 2%. PHEMA itself shows reasonably good elastic behaviour under eyelid load as illustrated in *Figure 3.5*.

Hydrogels whose deformational behaviour is characterized by large ($\approx$5%) and rapid initial deformation that does not reach equilibrium within one minute and shows poor recovery, invariably give rise to lenses whose visual stability is unacceptable. Some early, fragile, high water content hydrogel lenses tended to behave in this way.

Hardness tests

Hardness can be defined as resistance to penetration. In a hardness test an indicator is pressed on the surface of the material under test, and the extent to which it sinks in for a given pressure and time is an inverse measure of the hardness. In this respect the test is related to compression testing. There are many hardness testers available commercially and suitable for plastics and rubbers, including the Vickers indenter, the Rockwell hardness tester and the Shore durometers. They may be divided into three categories.

(1) Hardness tests that measure the resistance of a material to indentation by an indenting probe (e.g. Brinell, Vickers and Shore durometers). Some tests measure the indentation with the load applied and some measure the residual indentation after the load is removed.

(2) Hardness tests that measure the resistance of a material to scratching by another material (e.g. the Bierbaum scratch test, the Moh hardness test). Similar techniques are commonly used in paint testing and involve pulling the sample beneath a loaded indenter.

(3) Hardness tests that measure recovery efficiency or resilience (e.g. the various Rockwell testers). Many of the hardness tests are a combination of (1) and (3).

There is no common method of measurement in these tests. For example, the Rockwell α scale hardness test measures the depth of penetration with the load applied, whereas the Rockwell R, L, M and E scale tests measure depth caused by a spherical indenter after most of the load has been removed. In these methods the amount of rebound or recoverable deformation is important. The Vickers Microhardness test differs again, in that a microscope is used to measure the diagonals of the pits left by a diamond-shaped indenter on a square base. There is a linear relationship between the depth of impression and the hardness number. Each of the hardness methods uses an arbitrary scale and, although the scales can be approximately compared, precise correlation is not possible.

Hardness testing using these various instruments is a fairly convenient method for comparing the relative hardness of materials, and results are being increasingly quoted in overviews of contact lens materials. The plethora of methods and difficulty of comparing them mean that they can, realistically, only provide supplementary information to that obtained by micropenetrometry which provides direct indentation results and can also be used to calculate rigidity modulus.

Other mechanical tests: tear, flex, creep

Various additional types of mechanical test may be used, but in general they are less readily adapted to contact lens studies; some of these are briefly described here.

Tear strength test

Tear strength is the force required to propagate a tear in a notched specimen and is expressed as force per unit length of the resultant tear. The result depends on many factors such as depth of notch, mode of applying the tearing force, thickness of specimen and temperature of test. This property is particularly important for hydrogels but no satisfactory comparative technique for use on lens materials has yet been developed.

Flexural test

The specimen is flexed repeatedly until it fractures. The number of flex cycles to break measures the flexural resistance of the material. The flex can be repeated in linear extension, bending without tension, or with a combination of bending and extension. This property should not be confused with the resistance of a lens to flexural deformation. Behaviour of this type is related to the deformational tests previously described and its relationship to clinical performance has been reviewed by Fatt (1987).

Creep test

Plastics often tend to become distorted if they are constantly loaded. Creep tests are therefore important for polymeric materials in service. A creep test records deformation against time for a constant stress over a relatively long period of time, in contrast to the conventional tensile and compression testing techniques previously described which measure short-term response. Thus, when a load is applied to a polymer specimen, there is a short-term elastic deformation, followed by the relatively slow deformation or creep. A creep test is normally carried out in tension rather than compression. Creep is particularly important in polymers whose behaviour lies between truly elastic on one hand, and rigid and glassy on the other. In the contact lens field the so-called 'rigid gas permeables' frequently show poor rigidity and are subject to creep. This manifests itself in dimensional instability and occurs in response to internal or external stresses imposed on the lens. It has been reported that high plus and high minus lenses can behave quite differently and, additionally, there is a clear material dependence (Kerr and Dilly, 1988). Much of the dimensional instability in RGPs occurs upon hydration and is a consequence of the hydrophilic monomers that are incorporated to overcome the hydrophobicity of siloxy- and fluoromethacrylates. For this reason observation of differences between the tensile stress–strain curves of non-hydrated and hydrated lens materials provides a useful short-term method for creep prediction.

Surface properties: general principles

The wetting of contact lenses is important because the maintenance of a precorneal tear film in the form of a thin capillary layer has long been recognized as a primary requirement for the physiological compatibility of lens and patient. Defining in quantitative terms the surface characteristics that are necessary to produce this behaviour has, however, only relatively recently been attempted.

The terms 'hydrophilic' and 'hydrophobic' have been widely and often misleadingly used in this connection. When used to refer to bulk properties they mean simply water-loving and water-hating, respectively. In this sense a dehydrated hydrogel can be said to be hydrophilic since it imbibes water to form a gel. When the terms are used in connection with surfaces they have a more specific meaning. The term 'hydrophilic' used in this sense means that water will spread spontaneously on the surface, whereas 'hydrophobic' implies that water will not spontaneously spread on the surface. Many contact lens materials are referred to as hydrophilic when by this definition they are not so. The position is complicated by the fact that when contact lens materials are referred to, the implication is that they are wetted by tear fluid rather than by water itself. These then are some

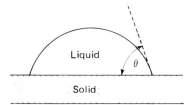

Figure 3.6 Droplet of liquid resting at equilibrium on a solid surface showing the contact angle (θ)

of the aspects of the subject that must be taken into account.

The most convenient way of assessing wettability is by the contact angle. The simplest method for measuring this is by observing the formation of a sessile drop of liquid (delivered, for example, by a hypodermic syringe) on the solid surface. The image of the droplet may be projected or photographed and the contact angle (θ) is the angle enclosed by the surface and the tangent to the droplet–surface interface (*Figure 3.6*). Thus, a liquid which spontaneously wets or spreads on a surface has a contact angle of zero. A hydrophilic surface then is one on which water exhibits a zero contact angle.

The wetting of the cornea by tear fluid can be treated in a similar way although it is a much more complex process — *see* Chapters 2 and 8. The epithelial surface is, itself, too hydrophobic to be spontaneously wetted by tears (Mishima, 1965) and is thought to be covered by a lipid layer (Ehlers, 1965). The resultant surface would itself be relatively hydrophobic and the most satisfactory hypothesis to explain the fact that tears wet the cornea is that the conjunctival glycoproteins also adsorb on the corneal surface thus rendering it wettable. Although the structure and function of tears are complex (Mishima and Maurice, 1961; Wolff, 1976), for the purpose of studying interactions with polymers we can consider the fluid to be an aqueous liquid whose surface tension has been reduced to approximately 46 dyn/cm by the presence of surfactants or wetting agents. It should be noted, however, that this value for the surface tension of tear fluid (Miller, 1969) has been thought by some workers to be too high (Lemp *et al.*, 1970). The surface tension of pure water by comparison is 72.8 dyn/cm.

Definitions

It was Thomas Young who first indicated that forces acting on the droplet (*Figure 3.6*) when it

has reached equilibrium may be resolved and expressed by the relationship:

$$\gamma_{sv} - \gamma_{sl} = \gamma_{lv} \cos\theta$$

where

γ_{sv} is the free energy or surface tension at the interface of solid and vapour

γ_{sl} is the free energy or surface tension at the interface of solid and liquid

γ_{lv} is the free energy or surface tension at the interface of liquid and vapour and

θ is the contact angle.

This provides a basis for the quantitative description of wettability of the substrate, together with the spreading of a liquid on that substrate, and their relation to the contact angle. As θ diminishes and approaches zero, the liquid approaches the condition where it will spread on the surface.

This condition is referred to as spontaneous wetting of the surface (in contrast to the situation where a mechanical force is used to induce spreading) and leads to the simplest relationship between the wettability of the surface and the ability of liquids of different surface tension to wet it. *Figure 3.7* shows such a relationship, and illustrates the concept of 'critical surface tension' of the substrate. Figures of this type are obtained by measuring the contact angle of a series of liquids of known surface tension on the substrate in question. The results are plotted in the form $\cos\theta$ (*y* axis) against surface tension of the wetting liquid (*x* axis), a function which is, in many cases, linear. This enables a line to be extrapolated on the graph to a point corresponding to spontaneous wetting, i.e. $\cos\theta = 1$. The value of the surface tension obtained in this way, which would correspond to that of a liquid just able to spontaneously wet the substrate, is known as the critical surface tension of the substrate. Liquids having surface tensions equal to, or less than, the critical surface tension of a given substrate would be expected to wet or spread on that surface.

A rather more precise description of surface properties arises from the analysis of the interaction of forces of different kinds across interfaces. Fundamental to this philosophy is the concept of the free energy of a surface. It is convenient to regard this as the equivalent of a solid or liquid surface tension, but being

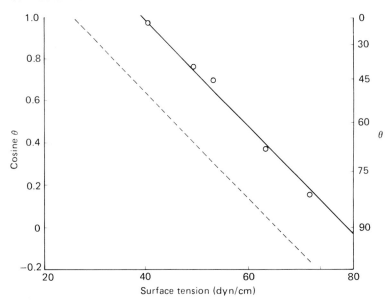

Figure 3.7 Determination of the critical surface tension of polymers by the method of Fox and Zisman illustrating the difference in wettability and critical surface tension of polymethyl methacrylate (——) and silicone rubber (----)

composed of two components. The first of these components is characteristic of the relatively non-polar background forces in molecules of the van der Waals type, and is known as the dispersive, or non-polar, component. The second originates principally from molecular dipoles and is known as the polar component.

Thus for a liquid

$$\gamma_l(\text{total}) = \gamma_l(\text{dispersive}) + \gamma_l(\text{polar})$$

and for a solid:

$$\gamma_s(\text{total}) = \gamma_s(\text{dispersive}) + \gamma_s(\text{polar})$$

The abbreviations γ_s^d, γ_s^p, γ_l^d and γ_l^p are normally used.

One very useful concept that arises from this treatment is that of interfacial tension between two liquids or between a liquid and a solid. The greater the interaction of forces of the same type across the interface, the lower will be the interfacial tension at that interface, and vice versa. For this reason, two liquids such as water and octane, which have very different balances of polar and dispersive forces, show little interaction at their interface and are thus immiscible. On the other hand, water and ethyl alcohol both have strong polar contributions which operate across an interface resulting in the miscibility of these two liquids. In the same way, the interfacial tension between a liquid and a solid is a measure of the interaction between

these materials. In the study of biocompatibility of materials with different biological environments, the desirability of achieving a low interfacial tension between the biomaterial and its environment is well recognized. The concept is equally valid in relation to ocular compatibility and will undoubtedly become more widely accepted as the limitations of currently quoted 'wetting angles' become recognized.

Two important equations must be quoted, the first of these illustrates the way in which the operation of forces across the interfaces are calculated, the basis of which is the so-called 'geometric mean' concept. Thus, for a solid and a liquid, the interfacial tension is given by:

$$\gamma_{sl} = \gamma_s + \gamma_l - 2(\gamma_s^d \gamma_l^d)^{1/2} - 2(\gamma_s^p \gamma_l^p)^{1/2}$$

Because the polar component of water is relatively high (51.0 dyn/cm) it is obvious from this equation that a low interfacial tension with water or with aqueous systems can only be achieved by solids that themselves have appreciable polar character.

The second equation, which was developed by Owens and Wendt, utilizes this principle in such a manner that measurements of contact angles with two different liquids enables the unknown polar and dispersive components of a given solid to be determined. This assumes that two liquids of known polar and dispersive components have been chosen. Owens and

Wendt's expression in the general form is shown below:

$$1 + \cos\theta = \frac{2}{\gamma_l}[(\gamma_s^d \gamma_l^d)^{1/2} + (\gamma_s^P \gamma_l^P)^{1/2}]$$

rearrangement enables two readily solved simultaneous equations to be generated and γ_s^d and γ_s^P thereby determined.

Measurement techniques

Some comments on the types of measurements that are made, the results that they yield and the problems associated with their measurement and interpretation are important. The most common method for measuring surface properties involves the use of a sessile droplet of liquid, introduced onto the surface of the material by a hypodermic syringe. The introduction and measurement are carried out in air, which means that the liquid will be in equilibrium with its vapour. This is essentially the condition described in Thomas Young's relationship, referred to above. Before considering the use that can be made of such information, some comments on factors that affect the form of the droplet and its contact angle on the material substrate are necessary.

In the first place, the liquid is responding to the *surface* forces in the polymer, emphasizing that this leads to the measurement of *surface* properties. The liquid–solid interaction is thus greatly influenced by minute traces of surface impurities, such as those caused by accidental handling, and accumulated during storage. Careful cleaning of the surface (using dilute surfactant followed by rigorous washing with pure water and careful drying under vacuum) is therefore essential. The techniques developed by Zisman (Fox and Zisman, 1950) in his extensive work on surface energetics provide a sound basis, for studies of this type.

Secondly, there is normally a difference between a contact angle produced as a droplet advances over the surface, on being dispensed from the hypodermic syringe, and the contact angle made with the surface asd the droplet recedes if it is drawn back into the syringe. These two angles, the so-called 'advancing' and 'receding' contact angles are often conceptually regarded as the advancing angle over a dry or unwetted surface and the receding angle as the

liquid withdraws over a previously wetted surface. The difference between them is referred to as contact angle hysteresis. The measurement normally used in surface characterization is referred to as the equilibrium advancing contact angle, and is taken immediately after the advancing droplet has been allowed to come to rest.

Other factors that can influence the experimentally determined contact angle are droplet size and surface roughness (or rugosity). The rule of thumb with respect to droplet size is that it is important to be consistent and not to use too large a droplet, otherwise distortion of the idealized droplet shape occurs. The effect of rugosity is rather more complex, but in essence a roughened surface will give a lower contact angle than a smooth surface of the same material. This emphasizes the necessity of ensuring that equally smooth surfaces are used when making comparisons. This can be quite difficult with fabricated articles such as contact lenses.

Inverted bubble or droplet measurement techniques are fundamentally different from those involving the measurement of a sessile drop in air. The inverted methods require the sample to be immersed in a liquid (usually water) and a droplet of a second liquid (or air) to be introduced beneath the sample surface. It is obviously essential that the droplet is of lower density than the immersion fluid. When the density difference is large, as in the case of air, the influence of droplet (i.e. bubble) distortion and the importance of droplet (bubble) size is much greater than in the case of the sessile drop experiment. The method is valuable in the study of hydrated surfaces, and has been cleverly adapted by Hamilton (1972) to the study of polar components of surface energy of solids. This is achieved in principle by choosing a liquid whose dispersive component is the same as that of water (e.g. octane, $\gamma^d = 21.8$ dyn/cm), thus allowing a direct correlation to be made between contact angle and polar component of surface free energy. One of the greatest difficulties of this method is that of exact determination of the tangent to the droplet at its point of contact with the solid, and thus measurement of the contact angle. When this technique is used with an air droplet (sometimes referred to as the captive air bubble technique), the contact angle is conceptually similar to that obtained when a 'receding' angle is measured by the sessile water droplet in air procedure. When a contact lens wetting or soaking solution is used instead of water the contact angle produced has no fundamental significance to either surface characterization, or to the prediction of eye–lens compatibility.

Additional variants of the two broad types of measurement technique outlined above involve the use of a vertically mounted specimen (lens or flat plate) which is immersed in, withdrawn from or contacted against the wetting liquid. The principle of these methods has long been recognized and their relevance to contact lens wetting phenomena described several years ago (Larke, Pedley and Tighe, 1973). More recently, attempts have been made to use them as a basis for 'new' methods of measuring the wetting behaviour of lenses in an attempt to achieve better correlation with behaviour *in vivo*. In reviewing their success in this respect, Pearson (1987) highlights variations both in magnitude of wetting angles obtained and even in rank order with a small group of RGPs.

Clinical significance

The information that can be obtained from these relatively simple techniques, if used with care and precision, is considerable. In the first place, sessile drop measurement in air with liquids of different surface tension can be used in the form of a Zisman plot (*see Figure 3.7*) to determine the critical surface tension of a solid. Ideally, four or five liquids should be used, none of which should interact strongly with the substrate. The critical surface tension gives an idea of the gross wettability of the substrate and is most useful in the case of solids that do not exhibit an appreciable polar component of total surface energy.

A more precise description of surface properties may be obtained by using two or more liquids whose surface tensions have known polar and dispersive components. Sessile drop measurement in combination with Owens and Wendt's analysis allows polar and dispersive components of surface energy to be determined. Water, methylene iodide and formamide are among the most commonly used liquids in this type of experiment. Inverted droplet measurements are very useful, but their interpretation is open to more debate. Even Hamilton's appar-

ently straightforward correlation of contact angle with polar surface energy component has been the subject of some doubt. The principal reason for this is the effect of mutual solubility of the liquids on their surface tensions and the extent to which this is important in what are almost instantaneous measurements. A more general problem with these methods is their conceptual similarity to receding angle techniques. Thus, the impinging droplet or bubble displaces water from the hydrated surface, and the extent to which the resultant interface is dominated by a residual interfacial water layer is not certain.

All these measurements have some part to play in the surface characterization of contact lens materials. On the other hand no single contact angle measurement can predict the complex interaction of a lens with tears. Furthermore, although critical surface tension (γ_c) is a useful parameter, the fact that lens materials need a degree of polarity in order to sustain the all important tear fluid layer suggests that it is not wholly adequate. It does, however, provide a useful basis upon which to discuss the susceptibility of a lens to the initial wetting process by tears. *Figure 3.7* enables polymethyl methacrylate and silicone rubber to be compared in this respect.

The figure illustrates the fact that tear fluid having a surface tension of 46 dyn/cm or slightly lower is only just able to wet the polymethyl methacrylate sample used in this experiment. The practice of using viscous wetting solution with methyl methacrylate lenses helps to establish the necessary continuous tear film on insertion. By contrast the silicone rubber sample shown on the same graph would require a liquid having a much lower surface tension ($\simeq 25$ dyn/cm) in order for it to be spontaneously wetted. The function of surface treatment of this type of polymer is to increase the critical surface tension of the material.

Variations in the slope and indeed the shape of plots of the type shown in *Figure 3.7* do occur especially when liquids capable of hydrogen bonding with the surface are used, as they must be in contact lens work. Failure to take this into account has resulted in calculated values for the critical surface tension of the cornea that are excessively low. Even when this fact is taken into account it will be seen that the critical surface tension of the cornea ($\gamma_c \simeq 35$ dyn/cm) is similar to, but somewhat lower than that of polymethyl methacrylate ($\gamma_c \simeq 39$ dyn/cm). There are several important observations that must be made on these figures.

The first point that requires clarification is the fact that these surfaces are unexpectedly wetted by a liquid of higher surface tension (46 dyn/cm). We can obviously take into account the fact that 46 dyn/cm is thought to be a conservatively high estimate of the surface tension of tear fluid and the unique nature of the corneal surface. The most important reason, however, since it applies to all surfaces, is the occurrence of a phenomenon known as contact angle hysteresis. This is the difference between the advancing contact angle observed when a liquid boundary advances over a clean dry solid surface and the receding contact angle observed when a liquid boundary recedes from a previously wetted surface. The former (advancing) value is used in experimental work *in vitro* because it is far more reproducible. The latter value, which is significantly lower is, however, important in the contact lens situation *in vivo*. This is because the establishment of the tear film, corresponding to the advancing contact angle, is assisted mechanically by the eyelid and sometimes by the use of wetting solutions. The receding angle, however, dictates whether the formed film will be stable or will break up on the lens surface.

It is important to note that this difference, although significant, is relatively small and is not sufficient to sustain tear films on polymers having critical surface tensions significantly lower than polymethyl methacrylate. This raises the second point. Although there are many alternative thermoplastic polymers that might compete with polymethyl methacrylate in contact lens use, there are very few (suitable in other respects) that share its similarity in critical surface tension to the cornea. This is probably the major single reason that polymethyl methacrylate occupied the unique position that it did for so long. Of the materials currently available, only cellulose acetate butyrate possesses similar surface properties. Early clinical studies in conjunction with surface treatment of polymers (Larke *et al.*, 1973; Pedley, 1976) indicate that for a material to be useful for contact lens fabrication it should have an equilibrium advancing contact angle (θ) with water of not greater than 65–70°. This is, in fact, a better

single criterion than the critical surface tension because of the aforementioned effects of polarity and hydrogen bonding on the determination of the latter.

It must be emphasized, however, that single 'wetting angle' or contact angle measurements are of very limited value in predicting clinical behaviour. Whereas they can provide a broad distinction between materials that are so nonwettable as to be clinically dangerous, and materials that are capable of sustaining a tear film, they give little guidance beyond that. Since they are so widely quoted some comment on differences in measurement protocol is appropriate. Although it may be argued that lenses are soaked and thus to a degree 'hydrated' before use, the tendency of the front lens surface to become partially dehydrated in wear is well known. Thus, the 'dry' contact angle will give a useful guide to initial tear film stability under the least advantageous conditions. The effect of soaking in saline and in proprietary wetting solutions illustrates the wettability of the lens under the most advantageous, but not necessarily most representative, conditions. The least physiologically representative method of measuring the 'wettability' of the lens is to pre-soak the material and then measure a receding contact angle using, not water, but a low surface tension wetting solution to make the measurement. The equivalent of this is to immerse the sample in wetting solution and use the inverted air bubble technique. Measurements of this sort are unrepresentative of any clinical or physiological situation but are commonly used by manufacturers to demonstrate how wettable their own materials are. In all these methods of measurement a $\pm 2°$ 'error bar' must be allowed, because this is the limit of reproducible measurement. It is plainly nonsensical therefore to quote values to an accuracy of 0.1° as is sometimes done, especially in commercial literature.

These points taken together illustrate the need for standardization in measurement of contact lens properties by materials scientists and materials manufacturers. In particular, they illustrate the need to define the measurement conditions accurately when quoting results. It is, unfortunately, common to read in manufacturers' literature claims for a particular wetting angle without any indication of the wetting liquid, the state of hydration or degree of pre-soaking of the material, or even the technique used to make the measurement. The difference between a sessile drop contact angle measured with water on a surface and a captive (inverted) air bubble contact angle measured in a proprietary wetting solution can be as much as 40–50°. Figures quoted in the absence of any definition of measurement conditions are therefore meaningless as a basis of comparing the behaviour of competitive materials.

The fundamental lack of correlation between a simple single contact angle, however measured, and behaviour during wear, relates to the fact that when the lens is inserted into the eye a 'biological interface conversion' process begins. The fact that lenses produce lower measured contact angles after wear illustrates this point (Madigan and Holden, 1986; Morris and Tighe, 1986). This conversion process in part relates to the structured way in which the tear film wets the cornea, a point previously discussed, and is very much dependent upon the interfacial tension established between tears and the polymer surface. It has already been demonstrated that the interfacial tension varies with both polar and non-polar interactions between the liquid and solid. It is not surprising, therefore, that simple 'wetting angle' correlations with clinical behaviour are so poor, since they take no account of these parameters. With contact lens research, as is already commonplace in other areas of biomaterials work, attention will undoubtedly turn to more complete surface energy characterization. Even so, it is difficult to achieve a match between biological processes, which take place at a molecular level, and the macroscopic probe techniques that are currently available for surface characterization.

Although it might be anticipated that hydrogel polymers would present no problems in relation to wettability, this is not the case and relates to a further point arising from critical surface tension data. Although hydrogels are readily wetted by tear fluid and are capable of sustaining a tear fluid layer, they present a considerable problem in their tendency to accumulate proteinaceous and other material on the lens surface during use. In addition to any specific interaction of such debris with functional groups on the surface of the polymer there is a general principle involved. This is the observation (Schonhorn, 1972) that the adhesion of a mobile phase to a solid substrate increases as the surface becomes more wettable (i.e. as its critical surface tension increases). There is then a desirable limit to the wettability of polymers for contact lens use. Hydrogels are not truly hydrophilic (in terms of the precise definition stated earlier) since they exhibit an equilibrium advancing contact angle of around 20°. If this value could be raised, however, it would be possible to retain wettability by tear fluid while decreasing the problems of lens cleaning. Perhaps the best analogy here is that of non-stick domestic pan linings. Scrambled egg, which in some respects resembles the proteinaceous debris in question, adheres strongly to high energy metal surfaces but relatively weakly to the low energy poly(tetrafluoroethylene) surfaces used as pan coatings. It has been fairly recently shown (Barnes et al., 1974; Pedley and Tighe, 1974; Tighe and Gee, 1984) that by structural modification it is possible to produce hydrogels whose critical surface tensions are substantially lower (i.e. less wettable by tear fluid) than would be predicted from their water contents and bulk structural considerations.

Oxygen permeability

The importance of oxygen to corneal metabolism is well known and the physiological consequences of oxygen deprivation in this respect are discussed elsewhere, particularly in Chapters 2 and 15. Notable contributions to our knowledge of the effect of contact lenses of different types have been made over a considerable period by R. M. Hill (Hill and Fatt, 1964; Hill, 1966; Hill and Schoessler, 1967; Hill and Augsburger, 1971). A great deal of confused information has been published, however, on the actual values of oxygen permeability for different contact lens materials, particularly hydrogels.

Two questions must be addressed. What level of oxygen permeability is required to satisfy the corneal requirements, and how can the permeability of the materials be reliably measured in a manner that reflects their use in the eye? The oxygen requirement of the cornea has been expressed in various ways, including a direct figure for oxygen consumption and, alternatively, the minimum partial pressure of oxygen required to maintain normal corneal metabolism. It must be pointed out that such quantities are impossible to measure in such a manner that the techniques used give unambiguous results and do not, in their use, influence corneal behaviour. Thus, the value widely accepted for many years as the minimum partial pressure of oxygen required to prevent corneal oedema (11–19 mmHg, Polse and Mandell, 1970) has been progressively updated to 23–37 mmHg (Mandell and Farrel, 1980), 40 mmHg (O'Neall, Polse and Sarver, 1984) and even 74 mmHg (Holden, Sweeney and Sanderson, 1984). Since the work on which the latter figure is based may also be interpreted as showing an exponential decline in corneal thickness, and yet the error bars on the relevant measurement are within the same order of magnitude, the difficulty in obtaining an absolute correlation can be appreciated. These comments are not intended as a criticism of the excellent work and contributions to scientific knowledge of the groups involved, but rather an indication of the problems in this difficult field. A useful overview of the history and current status of the topic has been compiled by Efron and Brennan (1987). Before this information can be translated into a property requirement for contact lens materials, some consideration of the principles and definitions involved in oxygen permeability is required.

Definitions

The important fundamental texts in modern membrane science are agreed upon the use of the simple fundamental definition:

$$P = DS \tag{1}$$

for the transport of the gas through a polymer membrane. In this expression, P is the permeability coefficient for a given polymer-permeant (i.e. gas) system, D is the diffusion coefficient of the gas through the polymer, and S is the solubility of the gas in the polymer. In order to correlate the permeability coefficient (P) with the rate at which the gas passes through a membrane of given dimensions (area and thickness) for a given gas pressure, the equation:

$$j = \frac{PA}{L}\Delta p \tag{2}$$

is used. Here j is the flux of the gas (volume passing through in unit time), A is the membrane area, L is the membrane thickness, and Δp is the pressure difference across the membrane. The flux, j, is sometimes expressed by the symbol Q, or F, or its components v/t (volume per unit time).

Since the oxygen passing through the contact lens is consumed by the cornea, it is apparent that, in principle, it should be possible to balance this consumption requirement with the oxygen flux through a contact lens of given dimensions and given conditions, and to define the required lens behaviour in terms of a permeability P. Among the people who have carried out this sort of analysis, Fatt's work (Fatt and St Helen, 1971) appears to have had the greatest long-term influence. He represented the previous equations as

$$j = \frac{Dk}{L}(p_{\mathrm{L}} - p_{\mathrm{o}}) \tag{3}$$

where p_{L} is defined as the oxygen pressure at the front surface of the lens, and p_{o} as the oxygen pressure behind the lens (i.e. at the corneal surface). It is apparent that p_{o} should correlate with the minimum oxygen tension for normal corneal function. Unfortunately, Fatt chose to use k to represent gas solubility instead of the more usual term S. For this reason, the contact lens literature favours the use of the term Dk whereas in membrane science, DS or more commonly P is used. Thus Dk (or more simply P) is the permeability coefficient for a given material, whereas Dk/L or P/L refers specifically to the permeability (transmissibility) of a sample of that material of a given thickness (such as a contact lens). The values of the permeability coefficient are frequently different when, on one hand, the membrane separates two gas phases and, on the other, the membrane separates two liquid phases. The difference between these values, referred to as P_{g} and P_{d} respectively, is associated with the so-called 'barrier effect' or 'boundary effect' and has considerable significance in contact lens work.

The first point to note is that conventional 'gaseous' oxygen permeability coefficients (P_{g}) obtained for the transport of oxygen from the gas phase through the polymer film to another gas phase are not applicable to contact lens work. Values determined in this way are of great value in the food packaging industry, for example, and commercial apparatus for this type of measurement is readily obtainable. Measurements made in this way are inapplicable in the present context because (1) materials such as hydrogels are progressively dehydrated under these conditions and will give completely erroneous results, and more important, (2) these methods do not simulate the actual situation of the contact lens on the eye. In order to do this it is necessary to measure the transport of oxygen dissolved in one aqueous phase through the polymer and into another aqueous phase. This value is referred to as the 'dissolved' oxygen permeability coefficient (P_d).

The experimental difficulties associated with these measurements on samples that are often fragile are quite severe. Although measurements on thermoplastics and elastomers are easier to make than on hydrogels, there is with all hydrophobic polymers a barrier effect resulting from the interfacial tension between the polymer and aqueous phase. In order to obtain P_d values on such polymers, therefore, measurements on samples of various thicknesses must be made. Because of this barrier effect, hydrophobic polymers transport oxygen much less efficiently from water phase to water phase (as on the eye) than from gas phase to gas phase. This has meant that over-optimistic predictions have been made for polymers such as ethyl cellulose, polystyrene and poly(4-methyl pent-1-ene) on the basis of their quoted gas–gas (P_g) permeabilities. When measurements of the 'dissolved' oxygen permeabilities have been made, however, the disappointing clinical performance of such materials is understood.

Measurement techniques

Several different experimental procedures for determining oxygen permeability may be distinguished. In each case, oxygen at a known effective concentration passes from the donor side of the cell through the membrane (of known thickness and cross-sectional area) to a receiver side, also of known volume, where it is sensed.

In a gas–gas transport system, the donor side is initially at a positive pressure with respect to the initially evacuated receiver side. The increase in pressure of the receiver side is monitored (usually manometrically) and the rate of transport of oxygen, and thus the permeability coefficient for the membrane, may be calculated.

In a liquid–liquid cell, the cell is preferably stirred on both sides of the membrane, the concentration on the donor side being initially set at some positive level relative to the receiver side. The increase in concentration on the receiver side is monitored and since the volume of liquid on the receiver side is known, the permeability coefficient is again calculated. The difference between gas–gas transport and this procedure is, of course, that the former method leads to the gaseous permeability coefficient (P_g) whilst the liquid–liquid cell yields the dissolved oxygen permeability coefficient (P_d). Since the sensitivity and accuracy of the measurement system used on the receiver side deteriorates as the receiver volume increases, attempts are made to minimize this volume. As a result, modified systems may advantageously be used in which the donor side is stirred and the receiver side is of minimal, but accurately known, volume and contains a built-in detector.

It has been shown to be particularly important to stir the high concentration side of the membrane in order to minimize surface layer effects. Studies have shown that although failure to stir the low concentration side of the membrane produces a drop of only some 3% in the measured transport properties of the membrane, this figure increases dramatically, and is associated with a great deal of irreproducibility, if the high concentration side is not stirred.

Thus, the least satisfactory, but in many ways most convenient system, forms the basis of the technique frequently used to measure the permeability coefficient (expressed as Dk, see above) of contact lenses. In this the lens is clamped directly onto the detector electrode. The system, referred to here as the polarographic electrode technique, has several shortcomings. First, the donor side is unstirred, secondly the thickness of the contact lens normally shows a centre-to-edge variation and thirdly, because the lenses vary in curvature, the volume of the receiver side is not accurately fixed. In practice, this last point should be less important in this system, because the technique is not usually operated in the manner that measures rate of increase in oxygen concentration on the receiver side of the cell, but rather the resultant equilibrium oxygen consumption by the electrode. The ability to do this relies on the assumption that oxygen transported to the receiver side is efficiently consumed by the electrode sensor, and that, as a result, the partial pressure of oxygen on the receiver side is always effectively zero. With very permeable samples, however, these assumptions are not justified. In all cell configurations, it is important to have an oxygen-tight seal of the membrane separating donor and receiver chambers, but this again is difficult to achieve with the format and samples involved in contact lens measurement.

The inherent problems associated with the polarographic technique and the use of the Dk (as distinct from the P_g, P_d approach) are illustrated in the recent controversies over the Dk values of RGP materials. Measurements by Fatt on a group of materials which appeared to have extremely high permeabilities, did not accord with either clinical observations or permeability measurements made by Brien Holden's group in Australia. Although the values were subsequently recalibrated downwards by Fatt, there is still disagreement on figures and interpretation (Andrasko, 1986; Brennan, Efron and Holden, 1986a,b; Fatt, 1986). It is clear that the polarographic electrode technique is very convenient for the determination of approximate values of oxygen permeability but is inadequate as a primary standard. The way in which the Dk term has been used to describe permeabilities has failed to take into account the difference between gaseous (i.e. P_g) and dissolved (i.e. P_d) values and the nature of the boundary layer effect (the nature and importance of which is described in the next section). Although belated attempts are now being made to do this (Fatt, 1986) the fundamental shortcomings of the polarographic electrode technique will always limit its accuracy. Further comments are contained in the section dealing with commercial RGP materials.

A description of suitable apparatus for 'dissolved' oxygen permeability measurements has been given (Ng, 1974; Ng and Tighe, 1976a) and its application to both hydrogels (Ng and Tighe, 1976b) and non-hydrogels (Ng, Pedley and Tighe, 1976) discussed. Measurements were made at both 25°C and 34°C, i.e. at room temperature and the temperature of the cornea respectively.

The boundary effect

The nature of the barrier or boundary effect and its experimental isolation was first effectively described by Hwang, Tang and Kammermeyer (1971). Past workers in these laboratories have

pointed out its relevance to contact lens materials (Ng, Pedley and Tighe, 1976), a point which has subsequently been repeated by others (Refojo, Holly and Leong, 1977; Refojo and Leong, 1979; Peppas, Smolen and Yang, 1981). When measurements are made in the gas phase, oxygen dissolves directly in the polymer at the membrane–gas interface and the permeability coefficients show no dependence on thickness. When measurements are made in the condensed liquid phase, oxygen dissolved in this phase is hampered in its subsequent dissolution in the membrane by the presence of a structured water layer at the aqueous interface with the polymer membrane. The presence of a stagnant boundary layer in unstirred systems is well known, but the residual effect described here is observed even when the liquid is agitated. As a result, when polymer membranes of progressively decreasing thickness are used, the proportional contribution of this barrier becomes greater, a point illustrated by plotting the inverse of the apparent permeability coefficient (P_d) against the inverse of the thickness (L). Extrapolating to infinite thickness (i.e. $1/L = 0$) produces permeability coefficients similar to those obtained in the gas phase. In this treatment increased slope corresponds with increased barrier effect, and zero slope implies the absence of such effect (as in gas–gas measurements). In summary, values of P_g are independent of sample thickness, whereas individual values of P_d vary with the thickness of the specimen used. The major consequence of this effect for RGP contact lens materials is a function of the fact that improved oxygen permeability has only been achieved at the expense of some sacrifice in wetting properties. As a result, attempts to improve transport properties of a contact lens by reducing centre thickness are with these, as with all non-hydrophilic materials, faced with the law of diminishing returns, because of the residual boundary layer effect. This point is illustrated by considering the relationship between corneal oxygen requirement and polymer permeability.

The relationship of corneal oxygen requirement to the thickness and dissolved oxygen permeability coefficient (P_d) of a material can be approached in various ways. The minimum partial pressure of oxygen (sometimes called oxygen tension) required at the anterior surface of the epithelium, for the purpose of calculation, may be taken to be somewhere in the range

11–19 mmHg quoted by Polse and Mandell (1970). Taking an average value (15 mmHg) it can be assumed that this is the minimum oxygen tension required behind a contact lens during both open and closed eye conditions. This value can then be inserted (as p_2) in a relationship (Fatt and St Helen, 1971) which enables the oxygen flux (F) across the epithelial surface under a tight fitting contact lens to be determined, i.e.

$$F = \alpha p_2^\beta$$

In this equation α and β are two empirical constants having the values $\alpha = 0.24 \times 10^{-6}$ [ml(STP)]/(cm^2 s mmHg$^{1/2}$) and $\beta = 0.5$. This calculation indicates that the critical (or minimum) oxygen flux through a contact lens should be 0.93×10^{-6} ml(STP)/cm^2 per s. In alternative units this is approximately 3.5×10^{-6} l/cm^2 per h. This value compares well with independently determined values which range from 2.8 to 7.8×10^{-6} l/cm^2 per h and can, therefore, be taken as a minimum but sufficient oxygen flux (F) to maintain corneal transparency. (For explanation of units see Addendum, I p. 119.)

One way in which this information can be used is by comparing it with values obtained from the equation relating oxygen flux, thickness and dissolved oxygen permeability coefficient for contact lenses.

$$F = \frac{P_d}{L} \times \Delta p$$

L is the contact lens thickness and Δp is the pressure difference across the lens. Since the minimum partial pressure of oxygen behind the lens has been taken as 15 mmHg and since the generally accepted values for open and closed eye in the absence of a lens (Fatt and Bieber, 1968) are 155 mmHg and 55 mmHg respectively.

Δp (open eye)   = 140 mmHg

Δp (closed eye)   = 40 mmHg

Pedley (1976) has pointed out, on good evidence, that these values could, in fact, be as low as 107 mmHg and 28 mmHg respectively, but for the present calculation the earlier values will be used.

Figure 3.8 shows the result of this calculation for various contact lens materials and must be

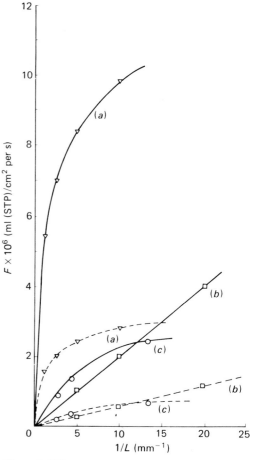

Figure 3.8 The correlation of oxygen flux (F) through the contact lens with inverse of lens thickness (L) at 34°C for various materials under open (——) and closed (----) eye conditions. (a) Silicone rubber; (b) PHEMA; (c) poly(4-methyl pent-1-ene)

used in conjunction with the 'critical' F value of 0.93×10^{-6} ml(STP)/cm^2 per s. The first point of interest is the boundary effect seen clearly here with the hydrophobic materials. It is because of this that the gaseous oxygen permeability coefficients give a misleadingly optimistic picture of the suitability of a polymer for contact lens use. In the case of a poly(4-methyl pent-1-ene) lens of 0.1 mm centre thickness the 'dissolved' permeability coefficient is about half the 'gaseous' figure. Using the latter figures one would predict that such a lens might just allow the cornea to respire normally even in the closed eye condition. Not only is this situation impossible with a lens of this thickness but as the figure shows, reducing lens thickness is of virtually no value since the boundary effect is the controlling factor at this point. Although silicone rubber shows a boundary effect its oxygen permeability is so high that this does not interfere with the oxygen flux requirements of the cornea.

PHEMA hydrogel having an equilibrium water content of 39% and a 'dissolved' oxygen permeability coefficient of 145×10^{-10} (ml O_2 mm)/(cm^2 s cmHg) at 34°C and in the form of a contact lens 0.2 mm thick would give an oxygen flux just sufficient for the corneal requirement in the open eye condition but quite insufficient in the closed eye situation. Bearing in mind that

PHEMA lenses are frequently thicker than this and Pedley's suggestion that the figure for the pressure difference across the lens should be reduced somewhat, the prediction is seen to be consistent with the fact that it is clinically desirable to avoid tight fitting for daily wear with these lenses. The material is of course unsuitable for extended wear with lenses of realistic centre thickness.

An alternative approach is to take the experimentally determined figures for the oxygen consumption of the cornea under normal conditions and calculate the relationship between oxygen permeability coefficient (P_g) and lens thickness. This has been done by Ng (1974) for both open eye and closed eye conditions and used as a basis for predicting continuous wear requirements (Ng and Tighe, 1976b). The relationship is shown in *Figure 3.9* for the range of corneal oxygen consumption figures suggested by various workers. This figure indicates that for lenses having a centre thickness of the order of 0.15 mm the minimum dissolved oxygen permeability coefficient (P_d) requirements for open and closed eye conditions are 80 and 320×10^{-10} (ml O_2 mm)/(cm^2 s cmHg) respectively. It is interesting to note that the latter figure is of the same order as values quoted for the oxygen permeability of corneal tissue.

It is important to realize that these calculations indicate the reasonableness of the concept of extended wear *in principle*. Equally, the magnitude of the predicted permeabilities of materials for successful use in extended wear depend upon many assumptions. Even when variables related to the design and fit of a lens are taken out of the equation many more uncertainties exist. These include the previously described debate relating to corneal oxygen consumption, the role of eyeball movement during sleep, the solubility of oxygen in tear fluid (as distinct from water) and the person-to-person variations, as well as the diurnal variations, that affect these factors. Whereas in the 1970s hydrogel polymers were the major group of materials to be considered in extended wear, in the 1980s the position has changed. Rigid gas permeable materials have been developed whose permeability exceeds that of conventional high water content hydrogels. Indeed, it has been suggested that the inherent 'upper ceiling' on hydrogel permeabilities, coupled with the problem of poor strength of

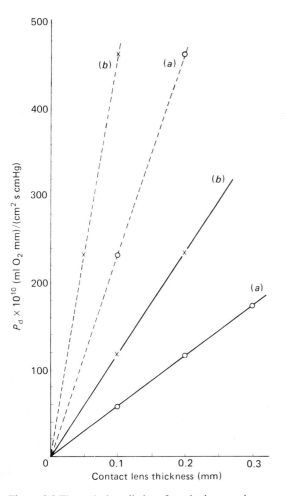

Figure 3.9 Theoretical prediction of required contact lens thickness from the 'dissolved' oxygen permeability coefficient for an oxygen flux of 3.5 or 7.0 μl/cm^2 per h under both open (———) and closed (----) eye conditions, at 34°C. (a) 3.5 μl/cm^2 per h; (b) 7.0 μl/cm^2 per h

ultrathin, high water content lenses makes hydrogels fundamentally unsuitable for safe extended wear. This viewpoint is challenged by the proponents of the use of hydrogels in this type of application, however, who point to the many unsatisfactory features of current RGP materials. The nature of these two groups of materials will now be explored in more detail, together with the characteristics of commercially available materials of each type.

Hydrogel polymers

It is simplest to regard hydrogels as 'washing line' polymers having a long (i.e. the 'washing line') backbone as described in an earlier section from which a variety of chemical groups may be suspended (the 'washing'). The function of the chemical groups in hydrogels is primarily to attract and bind water within the structure. Greater physical stability is achieved by fastening the 'washing lines' together at intervals by the use of cross-links. Some of the monomers used to achieve these structures have been previously described, to which the following may be usefully added.

2-Hydroxyethyl acrylate and methacrylate.
2- and 3-hydroxypropyl acrylate and
    methacrylate.
Acrylic acid and methacrylic acid.
Acrylamide and N-substituted acrylamides.
Methacrylamide and N-substituted
    methacrylamides.
N-Vinyl pyrrolidone and other N-vinyl lactams.
Glycidyl acrylate and methacrylate.
2-Aminoethyl acrylate and methacrylate.

These can be copolymerized in various combinations with each other and with hydrophobic monomers such as:

Methyl, ethyl or propyl acrylate or
    methacrylate.
Methoxyethyl or ethoxyethyl acrylate or
    methacrylate.
Styrene or substituted styrenes.

Some of these monomers have been mentioned previously. Of the others, the following are particularly important.

N-Vinyl pyrrolidone, Acrylamide, 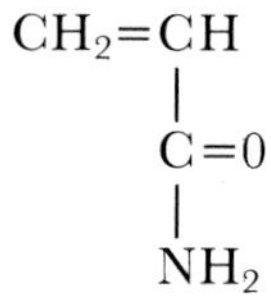 Methoxyethyl methacrylate structures; divinyl compound and ethylene glycol dimethacrylate structures shown.

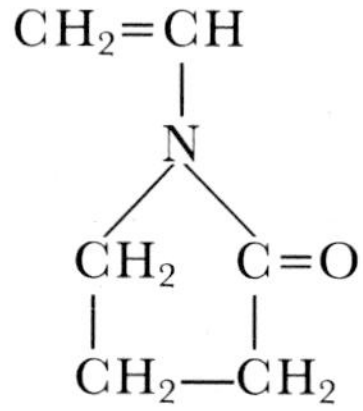

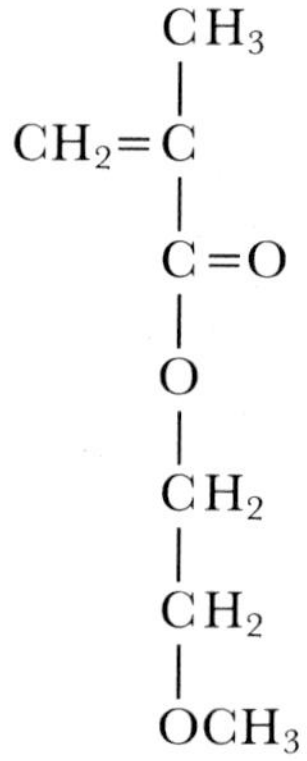

The incorporation of cross-links is usually achieved by copolymerizing small (of the order of 1%) quantities of divinyl compounds such as:

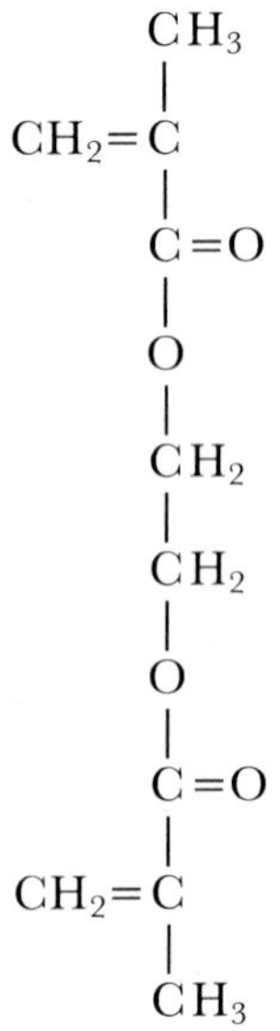

ethylene glycol dimethacrylate with the monomer mixture. Hydrogels formed in this way (i.e.

in which the network is linked together by primary chemical bonds) are the most satisfactory type for contact lens usage. There are, however, other classes of hydrogel (for example polyelectrolyte complexes and microcrystalline gels such as those of cellulose or collagen) which either because of fabrication difficulties or instability under conditions of changing pH and tonicity are less suitable for this application. A survey of the earlier literature on various types of hydrogels and its relevance to contact lens work can be found elsewhere (Larke, Ng and Tighe, 1971).

From the previous discussion on the desirable ranges of various properties under both open eye and closed eye conditions, available on the cornea and its possible use as a model structure, and a knowledge of the way in which the various available monomers govern the properties of the hydrogels that they produce, it should be possible to assess the feasibility of designing a hydrogel for use in both daily wear and extended wear lenses.

The patent literature

A useful picture of the development of commercial hydrogel lenses can be obtained by looking at the patent literature. The chemistry of most of the materials used commercially today is based on ideas described in patents that had been published by the early 1970s. A brief overview of these developments will provide a useful background to the information on commercially important material types, although little protection of the significant ideas seems to have been provided by the patents. The situation in RGP materials was similar, until recent successful patent litigation was undertaken. A comprehensive review of the patents in this field published up to 1981 has been compiled (Pedley, Skelly and Tighe, 1982) and the information relating to their assignment and publication is detailed therein. An abbreviated compilation is listed in Addendum II. The growth of the patent literature in this area has been affected by several factors. The extensive evaluation of novel hydrogel structures in the contact lens field in comparison to the almost unique dependence upon PHEMA in other biomedical areas is largely a result of the comparative ease of clinical investigation in the former case but

has also been greatly influenced by the fact that the consequences of biocompatibility problems in the eye are slight in comparison with those involving blood contact. In addition the specific permeability requirements for extended wear have led to the exploration of compositions that will produce relatively high equilibrium water contents. Another major feature has been the initial lack of restrictive legislation in either Europe or America followed in late 1968 by the decision of the Federal Food and Drugs Administration to classify soft contact lenses as a drug. This had the effect of limiting the exploratory clinical work carried out in the USA since that time and served as a result to curtail activity in the clinical field. In contrast patent activity in the UK began slowly but showed marked growth in the 1970s. Of the other countries showing activity, Japan has shown the most marked recent growth in published patent specifications.

The 1960s and the work of Wichterle

The earliest hydrogel patents are those of Wichterle and his co-workers, whose work has already been mentioned. In subsequent years, these have been expanded and enlarged covering both processes for lens production and the composition of materials. The claims of the original patents encompass the formation of sparingly cross-linked soft and elastic hydrogels both by polymerization of hydrophilic monomers and alternatively by the cross-linking of preformed hydrophilic (water-soluble) polymers. Although the latter method, which is typified by the cross-linking of polyvinyl alcohol with adipic acid, is a useful hydrogel-forming reaction, it is not readily adapted to the manufacture of contact lenses. The polymerization of hydrophilic monomers, such as 2-hydroxyethyl methacrylate (HEMA) in the presence of ethylene glycol dimethacrylate (EGDMA), however, is ideally suited to lens formation. The major lens-forming processes suggested by Wichterle included polymerization of the monomers *in situ* in a rotating contact lens mould as well as bulk polymerization in rod or button form followed by shaping of the polymer to lens form and then by hydration. It was not until the invention was taken up in the USA that commercial success was obtained. The success of this original work may be judged, however, from the fact that a major proportion of the soft lenses sold today are based, directly or indirectly, on Wichterle's patents.

Although Wichterle's original patents envisaged the use of monomers other than HEMA their primary concern is with the technique of manufacture of hydrogels *per se* and particularly with their application in the contact lens field. The specific advantages of monomers other than HEMA are not described and their role has been largely unexploited, except in the contact lens field. Thus although Wichterle's patents in the period 1961–68 mention the possible use of some other monomers (for example, acrylamide, methacrylic acid and dimethylaminoethyl methacrylate) no indication is given of the benefits that these might confer either in terms of the physical properties of hydrogels or improved characteristics of the lenses formed from them. It was not until the early 1970s that the patents began to appear in which such benefits were described. The major feature of the large number of claims published at this time was the use of *N*-vinyl pyrrolidone (usually referred to simply as vinyl pyrrolidone and abbreviated as NVP). Two methods of use of vinyl pyrrolidone in hydrogels can be distinguished. These are graft copolymers and random copolymers (more correctly called statistical copolymers). Using the washing line analogy, random copolymers consist of two or more types of washing attached in random (rather than perfectly alternating) sequence along the line, or polymer chain. In a graft copolymer a washing line is first assembled and additional pieces of washing attached so that they trail from the existing pieces in short secondary chains. The appearance is thus something like a comb with irregular and rather long teeth.

Vinyl pyrrolidone patents

The distinction of the first patent publication involving the use of a poly(vinyl pyrrolidone) (PVP) backbone onto which 2-hydroxyethyl methacrylate was grafted must go to H. R. Leeds whose American patent application was filed in October 1968 and published some 2 years later. Shortly afterwards (first filing July 1969, published February 1972) Maurice Seiderman in a series of patents described a similar process involving the use of polyvinyl pyrroli-

done backbone onto which, in addition to HEMA, vinyl pyrrolidone monomer was grafted. The use of other monomers such as lauryl methacrylate, cyclohexyl methacrylate, 2-aminoethyl methacrylate and methacrylamide as modifiers is also described and water contents as high as 87% are claimed.

The third group of workers whose contribution to the hydrogel patent literature in the polyvinyl pyrrolidone graft copolymer field must be considered are O'Driscoll and Isen. Although the date of first filing (November 1969) is slightly later than that of Leeds and Seiderman, the patents are important because they formed the basis both of the Griffin Lens and of later continuation patents assigned to Warner-Lambert and American Optical Corporation. The O'Driscoll and Isen patents are based on graft copolymers of a hydroxyalkyl methacrylate (such as HEMA) and polyvinyl pyrrolidone. The significant difference, however, between their patents and earlier ones covering polyvinyl pyrrolidone graft copolymers is a post-polymerization radiation treatment and treatment in the hydrated state with hydrogen peroxide. These steps are claimed to increase the toughness and elasticity of the final lens. The possibility (common to all polyvinyl pyrrolidone graft copolymers) of low-molecular-weight polyvinyl pyrrolidone being leached out over a period of time has caused problems with this type of hydrogel. There is a substantial amount of anecdotal information linking this phenomenon with grief cases encountered in the early use of the Griffin lens (which played a significant part in the development of early high water content lenses). For that reason direct copolymerization of vinyl pyrrolidone with other monomers has generally proved more satisfactory although a number of improved PVP/HEMA-based materials have maintained the commercial importance of graft copolymers.

Because of its great hydrophilicity the use of vinyl pyrrolidone offers the obvious advantage over simple PHEMA of increased water contents. In addition to the graft copolymers described above, NVP may be used to produce high water content gels by simple copolymerization of mixtures of monomers. The earliest patent to describe such copolymers and their advantages in the contact lens field is that of Robert Steckler (file date April 1969). The patent describes copolymerization of 60–90%

Table 3.2 Lenses and lens materials having water contents lower than PHEMA

Name	Manufacturer	Principal components	Water content (%)	USAN nomenclature
Durasoft	Wesley–Jessen	HEMA/2-ethoxyethyl methacrylate copolymer	30	Phemefilcon
AL-47	Alden Optical		36	Isofilcon
Flexol-35	Burton Parsons	HEMA copolymer	35	—
Gelflex	Dow Corning Ophthalmics	HEMA/MMA copolymer with TEGMA cross-links	36	Dimefilcon-A
Hoyasoft	Hoya Corporation	HEMA copolymer	35	—
Menicon Soft	Toyo Contact Lens	HEMA, vinyl acetate, pentyl methacrylate	29	Mafilcon

See also Tables 11.1 and 22.2.

by weight of an *N*-vinyl lactam (e.g. *N*-vinyl pyrrolidone) with 40–10% vinyl or acrylate ester (e.g. vinyl acetate, HEMA or methyl acrylate) to produce hydrogels with water contents ranging from 35 to 95%. Similar concepts are outlined, but with less detail, by Maurice Seiderman in one of his patents. Although Seiderman's poly(vinyl pyrrolidone) graft copolymers are disclosed in patents contemporary with that of Steckler his claims relating to monomer copolymerization are made some time later (file date November 1970).

A similar delay occurs before the filing of patents in the names of the two British workers who are associated with this particular area (namely John de Carle and Philip Cordrey). These patents (de Carle and Cordrey *et al.*) were in fact filed after the publication of Steckler's American patent and contain no new disclosures in terms of the monomers employed. Since they claim copolymers of vinyl pyrrolidone with HEMA (de Carle) and with methyl methacrylate (Cordrey), however, they jointly represent the first British work to be filed in this area. The patents do extend the ratio of monomers employed to encompass the possibility of using somewhat lower quantities of vinyl pyrrolidone. Later patents assigned to the American Optical Corporation pursue this trend to the extent of incorporating as little as 10–20% of vinyl pyrrolidone in copolymers with alkyl and hydroxyalkyl acrylates and methacrylates (e.g. methyl methacrylate or HEMA).

It is quite clear, however, that the credit for first description of this group of hydrogels, which play such a large part in current contact lens technology, must go to Robert Steckler. In the succeeding years over 100 hydrogel patents relating to contact lens materials have been published, covering novel monomers, novel cross-linking agents and modified methods of polymerization. Relatively few of these have achieved commercial significance, and none has had the influence of the key patents described above. This is clearly demonstrated by reference to the range of commercial materials that have been developed in the last two decades.

Commercial lenses, materials and their properties

It is virtually impossible to keep abreast of the worldwide position relating to the appearance

Table 3.3 Lenses and lens materials based principally on PHEMA

Name	Manufacturer or supplier	USAN nomenclature*
Alcon-38	Alcon Labs (UK)	—
Aoflex	American Optical	
AO Multivue	American Optical	Tefilcon
Duracon (Medigel-38)	Medicornea	—
Flexicon	Söhnges	—
Geltakt	Spofa-Ergon Co	
Hydroflex	Zeiss (Wöhlk)	—
Hydron	Hydron Europe	Polymacon
Profil-H	Essilor	
Semisoft-38	Toyko Contact Lens Research Institute	—
Snoflex-38	Smith & Nephew	
Soflens	Bausch & Lomb	Polymacon
Weicon	Ciba Vision (Titmus Eurocon)	

*USAN equivalents also include: Tefilcon (Cibasoft, Cibathin, Torisoft, Softint, Bisoft); Polymacon (CustomEyes 38, Vesoft, Synsoft, Cellusoft, Soform II, Omega, Nuview, Cooper 38, Metrosoft II). *See also Tables 11.1 and 22.2.*

Table 3.4 Lenses or lens materials with water contents greater than 40%

Name	Manufacturer/supplier	Principal components*	Water content (%)	USAN nomenclature†
Accugel	Strieter Labs	HEMA, PVP, MA	47	Droxifilcon-A
Accusoft	Ophthalmos Inc.	HEMA, PVP	47	Droxifilcon-A
Amsoft	Lombart Lenses	HEMA, BMA	43	Deltafilcon-A
AO-Soft	American Optical	HEMA, NVP, MMA	42.5	Tetrafilcon-A
Aquaflex	UCO Optics	HEMA, NVP, MMA	42.5	Tetrafilcon-A
Comfortflex	Capital Contact Lens	HEMA, BMA	43	Deltafilcon-A
CSI 38	Corneal Sciences	MMA, glyceryl methacrylate	40	Crofilcon-A
Custom Flex	Custom Contact Lens	HEMA, BMA	43	Deltafilcon-A
Duragel (=Permaflex)	Duralens/ CooperVision Optics	NVP/MMA	73	—
Flexol	Burton Parsons	HEMA, AMA, MA	72	—
Flexlens	Flexlens Inc.	HEMA, NVP	43	Hefilcon-A
Hydralens	Ophthalmos Inc.	HEMA, PVP	47	Droxifilcon-A
Hydrocurve (I)	Soft Lenses Inc.	HEMA, NVP	43	Hefilcon-A
Hydrocurve (II)	Soft Lenses Inc.	HEMA, diacetone acrylamide	55	Bufilcon-A
Hydrocon	Kontur Kontact Lens	HEMA, PVP	56	—
Hydromarc	Frontier Contact Lens (Automated Optics)	HEMA, MA	43	Etafilcon-A
Igel 68	Igel Optics	MMA/NVP/CMA	68	Xylofilcon-A
Lunelle	Essilor	AMA/NVP	70	
Naturvue	Automated Optics	HEMA, NVP	43	Hefilcon-A
Permalens	CooperVision Optics	HEMA, NVP, MA	71	Perfilcon-A
Permaflex 43	CooperVision Optics	HEMA, NVP, MMA	43	Tetrafilcon-A
Permaflex 74	CooperVision Optics	MMA, NVP	74	Surfilcon-A
Sauflon 50	Contact Lens Mfg	NVP, MMA	50	Lidofilcon-A
Sauflon 70	Contact Lens Mfg	NVP, MMA	70	Lidofilcon-A
Sauflon PW	Contact Lens Mfg	NVP, MMA	80	Lidofilcon-B
Scanlens	Scanlens	MMA/NVP	73	—
Snoflex 50	Smith & Nephew	MMA, NVP, MHPM	52	—
Sof-Form	Salvatori	HEMA, BMA	43	Deltafilcon-A
Softcon	American Optical	HEMA, PVP	55	Vifilcon-A
Soft Site	Paris Contact Lens	HEMA, NVP	46	Hefilcon-A
Theraflex	Union Optics	NVP, MMA, glycidyl methacrylate	60	—
Tresoft	Alcon Optics	HEMA, MA	46	Ocufilcon
Tripol 43	Capital Contact Lenses (Comfortflex Hydrophilics)	HEMA, BMA	43	Deltafilcon-A
Visimarc		HEMA/MA	43	Etafilcon
Vistagel A	Vista Optics	MMA/NVP	60	—
Welflex 55	Wöhlk	AMA/NVP	55	—

* HEMA = 2-hydroxyethyl methacrylate; NVP = *N*-vinyl pyrrolidone; PVP = polyvinyl pyrrolidone (i.e. graft copolymer); MA = methacrylic acid; MMA = methyl methacrylate; BMA = butyl (probably isobutyl) methacrylate; AMA = alkyl methacrylate; MPHM = 3-methoxy-2-hydroxypropyl methacrylate; TEGMA = triethylene glycol methacrylate; CMA = cyclohexyl methacrylate.
† USAN = United States Approved Name Council: many other USAN equivalents exist, e.g. Hefilcon (Bausch & Lomb Toric, Miracon); Deltafilcon (Aquasoft, Metrosoft, Soft Form Toric, Softics, Softflow, Softact); Lidofilcon (B&L 70, CV 70, Genesis 4, Hydrosight 70, Q&E 70, Lubrisof, PDC 70, N&N 70).
See also Tables 11.1 and 22.2.

and disappearance of commercial materials but it is instructive to take an overview of the range of materials that have been available in recent years. *Tables 3.2–3.4* show names, principal components, water contents and manufacture of various materials and lenses. The materials are divided into these, based substantially on PHEMA and having water contents around 40% (*Table 3.3*) together with those of lower (*Table 3.2*) and higher (*Table 3.4*) water content. Many of the properties of hydrogels are controlled predominantly by the amount of water in the gel. It is more convenient to describe the properties of hydrogels as a class of materials, noting how these are affected by the water and by the polymer matrix. Because of the importance of the water content of a hydrogel, it is appropriate to start with this.

Water content

This is the most important single property of hydrogel and is more correctly called the equilibrium water content (EWC). Some confusion has arisen between this term and 'water uptake'. If a dry polymer takes up its own weight of water its equilibrium water content, which is defined as:

$$\frac{\text{Weight of water}}{\text{Weight of hydrated gel}} \times 100\%$$

will be 50%. It is important to define the temperature at which the measurement was made and whether this was made in pure water or saline solution. It will become apparent that the water content of a gel measured in water at 20°C can be quite different from its value at eye temperature and in isotonic saline.

PHEMA hydrogel has an equilibrium water content of approximately 39% (depending upon conditions of measurement). This can be progressively reduced by copolymerizing with increasing amounts of a hydrophobic monomer such as methyl methacrylate or styrene. It can on the other hand be progressively increased by copolymerizing with increasing amounts of a more hydrophilic monomer such as vinyl pyrrolidone or acrylamide. Vinyl pyrrolidone and acrylamide can alternatively be copolymerized with, for example, methyl methacrylate. The water contents of the resultant polymers are dependent upon the relative proportions of hydrophilic and hydrophobic monomers. Leaving aside the sophistications of graft vs random copolymerization and spin-cast vs bulk polymerized materials we can use this as a basis for categorizing available lens material. Thus the three main groups of materials described above correspond to the three tables of commercial lenses (*Tables 3.2–3.4*). The compositional information taken together with earlier comments on the patents gives a useful overview of the ways in which a range of water contents may be achieved.

Dimensional stability

Since the linear swell and volume swell shown by hydrogels on hydration is a direct consequence of the volume of water absorbed, any phenomena that cause a change in water content will cause a change in lens dimensions.

PHEMA is an extremely stable hydrogel and variations in temperature, pH and tonicity have relatively little effect on its water content. The use of monomers that are more hydrophilic than HEMA invariably incurs some penalty in this respect, whether the monomer is more hydrophilic because of a basic nitrogen atom (as in *N*-vinyl pyrrolidone and acrylamide) or of an acidic hydrogen atom (as in methacrylic and acrylic acid). The precise combination of monomers used can have a marked effect on the stability of the material. This is illustrated with respect to temperature changes in *Figure 3.10*. Several features are noteworthy including (1) the uniquely regular behaviour of PHEMA, (2) the decrease in water content in other cases between 20°C and 40°C, which is attributable to an increase in hydrophobic interaction or bonding in the gel, and (3) the dramatic

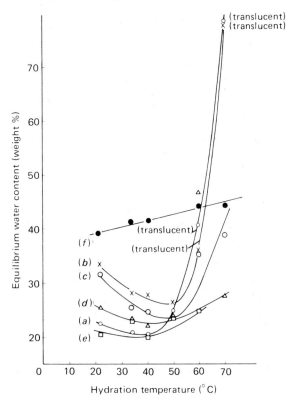

Figure 3.10 Effect of temperature on the equilibrium water contents of various hydrogels based on hydroxypropyl methacrylate (HPMA) and *N*-vinyl 2-pyrrolidone (NVP). (*a*) HPMA; (*b*) HPMA:NVP (80:20); (*c*) HPMA:NVP (80:20) + 1% EGDMA; (*d*) HPMA:NVP (80:20) + 5% EGDMA; (*e*) HPMA:NVP (80:20) + 10% EGDMA. The gels are cross-linked with ethylene glycol dimethacrylate (EGDMA). PHEMA (*f*) is shown for comparison

increase in water content with concurrent onset of translucency shown by some compositions at temperatures above 60°C. This type of instability would obviously be most undesirable in a lens that was to be heat sterilized since, although the behaviour is reversible, it leads to progressive deterioration of the polymer network. The figure also shows how increasing the cross-link density decreases the freedom of chains to rotate, thereby restricting the ability of the polymer network to expand with increasing temperature.

The sensitivity of water content to tonicity is similarly affected by monomer structure (*Figure 3.11*). In general, hydrogels show some small decrease in water content when the equilibration solution is changed from pure water to isotonic saline. It should be emphasized, however, that such a change, and others induced by changing the nature of the storage solution, are much greater than those brought about by

tonicity variations in the eye. Variations with respect to pH are much more marked and monomer dependent, as minima in water content are often observed with varying pH. The pH changes involved in such studies are vastly greater than those occurring diurnally or on a patient-to-patient basis on the eye, which lie well within one pH unit.

Mechanical properties

In its dehydrated state, PHEMA (and indeed most other hydrogel forming polymers) is hard and brittle. In this it resembles polymethyl methacrylate. When swollen in water, however, it becomes soft and rubber-like with a very low tear and tensile strength. This lack of mechanical strength has, of course, a profound effect on the lifetime of the lens. Although the water content has a marked effect on mechanical strength, the chemical structure of the polymer can also play a large part in determining its value. This point can be best illustrated by comparing the tensile strength of PHEMA with that of cellophane. Bixler and Michaels (1968) have reported that cellophane with a water content of 55% has a tensile modulus of nearly 5 times and an ultimate strength of over 50 times that of PHEMA.

Although water content plays a large part in controlling the mechanical properties in hydrogels it is, therefore, only one of several factors. It is possible to produce very stable high (>70%) water content gels. Considerable current interest centres on the preparation of synthetic hydrogels which more closely mimic the composite hydrophilic gels, such as articular cartilage and the cornea, which are found in nature.

The elastic behaviour and rigidity of hydrogels is, consequently, closely governed by monomer structure and effective cross-link density, which includes not only covalent cross-link but also ionic, polar and steric interchain forces. By use of modified monomer combinations and cross-linking agents, high water content polymers with reasonable stability and elasticity can be prepared. It will be apparent that there are now commercially available high water content lenses which are vastly superior in strength to the earlier generation of fragile gels of similar water content based on HEMA–vinyl pyrrolidone. In general,

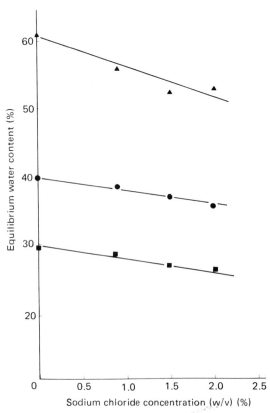

Figure 3.11 The equilibrium water contents of some hydrogels in hydrating solutions of various sodium chloride concentrations at 20°C. ▲ HEMA:NVP:styrene (47.5:47.5:5); ● PHEMA; ■ HEMA:styrene (95:5)

making hydrogels with good elastic response and reasonable rigidity is very much less of a problem than overcoming the poor tear strength of such materials. Unfortunately, however, the problem of poor tear strength is fundamental to these materials and, although interpenetrating network techniques have been used to produce optically clear 'composite' hydrogel wound dressings having high tear strength, the principles have not yet been extended to commercially available contact lenses.

Oxygen permeability

This topic has been discussed at some length and it is only necessary at this point to indicate that oxygen permeability of hydrogels is governed by the water content (W%). This is illustrated in *Figure 3.12* which demonstrates that permeability varies with water content according to the expression (at 34°C)

$$P_d = 24 \times 10^{-10}\, e^{0.0443W}\, \text{(ml (STP) mm)}/\text{(cm}^2\text{ s cmHg)}$$

Although the increase in oxygen permeability coefficient with this change in temperature is quite marked (a factor of approximately two, given the same water content at both temperatures), this may not be representative of the change in P_d for a given hydrogel. The reason for this is the previously discussed observation that many hydrogels decrease in water content with increasing temperature in this region. To calculate the oxygen permeability of a hydrogel at 34°C then, it is necessary to use the value of the water content determined at that temperature. Thus a value for P_d of 350×10^{-10} (ml O$_2$ mm)/(cm^2 s cmHg) at 34°C would be given by a gel having a water content of something over 60% at that temperature. The water content of that same gel at 25°C might, however, be nearer 70%. According to the more modest of the corneal requirement predictions discussed earlier, this would represent the minimum water content required for an extended wear lens having a centre thickness of around 0.15 mm.

PHEMA hydrogel having an equilibrium water content of 39% and a 'dissolved' oxygen permeability coefficient of 145×10^{-10} (ml O$_2$ mm)/(cm^2 s cmHg) at 34°C and in the form of a contact lens 0.2 mm thick would give an oxygen flux just sufficient for the corneal requirement in the open eye condition but quite insufficient in the closed eye situation. One advantage of

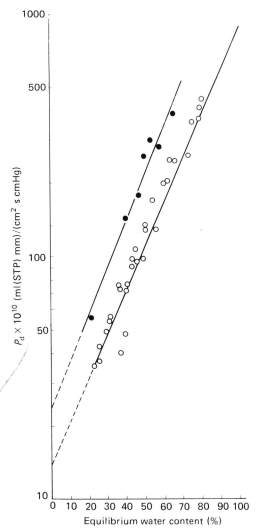

Figure 3.12 The variation of log dissolved oxygen permeability coefficient (P_d) as a function of water content for various hydrogels at 25°C (○) and 34°C (●)

hydrogels is the virtual absence of a boundary layer effect, because of the low interfacial tension with water. This means that thinner samples of the materials give progressively more effective net transport.

Optical transmittance

Transparency is obviously an essential requisite of a hydrogel for contact lens use, but not all hydrogels are optically transparent. Translucence and opacity in hydrogels is associated with microphase separation of water which thereby produces regions of differing refractive index within the gel. Although it is possible to synthesize hydrogels that show this type of behaviour (e.g. by making copolymers with large blocks or segments of hydrophobic and hydrophilic monomers rather then randomly dispersing them), in contact lens usage the unwanted onset of translucency assumes greater importance. This is usually associated with sudden or large changes in temperature which induce the gel to absorb excessive quantities of water. This point, which has been illustrated in *Figure 3.11* with respect to the thermal stability of hydrogels is, fortunately, normally reversible.

Density

The density of hydrogel polymers depends upon both the water content and the monomer composition. Very low water content (and fairly rigid) gels containing styrene as the hydrophobic monomer have the greatest densities of the common hydrogels. These are around 1.22 g/ml at 10% water content and 20°C. Typical copolymers containing HEMA and the more hydrophilic monomers decrease progressively from around 1.16 at 38% water content to around 1.05 at 75% water content (all at 20°C).

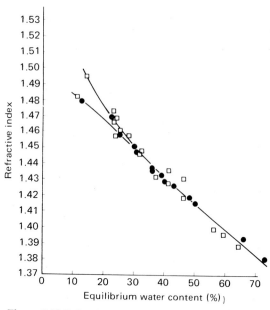

Figure 3.13 Refractive indices of various hydrogels as a function of their equilibrium water contents at 20°C (●) and 34°C (□)

Refractive index

Refractive index again decreases progressively with increasing water content. The variation is almost linear with water content, and the results for hydrogels of the various types indicated above lie within a fairly narrow, almost rectilinear band, decreasing from 1.46–1.48 at 20% water content to 1.37–1.38 at 75% water content. This point is illustrated in *Figure 3.13*. This figure also illustrates the point that refractive index measurement can be used as a rapid method of determining the approximate water content of an unknown gel. The method suffers from inherent inaccuracies, including the assumption that dehydrated hydrogels all have the same refractive index (whereas they can be very different). Despite this, the procedure is very convenient and enables the approximate water content of a lens to be determined quickly (*see* Chapter 13).

Surface properties

It is apparent that hydrogels do not suffer deficiencies in terms of inherent wettability. Indeed, it may be desirable to reduce their ability in this respect. One related factor that contributes to the comfort of hydrogels is the low coefficient between the lens and the eyelid. This frictional interaction is much greater with elastomers of similar bulk rigidity (such as ethylene propylene terpolymer and silicone rubber) even after surface treatment. Hydrogels are, however, not truly hydrophilic (in terms of the precise definition stated earlier) since they exhibit an equilibrium advancing contact angle of around 20°. If this value could be raised, however, it may be possible to retain wettability by tear fluid while decreasing the problems of lens cleaning.

The fact that such a variety of structures is possible in hydrogel chemistry, coupled with the fact that equilibrium water content, oxygen permeability, mechanical properties and surface characteristics are interrelated with structure in different ways make it possible, in principle, to design hydrogels to fulfil a wide range of functions. That range certainly includes contact lenses for both daily and extended wear. It is somewhat paradoxical that the hydrophilic nature of these materials, although overcoming the initial problems of the tear film instability, has given rise to a variety of surface-related problems associated with lens spoilation. These are dealt with in the following section.

The nature and occurrence of lens spoilation (*see also* Chapters 4 and 13)

The interaction of the hydrogels with biological fluids has been widely studied in recent years. Blood contact devices and blood interaction problems have undoubtedly commanded greatest attention, and the role of protein deposition has been recognized to be of paramount importance. Baker and Tighe (1981) have contrasted the nature of tears and blood on the basis of available literature and drawn attention to similarities and differences in factors affecting polymer compatibility, particularly with respect to the role of protein deposition in two cases. No account of hydrogels as contact lenses would be complete without an account of the range and nature of phenomena which are commonly collected together under the umbrella term 'spoilation'. A more complete overview has been compiled by Bowers and Tighe (1987a) where a detailed compilation of the primary references may be found. Ironically, this only became a major materials problem with the advent of soft hydrogel lenses providing as they did greater comfort and allowing extended wearing times.

The term 'spoilation' is used to encompass physical and chemical changes in the nature of hydrogel contact lenses and the various extraneous deposits which may impair the optical properties of the lens or produce symptoms of discomfort and often intolerance to the wearer. The extent of the situation may be appreciated by considering the reported incidence of lens spoilation which, in clinical records, varies from less than 10% to over 80% of extended wear lenses. Lens spoilation occurs in the majority of cases in some 3–6 months of daily or particularly extended wear, although it has been observed within 48 hours of wear. The degree of lens spoilation appears to be independent of the level of lens hydration but several workers have noted that there appear to be differences in the types of spoilation depending on the type of hydrogel lens used.

Although it is convenient in an overview to divide the observed types of spoilation into different classes, such a classification is largely artificial. There is considerable overlap between the classes and systematic analyses of the results of spoilation are rarely undertaken in conjunction with clinical reports relating to incidence. The classification is best regarded, therefore, as a grouping of various related types of clinically observed phenomena. An indication is given of the current view of the occurrence, chemical composition and potential aetiology for each clinically observed 'class' of lens spoilation.

Discrete elevated deposits

Probably the most chemically complex manifestations of ocular incompatibility are discrete elevated deposits, the so-called 'white spots' varying in diameter up to around 1 mm and found on the anterior lens surface (*see Plate 32*). They are also referred to in the contact lens literature as mucoprotein–lipid and mucopolysaccharide deposits. Ruben and others (e.g. Tripathi, Tripathi and Ruben, 1980) cite the deposition of mucoprotein–lipid deposits on lenses as a major cause of spoilation, with a reported incidence of up to 80% of patients fitted. Such a figure is, however, very much higher than the incidence in general clinical practice.

There is a considerable variation in the reports of the chemical composition of this group of deposits from patient to patient which has given rise to continued speculation as to their origin. Much of the variation arises from differences in quality and sensitivity of the analytical work. Tear solutes include proteins (principally albumin, globulin, lysozyme, but many others), amino acids, mucin, glycoproteins, glucose and lipids (phospholipids, neutral fats, fatty acids, cholesterol and its esters), calcium, potassium, chloride, bicarbonate, phosphate and urea. Individual variations do, however, exist, especially in the mucoprotein content and in the meibomian secretions, and this may be further influenced by the stimulus of contact lens wear. It is obvious, therefore, that the tears are a constantly available source for many of the components of deposit formation. To this, however, must be added the products of normally desquamating epithelial cells and, in pathological conditions, necrotic tissue as well as altered tear components.

Apart from the problem of lens decentring leading to poor fit, mucoprotein–lipid deposits lead to a decrease in visual acuity and give rise to injury of the cornea and palpebral conjunctiva. Patients with such deposits on their lenses often show clinical conditions such as giant papillary, follicular and other allergic conjunctivitis as depicted in *Plates 47–51* and *55–58*. It is thought that these conditions result either from mechanical irritation of the deposits on the conjunctiva or the absorbed proteins providing an antigenic stimulus initiating an autoimmune response (Allansmith, Korb and Greiner, 1977).

Lens coatings

A major class of spoilation involves surface films, coatings and plaques. One group of these, which are related to discrete deposits, although somewhat more geographically dispersed, are the so-called protein films. Such films are characterized by a thin, semi-opaque, white superficial layered structure which appears to consist of denatured protein. The films vary in their extent of lens coverage as seen in *Plates 25* and *45*, ranging from small patches to complete covering of the lens surface. The general accumulation of protein films on soft lenses leads to an increase in surface haziness and surface rugosity. A decrease in visual acuity results is due both to lens opacity and to poor lens movement on the eye. Red eye, increased irritation and conjunctivitis are typical patient responses to protein covered lenses. These deposits have been variously attributed to mucoproteins, albumin, globulins, glycoproteins and mucin.

Karageozian (1976) has reported that protein films consist mainly of denatured lysozyme. Since lysozyme comprises only 18% of the total tear protein in comparison with some 60% albumin and 22% globulin, selective adsorption was proposed. Hathaway and Lowther (1976), however, reported that albumin, as well as lysozyme, forms marked deposits in a short period of time. Not surprisingly, the incidence of proteinaceous films is higher on thermally disinfected daily wear lenses.

Inorganic films are similar in gross appearance to protein films although their incidence is lower. Heavy inorganic films often cause damage to the lens surface (*Plates 36–40*), since the material may penetrate into the lens matrix. They are frequently covered with protein that smoothes the underlying rough inorganic material, which is composed mainly of calcium phosphate. The deposit may well be hydroxy-apatite, the thermodynamically stable phase of calcium phosphate commonly encountered in biological conditions. Once nucleated, hydroxyapatite will grow directly from slightly supersaturated solutions like tears. The mechanism discussed by Bloomfield, David and Rubin (1978) which leads to corneal calcification, may contribute to hydrophilic lens calcification, although this has not been widely recognized. Briefly, the release of calcium and phosphorus from injured cells could increase the calcium–phosphorus product locally. The activation together with release of such cellular enzymes as alkaline phosphatase and adenosine triphosphatase which are present in corneal cells, also may lead to local calcification. These enzymes have pyrophosphatase activity, i.e. they cause the hydrolysis of pyrophosphate to phosphate. Pyrophosphates are inorganic compounds that are widely distributed in the body and act as physiological inhibitors of calcification in soft tissues. It is clear that phosphate-buffered contact lens solutions increase the probability of calcium phosphate formation on lens surfaces, especially if the solution contains a measurable calcium ion concentration.

Microbial spoilation

One of the most serious hazards of soft lens wear is spoilage due to invasion and contamination by microbial organisms. Separate studies have produced similar figures for the occurrence of this type of spoilation. They have indicated that in one set of patients some 24% of patient lenses showed problems related to the presence of pathogenic organisms and in another about 30% of patients fitted with soft lenses carry such organisms. Normally the lens surface can be expected to have traces of microorganisms due to the presence of harmless flora, including fungi of the conjunctival sac. Many species of fungi and yeasts have been identified on soft lenses (*see Plate 33*). Among these are the yeasts of the *Rodotonita* species, *Candida tropicales*, *fusarium* and *albicans* together with fungi such as *Aspergillus fumigatus*, *Aspergillus niger* and *Penicillium* sp. Additionally, the presence of the fungus *Cephalosporium acremonium* on and within a therapeutic soft lens has been noted. Factors which may influence soft lens infiltration by fungi include enzymatic activity, produced by the fungus, which leads to polymer degradation, thus providing a matrix and nutrient source for fungal growth. Protein deposits and other debris are thought to predispose lenses to fungal invasion. Prevention through adequate cleaning and disinfection procedures must be practised because microbial colonies, once established, are extremely difficult to eradicate.

Several workers have reported the presence of bacteria on both the anterior and posterior surfaces. Fowler, Greiner and Allansmith (1979) found bacterial cells on the anterior surface of several lenses; each lens surface was found to be contaminated with dried mucus. Some bacteria were scattered randomly over the surface, with no apparent attachment to the surface of the lens, whereas others were attached to the coated surface by thin, flagella-like pseudopodia $0.1-1.3\,\mu m$ in diameter. The distal ends of these structures were free and unattached to the surface. Several bacteria were actually embedded in the surface coating, whilst others were aggregated around clumps of mucus. It would therefore appear that bacteria may use the lens coating as a nutrient source, and as a result of their attachment and proliferation may provide antigenic mass.

Lens discolouration

The discolouration of hydrogel contact lenses appears to be a major drawback in the use of such materials although the frequency of its occurrence is not well documented. An increase in incidence of discolouration or loss of lens transparency has been linked with several factors including nicotine from cigarettes, topical adrenaline and topical vasoconstrictors as well as components from the tear fluid. The possible nature of discolouration is described in various papers of which the most noteworthy is that of Kleist (1979). Yellow or brown discoloured lenses (*Plate 35*) have been found to contain granular particles deposited just below the lens surface. In summary, this is believed to be structurally similar to melanin, the skin pigment and to be immobilized within the hydrogel matrix. Adrenaline and other similar compounds used in eye medications may play a potential role in lens discolouration since they may be taken up by the lens. Additionally, adrenochrome is believed to be a possible precursor of melanin. Therefore the presence of adrenochrome in eye medications may enhance the natural production of melanin. Similarly, melanin production is stimulated by nicotine and the other polycyclic aromatic compounds in tobacco smoke. Thus it is not a direct discolouration but a nicotine-stimulated biochemical mechanism. Some preservatives, notably chlorhexidine derivatives and sorbic acid, appear to enhance discolouration in some circumstances. This is discussed further in Chapter 4.

Summary

From this brief overview certain obvious conclusions may be drawn. The chemical composition of lens deposits is extremely complex and nearly all chemical components found to be present in lens deposits are contained within the tear film. It has been noted by several workers that differing hydrogel polymeric compositions appear to highlight relatively specific deposit types. Another variable in what appears to be a multifactoral problem is the composition of the tear film — great differences in component concentrations have been noted from one individual to another. In summary, therefore, hydrophilic soft lens spoilation results primarily from the interaction of the polymer with the microenvironment of the eye. Differing degrees of spoilation from one polymeric composition to another result not only from differences in surface chemistry of the material but also differences in the patient tear film together with the design and fit of the lens.

A series of recent papers in the journal *Biomaterials* describes work carried out in these laboratories using a novel array of analytical techniques in conjunction with lenses worn under clinical supervision. This work (e.g. Bowers and Tighe, 1987b,c) has established the importance of the role of lipids in the initiation of 'white spot' formation, and the existence of a common biological interface conversion process. This means that in cases where white spots are formed they have a very similar morphology and composition. Additionally, changes in the surface chemistry of lens materials affects the rate of white spot formation, rather than the ultimate fate of the lens. By changing the wear protocol, method of sterilization and composition of storage solutions the path of spoilation can be completely changed. In such cases the comments relating to white spot formation still apply but its importance is eclipsed by the more rapid onset of other types of spoilation process such as calcium or protein film formation which effectively terminate the wearing schedule for that particular lens.

RGP materials

History and patent literature

Scientists have studied the interrelation of polymer structure and polymer properties for many years. When the need to modify poly(methyl methacrylate) or PMMA to improve its oxygen permeability arose, there was therefore no difficulty in knowing where to look for polymers having high permeabilities. The problems lay in combining such polymers (silicone rubber, for example) with PMMA to achieve a balance of properties. This problem arose because quite different types of reactions are used in the formation of the two materials. This can be illustrated by using the picture of polymers such as PMMA and hydrogels as 'washing line' polymers. They have a long backbone (i.e. the string or 'washing line') from which a variety of chemical groups may be suspended (the 'washing'). The function of the chemical groups in hydrogels is primarily to attract and bind water within the structure. PMMA has much less hydrophilic 'washing' and remains glassy in water because it has very little appetite for moisture. Greater physical stability is achieved by fastening the 'washing lines' together at intervals by the use of cross-links. In order to incorporate an individual 'monomer' unit into such a structure it is necessary that the monomer shall have a carbon-to-carbon double bond. Some (fairly exotic) examples are shown in *Figure 3.14b–f*. Without the double bond the washing cannot be pegged onto the washing line and when it is pegged onto the line the double bond is converted into a normal single bond.

Other types of polymer, of which silicone rubber is one example, can be regarded as 'poppet bead' polymers. The individual units are joined just like the individual beads on a 'poppet bead' necklace. There is no 'washing' hanging from the chain and the properties of the polymer are controlled by the structure of the poppet beads themselves. *Figure 3.14a* provides an illustration of this type of polymer chain. The

fundamental problem that prevented simple PMMA–silicone rubber combinations from being prepared is that the 'washing line' and 'poppet bead' chemistries are incompatible and beads cannot be inserted into the washing line. The siloxymethacrylates that form the basis of current gas permeable technology get round this problem in a well recognized, but nevertheless quite ingenious, way. Short segments of the poppet bead chain are turned into 'washing' by attaching them to a chemical intermediate that contains the necessary double bond. This can be seen in the structure of the siloxymethacrylate monomer (*Figure 3.14b*) which in essence consists of the individual units of silicone rubber structure pasted onto a modified methyl methacrylate molecule. On the basis of this simple picture, the story of the gas permeable patents can be unfolded. An abbreviated compilation is listed in Addendum II.

Silicone rubber

Among the earliest non-hydrogel polymers that offered any competition to PMMA was silicone rubber itself. This material, which is substantially poly(dimethylsiloxane) (*Figure 3.14a*) has the highest oxygen permeability of any commercially available polymer (being around 1000 times more permeable to oxygen than PMMA). It is furthermore softer and flexible, and in this respect resembles hydrogels, but unlike hydrogels is exceptionally hydrophobic. Silicone rubber is such an important precursor to many of the current RGP materials that the appropriate technology as disclosed in the patent literature must be taken as a basis for later developments.

The earliest silicone rubber patents were concerned with methods of lens manufacture, particularly the use of compression moulding techniques together with questions of mould design, that were able to produce finished lenses with high quality edges. Similarly, attention was paid to methods for improvement of the mechanical strengths of poly(dimethylsiloxane)-based compositions. Many of these patents resulted from the work of the Dow Corning Corporation.

The major stumbling-block to the successful use of silicone rubber-based lenses has, however, been inadequate wetting properties rather than lack of toughness or durability. This is reflected in a large number of patent specifications that

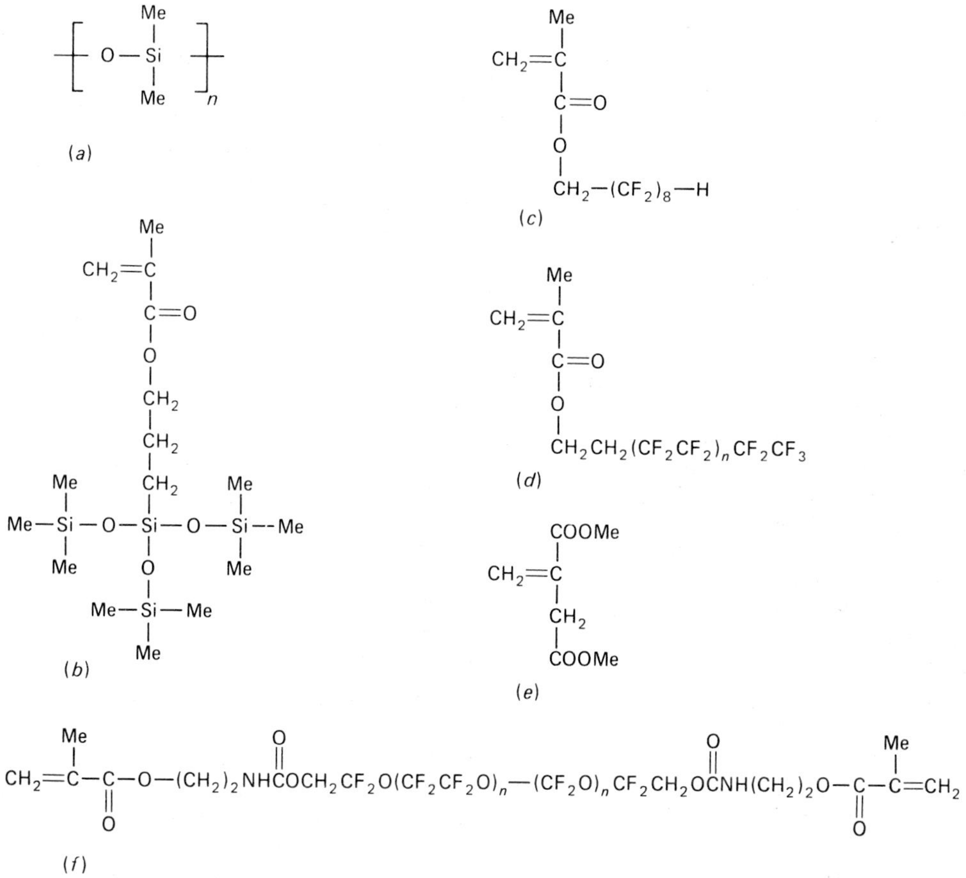

(a)
$$\left[\!-\!O\!-\!\underset{\underset{Me}{|}}{\overset{\overset{Me}{|}}{Si}}\!-\!\right]_n$$

(b)
$$CH_2\!=\!\underset{\underset{\substack{C=O\\|\\O\\|\\CH_2\\|\\CH_2\\|\\CH_2}}{|}}{\overset{\overset{Me}{|}}{C}}$$

$$Me\!-\!\underset{\underset{Me}{|}}{\overset{\overset{Me}{|}}{Si}}\!-\!O\!-\!\underset{\underset{O}{|}}{\overset{\overset{CH_2}{|}}{Si}}\!-\!O\!-\!\underset{\underset{Me}{|}}{\overset{\overset{Me}{|}}{Si}}\!-\!Me$$

$$Me\!-\!\underset{\underset{Me}{|}}{Si}\!-\!Me$$

(c)
$$CH_2\!=\!\underset{\underset{\substack{C=O\\|\\O\\|\\CH_2-(CF_2)_8-H}}{|}}{\overset{\overset{Me}{|}}{C}}$$

(d)
$$CH_2\!=\!\underset{\underset{\substack{C=O\\|\\O\\|\\CH_2CH_2(CF_2CF_2)_nCF_2CF_3}}{|}}{\overset{\overset{Me}{|}}{C}}$$

(e)
$$CH_2\!=\!\underset{\underset{\substack{CH_2\\|\\COOMe}}{|}}{\overset{\overset{COOMe}{|}}{C}}$$

(f)
$$CH_2\!=\!\underset{\underset{O}{\|}}{\overset{\overset{Me}{|}}{C}}\!-\!C\!-\!O\!-\!(CH_2)_2NH\overset{O}{\overset{\|}{C}}OCH_2CF_2O(CF_2CF_2O)_n\!-\!(CF_2O)_nCF_2CH_2O\overset{O}{\overset{\|}{C}}NH(CH_2)_2O\!-\!C\!-\!\underset{\underset{O}{\|}}{\overset{\overset{Me}{|}}{C}}\!=\!CH_2$$

Figure 3.14 RGP material structures: (a) poly(dimethylsiloxane); (b) tris(trimethylsiloxy)-γ-methacryloxypropylsilane; (c) 1,1,9-trihydroperfluoronyl methacrylate; (d) perfluoroalkylethyl methacrylate; (e) dimethyl itaconate; (f) typical perfluoroether dimethylacrylate

describe the methods of producing hydrophilic silicone rubber surfaces. The difficulty in obtaining clinically acceptable and permanent hydrophilic surfaces, however, is reflected in the relative lack of success of silicone rubber as a contact lens material. The earliest methods of surface treatment described involved direct chemical attack by alkyl titanate or chlorosulphonic acid followed by hydrolysis. More sophisticated treatments involving a range of both ionizing and non-ionizing forms of radiation soon followed, often in conjunction with N-vinyl pyrrolidone (NVP) or 2-hydroxyethyl methacrylate (HEMA), to assist in achieving a hydrophilically modified substrate. Although the methods differ in detail and complexity, they are all essentially free radical reactions.

It is apparent, therefore, that the extremely high oxygen permeability of silicone rubber is exceptionally difficult to harness in the form of a clinically acceptable contact lens because of the hydrophobic nature of the polymer and the great difficulty experienced in generating a hydrophilic surface on the material with any degree of permanence (see Plates 44 and 45). A series of patents describe attempts to overcome this latter difficulty with some compromise in oxygen permeability by utilizing other flexible polymers that are more readily and permanently surface treated. The first group of these are the carbon-based elastomers such as ethylene–propylene–terpolymer, cis-polyisoprene, styrene–butadiene copolymers, cis-polybutadiene, polyurethane elastomers and natural rubber. A very broad and early patent filed by the Dow Corning Corporation seeks coverage for the use of these materials in contact lenses. The technique subsequently used for final lens production is compression moulding.

Some flexible thermoplastics materials have been suggested as being suitable for contact lens manufacture in the patent literature, but none of these has achieved clinical significance. One interesting proposal involves the heating and subsequent quenching of polyethylene to reduce crystallinity and thereby increase optical clarity. Another describes the use of thermoplastics in general and polyvinyl chloride in particular to produce lenses of complex laminated design with a flexible central portion.

The Gaylord patents — harnessing silicon

A major advance in the development of RGP contact lens materials that are susceptible to the conventional lathing and lens polishing processes, is found in the work of Gaylord. There are two distinct aspects of this work. The first encompasses the use of siloxy derivatives of methacrylate monomers (e.g. tris(trimethyl-siloxy)–γ-methacryloxypropylsilane (*Figure 3.14b*) and the second the use of fluoroalkyl methacrylates (e.g. 1,1,9-trihydroperfluoro-nonyl methacrylate — *Figure 3.14c*). Both these lines of work have been subsequently developed and form the basis of most existing commercial gas permeable contact lens materials. *Figure 3.14b* is often referred to as 'tris monomer' and has been the most widely used monomer in siloxymethacrylate contact lens materials. The widely used fluoromethacrylate monomers are much simpler than that shown in *Figure 3.14c*, however.

In the event, the Gaylord patent describing the copolymerization of series of fluoroalkyl acrylates and methacrylates with methyl methacrylate is not unique. It was pre-dated by three quite significant patents describing the use of chemically similar materials in contact lens applications. The first of these was filed in 1967 and assigned to Du Pont by Girard, Sampson and Soper. In particular, it describes the advantages of contact lenses prepared from polymers derived from perfluoroalkylethyl methacrylates (*Figure 3.14d*) in terms of its relatively low refractive index (1.39) in comparison to the value of 1.49 for methyl methacrylate. In a subsequent patent, also assigned to Du Pont by A. E. Barkdoll, a wider range of

polymers based primarily on various per-fluoro(methyl vinyl ether) tetrafluoroethylene copolymers are described together with means of rendering them hydrophilic. The main thrust of the patent is the production of soft flexible materials processable by compression moulding, but significantly attention is drawn to the fact that the lenses thus produced are appreciably more oxygen permeable than PMMA. At the same time, a third Du Pont patent filed in the name of C. S. Cleaver draws together some of the features of the Barkdoll and the Girard patents. Thus Cleaver describes copolymers of fluoroalkyl methacrylates with methyl methacrylate, the production of lens blanks which were then machined and polished to prescription lenses and the advantageously high oxygen permeability of the resultant lenses. These lenses were not only described in patent literature, but were used with apparently favourable results in a preliminary clinical trial of the so-called CLP-2A lens (Miller, White and Hodd, 1975).

Although Cleaver's concept of the fluorine-containing contact lens was first filed in mid-1971 (a full year before the date of filing of the Gaylord patent), over a decade elapsed before significant commercial use was made of fluorocarbon-based contact lenses. The reason appears to be fairly straightforward and to reflect the immediate advantage in oxygen permeability of the siloxymethacrylates over the relatively simple fluorinated methacrylate esters described by Gaylord or the Du Pont workers. This is illustrated in their permeabilities, quoted by Gaylord in his two patents. Whereas the oxygen permeabilities claimed for materials described in the fluoroalkyl methacrylate patent are some three to four times greater than that of PMMA, typical examples described in the siloxymethacrylate patent are claimed to have permeabilities 15–20 times greater than PMMA. There is internal evidence in these Gaylord's patents that the baseline value of PMMA taken may be some three times too high. If this is the case, as seems likely, some revision of the permeabilities claimed is necessary. Thus, the fluorinated materials would become some 10 times more permeable than PMMA, whereas the siloxy copolymers would be around 50 or so times more permeable than PMMA.

On the other hand, it has to be said that the permeabilities quoted by Du Pont workers, reflected in values claimed by Cleaver, are probably unduly optimistic. In this patent, compositions broadly similar to those described by Gaylord are claimed to produce materials some 200 times more oxygen permeable than PMMA! The long delay in commercial use of fluorine-based gas permeable materials is a consequence of the fact that more complicated structures than those described in any of these early patents are required to achieve oxygen permeabilities as commercially attractive as this. On the other hand, the relative simplicity and effectiveness of the siloxymethacrylate concept resulted in direct commercial utilization of this group of materials.

It was, however, some 3 or 4 years after the publication of Gaylord's first patents before the so-called siloxymethacrylate gas permeable contact lens materials began to achieve significant market penetration in the contact lens world. This time period corresponds, coincidentally, to the appearance of the third Gaylord patent in late 1978, which is a continuation-in-part, following a series of interim abandonments of various of the original siloxanyl–methacrylate patents. Its claims are somewhat more restricted than those of the original; its scope is limited to a method for correcting visual defects rather than the new composition of matter of the original. In addition, the maximum percentage of siloxymethacrylate in the compositions described has been reduced from 70% to 60%. A new assignee also appears on this patent, this being Syntex (U.S.A.) Inc. who in the next few years gained control of the major proportion of key patents in this area. This property changed hands in the mid-1980s when Syntex were acquired by Pilkington, who already had extensive interests in the general optical field.

After Gaylord — copies and court cases

It is relevant to note that although Gaylord's work marks the beginning of the use of siloxymethacrylates as contact lens materials, the underlying chemical concepts had been previously known and discussed in various different contexts. Thus the synthesis and polymerization of siloxymethacrylate monomers is described in the chemical literature and reference is even made to their use as biomaterials, but not in the field of contact lenses. It was this aspect of the patents that led to their being

upheld in the court cases that began in the late 1980s, a topic that will be discussed in the light of the technical developments that were described in what we might call the 'post-Gaylord patents'.

Within a 12-month period in 1978 and early 1979, at about the time of appearance of Gaylord's third patent, three workers began to file their separate series of patents related to siloxymethacrylate-based contact lens materials. These were, in advancing order of the priority date for the first written filing, Kyoichi Tanaka (Toyo Contact Lens Co. Ltd), Edward Ellis (Polymer Technology Corporation), and Nick Novicky whose later patents (and presumably rights to the earlier) were assigned to Syntex (U.S.A.) Inc. The Ellis and Novicky patents form a clear line of continuation from early Gaylord's work and, because of this, are best considered together. Tanaka's work, for which parallel filings exist in Japan and the USA, has some slight and significant differences mainly concerned with the inclusion of a hydroxyl group into the siloxy monomer to improve wettability.

Early in 1978, two patents were filed in the names of Edward Ellis and Joseph Salamone that used Gaylord's basic concept with slight but significant modification. The first of these described the electrostatic binding of a polyelectrolyte complex coating to the surface of an otherwise hydrophobic contact lens in order to render the material hydrophilic. Although the patent in question failed to deal effectively with the question, it highlights a very real problem associated with the incorporation of substantial proportions of hydrophobic organosilicone monomers into materials for contact lens use. The second patent again uses Gaylord's basic composition based on *Figure 3.14b* but claims novelty in the additional use of methacrylic acid (a hydrophilic monomer referred to but not exemplified by Gaylord) to improve surface wettability, and by the incorporation of an itaconate ester (e.g. dimethyl itaconate — *Figure 3.14e*). This composition forms the basis of the Boston range of gas permeable materials.

Novicky's first patent describes the shortcomings of the prior art contact lenses based on siloxy monomers in terms of their inadequate mechanical properties, inadequate resistance to ocular spoilation and modest oxygen permeability. The advantages that he claims for his disclosure fall into two areas. The first is an improved synthesis of the siloxane intermediates and the second the use to which such an intermediate may be put in the preparation of more highly branched siloxanyl methacrylates than are described in Gaylord's original patent. A further feature of the patent is the importance attributed to the use of methacrylic acid and N-vinyl pyrrolidone (rather than 2-hydroxyethyl methacrylate) and cyclohexyl methacrylate as co-monomers. Although the use of the former compounds which are incorporated to improve hydrophilicity is described (but not exemplified) by Gaylord, he makes no specific mention of cyclohexyl methacrylate among the many other alternatives to methyl methacrylate that he lists. Furthermore, Gaylord specifically refers to the advantages associated with the use of lower rather than higher degree of branching in the siloxy substituents. It has to be said that the evidence currently available suggests that the claims made by many of the 'post-Gaylord' patents are not upheld by subsequent events. Although minor components may assist in the achievement of some improvement in mechanical properties and in wettability, the most widely used siloxy monomer in current commercial materials was exemplified by Gaylord in his original patent. This is the so-called 'tris monomer' shown in *Figure 3.14b*.

In this respect the recent US court case involving Pilkington–Sola–Syntex (who hold the Gaylord patents) on one hand, and the manufacturers of Optacryl and of Paragon materials on the other, was of considerable interest. The questions of relevance here are whether the Gaylord patent is valid (in view of the fact that the chemistry was already known) and whether Paragon and Optacryl materials depend upon the Gaylord invention. In the event the judge ruled that Gaylord's patent is valid because the use of siloxymethacrylates to produce oxygen-permeable contact lens materials constituted a non-obvious solution to a problem that many others had unsuccessfully tackled.

Furthermore, it was clear from evidence produced during the case that the siloxy monomers disclosed in Gaylord's patent have not, in practice, been superseded by improved siloxy components. None of the minor components for which advantage was claimed could be shown to produce improved materials. This

supports the widely held view that the 'tris monomer' (*Figure 3.14b*) is the only siloxy monomer of commercial significance in current materials. Improved oxygen permeability in the siloxymethacrylate materials has been achieved by simply increasing the proportion of 'tris monomer' used rather than employing the supposedly superior siloxy monomers described in the large number of post-Gaylord patents, of which only a small number have been mentioned here.

US patents — 1980 and beyond

In addition to the increasingly complex siloxy methacrylate derivates (which are, in general, so difficult to prepare in pure form that they have yet to become commercially significant), other lines of work have been described. Two significant ideas emerged at the end of the 1970s both naming Mitchel Shen as a co-inventor. The first of these, assigned to Wesley–Jessen Inc., encompassed the use of alkyl-substituted polystyrenes, and the second (Biocontacts Inc.) described the way in which the ester interchange reactions could be employed to convert a hard lens (manufactured therefore by conventional lens techniques) to a lens with a lower glass transition temperature. In the Wesley–Jessen patents the introduction of progressively more bulky alkyl groups as in the series vinyl toluene, isopropyl styrene, and t-butyl styrene is shown to produce a progressive improvement in oxygen permeability. This has led to the development of the Airlens. Although the second of the patent areas envisaged the physiological compatibility associated with lower glass transition temperature as the main advantage of the materials produced, subsequent work indicates that the oxygen permeabilities compare well with those of other commercial gas permeable contact lenses. The essence of the invention involves copolymerization of butyl methacrylate and acrylic acid (or anhydride) followed by the use of direct and/or indirect esterification reactions with butanol, pentanol or propanol to form a substantially complete esterification. Both the Revlens and Japanese Ricky lenses seem to be based on this approach.

The now well-known patents from the 3M Co. take a series of ideas that have been previously disclosed in patent literature, and assemble them to produce materials that are in some way novel. Both patents use the concept of a long flexible oxygen-permeable chain with polymerizable acrylate or methacrylate groups at each end. Two candidates were chosen for this flexible, permeable chain. One of these is the siloxane backbone that has formed the basis of so many patents in this area, and the other a perfluoropolyether segment. It is the perfluoropolyether that has been used as the basis of the 3M contact lens material. An example of the precursor dimethacrylate described in the patent is shown in *Figure 3.14f*, although it is not a requirement of the claim that the urethane group be included. The values of n in *Figure 3.14f* can vary quite widely and independently but might, for example, be in the region of 20. The thinking behind compounds of this type clearly goes back to much earlier 3M patents and connected not with contact lens materials but concerned with perfluoroalkylene oxide elastomers and urethane derivatives of these. Similarly, work on fluorine-containing contact lens materials can be traced back to the work of Barkdoll, Girard, Cleaver and Gaylord which has been described earlier. One of these (the CLP-2A lens) gave very satisfactory results in early clinical trials, but the manufacturer, Du Pont, decided not to pursue the project. Unlike the earlier material, lenses based on the 3M patent are not susceptible to lathe-cutting, being too soft and flexible. They are typically based on combinations of the fluoromonomer (e.g. *Figure 3.14f*), methyl methacrylate and a hydrophilic monomer such as *N*-vinyl pyrrolidone. The material is claimed to have extremely high permeability (600 times greater than PMMA) and has been given the USAN name Fluorofocon A. The general availability and results of more widespread clinical experience of this material are awaited with interest.

The Japanese patents

The first Japanese patent in this field has already been referred to. It describes the work of Tanaka for the Toyo Contact Lens Company and appeared at the same time as the disclosures of Ellis and of Novicky. Although not vitally significant in its own right it marks the beginning of a growing number of patents based on Japanese work. These are worth considering here in some detail since most of them are not easily accessible (being in the original Japanese)

but, additionally, they do contain some interesting ideas and a wealth of information. In the post-1980 period, a very marked expansion in Japanese patent coverage emerged, principally as a result of work assigned to Hoya Lens K.K. and Toyo Contact Lens Co. Ltd, with the significant additional incursion of Syntex and Paragon Optical into the Japanese patent literature. Many of this substantial group of patents deal with concepts that have been outlined above in connection with the development of ideas in the US patent literature. A significant number of original ideas have emerged during this period, however, which may form the basis for new and interesting contact lens materials. These include silyl acetylene polymers, pentafluorostyrenes, urethane siloxanol acrylates and polyperfluoroalkylene oxide copolymers.

The Japanese patents assigned to Hoya and Toyo provide valuable information on the use of fluoroalkyl methacrylates in conjunction with siloxymethacrylates, and the properties of fluoroalkyl methacrylates themselves. Here again the nature of the work is not novel since fluoroalkyl methacrylates are referred to in the early groups of Gaylord and related patents, which have been previously mentioned. The properties, specifically the permeabilities of the individual homopolymers, are carefully described in preparation for their use in the later mixed-monomer patents. It is interesting to compare the increase in relative permeability along the series of homopolymers methyl methacrylate, trifluoroethyl methacrylate, hexafluoroisopropyl methacrylate (1:60:100). The ground is clearly seen in this patent for the development of fluorine-containing siloxymethacrylate gas permeable materials (e.g. Equalens, Fluoroperm, Menicon SP) which penetrated the UK and American markets towards the mid-1980s. It is in the Japanese patents, however, that the relationship between composition and permeability of these materials is clearly described. Patents filed by American companies appeared later and contained less information.

The readily discernible trend in methacrylate-based contact lens materials described in the patent literatures and discussed here is one of increasing oxygen permeability. Although a range of variants has been disclosed, the essential structural developments have centred around the incorporation of higher proportions of more highly branched siloxy derivatives, and the use of fluorocarbon in the place of hydrocarbon substituents. Much attention has been paid in the patent literature to the comprehensive coverage of all possible structural variants of Gaylord's original disclosures, published in 1974. Despite this, little that is truly new has appeared since then, although the number of 'new' materials continues to grow steadily. A brief overview of the commercially available gas permeable materials illustrates this.

Commercial RGP materials and their properties

The influence of the disclosures, previously outlined and contained in the patent literature, is reflected in the nature and the properties of commercially available contact lens materials. *Table 3.5* gives an overview of commercially available RGP materials together with information on chemical type, oxygen permeability, wettability, mechanical properties and refractive index. This information has been compiled from various sources including manufacturer's literature, reviews and results compiled by other workers, and measurements made in these laboratories. In addition, values for PMMA and cellulose acetate butyrate are included for comparison. A variety of additional materials exist, all based on various aspects of the principles discussed in the previous section. These include OTC V and VII (Ocular Technology), Siloxycon 14 (Neefe), Medicon (A.I.T.), Oxycon and Oxycon 32 (Biomedic Polymers) together with Revlens (Biocontacts), based on butyl acrylate, Hydex (Glasflex) and Opus III (Frigitronics). The last two named make use of a combination of siloxymethacrylate with *t*-butyl styrene, which forms the basis of the Wesley–Jessen Airlens.

The major problem in making comparisons between materials and particularly in comparing manufacturers' claims is that there is no rigid standardization of experimental techniques to provide a basis for such comparisons. These factors, coupled with the debatable relevance of existing measurements *in vitro* to the clinical performance of materials, present a major problem to the clinician in selecting materials on the basis of manufacturers' literature.

The first point to consider is the range and reliability of oxygen permeability measurements. Complications in making true permeability measurements on materials arise from the curvature and varying thickness of individual contact lens samples, the thickness dependence, and the lack of widely available standards for instrument calibration especially in the high *Dk* region in which many of the recently developed materials are claimed to lie.

The problems associated with the use of increasing quantities of siloxymethacrylates to achieve high oxygen permeabilities are two-fold. First, incompatibility, phase separation and deterioration in mechanical properties limit the amount of such monomers that can be incorporated. Secondly, their use requires the incorporation of hydrophilic monomers containing hydroxyl, carboxyl, amide or lactam groups to improve wettability. It is well recognized that developments that have produced higher oxygen permeabilities have led to problems with mechanical properties, and that such problems are quite common. Despite this, the currently used mechanical property measurements do not indicate any clear distinction between materials. There is certainly no accepted basis upon which the durability of existing materials can be correlated with presently used mechanical property measurements.

Similar problems arise with the measurement of wettability by contact angle techniques. In this case, contact angle hysteresis, the effect of soaking on water uptake and thus the wettability of materials, coupled with the use of the inverted or captive air bubble technique in solutions other than water, combine to produce wide variations in the reported values for a given material. On the other hand use of a low surface tension wetting solution in combination with the captive air bubble technique produces a low contact angle with almost any polymer. Such measurements are of no clinical significance, nor do they provide any rational basis for comparing the surface properties of different candidate materials.

The properties listed in the table reflect these points. The variation in values quoted at various times and from various sources for some materials is quite alarming. It is possible to imagine the indignation that would be caused among the motoring fraternity if the top speed, acceleration, engine capacity and fuel consump-

Table 3.5 Some commercial RGP materials and their properties

Name of lens and manufacturer	Material type	$Dk \times 10^{11}$ (standard units)	Contact angles (°)		Hardness	Refractive index (n)
			Dry	Soaked		
Airlens (Wesley–Jessen)	Butyl styrene polymer	21‡	64, 76†	12, 19†	86 SD†	1.53
Alberta N (Calgary Corneal Contact)	Fluoroalkyl itaconate – siloxane copolymer	42‡; 25†	85†	40, 52†	120 R†	1.445
Alberta XL 30 [GP IV, = Sil-O₂-Flex]	Siloxymethacrylate copolymer	12.8*; 22‡	65*	28†		1.48
Boston II (Polymer Tech. Corp.)	Siloxymethacrylate – itaconate copolymer	10*; 12–14†,‡	65*; 80†	33, 42†	85 SD, 83 SD†	1.46
Boston IV	Siloxymethacrylate – itaconate copolymer	14*; 19, 24†; 26‡	79*; 90†	30†; 17‡	119 R†	1.468
Equalens (Polymer Tech.)	Fluoromethacrylate – siloxy copolymer	72‡	55*; 94†	30‡; 60†		1.439
Fluorofocon A (3M)	Perfluoropolymer	95†; 90‡; 70(20°C)‡		44†		1.40
Fluoroperm (Paragon)	Fluoromethacrylate – siloxy copolymer	92‡		16‡	81 SD	1.471
GP 26 (Bausch & Lomb) [=Boston IV]	Siloxymethacrylate– itaconate copolymer	26‡		17‡	118 R, 85 SD†	1.468
Hyperm (Hydron Europe)	Siloxymethacrylate copolymer	12*; 18‡	71*	24‡	84 SD†	1.47
Menicon O₂ (Toyo)	Siloxymethacrylate copolymer	5–8†; 10‡		16†	82 SD†; 7.6 V‡	1.481
Menicon Super O₂	Siloxymethacrylate copolymer	52‡				1.47
Menicon SP	Fluoromethacrylate – siloxy copolymer	32‡		20†		1.48
Optacryl 60 (Optacryl Inc.)	Siloxymethacrylate copolymer	9*; 12‡; 18‡	65*; 76†	25†	85 SD†; 88 SD‡	1.467
Optacryl K	Siloxymethacrylate copolymer	21†; 32‡	82†	25–30†	83 SD†; 86 SD‡	1.467
Optacryl EXT	Siloxymethacrylate copolymer	54†; 59‡	92†	<30‡	81 SD†; 82 SD‡	1.464
Optacryl Z	Siloxymethacrylate copolymer	67, 70†; 84‡	91†	25–30†,‡	78 SD†; 80 SD‡	1.461
Oxyflow (Contact Lens Supp.)	Siloxymethacrylate copolymer	20*; 28‡	72*	35†	84 SD†	
Polycon I (Pilkington/Sola-Syntex)	Siloxymethacrylate copolymer	3.1†; 5‡	67*; 83†	30†; 34†	83 SD†	1.49
Polycon II	Siloxymethacrylate copolymer	6.5*; 6.5†; 12‡	77†	25†; 32†; 15‡	84.5 SD†	1.473
Polycon HDK	Siloxymethacrylate copolymer	50‡		25†	85 SD‡	1.465
Paraperm O₂ (Paragon Optical Inc.)	Siloxymethacrylate copolymer	8†; 12‡	80†	46†; 23†	85 SD†; 86 SD‡	1.48
Paraperm EW	Siloxymethacrylate copolymer	32,49†; 56‡	68*; 92†	26†	10.6 V†; 82 SD‡	1.475
Paraperm O₂ Plus	Siloxymethacrylate copolymer	31†; 39‡	91†		11.3 V†; 84 SD‡	
Paraperm EW2	Siloxymethacrylate copolymer	92†; 97‡		16‡	81 SD‡	1.471
Silcon (Dow Corning)	Silicone polymer	10*; 17‡	92†	31†	82 SD†	
Silperm	Silicone polymer	12*	90*	50†; 15†		
PMMA	Polymethyl methacrylate	0.1*	63–67*,†	15–35*,†	88.5 SD†	1.49
CAB (=Cabcurve; GP II; Meso; Paracab; Persecon)	Cellulose acetate butyrate	4–8*,†	62–65*,†	12–31*,†	77.5 SD†	

*These laboratories; †various published sources; ‡manufacturers' literature; *Dk* values at *20°C, †‡35°C; hardness, V=Vickers, SD=Shore, R=Rockwell (R).
See also Table 10.11.

tion of cars were quoted with such unreliability. To make the analogy more realistic it is necessary to imagine that the manufacturers' performance figures are obtained on a hill of undisclosed slope. This is not to suggest that the manufacturers are guilty of misrepresentation but rather that no concensus view on standardized test procedures has emerged.

The need for improved test methods

Whereas biomaterials research has been advancing, the methodology commonly used for testing contact lenses has stood still. One of the problems is that the questions that were asked about the properties of materials 15 years ago are not sufficiently discriminating today. As a result we have inherited a mixture of concepts and methodologies that are inappropriate to present day requirements. It is important that steps are taken to remedy the situation. It is in the interests of both practitioners and manufacturers to produce methods of test that reflect the relative merits and shortcomings of different RGP materials. Some of the current problems and potential improvements are outlined below.

Oxygen permeability

In the early 1970s, for example, it was sufficient to know whether the oxygen permeability of a hard lens material was appreciably greater than that of PMMA or about the same. The scale of values for available materials was very limited. It was very convenient to use a technique in which a lens could be placed on a polarographic electrode and measured directly. As the available materials have increased in permeability, however, so has the relative importance of the many errors associated with this technique. Brien Holden's group in Australia have, quite rightly, put the permeability values obtained by the method under close scrutiny. The truth of the matter is that the technique is extremely convenient but never was, and never will be, an acceptably scientific basis for a standard method. This point was made in the national responses to the ISO draft proposal that sought to use it in this way.

There are many areas of membrane science in which the oxygen permeability of materials is studied. The understanding of the difference between gas phase transport and that in the aqueous phase, together with the effect of thickness and of boundary layer phenomena has been in place for many years. These problems are shared by the contact lens community, but are by no means peculiar to them. In fact the only feature that is peculiar to the contact lens community is the strange adoption of the term Dk (for the product of diffusion and solubility). No attempt is made to distinguish between the contribution of D and k in the permeabilities of individual contact lens materials; indeed the use of Dk seems to be a bizarre sophistication in view of the more common use in other fields of the simple term 'P'. The situation will become more complex if subscripts to indicate more precisely the conditions of measurement are adopted.

It is logical that a series of 'Gaylord' compositions should be prepared and their permeability characteristics determined using sound and well-established experimental techniques. These would then provide calibration standards for the simple polarographic electrode cell used in contact lens work. This would mean that the polarographic electrode method would cease to be a candidate for a role that it cannot fulfil — that of a primary standard technique. The difficulties associated with such a proposal are far fewer than those involved with the direct determination of a fundamental materials property by the use of a polarographic electrode and cigarette paper!

Surface properties

The field of contact lens surface properties has also become more complex with the passage of time. The water wettability of materials provides a good primary indication of the ability of tears to form a coherent and stable layer on the surface of the material. It tells nothing of the compatibility of the material with tears. Unfortunately the inverted air bubble technique has recently been used as a standard in contact lens work. The measurement is made after an air bubble is allowed to impinge, from underneath, onto the surface of the sample, which is suspended in an aqueous liquid. This is the most difficult type of contact angle to measure correctly since it involves judging where the base of a distorted sphere just impinges on a surface. More importantly, the air bubble has to displace water from the surface of the sample, which is frequently pre-soaked. Since all the siloxymethacrylate gas permeable materials contain appreciable amounts of hydrophilic monomer to improve surface wettability they all retain a strongly adsorbed water layer at the surface under these conditions. Not surprisingly, therefore, very similar and very low so-called 'wetting angles' are obtained with current gas permeable materials. What is measured in each case is the value for a diffuse layer of water on a polymer surface. The values obtained are similar to those obtained by this technique with hydrogels. The biological and biochemical events at surfaces, on the other hand, occur at a molecular level and do not recognize the diffuse water layer 'barrier' that is sensed by macroscopic 'droplet' techniques. This is the underlying reason for the lack of relevance to clinical practice of the 'wetting angle', as presently measured. Characterization of polymer surfaces has developed a great deal in the last decade or so. In addition well-established techniques exist which enable the detailed surface energy components, rather than a single 'wetting angle', to be determined. Biomaterials science makes widespread use of such methods; the contact lens community could profitably do the same. Predicting compatibility *in vivo* from tests *in vitro* is never entirely successful. Increasingly, however, it enables differences between the performance of materials to be successfully predicted. In addition the use of biological probes, such as animal cells, and interaction with biological sera provide useful information in the development of new biomaterials. The area is complex, but offers several approaches that will improve considerably on the captive air bubble technique, and will have some relevance to clinical performance.

Mechanical properties

Little organized work is done on mechanical properties at present, but the values quoted are almost invariably related to the hardness of the material. Although hardness tests have some place in contact lens characterization, they do not reflect the type of mechanical failure or problems that normally arise. Such problems are usually associated with fracture, chipping or splitting (*Plates 27* and *30*) on one hand and distortion of one sort or another, on the other. Mechanical properties of polymers are of paramount importance in many fields. A vast number of testing methods have been devised for different applications. It would be a relatively straightforward procedure to adapt suitable methods for measuring resistance to fracture and to distortion. One immediately useful way of comparing lenses is by use of tensile stress–strain analysis on both dry and soaked lenses or discs. With care, reproducible stress–strain curve parameters can be obtained which tell a great deal about the behaviour of individual materials.

Conclusions

The contact lens literature is vast and expanding rapidly. The subject is now recognized as an important aspect of biomaterials science and, given the length of time that work has been carried out on contact lenses, is one of the oldest branches of the subject. It is clear that several areas of chemistry, physics and biology underpin the work, and that future progress depends upon the application of principles from all of these disciplines. Although it is unlikely that the search for the 'ideal' contact lens will produce a material that satisfies all requirements and is suitable for all applications, marked advances can be expected. In the face of all these points one aspect of the subject is woefully inadequate and has made little progress in the last decade. The aspect in question is the adoption of standard measurement techniques that would enable important materials properties to be reproducibly measured in the laboratory and which would have some relevance to clinical performance. This requires joint pressure from both clinicians and manufacturers. It may be a difficult task, but it is vital to the future success of this important interdisciplinary field.

Acknowledgements

I am grateful to past and present research students for excellent research work and stimulating discussions.

Addendum I
Units and terms in permeability measurements

Manufacturers' literature and, indeed, work by independent authors express properties in a variety of terms and units. This addendum provides some explanatory notes and conversion factors.

Oxygen permeability

The most important term in this work is the oxygen permeability coefficient, P, which is the amount of gas passing in unit time through a unit area of membrane subjected to a unit gas pressure gradient (i.e. pressure difference per unit thickness) across the membrane. The difference between 'dissolved' and 'gaseous' coefficients (P_d and P_g) is discussed in the text (see p. 93). The units in both cases are (ml(STP) mm)/(cm^2 s cmHg) or one of the equivalents listed below. The oxygen permeability coefficient is equal to the product of the oxygen diffusion coefficient (D) and its solubility (S), i.e. $P = D \times S$. The units of D are simply cm^2/s and those of S, ml/cm^3 per cmHg, e.g. ml O$_2$/cm^3(H$_2$O) per cmHg.

Two additional terms that are sometimes used are oxygen flux (F), which is the volume of gas passing per unit time through unit area of a membrane under given experimental conditions (for example, pressure difference, temperature) and oxygen transmission rate (TR) which is the amount of gas passing in unit time through a unit area of a membrane of given thickness under unit gas pressure gradient. The units of F are typically ml/cm^2 per s and those of TR, ml(STP)/(cm^2 s cmHg). In order to convert transmission rates (sometimes referred to as transmissibility, see Chapter 11, p. 386) to permeability coefficients the value is simply multiplied by sample thickness; for example, TR × sample thickness = P.

To convert oxygen flux values to permeability coefficients it is first necessary to change the volume of gas to its value under conditions of standard temperature and pressure (STP) and then to multiply by sample thickness and divide by the oxygen pressure gradient across the sample; for example, F (converted to STP) × sample thickness × 1/oxygen pressure gradient = P.

The units of P are preferably (ml(STP) mm)/(cm^2 s cmHg) but may contain alternative terms for thickness (cm, mm), time (min^{-1}, h^{-1}, day^{-1}), volume (cm^3), area (m^2, 100 in^2) or pressure gradient (atm^{-1}, mmHg^{-1}). In addition, units are sometimes 'simplified' by dividing or multiplying top and bottom by a common

factor such as cm or mm. One of the most common examples is the conversion:

$$\frac{\text{ml(STP) cm}}{\text{s cm}^2\,\text{mmHg}} \times \frac{\text{cm}}{\text{cm}} = \frac{\text{ml(STP) cm}^2}{\text{s cm}^3\,\text{mmHg}}$$

The two sets are identical but the right-hand units may now be expressed as:

$$\frac{\text{ml O}_2\,\text{cm}^2}{\text{s ml mmHg}}$$

or   (cm^2/s)(ml O$_2$/ml × mmHg)
       as used by Fatt (see Chapter 11)

When dealing with strange or unrecognizable units it is advisable to (1) change millilitres to cubic centimetres and (2) try multiplying both top and bottom of the equation by the same factor, for example

$$\frac{\text{cm}}{\text{cm}}$$

until one of the recognizable forms of units listed below is reached. Remember also that the value quoted may be an oxygen flux or transmission rate, especially if the determination was carried out on a lens. In such cases the quoted figure must be multiplied by sample thickness, or thickness and pressure gradient, as indicated above.

The more commonly encountered units of oxygen permeability are related as shown below.

1 (ml(STP) mm)/(cm^2 s cmHg)
or ml(STP) mm cm^{-2} s^{-1} cmHg^{-1}
or (cm^3(STP) mm)/(cm^2 s cmHg)
or cm mm s^{-1} cmHg^{-1}

is equivalent to

0.1 (ml(STP) cm)/(cm^2 s cmHg)
or ml(STP) cm cm^{-2} s^{-1} cmHg^{-1}
or (cm^3(STP) cm)/(cm^2 s cmHg)
or cm^2/s per cmHg
or (cm^3(STP)/(cm s cmHg)

is equivalent to

0.1 (ml(STP) mm)/(cm^2 s mmHg)
or ml(STP) mm cm^{-2} s^{-1} mmHg^{-1}
or (cm^3(STP) mm)/(cm^2 s mmHg)
or (cm mm)/(s mmHg)
or (cm^2/s)(ml O$_2$/ml mmHg) as illustrated in the example above

is equivalent to

0.01 (ml(STP) cm)/(cm^2 s mmHg)
or (cm^3(STP) cm)/(cm^2 s mmHg)
or cm^2/s per mmHg
or (cm^3(STP))/(cm s mmHg)

is equivalent to

$7.6 \; (ml(STP) \; cm)/(cm^2 \; s \; atm)$
$or \; (cm^3(STP) \; cm)/(cm^2 \; s \; atm)$
$or \; cm^2/s \; per \; atm$
$or \; (cm^3(STP))/(cm \; s \; atm)$

is equivalent to

$2.59 \times 10^{12} \; (ml(STP) \; ml)/(day \; m^2 \; atm)$
$or \; (cm^3(STP) \; ml)/(day \; m^2 \; atm)$

is equivalent to

$16.5 \times 10^{10} \; (ml(STP) \; ml)/(day \; (100 \; in)^2 \; atm)$

is equivalent to

$1.02 \times 10^{10} \; (in^3 \; ml)/(day \; (100 \; in)^2 \; atm)$

is equivalent to

$7.69 \times 10^{-6} \; cm^4/s \; per \; dyn.$

Addendum II

A bridged patent compilation: hydrogel materials

The work of Wichterle

WICHTERLE, O. and LIM, D. (1961). Method for producing shaped articles from three dimensional hydrophilic high polymers. US Patent 2 976 576

WICHTERLE, O. and LIM, D. (1965). Cross-linked hydrophilic polymers and articles made therefrom. US Patent 3 220 960

WICHTERLE, O. (1968). (to Ceskoslovenska Akademia Ved) Reshaping a hydrogel by mechanical removal and swelling to form a hydrogel contact lens. US Patent 3 361 858

WICHTERLE, O. (1968). (to Ceskoslovenska Akademie Ved) Method for centrifugal casting a contact lens. British Patent 3 408 429

WICHTERLE, O. (1970). (to Ceskoslovenska Akademie Ved) Method of manufacturing soft and flexible contact lenses. US Patent 3 496 254

WICHTERLE, O. (1970). (to Ceskoslovenska Akademie Ved) Method of preparing shape retaining bodies of organic polymer hydrogels. US Patent 3 499 862

WICHTERLE, O. (1971). (to Ceskoslovenska Akademie Ved) Method of centrifugally casting a layered contact lens. US Patent 3 557 261

WICHTERLE, O. (1972). (to Ceskoslovenska Akademie Ved) Anhydrous sparingly cross-linked hydrophilic copolymers. US Patent 3 699 089

WICHTERLE, O. (1974). (to Ceskoslovenska Akademie Ved) Contact lens blank or replica made from anhydrous sparingly cross-linked hydrophilic copolymers. US Patent 3 822 089

Vinyl pyrrolidone-based patents

LEEDS, H. R. (1971). Hydrophilic graft copolymers. US Patent 3 621 079

SEIDERMAN, M. (1972). Hydrophilic gel polymers insoluble in water from polyvinyl pyrrolidone with N-vinyl pyrrolidone and methacrylic modifier. US Patent 3 639 524

SEIDERMAN, M. (1973). Hydrophilic gel polymers of N-vinyl pyrrolidone and hydroxyalkyl methacrylates. US Patent 3 721 657

SEIDERMAN, M. (1973). Contact lenses from hydrophilic gel polymers of polyvinyl pyrrolidone monomeric vinyl pyrrolidone and methacrylic modifier. US Patent 3 767 731

SEIDERMAN, M. (1974). Hydrophilic gel polymers of N-vinyl pyrrolidone and hydroxyalkyl methacrylates. US Patent 3 792 028

SEIDERMAN, M. (1976). Contact lenses from hydrophilic gel polymers of polyvinyl pyrrolidone and hydroxyalkyl methacrylates. US Patent 3 966 847

SEIDERMAN, M. (1970). Hydrophilic plastic contact lens. US Patent 3 503 942

O'DRISCOLL, K. F. and ISEN, A. A. (1971). (to Griffin Laboratories Inc.) Fabrication of soft plastic contact lens blank. US Patent 3 700 761

O'DRISCOLL, K. F. and ISEN, A. A. (1974). (to Warner-Lambert Company) Fabrication of soft plastic lens. US Patent 3 816 571

O'DRISCOLL, K. F. and ISEN, A. A. (1974). (to Warner-Lambert Company) Fabrication of soft plastic contact lens blank and composition thereof. US Patent 3 822 196

O'DRISCOLL, K. F. and ISEN, A. A. (1974). (to Warner-Lambert Company) Irradiated composition for soft contact lens. US Patent 3 841 985

EWELL, D. G. (1972). (to Kontur Kontact Lens Company Incorporated) Hydrophilic contact lens materials. US Patent 3 647 736

STECKLER, R. (1970). Hydrogels from cross-linked polymers of N-vinyl lactams and alkyl acrylates. US Patent 3 532 679

DE CARLE, J. T. (1972). Improvements in or relating to hydrophilic polymers and contact lenses manufactured therefrom. British Patent 1 385 677

CORDREY, P. W. and MIKUCKI, W. (1975). (to Contact Lens Manufacturing Limited) Hydrophilic copolymers and articles formed therefrom. British Patent 2 391 438

A bridged patent compilation: RGP and related materials

Silicone rubber-based materials

BURDICK, D. F., MISHLER, J. L. and POLMANTEER, K. E. (1967). (to Dow Corning Corp.) Blends of two polysiloxane copolymers with silica. US Patent 3 341 490

McVANNEL, D. E., MISHLER, J. L. and POLMANTEER, K. E. (1967). (to Dow Corning Corp.) Hydrophilic contact lens and method of making same. US Patent 3 350 216

POLMANTEER, K. E. (1970). (to Dow Corning Corp.) Optical compositions of silicone rubber. US Patent 3 518 324

TRAVNICEK, E. A. (1976). (to American Optical Corp.) Optically clear filled silicone elastomers. US Patent 3 966 189

WAJS, G. (1978). (to Essilor International) Grafted silicon polymers and their use for contact lenses. Ger Offen 2 813 558

Siloxymethacrylate and fluoropolymers: Gaylord and precursor patents

BARKDOLL, A. E. (1974). (to E. I. Du Pont de Nemours & Co) Low refractive index contact lenses. British Patent 1 367 846

CLEAVER, C. S. (1974). (to E. I. Du Pont de Nemours & Co) A contact lens having an optimum combination of properties. US Patent 3 950 315

GAYLORD, N. G. (1974). (to Polycon Lab Inc) Oxygen-permeable contact lens composition methods and article of manufacture. US Patent 3 808 178

GAYLORD, N. G. (1978). (to Syntex USA Inc) Method of correcting visual defects; compositions and articles of manufacture useful therein. US Patent 4 120 570

GIRARD, L. J., SAMPSON, W. G. and SOPER, J. W. (1970). (to E. I. Du Pont de Nemours & Co) Contact lens having an index of refraction approximating that of human tears. US Patent 3 542 461

Post-Gaylord siloxy patents

ELLIS, E. J. and SALAMONE, J. C. (1979). (to Polymer Technology Corp) Contact lens with a hydrophilic, polyelectrolyte complex coating and method for forming same. US Patent 4 168 112

ELLIS, E. J. and SALAMONE, J. C. (1979). (to Polymer Technology Corp) Silicone-containing hard contact lens material. US Patent 4 152 508

NOVICKY, N. N. (1980) Oxygen permeable hard and semi-hard contact lens compositions, methods and articles of manufacture. US Patent 4 242 483

TANAKA, K., TAKAHASHI, K., KANADA, M. and TOSHIKAWA, T. (1979). (to Toyo Contact Lens Co Ltd, Japan) Methyl-di(trimethylsiloxy)silyl propylglycerol methacrylate. US Patent 4 139 548

New ideas in US patents

LOSHAEK, S. and SHEN, C. M. (1980). (to Wesley-Jessen Inc) Contact lenses of high gas permeability. US Patent 4 228 269

RICE, D. E. and IHLENFELD, J. V. (1984). (Minnesota Mining & Manufacturing Co) Contact lens containing a fluorinated telechelic polyether. US Patent 4 440 918

SHEN, C. M., MANDELL, R. B. and STARK, L. (1974). (to Biocontacts Inc) Physiologically compatible plastic contact lenses and a method for their production. US Patent 3 850 892

Selected Japanese patents

TANAKA, K., NAKAJIMA, T., NAKADA, K., TOSHIMA, N. and SHIKAMI, S. (1983). (to Toyo Contact Lens Co Ltd) Hard contact lens having hydrophilic surface. Jap Kokai 58-17412

TARUMI, N. and KOMIYA, S. (1982). (to Hoya Lens KK) Contact lens with high oxygen permeability. Jap Kokai 57-182718

TARUMI, N., HIRAYAMA, N., KOMIYA, S., TSUCHIYA, M., MASUHARA, E. and NAKABAYASHI, N. (1980). (to Hoya Lens KK) Acrylic polymers for contact lenses. Jap Kokai 55-69606

YOKOYAMA, K., MASUHARA, E. and TSUCHIYA, M. (1984). (to Hoya Lens KK) Oxygen-permeable contact lens. Jap Kokai 59-214822

References

ALLANSMITH, M. R., KORB, D. R. and GREINER, J. V. (1977). Giant papillary conjunctivitis in contact lens wearers. *Am. J. Ophthal.* **83**, 697–708

ANDERTON, J. (1973). Consideration of the cornea as a model for the design and synthesis of polymers for continuous-wear contact lenses. *MSc Thesis*, University of Aston, Birmingham

ANDRASKO, G. (1986). Corneal deswelling response to hard and hydrogel extended wear lenses. *Invest. Ophthal. Vis. Sci.* **27**, 20–23

BAKER, D. and TIGHE, B. J. (1981). Polymers in contact lens applications (VIII) the problem of biocompatibility. *Contact Lens J.* **10**(3), 3–14

BARNES, A., ENSOR, R., NG, C. O., PEDLEY, D. G. and TIGHE, B. J. (1974). Wettability phenomena in synthetic hydrogels for contact lens applications. Paper presented at 5th European Symposium on Fluorine Chemistry, Aviemore, Scotland

BECKER, W. E. (1966). Corneal contact lens fabricated from silicone rubber. US Patent 3 228 741

BITONTE, J. L. and KEATES, R. H. (1972). *A Symposium on the Future of Flexible Lenses vs Rigid Lenses.* St Louis: Mosby

BIXLER, H. J. and MICHAELS, A. S. (1968). Polyelectrolyte complexes. In *Kirk-Othmer Encyclopaedia of Chemical Technology*, 2nd edn, Vol. 16. New York: Interscience

BLOOMFIELD, S. E., DAVID, S. D. and RUBIN, A. L. (1978). Acute corneal calcification. *Ann. Ophthal.* **10**, 355–360

BOWERS, R. W. J. and TIGHE, B. J. (1987a). Studies in the ocular compatibility of hydrogels (I). A review of clinical manifestations of spoilation. *Biomaterials* **8**, 83–88

BOWERS, R. W. J. and TIGHE, B. J. (1987b). Studies of the ocular compatibility of hydrogels (II). White spot deposits — incidence of occurrence, location and gross morphology. *Biomaterials* **8**, 89–93

BOWERS, R. W. J. and TIGHE, B. J. (1987c). Studies of the ocular compatibility of hydrogels (III). White spot deposits — chemical composition and geological arrangement of components. *Biomaterials* **8**, 172–176

BRENNAN, N. A., EFRON, N. and HOLDEN, B. A. (1986a). Oxygen permeability of hard gas contact lens materials. *Clin. expl Optom.* **69**, 82–89

BRENNAN, N. A., EFRON, N. and HOLDEN, B. A. (1986b). Further developments in the RGP *Dk* controversy. *Int. Eyecare* **2**, 508–509

BURNS, R. P., ROBERTS, H. and RICH, L. F. (1971). Effect of silicone contact lenses on corneal epithelial metabolism. *Am. J. Ophthal.* **71**, 486–489

CURETON, G. L. (1973). New perspectives on solutions for hard and soft contact lenses. *Mfg Optics Int.* **26**, 503–511

DOW CORNING CORPORATION (1967). Hydrophilic silicone rubber. *British Patent* 1 229 608

E. I. DUPONT DE NEMOURS AND COMPANY (1971). Contact lenses. *British Patent* 1 254 567

EFRON, N. and BRENNAN, N. A. (1987). In search of the oxygen requirement of the cornea. *Contax* July, 5–11

EHLERS, N. (1965). The precorneal film. Biomicroscopical histological and chemical investigations. *Acta ophthal.* Suppl. 81

FATT, I. (1986). Now do we need 'effective permeability'? *Contax* July, 6–17

FATT, I. (1987). Flexure of hard contact lenses. *Contax* September, 12–16

FATT, I. and BIEBER, M. T. (1968). The steady state distribution of oxygen and carbon dioxide in the *in vivo* cornea. 1: The open eye in air and the closed eye. *Expl Eye Res.* **7**, 103–112

FATT, I. and ST HELEN, R. (1971). Oxygen tension under an oxygen-permeable contact lens. *Am. J. Optom.* **48**, 545–555

FOX, H. W. and ZISMAN, W. A. (1950). The spreading of liquids on low energy surfaces. *J. Colloid Sci.* **5**, 514–531

FOWLER, S. A., GREINER, J. V. and ALLANSMITH, M. R. (1979). Attachment of bacteria to soft contact lenses. *Archs Ophthal.* **97**, 659–660

HAMILTON, W. C. (1972). A technique for the characterisation of hydrophilic solid surfaces. *J. Colloid Interface Sci.* **40**, 219–222

HATHAWAY, R. A. and LOWTHER, G. E. (1976). Appearance of hydrophilic lens deposits as related to chemical etiology. *Int. Contact Lens Clin.* **3**, 27–35

HILL, R. M. (1966). Effects of a silicone rubber lens on corneal respiration. *J. Am. optom. Ass.* **37**, 1119–1121

HILL, R. M. and AUGSBURGER, A. (1971). Oxygen tensions at the epithelial surface with a contact lens *in situ*. *Am. J. Optom.* **48**, 416–418

HILL, R. M. and FATT, I. (1964). Oxygen measurements under a contact lens. *Am. J. Optom.* **41**, 382–387

HILL, R. M. and SCHOESSLER, J. (1967). Optical membranes of silicone rubber. *J. Am. optom. Ass.* **38**, 480–483

HOLDEN, B. A., SWEENEY, D. F. and SANDERSON, G. (1984). The minimum pre-corneal oxygen tension to avoid corneal edema. *Invest. Ophthal. Vis. Sci.* **25**, 476–480

HWANG, S. T., KAMMERMEYER, K. and TANG, T. E. (1971).

Transport of dissolved oxygen through silicone rubber membrane. *J. macromol. Sci. Phys. (B)* **5**, 1–10

KAMATH, P. M. (1969). Physical and chemical attributes of an ideal contact lens. *Contacto* **13**(4), 29–34

KAMATH, P. M. (1970). Rigid gas permeable plastic contact lens. US Patent 3 551 035

KARAGEOZIAN, H. L. (1976). Use of the amino acid analyser to illustrate the efficacy of an enzyme preparation for cleaning hydrophilic lenses. *Contacto* **20**, 5–10

KERR, C. and DILLY, P. N. (1988). Problems of dimensional stability in RGPs. *Optician* **195**(5134), 21–23

KLEIST, F. D. (1979). Appearance and nature of hydrophilic contact lens deposits. *Int. Contact Lens Clin.* **6**, 120–130

LARKE, J. R., NG, C. O. and TIGHE, B. J. (1971). Hydrogel polymers in contact lens applications: Parts I and II. A survey of existing literature. *Optician* **162**(4206), 12–16 and (4207), 12–16

LARKE, J. R., PEDLEY, D. G. and TIGHE, B. J. (1973). Polymers in contact lens applications: Parts III and IV, Wettability phenomena. *Optician* **166**(4300), 32–39 and (4301), 21–30

LARKE, J. R., PEDLEY, D. G., SMITH, P. and TIGHE, B. J. (1973). A semi-rigid contact lens. *Ophthal. Optician* **13**, 1065–1067

LEMP, M. A., HOLLY, F. J., IWATA, S. and DOHLMAN, C. H. (1970). The precorneal tear film: I. Factors in spreading and maintaining a continuous tear film over the corneal surface. *Archs Ophthal.* **83**, 89–94

MAIGAN, M. B. and HOLDEN, B. A. (1986). Lens wear and its effect on wetting angle. *Int. Eyecare* **2**, 36–44

MANDELL, R. B. and FARREL, R. (1980). Corneal swelling at low atmospheric oxygen pressures. *Invest. Ophthal. Vis. Sci.* **19**, 697–702

MILLER, D. (1969). Measurement of the surface tension of tears. *Archs Ophthal.* **82**, 386–371

MILLER, D., WHITE, P. and HODD, D. B. (1975). Preliminary results of the CLP-2A corneal contact lens clinical trial. *Contact intraoc. Lens Med. J.* **1**(4), 24–33

MISHIMA, S. (1965). Some physiological aspects of the precorneal tear film. **73**, 233–241

MISHIMA, S. and MAURICE, B. M. (1961). The effect of normal evaporation on the eye. *Expl Eye Res.* **1**, 46–52

MORRIS, J. A. and TIGHE, B. J. (1986). Study of patients fitted with materials of different wetting angle. *Transactions of the British Contact Lens Association Conference*, pp. 72–75

NG, C. O. (1974). Hydrogel polymers in contact lens applications. *PhD Thesis*, University of Aston, Birmingham

NG, C. O. and TIGHE, B. J. (1976a). Polymers in contact lens applications: V. Design and calibration of a technique for dissolved oxygen permeability measurements. *Br. Polymer J.* **8**, 78–82

NG, C. O. and TIGHE, B. J. (1976b). Polymers in contact lens applications: VI. The dissolved oxygen permeability of hydrogels and the design of materials for use in continuous-wear lenses. *Br. Polymer J.* **8**, 118–123

NG, C. O., PEDLEY, D. G. and TIGHE, B. J. (1976). Polymers in contact lens applications: VII. Oxygen permeability and surface hydrophilicity of poly(4-methylpent-1-ene) and related polymers. *Br. Polymer J.* **8**, 124–130

O'NEAL, M. R., POLSE, K. A. and SARVER, M. D. (1984). Corneal response to rigid and hydrogel lenses during eye closure. *Invest. Ophthal. Vis. Sci.* **25**, 837–842

PEARSON, R. (1987). Rigid gas permeable wettability and maintenance. *Contax* September, 8–11

PEDLEY, D. G. (1976). Hydrophilic polymers. *PhD Thesis*, University of Aston, Birmingham

PEDLEY, D. G. and TIGHE, B. J. (1974). Hydrogel-forming polymers. British Patent Prov. Spec., 40464/74

PEDLEY, D. G., SKELLY, P. J. and TIGHE, B. J. (1980). Hydrogels in biomedical applications. *Br. Polymer J.* **12**, 99–110

PEPPAS, N. A., SMOLEN, V. F. and YANG, W. M. H. (1981). Oxygen permeability coefficients of polymers for hard and soft contact lens applications. *J. Memb. Sci.* **9**, 53–67

POLSE, K. A. and MANDELL, R. B . (1970). Critical oxygen tension at the corneal surface. *Archs Ophthal.* **84**, 505–508

REFOJO, M. F. and LEONG, F. L. (1979). Water-dissolved oxygen permeability coefficients of hydrogel contact lenses and boundary layer effects. *J. Memb. Sci.* **4**, 415–426

REFOJO, M. F., HOLLY, F. J. and LEONG, F. L. (1977). Permeability of dissolved oxygen through contact lenses I. Cellulose acetate butyrate. *Contact Intraoc. Lens Med. J.* **3**(4), 27–33

ROSEN, H. (1969). Contact lens with flexible central portion. US Patent 3 468 602

SCHONHORN, H. (1972). Wetting phenomena pertaining to adhesion. In *Progress in Membrane and Surface Science*, pp. 121–137. New York: Academic Press

STUDIES INC. (1969). Flexible polyethylene contact lens. US Patent 3 431 046

TIGHE, B. J. (1976). The design of polymers for contact lens applications. Based on paper at symposium entitled: Polymers in biomedical applications. Presented at Brunel University, May, 1974. *Br. Polymer J.* **8**, 71–77

TIGHE, B. J. and GEE, H. J. (1984). (to Kelvin Lenses Ltd, Manchester) Fluorine-containing hydrogel-forming polymeric materials. US Patent 4 433 111, Feb. 21st 1984

TRIPATHI, R. C., TRIPATHI, B. J. and REUBEN, M. (1980). The pathology of soft lens spoilage. *Ophthalmology* **87**, 365–372

WICHTERLE, O. and LIM, D. (1960). Hydrophilic gels for biological use. *Nature* **185**, 117–118

WICHTERLE, O. and LIM, D. (1961). Method for producing shaped articles from three-dimensional hydrophilic high polymers. US Patent 2 976 576

WICHTERLE, O. and LIM, D. (1965). Cross-linked hydrophilic polymers and articles made therefrom. US Patent 3 220 960

WOLFF, E. (1976). *Anatomy of the Eye and Orbit*, 7th edn. London: H. K. Lewis

Chapter 4

Drugs and solutions in contact lens practice and related microbiology

J. H. Stewart-Jones, G. A. Hopkins and A. J. Phillips

Formulation

Although contact lens solutions and eye drops are both pharmaceutical products, the way in which they are used puts different requirements on their formulation and presentation. As distinct from contact lens solutions which may remain in use for 3–4 weeks, eye drops in contact lens practice are for single diagnostic or prophylactic use only. Any problems that could arise from the long-term use of drops are most unlikely to appear because their use will be short. Small, single-use containers are the ideal presentation for eye drops but would not always be cost effective for contact lens solutions.

However, contact lens solutions and eye drops do have some requirements in common, e.g. sterility, safety, efficacy.

Sterility is not only important when the solution is first manufactured, but also because it should remain sterile for its recommended useful life. Single-use containers do not require the presence of a preservative as they are disposed of immediately after first use. Multi-use containers (eye drops and solutions) will need an antimicrobial preservative to prevent microorganisms invading the sterile environment of the solution. These will be discussed below.

Two other factors that are important when considering the formulation of ophthalmic solutions are pH and tonicity. The pH of an ophthalmic solution can affect its therapeutic effect, comfort, stability, sterility and viscosity (Hind and Goyan, 1947).

Ophthalmic drugs are, in most instances, alkaloid salts, salts of weak bases and strong acids, which at a pH of above 7 (i.e. an alkaline pH) become free bases, insoluble in water but soluble in lipids. The corneal epithelium (*Figure 2.1*) is a cellular layer whose cells are joined by desmosomes. There are minimal intracellular spaces, and so to pass the epithelium, drugs must pass through the lipoprotein cell membranes, i.e. they must be lipid soluble. Thus, a high pH will facilitate passage through the epithelium. The stroma, containing few cells, favours water-soluble substances while the endothelium again is more permeable to substances soluble in lipids.

Thus, for a drug to pass through the cornea, its solubility must swing from lipid soluble to water soluble, to lipid soluble, and back to water soluble again to dissolve in the aqueous.

A high pH, therefore, although increasing passage through the epithelium, may inhibit passage through the stroma. Also, a high pH is irritating and the drug may precipitate from the eye drops or may become unstable and be hydrolysed. Brawner and Jessop (1962) found that contact lens solutions with a neutral pH were less irritating than those with acid reactions.

Tears contain one or more buffer systems which will keep the pH between 7.2 and 7.6. When a drop is applied to the eye it will be buffered to this range irrespective of its normal pH unless it is highly buffered itself. It is therefore questionable whether buffering eye drops is useful.

The eye can tolerate solutions with osmotic pressures between the equivalent of 0.5 and 2.0% sodium chloride (0.9% is isotonic) with little or no discomfort, and there is no justification for raising the tonicity of hypotonic solutions (solutions with an osmotic pressure less than the tears) to an isotonic value. Solutions of eye drops, as normally prepared, are generally hypotonic, i.e. they have an osmotic pressure less than tears. Notable exceptions are 10% phenylephrine and 30% sulphacetamide sodium which are hypertonic and therefore cause some stinging, initially, on instillation. Eye lotions, however, because of the larger amounts used, should be isotonic.

Microbiology

In its exposed position, the eye is susceptible to infections from a variety of microorganisms such as bacteria, fungi and viruses. This risk may be increased by the placing of pieces of plastic (contact lenses or shells or drug release devices) in the conjunctival sac which may not be sterile and may interfere with the tears, the carrier for many of the eye's defences against infection. The tear film contains an armoury of antimicrobial agents in order to cope with the challenge of invading organisms and to maintain the conjunctival sac at a relatively low level of infection. Tears contain immunoglobulins A and G (IgA and IgG) in different proportions to those found in plasma. In addition, tears contain β-lysin and lysozyme, an enzyme capable of dissolving the cell wall of Gram-positive bacteria such as staphylococci. β-Lysin acts principally on the cell membrane.

The result of an infection depends more on the site of infection than on the infecting organism. Some microbes, however, do produce very distinctive results, e.g. herpes simplex.

It is important therefore, to know something of the structure of microorganisms, especially fungi, bacteria and viruses.

Fungi are composed of large cells with a well-defined, multichromosomal nucleus surrounded by a nuclear membrane. Bacteria are smaller, simpler cells with only one chromosome and no nuclear membrane, while virus particles are not really cells at all. By far the most important group as far as the practitioner is concerned is bacteria.

The normal diameter of a bacterial cell is of the order of 1 micrometre (μm), bounded by a rigid cell wall. This is an important structure because it can account for up to 25% of the volume of the cell and is responsible for many of the properties of the cell. It determines the shape of the cell and allows it to withstand an extreme range of hostile environments as well as

determining some of the biochemical differences between species. Some of the bacteria have a structureless, gel-like capsule surrounding the cell wall which further protects the cell, especially from phagocytosis. Such bacteria are therefore more virulent than species without one. Below the cell wall is the protoplast which is the living part of the cell, surrounded by the cell membrane and containing many cytoplasmic structures such as ribosomes and the single bacterial chromosome.

Bacteria multiply by binary fission or the splitting of the cell into two equal daughter cells. Unlike the cell division in higher animals, there is no mitosis.

There are many characteristics which are used to classify or 'type' bacteria. One of the most common of these is the shape and form of aggregation. Spherical bacteria are referred to as cocci. When they are found in pairs they are called diplococci; if in fours, tetrads. Streptococci are formed of chains of cocci while staphylococci have the form of bunches of grapes.

Rod-shaped bacteria are called bacilli. Coccobacilli are short and stumpy in appearance, while fusiform and filiform bacilli are longer and thinner. If the cell is curved or spiral in form then they are called vibrios and spirillas, respectively.

Biochemical differences also assist the typing of bacteria. For example, the form of respiration of any bacterial species can fall into one of three groups: aerobes, which can exist only in the presence of air; anaerobes, which can exist only in the absence of air; facultative anaerobes, which can exist under either condition.

The permeability of the cell wall determines the bacterial cell's reaction to certain histological stains. Most important is the Gram stain which involves treatment with two different stains, and organisms are designated Gram-positive and Gram-negative depending on the stain that they retain.

Bacteria and disease

Not all bacteria cause disease. In fact, many bacteria are responsible for maintaining the fertility of the soil by nitrogen fixation. However, many diseases result from the invasion of bacteria into tissues.

Bacteria cause disease by two mechanisms:

(1) Invasion and destruction of tissues when only the infected part shows lesions.
(2) The production of toxins which are carried by the blood and lymph systems to all parts of the body and produce widespread effects.

Toxins are of two types: exotoxins and endotoxins. Exotoxins are proteins, produced principally by the Gram-positive bacteria and are released without damage to the bacterial cell. They are very potent and tend to be specific for certain tissues (botulinum toxin attacks the nervous system). Endotoxins are non-protein substances, produced by many Gram-negative organisms and are only produced if the cell breaks down. These are less potent and tissue specific than the exotoxins.

Invasiveness of bacteria depends on the organism's resistance to phagocytosis and its survival in cells. If the organism, by having a thick capsule, can resist phagocytosis, then it will behave as an extracellular parasite. If it becomes ingested by the phagocytes but stays alive inside the cell, then it will become an intracellular parasite.

The virulence of an organism depends on both the toxicity and the invasiveness of the cells. It is measured in terms of the LD_{50}, i.e. the number of organisms needed to kill 50% of a test group of animals.

Fungi

Fungi are composed of more complex cells than bacteria. They grow either as single cells (yeasts) or as multicellular filamentous colonies (moulds or mushrooms).

Yeast cells are oval cells of about 3–5 μm in diameter surrounded by a cell wall. Beneath the cell wall is the cell membrane containing a nucleus with a nuclear membrane and several chromosomes. The cytoplasm contains mitochondria and an endoplasmic reticulum, structures which are absent from bacteria.

Some fungi exhibit the property of dimorphism, i.e. they can exist either in the form of yeast cells or as mould hyphae dependent on conditions. Some pathogens appear in tissues as cells while others grow *in vitro* as hyphae. There are four main classes of fungi: the Phycomycetes (including *Mucor* sp., the bread mould), the Ascomycetes (including *Penicillium* sp., the

penicillin producer), the Basidiomycetes (the mushrooms) and the Deuteromycetes (which include most of the human pathogens).

The first three classes can reproduce by a sexual method as well as asexually while the Deuteromycetes have no sexual phase and because of this are called the fungi imperfecti.

Fungi are less important than bacteria in causing diseases in man although their harmful effects can have far-reaching results on the food supply and can produce substances which are extremely toxic, for example, muscarine and ergotamine. However, fungi can produce several diseases which range from the just irritating (athletes' foot) through to very serious and possibly lethal conditions (Madura foot). Fungal infections predominantly affect the skin and mucous membranes, but systemic infections can occur which threaten all systems of the body. All fungi are aerobes or facultative anaerobes.

Viruses

Viruses consist of a single type of nucleic acid surrounded by a protein sheath and lack the fundamental mechanisms for growth and multiplication (ribosomes, enzymes and energy-generating systems). They multiply by invading a host cell and using its replication machinery to produce new viral nucleic acid and protein, involving the death of the host cell. Their peculiar 'life-cycle' makes them behave as obligate intracellular parasites.

Viruses are extremely small, the largest virus being approximately the same size as the smallest bacterium. Their smallness of size accounts for the term 'filtrable viruses' indicating that they can pass through filters which will retain other microorganisms.

There are three main types of virus distinguished by the type of host they invade: animal viruses, plant viruses and bacterial viruses or bacteriophages. The diseases resulting from infection by viruses include many common conditions ranging from the childhood diseases such as mumps and measles to several serious and notorious illnesses such as smallpox and rabies.

Microbiology of the eye

While a microorganism resides in the tear film of the conjunctival sac, it is unlikely to cause problems. It is only when it gains access to the tissues of the eye or adnexa, that problems are encountered. Organisms can be invasive or opportunistic. Invasive organisms, such as *Neisseria gonorrhoeae*, will penetrate the normal protective epithelium in order to set up an infection. Opportunists such as *Pseudomonas aeruginosa* require a break in the surface layers to gain access to the inner sterile layers where they will face no competition from other microorganisms.

Any foreign body placed on the cornea introduces the risk of corneal damage whether it is a piece of grit, a contact lens or an ophthalmic instrument such as a tonometer head. Whereas it is impossible to guarantee that a piece of grit will be sterile, it should be part of normal practice that the other two should be disinfected prior to use.

It should be emphasized that the use of prophylactic antimicrobial agents will not necessarily safely compensate for the use of infected lenses and instruments.

Much of this chapter is linked with the prevention of infected lenses. Serious infection has been reported from contact lenses (Josse, 1984; Weissman *et al.*, 1984) involving *Ps. aeruginosa*, a notorious ocular opportunistic pathogen.

However, in one study, the number of bacteria found in the conjunctival sac was reduced compared with non-lens-wearing patients (Hovding, 1981). The principal decline was in the numbers of *Staphylococcus epidermidis* (normally considered a non-pathogen).

Once the organism has gained access to the corneal tissue, it will multiply and spread. This presence of foreign material should engender some host inflammatory response. Tissue damage will occur followed, hopefully, by tissue repair and recovery.

Spread of the infection and release of toxic substances, are the principal causes of tissue damage. Microorganisms in this situation are essentially parasites and take away from the host cell nutrients and perhaps oxygen. Digestion of the corneal substance to provide a medium for the organism can be brought about by the release of enzymes.

There are many microorganisms that have produced infections of the eye. The following are the major ones:

(1) Gram-positive cocci:
   streptococci

(2) Gram-negative cocci:
   Neisseria gonorrhoeae
   Neisseria meningitidis
(3) Gram-positive rods:
   Corynebacterium diphtheriae
(4) Gram-negative rods:
   Pseudomonas aeruginosa
   Klebsiella pneumoniae
   Moraxella lacunata
   Haemophilus influenzae
   Haemophilus aegyptius
(5) Fungi:
   Candida albicans
   Aspergillus niger
(6) Viruses:
   adenovirus B
   herpes simplex
   molluscum contagiosum
(7) Protozoans:
   Acanthamoeba sp.

As well as causing eye infections, some pathogens could use the eye as an entry route to the whole body. The recently discovered human immunodeficiency virus (HIV — the virus for acquired immune deficiency syndrome or AIDS), has been found in tears, along with infected cells. This has led to concern that trial lenses could cause fomite transmission from one patient to another. This is extremely unlikely and there are no recorded cases of HIV being transmitted to patients or practitioners by contaminated contact lenses. It is not necessary to go to the lengths of having disposable trial lenses, because HIV is not a particularly hardy type and is destroyed by many of the routine soft lens disinfecting procedures, i.e. heating in saline above 60°C and oxidative processes such as hydrogen peroxide or chlorine release systems. For hard lenses, it may be necessary to modify the disinfection of trial lenses following fitting. The normal disinfecting solutions have less effect on HIV than the systems mentioned above. Protein-removing agents such as papain will assist in the destruction of virus particles by interfering with their capsid (surrounding protein sheath).

Jacobs (1986) recommends 70% alcohol solution for PMMA and holding RGP lenses at 60°C for one hour after thorough cleaning. Soaking hard and rigid gas permeable (RGP) lenses in 3% hydrogen peroxide solution for a minimum of 20 minutes is also effective.

Multidose eye drops should be avoided as far as possible.

Tonometers could possibly transfer contaminated tears and should be disinfected with 70% alcohol as should trial frames.

Infections directly or indirectly caused by contact lens wear are most likely to involve the cornea and conjunctiva. Fungal growth has been found on soft lenses and, therefore, the possibility of fungal as well as bacterial and viral infections should always be considered. The appropriate aspects of after-care and management are dealt with in Chapter 19. Any infection or suspected infection or allergic response requires medical treatment, preferably by an ophthalmologist who is conversant not only with contact lens fitting but also with the implications of prolonged ocular contact with the various constituents of contact lens solutions and materials.

Readers wishing to pursue further the subject of microbiology and the eye are referred to the work of Locatcher-Khorazo and Seegal (1972).

Antimicrobial agents

Antimicrobial agents can be usefully divided into physical and chemical agents. Their function is to produce either sterilization, which is removal or killing of all viable organisms, or disinfection which is the elimination of the possibility of infection from a material (and may not involve the removal of all viable organisms).

Physical agents

The mode of action of all these agents (with the exception of filtration) is to subject the organisms to sufficient energy to produce lethal protein denaturation and cell changes. The most common physical agent is heat. While a temperature of 70°C will kill most vegetative organisms in a few minutes (Dallos and Hughes, 1972, reported that *Ps. aeruginosa* and *Streptococcus faecalis* are killed at 70°C in 5 minutes), spores are resistant to boiling, even for hours. To ensure complete sterilization, the autoclave is now the method of choice, exposing the material to a temperature of 121°C for 15–20 minutes. The medium in which the material is heated is steam, as moist heat is much more effective than dry heat in killing bacteria. To sterilize by dry heat requires a temperature of 160°C and a time

of 2 hours and is clearly only suitable for glass or metal objects. Thermolability is always a disadvantage in heat sterilization and for some materials such as milk or wine a much lower temperature than 121°C is used to avoid breakdown of the material being treated. Pasteurization of milk consists of heating the milk to 62°C for 30 minutes.

At the other end of the temperature scale, freezing only slightly lowers the viable count of bacteria and, indeed, freezing is a method of preserving cultures. It never produces sensitization.

Irradiation by ultraviolet light is a method useful in reducing the level of airborne contamination by acting on the DNA molecules in bacteria. Apart from air sanitation, ultraviolet radiation can be used for sterilizing surfaces, but is of little use for sterilizing solutions contained in ultraviolet absorbing containers. Irradiation by gamma rays is a popular method for sterilizing single-dose containers of eye drops. The method of kill produced by these rays is markedly different from that produced by ultraviolet rays, involving irradiation at much higher energies. Free hydroxyl radicals are produced which are highly oxidizing and cytotoxic.

Waves of a different nature, i.e. sound waves, also have a disruptive effect on bacteria — *see* p. 151. Frequencies of between 15 kHz and MHz are bactericidal, but this effect has little practical application as yet.

One method of removal of bacteria from suspensions without killing, is filtration, using filters with a maximum pore size of 0.22 μm. This is the method of choice for heat-labile materials.

Chemical agents

Chemical agents can be divided into two different groups: the non-specific bactericidal, disinfecting agents which are mostly used *in vitro*, and the more specific bactericidal or bacteriostatic chemotherapeutic agents which are used *in vivo* to treat established infections or to act as prophylactic agents to prevent the occurrence of infections.

Disinfecting agents

There are a large number of compounds which can be lethal to microorganisms if applied in sufficiently high concentrations. However, it is a property of the common disinfecting agents that they have an antibacterial effect in low concentrations. Their effect is dependent on their concentration and the temperature. Hence, the sterilizing technique of heating with a bactericide.

Although disinfectants cover a wide group of compounds, there are two major mechanisms of action: the dissolving of lipids from the cell membranes, and the alteration by denaturation of proteins essential to the cell's life.

Before any antimicrobial substance is used for disinfecting or keeping solutions sterile it must, of course, be subjected to stringent tests *in vitro* to determine its potency and spectrum of activity (i.e. how many different types of bacteria will be inactivated by it). Any test *in vitro* applied must bear some relationship to the actual use to which the substance is to be put; for example, a substance which is to be incorporated into contact lens solutions must be tested in a way that will to some extent mirror its practical use.

Davies and Norton (1975) suggest that the activity of an antimicrobial substance, determined by a test *in vitro*, will depend on several criteria, as follows:

(1) The organism used and the conditions under which it is grown.
(2) The method of harvesting the cells (preparing the inoculum).
(3) The volume of test solution and the size of the inoculum.
(4) The temperature of holding the experimental solution and the frequency of sampling.
(5) The recovery medium to be used and the time and temperature of incubation.
(6) The criterion of antimicrobial activity to be considered acceptable.

Brown (1968), while investigating the survival of *Ps. aeruginosa* in fluorescein sodium solutions containing phenylmercuric nitrate, found that when cells were inoculated direct from the nutrient they retained their activity longer than cells which were washed in water before inoculating into the test solution. The broth had a protective effect. Riegelman, Vaughan and Okumoto (1956) state that tests *in vitro* sometimes give a false result because of 'carry-over' from the test solution to the recovery medium.

It is apparent since the reports of Norton *et al.* (1974) and McBride and Mackie (1974) that the antimicrobial performance of some contact lens solutions is open to question. Of 14 contact lens soaking solutions only seven inactivated the four test strains (three bacteria and one fungus) within 4 hours. They recommend some form of standard test for contact lens solutions. The mere presence of an antimicrobial substance in the formulation is no guarantee of adequate disinfecting ability.

Ganju (1974), however, felt that the tests applied by Norton *et al.* (1974) were too rigorous and a solution containing sufficient antibacterial substance to pass their tests would be too irritating to ocular tissues. He applied tests to soft contact lens-soaking solutions using smaller numbers of bacteria.

Recently, Lindeman-Meester (1974) has applied the tests of Kelsey and Sykes (1969) and Maurer (1969) for soft contact lens-soaking solutions.

Mercurial antibacterials (thimerosal*, phenylmercuric nitrate)

These compounds owe their activity to the binding of mercury ions to sulphydryl groups of enzymes and other proteins. Fear has been expressed in the past about the absorption of mercury into the eye. This has been demonstrated by Winder *et al.* (1980). Thimerosal and other mercurials have been implicated in allergies to contact lens solutions (Shaw, 1980; Wilson, McNatt and Reitschel, 1981; Wright and Mackie, 1982). Cytotoxicity has been demonstrated by Takahashi (1982) but this is less than for other preservative systems (Gasset *et al.*, 1974).

With regard to antimicrobial activity, mercurial compounds compared badly with chlorhexidine (Tragakis, Brown and Pearce, 1973). Thimerosal 0.004% required 24 hours to kill an innoculum of *Ps. aeruginosa* (Norton *et al.*, 1974). However, it has marked antifungal activity. Its antimicrobial activity is reduced with EDTA (Morton, 1985).

*Thimerosal is the American USAN solution equivalent to the British solution thiomersal or thiomersalate and because thimerosal is used almost universally in solutions this name will be used throughout this chapter.

Benzalkonium chloride

This substance is a cationic detergent which even in low concentrations is active against a considerable range of bacteria. In higher concentrations it can be irritating (Sussman and Friedman, 1969) and has been reported to cause significant corneal damage (Gasset *et al.*, 1974). It has been reported to lose its activity in the presence of cotton, polyvinyl alcohol and methylcellulose (Strachan, 1971). In concentrations above 0.01% it has the disadvantage in contact lens solutions of interfering with the wetting effect of these solutions. This is because the cationic hydrophilic group binds with the lens surface leaving the hydrophobic chain sticking out' (Dabezies, 1970).

The concentration used in contact lens solutions varies between 0.004% and 0.01%. The differences in these concentrations will have a great effect on the rate of bacterial kill. Wetting solutions normally contain 0.004% to avoid adverse effects on the eye, while 0.01% is used in soaking solutions where much greater antibacterial effect is required.

The critical value of concentration must be put into question particularly when considering the advisability of all-in-one solutions, as 0.01% benzalkonium chloride causes instability of the tear film (Wilson, Duncan and Jay, 1975).

Cetrimide (Cetavlon, ICI)

Like benzalkonium chloride, this is a cationic detergent, producing its bactericidal effect by dissolving the lipoprotein membrane of the bacterial cell and denaturing proteins. Some patients show a sensitivity reaction to this compound (Strachan, 1971) and the activity can be lost if the solution comes in contact with bark corks (Anderson and Keynes, 1958). In fact, Lowbury (1958) found cultures of *Ps. aeruginosa* growing in solutions of cetrimide that had been stoppered with a cork. It is often used in combination with chlorhexidine (Hibitane).

Chlorhexidine (Hibitane)

Chlorhexidine (a biguanide germicide) is found in many soft contact lens solutions either on its own or in combination with thimerosal. It has a better antibacterial action than thimerosal and leads to less allergic effects. It is effective in high dilution against a range of microorganisms.

Although it is toxic to the endothelium at a low concentration (20 µg/ml), this level will not be achieved by topical use and the epithelium is far more resistant requiring a much higher level to cause cellular damage (Green *et al.*, 1980).

Hydroxybenzoates

These compounds have fallen from use since it was found that they were inactive against *Ps. aeruginosa*. Hugo and Foster (1964) found that strains of *Pseudomonas* could grow in solutions of hydroxybenzoates without previous adaptation. Barkmar *et al.* (1969) found them very irritating. However, they are being re-introduced in the form of Nipastat in soft contact lens soaking solutions (*see* p. 149).

Chlorbutol

Chlorbutol is found in some eye drop formulations and contact lens solutions but has apparently fallen out of favour in recent years. This volatile antimicrobial agent has antifungal and antibacterial effects.

Sodium edetate (EDTA)

Ethylenediamine tetraacetic acid (EDTA) is a chelating agent which produces its effect by removing calcium ions from solution and disrupting the cell wall (MacGregor and Elliker, 1958; Brown and Richards, 1965). It is especially used with benzalkonium chloride with which it has a synergistic action. Since mercurial antimicrobials depend for their action on mercury, it would seem likely that EDTA would antagonize the action of thimerosal. Brown (1968) found that a mixture of PMN (phenylmercuric nitrate) and EDTA was less effective than PMN alone. However, Richards and McBride (1972) found an opposite effect. Further work needs to be carried out to determine the reaction of EDTA with mercurial antimicrobials, because many contact lens solutions contain a mixture of these two substances.

Solutions for hard (PMMA) lenses

The various solutions and drops available in the UK and elsewhere for use with hard lenses are given in Appendix F, *Table F.I.*

Historically the large majority of corneal lenses were manufactured from polymethyl methacrylate (PMMA) which is still used today but to a lesser extent. This material has good optical and mechanical properties which make it very suitable as a contact lens material. In addition the material is inert as far as the eye is concerned and rarely, if ever, produces an allergic response. Unfortunately, polymethyl methacrylate is hydrophobic in nature as it contains a large number of hydrophobic methyl groups in proportion to its hydrophilic carboxy ester groups. This means that the lens surface is not readily wetted by tear fluid. In order to avoid patient discomfort, therefore, the lenses need to be wetted before being placed on the eye. A second consequence of the hydrophobic nature of the plastics is that hydrophobic substances present on the eye, on the fingers, in soaps and cosmetics, readily adhere to the lens surface. These substances are therefore likely to irritate the eye by disruption of the tear film and are also likely to be present on the lenses when they are removed from the eye. Rewetting solutions for use with lenses *in situ* are often therefore necessary and, further, the lenses should always be cleaned immediately after removal from the eyes.

Despite being hydrophobic in nature, polymethyl methacrylate is, nevertheless, capable of absorbing a small quantity of liquid (around 2%). This small amount of liquid has two particular effects on corneal lenses (Phillips, 1969). First, complete hydration of the lens improves its wettability. This in turn improves both patient comfort and reduces adherence of mucus to the lens. Secondly, due to surface expansion, the curvature of a dehydrated corneal lens alters significantly (depending on power and thickness) over the first few hours of wear as it becomes hydrated. This again may affect patient comfort (as the fit is temporarily incorrect) and vision (as an incorrect tear lens is introduced). Further, when not on the eye there is a high risk of bacterial contamination of the lenses if they are left to dry out, and traces of mucus not cleaned from the lens provide an excellent bacterial breeding ground.

The hydrophobic nature of the lens material plus the effect of the liquid content when hydrated has necessitated the formulation of four types of contact lens solutions and gels, each with its own specific functions: wetting solutions; cleaning agents; storage (soaking) solutions; and rewetting solutions.

Each group, however, must nevertheless conform to the following prerequisites of all contact lens solutions.

(1) They must be sterile, stable and transparent.
(2) All solutions must be harmless to the eye if instilled undiluted.
(3) They must have no adverse effect on the contact lens material for which they are intended.
(4) They must be compatible with all other solutions used for the same lens material.
(5) In addition to being sterile, if presented in multidose form, all solutions should be self-sterilizing.

Wetting solutions

Following the discussion above, the functions of a wetting solution may be listed as follows:

(1) By acting as a lubricant between the surfaces of the lens and of the cornea and lids, its cushioning effect minimizes discomfort to the patient during initial insertion of the lens and subsequent wearing. This, in turn, encourages the prolonged wearing of lenses.
(2) By its action of encouraging even distribution of tears over the lens, it improves the optical performance.
(3) It acts as a mechanical buffer between lens and finger during the act of lens insertion and thus prevents lens contamination. This same buffer action prevents discomfort and possible corneal insult should the lens be inserted too rapidly.
(4) The wetting agents within the solution make it a suitable daily cleaning solution for many wearers for use following lens removal.

There is available to the practitioner a very wide choice of commercially produced wetting solutions. Some have fairly simple formulations, others appear more complex. However, all wetting solutions should have the following essential properties in addition to the criteria already listed above:

(1) They must have an adequate wetting effect on polymethyl methacrylate, even in high dilution.

(2) They must contain a viscous additive so that the solution adheres to the lens while it is being inserted and creates a protective cushion effect.

The constituents of a wetting solution vary with different proprietary brands, but the following include those main ingredients normally incorporated.

Preservative(s)

Those commonly used to maintain solution sterility include benzalkonium chloride (0.004–0.01%), chlorbutol (0.4%), phenylmercuric acetate or nitrate (0.002–0.01%), thimerosal (0.01–0.01%), chlorhexidine digluconate (0.002–0.01%), and cetylpyridinium chloride (0.001–0.01%). Ethylenediamine tetraacetate (EDTA; 0.01–0.1%), a chelating agent, may also be incorporated to enhance the antimicrobial activity of the bactericide in the wetting solution. It was demonstrated by Gould and Inglima (1964) that solutions containing either benzalkonium chloride or chlorbutol, when compounded with a 0.1% EDTA solution, displayed a marked increase in activity against *Ps. aeruginosa*. Further, by removal of metal ions from the bacterium cell wall, resistance to the bactericidal agent was prevented from building up. As previously stated (p. 131) there is some doubt if the enhancing effect of EDTA is as effective with phenylmercuric nitrate (Brown, 1968). Richards and Reary (1972) showed a reduction in the efficacy of thimerosal when EDTA was added in acid media.

Details of preservatives are given in Appendix F, *Table F.1*, at the end of the book.

Viscosity-building agent(s)

Methylcellulose, polyvinyl alcohol, hydroxypropylmethylcellulose (hypromellose) and hydroxyethylcellulose may be used to increase the viscosity of the solution and act as lubricant and clinging agents.

Wetting agent(s)

Polyvinyl alcohol, as well as having good viscosity-building properties is also often used for its good adhesive and wetting properties. Krishna and Brow (1964), using 1.4% polyvinyl alcohol in isotonic saline solution, found it had a greater surface contact time than 0.5% methylcellulose in isotonic saline solution. They also found that, unlike methylcellulose, polyvinyl alcohol does not retard regeneration of corneal epithelium. The liquid polymer polyvinyl pyrrolidone is also often used for its good spreading and wettability on the eye and lens surfaces (Hill and Terry, 1974).

Isotonic and buffering agents

Sodium and potassium chloride may be added to make the solution isotonic with tears. However, the importance of isotonicity has been over-emphasized in the past — especially for the small quantities involved on a contact lens — and a range of 0.7–1.2% sodium chloride solution equivalents is acceptable.

The normal range of tear liquid pH is from 7.0 to 8.5. Not only does this vary from person to person but there is also a daily temporal variation within the same individual (Carney and Hill, 1975). For this reason, a solution may show a pH range of 6.0–8.5 with greater initial comfort nearer to the physiological average of 7.2 (Brawner and Jessop, 1962). The solution should either not be buffered or only weakly buffered in order to allow the solution to adjust to the pH of the tear liquid as quickly as possible. Borate, bicarbonate and particularly phosphate buffers are those commonly used.

Colouring agents

There has recently been a move away from the inclusion of colouring agents. Apart from the easier differentiation between, for example, a soaking and wetting solution, they serve little use, and may act as an irritant or give rise to an allergic response.

Water

The water that is used in pharmaceutical products is purified water. This is similar to distilled water but is produced either by distillation or by passing water through an ion-exchange column. It still causes some confusion to patients who request distilled water and receive a bottle marked purified water. Another potentially dangerous source of confusion is that neither purified nor distilled water is necessarily sterile, being 'pure' of minerals but not of microorganisms. Unless supplied as sterile, it is safer to assume that it is not.

The inclusion of a bactericidal agent is obviously essential in most solutions used in contact lens practice. But of equal importance is the hygiene observed by the individual in making sure that his hands are washed thoroughly (*see* Plate 1), and are free of all traces of creams and nicotine prior to the handling of the lenses.

Cleaning agents

One of the most important aspects of any lens care regimen is the use of a prophylactic cleaning step in the normal daily hygiene routine to remove mucus, dirt, cosmetics and other environmental contaminants prior to overnight storage of the lens in a disinfectant solution. From a microbiological point of view, a clean lens is far easier to disinfect than a dirty lens as the removed contaminants cannot inactivate the preservative. Furthermore, these deposits can build up in time to levels sufficient to interfere with vision, lens wettability, and wearing comfort unless adequate prophylactic cleaning is carried out daily. As lens cleaning is accomplished outside the eye and the cleaning product used to effect the cleaning is not meant for direct instillation, it is possible to use slightly stronger cleaning agents than could normally otherwise be tolerated.

Although anionic, non-ionic, and amphoteric (balanced positive and negative constituents) surfactants are currently used in contact lens cleaning products, preference seems to favour non-ionic and amphoteric cleaners (Shively, 1975a). These cleaning agents emulsify lipids, solubilize debris and remove accumulated contaminants most favourably in an alkaline (pH 7.4 and above) environment. Following rinsing under cold running tap water the lens surface is clean and ready for overnight storage. It should be mentioned that cleaning hydrophobic and semi-hydrophobic lenses with various household cleaners such as laundry detergents, dishwashing compounds, skin cleansers and hair shampoos cannot be recommended because of their offensive and harsh actions on the lens surface or potential for damage to the cornea. This group of cleaners normally contains strong anionic detergents, caustic chemicals or detrimental solvents. Additionally, it is well known that *ani*onic detergents interact with commonly used *cati*onic preservative agents such as benzalkonium chloride, chlorhexidine digluconate or acetate, and cetylpyridinium chloride resulting

in deposition of a water-insoluble film on lenses with resultant discomfort for the wearer.

Specific itemization of constituents in various cleaning products cannot be given as most of these agents are regarded as proprietary to the lens solution manufacturer. Where these details are not available, manufacturers should be requested to provide information to support claims made for their cleaning products.

Even though cleaning products are not meant for use on the eye, it is important that they be packaged sterile and be self-disinfecting due to repeated exposure to the environment during use. This is normally accomplished by the use of preservative agents as described in the discussion on wetting solutions.

Isotonicity is not considered necessary in cleaning products as these products are not meant for direct instillation. Viscosity agents are incorporated by some manufacturers although their function in this context is not apparent.

Finally, although these products are meant for use outside the cornea, it is important that no irreversible ocular insult occur should they be accidentally transferred to the eye.

Cleaning products are routinely used by rubbing the solution on the lens surfaces and massaging the debris and contaminants off the lens surfaces with the fingers. This is then followed by a water rinse to remove the contaminants. However, various mechanical lens cleaning devices for wearer usage have emerged, mainly in the USA, which appear to facilitate this cleaning process. The use of an adjunctive cleaning solution is still, of course, required. The advantage of these devices appears to be for those wearers with poor manual dexterity and to reduce the continual surface scratching through the use of the fingers.

Soaking solutions

On removal from the eye and after cleaning, corneal lenses should be stored in a specially formulated soaking solution. This serves the following functions:

(1) By means of the bactericidal agent it contains, it should sterilize the lens and maintain its sterility.
(2) Maintenance of the hydrated equilibrium of the lens while it is not being worn.
(3) Prevention of the hardening of any ocular secretions remaining on the lens and to

loosen the adhesion of any accumulated mucus.

Phillips (1969) has reviewed the arguments in favour of storing a corneal lens in a soaking solution. The advantages of this form of storage over dry storage include improved lens surface wetting, visual performance and patient comfort, less corneal staining and lens abrasion and greater evidence of freedom from bacterial contamination. Further, due to hydration and dehydration, the curvature of a lens stored dry fluctuates every time it is placed on or removed from the eye. A lens stored in a soaking solution retains a constant curvature.

Soaking solutions also contain the antibacterial agents listed under Wetting solutions (p. 132). Slightly higher concentrations or two synergistic agents are often employed because decontamination is one of the major functions of the storage solution. Solubilizing agents are also often incorporated to loosen the attachment of any debris still attached to the lens. Soaking solutions should preferably irritate either minimally or not at all if transferred to the eye, although some manufacturers recommend that the solution be rinsed from the lens prior to the application of a wetting solution.

It is important to realize that the capability and efficacy of the solution to disinfect lenses is related to the regular changing of the storage solution every 2 or 3 days. The solution in the storage case will deplete with use as solution is removed with the lens. Further, the effectivity of the preservative will be reduced with each disinfection cycle by contaminants adhering to the lens surface such as mucus, atmospheric dust etc., and even cellular constituents released from dead and dying cells. If too many cycles of disinfection are carried out in the same volume of solution, the concentration of bactericide may be reduced to an inefficient level or worse, to such an extent that, for example, a resistant pseudomonad may actually grow in the solution. Responsibility for correct instruction of the lens wearer in this aspect of lens hygiene rests with the practitioner.

The importance of proper storage cases for use with soaking solutions must also be emphasized. Sufficient fluid volume must be contained to enable adequate diffusion of adsorbed contaminants into the solution and also to provide sufficient quantities of available preservative. Identification for each right and left lens must

be provided, preferably also with tactile projections. Colour coding of container caps is also helpful.

Caps should be screw threaded to prevent solution loss even under such conditions as pressurized aeroplane cabins. Storage cases should not contain any materials which may be irritant to the eye such as plasticizers found in the sponge rubber inserts sometimes used. For the reasons listed above, it is not sufficient to issue the patient with lens mailing containers for permanent use as storage cases.

Artificial tears/rewetting agents

When no contact lens is present the precorneal film has the primary role of resurfacing the cornea with a hydrophilic coating with every blink, because there is no actual flow of tears across the cornea. Introduction of the lens disturbs this corneal resurfacing process and the lens itself becomes the surface which the precorneal film must coat with a hydrophilic layer. Further, this fluid film easily ruptures when adjacent to the boundary of a solid object such as a contact lens placed in the film. When this phenomenon is associated with incomplete blinking, corneal staining in the peripheral–horizontal (3 and 9 o'clock) regions can often be detected, presumably indicating areas of localized corneal dessication. When the precorneal film is unable to spread over the lens due to lipid contamination (presumably arising from meibomian gland hyperactivity due to irritation of the inner lid margins), then decreased visual acuity and possible patient discomfort results.

In view of the above problems, rewetting solutions* have been designed for use with the lens *in situ*. These solutions contain wetting agents such as polyvinyl alcohol or Polysorbate 80, or highly viscous solutions containing polyvinyl pyrrolidone. Some are intended for use with hard lenses and some with soft lenses (as indicated in the footnotes), but those for use with soft lenses are really suitable for both types.

An artificial tears solution is indicated in conditions where natural tear liquid is reduced (*see* Chapter 8). A number of proprietary preparations* are available to the practitioner. Such solutions may contain benzalkonium

---

*Appendix F, *Tables F.I* and *F.II*, at the end of the book, give more details of these preparations for hard and soft lenses.

chloride (0.004–0.01%), chlorbutol (0.5%), thimerosal (0.02%), EDTA (0.05–0.1%) as preservatives; polyvinyl alcohol, hypromellose or hydroxyethylcellulose as wetting and viscosity-building agents; and sodium, potassium or magnesium chloride to provide solution isotonicity. Again, depending on the preservative, some of these are not suitable if soft lenses are worn. This rules out those containing chlorbutol and benzalkonium chloride.

Some cellulose acetate butyrate lenses should not be stored in solutions containing benzalkonium chloride as a slow reaction occurs with the material over a period of several months. The lens takes on a light straw colour, fluoresces a light blue under ultraviolet light, and a change in back optic zone radius (BOZR) results.

Multifunctional solutions

Multifunctional solutions are generally intended to combine the actions of cleaning and storage — or wetting, cleaning and storage — in one single product. The rationale behind the manufacture of such solutions is that some wearers will not carry out correct lens hygiene procedures due to the confusion of the multiplicity and expense of the solutions they must use. Most contact lens practitioners come across patients who omit one or more steps of the hygiene regimen simply because they run out of the appropriate solution. Often this step is then permanently omitted.

The basic components of combination cleaning and storage solutions are similar to the individual solutions with these functions. Most cleaning ingredients are non-ionic or amphoteric (Shively, 1975a) for the reasons mentioned earlier. Most combination wetting and storage solutions are similar in formulation to wetting solutions but with a lower viscosity. The authors have found that patients with lens mucus problems have sometimes benefited by storage of the lenses in combination solutions containing wetting agents such as polyvinyl alcohol, presumably due to surface adsorption of the wetting agent.

As might be expected, the combination of different lens hygiene functions into multifunctional solutions has elicited discussion about a possible compromise of efficacy in these products. For example, the relatively high viscosity required for a mechanical buffer action is contrary to the low viscosity required for

diffusion of surface contaminants into the storage solution. Further, solution viscosity of any degree would appear to retard bactericidal activity as was shown by the poorer performance of all combination wetting and soaking solutions tested by Norton et al. (1974) compared to soaking solutions alone. While acknowledging some compromise, the practitioner may feel that certain patients, for example, through lack of mental ability, application or responsibility, or simply because of occupational factors such as large amounts of travelling or when on holiday, should be advised to use multifunctional products.

Solutions for rigid gas permeable lenses

The advent of rigid gas permeable (RGP) (or gas permeable hard) lenses of varying types has led to additional problems for the practitioner and solution manufacturer.

Cellulose acetate butyrate (CAB) lenses appear prone to lipid deposits but only minimally to protein deposits. The negative surface charge of the silicone–acrylate group of materials attracts both protein and lipid deposits so that a denatured surface layer of protein may build up on the lenses of some patients as with hydrogel lenses (see below).

The majority of hard and soft lens solutions appear suitable for use with RGP lenses. However controversy exists as to whether benzalkonium chloride is bound to silicone–acrylate material surfaces or not (Rosenthal et al., 1986). Rosenthal et al. (1986), utilizing highly sensitive fluorescence spectroscopy, have shown minimal absorption of chlorhexidine digluconate to silicone–acrylate surfaces, but below a clinically significant level. They postulated that the positively charged chlorhexidine molecules probably bind to free carboxylate groups on the lens surfaces by electrostatic attraction and behave like a classic surface agent that forms a typical monolayer (see below). When the anionic binding sites of the silicone–acrylate polymer become saturated, no further uptake occurs. This explains their observation that chlorhexidine adsorption reached a plateau at a relatively low surface concentration.

In contrast, the continuing uptake of benzalkonium chloride found by these workers, beyond that which would be expected to occur if it was adsorbed as a monolayer, suggests that the mechanism of adsorption is one of self-aggregation whereby molecules of benzalkonium chloride bind to each other in layers. Like the chlorhexidine molecules, benzalkonium is positively charged and its initial adsorption may be the result of similar electrostatic forces. However, its longer hydrophobic chain may orient itself on the lens surface so as to create a template to which the hydrocarbon tails of adjacent benzalkonium molecules can adhere by the mechanism of hydrophobic interaction. As a result, benzalkonium, unlike chlorhexidine, can continue to form adherent layers on the lens surface with a potential for eventually reaching toxic concentrations, especially with sensitive individuals. Furthermore, because of its longer hydrocarbon chain, the binding strength of benzalkonium chloride to silicone–acrylate polymers due to hydrophobic interaction is greater than that of chlorhexidine digluconate and it resists removal even by vigorous cleaning. Further, in addition to its potential toxicity, adsorbed benzalkonium chloride intensifies the hydrophobicity of the lens surfaces. This reduced wettability may facilitate the adhesion of other hydrophobic elements present in tears and thereby accelerate the formation of surface deposits. Clinical findings appearing to confirm these laboratory findings were reported by Herskowitz (1987).

One RGP storage solution (Boston/Bausch & Lomb Conditioning Solution) has been formulated to take advantage of the electrostatic interaction postulated above. A cationic hydrophobic polyelectrolyte component competes with both chlorhexidine and lipid molecules for the anionic binding sites on the polymer thus theoretically reducing the concentration of adsorbed chlorhexidine and minimizing lipid deposition.

In contrast, Wong, Dziabo and Kiral (1986) found clinically insignificant levels of benzalkonium chloride adsorbed to silicone–acrylate lenses after 16 days' continuous exposure to a wetting and soaking solution preserved with benzalkonium chloride (Allergan's Wet-n-Soak). Furthermore, they pointed out that the effectiveness of benzalkonium chloride is readily decreased by serum and proteins so that, whatever small amount is accumulated on the lens, is inactivated within the tear environment

and therefore is of no consequence. In addition, any small amount of benzalkonium chloride left on the lens will be inactivated upon cleaning with detergent cleaners provided this cleaning is carried out. Similar results were reported by Hoffman (1987), and Richardson, Gee and Meakin (1980) for CAB material.

While controversy still exists over the use of this preservative for silicone–acrylate materials, it is pertinent to report the increase in problems found by UK practitioners when the thimerosal preservative in Alcon's Soaclens was temporarily replaced with benzalkonium chloride (Anon, 1985). As with hydrophilic lenses, practitioners should be constantly alert to the potential problems of preservative sensitivity and also the importance of lens cleaning because preservative binding to surface deposits may also occur.

Manufacturers claim improved wettability following the use of various storage and cleaning regimens (Benjamin and Simons, 1984). However, most studies are carried out on new lenses and highly variable results are obtained on worn and therefore deposited lenses. Because of their susceptibility to protein and lipid deposits described above, silicone–acrylate will often, but not always, develop a layer of denatured protein which may be difficult to remove and cause loss of tolerance and vision. Both soft and hard lens surfactant cleaners can be used on a daily prophylactic basis. Those utilizing hypertonicity as a cleaning method will have no effect although others, such as Alcon's Polyclens (Opti-Clean), will work equally well for RGP as well as PMMA and hydrogel materials. Other cleaners are formulated specifically for RGP lenses such as the Boston/Bausch & Lomb Intensive Cleaner. This contains a very fine, soft abrasive in suspension with friction enhancing agents that mechanically break the bond between the lens surface and debris.

In addition to daily cleaning, many patients are also advised to utilize protease enzymes to remove denatured protein, although not usually at the same frequency as hydrogel lens wearers (see below).

Some RGP materials are recommended to be used with one solution specifically designed for the lens material, e.g. Menicon O_2 solution for use with the Menicon O_2 lens. Chlorhexidine-preserved solutions should not be used with styrene lens materials as surface wettability is reduced.

Lenses made largely from pure silicone are no longer commonly available due to problems of poor surface wettability. However, their high oxygen permeability still makes them useful for very high prescriptions, e.g. lenses for aphakic neonates. Additionally, a technological break-through in improving wettability or surface treatment may lead to a resurgence of these lenses.

Silicone rubber lenses are manufactured from approximately 40% cross-linked dimethyl poly-siloxane (silica) mixed with siloxane polymer as a filler, and the entire mixture heated at a high pressure in order to achieve further polymeriza-tion and cross-linking. The silica helps to determine the refractive index of the final lens which lies somewhere between 1.49 and 1.56. Although the material is highly transmissive to oxygen and other gases, water adsorption is negligible (0.4% compared with 1.5–2.0% for PMMA) and lens parameters are not normally affected by the storage solution characteristics (Phares, 1972a), the solution being used for its antibacterial function only. The extremely hydrophobic nature of silicone lenses makes them difficult to wet and maintain wettable during wear (see Plates 44 and 45). Wetting solutions containing polyvinyl alcohol or cellu-lose derivatives and formulated for conventional PMMA lenses are not adequate wetting agents for silicone lenses (Krezanoski, 1972a). They may be used with safety, however, with the exception of solutions containing chlorbutol as this is bound or adsorbed onto the lens surface. This concentrating effect of the preservative causes marked ocular discomfort. To overcome its hydrophobic nature, silicone lenses have been surface coated with a more hydrophilic material (although this suffers from the expected disadvantage that it eventually wears off) or treated to produce surface molecular reorienta-tion (Shively, 1975a). Special wetting agents were also investigated in an attempt to over-come the wetting problem (Krezanoski, 1972a). Most cleaners designed for PMMA lenses are only partly effective in maintaining silicone lens surfaces in a clean state. Two manufacturers produced solutions specifically for storing sili-cone rubber lenses although these are no longer available.

Combinations of differing classifications of material into a single lens have also been achieved, for example a hard gas permeable optic portion with a polyhydroxyethyl metha-crylate (PHEMA) periphery. This appears to allow the optical quality of a rigid lens to be partly combined with the comfort of a soft lens although, of course, it raises potential problems from the lens sterility and wetting point of view.

In each instance the practitioner must consult the manufacturers' literature extremely careful-ly to decide which solutions may or may not be used with each material. Both verbal and written instructions must be given to each patient who should also be advised not to use any unlisted solutions without first checking with the prescribing practitioner. The constant development of new materials requires practi-tioners to be always up to date with current literature and constantly aware of potential toxic or hypersensitivity problems.

Solutions for hydrophilic lenses

Details of the drops and solutions available in the UK (and elsewhere) for soft lenses are given in Appendix F, Table F.II.

During the early stages in the development of hydrophilic lenses it was thought that the hydrophilic nature of the surface would obviate the need for most solutions because wetting agents were obviously unnecessary, and for the same reason it was thought that cleaning would also be unnecessary. However, as experience has been gained over the last few years, the complexities of dealing with new materials for use in contact with the eye has become increasingly apparent. Further, while the large majority of hydrophobic lenses are made from relatively few materials, hydrophilic lenses are made from many materials, include differing additives and have widely varying physical and physiological properties.

Perhaps the most difficult problem that has arisen with hydrophilic lenses is that of disinfec-tion. Fortunately a considerable number of conjunctival sacs do not contain pathogenic bacteria. Smith (1954) reported 5000 cases in which swabs were taken from the conjunctival sacs of apparently normal eyes. Of these cases, 47% showed no bacterial contamination in the sac. Other authors quote between 20 and 70% as the incidence of sterile conjunctival sacs (Duke-Elder, 1965). In general, the majority of the conjunctival flora are harmless saprophytes involved in the destruction of dead cells. Only 25% of conjunctival sacs appear to contain potential pathogens (Smith, 1954). Bacteria such as *Ps. aeruginosa* are rarely found in the sac. *Staph. aureus* is found more often but still only in a minority of cases (2–15%). Even if an organism is a potential pathogen, it has been established that the conditions in the sac are likely to reduce the virulence of the organism. This is due in part to its relatively low temperature, in part to the action of the lysozyme of the tears, and in part to the mechanical action of blinking and the sluicing effect of the lacrimal secretion. In addition to the physical and chemical factors inhibiting the pathogens, non-pathogens also contribute to the protection of the eye by competing with the pathogens for nutrients. These factors combine to provide a relatively stable protective system for the eye against infection.

There are, however, many examples of how changes in the prevailing conditions can disrupt this balance: for example, keratoconjunctivitis sicca due to insufficient or inadequate tears; exposure keratitis due to the inability of the lids to sweep the cornea, and even bandaging the eye which causes an increase in the number and virulence of organisms, discharge often being noted. Contact lenses unfortunately interfere with the eyes' defence mechanisms. Hydrophilic lenses in particular prevent the lids from sweeping the cornea and interfere with the tears washing the cornea. They probably raise the corneal temperature and can also induce breaks in the corneal epithelium. In reports that appear in the literature of corneal infection occurring in otherwise 'normal' contact lens wearers, one of the main causes has been found to be the introduction of significant bacterial contamination either on the lens or via contaminated solutions. While bacteria appear unable to penetrate the intermolecular 'pores' of hydrophilic lenses; (Knoll, 1972; Matas, Spencer and Hayes, 1972) except possibly into defects in older lenses (Poster, 1972; Tripathi and Ruben, 1972), the tear liquid absorbed by the lenses serves as an excellent bacterial culture medium.

Further, surface irregularities in the lens occurring during manufacture (Matas, Spencer and Hayes, 1972; Filppi, Pfister and Hill, 1973) and eye secretions adhering to the lens surface may permit a nidus to form where bacteria can aggregate and possibly be protected from

disinfection processes (*see Figures 13.30* and *13.31*).

It was also pointed out by Ruben (1966) that fungi can grow into hydrophilic lenses and Filppi, Pfister and Hill (1973) have shown penetration by *Aspergillus fumagatus*, and Dallos and Hughes (1972) penetration by *Thrichotecium roseum* (this latter mould sometimes being found in tap water). The mechanism of penetration is probably by means of enzymes which cause degradation of the lens material and permit entry of the fungal hyphae (*Plate 33*).

Lenses which show spots on or within the lens substance should not be dispensed even though they may not necessarily be fungal growth and could, for example, be rusting ferrous particles (Loran, 1973). Even though there is no apparent damage to the lens there is always a possibility that endotoxins synthesized by the fungus are bound within the plastics. Fungi will quickly overcome the preservative in any disinfecting solution unless the solution is replaced at daily intervals. Thus, as well as antibacterial activity, any methods of soft lens disinfection must also have a high fungicidal capability.

A further problem occurring with hydrophilic lenses is that of deposits adhering to the lens surfaces (*Plates 31, 32, 36–40*). The main sources of these deposits are ocular secretions, tap water contaminants which may have been absorbed by the lenses, eye drops, finger dirt, eye make-up and contaminants introduced during manufacture and from the atmosphere (*see Figures 13.27* and *13.28*). The bulk of deposits, however, are mucoproteins from the tear liquid. Also found are calcium (Ruben, Tripathi and Winder, 1975), iron and other insoluble divalent and trivalent metal salts if impure water for storage or rinsing solutions has been used. Environmental and occupational factors also affect the cleanliness of lenses. Rusting ferrous particles are commonly seen in the surface of the lenses or deeper if introduced during manufacture (or possibly from high speed projectile particles) (*see Plate 40* and *Figure 13.29*). Some eye drops containing phenylephrine, adrenaline or berberine cause discolouration and some preservatives from sterilizing and hydrating solutions may concentrate in the matrix of soft lenses causing either discolouration (*Plate 35*) or surface filming and consequently discomfort to the patient (Ganju and Cordrey, 1975). Handling the lenses may transfer a variety of contaminants such as lipstick, mascara, oily creams, detergents and nicotine to the lenses if strict personal hygiene is not observed. Further, Wilson *et al.* (1971) found fungal contamination in 12% of eye make-up samples and bacterial contamination in as high as 43% of samples.

Repeated disinfection by boiling and to a lesser extent with chemical disinfecting solutions denatures the surface mucoprotein, slowly building up a tenacious irregular surface layer. This may cause symptoms of discomfort, lowered acuity, lens discolouration and conjunctival injection and possibly an apparent change in fitting and power. For these reasons the development has taken place of daily cleaning solutions to prevent surface deposits from building up and rejuvenating products to remove deposits already present.

Because of the gradual build-up of deposits on the lenses, a more effective cleaning treatment is required at periodic intervals depending on the patient, lens material, method of disinfection etc. Ganju and Cordrey (1975) and Gasson (1975) have shown measurable drops in ultraviolet and visible light transmission through many lenses only a few months old which had not been correctly cleaned. Typically this was around 15% for visible light, and Gasson noted that some 15% of soft lens wearers noted a reduction in acuity after 6 months wear (although approximately twice as many reported an improvement). Because of the nature of the material most lenses cannot be repolished as with hard lenses, and the development of enzymatic and oxidative systems has emerged, some for use by the patient and others for use by the practitioner.

Finally, it is not uncommon for hydrophilic lens wearers to experience some discomfort or temporary drop of vision while the lenses are worn. Ignoring physical causes such as lens movement or distortion, the cause may vary from inadequate tear formation and a dirty lens, to personal idiosyncrasies. To overcome the problem, products have been developed which rehydrate and clean the lens *in situ*. These products are especially helpful in cases where the front surface of the lens has become dehydrated, for example, due to low environmental humidity, causing a change in lens curvature resulting in discomfort and impairment of vision.

The usual sequence of events during soft lens wear and care is for the lens to be cleaned on removal from the eye with a special cleaning solution. This is rinsed off with a suitable saline rinsing solution. The lens is then disinfected or sterilized by one means or another. It is then ready to wear, but sterile or preserved physiological saline solution may be used to rinse the soaking solution off the lens in some cases. Also, prior to or during wear a rewetting solution may be used. From time to time special cleaning or rejuvenating procedures become necessary, utilizing further special solutions or compounds.

The problems of disinfection, cleaning, rinsing, restoring and rehydrating hydrophilic lens materials has led to the development of four specific groups of systems and solutions: disinfecting solutions or systems and rinsing solutions; cleaning solutions and methods; rejuvenating systems; lens conditioning and tear replacement solutions.

Methods of disinfection

Heating methods

The American Food and Drugs Administration (FDA) regulations state that methods for soft lens hygiene should fulfil the requirements for disinfection. This is defined as 'the physical or chemical process producing destruction of pathogenic microorganisms' (United States FDA, 1973). This definition does not imply the destruction of bacterial spores because these are at a resistant stage, but only of vegetative microorganisms. Mould spores are considered to be reproductive stages and resist heat only slightly better than vegetative forms of bacteria. Total sterility is only achieved by autoclaving for 15 minutes at 120°C and 15 lb/in^2 (103.5 kPa) pressure and for this reason moist heat units which destroy vegetative microorganisms are often described as 'asepticizors' rather than 'sterilizers'.

Heating was suggested some years ago by Ruben (1966) and Morrison (1966) and was recognized by the FDA in 1972 as the first approved method of disinfection for use with soft lenses. Although the physical requirement for disinfection is 80°C for 10 minutes, the temperature achieved inside the Bausch & Lomb lens carrying case during a normal asepticizing cycle is 96°C for approximately 20 minutes (Mote, Filppi and Hill, 1972). Typical heating units are

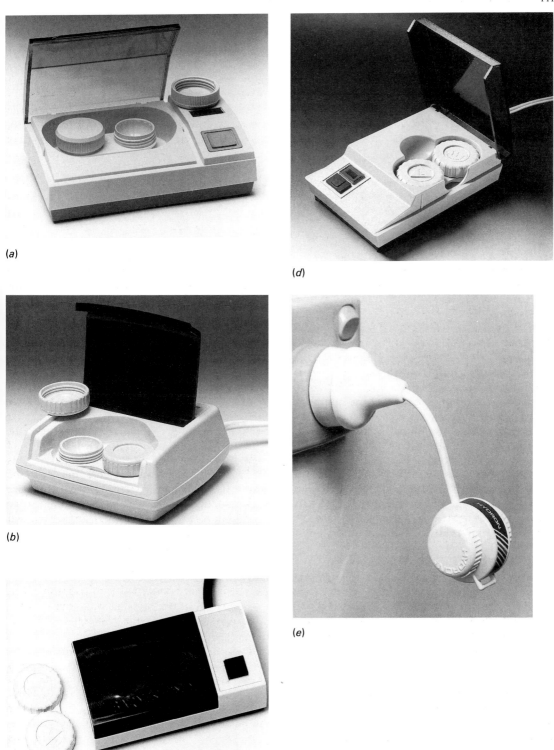

(a)

(b)

(c)

(d)

(e)

Figure 4.1 Various thermal units for hydrogel lens disinfection: (*a*) Alcon; (*b*) Allergan; (*c*) Pilkington Barnes–Hind; (*d*) Bausch & Lomb; (*e*) Allergan Hydron

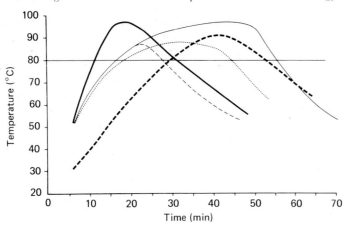

Figure 4.2 Time–temperature cycle of the saline contained within the contact lens cases produced by several different manufactuers. — Allergan; ..... Alcon Micro-Therm; --- Pilkington Barnes–Hind; —— Bausch & Lomb, long cycle; ---- Bausch & Lomb, short cycle. (Reproduced by kind permission of Bausch & Lomb)

shown in *Figure 4.1* and a typical heating cycle is shown in *Figure 4.2*.

Boiling, and particularly repeated boiling, may possibly cause molecular breakdown or degradation of the lens material over a period of time thereby shortening the life of the lens. Mandell (1974), however, states that the temperature at which this occurs rapidly for HEMA material is probably about 30°C higher than that normally used in the asepticizing process so that any breakdown of the molecular structure probably occurs at an extremely slow rate. Because all current lens materials are stable below 85°C, Dallos and Hughes (1972) tried to achieve sterilization by pasteurization at 70–73°C. They found that representative samples of heat-resistant pathogenic bacteria were killed after heating for 2 minutes at 70°C. These writers recommended daily pasteurization with the unit heating up to 72°C (i.e. slightly higher than required) over a 2–3 hour period and remaining at 72°C for 30 minutes.

As stated above, units used in practice immerse the lens storage container, which keeps the lenses in a suitable saline solution (*see* p. 133), in steam from boiling water. The temperature reached inside the lens case is typically around 96°C for 20 minutes. The efficacy of these asepticizing units has been demonstrated by Knoll (1972) using bacteria, a fungus and virus; Mote, Filppi and Hill (1972) using Gram-positive and Gram-negative bacteria, a spore former, and a fungus; Hydron Lens Ltd (1972) using a selection of pathogenic bacteria; Filppi and Pfister and Hill (1973) using the fungus *A. fumagatus*; and Busschaert *et al.* (1974) using a selection of bacteria, fungi and bacterial spores. Ludwig, Meisler and Rutherford (1986) reported thermal disinfection as being more effective against the protozoa *Acanthamoeba* sp. than chemical disinfecting methods. Busschaert and his co-workers found, however, that bacterial spores were occasionally able to survive the asepticizing cycle; Tragakis, Brown and Pearce (1973) also found the fungus *A. fumagatus* sometimes survived asepticization (possibly by sporulating) and Bernstein, Stow and Maddox (1973), in contrast with the other workers listed above, found 20% of unopened Soflens cases to be contaminated after asepticization by the patient. This number increased to 86% contamination of the cases a few hours after opening, although presumably the lenses would normally be in the wearers' eyes by this time.

In their study, one patient showing bacterial contamination of her container and an eye infection admitted to changing the saline solution only every 2–3 days. The importance of daily asepticization and the use of fresh solution must therefore be greatly impressed on the patient. Some manufacturers produce pre-prepared saline solution containing thimerosal or sorbic acid, as an added method of disinfection following asepticization should the container be opened and bacteria inadvertently allowed to enter. Bacteria may also be sucked in from the outside as the container cools and patients must be advised to use the correct screw-cap container and to make sure it is firmly tightened. Similarly, a loose cap may allow loss by evaporation of the water within the container causing hypertonicity of the saline solution, alteration of the lens dimensions and subsequent discomfort on lens insertion.

In some countries sterile, unpreserved, physiological saline is available in 500 ml bottles with jet dispenser nozzles, and compressed-air powered saline aerosols are now widely available. It may also be prepared from specially manufactured salt tablets or granules shaken up with the correct quantity of purified or distilled water — but this is not sterile. It is important that this solution is not used for rinsing the lenses prior to their insertion in the eye, for neither purified nor distilled water is sterile and is often very far from it (Jenkins and Phillips, 1986). In addition there are increasing reports of stromal keratitis and ulceration in patients using home-made saline due to the presence of *Acanthamoeba* sp. in the water (Epstein *et al.*, 1986). Also available are sterile (unpreserved) unit dose saline solutions such as Salettes, as detailed in Appendix F, *Table F.II*, as well as 0.9% sodium chloride solution available in 1 litre and 500 ml bags intended for intravenous saline drips. Physiological saline solution preserved with thimerosal and EDTA or sorbic acid is also suitable for the boiling of lenses. The commercially available brands of preserved saline solution are also included in Appendix F, *Table F.II*. However, the use of preserved salines in thermal units increases the risk of hypersensitivity to preservatives bound to the lens surface deposits (because of the greater incidence of bound surface deposits generally found with heat disinfection methods) and lens discolouration if thimerosal is used as the preservative.

One major problem with boiling is that mucoproteins present on the lens become coagulated or denatured on the lens surface by the asepticizing process. The film thus formed may cause lens discomfort, loss of acuity, loss of transparency, conjunctival injection and possibly a change in lens fitting and power. It may also reduce lens porosity and thereby aid the formation of corneal oedema. For this reason daily cleaning is a necessity prior to boiling (*see below*).

A modified form of pasteurization is provided by the Bausch & Lomb and Pilkington Barnes–Hind Softmate low heat disinfecting units. These utilize a short cycle thermal unit which heats to only around 80°C and maintains a temperature above 70°C for approximately 15 minutes (*see Figure 4.2*) (Liubinas, Swenson and Carney, 1987).

Since some of the newer lens materials, especially polymers containing methacrylic acid, absorb up to 38 times more protein than PHEMA (Stone, Mowrey-McKee and Kreutzer, 1984), normal heat disinfection methods will cause considerable denaturation and lens discolouration in some cases. The lower heat temperatures utilized are claimed to reduce this problem and yet provide adequate disinfection even against heat-resistant organisms such as *Streptococcus faecalis*.

Lenses may also be pasteurized by utilizing an ordinary household vacuum flask. The flask is pre-heated with boiling water then refilled with boiling water. The lenses, in their tightly capped container and stored in saline, are then carefully dropped into this flask which is left uncapped overnight.

The instructions to be given to the patient regarding asepticizing are given in Chapter 9. Practitioners using trial lenses stored in saline solution should boil them at frequent intervals once they have been used and re-sealed in order to kill bacteria which may have survived earlier boiling by sporulating. Lenses received from the manufacturer should ideally have been auto-claved and therefore be sterile. Lenses which have been used on a patient's eye should be boiled or preferably autoclaved (Litvin, 1977), before being returned to the lens rack.

The use of autoclaving by laboratories to achieve lens sterilization would not, however, appear to be without its drawbacks. Larke (1974) has noted that the pH of lens storage saline solution is usually acidic in the region of 5.5–6.5 following autoclaving and often therefore gives rise to ocular irritation. In addition, should the lens vial remain unopened for a matter of weeks or months, the pH will continue to fall and may reach 4.0–4.5. The absorption of atmospheric carbon dioxide with the formation of weakly dissociated carbonic acid would seem a possible mechanism and this seems to be a problem in lens vials which have gas permeable silicone rubber stoppers.

The advantages of boiling or asepticizing as a method of lens disinfection may therefore be summarized as follows:

(1) It is generally accepted as an effective method of lens disinfection and is recognized as such by health authorities throughout the world.
(2) After the initial purchase of the boiling unit it is the least expensive method.

(3) Where unpreserved saline solution is used (*see* earlier paragraph) there is no risk of allergy or hypersensitivity to any preservative.

The disadvantages may be summarized as follows:

(1) After the fees for the fitting and supply of soft lenses, the additional cost of the asepticizor often makes it initially prohibitive.
(2) There is a fairly high risk of microorganism build-up if the procedure is not carried out daily and fresh saline solution prepared daily (Brown *et al.*, 1974).
(3) Certain bacterial spores may survive asepticizing and may cause lens damage if the boiling is not carried out daily to destroy vegetative forms of the organism.
(4) Since some aseptors use saline solution which does not contain a preservative, there is a slight risk of microorganisms being transferred onto the lens from the fingers. Such a possible case has been cited by Storey (1973).
(5) Of the various methods of hydrogel disinfection, heating methods cause the greatest denaturing effect of ocular secretions remaining on the lens surface with the accompanying disadvantages mentioned above and greater risk of problems such as giant papillary conjunctivitis (*see* Chapter 19).
(6) Repeated heat disinfection may cause slow degradation of the polymer structure thereby reducing the life of the lens. It should be emphasized that this effect undoubtedly varies from material to material and that to the authors' knowledge no experimental work has yet been undertaken on this aspect. Nevertheless it is generally accepted that thermal methods shorten the life of most hydrogel lenses by around 25%, largely because of exacerbated deposit formation.
(7) Following from the above, the technique is not a universal one suitable for all lens materials and some materials degrade very quickly with repeated heat sterilization.
(8) Although not as slow for lens disinfection as soft lens storage solutions (*see below*) the method is not rapid, taking approximately one hour and possibly a further hour for cooling and for the lens dimensions to return to normal (Loran, 1974). Again, although quicker than some hydrogen peroxide disinfection procedures, the method is slightly more time consuming for the patient than the use of soft lens storage solutions.
(9) There are occasions when it is impossible to asepticize by boiling, for example, while travelling.

Chemical disinfection

Hydrogen peroxide

The first method of chemical disinfection was by means of 3% hydrogen peroxide (Isen, 1972). The need for an alternative to heating methods arose because the lens material currently used by Isen did not stand up well to repeated boiling. Although tending to fall out of favour after its initial introduction because of the prolonged nature of the neutralizing step (*see below*), it has been revived in recent years.

The antimicrobial efficacy of hydrogen peroxide has been well known for over 100 years. The 3% solution is possibly the most effective disinfecting agent available in contact lens practice today and will kill large numbers of microorganisms very quickly (Levine, Litsky and Lamm, 1981; Penley *et al.*, 1985). It has a broad antibacterial spectrum but exposure times of 1 hour (Penley *et al.*, 1985) and 4 hours (C. Jenkins, 1986, personal communication) have been recommended to ensure adequate antifungal and antiprotozoan activity.

The stability of dilute solutions is highly pH dependent (Schumb, Satterfield and Wentworth, 1955) and for this reason the 3% solutions used in contact lens practice are now adjusted to an approximate pH of 4–5. In addition 'stabilizers' are also necessary, e.g. phosphates, which complex iron. As the pH rises so more stabilizer is required to prevent peroxide breakdown.

In the original method described by Isen, the lenses were soaked for 5 minutes in 3% hydrogen peroxide which is highly acidic having a pH of 3.0–4.0. This was therefore neutralized by exposure to 0.5% sodium bicarbonate in 0.9% sodium chloride for 1 minutes and the lenses then immersed in 0.9% sodium chloride for 15 minutes. The lenses were then stored overnight in isotonic saline solution. Feldman

(1971) and Gasset, Ramer and Katzin (1975) described modifications to the neutralizing step but all involved several time-consuming neutralizing steps.

The technique underwent a revival during the late 1970s with the introduction by American Optical of a platinum catalyst to break down residual hydrogen peroxide:

$$Pt + 2H^+ + H_2O_2 \rightarrow Pt^{2+} + 2H_2O$$

$$Pt^{2+} + H_2O_2 \rightarrow Pt + 2H^+ + O_2$$

Lenses are first soaked in 3% hydrogen peroxide (Lensept) for 10–15 minutes as the disinfection step, and then placed in a second container, in preserved salined (Lensrins) to maintain sterility, and containing a platinum-coated plastic disc as catalyst. The technique has the advantage that it eliminates the time-consuming elution/neutralizing steps of earlier methods because this is done, usually overnight, by the catalyst. The major disadvantages are the slow action of the catalyst (4 hours for complete neutralization) should patients forget to transfer lenses to the second container before retiring at night and the fact that platinum is easily poisoned so that the catalyst needs replacing after approximately every 100 uses.

As a further simplification of the system, American Optical have introduced the AOSept system where the hydrogen peroxide is mixed with physiological saline and the combined mixture placed directly in the container with the platinum disc. Because of the slow action of the platinum catalyst, the lenses are disinfected before the hydrogen peroxide is broken down. The method thereby becomes a 'one-step' system eliminating the need for a separate neutralizing step and the risk of severe ocular stinging if patients forget this step. A further advantage is the elimination of the need for preservatives in the saline. Stability of the hydrogen peroxide at the relatively high pH (6.5) necessitated by this method is maintained by the higher level of stabilizers incorporated.

In the Allergan 'Oxysept' system a preserved saline containing the catalyst 'catalase' is used. Catalase, present in blood, potatoes and other plant and animal tissues, is an enzyme, a specific biochemical catalyst, that rapidly increases hydrogen peroxide decomposition (Gyulai *et al.*, 1986). Commercial material is derived from bovine or canine liver or fungal tissue. The major advantage of the system is the rapid neutralizing step (10 minutes) and the biocompatibility of the catalyst. The disadvantages are the relative instability of catalase and the need for a preservative (thimerosal) in the neutralizing solution.

Hydrogen peroxide can also be neutralized by reaction with various chemical agents in the second, neutralizing agent:

(1) Sodium pyruvate (Cooper Vision)
$$CH_3COCOONa + H_2O_2 \rightarrow$$
(Sodium pyruvate)
$$CH_3COONa + CO_2 + H_2O$$
(Sodium acetate)

(2) Sodium sulphite (Pilkington Barnes–Hind)
$$Na_2SO_3 + H_2O_2 \rightarrow H_2O + Na_2SO_4$$
(Sodium sulphite)   (Sodium sulphate)

(3) Sodium thiosulphate (Bausch & Lomb)
$$2\,Na_2S_2O_3 + H_2O_2 \rightarrow Na_2S_4O_6 + 2\,NaOH$$
(Sodium thiosulphate)   (Sodium tetrathionate)

All three methods have the advantage that neutralization is achieved fairly rapidly (10–30 minutes) and they are relatively stable with biocompatible by-products. All suffer the disadvantage of requiring separate disinfection and neutralization steps and the need for a preservative in the neutralizing medium to maintain lens and solution sterility. Some manufacturers are now producing unit dose neutralizing solutions to provide preservative-free systems.

Failure to neutralize the hydrogen peroxide in the lens will cause severe transient discomfort and the need for immediate lens removal! The eye may remain hyperaemic and show mild corneal superficial punctate staining to sodium fluorescein for several hours. Serious eye damage has not been reported, although Knopf (1984) has reported recovery taking several days in a patient with a previous history of blepharoconjunctivitis.

Because no gas is released in the thiosulphate and sulphite reactions, a pressure vent is not required in the lens storage case. Carbon dioxide is formed during the pyruvate reaction but a special case is not required because the gas dissolves in aqueous solution producing a bicarbonate ion. The oxygen produced in the catalytic neutralization of the platinum and catalase methods restricts the case usage to the domestic situation because solution leaks from the vents when it is used as a transportation vessel.

The CooperVision (Titmus Eurocon) system utilizes a lower level of peroxide (0.6%) than all other manufacturers. For this, a minimum disinfection time of 2 hours is recommended.

Because of its good antimicrobial activity, its mild cleaning action, and ability to prevent or reduce lens discolouration, hydrogen peroxide methods of lens disinfection have become increasingly popular.

Chlorhexidine and thimerosal preserved saline storage solutions

The inconvenience of the boiling and early hydrogen peroxide disinfection routines meant that alternative methods were looked for with emphasis on the search for simple storage and rinsing solutions which would be non-irritant to the eye and harmless to lens materials.

The first and major problem was that of the adsorptive or binding ability of most hydrogel materials. Because hydrophilic lenses have the ability to take up water, they will of necessity absorb an aqueous solution of chemical which might be presented to them. This should not create a problem if the solution by itself is safe on the eye. A potential problem arises, however, if the soft lens adsorbs (or loosely complexes with certain molecules on the lens surface) the preservative from the solution, because this will then be concentrated on the surface. Unfortunately, many of the commonly used hard lens solution preservatives are strongly bound by hydrogel materials. These preservatives are harmful to living bacterial cells and will generally be damaging to the corneal epithelial cells if present in higher than normal concentrations.

Benzalkonium chloride (a cationic preservative) has been shown to be a strong soft lens binder whereas thimerosal (an anionic preservative) is not (Sibley and Yung, 1973). It would appear, therefore, that electrostatic forces are involved. Chlorhexidine as a cationic preservative is also bound (Sibley, 1973, cited by Browne, Anderson and Charvez, 1974) but as it has a large molecular structure and a very weak cationic action its binding capacity is about one-sixth that of benzalkonium chloride (Hind, 1975). Various authors have shown that for most patients the amount of preservative bound

to the lens is insufficient to cause ocular irritation (Krezanoski, 1972a; Phares, 1972b; Brown et al., 1974; Hind, 1975). Other workers have mentioned the binding ability of the other commonly used hard lens preservatives, phenyl-mercuric nitrate and chlorbutanol (Krezanoski, 1972b; Ganju, 1974), but EDTA does not appear to be bound to any significant degree. Surprisingly, Lerman and Sapp (1971), from laboratory and clinical experiments, determined that the concentration of benzalkonium chloride and chlorbutol normally used in ophthalmic preparations was bound to an insufficient degree to cause ocular irritation. This unexpected result may be due to the fact shown by Otten and Szabocsik (1976) that the final formulation of the solution has a significant effect on the binding ability of the preservative, although they were unable to offer any explanation for this.

Although chlorhexidine is only minimally bound to clean lens material, it is very effectively bound to protein deposits on the lens surface and, unfortunately, this exacerbates the binding effect. Not only does this reduce the efficacy of the solution but the increased concentration of bound preservative causes symptoms of ocular discomfort over a period of time as the lens contaminants build up, often leading to lens rejection (Hind, 1975). Further, there is the danger of a sudden release of preservative from the lens to the cornea if there is a pH change, fluid movement across the lens or replacement by ions present in the tear liquid (Ganju, 1974). Daily cleaning of the lens is therefore of paramount importance.

Most of the soft lens storage or soaking solutions* may also be used for rinsing lenses following lens cleaning. However, any solution of physiological saline is suitable for this rinsing procedure. Ideally, unpreserved sterile saline solution should be used but non-sterile saline solution (made up from salt tablets and purified or distilled water) is permissible provided that the lens is to be boiled or disinfected by some other means, directly afterwards. Preserved saline solutions* specially formulated for lens rinsing are also available.

For the reasons discussed above it is obviously essential that patients with soft lenses must be advised not to use any solutions intended for

*See Appendix F, *Table F.II*, for examples.

hard lenses or other therapeutic eye drops without discussing it with their practitioner (*see below*). It is also important that soft lens solutions contain the least possible amount of preservative in order to minimize any binding effect to the lens material or contaminants. The use of minimal quantities of preservative has led to criticism of the antibacterial efficacy of these solutions.

Norton *et al.* (1974), using proprietary soft lens storage solutions, found that none was able to disinfect a standard laboratory contamination of 10^6 organisms/ml of *Ps. aeruginosa*, *Staph. aureus*, *M. luteus* and *C. albicans* in less than 24 hours, many taking 48 hours. These workers also found discrepancies between different solutions containing similar quantities of the same preservatives and postulated two reasons for this. First, that all the solutions were packaged in plastics containers and some preservatives may be adsorbed by the plastics. This could result in reduced concentration of preservative available in the solutions and would depend on such factors as the type of plastics used and the time stored (indicating the need for manufacturers to date-stamp solution bottles). Secondly, that the solutions used are complex and usually contain viscolizers such as hydroxyethylcellulose and polyvinyl alcohol, buffering agents, electrolytes and surfactants, all of which may influence the antibacterial performance of the preservative.

Holden and Markides (1971) found that a solution of 0.001% thimerosal took over 24 hours to kill an inoculum of *Staph. aureus*, and 6–24 hours for an inoculum of *Ps. aeruginosa*. Grosvenor, Charles and Callender (1972) and Baker and Remington (1972) all found that lenses stored in the same solution and supplied by manufacturers were often received highly contaminated. Charles (in Davies *et al.*, 1973) noted that this solution was also ineffective against clumped groups of bacteria. Similar results to those of Holden and Markides (1971) were found for *Staph. aureus* by Lindeman-Meester (1974) using 0.002% thimerosal plus 0.1% EDTA. Tragakis, Brown and Pearce (1973) found that high concentrations (10^7/ml) of *Pr. vulgaris* were able to survive 24 hours exposure to 0.005% chlorhexidine. Feldman (1971) found this concentration of chlorhexidine to be effective against several bacteria but to be ineffective against the fungus *A. fumagatus*.

Similar results against fungi were stated by Charles (in Davis *et al.*, 1973).

It would appear from the above, and the results of other workers, that of the two commonly used preservatives suitable for soft lens storage solutions — chlorhexidine and thimerosal — chlorhexidine is the more effective but has poor fungicidal capacity. Thimerosal is slower acting but is known to be more effective as an antifungal. For this reason many but not all solutions utilizing these preservatives make use of both agents, chlorhexidine at 0.0005–0.005% and thimerosal at 0.001–0.0025% strengths, and they may also incorporate EDTA at 0.01–0.1%. The incorporation of EDTA is both for enhancement of the bactericidal effect of the main preservative, and the postulated, but unproven, advantage of reducing calcium ions which may eventually form deposits on the lens. However, Morton (1985) found a reduction in antimicrobial activity when EDTA and thimerosal were used in combination.

The solutions are made isotonic and may contain liquid polymers such as polyvinyl pyrrolidone, and possibly surfactants to act as cleaning agents. Hampson (1973) states that lenses stored in an acidic pH solution take two to three times as long to settle and become comfortable as those stored in a slightly alkaline pH solution. For this reason most manufacturers moderately buffer solutions to a neutral or slightly alkaline pH.

As stated earlier, Holden and Markides (1971) found that a solution of 0.001% thimerosal alone took 24 hours to kill high concentrations of *Staph. aureus* and *Ps. aeruginosa*. Using a combination of 0.005% chlorhexidine and 0.001% thimerosal the killing time was reduced to 2–15 minutes. Similar results were found by Toxicol Laboratories (1972) using a different proprietary solution with similar constituents. Feldman (1971) gives a decontamination time for a similar chlorhexidine–thimerosal combination of less than 1 hour for all bacteria tested except *Staph. aureus* which was killed in under 2 hours. Phares (1972b) found a sterilizing time of 15 minutes to 3 hours for an inoculum of *Ps. aeruginosa*, *Staph. aureus* and *E. coli* using 0.005% chlorhexidine alone. Tragakis, Brown and Pearce (1973), using bacteria and fungi, gave a sterilizing time of 8 hours for inocula of bacteria and fungi. Grosvenor, Charles and Callender

(1972) took cultures from the cases and chlorhexidine–thimerosal storage solutions of 125 patients wearing soft lenses. In only one case was a positive culture found and here there was serious doubt that the wearer in question was following the practitioner's instructions.

From the accumulated evidence it would appear that chlorhexidine–thimerosal disinfecting solutions are able to cope with all levels of bacterial and fungal contamination normally encountered. There is evidence that very large levels of contamination may take several hours for disinfection, although even this should be coped with during the overnight storage period. Higher levels of contamination should be greatly reduced by cleaning and rinsing prior to storage (*see below*).

The major disadvantage of the chlorhexidine–thimerosal combination has been the relatively high incidence of reported patient hypersensitivity or toxic reaction cases, with thimerosal as the major culprit (Rèetschel and Wilson, 1982; Mondino and Groden, 1986). Nevertheless, chlorhexidine–thimerosal preserved solutions have been used successfully by millions of hydrogel wearers for over a decade.

Other chemical disinfection systems

Because of some of the disadvantages associated with chlorhexidine–thimerosal storage solutions, alternative methods of lens disinfection have been examined. Specificity, greater antibacterial and antifungal activity, reduced incidence of ocular reaction, reduced binding to lens materials and protein, and additional cleaning action have been sought. These are summarized below in alphabetical order.

Alkyl triethanol ammonium chloride

This solution combines thimerosal with a quaternary ammonium compound, alkyl triethanol ammonium chloride, to provide the disinfecting action. The disinfecting action reported by the manufacturer (Allergan) is slow but effective and is reported not to concentrate in the lens (Shively, 1975a). However, the disadvantages are the relatively high concentrations of thimerosal used and the fact that some patients complain of stinging on lens insertion (Morgan, 1979).

In addition to acting as an antimicrobial agent, the alkyl triethanol ammonium chloride is also used for its surfactant properties, and two other surfactants — Polysorbate 80 and propylene glycol — are also included to give the solution a cleaning as well as a disinfecting action.

Benzyl alcohol (phenylmethanol)

Although first introduced as a bactericide in 1947, benzyl alcohol has only recently been used as a preservative in contact lens solutions.

In higher concentrations, it is used for its anaesthetic as well as its bactericidal properties, for example in dental cavity work. However, there is no apparent anaesthetic effect at the 0.1% level used in current contact lens preparations.

Benzyl alcohol is claimed to be non-cytotoxic but effective as a bactericidal and viricidal agent (Anon, 1987). It is also claimed to have a low affinity to rigid gas permeable lens materials and lower ocular sensitivity reactions compared to benzalkonium chloride, chlorhexidine, and thimerosal. However, Klein, Millwood and Walther (1954) warned against dangers from *Ps. aeruginosa* infections in eye drops by permitting concentrations below 0.9%. For this reason current products also incorporate either EDTA or sorbic acid as co-preservatives.

Dymed

Dymed is the proprietary name for the preservative polyhexanide [poly(1-hexamethylenebiguanide hydrochloride)]. Dymed is currently used by Bausch & Lomb in a range of products and is claimed to show very low patient reactivity.

Polyhexanide was originally developed by ICI in the UK and is used as the swimming pool bactericide and algaecide, Baquacil. Its particular application in this usage is its antimicrobial action even in high dilution. In contact lens solutions it is commonly used at a strength of 0.00004%.

As a biguanide, polyhexanide belongs to the same pharmaceutical family as chlorhexidine. Both are cationic disinfectants which adsorb onto the often negatively charged bacterial cell surface, disrupt the cytoplasmic membrane releasing potassium ions and other cytoplasmic constituents, cause precipitation of cell contents and the death of the cell. Ikeda, Yamaguchi and

Tazaka (1985) report greater activity of this group against Gram-positive bacteria and less against Gram-negative bacteria.

Halazone

Marketed under the name Aerotabs (Sauflon), this product resembles Softabs (*see below*) in that it is a chlorine-release tablet system.

Halazone [4-(dichlorosulphamoyl)benzoic-acid] is commonly used in the disinfection of drinking water by virtue of its chlorine release. Indeed its first usage for this purpose was in the trenches in World War I (Sykes, 1965)! In the Aerotab form approximately 8 parts per million available chlorine is present when dissolved in saline, a slightly higher figure than the comparative Softab value. However, bactericidal activity is also dependent on pH and organic load and chlorine-based systems are very dependent on these additional factors. Little or no ocular irritancy is claimed even if the solution is inserted directly into the eye immediately after dissolving the tablet. Tablets should be protected from the light.

Iodophors

Alternative lens disinfection systems based on an iodophor in an isotonic polymeric vehicle appeared to show good clinical results (Johnson and Littlewood, 1975). When the iodophor (in a phosphoric or citric acid diluent) is placed in combination with a complementary neutralizing medium preserved with sorbic acid, EDTA and sodium borate, the iodine is reduced to the iodide ion. Unique to this system is the colour indicating a disinfecting action. When the solution and the lenses have become colourless there is a remaining preservative action, but the lenses may be safely inserted direct from the solution. Disinfecting time is stated by the manufacturer to be 2 hours. The concentration of active (diatomic) iodine is 0.005%, and there appears to be the definite advantage of no binding effect of the preservative (although J. Stone, 1976, personal communication, reported pronounced stinging if first used on old, and therefore probably contaminated, lenses when disinfection should be followed by boiling to prevent this problem). Slightly more attention and cooperation is required on the part of the patient in the correct preparation of the disinfecting solution because neutralization is

essential, the diluent having a pH of less than 5.0. A further disadvantage is that the cost of iodophors is high compared to other disinfectant methods. For these reasons the system is no longer available.

Microwaves

Preliminary work has shown that domestic microwave ovens are able to sterilize hydrogel lenses (Anon, 1986). However, for true sterilization the lenses must be in the dry state, rotated to avoid 'cold spots' in most ovens, and then rehydrated with sterile (unit dose or preserved) saline afterwards. At the present time this is impractical for most patients.

Kerr (1985) has described the use of domestic microwave ovens as a heating unit to pasteurize lenses by placing them in 15 ml saline in open containers and then bringing the saline to boiling point. The unit should then be shut down, the lenses allowed to cool, and the caps replaced. Patients should be warned of the dangers of leaving caps screwed firmly on the container when using a microwave oven because container explosion may occur when saline boiling occurs.

Rohrer *et al.* (1986) obtained lens dehydration in 2 minutes, viral inactivation in 4 minutes and complete sterilization in 8 minutes using a rotating 'rotisserie' to avoid 'cold spots' in the microwave oven.

p-Hydroxybenzoic acid (Nipastat)

The hydroxybenzoates are active against moulds, fungi and yeasts but less active against bacteria. The higher esters are the most effective but are limited by lower solubility. Unlike sorbic acid, the hydroxybenzoates are active at pH 7–9. Mixtures of two or more esters are likely to be more effective than the use of a single ester, because in this way a higher total concentration of preservative can be obtained in the solution and, in addition, the mixture may be active against a wider range of organisms.

Ganju and Thompson (1975) reported a solution (*see* Appendix F, *Table F.II*) containing a mixture of methyl, ethyl, propyl and butyl esters of *p*-hydroxybenzoic acid (Nipastat) in combination with a water-soluble polymer complex and reported success in its use as a lens disinfectant. It should be noted, however, that the numbers of microorganisms challenged were low compared with other workers and that the first subculture was not taken until after 8 hours exposure to the preservative. The work of Hugo and Foster (1964) has also shown that it is not always entirely effective in eliminating contamination by *Ps. aeruginosa*. *Martindale's Pharmacopoeia* (Anon, 1982) reports that concentrations of 0.2% are necessary for safe bactericidal concentration but that at this level the solution may be irritant to the eye. As its name would suggest therefore, the solution should be regarded as bacteriostatic and it should not therefore be presented with high microbial challenges.

The *p*-hydroxybenzoates show a very slight tendency to concentrate on hydrophilic lens surfaces in a similar manner to chlorhexidine. The great advantage of this preservative is that it is non-mercurial and contains no quaternary ammonium compound, thereby providing a very useful alternative for patients showing a possible allergy or sensitivity to chlorhexidine–thimerosal preserved solutions.

Polyquad

Polyquad (Alcon) is a relatively new preservative in the contact lens solution field. Its large polymeric molecule* resists diffusion into the lens matrix minimizing the toxic or hypersensitivity reaction found with chlorhexidine–thimerosal preserved solutions. Greater antibacterial and antifungal activity is claimed by the manufacturer than thimerosal, alkyl triethanol ammonium chloride plus thimerosal, or sorbic acid.

As a cationic detergent, the preservative is bound ionically to the methacrylic acid used in some hydrogel materials and toxic keratitis may result. Polyquad preserved solutions were initially therefore reserved for materials with a water content of 45% or less which did not contain methacrylic acid. Reformulation has eliminated this problem and the preservative is now considered suitable for use with lenses of any material or water content.

Potassium sorbate/sorbic acid

Sorbic acid is used by several solution manufacturers as an alternative preservative to the chlorhexidine–thimerosal combination. It is

*The molecular weight of polyquad is 5000 compared to chlorhexidine 359, polyhexanide (Dymed) 1300, sorbic acid 112 and thimerosal 405.

commonly used as the potassium salt because this is considerably more water soluble and has identical actions.

Sorbic acid has antibacterial and antifungal properties. It is active against moulds and yeasts and, to a lesser degree, against bacteria, the fungistatic activity being increased in saline solution. It is not effective above about pH 6.5 with an optimum pH of around 4.5. Solutions of 0.1% sorbic acid stored in polypropylene, polyvinyl chloride, polyethylene or glass containers showed a marked loss of potency except when refrigerated or when an antioxidant such as sodium metabisulphite was also present (McCarthy, 1973). Sorbic acid solutions should also be protected from the light.

Although popular with many practitioners and patients, it will, as with all preservatives, cause reactions in some patients. Josephson and Caffrey (1986) report a sensitivity reaction in 15% of patients using a 0.1% preserved solution. *Martindale's Pharmacopoeia* (Anon, 1982) specifically mentions its potential for ocular irritancy in topical solutions. Callendar *et al.* (1986) report poorer lens disinfection results with sorbic acid-preserved solutions than alkyl triethanol ammonium chloride combined with thimerosal.

Sodium dichloroisocyanurate (Halane)

Marketed under the name 'Softabs' (Alcon) this product breaks down in water to form hypochlorite. Because hypochlorite is not stable in aqueous solution it will spontaneously break down to form chlorine and sodium chloride. The 3–5 parts per million (ppm) chlorine liberated is adequate to disinfect the solution in approximately 4 hours as well as providing a mild cleaning action (Brewitt and Conrads, 1986). At 3–5 ppm the chlorine level is already below the ocular irritation level and this is further reduced after the overnight soaking period (Parker, 1983).

The main advantages of the system are minimal risk of patient sensitivity, simplicity in use and minimal risk in cases of poor compliance (compared to hydrogen peroxide), portability when combined with unit dose saline, ability for use with hypotonic saline in patients showing marginal dry eye problems, and the mild cleaning action in addition to its disinfection properties.

Sonification

Ultrasound is the range of sound waves of higher frequency than those to which the human ear is sensitive. The auditory range is approximately from 100 cycles/second (100 Hz) to 15 000 or 16 000 cycles/second (15 or 16 kHz). Above 16–20 kHz, the sound waves result in no sense of hearing in the human ear and are referred to as ultrasound.

The cleaning action of ultrasound units is produced by a process known as cavitation. The ultrasound waves produced by transducers in the unit create frictional forces within the liquid medium. This produces both heat and the liberation of microscopic bubbles. These bubbles re-dissolve almost immediately, producing an implosion or 'cavitation' effect. Because most cavitation occurs at, or very close to, solid surfaces, contact lenses immersed in a cleaning tank are claimed to benefit from boundary or surface cavitation.

The microbiological action of ultrasound arises by three mechanisms:

(1) The purely mechanical strain put on the cell wall by the sudden application, and the equally sudden release, of pressure.
(2) The cavitation effect of fluid within the cell.
(3) The rise in temperature produced by ultrasound.

Charles (1975) first pointed out the possibility of using sonic oscillation for cleaning and disinfecting hydrogel lenses. However, his tests showed that sonification for as long as 2–3 hours was necessary to kill an inoculum of *Ps. aeruginosa*. Spores were also somewhat resistant to this procedure. Because only small volumes can be treated at a time, ultrasound has found little use in conventional microbiology and therefore little evidence exists as to its efficacy and what evidence exists is often contradictory. Nevertheless it can be stated that:

(a) The efficacy of antimicrobial activity is more related to the *intensity* of wave emission than to its frequency.
(b) Cavitation becomes more difficult and less intense as the frequency is increased, thus requiring a higher power input to produce any effect.

These points therefore place a limitation on the manufacturer of patient units where size, weight, cost and heat generation must all be balanced against the desired cleaning and antimicrobial activities.

At least two ultrasonic contact lens units are currently available. The 'Lenso Clean' utilizes a 33 kHz unit over a 10-minute cycle (Anon, 1984). Both cleaning and low temperature disinfection are claimed. Examination of the Mark I 'Sonasept' unit (SMC Metal Tech Co.) by C. Jenkins (1986, personal communication) showed a saline temperature rise to 71°C in the lens containers indicating lens disinfection by pasteurization. Jenkins considers it unlikely that small patient units can provide sufficient energy to disinfect lenses by sonification alone so that they should be regarded as low heat units. The Aquasterile unit (specialist optical source) combines ultrasonic vibration with ultraviolet light in a 22-minute cycle. Its efficacy has so far not been independently assessed.

Little independent evidence exists on the cleaning capability of patient ultrasonic units. Erikson (1985) claims that ultrasonic devices can markedly increase the effectiveness of Allergan's enzyme cleaner on soft lenses. Kerr (1988) reports surface calculi reduced smoothly down to the level of the lens surface with Miraflow (Cooper) in the unit as cleaning agent. Liprofin (Alcon) is also likely to work effectively at the temperature induced by current ultrasonic units. Kerr also reports that most RGP lenses (including fluoropolymers) appear to be effectively cleaned and dimensionally unchanged.

Further work is now awaited on the full antimicrobial safety and long-term cleaning action of ultrasonic units, particularly if inexpensive, unpreserved saline alone is utilized. The use of relatively expensive, larger volumes of cleaners would negate the advantages of these fairly expensive units and restrict them to practitioner usage. The use of preserved saline to enhance antimicrobial activity would provide no advantage over current chemical disinfection methods, unless a significant cleaning action was also obtained.

Trimethoprim

Trimethoprim has been used for many years in the treatment of urinary tract disorders. Its antibiotic-like action specifically inhibits bacterial dihydrofolate reductase (an enzyme essential to bacterial growth), while exhibiting very little effect against the mammalian enzyme. Studies done with this drug show that at dosages lower than the therapeutic level, it is an effective preservative for contact lens solutions (Feldman, 1985). In addition, the bactericidal properties are enhanced by such agents as EDTA and sorbic acid giving a synergistic effect. Initial studies appear to show minimal binding to the lens surface or deposits, or incidences of hypersensitivity. The future of this preservative will depend upon the reaction of the various regulatory bodies to the use of a systemic drug as a contact lens preservative and fears that its widespread use will enable the build-up of bacterial immunity (Anon, 1980).

A further disadvantage is that it is stated in *Martindale's Pharmacopoeia* (Anon, 1982) to have little activity on its own against *Ps. aeruginosa* presumably indicating its usage in combination with sorbic acid and EDTA.

The advantages of chemical disinfecting solutions may therefore be summarized as follows:

(1) Generally they are convenient, and for the patient who may already have had hard lenses, they fit into a similar pattern.
(2) The initial cost is low.
(3) They are portable.
(4) They are generally effective for all microorganisms normally encountered and this will still apply even if the wearer occasionally omits to change the solution daily or does not wear his lenses for a few days.
(5) Sporulating bacteria are destroyed if they revert to their vegetative form.
(6) There appears to be no effect on the life of the lenses.
(7) There is less coagulation of mucoprotein left on the lens than with heat sterilization.

Set against these are the following disadvantages:

(1) Chemical disinfecting solutions are more expensive in the long term.
(2) There is a risk of some binding with certain antimicrobial agents and this applies particularly if the lens is not cleaned prior to being placed in the solution.
(3) There is some risk of ocular irritation by solution constituents. Hind (1975) has estimated this to be 5–10% for one proprietary solution, and 4% for another as estimated by Trager (Davis *et al.*, 1973).
(4) The solutions cannot generally cope with large influxes of microorganisms.
(5) The solution method is slow, often taking 6–8 hours to be certain of complete disinfection.
(6) Many preservatives still cause slight coagulation of any mucoprotein remaining on the lens surfaces.
(7) Most solutions have no cleaning action and still necessitate the use of separate cleaning compounds.
(8) The possibility exists that solutions may be suitable for use with only specified lens materials.

Practitioners occasionally find that patients using heating methods of disinfection will change to chemical disinfection, for example, on holiday when mains electricity may not be available or may be the wrong voltage. While many patients experience no difficulties with alternating disinfection methods it can sometimes give rise to problems. First, it has already been mentioned above that heating methods of disinfection accelerate the denaturation of proteinaceous deposits on the lens surface. Chlorhexidine then binds more strongly to these deposits than to the lens surface and gives rise to a toxic or allergenic response. Secondly, there is good evidence that tear protein bound to contact lens surfaces can cause an immune response (Allansmith *et al.*, 1977; Refojo and Holly, 1977). The present understanding of this process is that the adsorbed protein molecule undergoes changes that may be accelerated by alternating dry/wet and hot/cold conditions, as well as by mechanical rubbing from fingers and lids. The altered denatured protein may then no longer be recognized as 'self' and be capable of provoking an autoimmune response (McMonnies, 1978).

Conversely, practitioners may wish their patients to change from chemical disinfection of their lenses to heat disinfection, or from one chemical disinfection method to another, as may be done if a patient is thought to have developed an adverse reaction to a particular preservative. Before doing so all traces of the existing preservatives should be removed from the lenses by:

(1) Soaking the lenses in at least three changes of unpreserved physiological saline solution at room temperature during a period of 24 hours.

(2) Boiling the lenses in distilled water followed by an overnight soak in unpreserved physiological saline solution, replenishing the latter and then re-boiling.
(3) Boiling in unpreserved physiological saline solution, replenishing and then re-boiling.

The properties of a soft lens disinfecting solution may therefore be listed as follows (modified from Cureton and Sibley, 1974):

(1) The solution should be capable of disinfecting the lenses in 4–6 hours or less.
(2) The antimicrobial agents used should not easily be inactivated by small amounts of proteins, lipids or other tear components.
(3) The solution should be isotonic and either non-buffered or lightly buffered to a pH approximating that of the average tear liquid.
(4) The antimicrobial agents used should not bind to protein or other lens surface deposits from the eye.
(5) The solution should not react with or adsorb to soft lens materials, or the container materials.
(6) The solution should be non-irritating and non-toxic to the ocular tissues.
(7) The cost of the regimen should encourage good compliance.

Two additional useful but not essential properties may also be listed:

(1) The solution should be capable of withstanding boiling without degrading.
(2) The combination of a cleaning action with the disinfectant/storage action would be helpful.

Cleaning solutions and methods

While the lens is on the eye, the mucin in the tear fluid is adsorbed onto the surface of the lens in the same way that it is adsorbed onto the epithelium of the cornea. Mucin and other proteins of the tears such as lysozyme remain in their natural state when attached to the soft lens surface in the eye. As long as the soft lens remains in the environment of the tear fluid, the eye will usually accommodate the lens without excessive protein film build-up. However, as mentioned earlier, daily removal of the lens, over a period of time, results in the denaturing of adsorbed proteins. This process occurs very slowly when the lenses are stored in a cold sterilizing solution but more rapidly when they are boiled. The problem is compounded by lipid secretions from the meibomian glands which can also bind to the lens surfaces, forming a lipoprotein film that is difficult to remove and which can impair visual acuity and cause discomfort. Further, chlorhexidine and other preservatives will bind to this film increasing both their concentration and contact time with the eye and causing a burning sensation (Hind, 1975). As mentioned earlier, sudden release of adsorbed preservative may also cause marked irritation.

In addition, the bound preservative loses its disinfecting ability so that the solution takes longer to sterilize the lens. The surface film may itself serve as a growth medium for bacteria and fungi and may actually protect microorganisms trapped within it. Cureton and Hall (1974), Hind (1975) and Thompson and Mansell (1976) have shown a marked improvement in the time taken for disinfection where lenses have been cleaned prior to storage. This has presumably arisen from the combined effect of physically reducing the number of microorganisms by cleaning and rinsing, and also by removing or reducing surface contaminants and thereby enhancing the disinfectant action of the boiling or chemical solution.

In addition to the lipoprotein surface film, various salts, divalent or trivalent ions (for example calcium) and other contaminants such as environmental pollutants, chemical vapours, cosmetic ingredients, water impurities, nicotine, oils and dirt from the fingers, and preservative and active ingredients from ophthalmic products may be present in the adsorbed or absorbed state.

The cleaning problem is further complicated by the fact that different lens materials are affected by contaminants in different ways. Some lens materials become cloudy and hazy and accumulate rough deposits which are sometimes impervious to ordinary cleaning procedures. Other lens materials become discoloured and occasionally form deposits in the form of white spots (Ganju and Cordrey, 1975). Contaminants are often visible to both patient and practitioner with the naked eye, and the patient should be instructed to cease wearing any lens showing any opaque area on its surface.

Surface deposits are often seen with the slit

lamp and usually take the form of roughness of the lens surface appearing between blinks. Removing the lens from the eye, holding it with a suitable pair of tweezers, and allowing it to air dry will often disclose previously invisible deposits.

Cleaning methods have therefore been developed for daily and/or periodic use and fall into three categories: surfactants, enzymatic systems and calcium preventing solutions.

Surfactants

This is the largest group of products. Their cleaning property depends upon their ability to lower the surface tension of oil or solid–water interfaces. Surfactant cleaners will help remove lipids, mascara, some types of aerosol spray, lipstick, facial make-up, calcium salts before deposition, and protein before it becomes denatured. Because of the porous nature of hydrophilic lenses and their interaction with many ionic compounds, the selection of a surfactant is limited to a non-ionic block copolymer (Ganju and Cordrey, 1975). Surfactant cleaners should be designed to be safe and cause minimal or no ocular discomfort if accidentally instilled into the eye, to be readily rinsed off the lens by the rinsing or storage solution, and to be compatible with all hydrophilic lens materials and accessories. Solutions are often made slightly viscous to facilitate handling and possibly formulated at an alkaline pH to maximize protein removal (Hind, 1975). Phillips (1980) found few surfactants formulated at an alkaline pH, however, and presumably the need for differing pH values for maximum surfactant or preservative activity becomes an overriding factor.

In using a surfactant cleaner, oil droplets are first broken up by physical dispersion. These would then normally coalesce on contact. However, the surfactant forms a surface monolayer with the ions, oriented with the polar end 'buried' in the surface of the oil droplet. Thus a surface electrical charge is established which causes mutual repulsion (*Figure 4.3a*) between any two droplets that approach one another and coalescence is prevented. It should be stressed that the essential act of cleaning, however, is the initial mechanical dispersion.

A similar effect — of the detergent forming a surface monolayer in an aqueous environment

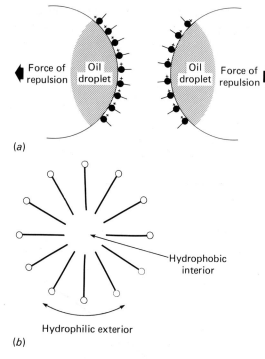

Figure 4.3 (*a*) Orientation of surfactant molecules on lipid droplets. (*b*) Typical micelle structure

— is what lowers the surface tension and hence gives rise to the term 'surfactant'.

It is important to realize that the formation of a monolayer is not an energetically stable structure. Detergents will, at a certain concentration, form molecular arrangements known as micelles in the solution (*Figure 4.3b*) and it is these structures that are energetically more favourable, i.e. they use less energy to accomplish the same objective.

Thus surfactant cleaners aim at using a concentration of detergent which achieves its critical micelle concentration or CMC. This is, in practice, very difficult as several excipients of the formulation will interfere with the formulation of the CMC. Equally, increasing the surfactant concentration beyond that necessary to form its CMC will not improve the efficacy of the solution and may increase the risk of ocular irritancy. Little evidence exists in comparing the efficacy of different surfactant cleaners and patients generally use that advised by their practitioner or select on a basis of availability, cost or preference for a particular solution viscosity.

In order to improve or enhance the efficacy of normal surfactants several laboratories have marketed modified or 'improved' surfactant cleaners.

Hypertonic solutions

Two such solutions, Sterisolv (Sauflon Pharmaceuticals), and the in-eye cleaner, Clerz (Cooper), incorporate a hypertonic saline element (2.5% and 1.2%, respectively) so that deposits in the lens surface matrix are drawn out by osmotic pressure before emulsification by the surfactant.

Combined storage solution and cleaner

Allergan's Hydrocare solution incorporates surfactants into the disinfecting solution itself so that this may be used for both cleaning and disinfecting purposes. The main preservative, alkyl triethanol ammonium chloride, has surfactant properties. In addition Polysorbate 80 and propylene glycol are incorporated for surfactant and cushioning functions.

Incorporation of alcohol

Miraflow (Cooper) incorporates 20% isopropyl alcohol as a lipid solvent as well as a surfactant. The cleaner is also hypertonic which further aids the cleaning action (Brezinski, Carney and Hill, 1986).

Incorporation of polymeric beads

Alcon's Polyclens (Opti-Clean) is a multipurpose cleaner suitable for hard, gas permeable hard, and hydrogel lenses. It combines a surfactant and fine polymeric beads of ground plastic. As the 'beads' of plastic are from a soft material and are combined with a surfactant there appears to be minimal or no abrasive effect on the lens surface material (*Figure 4.4*).

The beads are claimed to have an abrasive effect on surface deposits without affecting the lens material. Phillips and Czigler (1985) demonstrated the effectivity of the cleaner with hydrogel lenses and the reduced need for enzymatic cleaners (*see below*). The disadvantages of the cleaner found were its slightly greater cost, stinging if not adequately rinsed from the lens, and the greater quantities of rinsing fluid needed.

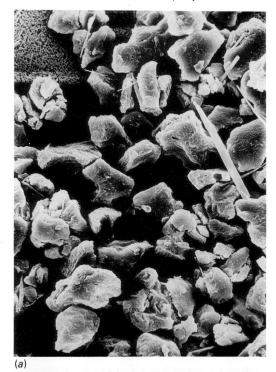

(a)

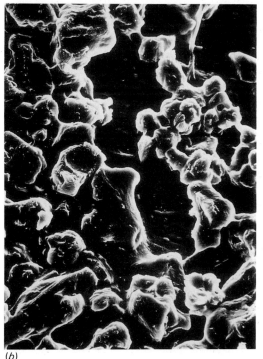

(b)

Figure 4.4 Polymeric beads contained in Polyclens (Opti-Clean). (*a*) Rinsed; (*b*) coated with surfactant. (From Phillips and Czigler, 1985, and reproduced by kind permission of *Clinical and Experimental Optometry*)

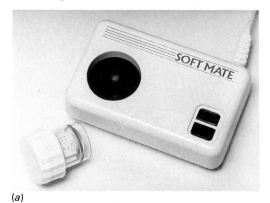

(a)

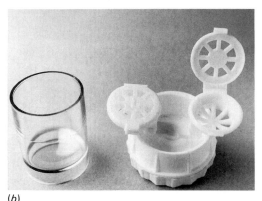

(b)

Figure 4.5 (*a*) Pilkington Barnes–Hind mechanical agitator for soft lens cleaning; (*b*) lens container

'Extra-strength' cleaners

Pilkington Barnes–Hind's Softmate 'Weekly Cleaner' (Intensive Cleaner) is claimed as 'extra-strength' and contains three surfactants.

From the foregoing discussion it has already been stated that the effectivity of a surfactant does not increase once the CMC has been reached and therefore there is no such thing as an 'extra-strength' surfactant. However, the manufacturers claim (V. Zuccaro, 1979, cited by Phillips, 1980) that most other manufacturers use a single surfactant only and in low concentration so that the terminology is a relative one. Further, it is claimed that the three surfactants have been selected to provide a wide range of activity against lens soilants.

A mechanical agitator (*Figure 4.5*) is available to assist in the use of this cleaner and is also useful for those patients with rough skin or poor dexterity who may have problems with normal digital cleaning.

Enzymatic systems

An enzyme is an organic catalyst, i.e. it aids a chemical change in other bodies without undergoing change in itself, and is formed by living cells but is not dependent on their presence for its action. However, a number of enzymes require simple ions as activators and will not function in their absence. All enzymes are proteins, but not all proteins are enzymes. There are currently four types of enzyme preparation available.

Papain tablets (Hydrocare and Prymecare)

Papain is derived from the dried and purified latex of the pawpaw fruit (*Carica papaya*) tree and normally used as a meat tenderizer and in the manufacture of chill-proof beer.

Papain is an endopeptidase, i.e. it catalyses the cleavage of peptide bonds in the interior of a protein molecule (*Figure 4.6*) and has a broad substrate specificity, i.e. will act upon peptides, amides, esters and thioesters. Proteins are thereby broken down to shorter peptide chains, e.g. dipeptides, tripeptides etc. It can be seen that an important step with the use of enzymatic cleaners is the use of a surfactant cleaner to disperse these molecules and residual enzyme *after* the cleaning procedure. Lens structure is not affected because the enzymatic activity is specific for peptide linkages (Blanco, Curry and Boghosian, 1975).

Numerous studies exist on the efficacy of papain. The following serves to emphasize important points. Tsuda, Ando and Anan (1977) reported the incidence of deposits on Toyo material lenses which were cleaned daily with a surfactant cleaner.

(1) After 3 months 59% showed obvious surface deposits.
(2) After 3–5 months 78% showed obvious surface deposits.

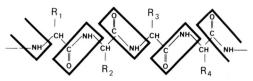

Figure 4.6 The basic primary structure of a protein molecule. R = residue of each amino acid; ☐ = peptide bond

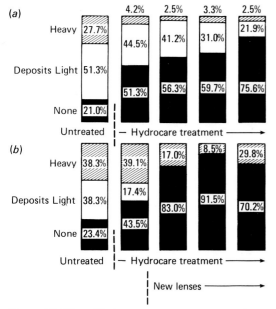

Figure 4.7 Effect of Hydrocare enzyme treatment used weekly as seen at approximately 2-monthly intervals; (*a*) on heavily deposited lenses; (*b*) lenses were replaced at the third visit. (Modified after Tsuda, Ando and Anan, 1977 and reproduced by kind permission of *Optometry Today*)

(3) After 6–8 months 82% showed obvious surface deposits.

(4) After 9–11 months 89% showed obvious surface deposits.

Patients were then put onto weekly papain treatment (*Figure 4.7*). it can be seen from *Figure 4.7a* that even with badly coated lenses the incidence of both heavy and light deposits was significantly reduced. From *Figure 4.7b*, it can be seen that new lenses were not kept free of heavy deposits entirely. However, it should still be noted that after approximately 6 months, almost a third of all patients still showed slight deposits. In other words the technique, along with all other patient cleaning methods, is not 100% effective.

In another study by Karageozian, Walden and Boghosian (1976), ultraviolet absorption spectra of human-worn hydrophilic lenses were measured after cleaning with a commercially available surfactant and with papain enzyme cleaner (*Figure 4.8*).

The disappearance of the ultraviolet absorbing protein after a single enzyme treatment is striking. While the paper was critical of the cleaning value of surfactant cleaners, the de-

posits were *denatured* protein and, from earlier discussion, it would be surprising if there was any cleaning effect at all. The slight cleaning effect shown by the surfactant in the figure is presumably the abrasive effect of palm cleaning which has *physically* removed some of the surface film.

McClure *et al.* (1977) showed the effect of weekly papain cleaning on lenses which had been worn for varying periods without cleaning (*Figure 4.9*). The improvement in visual acuity once enzymatic treatment had begun is again striking. However, it is interesting once more to note that the acuity recovery with the older, more heavily deposited lenses, was not to the original level and presumably indicated the inability of the enzyme to remove *all* the residual deposits. In addition, it shows the importance of starting patients on the regimen from the very beginning of lens wear.

One potential disadvantage of papain is that some patients experience discomfort or mild conjunctival hyperaemia after its use (Fichman,

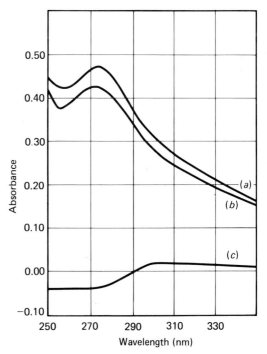

Figure 4.8 Ultraviolet absorption spectra of human worn hydrophilic lenses. (*a*) Absorbance of uncleaned lens. (*b*) After ×8 cleanings with a surfactant cleaner. (*c*) After a single cleaning with papain enzyme. (After Karageozian, Walden and Boghosian, 1976, and reproduced by kind permission of *International Contact Lens Clinic*)

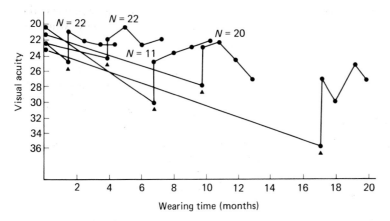

Figure 4.9 The effect of soft lens wearing time and weekly papain cleaning on visual acuity. Graph describes mean visual acuity as a function of wearing time. Weekly enzyme cleaning was begun at ▲. Separate groups of patients were used for each of the five categories. (After McClure *et al.*, 1977)

Baker and Horton, 1978; Bernstein *et al.*, 1984). It is essential that the lenses are not soaked for more than 2–3 hours in the enzyme solution (less for some patients) and that careful surfactant cleaning is carried out after the treatment. This cleaning is also important in removing enzyme by-products which may otherwise reattach to the lens surface. Because enzymatic treatment does not disinfect the lenses, they should be put through a disinfection cycle after the cleaning procedure. For lenses disinfected by thermal methods, this will also destroy any residual enzyme.

In order to avoid patent restrictions and to attempt to gain greater cleaning efficacy, and provide an alternative to those patients sensitive to papain, differing enzymes have been gradually introduced.

Pronase (Amiclair)

Amiclair tablets (Abatron) contain a mixture of three enzymes: a bacterial protease isolated from *Bacillus subtilis* (subtilisin?); a lipase isolated from *Rhizopus arrhizus* var. *delomar*; and pronase, a proteolytic enzyme obtained from *Streptomyces griseus* which is stated to remove mucus. Additionally, the product contains EDTA which is stated to aid in reducing calcium deposit formation.

Interestingly, pronase is itself a protease so that the system contains two proteases, presumably to attempt to cover the range of protein or protein-containing deposits. Pronase was first isolated from *Streptomyces griseus* as a by-product from the industrial production of streptomycin (D. Lloyd, 1979, cited by Phillips, 1980). It exhibits an extremely broad specificity and is able to effect a 60–80% hydrolysis of many proteins. Normally the extent of protein hydrolysis by any protease is limited to 10–30% and even then almost all of the resulting digestion products are polypeptides. Pronase was found to be capable of hydrolysing various kinds of peptide bonds in protein until the majority of amino acids making up the protein were liberated as individual free amino acids. It is essentially a peptidase of a relatively new type because it is capable of splitting not only terminal peptide bonds, but also internal peptide bonds of proteins and so does not fall into the traditional classification, i.e. exopeptidase or endopeptidase. Presumably the claim that pronase removes mucus from soft lenses is because mucus contains albuminous substances such as mucin and albumin, collectively known as the glycoproteins (proteins covalently linked to carbohydrates), and found in deposits on soft lenses.

Lipases are enzymes widely distributed in plants and present also in the liver, gastric and pancreatic secretions which break down fats to the constituent fatty acids and glycerol by a hydrolysis reaction. Lipids can be generally classified as:

Lipids

Triglycerides — fats/oils, based on physical difference

Phospholipids — e.g. lecithin

Sphingolipids

Steroids — e.g. cholesterol/cholesteryl esters

Structurally speaking lipids are esters. In the triglycerides the alcohol is glycerol which is esterified with fatty acids. Thus:

$$
\begin{array}{ccc}
& & \text{ester linkage} \\
& & \downarrow \\
\mathrm{CH_2OH} & & \mathrm{CH_2O-CO-R_1} \\
| & & | \\
\mathrm{CHOH} & \xrightarrow[\text{Three fatty acids}]{\text{Esterification}} & \mathrm{CHO-CO-R_2} \\
| & & | \\
\mathrm{CH_2OH} & & \mathrm{CH_2O-CO-R_3} \\
\\
\text{Glycerol} & & \text{Triglyceride}
\end{array}
$$

(where R_1, R_2 and R_3 are fatty acids)

Various fatty acids combine to form a variety of triglycerides which are the most abundant lipids found in both plants and animals. They are commonly designated as the neutral fats. If the fatty acid is esterified with an alcohol of higher molecular weight than glycerol then the resulting compound is called a wax.

The action of lipases may be summarized as:

(1) Lipases attack the ester linkage (*see above*) of triglycerides (fats) breaking them first to diglycerides, then to monoglycerides and subsequently to glycerol with the liberation of fatty acids at each step. The rate of reaction will decrease as the degradation tends towards completion.

(2) The ultimate breakdown product, glycerol, is freely soluble in water but fatty acids, monoglycerides and diglycerides are either sparingly soluble or totally insoluble. For this reason surfactant cleaning following lipase action is also essential.

(3) It has already been stated that lipases will only attack the triglyceride fraction of lens deposits. With the different classes of lipids which may be present in human tears, it would not be too presumptious to assume that these other classes would not be affected by lipase, e.g. phospholipids are only degraded by phospholipase, lipoproteins are only degraded by lipoprotein lipase. This latter enzyme catalyses the hydrolysis of triglycerides only when in association with protein.

Thus considering the specificity of lipases one may require a 'cocktail' of enzymes to remove all lipid deposits on lenses. For this reason the current name of 'lipase' is 'glycerol ester hydrolase' which is a more acceptable and accurate description of the enzyme's function. Nevertheless, it can be argued that the incorporation of a lipase can only add to the cleaning process albeit by a debatable amount.

Pancreatin tablets (Alcon Enzymatic and Sauflon Effervescent)

Pancreatic extract tablets may be expected to contain the following: trypsin, chymotrypsin and carboxypeptidase as proteases; amylase (to break down polysaccharides (mucins); deoxyribonuclease; lipase.

Schachet (1983) found an improvement with the use of the multi-enzyme, although the opposite was found by Kjellsen, Kiral and Erikson (1984). Because lipids and mucins are easily removed by surfactant cleaning, the only stubborn lipid deposit is that found in the white calculi seen occasionally on lens surfaces. These are not removed by either surfactant or enzymatic cleaning probably due to the presence of calcium salts of fatty acids. It would appear therefore that differences are most likely to revolve around the efficacy and speed of the various proteases present. Unfortunately, few independent assessments are currently available and the main advantage to the practitioner is in the choice of products now available so that alternatives are available where patients show sensitivity to specific enzymes.

Subtilisin (Ultrazyme and Bausch & Lomb Sensitive Eyes)

The subtilisins are alkaline serine proteases (i.e. proteases having a particularly reactive serine amino acid at their catalytic site) produced by various species of *Bacillus*, in particular *B. subtilis* and *B. licheniformis*. Due to its thermostability the enzyme is industrially very important and is produced in large quantities for this purpose. Nevertheless, its use in the contact lens area is relatively new. The enzyme functions optimally at around pH 8–11 (Vita, Dalzoppo and Fontana, 1985) and has an action similar to chymotrypsin but broader specificity.

The advantages claimed for subtilisin are minimal binding or adsorption property to hydrogel lens material, longer peak action time allowing cleaning to continue during the overnight period, minimal evidence of subsequent ocular irritation due to residual enzyme and, in the case of the Allergan product (Subtilisin A), the enzyme is formulated to work in the acidic environment of hydrogen peroxide. In practice this is likely to be achieved by the incorporation of a suitable agent to raise the solution pH to an optimum alkaline level for maximum enzymatic activity. Not only does this reduce the number of cleaning steps for the patient because enzyme cleaning and disinfection are carried out simultaneously, but subtilisin has a synergistic antimicrobial effect with hydrogen peroxide significantly reducing kill times for the yeast *C. albicans* which normally has a slow kill time in hydrogen peroxide (C. Jenkins, 1986, personal communication). In addition, hydrogen peroxide acts as a 'substrate modifier', i.e. it exposes more peptide linkages to the enzyme, so that a more efficient cleaning action is produced. Other enzymatic cleaners also incorporate substrate modifiers, e.g. cysteine in papain enzyme.

Finally, the Allergan enzyme has *N*-acetylcysteine incorporated. This product is well known for its mucolytic properties.

From the discussion above it can be seen that after removal of the lenses, whatever the chosen method of disinfection, the patient should be strongly advised to carry out a prophylactic daily surfactant cleaning step prior to the disinfection procedure. This reduces the majority of loosely bound surface deposits and significantly reduces microbial contamination. In addition, surfactant cleaning is essential after enzymatic cleaning to remove the enzyme breakdown products. Because surfactant cleaners are largely effective for lipids and unbound protein, most practitioners also advise weekly or fortnightly enzymatic (or equivalent) cleaning in addition to remove or reduce bound denatured protein. Patients using heat disinfection must be advised to carefully rinse cleaning solutions from the lens prior to being placed in the asepticizor unit, because certain cleaners

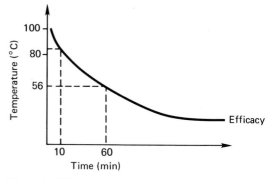

Figure 4.10 Time–temperature efficacy curve of Allergan's Calcium Deposit Preventer solution

may be baked on, forming a white film and making the lens unwearable (Davis *et al.*, 1973).

Although largely used with hydrogel lenses due to their greater affinity to bind protein, enzymatic cleaning can be used with any type of contact lens as a means of removing bound protein and is particularly applicable in those patient groups susceptible to deposit related problems such as giant papillary conjunctivitis (Korb *et al.*, 1983).

Calcium preventing solutions

Some patients are prone to lay down areas of calcium carbonate or phosphate in the lens structure. In addition, the white calculi sometimes seen on (especially) high water content hydrogels are lipids often combined with calcium salts. These salts will not be removed by surfactant or enzymatic cleaners.

Allergan's Sorbisal and Calcium Deposit Preventer contains a heat-activated chelating agent (sodium hexametaphosphate) which removes calcium ions present in or on the lens matrix. The time–temperature curve is shown in *Figure 4.10*.

It can be seen that the solution can only be used by patients using a thermal disinfection method. However, it may be used by practitioners as a rejuvenating method in a heat-controlled bath with a magnetic stirrer at 60°C for 1 hour. The effectivity of this method is shown in *Figure 4.11b*.

Rejuvenating systems

As lenses age, deposits accumulate both on the surface and within the surface matrix of the lens.

these are more obvious as the lens cools and dries off the eye. In addition, the lens appears to tighten in fitting as protein displaces water from the surface matrix. Irregular protein deposition may cause a 'pie-crust' effect of the lens edge and limbal injection and superficial corneal staining may occur due to the tighter fitting and possible reduced oxygen transmission. In this situation the practitioner must decide whether to replace or attempt to rejuvenate the lens. This, in turn, will depend upon the patient's financial status, the age of the lens, the lens replacement cost and the degree of deposition.

Due to the high overhead costs of producing relatively small quantities of practitioner rejuvenating cleaners, only two are now currently available. Both are oxidizing agents but are stronger than that available as patient cleaning systems described above.

Oxidation was originally defined as the addition of oxygen to a compound. This definition was later extended to include the removal of hydrogen from a compound. Better understanding of the principles involved has led to the current definition in which oxidation is defined as 'a process in which electrons are removed from a species'. Reduction is the opposite process, i.e. electrons are added. Both processes must occur simultaneously and are hence often known as redox reactions.

In the cleaning of hydrogel lenses we are interested in the fact that the end products of the oxidation of proteins (and most other deposits) are of low molecular weight (i.e. are small), and are often water soluble (i.e. they are easily dispersed). It can be seen that the effect is, in fact, the same as for an enzyme. The difference is the mode, speed and/or degree of reaction, plus the fact that the reaction is not specific for proteins, and many other lens contaminants may also be broken down by the oxidation process. The main advantage, therefore, of oxidizing systems is the broad range of activity against lens deposits.

Liprofin (Alcon)

Liprofin is an inorganically based active substance, largely sodium perborate, which is water soluble. On being heated it evolves reactive oxygen which decomposes both organic and inorganic substances. If the solution is heated to boiling point, the oxygen radicals are liberated

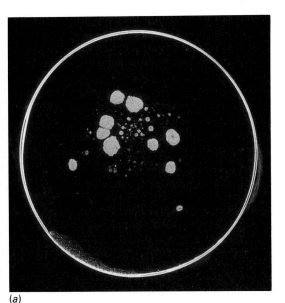

(a)

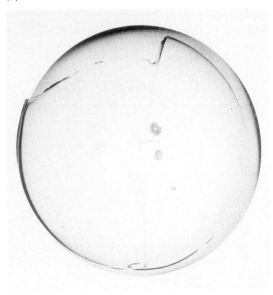

(b)

Figure 4.11 (a) Hydrogel lens showing cluster of large calculi deposits. (b) Same lens cut in half (and damaged in the process). The left half was cleaned with Calcium Deposit Preventer and the right half with Liprofin

Great individual variation is found in both speed and degree of deposit accumulation although patient thoroughness in following their practitioner's instructions plays a major role. Patients complain of reducing comfort, vision, decreasing tolerance and possibly discoloured lenses. The practitioner may see the surface deposits by slit lamp examination although

very rapidly and only partial removal of heavy deposits occurs. From experimentation, a temperature of 50–60°C over a period of 2–4 hours has been found to produce a highly efficient cleaning ability and to cause no change in lens dimensions. To improve cleaning ability, constant agitation is preferable and for simplicity this can be done by means of a magnetic stirrer.

After Liprofin cleaning, the lens should be rinsed thoroughly, cleaned with a surfactant cleaner and then soaked in a saline solution for at least 30 minutes. The method is highly effective as a sterilizing method being effective against bacteria, fungi and even viruses. Care should be taken in the cleaning of high water content lenses as parameter changes may occur with this product.

Monoclens (Sauflon Pharmaceuticals)

Monoclens is a mixture of two groups of substances: a non-ionic preparation of ethylene oxide and propylene oxide as a block copolymer plus sodium perborate acting as an oxidizing agent.

The copolymer is thought to act by presenting a stronger ionic attraction for the protein deposits and other organic impurities so that they detach themselves from the lenses and move to the copolymer. The oxidizing agent helps break down both organic and inorganic deposits.

The method used is that the lens is boiled in a solution made up with saline and the copolymer oxidizing agent for 10 minutes and then shaken gently. It should then be allowed to simmer for a further 2 hours at a constant temperature of 70–80°C or simply left at room temperature overnight without either of which treatments cleaning is incomplete. The lens is then removed, rinsed with saline and boiled for half an hour with fresh physiological saline to remove all traces of the copolymeric agent and to disinfect it.

As an alternative, the lens may simply be soaked in the Monoclens solution for 2 hours or more although the cleaning efficacy is not as great.

The theory of the electrical 'pull' effect of the copolymer is used in the supplementary cleaner 'C40' which incorporates the copolymer only, i.e. there is no oxidizing agent present. The lens is stood in a vial of Monoclens C40 for a few

hours, or left overnight, after which it is boiled in saline for 30 minutes and finally cooled.

Oxidative cleaning and changes in lens parameters

One of the first oxidative cleaning solutions used for soft lenses was sodium hypochlorite (Milton). This bleach removed all discolouration and traces of mucoprotein within 15 minutes. However, after two to three such treatments lenses began to alter in curvature and/or power. Diluting the solution reduced the problem although it still occurred more slowly and occasionally lenses became distorted. De Carle (J. T., 1979, cited by Phillips, 1980) reported that this change took place even with a 10 times dilution (i.e. 0.10% sodium hypochlorite). In the case of Permalenses the lens total diameter increased by about 0.2 mm per cleaning.

There appears to be little doubt that excessive or prolonged use of stronger oxidizing agents will result in breakdown or alteration of the lens polymer. Lenses with small cracks or nicks or even relatively old lenses will probably be damaged by oxidative cleaning methods. Where inorganic deposits, such as calcium, are removed, a small pit may be left in the lens.

However, provided they are used minimally to 'rescue' lenses not responding to other cleaning techniques, there appears to be no significant change in lens dimensions (Phillips, 1980). In a study of three hydrogels cleaned with Monoclens, Ganju (1977) found a very small flattening of back optic zone radius (BOZR), a small reduction in negative power, and a small increase in total diameter (TD), but all at clinically insignificant levels.

Tighe (B. J., 1979, cited by Phillips, 1980) believes the reasons for the small parameter changes are as follows: any polymer containing HEMA is likely to contain carboxyl (-COOH) groups as a result of the presence of methacrylic acid. When these are treated with salts of weak acids (e.g. sodium bicarbonate), or any solution of a salt that has become alkaline, the carboxyl groups are partially converted to their appropriate salt. Even a small amount of this type of change produces a measurable increase in water content — hence the increase in diameter plus some slight flattening of the lens. Permalens and several other lens materials do this. In Permalens the presence of vinyl pyrrolidone aggravates the situation because the nitrogen can 'quaternize' and stabilize the effect. In summary, Tighe argues that:

(1) It is an effect of an alkaline salt, especially a sodium salt, and not oxidation that causes the parameter changes.
(2) All HEMA-containing polymers will do it to some extent.
(3) The purity of the HEMA monomer used is important.
(4) It is worse with high water content vinyl pyrrolidone containing materials.

Factors influencing the prescribing of hydrogel disinfection and cleaning procedures

Over the last decade, prescribing habits have swung backwards and forwards from thermal to chemical disinfection methods and vice versa. Many practitioners still prescribe one single technique to the exclusion of all others. Gradually this attitude is changing and practitioners are prescribing methods most applicable to each individual patient. The following points may provide guidance:

(1) Lens material: chemical disinfection techniques are indicated where a particular material, particularly the high water content ones, is affected by heat. Materials prone to discolouration should be disinfected with a hydrogen peroxide method.
(2) Daily or extended wear lenses: the relatively infrequent cleaning of an extended wear lens indicates a more thorough cleaning procedure, e.g. improved surfactant plus enzymatic cleaner. A hydrogen peroxide procedure is also commonly used for its additional mild cleaning effect.
(3) History of general or ocular allergies, or other factor which may indicate a patient likely to show a solution allergic or toxic reaction. The following patients may be considered as possible candidates to show sensitivity to chemical disinfection preservatives:
  (a) strong history of general allergies;
  (b) history of eyes that overreact to ordinary stimuli, e.g. tiredness, alcohol, cigarette smoke;
  (c) signs of overly reactive or sensitive eyes by external examination, e.g. injected

conjunctiva, engorged limbus;
  (d) dry eyes or tear film abnormality;
  (e) former hard or RGP lens wearers, i.e. previous exposure to certain preservatives;
  (f) high water content lenses worn on daily basis, i.e. regular exposure to high preservative levels;
  (g) sensitivity exhibited by special tests, e.g. conjunctival smears, skin scratch or patch testing.

In these cases, the practitioner should be prepared to transfer the patient to a different preservative system or possibly prescribe a thermal disinfection method. However, in a retrospective study, Young (1985) was unable to identify patients who showed solution sensitivity from an investigation of their allergic history alone.

(4) Tear flow and type of lacrimal fluid: as mentioned above the dry-eyed patient is often more prone to preservative reactions. Additionally, the dry-eyed patient is more susceptible to deposit formation. The patient exhibiting a high tear lipid level should be prescribed an enzymatic cleaner containing a lipase and use an improved lipid solvent surfactant, e.g. Miraflow.
(5) Patient's occupation and hobbies: occupations which involve travelling or patients who go camping, for example, are better advised to use chemical disinfection. Certain industrial occupations may indicate specific regimens, e.g. patients experiencing a high incidence of rust spots will find their appearance minimized if chemical rather than thermal disinfection is used.
(6) Patient's personality and intelligence: it usually becomes apparent to practitioners very quickly, the degree of cooperation and conformity to instructions that they are likely to experience from each patient. At the extreme end some patients should be rejected as contact lens candidates if they are not likely to fully cooperate or understand instructions. However, for less intelligent groups practitioners may feel an automated thermal unit or simple chemical disinfection regimen is ideal. In such cases, the protease cleaning may be omitted and hydrogen peroxide systems are best avoided.
(7) Patient's general health and current sys-

temic or ocular medication: practitioners are increasingly becoming aware of the relevance of general health and systemic medication on contact lens wear and deposit formation. For example the dry eye found in certain arthritis cases will commonly exacerbate a deposit problem. The hyperlipid secretion in acne vulgaris will produce differing deposits. In such cases the cleaning regimen must be modified or strengthened as appropriate. The effect of systemic medication is discussed below.

(8) Climate: patients living in tropical and subtropical climates should be warned that many contact lens solutions are not stable above 25°C. Heat disinfection possibly using preserved or unit-dose saline may be preferable. Surfactant cleaners and any other solutions should be stored in a refrigerator when not in use.

(9) Previous deposit problem and type: in spite of all possible care many problems with solution reactions and deposit problems are found only once wear has begun. It becomes extremely important that practitioners are prepared to monitor each patient and modify cleaning and disinfection procedures when appropriate. Patients should be warned in advance that this may become likely to avoid concern if problems do, in fact, occur.

Practitioners should be capable of recognizing solution allergic or toxic reactions and, in the case of deposit problems, recognizing the type of deposit problem and being able to prescribe the appropriate remedy.

The following signs and symptoms are commonly found in cases of adverse solution reactions:

(1) Discomfort on insertion, possibly slowly improving if wear is continued.
(2) Photophobia.
(3) Epiphora.
(4) Conjunctival hyperaemia, especially limbally.
(5) Decreased wearing time.
(6) Possible mild diffuse superficial punctate keratitis staining with sodium fluorescein.
(7) Possible intraepithelial microcysts and/or perilimbal infiltrates if the condition has been present for some time.

Deposits are laid down on hydrogel lenses almost as soon as the lens is placed in the eye. The main source of deposit is lysozyme protein (Karageozian, 1974). Lipid may also be present from the meibomian glands and by finger contact. Mucus will be present secreted by the conjunctival goblet cells and calcium salts may also be deposited from the lacrimal fluid. In addition, make-up, aerosol sprays of hair lacquer and deodorant etc., may contaminate the lens. These deposits will gradually increase, in spite of patient cleaning, until symptoms occur.

Patients experiencing a clinically significant deposit problem may complain of mild discomfort, poorer vision, slight photophobia and loss of tolerance. The practitioner may find a myopic shift in the prescription, a fall in best acuity, a 'roughened' lens surface appearance visible by slit lamp microscopy, a tighter fitting lens and possible lens discolouration (see Plates 25, 31 and 36). Some deposits are best identified in the eye by slit lamp microscopy; others are best seen by removing the lens, air drying and cooling it, and then examining it against a diffuse light source. Scanning electron microscopy, morphological stains and dark field microscopy provide further means of identification although these are not commonly available to the practitioner.

There are two types of protein film, the most common of which produces a white, partially opaque layer covering all or part of the lens (Figure 4.12). Alternatively protein may be almost invisible, often not being recognized by slit lamp examination until it begins to crack. It may sometimes be visible by air drying. In such cases, the subjective symptoms are often the main guide to the presence of the protein.

Lipid appears as greasy or smeary deposits on the lens surface that change in pattern on blinking (see Plate 26). Lipid deposition is sometimes worse in patients using chlorhexidine-preserved solutions because this induces surface hydrophobicity.

Pigment deposits in soft lenses are usually yellow to brown, the discolouration gradually increasing with lens age (see Plate 35). They appear to be made up of a melanin-like polymer derived from the polymerization of aromatic compounds in the tears (Ruben, 1976). Because melanin is formed by oxidative polymerization, the rate of melanin formation may be increased by thermal disinfection procedures. Pigmentary

165

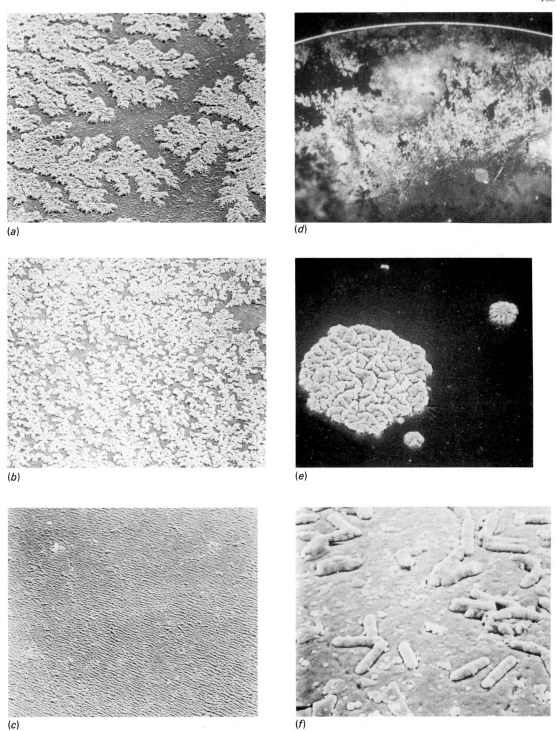

(a)

(d)

(b)

(e)

(c)

(f)

Figure 4.12 Protein film on a hydrogel lens. (*a*) Early stages spreading across the lens surface. (*b*) Later stage now covering most of the lens surface. (*c*) Final stage where the lens surface is completely covered. (*d*) Deposits as seen by dark field microscopy. (*e*) Isolated protein deposit as seen by scanning electron microscopy showing the convoluted surface shapes commonly seen. The polishing marks on the lens surface can clearly be seen. (*f*) Rod-shaped bacteria on top of a protein film (Flinders Medical Centre)

deposits may fluoresce slightly under ultraviolet light.

Microorganisms such as fungi and yeasts can grow on and into hydrogel materials if proper lens disinfection is not carried out. They may be observed as white or coloured filamentary growths that grow through the lens polymer. The fungal hyphae may extend from one lens surface to the other and cannot be removed so that the lens damage is permanent (*see Plate 33*).

Calcium salts form a hazy white surface layer often resembling protein (*see Plate 36*). The main cause of inorganic films appears to be precipitation and growth of calcium phosphates from tears while the lens is in the eye. Tear chemistry and tear production are important factors. Poor blinking, insufficiency of tears, or low tear film break-up time seem to be associated with these deposits (Koetting, 1976). The presence of protein films may also predispose the lens to the build-up of inorganic materials because the protein-covered lens surface becomes more hydrophobic and more likely to dry between blinks. The end result seems to be alternate layers of protein and calcium so that cleaners for both types of deposit are necessary and removing the protein merely exposes the rough underlying inorganic material. Calcium phosphate may form as a result of interaction between free calcium ions in the tears and phosphate buffers used in certain solutions. The resulting calcium phosphate is insoluble and is precipitated out within the lens matrix.

Another calcium-containing deposit is composed of insoluble crystalline growths known as lens calculi. They are also referred to as jelly bumps, barnacles and mulberry-like growths and appear as small white elevations on the lens surface (*Figure 4.11a* and *Plate 32*). Careful examination will often reveal that these deposits are an annulus, the central 'hole' of which is filled with mucus (*see Plates 38* and *39*). Because the outer annulus can be demonstrated to be mainly lipid on which secondary calcium salts have deposited, it can be postulated that they originate from lipid build-up around dry spots on the lens surface. This lipid ring builds up until it eventually protrudes through the tear film. Formation is largely a matter of the lens wearer's tear chemistry. Certain wearers are susceptible to the formation of this deposit and will rapidly form it again on replacement lenses. They are more commonly seen on extended wear lenses. Their effect on the eye is minimal until they reach a fairly large size. Removal (described below), unless done early, commonly leaves a pit in the lens surface. Roth (1987) notes that calculi may appear following systemic antibiotic therapy indicating a change in tear chemistry.

Mercurial deposits are grey to black discoloured patches. They are more commonly seen in thermally disinfected lenses utilizing thimerosal-preserved saline and less commonly in chemically disinfected lenses. The primary cause of mercurial deposits in well-documented cases appears to be due to the re-use of the same preserved saline or cold disinfection solution. As the contaminant load of the solution increases with each re-use, the thimerosal decomposes to a greater extent and finally mercurial decomposition products begin to precipitate in the lens matrix (Petricciani and Kreszanoski, 1977). Although these deposits would appear to be non-toxic to the eye, they consist of insoluble compounds, probably the very insoluble black mercuric sulphide, and are difficult to remove. The answer lies in their prevention.

Rust-coloured spots are small, discrete red-to-orange spots seen within the lens matrix (*see Plate 40*). Occasionally discomfort is caused but generally the patient is asymptomatic. They are generally related to penetration of iron-containing foreign bodies into the lens. These rapidly oxidize to form ferrous oxide which spreads over a small area within the lens matrix.

Once deposits have been identified, the patient's regimen should be modified as follows. Alternatively, a more frequent lens replacement scheme should be used. In practice both tactics may be adopted.

For protein deposits

(1) Chemical disinfection is better than heat.
(2) Use 'improved' surfactants, e.g. Polyclens (Opti-Clean), Sterisolv etc.
(3) Use a hydrogen peroxide system with the lens in peroxide overnight if possible e.g. Oxysept, Mirasept systems etc.
(4) Use proteolytic enzyme weekly.
(5) If thermal disinfection is indicated for other reasons, a low heat unit may be preferable or pasteurization.
(6) Prescribe a non-ionic lens material as these are generally more protein resistant, e.g. the

HEMA group, CSI, Permaflex, Sauflon, Softcon etc.

(7) Prescribe a 'deposit resistant' lens, for example Pilkington Barnes–Hind's Elite and Kelvin's (CooperVision) X-Ten, where lenses of these water contents (medium and high respectively) are required.

For lipid deposits

(1) Less of a problem with thermal disinfection.
(2) Avoid chlorhexidine-preserved solutions because this increases surface hydrophobicity and allows lipid adhesion.
(3) Use specific lipid cleaners, e.g. Miraflow.
(4) Use in-eye cleaners, e.g. Clerz, Adapettes, Soft Comfort etc.
(5) Utilize enzyme cleaners containing a lipase, e.g. Amiclair, Alcon Enzyme etc.

For calcium deposits

(1) Less with thermal disinfection.
(2) Use hydrogen peroxide (low pH dissolves calcium).
(3) Use proteolytic enzyme weekly as sometimes secondary to protein.
(4) Check blink action; advise accordingly; use in-eye lubricants if necessary.
(5) Use sequestering agent, e.g. Sorbisal plus Calcium Deposit Preventer. Only activated in thermal disinfection.
(6) May be worse with tight fitting lenses.
(7) Prescribe glyceryl methyl methacrylate (CSI) material lenses (Levy, 1984).

For calculi

(1) Use lipid solvent cleaner, e.g. Miraflow.
(2) Use lipase-containing enzyme.
(3) Use weekly intensive surfactant cleaner.
(4) Utilize in-eye lubricants in extended wear-cases and remove and clean more frequently.
(5) Often worse in tear potassium deficiency cases (*see below*), e.g. patients on systemic antihypertensives or diuretics with no potassium supplements; some cases of renal stones etc. Possibly helped if potassium sorbate preserved solutions are used. Refer to general practitioner if necessary.
(6) Check blink action.

For rust spots

(1) Less visible with chemical disinfection.
(2) Hydrogen peroxide disinfection systems may reduce visibility.

For discoloured lenses

(1) Switch lens material if NVP-containing polymer being used with thermal disinfection, or switch to chemical disinfection.
(2) If considered due to nicotine from smoking, the patient should be advised accordingly.
(3) If considered due to heavy protein deposition refer to the appropriate section above.
(4) Utilize non-thimerosal preserved saline if thermal disinfection used.
(5) Use hydrogen peroxide system for disinfection.
(6) Check systemic medication (*see below*).

For dry-eyed patients

Since deposit problems are exacerbated for the dry-eyed patient the following advice may be helpful. It should be emphasized that there is no panacea for this group of patients.

(1) Use Softab or Aerotab system and dilute the saline by 20–50%. This temporarily increases the water content of the lenses which is then slowly released onto the eye.
(2) Saline dilution may also be utilized with thermal disinfection, but thermal disinfection is best avoided since this exacerbates the deposit problem to which dry-eyed patients are particularly prone.
(3) Use in-eye lubricants frequently. Rengstorff (R., 1987, personal communication) reports significant help with the use of vitamin A-containing eye drops.
(4) Resoak lenses for 15–30 minutes during the day or swap to presoaked spare pair.
(5) Improve cleaning routine because deposits are more likely in this group which in turn exacerbates the dryness symptoms.
(6) Refit with a lens material containing a high percentage of 'bound' to 'free' water (see Chapter 11). A non-ionic, low water content lens appears to perform best.
(7) Refit with a 'deposit resistant' lens.

Deposits, lens discolouration and systemic and ocular medication

Practitioners are becoming increasingly aware of the effect of drugs and solutions on soft lens deposits and discolouration. As knowledge increases so special advice can be given prior to lens issue and in solution prescribing. The following is a summary of the limited information currently available.

Sympathomimetic eye drops

Repeated instillation of eye drops containing substances such as adrenaline (epinephrine), phenylephrine (neosynephrine) or other readily oxidized sympathomimetics can cause brown, grey or black lens discolouration and lens stiffening (Miller, Brooks and Mobilia, 1976).

Hydrogen peroxide will cleave the melanin particles produced and soften the lens again.

Tetrahydrozoline (Visine) may also cause lens discolouration.

Alcohol

Dean Hart (1986) reports from retrospective analysis that lens wearers who consume more than four alcoholic drinks a week are 10 times more likely to experience lens lipid deposits. This may possibly arise from the diuretic effect of alcohol (see below).

Diagnostic eye drops

Both sodium fluorescein and rose bengal can concentrate in hydrogel lenses. Natural diffusion out is reasonably quick in high water content lenses. Hydrogen peroxide, Liprofin, or boiling in distilled water (a form of purging) all help speed up the process.

High-molecular-weight Fluorexon still diffuses into hydrogel lenses but more slowly.

Diet

Calculi deposits, mainly lipid, are commonly found in patients who regularly ingest cholesterol-rich foods (Hill and Terry, 1976).

Hypokalaemia

Hypokalaemia is the condition of low blood potassium levels. The patient may experience arrhythmia (destabilized cardiac rhythm) and/or muscle cramps. It commonly occurs if a diuretic is prescribed, e.g. frusemide (Lasix) (which increases potassium excretion) with no potassium ion compensation also prescribed, e.g. Slow-K.

Patients exhibiting hypokalaemia have been observed to show hyperlipidaemia (Knochel, 1984), higher tear lipid levels (Hart, 1986), and increased lens calculi.

Norwood (1983) reports patients with kidney stones also showing lens calculi. Many people who form calcium stones have excess urinary calcium. In addition, certain clinical states may diminish stone inhibitor excretion, one of which is hypokalaemia (Kanig and Conn, 1985).

Hart (1986) has measured low tear potassium levels in patients who show definite tear lipid problems and postulates that the use of potassium sorbate-preserved solutions for lens storage may help.

Nasal decongestants

Brompheniramine, phenylephrine and phenylpropanolamine have been reported (Banes, 1985) as causing increased sensitivity to contact lens wear, although it is not stated if this is due to reduced tear secretion or not. As mentioned above, adrenaline and phenylephrine in nasal decongestants may turn soft lenses grey, black or brown if repeatedly instilled into the eye (Sugar, 1974).

Nicotine

Soft lenses have been reported to turn yellow or yellow-brown in wearers who are heavy smokers (Kleist, 1979), although it is not clear if this is from finger or atmospheric contamination. Hicks (1985) reports a nicotine-stained lens from a tobacco chewing patient. Regurgitation through the canaliculi is postulated as the causative mechanism (see also Chapter 3, p. 109).

Nitrofurantoin

Available as tablets, capsules or suspension (Furadantin and Macrodantin), this drug is a synthetic antibacterial used almost exclusively for urinary tract infections. It increases tear flow and turns the urine and soft lenses brown. The profuse lacrimation and ocular irritation can easily be confused with a contact lens problem (Hopkins, 1985).

Oral contraceptives

Farrall (1976) has shown that a reduction in tear output with associated drop in lysozyme and relative increase in globulin-type protein is to be expected when women first take oral contraceptives, or change to another type, or cease to take it. The effects of increased corneal oedema, reduced lacrimal secretion and increased mucus and lipid content of the tear film may last a few weeks but will gradually subside. Fortunately modern, low oestrogen dose tablets produce only infrequent problems to the contact lens wearer.

De Vries (1985) also reports a higher frequency of calcium deposit problems in women taking oral contraceptives, the problem being greater in the higher oestrogen dosage group.

Phenolphthalein

Available as Agarol (suspension), Veracolate (tablets), Alophen (pills) and Ford pills, phenolphthalein is used as a purgative in malabsorption syndromes such as pancreatic dysfunction etc. Because the products are mainly available as over-the-counter preparations, they are unfortunately often used as slimming aids by virtue of the diarrhoea produced. The urine and faeces are turned pink to red and contact lenses pink (Aucamp, 1980).

Preservatives in therapeutic eye drops

Contrary to earlier thinking, the preservative used in the common and relatively infrequently administered therapeutic eye drops appears unimportant. Although preservatives may be used which theoretically bind and concentrate in hydrogel lenses, this does not cause an observed clinical problem in practice due to the small amount of preservative present and the short contact time (Lemp, 1978).

However, many therapeutic eye drops cause stinging in *hard* lens wearers, possibly due to pre-existing corneal insult, oedema, or the effect of the solution on the tear film and its break-up time (BUT).

Phenazopyridine hydrochloride

Phenazopyridine (Pyridium) produces a topical anaesthetic effect on the mucosa of the urinary tract. It is used as palliative therapy in cystitis, prostatitis and urethritis. Phenazopyridine turns urine reddish-brown and may also discolour soft lenses this colour (Aucamp, 1980). One report has been made of a lens turning grey when a patient taking this drug used a thermal disinfection routine (Barnard, 1984).

Phenazopyridine produces keratitis sicca in dogs (Slatter, 1973).

Reduced tear secretion

Drugs that cause reduced tear secretion may affect lenses of all types but, in particular, hydrogel lenses. Drugs affecting tear flow may be divided into the following categories:

(1) Anticholinergic drugs such as atropine and hyoscine (scopolamine). These are often sold as over-the-counter cold and 'flu preparations, antidiarrhoeals (diphenoxylate hydrochloride, Lomotil) and some sedatives.
(2) Antihistamines: these reduce both aqueous and mucous secretions. Most antihistamines have, to some extent, antimuscarinic actions. It is this which produces any side effects that occur. Typical examples are promethazine (Phenergan), chlorpheniramine (Piriton) and trimeprazine (Vallergan).
(3) Psychotropic drugs with an anticholinergic action, for example tricyclic antidepressants, e.g. amitriptyline (Tryptanol), imipramine (Tofranil), doxepin (Sinequan), and neuroleptics, e.g. benztropine (Cogentin) and benzhexol (Artane).
(4) Diuretics.
(5) Beta-blockers, e.g. practolol (now discontinued) and in some cases, atenolol, and oxprenolol (Banes, 1985).
(6) Certain general anaesthetics: tear flow may be reduced 30 minutes after the inhalation of nitrous oxide, halothane or enflurane (Krupin, Cross and Becker, 1977).
(7) Phenazopyridine (Pyridium).
(8) Higher dose oestrogen oral contraceptives.
(9) Appetite suppressants: diethylpropion (Tenuate Dospan).

(10) Anti-allergic: sodium cromoglycate (Opticrom) (Bates, 1985).
(11) Anti-parkinsonism drugs.
(12) Although not listed as a known side effect, Bergmanson and Rios (1981) reported dry eye symptoms and the adherence of a hydrogel lens to the cornea in a patient prescribed the mild analgesic Darvocet-N 100.

Darvocet-N 100 is a combination of dextropropoxyphene 100 mg and 650 mg. Dextropropoxyphene is used as the napsylate or hydrochloride salt and, although structurally related to the narcotic analgesic methadone, does not compare to it in analgesic potency. The combination with paracetamol or aspirin is reported to produce greater analgesia than either drug administered alone.

The various drug combinations may be supplied as Capadex, co-proxamol, Di-Gesic, Doloxene, Paradex and Paxalgesic, and are used for the symptomatic relief of pain associated with neuralgia, dysmenorrhoea, rheumatism, arthritis, sciatica, lumbago, toothache and other types of nervous or muscular pain; and to reduce fever in common cold and influenza.

(13) Isotretinoin (Roaccutane or Accutane) is a synthetic vitamin A compound used for the treatment of recalcitrant cystic acne. It has numerous toxic ocular side effects which include anterior segment inflammation, dry eye syndrome, contact lens intolerance, altered refraction, photophobia and reduced night vision (Caffery and Josephson, 1988).

Respiratory drugs

Beclomethasone (Becotide) and salbutamol (Ventolin) have been reported to occasionally cause increased sensitivity to contact lenses and solutions (Banes, 1985).

Rifampin or rifampicin

Available as Rifadin and Rimactane, this is a semisynthetic antibiotic, bactericidal to both Gram-positive and some Gram-negative bacteria. Its use is mainly in tuberculosis and ocular chlamydial cases and has been reported to turn soft lenses orange (Lyons, 1979).

Skin creams

Some skin creams such as Oxywash for teenage spots and pimples contain benzyl peroxide which may bleach or discolour Cibatint lenses (see Plate 37).

Other hand creams such as Vaseline Intensive Care and Skin Repair may remain on the hands after several washes and, if brought into contact with a hydrogel lens surface, are extremely difficult to remove (see Plate 26). Liquid soaps not fully rinsed from the hands may produce a similar but lesser effect.

Johnson's Baby Lotion may discolour soft lenses pink if not carefully washed from the hands. Eye make-ups are also likely to discolour hydrogel lenses if misused.

Sulphasalazine

Prescribed as Salazopyrin, this drug is used for ulcerative colitis, especially for maintenance therapy following corticosteroid treatment, and also for treatment of active Crohn's disease especially in patients with colonic involvement.

The alkaline urine and contact lenses may be discoloured orange-yellow (Riley, Flegg and Mandal, 1985).

Tetracyclines

Available in a wide range of products, such as tetracycline (Achromycin), Mysteclin (tetracycline + nystatin) oxytetracycline (Terramycin), doxycycline (Vibramycin) etc., the tetracycline group has a wide range of antimicrobial activity against Gram-positive and -negative organisms and often to microorganisms insensitive to other chemotherapy, e.g. rickettsiae, Chlamydia trachomatis etc. It is commonly prescribed in bronchitis, sinusitis, prostatitis, teenage acne, blepharitis etc.

Tetracycline is known to discolour teeth brown if used with young children, the teeth fluorescing yellow at first and then, later, permanently brown. This is probably due to a tetracycline–calcium orthophosphate compound or perhaps an oxidation product. Presumably similar compounds are formed in the tears and the lens ultimately discolours yellow-brown.

Current medical trends are to use tetracyclines such as doxycycline which appears not to cause dental (and possibly contact lens) discolouration to the same extent. However, Banes (1985) reports a case of marked photophobia and contact lens sensitivity on a patient taking doxycycline.

Some evidence has been put forward to claim an increased sensitivity to thimerosal-preserved solutions in patients taking systemic tetracycline (Crook and Freeman, 1983).

Topical medication and pharmacological effects

Hydrogel lenses may have the following effects:

(1) Increase the contact time of the drug. For example corneal anaesthesia is prolonged if a soft lens is reinserted over a cornea anaesthetized for applanation tonometry.
(2) Adsorb, concentrate and gradually release certain drugs. The effect of certain cycloplegics, pilocarpine, phenylephrine, idoxuridine, possibly steroids and other high-molecular-weight, water-soluble drugs may be enhanced by the use of a hydrogel delivery system provided they are preservative free or use appropriate preservative systems (*see* Chapters 21 and 24). However a minimum 2-hour soak in the appropriate solution is necessary for maximum effect.

In a similar manner, swimming pool chlorine may be concentrated in hydrogel lenses and subsequently released onto the cornea causing tissue damage after a prolonged open-eye swimming session in heavily chlorinated pool water. Nevertheless, protection is afforded to the eye during swimming and adverse effects from the chlorine may be avoided if the lenses are removed straight after swimming and rinsed thoroughly. Disinfection is also advisable to minimize any risk of subsequent infection from contaminated pool water.

The vapour from trichlorethylene can be concentrated in soft lenses with severe adverse ocular effects.
(3) An exaggerated response may be seen, possibly due to a compromised cornea, in long-term wearers. A mydriatic response has been reported with as little as a 0.125% phenylephrine hydrochloride solution (Krezanoski, 1981).

(4) Effect of the vehicle used for the medication. Clear vehicles create the least problems. Oleaginous composition or suspensions can lead to discomfort or lens intolerance but fortunately are little used nowadays (Krezanoski, 1981).

Topical medication and pH

Low (acidic) pH therapeutic solutions, e.g. some adrenaline solutions, can cause water loss from hydrogels, shrinkage and steepening. High (alkaline) pH solutions cause the opposite. Methacrylic acid-containing materials are the most prone to this effect (Krezanoski, 1981).

Topical medication and tonicity

Hypertonic solutions such as 10% sodium sulphacetamide or 6–8% pilocarpine hydrochloride can cause lens dehydration and temporary parameter changes if administered to hydrogel lens wearers. High water content lenses are the most prone to this effect (Krezanoski, 1981).

Trandate (labetalol)

Labetalol (Trandate) is an antihypertensive agent exhibiting both α- and β-adrenergic blocking properties. The β-blocking agents in general lower blood pressure by reducing heart rate and contractability. Norwood (1983) observed lens calculi on patients taking labetalol which did not occur when methyldopa (Aldomet) was prescribed as an alternative. Although marked xerophthalmia and keratoconjunctivitis occurred with earlier β-blockers, such as practolol, this has not been observed with labetalol. However, the calculi are probably caused by some subtle interference with or reduction of the tear liquid. Banes (1985) has indeed reported dry eyes in some patients prescribed atenolol (Tenormin) and oxprenolol (Trasicor).

Summary of lens deposits and discolouration

The following may serve as a useful practitioner's reference list. Soft lenses are generally referred to unless otherwise stated. It should be emphasized that discolouration is only likely with prolonged use of many of the medications listed.

Deposits

Protein
- Usually natural, high lysozyme levels in tears
- Pseudoprotein following conjunctivitis
- Giant papillary conjunctivitis
- Exacerbated by thermal disinfection methods

Lipid
- Natural hyper-meibomian secretion
- High cholesterol diet
- Low tear potassium levels
- Regular alcohol drinker
- Pseudolipid with intensive hand creams and unrinsed liquid soaps
- Loss of coating with certain RGP materials
- Acne

Calcium
- Natural high tear levels
- Poor blinkers/dry eyes
- High oestrogen dose contraceptive pills
- Calcium phosphate resulting from phosphate buffers in solutions used
- Use of tap water for rinsing

Calculi
- Natural for some individuals
- Beta-blockers, e.g. labetalol
- Low system or tear potassium levels
- Higher oestrogen dose contraceptive pills
- Poor blinkers/high water contact lenses
- May be worse after antibiotic therapy (Roth, 1987)

Discolouration

Grey
- Phenazopyridine
- Adrenaline (epinephrine)
- Phenylephrine
- Prolonged thimerosal preservative use
- Tetrahydrozoline (Visine)
- Repeated thermal disinfection with same saline
- Swapping lenses soaked in chlorhexidine/thimerosal to sorbic acid solutions

Brown
- Adrenaline (epinephrine)
- Phenylephrine
- Nitrofurantoin
- Tetrahydrozoline
- Nicotine
- Tetracycline
- Boiling in old sorbic acid-preserved solutions
- Boiling NVP-containing materials

Reddish-brown
- Phenazopyridine
- Iodine-liberating disinfecting systems used with old or high water content lenses

White
- Calcium deposits
- Boiling in Mirasol
- Boiling in Flexsol

Yellow
- Nicotine
- Tetracyclines
- Boiling in old sorbic acid-preserved solutions
- Old lenses in chlorhexidine solutions

Orange
- Rifampicin
- Duragel disinfecting tablets with old or chlorhexidine-soaked lenses. Product now discontinued but could apply to other chlorine release systems
- Sulphasalazine
- Fluorescein

Pink
- Phenolphthalein
- Commercial metabisulphite as antioxidant in adrenaline eye drops
- Some antioxidants in commercially used hydrogen peroxide
- Johnson's baby lotion
- Antioxidant used in commercial hydrogen peroxide (phenacetin?)

Red
- Rubber stamp ink
- Rose bengal

Black
- Adrenaline (epinephrine)
- Phenylephrine
- Tetrahydrozoline

Blue
- Rubber stamp ink

Purple   Heating protein deposits in old
             sorbic acid-preserved
             solutions

Green   Pale-green or brown reported
             in some cases after usage of
             Bausch & Lomb Thermal
             Enzyme Tablets

Solution misuse and incompatibility

The following summarizes some of the more common patient mistakes and misuses of soft lens solutions and serves to emphasize the need for careful patient instruction.

(1) Tints: Cibatints are reduced or removed by strong oxidants such as chlorine (Softabs or Aerotabs) or sodium perborate (Liprofin).

(2) Preservatives and discolouration: thimerosal has been reported as causing grey-black discolouration of soft lenses and containers. Chlorhexidine has been blamed for causing lens yellowing.

(3) Hydrogen peroxide: proprietary pharmaceutical and supermarket hydrogen peroxides contain stabilizers. Phenacetin, one such product, may cause some lenses to turn pink.

(4) Daily soft lens cleaners used as soaking solutions may cause a gummy residue, opaque or discoloured lenses, and ocular irritation.

(5) Cold disinfection solutions used in thermal units, not thoroughly rinsed and re-used. A gummy residue and lens discolouration may result.

(6) Enzyme misuse. Lenses soaked in papain for longer than 1–2 hours may cause irritation in some wearers on subsequent lens insertion.

(7) Barnes–Hind Weekly Cleaner insufficiently rinsed from the lens after use. An irritation reaction is caused.

(8) Polyvinyl alcohol-containing solutions mixed with boric acid-containing solutions. A gummy gelatinous precipitate is formed.

(9) Misuse of thermal unit. Repeated use of the same saline has been reported to turn lenses grey to grey-black (Sibley, 1984).

(10) Use of high-molecular-weight containing solutions, e.g. polyvinyl alcohol in a thermal unit (Sibley, 1984). This can cause whitish-coloured gummy residues that can ruin hydrogel lenses, e.g. Alcon's Flexsol contains adsorbase which forms a white film on the lens if heated. Flexcare is the same formula with no adsorbase and which does not form the residue on heating. Cooper's Mirasol produces a similar effect on heating.

(11) Changing preservatives: soaking chlorhexidine–thimerosal disinfected lenses in sorbic acid-preserved solutions without purging may cause lenses to discolour grey to black (Sibley, 1984).

(12) Use of old (expired) solutions may cause discolouration and precipitation (Sibley, 1984).

(13) Use of old sorbic acid-preserved solutions and deposited lenses. Sorbic acid slowly breaks down with oxidation to form small amounts of aldehydes. The effect is speeded up by low pH, temperature, light, oxygen and trace metal ions. Amine in protein on the lens surface combines with the aldehyde to produce a yellow-brown discolouration (Sibley and Chu, 1984). This can usually be removed by Liprofin or hydrogen peroxide cleaning.

(14) Sorbic acid concentration: concentrations greater than 0.15% have been reported to turn lenses grey-green if used with heat or hydrogen peroxide (Greco, 1984).

(15) Heating high water content lenses containing NVP will gradually induce a brown discolouration (Lubert and Caplan, 1984).

(16) Storage of hydrogels in hard lens solutions. Marked discomfort can be produced especially if benzalkonium chloride or chlorbutanol-preserved solutions were inadvertently used. Purging and use of a strong oxidizing cleaner, e.g. Liprofin, may remove the preservative.

Lens conditioning, tear replacement and similar solutions

Some soft lens wearers experience occasional discomfort or loss of acuity while the lens is in the eye. Assuming that no fitting problems exist, the cause may be partial dehydration of the lens or the build-up of meibomian secretion on the lens surface. To overcome these problems solutions have been developed which clean and rehydrate lenses *in situ* (*see* Appendix F, *Table F.II*, at the end of the book). One manufacturer has also developed a solution (Hydrosol, *Contactasol*) to be rubbed into the lens surface prior to insertion and which is stated to aid initial comfort and to reduce the build-up of surface deposits during subsequent wear.

Rehydration and lens cleaning *in vivo* are needed by the extended wear patient on waking. Solutions such as Clerz (Cooper) have been developed for this purpose. Similar products are listed in Appendix F, *Table F.III*. Clerz is a hypertonic saline combined with a surfactant. The hypertonicity will 'draw out' surface contaminants and possibly temporarily flatten the lens front surface thereby stimulating movement of a possibly slightly dehydrated (and therefore tight-fitting) lens. Such lubricating drops are often needed during the day especially if the patient is located near heaters, air-conditioners or has been in a windy environment.

Soft lenses are still developing at a rapid pace and coupled with this has been the development of related solutions. Practitioners must accept the fact that no particular solution or technique will be ideal for every patient or lens material. In the same way that careful investigation will indicate the optimum lens material and parameters for a particular patient, the practitioner must equally carefully ensure that the method of disinfection selected is both appropriate to his individual patient's temperament, occupation and available facilities as well as to the lens material to be used.

Similarly, care must be taken in choosing the lens storage case or container. Particularly with asepticizor units the practitioner may have no choice since only the one design of case will fit the unit. Where a choice is possible, the practitioner should choose a container which conforms to the following ideals.

(1) A transparent container will allow the quantity of solution to be seen.
(2) The container should have to be everted to remove the lenses thereby ensuring that the solution is changed at least each time the lens is worn.
(3) It should be clearly marked 'Left' and 'Right', preferably also colour-coded, possibly with identifying tactile projections.
(4) The storage solution volume should not be so small that insufficient quantities of preservative are contained (where chemical disinfecting solutions are used). It should be large enough to allow adequate diffusion and dilution of contaminants into the solution. Conversely the container volume should not be so large that excessive quantities of solution are used which may discourage daily changing of the solution because of the cost.
(5) The container material must be compatible with lens materials and solution constituents.
(6) The container material must be capable of withstanding regular boiling and have leak-proof caps.

Scleral lens solutions

For a sealed scleral lens, a solution of 2% sodium bicarbonate, with 0.2% chlorbutol can be used. It is important to avoid the use of hydrobenzoates, or phenylmercuric nitrate or acetate in a sealed scleral lens solution, as they cause intense irritation to the eye.

Ophthalmic preparations*

Eye drops are either dispensed in multiple-dose containers or in a single-dose disposable unit (*Figure 4.13*), the latter having the advantage of ensuring that a sterile solution is always available for use. Unfortunately, at the present time not all the preparations required are available in this form (*see* Appendix F, *Table F.III*).

Substances in solution are more likely to break down than those in a dry state. Therefore, a limit must be put on the time for which eye drops may be used. An expiry date is shown on the labels of some preparations. This refers only to unopened bottles, stored according to the manufacturers' instructions. Usually, this

---

*More details of the following ophthalmic preparations mentioned on pp. 176–180 are obtainable from *Mims*, published monthly by Haymarket Publishing Limited, Medical Division, 76 Dean Street, London W1A 1BU, and the *Data Sheet Compendium* published yearly by the Association of the British Pharmaceutical Industry (Pharmind Publications). These publications give brand names and the names of the various manufacturing drug houses, as well as strengths, dosages, legal categories, contra-indications side effects etc.

means in a cool dark place. If no expiry date is shown, eye drops can usually be stored for about one year without the need for discarding. However, once a bottle has been opened, the drops become susceptible to contamination and oxidation from the air. The storage time for opened bottles of eye drops is therefore much less, and it is valuable to have a guide as to how long partly used bottles may be kept. The British Pharmaceutical Codex (1973) recommends that eye drops for domiciliary use may be used for about one month after opening, while those for use in hospital wards require not only a separate container for each patient but when both eyes are being treated a separate container for each eye. Further, these eye drops should be discarded not later than one week after opening. These recommendations do not apply to multiple-dose containers of fluorescein which should be discarded after having been used only once.

The single-dose form contains about 0.5 ml of the particular eye drop and no preservatives, bactericidal or fungicidal agents are incorporated into these preparations. Hence, these preparations must only be used for one patient and must not be stored after use. Irrespective of container form or time, any eye drops which become discoloured or cloudy should not be used.

When using the orthodox method of instilling drops into the conjunctival sac, great care must be taken not to contaminate the end of the dropper tube by touching the lids or lashes. If this does accidentally occur, then the dropper must either be re-sterilized or discarded and replaced. This is an obvious disadvantage of the plastic-type multidose container, which has its dropper permanently fixed and cannot be satisfactorily sterilized if contaminated. The method using a glass rod for instillation is particularly suitable for use with fluorescein solution. The glass rod should only be used for one patient, then re-sterilized before subsequent use. Care must be taken not to damage the bulbous instilling end of the glass rod by careless handling.

Eye ointments are also frequently used, and the danger of contamination is just as great as with the use of eye drops — particularly since no preservatives can be incorporated in these ointments. The 1973 British Pharmaceutical Codex recommends that every care should be taken to keep eye ointment in a sterile state. Whenever possible, single-dose containers

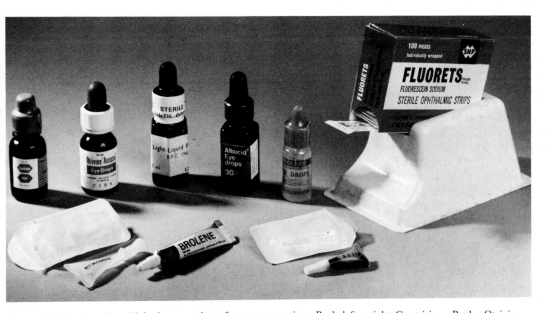

Figure 4.13 Single- and multiple-dose containers for eye preparations. Back, left to right: Gantrisin — Roche; Otrivine, Antistin — Ciba; Light Liquid Paraffin BPC; Albucid — British Schering; Brolene — May & Baker; Fluorets — Smith & Nephew Pharmaceuticals. Front, left to right: Proparacaine Uni-Min — Pilkington Barnes–Hind; Brolene ointment — May & Baker; Rose Bengal Minim — Smith & Nephew Pharmaceuticals

should be used and the ointment can be administered either direct from the tube into the lower conjunctival sac (providing it is being used for only one patient) or by the glass rod method.

Hydrophilic lenses should be removed before any ophthalmic drugs are administered, as some therapeutic agents and preservatives can be concentrated in these lenses. This is particularly necessary with multiple-dose eye drops containing preservatives which, when released from the lens, can have an irritant effect on the eye.

The following topical ophthalmic preparations are the ones most commonly used in contact lens practice: topical anaesthetics, conjunctival decongestants, diagnostic staining agents, and chemotherapeutic agents.

Topical anaesthetics

Topical anaesthetics are used in contact lens practice to produce surface anaesthesia of the cornea and conjunctiva by reducing the sensitivity of their sensory nerve endings. Their action, which is reversible, prevents the transmission of impulses along the nerve fibres.

The ideal requirements of a surface anaesthetic are:

(1) Rapidity of action.
(2) Adequate depth of anaesthesia.
(3) Short duration.
(4) Non-toxic.
(5) Non-irritant.
(6) No subsidiary actions such as cycloplegia, mydriasis or vasoconstriction.
(7) Stability.

The depth and duration of anaesthesia depends on the strength of the drug used and the number of drops instilled at regular intervals. For this reason, onset and duration times of anaesthesia can sometimes be misleading.

All the topical anaesthetics have some effect on the corneal metabolism and increase its permeability to other drugs. Hence, 0.1% adrenaline instilled into the eye normally causes no mydriatic effect, while if instilled after a topical anaesthetic some dilatation of the pupil may occur. This should not be confused with the pupil dilatation which occurs following the instillation of 0.1% adrenaline in patients with hyper-excitability of the sympathetic system,

known as Loewi's adrenaline eye test used in the diagnosis of thyrotoxicosis. Another effect on the cornea which is frequently encountered is desquamation of the superficial epithelium, cocaine being one of the chief offenders. But all local anaesthetics have some deleterious effect on the corneal epithelium due to the insensibility produced.

The three most commonly used topical anaesthetics are amethocaine (tetracaine, pantocain, Pontocaine, Decicain), proxymetacaine (Ophthaine, Squibb Proparacaine, 'Uni-Mins', Pilkington Barnes–Hind), and oxybuprocaine hydrochloride (Benoxinate, Smith & Nephew Pharmaceuticals; dorsacaine, Novesine, Wander). All have the advantage of causing no subsidiary actions such as cycloplegia, mydriasis or vasoconstriction. Their legal category is indicated in Appendix F, *Table F.III.*

Amethocaine hydrochloride

Solutions of 0.5 or 1% cause some initial discomfort on instillation, due to a stinging sensation. Onset time of anaesthesia is 10–30 seconds and duration of anaesthesia is about 10 minutes. It has no subsidiary actions, and only very rarely does it cause any toxic effects.

Amethocaine is incompatible with alkalis, bromides, silver salts and oxidizing agents, and solutions should be protected from light.

Proxymetacaine hydrochloride

A 0.5% solution is a very satisfactory all-round anaesthetic, pleasant, non-irritant, safe, effective and free from subsidiary actions (Rycroft, 1964). With a single instillation, the onset of anaesthesia occurs in an average of 13 seconds and persists for an average of 15.2 minutes (Boozan and Cohen, 1953). Its initial discomfort is considerably less than with amethocaine, and allergic manifestations have occurred only rarely. In a clinical evaluation of cocaine, dorsacaine (Novesine), proxymetacaine (Proparacaine), Pontocaine and Butyn, Jervey (1955) found that proxymetacaine seemed to produce the least discomfort. It is recommended that proxymetacaine should be stored in a refrigerator after opening, to prevent discolouration. Once discoloured, it should be discarded.

Oxybuprocaine hydrochloride (Benoxinate)

Oxybuprocaine hydrochloride 0.4% is a synthetic *p*-aminobenzoic acid derivative incompatible with alkalis and silver salts. Onset time of anaesthesia is about 30 seconds and duration of anaesthesia about 10–15 minutes. Emmerich, Carter and Berens (1955) compared 0.4% oxybuprocaine with 0.5% Pontocaine and found that sensations of irritation were significantly less with oxybuprocaine, and that the microscopic changes in the epithelium of the cornea were significantly less after the application of oxybuprocaine.

Topical anaesthetics are used primarily in contact lens practice prior to taking eye impressions. For this purpose, usually two to three drops are instilled — the first into the lower conjunctival sac, and the subsequent drops onto the superior limbal region, so allowing the anaesthetic to run gently over the whole cornea. This ensures that the whole cornea is effectively anaesthetized. One drop can also be instilled in the other eye to inhibit the blink reflex. Regardless of the particular anaesthetic which is used, it is of the utmost importance to ensure that either the corneal sensitivity has returned or that the eye is adequately protected by an eyepad or shade before the patient leaves the practice. The possible hazard of a foreign body becoming embedded in an insensitive cornea must not be overlooked.

Following the instillation into the conjunctival sac of a local anaesthetic, lacrimation may be reduced and, to prevent corneal epithelial drying from occurring (which is liable to cause a rapid and severe drop in vision), patients should be encouraged to blink frequently until normal sensitivity returns (about 15–20 minutes). Alternatively, an artificial tears solution may be instilled. This keeps the cornea moist. Eye rubbing should be discouraged as the surface epithelial cells may be damaged or dislodged.

Conjunctival decongestants

These are drugs which may be used to prevent conjunctival injection during the impression process or during prolonged fitting procedures. The two preparations most frequently used are adrenaline (epinephrine) and naphazoline, the former being the more widely used. Both are sympathomimetics, acting as vasoconstrictors, producing only slight, if any, mydriatic effect, depending on the pigmentation of the iris, a dark iris being least affected.

More details are given in Appendix F, *Tables F.I* and *F.III* at the end of the book.

Adrenaline acid tartrate BP

This is the form generally used for preparing eye drops, although adrenaline hydrochloride is also sometimes used. Solutions are sterilized by autoclaving, with the addition of sodium metabisulphite. Adrenaline solutions must, however, be kept in well-secured amber-coloured bottles protected from the light and air. If the solution does become discoloured, it should be discarded. As a conjunctival decongestant, 0.1% adrenaline is used, one or two drops being instilled into the lower conjunctival sac, which has a time course of about 1 hour.

Adverse systemic effects from its topical administration are rare but include skin pallor, tremors, marked nervousness and increased respiratory and heart rate and blood pressure. Pupil dilatation may occur if instillation follows the use of a topical anaesthetic or, probably more likely, when there is damage to the corneal epithelium. A miotic should be used if there is considered to be any risk of precipitating an attack of acute narrow-angle glaucoma.

Naphazoline

This is available as the nitrate or hydrochloride, the nitrate being most frequently used as it is compatible with silver nitrate. It is a quick-acting, powerful and prolonged vasoconstrictor, used as a 1:1000 or 1:2000 aqueous solution, the latter strength usually being considered adequate. In action it is similar to adrenaline, but they are not chemically related. It has the advantage over adrenaline of being more stable to heat, light and air.

Adverse side effects are not common and it has no marked effect on pupil size, amplitude of accommodation or on the ocular tension. Hurwitz and Thompson (1950), using 0.1% naphazoline hydrochloride, found only a slight mydriatic effect, this occurring mainly in those subjects with lightly pigmented irides. They also found a negligible effect on accommodation.

One or two drops instilled into the lower conjunctival sac are adequate and it has a time course of about 4 hours. As with all vasoconstrictors, excessive use over long periods, particularly in chronic conditions, is not advised as the blood vessels gradually cease to react to it, and hyperaemia will persist.

A preparation which contains a vasoconstrictor (decongestant) and an antihistamine (anti-allergic) is suitable for contact lens practice, where in general the injection of the conjunctiva is due to a non-inflammatory cause. One such preparation (*see* Appendix F, *Table F.III*) contains 0.05% w/v xylometazoline hydrochloride (vasoconstrictor) and 0.5% w/v antazoline sulphate (antihistamine). Following instillation the effects last about 8 hours.

In addition to the preparations already mentioned there are a number of proprietary brands of decongestant solutions containing phenylephrine hydrochloride, 0.12–0.25%, which have a time course of about 4 hours. These solutions (*see* Appendix F, *Table F.I* at the end of the book) are not listed in the Poisons Rules and are therefore freely available to the general public.

The advisability of their indiscriminate use must be questioned, particularly with the inherent, if rare, danger of precipitating an attack of closed-angle glaucoma in a susceptible subject. Also, if a patient has an injected eye from wearing a contact lens, it is preferable that he seeks the advice of his practitioner so that the cause can be remedied. To instil a decongestant agent only masks the primary cause of the injection. These preparations can also cause discolouration of a hydrophilic lens if instilled into the eye with such a lens *in situ*.

Diagnostic staining agents

Fluorescein

Fluorescein stains damaged living tissue of the cornea and conjunctiva green and yellow, respectively. It is used as a means of checking the contact lens fit and for detecting corneal abrasions (*see Plates 10–20*). It may also be used to demonstrate patency of the lacrimal drainage channels into the nose, which is essential if contact lenses are to be fitted. A few minutes after instillation of fluorescein into the conjunc-

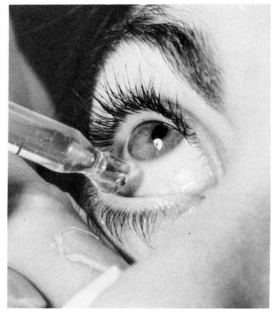

Figure 4.14 One drop of physiological saline is instilled into the conjunctival sac prior to examination. Care is taken not to touch the globe, lids or lashes with the dropper tip

tival sac of one eye only, the nose should be blown into a paper tissue which should show green staining under ultraviolet light. The other side may then be checked.

The official salt is fluorescein sodium BP either as a 1 or 2% solution, or as fluorescein-impregnated paper strips. It is essential that all solutions (other than single-dose units) are adequately protected with a bactericidal agent as *Ps. aeruginosa* can readily thrive in fluorescein (Chatoo, 1963; Doris, 1964). The impregnated strips have the advantage that they can be stored for an indefinite period without fear of deterioration or contamination, provided that they are kept dry. Paper strips also deliver in smaller amounts than from drops.

There is nothing more unsightly than the excess stain sometimes seen surrounding the eyes and/or the faces of patients after its use. Following the instillation of fluorescein for detection of abrasions, it is usually advisable to instil a drop of physiological saline solution to wash away any excess fluorescein from the normal tear film (*Figure 4.14*), which might otherwise mask any damaged areas. Such areas, if present, may then be observed with ultraviolet light, an ordinary corneal loupe, or a slit lamp biomicroscope.

Fluorescein sodium (molecular weight 376) has been used routinely for many years in contact lens practice for evaluating the fit of a hard contact lens. However, it is unsuitable for evaluating the fit of a hydrophilic lens because of its absorption and binding to the lens. If fluorescein has been instilled into the eye there should be a delay of at least 1 hour (and preferably 2) before a hydrophilic lens is inserted or the eye thoroughly irrigated before re-insertion).

A fluorescent water-soluble dye, Fluorexon, has been described by Refojo, Miller and Fiore (1972) and Refojo, Korb and Silverman (1972). It is a derivative of fluorescein but has a molecular weight of 710 and is absorbed much more slowly than fluorescein. The stain is reversible and washes out of the lens by boiling it in a saline solution. Fluorexon can be used as a 0.5% solution and stains damaged epithelium of the cornea and conjunctiva, but the fluorescence is not as effective as fluorescein. Also, solutions of Fluorexon are just as vulnerable to contamination as fluorescein (Refojo, Korb and Silverman, 1972) hence, single-dose eye drops are advocated.

Rose bengal

This is a fat-soluble stain and is used as a 1% solution to determine the presence of dried areas of corneal and conjunctival epithelium, prior to contact lens fitting, as well as the influence of facial skin conditions on contact lens tolerance. Its action differs from fluorescein in staining dead or desquamated tissue red when viewed under white light (see Plate 9), the presence of excess desquamation being an indication of an abnormal ocular condition or skin disease, either clinical or subclinical. It is, unfortunately very irritating to the eye.

The conjunctiva and skin are of the same origin; and if the palpebral or bulbar conjunctiva stain red, it is advisable to reject the patient for contact lenses until medical advice on the ocular or facial skin condition has been obtained. Otherwise, the wearing of contact lenses may only aggravate matters. Conditions in which positive staining occur are: keratoconjunctivitis sicca (Sjögren's syndrome), seborrhoeic eczema, acne vulgaris and acne rosacea.

A mixed stain of 1% fluorescein and 1% rose bengal has been suggested by Norn (1964) as serving a useful dual purpose in determining both epithelial lesions and degenerate epithelial cells. As mucus is also stained red by rose bengal, it can be differentiated if necessary by instilling one drop of 1% alcian blue (Norn, 1964) which stains the mucus blue. Rose bengal strips are available in some but not all countries.

Chemotherapeutic agents

The most effective of the chemotherapeutic agents are the broad spectrum antibiotics which with one exception (framycetin), however, are not available to the optometrist in the UK. As the use of a topical chemotherapeutic agent is purely prophylactic in contact lens practice, there are a number of preparations which meet this requirement. They are mainly preparations which belong to the sulphonamide group of drugs and, as a few patients are allergic to sulphonamides, it is advisable to exclude this possibility by questioning the patient before their use. Their legal categories are indicated in Appendix F, *Table F.III*.

Framycetin sulphate

Framycetin is available as 0.5% drops or ointment. It is active against many strains of Gram-positive and Gram-negative bacteria, for example *Staph. aureus*, *E. coli*, and some strains of *Ps. aeruginosa* and *Proteus vulgaris*. It is not inactivated by pus or bacteria. Resistant strains can develop with indiscriminate use. Framycetin is very similar in properties to neomycin.

Mafenide propionate

This is available in 5% solution only, the recommendation for its use being 3 or 4 drops, 3–4 times daily. It is relatively insoluble but has the general properties of sulphonamides and has the same spectrum of action.

Sulphacetamide sodium

This is the sulphonamide most frequently used in ophthalmic practice. It is available as 10, 15, 20 or 30% eye drops, or as a 2.5, 6 or 10% eye ointment. The eye drops must be protected from light, otherwise they deteriorate and show signs of precipitation.

Sulphacetamide sodium and zinc sulphate

This contains 5% sulphacetamide and 0.10% zinc sulphate in an aqueous solution. Its antibacterial activity is considered equal to that of a 30% solution of sulphacetamide sodium.

The range of activity of these chemotherapeutic agents is confined to the sulphonamide-sensitive organisms, which include many of the Gram-positive and some of the Gram-negative organisms.

Propamidine isethionate

This is another useful chemotherapeutic agent; it is available as an eye ointment containing 0.15% dibromopropamidine isethionate, or as eye drops containing 0.1% propamidine isethionate. The range of activity is against pyogenic cocci and some Gram-negative organisms, *E. coli* and *Pr. vulgaris*; some activity is also shown *in vitro* against *Ps. aeruginosa*. It is also liable to cause an allergic reaction in a few patients.

Care must be taken not to fall into a false sense of security in thinking that a single application of any one of these agents necessarily prevents an infection of the eye becoming established. Only repeated applications may be able to resolve an infection, then it becomes a therapeutic rather than a prophylactic measure (the former being the responsibility of a medical practitioner).

Miscellaneous agents

Hypertonic saline solution

This is useful for the relief of corneal oedema. Its continued use for therapeutic purposes to relieve corneal oedema during extended soft lens wear, necessary for some pathological ocular conditions, should be carried out under medical supervision (*see* Chapter 21).

UK statutes and regulations

The Medicines Act was enacted in the UK in 1968 but the orders relating to the sale and supply of drugs were not made until 1978. The appointed day was 1st February 1978, but because of the impact of the legislation a deferment of some of its effects was made until 1st August of the same year.

The Medicines Act covers all aspects of the manufacture, testing and sale of medicinal agents and it is proposed to concentrate here on Part III which specifically deals with the sale and supply of medicinal substances.

The effect of this part of the Act is to divide products into three groups. There is a provision for setting up a General Sales List, which contains all those drugs and agents which it is thought can be safely sold to the general public without the supervision of a pharmacist. The General Sales List was published in 1978 and contains some of the pharmaceutical agents used by optometrists, for example, hypromellose. However, in Schedule 6 of the order there is a specific exclusion from the General Sales List of all eye drops and eye ointments.

The other list of drugs is the Prescription Only Medicines (POM) List which contains those drugs, only obtainable on the prescription of a doctor, dentist or veterinary surgeon. As with all of this type of legislation there are exemptions and special cases. However, again, eye drops are singled out as requiring special control. For example, amethocaine hydrochloride is POM only when injected or applied to the eye.

Substances which appear on neither list are referred to as pharmacy medicines and although available for sale to anyone can only be sold under the supervision of a pharmacist. Thus, if an eye drop is not on the POM list it is automatically a pharmacy medicine (designated as P).

The lists published in 1978 make specific provision for the use of drugs by the optometrist. In the POM list there is a provision for the registered optometrist to obtain and supply certain drugs. (The original list as published has been modified by further statutory controls and some agents have been deleted and some added.) The agents listed include mydriatic/cycloplegics, miotics and sulphonamides. There is a separate order allowing the optometrist to obtain but not supply local anaesthetics and oxyphenbutazone ointments. Appendix F, *Tables F.I–F.III* at the end of this volume, give details of the drugs and eye drops used in association with contact lens fitting and wearing.

Contact lens solutions and contact lenses were brought under the Medicines Act by an order made in 1976. However, this particular order was mainly concerned with the manufacture and labelling and made no provision for subjecting them to control of sale.

In 1980, several important rules were applied to contact lens solutions which can be summarized as follows. With effect from January 1st 1980 no new solution, not previously on the market, could be sold without a product licence. Existing solutions were given a transitional exemption.

Full product licences were issued for most products on 1st July 1983. As a result of the licencing procedure, sales were restricted to registered optometrists, dispensing opticians and registered pharmacies.

The product licence ensures that products are fully tested for safety (but *not* efficacy) and approved by the DHSS prior to general release.

Acknowledgements

The authors wish to express their sincere thanks to the many laboratories and individuals who contributed information for use in this chapter.

References

ALLANSMITH, M. R., KORB, D. R., GREINER, J. K., HENRIQUEZ, A. S., SIMON, M. A. and FINNEMORE, V. M. (1977). Giant papillary conjunctivitis in contact lens wearers. *Am. J. Ophthal.* **83**, 697–708

ANDERSON, K. and KEYNES, R. (1958). Infected cork closures and apparent survival of organisms in antiseptic solutions. *Br. med. J.* **2**, 274–275

ANON (1980). Bacterial resistance to trimethoprim. *Br. med. J.* **6240**, 571–572

ANON (1982). *Martindale — The Extra Pharmacopoeia*, 27th edn. p. 1485. London: Pharmaceutical Press

ANON (1984). LensoClean ultrasonic contact lens cleaning system. *Contact Lens Forum* **8**(6), 83

ANON (1985). Contact lens commentary. *Optom. Today* **25**(24), 814

ANON (1986). Microwaving — the disinfection system of the future? *Int. Eyecare* **2**(4), 200

ANON (1987). *Fluor-o-stat and Fluor-o-wet.* Leaflet produced by Luxocon Products Inc. 2pp.

AUCAMP, A. (1980). Drug excretion in human tears and its meaning for contact lens wearers. *S. Afr. Optom.* **39**, 128–136

BAKER, S. R. and REMINGTON, J. S. (1972). Contamination of soft gel lenses. *Contacto* **16**(3), 4–6

BANES, S. (1985). Adverse ocular drug reactions. *Optom. Today* **25**(17), 557–559

BARKMAR, R., GERMANIS, M., KARPE, G. and MALMBORG, A. S. (1969). Preservatives in eye drops. *Acta ophthal.* **47**, 461–475

BARNARD, N. A. S. (1984). Discolouration of soft contact lenses as a side-effect of systemic drugs. *Ophthal. Optician* **24**(22), 802

BENJAMIN, W. J. and SIMONS, M. H. (1984). Contact angle update. Care regimens and their effect on a rigid silicone-acrylate surface. *Int. Contact Lens Clin.* **11**(8), 500–506

BERGMANSON, J. P. and RIOS, R. (1981). Adverse reaction to painkiller in hydrogel lens wearer. *J. Am. optom. Ass.* **52**(3), 257–258

BERNSTEIN, H. N., STOW, M. N. and MADDOX, Y. (1973). Evaluation of the asepticization procedure for Soflens hydrophilic contact lens. *Can. J. Ophthal.* **8**, 575

BERNSTEIN, D. I., GALLAGHER, J. S., GRAD, M. and BERNSTEIN, I. L. (1984). Local ocular anaphylaxis to papain enzyme contained in a contact lens cleansing solution. *J. Allergy Clin. Immunol.* **72**, 258–260

BLANCO, M., CURRY, B. and BOGHOSIAN, M. P. (1975). Studies of the effect of enzymatic cleaning on the physical structure of hydrophilic lenses. *Contacto* **19**(5), 17–20

BOOZAN, W. C. and COHEN, I. J. (1953). A new topical anaesthetic for the eye. *Am. J. Ophthal.* **36**, 1619–1621

BRAWNER, L. and JESSOP, D. G. (1962). A review of contact lens solutions. *Contacto* **6**, 49–51

BREWITT, H. and CONRADS, S. (1986). Experiences with the new contact lens disinfecting and cleaning compound dichloroisocyanurate sodium. *Z. prakt. Augenheilkd.* **7**, 67–70

BREZINSKI, S. D., CARNEY, L. G. and HILL, R. M. (1986). 'Salt balance' questions in contact lens solutions. *Contact Lens Spectrum* August, 29–32

BROWN, M. R. W. (1968). Survival of *Pseudomonas aeruginosa* in fluorescein solution. Preservative action of PMN and EDTA. *J. Pharm. Sci.* **57**, 389–392

BROWN, M. R. W. and RICHARDS, R. M. E. (1965). Effect of ethylenediaminetetra-acetate on the resistance of *Pseudomonas aeruginosa* to antibacterial agents. *Nature* **207**, 1391

BROWN, S. I., BLOOMFIELD, S., PEARCE, D. B. and TRAGAKIS, M. (1974). Infections with the therapeutic soft lens. *Archs Ophthal.* **91**, 275–277

BROWNE, R. K., ANDERSON, A. N. and CHARVEZ, B. W. (1974). Solving the solution problem. *Optician* **167**(4325), 19–24

BUSSCHAERT, S. C., SZABOCIK, J. M., GOOD, R. C. and WOODWARD, M. R. (1974). Challenging the efficacy of the Soflens Aseptor. *J. Am. optom. Ass.* **45**, 700–703

CAFFERTY, B. E. and JOSEPHSON, J. E. (1988). Ocular side effects of isotretinoin therapy. *J. Am. optom. Ass.,* **59**, 221–224

CALLENDAR, M. G., TSE, L. S., CHARLES, A. M. and LUTZI, D. (1986). Bacterial flora of the eye and contact lens cases during hydrogel lens wear. *Am. J. Optom.* **63**(3), 177–180

CARNEY, L. G. and HILL, R. M. (1975). pH profiles: part 1 — one pH, or many? *J. Am. optom. Ass.* **46**, 1143–1145

CHARLES, A. M. (1975). A comparison of some commercial methods for asepticizing and cleansing hydrogel lenses. *Contacto* **19**(3), 4–11

CHATOO, B. A. (1963). Fluorescein in ophthalmic practice. *Ophthal. Optician* **3**, 723–735

CROOK, T. G. and FREEMAN, J. J. (1983). Reactions induced by the concurrent use of thimerosal and tetracycline. *Am. J. Optom. physiol. Optics* **60**(9), 759–761

CURETON, G. L. and HALL, N. C. (1974). The separate functions of cleaning and sterilising soft contact lenses. *Am. J. Optom.* **51**, 406–411

CURETON, G. L. and SIBLEY, M. J. (1974). Soft contact lens solutions, past, present and future. *J. Am. optom. Ass.* **45**, 285–291

DABEZIES, O. H. (1970). Contact lens hygiene, past, present and future. *Contact Lens med. Bull.* **3**(2), 3–15

DALLOS, J. and HUGHES, W. H. (1972). Sterilisation of hydrophilic contact lenses. *Br. J. Ophthal.* **56**, 114–119

DAVIES, D. J. G . and NORTON, D. A. (1975). Challenge tests for antimicrobial agents. *J. Pharm. Pharmac.* **27**, 383–384

DAVIS, H., CHARLES, A. M., TRAGER, S. and PHARES, R. E. (1973). The soft lens situation: solutions, sterilization and contamination. *Contacto* **17**(4), 8–32

DE VRIES, K. (1985). Contact lenses and the pill. *Contact Lens Forum* **1**(6), 21–23

DORIS, J. A. (1964). Maintenance of sterility of eyedrops in opthalmic practice. *Ophthal. Optician* **4**, 12–14, 19

DUKE-ELDER, S. (1965). *System of Ophthalmology. Vol. VIII.* pp. 141–143. *Diseases of the Outer Eye, Part 1 — Diseases of the Conjunctiva and Associated Diseases of the Corneal Epithelium.* London: Kimpton

EMMERICH, R., CARTER, G. Z. and BERENS, C. (1955). An experimental clinical evaluation of Dorsacaine hydrochloride (Benoxinate, Novesine). *Am. J. Ophthal.* **40**, 841–848

EPSTEIN, R. J., WILSON, L. A., VISVESVARA, G. S. and PLOURDE, E. G. (1986). Rapid diagnosis of Acanthamoeba keratitis from corneal scrapings using indirect fluorescent antibody staining. *Archs Ophthal.* **104**, 1318–1321

ERIKSON, S. (1985). Cited by N. Bailey (1985) in *Contact Lens Forum* **10**(5), 11

FARRELL, H. (1976). Some effects of oral contraceptive steroids on the eye related to contact lens wear. *Optician* **171**(4423), 8–9, 13

FELDMAN, G. L. (1971). Sterility with soft lens solutions. Lecture presented to the Canadian Guild of Dispensing Opticians, October 23rd, Toronto, Ontario

FELDMAN, G. (1985). The trimethoprim solution. *Contact Lens Forum* **10**(7), 40–41

FICHMAN, S., BAKER, V. V. and HORTON, H. (1978). Iatrogenic red eyes in soft contact lens wearers. *Int. Contact Lens Clin.* **5**, 202–206

FILPPI, J. A., PFISTER, R. M. and HILL, R. M. (1973). Penetration of hydrophilic contact lenses by *Aspergillus fumagatus. Am. J. Optom.* **50**, 553–557

GANJU, S. N. (1974). The disinfection of hard and soft contact lenses. *Ophthal. Optician* **14**, 1202–1208

GANJU, S. N. (1977). Deposits on and discolouration of soft contact lenses. In-house paper prepared for Sauflon Pharmaceuticals

GANJU, S. N. and CORDREY, P. (1975). The physical contamination of hydrophilic contact lenses and their restoration. *Optician* **170**(4398), 19–25

GANJU, S. N. and THOMPSON, R. E. M. (1975). A new cold sterilising system for soft contact lenses. *Contacto* **19**(1), 19–23

GASSET, A. R., ISHIR, Y., KAUFMAN, H. E. and MILLER, T. (1974). Cytotoxicity of ophthalmic preservatives. *Am. J. Ophthal.* **78**, 98–105

GASSET, A. R., RAMER, R. M. and KATZIN, D. (1975). Hydrogen peroxide sterilisation of hydrophilic contact lenses. *Archs Ophthal.* **93**, 412–415

GASSON, A. P. (1975). Visual consideration with hydrophilic lenses. *Ophthal. Optician* **15**, 439–448

GOULD, H. L. and INGLIMA, R. (1964). Corneal contact lens solutions. *Eye Ear Nose Throat Mon.* **43**, 39–49

GRECO, A. (1984). A review and update of contact lens care systems. *Int. Contact Lens Clin.* **11**(5), 266–272

GREEN, K., LIVINGSTON, V., BOWMAN, K. and HULL, D. S. (1980). Chlorhexidine effects on corneal epithelium and endothelium. *Archs Ophthal.* **98**, 1273–1278

GROSVENOR, T., CHARLES, A. and CALLENDER, M. (1972). Soft contact lens bacteriological study. *Ophthal. Optician* **12**, 1083–1091; *Can. J. Optom.* **34**, 11–18

GYULAI, P., DZIABO, A., KELLY, W. and KIRAL, R. (1986). Efficacy of catalase as a neutraliser of a hydrogen peroxide disinfecting solution for soft contact lenses. *Int. Contact Lens Clin.* **2**(8), 418–422

HAMPSON, R. M. (1973). Considerations in the checking and predictability of hydrophilic lenses. *Optician* **165**(4328), 4–16

HART, D. (1986). Diet and lipid deposits. *Int. Eyecare* **2**(1), 30

HERSKOWITZ, R. (1987). Solution interaction and gas permeable lens performance. *Contact Lens J.* **15**, 3–8

HICKS, J. (1985). Unusual contact lens stains. *Contemporary Optom.* **4**(3), 13

HILL, R. M. and TERRY, J. E. (1974). Ophthalmic solutions: viscosity builders. *Am. J. Optom.* **51**, 847–851

HILL, R. M. and TERRY, J. E. (1976). Human tear cholesterol levels. *Archs Ophtal. (Paris)* **36**, 155–160

HIND, H. W. (1975). Various aspects of contact lens solutions for hard and soft lenses. *Optician* **169**(4380), 13–29

HIND, H. W. and GOYAN, F. M. (1947). A new concept of the role of hydrogen ion concentration and buffer systems in the preparation of ophthalmic solutions. *J. Am. pharm. Ass.* **36**, 33

HOFFMAN, W. C. (1987). Ending the BAK-RGP controversy. *Int. Contact Lens Clin.* **14**(1), 31–35

HOLDEN, B. A. and MARKIDES, A. J. (1971). On the desirability and efficacy of chemical sterilisation of hydrophilic contact lenses. *Aust. J. Optom.* **54**, 325–336

HOPKINS, G. (1985). Systemic drugs and their ocular side-effects. *Optician* **189**(4996), 33–42

HOVDING, (1981). The conjunctival and contact lens bacterial flora during lens wear. *Acta ophthal.* **59**, 387–401

HUGO, W. B. and FOSTER, J. H. S. (1964). Growth of *Pseudomonas aeruginosa* in solutions of esters of *p*-hydroxybenzoic acid. *J. Pharm. Pharmac.* **16**, 209

HURWITZ, P. and THOMPSON, J. M. (1950). Uses of naphazoline (Privine) in ophthalmology. *Archs Ophthal.* **43**, 712–717

Hydron Lens Ltd (1972). *Hydron Soft Lens Technical Report*, p. 19. Hydron Lens Ltd, Harold Hill, Romford, England

IKEDA, T., YAMAGUCHI, H. and TAZUKE, S. (1984). New polymeric biocides: synthesis and antibacterial activities of polycations with biguanide groups. *Antimicrob. Agents Chemother.* **26**(2), 139–144

ISEN, A. A. (1972). The Griffin lens. *J. Am. optom. Ass.* **43**, 275–286

JACOBS (1986). Infection control guidelines for optometrists and contact lens practitioners. *Clin. exp. Optom.* **69**, 40–45

JENKINS, C. and PHILLIPS, A. J. (1986). How sterile is unpreserved saline? *Clin. exp. Optom.* **69**(4), 131–136

JERVEY, J. W. (1955). Topical anaesthetics for the eye. *Sth. med. J.* **48**, 770–774

JOHNSON, D. G. and LITTLEWOOD, T. (1975). A clinical study to determine patient acceptance and efficiency of a new regimen of soft lens care. Submitted to *Can. J. Ophthal.* Cited by Shiveley (1975a)

JOSEPHSON, J. E. and CAFFREY, B. (1986). Sorbic acid revisited. *J. Am. optom. Ass.* **57**(3), 188–189

JOSSE, E. (1984). Corneal abscesses from soft contact lenses. *Nursing Times Supplement*, 3–4

KANIG, S. P. and CONN, R. L. (1985). Kidney stones. *Postgrad. Manag.* **78**(6), 38–51

KANSKI, J. (1987). Ocular manifestations of AIDS. *Optician* **193**(5090), 24–25

KARAGEOZIAN, H. L. (1974). Use of the amino acid analyser to illustrate the efficacy of an enzyme preparation for cleaning hydrophilic lenses. *Contacto* **20**, 5–10

KARAGEOZIAN, H. L., WALDEN, F. A. and BOGHOSIAN, M. P. (1976). Evaluation of the cleaning activity of various commercial cleaning regimens using human worn hydrophilic lenses. *Int. Contact Lens Clin.* **3**(2), 78–86

KELSEY, J. C. and SYKES, G. (1969). A new test for the assessment of disinfectants with particular reference to their use in hospitals. *Pharm. J.* **202**, 607–609

KERR, C. (1985). In 'Contact Us'. *Optician* **189**(4980), 13

KERR, C. (1988). Decontaminating lenses. *Optician* **195**(5129), 29

KJELSSEN, T., KIRAL, R. and ERIKSON, S. P. (1984). Single enzyme versus multi-enzyme contact lens cleaning system. *Int. Contact Lens Clin.* **11**(11), 660–671

KLEIN, M., MILLWOOD, E. G. and WALTHER, W. W. (1954). On the maintenance of sterility in eye drops. *J. Pharm. Pharmac.* **6**, 725–732

KLEIST, F. D. (1979). Appearance and nature of hydrophilic contact lens deposits. Part 1. *Int. Contact Lens Clin.* **6**, 120–130

KNOCHEL, G. P. (1984). Diuretic-induced hypokalemia. *Am. J. Med.* **77**(5), 18–27

KNOLL, H. A. (1972). Microbiology and hydrophilic contact lenses. *Am. J. Optom.* **48**, 840

KNOPF, H. L. (1984). Reaction to hydrogen peroxide in a contact lens wearer. *Am. J. Ophthal.* **97**(6), 796

KOETTING, R. A. (1976). Tear film break-up time as a factor in hydrogel lens coating — a preliminary study. *Contacto* **20**(3), 20–23

KORB, D. R., GREINER, J. V., FINNEMORE, V. M. and ALLANSMITH, M. R. (1983). Treatment of contact lenses with papain. Increase in wearing time in keratoconic patients with papillary conjunctivitis. *Archs Ophthal.* **101**, 48–50

KREZANOSKI, J. Z. (1972a). Pharmaceutical aspects of cleaning and sterilizing flexible contact lenses. *Ophthal. Optician* **12**, 1035–1091

KREZANOSKI, J. Z. (1972b). The significance of cleaning hydrophilic contact lenses. *J. Am. optom. Ass.* **43**, 305–307

KREZANOSKI, J. Z. (1981). Topical medications. *Int. Ophthal. Clin.* **21**, 173–176

KRISHNA, N. and BROW, F. (1964). Polyvinyl alcohol as an ophthalmic vehicle. *Am. J. Ophthal.* **57**, 99–106

KRUPIN, T., CROSS, D. A. and BECKER, B. (1977). Decreased basal tear production associated with general anaesthesia. *Archs Ophthal.* **95**, 107–108

LARKE, J. R. (1974). Some bacteriological considerations of soft lens wear. *Br. J. physiol. Optics* **29**, 66–91

LARKE, J. R., SMITH, P. G., PEDLEY, D. G. and TIGHE, B. J. (1973). A semi-rigid contact lens. *Ophthal. Optician* **13**, 1065–1067

LEMP, M. (1978). Bandage lenses and the use of topical solutions containing preservatives. *Ann. Ophthal.* **10**(10), 1319–1321

LERMAN, S. and SAPP, G. (1971). The hydrophilic (Hydron) corneoscleral lens in the treatment of corneal disease. *Can. J. Ophthal.* **6**, 1–8

LEVINE, W. L., LITSKY, W. and LAMM, R. A. (1981). Disinfection of hydrophilic contact lenses with commercial preparations of 3% and 6% hydrogen peroxide. *Dev. Indust. Microbiol.* **22**, 813–819

LEVY, B. (1984). Calcium deposits on glyceryl methyl methacrylate and hydroxyethyl methacrylate contact lens. *Am. J. Optom. physiol. Optics.* **6**, 605–607

LINDEMAN-MEESTER, H. H. M. (1974). Fluids for soft contact lenses tested by the Kelsey-Sykes test and Maurer test. *Contact Lens* **4**(6), 27–29

LITVIN, M. W. (1977). The incidence of eye infections with contact lenses. *Optician* **174**(4496), 11–14

LIUBINAS, J., SWENSON, G. and CARNEY, L. G. (1987). Thermal disinfection of contact lenses. *Clin. exp. Optom.* **70**(1), 8–14

LOCATCHER-KHORAZO, D. and SEEGAL, B. (1972). *Microbiology of the Eye.* St Louis, Missouri: Mosby

LORAN, D. F. C. (1973). Surface corrosion of hydrogel contact lenses. *Contact Lens* **4**(4), 3–10

LORAN, D. F. C. (1974). Determination of hydrogel contact lens radii by projection. *Ophthal. Optician* **14**, 980–985

LOWBURY, E. J. L. (1958). Contamination of cetrimide and other fluids by *Ps. pyoceanea. Br. J. industr. Med.* **8**, 22

LUBERT, G. P. and CAPLAN, L. (1984). Comparing thermal and chemical disinfection systems for the Etafilcon A 58% water content contact lens. *Am. J. Optom.* **61**(11), 683–688

LUDWIG, I., MEISLER, D. and RUTHERFORD, I. (1986). Susceptibility of Acanthaemoeba to soft contact lens disinfection systems. *Invest. Ophthal. Vis. Sci.* **27**(4), 626–630

LYONS, R. W. (1979). Orange contact lenses from rifampin. *N. Engl. J. Med.* **300**, 372–373

McBRIDE, R. J. and MACKIE, M. E. L. (1974). Evaluation of the antibacterial activity of contact lens solutions. *J. Pharm. Pharmac.* **26**, 899–900

McCARTHY (1973). *Cosmet. Perfum.* May, 88, 43

McCLURE, D. A., OHOTA, S., ERIKSON, S. P. and RANDERI, K. J. (1977) The effect on measured visual acuity of protein deposition and removal in soft contact lenses. *Contacto* **21**(2), 8–12

MacGREGOR, D. R. and ELLIKER, P. R. (1958). A comparison of some properties of strains of *Pseudomonas aeruginosa* sensitive and resistant to quaternary ammonium compounds. *Can. J. Microbiol.* **4**, 499–503

McMONNIES, C. M. (1978). Allergic complications in contact lens wear. *Int. Contact Lens Clin.* **15**, 182–189

MANDELL, R. B. (1974). *Contact Lens Practice, Hard and Flexible Lenses.* p. 819. Springfield, Ill: Thomas

MATAS, B. R., SPENCER, W. H. and HAYES, T. L. (1972). Scanning electron microscopy of hydrophilic contact lenses. *Archs Ophthal.* **88**, 287–295

MAURER, I. C. (1969). A test for stability and long term effectiveness in disinfectants. *Pharm. J.* **203**, 529–534

MEAKIN, B., WALTERS, K. A. and GEE, H. (1983). Interaction of benzalkonium chloride with Boston contact lens material. *Br. Contact Lens Ass.* **6**(2), 42–50

MILLER, D., BROOKS, S. M. and MOBILIA, E. (1976). Adrenochrome staining of soft contact lenses. *Ann. Ophthal.* **8**, 65–67

MONDINO, B. J. and GRODEN, L. R. (1980). Conjunctival hyperemia and corneal infiltrates with chemically disinfected soft contact lenses. *Archs Ophthal.* **98**, 1767–1770

MORGAN, J. F. (1979). Complications associated with contact lens solutions. *Am. J. Ophthal.* **86**, 1107–1119

MORRISON, R. J. (1966). Hydrophilic contact lenses. *J. Am. optom. Ass.* **37**, 211–218

MORRISON, R. J., TRESSER, A., VIGODSKY, H. S. and POLLAN, S. (1973). The effectivity of hygiene procedures upon soft contact lens material. *Contacto* **17**(1), 23–27

MORTON, D. J. (1985). EDTA reduces antimicrobial efficacy of thimerosal. *Int. J. Pharm.*, **23**, 357–358

MOTE, E. M., FILPPI, J. A. and HILL, R. M. (1972). Does heating arrest organisms in hydrophilic cases? *J. Am. optom. Ass.* **43**, 302–304

NORN, M. S. (1964). Vital staining in practice using a mixed stain and alcian blue. *Br. J. physiol. Optics* **21**, 293–298

NORTON, D. A., DAVIES, D. J. G., RICHARDSON, N. E., MEAKIN, B. J. and KEALL, A. (1974). The antimicrobial efficiencies of contact lens solutions. *J. Pharm. Pharmac.* **26**, 841–846. Also reproduced in *Optician* **168**(4360), 14–16

NORWOOD, C. (1983). Paper read to the Fifth Australian International Contact Lens Congress, Surfers Paradise, Queensland, Australia

OTTEN, M. and SZABOCSIK, J. M. (1976). Measurement of preservative binding with Soflens (polymacon) contact lens. *Aust. J. Optom.* **59**, 277–283

PARKER, J. H. (1983). The influence of material structure on contact lens cleaning. *Contact Lens Forum* **8**(6), 27–44

PENLEY, C. A., LLABRES, C., WILSON, L. A. and AHEARN, D. G. (1985). Efficacy of hydrogen peroxide disinfection systems for soft contact lenses contaminated with fungi. *Contact Lens Ass. Ophthal. J.* **11**(1), 65–68

PETTRICCIANI, R. and KRESZANOSKI, J. (1977). Preservative interaction with contact lenses. *Contacto* **21**(3), 6–10

PHARES, R. E. (1972a). Soft lens care. *J. Am. optom. Ass.* **43**, 308–313

PHARES, R. E. (1972b). Microbiology and hygienic care of hydrophilic lenses. *Contacto* **16**(3), 10–12

PHILLIPS, A. J. (1969). Contact lens plastics, solutions and storage — some implications. *Ophthal. Optician* **9**, 75–79

PHILLIPS, A. J. (1980). The cleaning of hydrogel contact lenses. *Ophthal. Optician* **20**(11), 375–388

PHILLIPS, A. J. and CZIGLER, B. (1985). Polyclens (Opti-Clean) — a further study. *J. Aust. Optom.* **68**(1), 36–39

POSTER, M. G. (1972). A preliminary study of the service life of the 'Soflens'. *Am. J. Optom.* **49**, 868–870

QUINN, L. H. and BURNSIDE, R. M. (1951). Gantrisin in the treatment of conjunctivitis. *Eye Ear Nose Throat Mon.* **30**, 81–82

RÈETSCHEL, R. L. and WILSON, L. A. (1982). Ocular inflammation in patients using soft contact lenses. *Archs Dermatol.* **118**, 147–149

REFOJO, M. F., KORB, D. R. and SILVERMAN, H. I. (1972). Clinical evaluation of a new fluorescent dye for hydrogel lenses. *J. Am. optom. Ass.* **43**, 321–326

REFOJO, M. F., MILLER, D. and FIORE, N. S. (1972). A new fluorescent stain for soft hydrophilic lens fitting. *Archs Ophthal.* **87**, 275–277

REFOJO, M. F. and HOLLY, F. J. (1977). Tear protein adsorption on hydrogels: a possible cause of contact lens allergy. *Contact Lens J.* **3**(1), 23–25

RICHARDS, R. M. E. and McBRIDE, R. J. (1972). The preservation of ophthalmic solutions with antibacterial combinations. *J. Pharm. Pharmac.* **24**, 145–148

RICHARDS, R. M. E. and REARY, J. M. E. (1972). Changes in antibacterial activity of thiomersal and P.M.N. on autoclaving with certain adjuvants. *J. Pharm. Pharmac.* **24** (Suppl.), 84–89

RICHARDSON, N. E., GEE, H. J. and MEAKIN, B. J. (1980). The compatibility of benzalkonium chloride with a CAB lens material. *J. Br. Contact Lens Ass.*, **3,** 120–124

RIEGELMAN, S., VAUGHAN, D. G. and OKUMOTO, M. (1956). Antibacterial agents in *Pseudomonas aeruginosa* contaminated ophthalmic solutions. *J. Am. pharm. Ass. (Sc.Ed.)* **45**, 93–98

RILEY, S. A., FLEGG, P. J. and MANDAL, B. K. (1985). Contact lens staining due to Sulphasalazine. *Lancet* **i**, 972

ROHRER, M. D., TERRY, M. A., BULARD, R. A., GRAVES, D. C. and TAYLOR, E. M. (1986). Microwave sterilization of hydrophilic contact lenses. *Am. J. Ophthal.* **101**, 49–57

ROSENTHAL, P., CHOU, M. H., SALAMONE, J. C. and ISRAEL, S. C. (1986). Quantitative analysis of chlorhexidine gluconate and benzalkonium chloride adsorption on silicone/acrylate polymers. *Contact Lens Ass. Ophthal.* **12**(1), 43–50

ROTH, H. W. (1987). Aetiology and composition of extended wear lens deposits. *Contact Lens J.* **15**(3), 3

RUBEN, M. (1966). Preliminary observations of soft (hydrophilic) contact lenses. *Proc. R. Soc. Med.* **59**, 531–532

RUBEN, M. (1976). Biochemical aspects of soft lenses. *Contact Intraoc. Lens Med. J.* **2**(4), 39–51

RUBEN, M., TRIPATHI, R. C. and WINDER, A. F. (1975). Calcium deposition as a cause of spoilation of hydrophilic soft contact lenses. *Br. J. Ophthal.* **59**, 141–148

RYCROFT, P. V. (1964). Ophthaine (proparacaine hydrochloride) a local anaesthetic for ophthalmic surgery. *Br. J. Ophthal.* **48**, 102–104

SCHACHET, J. L. (1983). Alcon's enzyme cleaner: a clinical study. *Contact Lens Forum* **8**(6), 67–82

SCHUMB, W. C., SATTERFIELD, C. N. and WENTWORTH, R. L. (1955). *Hydrogen Peroxide.* Monograph Series, American Chemical Society, No.128

SHAW, E. I. (1980). Allergies induced by contact lens solutions. *Contact Lens* **6**, 273–277

SHIVELY, C. D. (1975a). *Accessory Solutions Utilized in Contact Lens Care and Practice.* Private monograph published by Alcon Universal Ltd, Forth Worth, Texas

SHIVELY, C. D. (1975b). Hydrophilic flexible lens cleaning and chemical disinfection systems. *Contacto* **19**(3), 33–37

SIBLEY, M. J. (1984). Contact lens solutions incompatibilities. *Contact Lens Forum* **9**(5), 67–71

SIBLEY, M. J. and CHU, V. (1984). Understanding sorbic acid-preserved contact lens solutions. *Int. Contact Lens Clin.* **11**(9), 531–542

SIBLEY, M. J. and YUNG, G. (1973). A technique for the determination of chemical binding to soft contact lenses. *Am. J. Optom.* **50**, 710–714

SLATTER, D. H. (1973). Keratoconjunctivitis sicca in the dog produced by oral phenazopyridine hydrochloride. *J. Small Anim. Pract.* **14**, 744

SMITH, C. H. (1954). Bacteriology of the healthy conjunctiva. *Br. J. Ophthal.* **38**, 719–726

SNYDER, A. C., HILL, R. M. and BAILEY, N. J. (1977). Home sterilization: fact or fiction? *Contact Lens Forum* February, 41–43

STONE, R. P., MOWREY-McKEE, M. and KREUTZER, P. (1984). Protein — a source of lens discolouration. *Contact Lens Forum* **13**(9), 33–41

STOREY, K. (1973). Question corner. *Ophthal. Optician* **13**, 1219

STRACHAN, J. P. (1971). Physiology, pharmacology and contact lenses. *Aust. J. Optom.* **54**(1), 3–14

SUGAR, J. (1974). Adenochrome pigmentation of hydrophilic lenses. *Archs Ophthal.* **91**, 11–12

SUSSMAN, J. D. and FRIEDMAN, M. (1969). Irritation of rabbit eyes caused by contact lens wetting solutions. *Am. J. Ophthal.* **68**, 703–706

SYKES, G. (1965). *Disinfection and Sterilization. Theory and Practice*, 2nd edn, p. 384. London: E. & F. N. Spon

TAKAHASHI (1982). Cytotoxicity of mercurial preservatives in cell culture. *Ophthal. Res.* **14**, 63–69

THOMPSON, R. E. M. and MANSELL, P. E. (1976). The cleansing and decontamination of hydrophilic contact lenses — an improved standard chemical method. *Optician* **171**(4419), 11–15

TOXICOL LABORATORIES LTD (1972). Hydrosoak and Hydrosol — a comprehensive study. p. 2. Independent study carried out for Messrs Contactosol Ltd, Esher, Surrey

TRAGAKIS, M. P., BROWN, S. I. and PEARCE, D. B. (1973). Bacteriological studies of contamination associated with soft contact lenses. *Am. J. Ophthal.* **75**, 496–499

TRIPATHI, R. C. and RUBEN, M. (1972). Degenerative changes in a soft hydrophilic contact lens. *Ophthal. Res.* **4**, 185–192

TSUDA, S., ANDO, N. and ANAN, N. (1977). Fitting and analysis of the Menicon soft lens. *Int. Contact Lens Clin.* **4**(5), 24–31

UNITED STATES FOOD AND DRUGS ADMINISTRATION (1973). *Microbiological Guidelines for New Contact Lenses.* May, 1973

VITA, C., DALZOPPO, D. and FONTANA, A. (1985). Limited proteolysis of thermolysin by Subtilisin: isolation and characterisation of a partially active enzyme derivative. *Biochemistry* **24**, 1798–1806

WEISSMAN, B. A., MONDINO, B. J., PETTIT, T. H. and HOFBAUER, J. D. (1984). Corneal ulcers associated with extended-wear soft contact lenses. *Am. J. Ophthal.* **97**, 476–481

WILSON, L. A., McNATT, J. and REISTSCHEL, R. (1981). Delayed hypersensitivity to thimerosal in soft contact lens wearers. *Ophthalmology* **88**, 804–809

WILSON, W. S., DUNCAN, A. J. and JAY, J. L. (1975). Effect of benzalkonium chloride on the stability of the precorneal tear film in rabbit and man. *Br. J. Ophthal.* **59**, 667–669

WILSON, L. A., KUEHNE, J. W., HALL, S. W. and AHEARN, D. G. (1971). Microbial contamination in ocular cosmetics. *Am. J. Ophthal.* **71**, 1298–1302

WINDER, A. F., ASTBURY, N. J., SHERAIDAH, G. A. K. and RUBEN, M. (1980). Penetration of mercury from ophthalmic preservatives into the human eye. *Lancet* **ii**, 237–239

WONG, M. P., DZIABO, A. J. and KIRAL, R. M. (1986). Adsorption of benzalkonium chloride by RGP lenses. *Contact Lens Forum* **11**(5), 25–32

WRIGHT, P. and MACKIE, I. (1982). Preservative-related problems in soft contact lens wearer. *Trans Ophthal. Soc. UK* **102**, 3–6

YOUNG, G. (1985). Predicting soft lens solution hypersensitivity. *J. Br. Contact Lens Ass.* **7**(3), 126–129

Chapter 5

Practical optics and computer design of contact lenses

W. A. Douthwaite, M. W. Ford, J. L. Francis and Janet Stone

This chapter was enlarged in the second edition of the book to include several features which had been requested by interested readers. These included aspects of soft contact lenses and worked numerical examples to illustrate suitable methods of calculation. The work of Francis (1968) was also included, both in the chapter and in Appendices A–D at the end of the book. Examination questions (with answers) from past visual optics papers were also added for the benefit of examination candidates, and a section on contact lens design was incorporated illustrating both the mathematical approach using sagitta values and the method of drawing to scale to determine lens radii and other parameters.

Because these topics have an underlying mathematical basis, they are amenable to treatment by computer and it is appropriate that in this third edition of *Contact Lenses* there should be a section on the use of computers to assist resolution of problems in both optics of contact lenses and in their design. This section, which now forms Appendix E at the end of the book, is briefly mentioned towards the end of the chapter and has been written by two new and welcome contributors, Morley Ford and Bill Douthwaite. It consists of a series of interconnected computer programs with explanation and illustration of their use, enabling certain aspects of contact lens optics and design to be studied and numerical results quickly achieved. Because of the close relationship between the design and fitting of a contact lens and its optical effect on the eye, those readers with access to personal computers should study Appendix E in conjunction with this chapter and Chapters 10, 11 and 14. Elsewhere in the book reference to

Appendix E is given where appropriate.

There are two main aspects to be considered when dealing with the optics of contact lenses — the effects on the wearer of the optical differences from spectacles, and the necessity for the practitioner to understand the components which affect the back vertex power of the contact-lens/liquid-lens system. There is some overlap of these two aspects, but for the sake of convenience they are discussed separately in the first two sections of the chapter. In the second section a set of approximate rules is included, the use of which should permit contact lens practitioners to make quick and reasonably accurate estimates of changes in power caused by altering certain lens parameters. In all sections it is assumed that the reader has an understanding of basic optics and vergence considerations. The Cartesian sign convention is used throughout. For further understanding of the basic principles involved readers are referred to the works of Fincham and Freeman (1980), Obstfeld (1982), Bennet and Rabbetts (1984), Bennett (1985) and Douthwaite (1987).

It is hoped that the practical approach presented in the first two sections of this chapter will not dissuade readers from the study of more erudite mathematical methods of using schematic eye models to evaluate the optical effects of contact lenses. Readers are particularly encouraged to consider the latest and most realistic schematic eye data suggested by Bennett and Rabbetts (1988) which takes account of up-to-date research into the ocular components of the eye, and which it is hoped will be used in future editions of *Clinical Visual Optics* by Bennett and Rabbetts.

The practical effects of optical differences between contact lenses and spectacles

Again, it is convenient to subdivide this section, but it will be apparent to the reader that there is an overlap between the subdivisions. For example, a myope's eyes look bigger without negative spectacle lenses for the same reason that the myope himself sees objects larger than with spectacles — because the minifying effect of the spectacle lenses is removed.

The various differences, and similarities, between contact lenses and spectacles will now be considered.

Cosmetic appearance

Aside from the generally improved appearance that is usually achieved by doing away with spectacles, the magnification of the spectacle lenses is also eliminated. An observer therefore sees the eyes looking their normal size — smaller than with spectacles for a hypermetrope and bigger for a myope. Ugly appearances due to the prismatic effects and surface reflections of spectacle lenses are also removed.

Field of view or field of fixation, and field of vision

The wearer of a pair of centred contact lenses has a field of view equal in size to his field of fixation, i.e. limited only by the extent to which he can move his eyes. This normally gives a clear field of view of about 100°.

By comparison, the clear field of view of the spectacle wearer is limited by the size and vertex distance of the spectacle lens and is restricted to an apparent field of about 80° (although blurred vision is possible beyond the limits of the spectacle lens or frame as far as the eyes can rotate). *Figure 5.1* shows that in fact the myopic spectacle wearer has a much larger real field of view than this, depending on the power of the spectacle lens. On the other hand, the hypermetropic spectacle wearer (*Figure 5.2*) has a real field of view smaller than 80°. This means that, on transferring to contact lenses, the myope must move the eyes about more to see the same area of the visual field as he saw with his spectacles. The reverse applies to the hypermetrope.

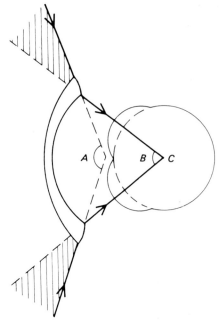

Figure 5.1 Field of view of a myope through a spectacle lens. A = actual macular field of view; B = apparent macular field of view; $A > B$; C = centre of rotation of eye. Hatched area is seen double due to prismatic effect (doubling is minimized by the spectacle frame, if present)

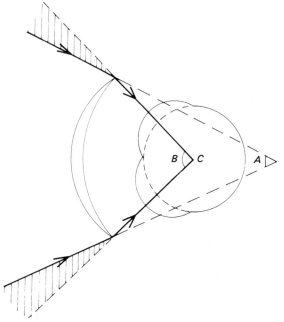

Figure 5.2 Field of view of a hypermetrope through a spectacle lens. A = actual macular field of view; B = apparent macular field of view; $A < B$; C = centre of rotation of eye. Blind area due to prismatic effect (and spectacle frame when present) is shown hatched

The sizes of the real and apparent fields of view through the spectacle lens are easily calculated. The angular subtense of the spectacle lens at the eye's centre of rotation, C, gives the apparent macular field of view, B. For example, size of spectacle lens, 50 mm. Thus, the semi-diameter is 25 mm. Distance from spectacle lens to C is 25 mm. Therefore $\frac{1}{2}B = \tan^{-1}(25/25) = 45°$. And thus $B = 90°$.

To obtain the size of the real macular field of view, A, requires that the position of the image of C, as formed by the spectacle lens, be found. Then A is the angular subtense of the spectacle lens at that point. Using the same example as above, if the lens has a power of -10.00 D, and making use of the usual nomenclature for object and image distances, then: $l = -25$ mm. Therefore, $L = -40.00$ D, $F = -10.00$ D; thus, $L' = L + F = -50.00$ D, $l' = 1000/L' = -20$ mm. C is thus imaged 20 mm from the spectacle lens, on the same side as C. Therefore, $\frac{1}{2}A = \tan^{-1}(25/20) = 51°\ 20'$. And thus $A = 102°\ 40'$.

In addition, the prismatic effects of the spectacle lenses cause blind areas in the peripheral visual field of the hypermetrope and areas of doubled vision for the myope, as illustrated in *Figures 5.2* and *5.1* respectively. The blind area experienced by a hypermetrope is enlarged due to the thickness of the spectacle frame. This prismatic effect and the blind area are particularly troublesome to aphakics owing to the high power of the spectacle lenses. Contact lenses afford great relief.

Whereas the average spectacle wearer accustoms himself to the presence of a spectacle frame in his peripheral visual field, the contact lens wearer must get used to an effect similar to some entoptic phenomena. In wearers of rigid corneal lenses, this effect may appear as a halo or partial halo in the peripheral visual field caused by refraction of light through the peripheral zone of the lens, including transitions, and through the surrounding tear film. The wearer of fenestrated scleral lenses experiences a similar effect due to the bubble, which gives rise to unusual reflections and refraction of light. In both cases the effect subsides as the lenses settle and lacrimation decreases. However, a slight effect may always remain, particularly if the pupil is large and the anterior chamber deep (Stone, 1959). *Figure 5.3* illustrates the optical reasons for these effects.

Soft lens wearers and, to a lesser extent, rigid lens wearers also experience visual disturbances due to contamination of the lens surfaces by deposits and interruption to the tear film on the front surface of the lens. Such effects may be compared to a dirty spectacle lens, but deposits on a contact lens obscure a proportionately larger area of the pupil because they are situated closer to it than deposits on a spectacle lens; also they remain in the same position relative to the visual axis as the eye moves, whereas the eyes can move to avoid deposits on a spectacle lens.

Oblique aberrations

Even best-form spectacle lenses allow objects viewed through their periphery to suffer from the effects of oblique aberrations — these being oblique astigmatism, coma, distortion, transverse chromatic aberration and curvature of field. Contact lenses remain almost centred in all directions of gaze, and any imperfections they impart to the retinal image are therefore

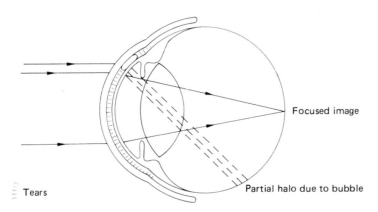

Tears

Focused image

Partial halo due to bubble

Figure 5.3 A partial halo in the visual field caused by the bubble behind a scleral lens. Similar effects occur with corneal lenses and deposits on a lens may give rise to scattering of light of a more general nature

kept to a minimum. By contrast, the visual acuity of a person wearing high-powered correcting spectacle lenses may drop slightly when the eyes are rotated to look through the most peripheral zones of the lenses.

The higher the prescription the greater these aberration effects are. Many aphakic spectacle wearers are extremely disturbed by pincushion distortion, and even medium to low hypermetropes wearing large spectacle lenses notice the same effect. Myopes, too, often suffer the disorientation of barrel distortion, and again the larger the lens and the higher the power the more noticeable it is. The relief afforded by contact lenses is then considerable.

Prismatic effects

Apart from the prismatic effects of spectacle lenses already mentioned, which affect both the appearance of a person and the field of view, two other factors must be considered. These are the prismatic effects of spectacle lenses during convergence and those due to the anisometropic spectacle correction, when the eyes make version movements.

Convergence

Spectacles optically centred for distance vision but which are used for all distances of gaze differ from contact lenses, which move with the eyes and thus remain centred (or nearly so) for all distances and positions of gaze.

Thus, during near vision, a spectacle-wearing myope experiences a base-in prism effect and a spectacle-wearing hypermetrope a base-out effect, as shown in *Figure 5.4*. Provided that contact lenses remain optically centred, no such prism effect is experienced by the contact lens wearer. Therefore, for a given object distance, the contact-lens-wearing myope exerts more convergence and the hypermetrope less convergence than with spectacles.

Table 5.1 gives the amount of convergence in prism dioptres (Δ) exerted by both eyes in various degrees of ametropia, assuming spectacles centred for a distance CD of 60 mm and

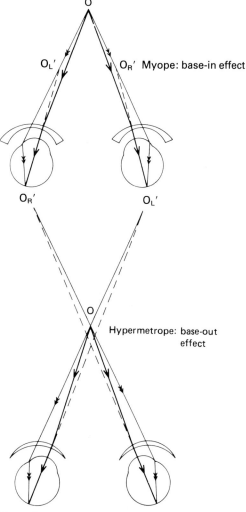

Figure 5.4 Spectacles centred for distance vision give prismatic effects when the eyes converge

Table 5.1 Comparison of convergence with spectacles and contact lenses

Spectacle refraction (D)	Convergence (Δ) at			
	0.33 metre from spectacle plane		0.25 metre from spectacle plane	
	Spectacles	Contact lenses	Spectacles	Contact lenses
−20	11.11	16.66	14.56	21.66
−15	12.11	16.66	15.87	21.66
−10	13.33	16.66	17.56	21.66
−5	14.80	16.66	19.31	21.66
0	16.66	16.66	21.66	21.66
+5	19.03	16.66	24.67	21.66
+10	22.19	16.66	28.63	21.66
+15	26.64	16.66	34.14	21.66

worn 27 mm in front of the eyes' centres of rotation, and contact lenses giving an equivalent power, remaining centred for all distances of gaze and worn 15 mm in front of the centres of rotation of the eyes. *Table 5.1* is used as a basis for the graph in *Figure 5.5*.

The significance of this difference in convergence must be considered in association with changes in accommodation (*see* Accommodation, p. 201, where it is shown that the ratio between accommodation and convergence remains the same with spectacles and contact lenses). The effect of the change in convergence alone, when transferring from spectacles to contact lenses, is only likely to be unfortunate in a myope whose near point of convergence is abnormally remote, when the removal of the base-in prism may be sufficient to disrupt binocular vision at near.

The general effect of transferring from spectacles to contact lenses for near vision, is as if the

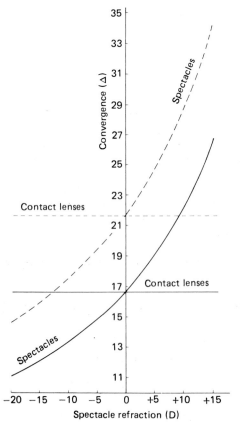

Figure 5.5 Convergence with spectacles and contact lenses. - - - - at 0.25 metre; —— at 0.33 metre. (Compare this with *Figure 5.18*)

myope had brought his near task a little closer, for he must converge and accommodate more, whereas for the hypermetrope the reverse applies and it is as if he had increased his working distance.

Anisometropia

Since contact lenses move with the eyes, the visual axes always pass through their optical centres — or very close to them. Thus, differential prismatic effects which can create difficulties for anisometropic spectacle wearers are virtually removed. (The effects of contact lens movement on the eyes are considered in the section on Incorporation of prism.)

An example will serve to illustrate this:

Spectacle correction: R −4.00 DS
L +1.00 DS

Prismatic effect when looking down at an object 10 cm below the horizontal and 25 cm in front of the spectacle plane (assumed to be 25 mm in front of the centres of rotation of the eyes):

R 3.33 Δ, base-down.
L 1.00 Δ, base-up.

Difference between the two eyes in the vertical meridian is over 4 Δ, which is too great for the patient to obtain comfortable binocular single vision. This spectacle correction would therefore necessitate vertical head movements rather than eye movements. *Figure 5.6* illustrates the difference in vertical eye rotation that would be required with this spectacle correction, in use as described, as well as the difference in magnification (*see* Relative spectacle magnification, p. 197).

Calculation of the prismatic effect is simple. The positions and sizes of the images O_R' and O_L' formed by the spectacle lenses are first found (*Figure 5.6*).

Thus, for the right eye, $l = -25$ cm.

Therefore, $L = -4$ D

Now $F = -4$ D, and since $L + F = L'$, $L' = -8$ D

Therefore $l' = -12.5$ cm

Since $\dfrac{h'}{h} = \dfrac{L}{L'}$, $h_R' = 10 \times \dfrac{-4}{-8}$ cm $= 5$ cm

And for the left eye, $l = -25$ cm. Therefore, $L = -4$ D

Myopic eye: base-down effect

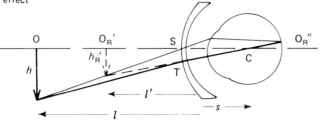

Hypermetropic eye: base-up effect

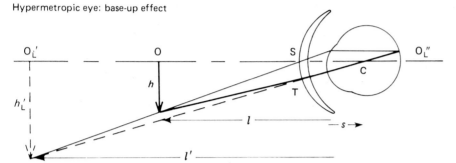

Figure 5.6 Anisometropia: during near vision when wearing spectacles the visual axis of the hypermetropic eye is depressed more than that of the myopic eye. The image seen by the hypermetropic eye is also larger than that seen by the myopic eye. O = object. O_R' and O_L' = images of O formed by the spectacle lenses. O_R'' and O_L'' = retinal images

Now $F = +1\,D$, and therefore $L' = -3\,D$

Therefore, $l' = -33.33\,cm$

and $h_L' = 10 \times \dfrac{-4}{-3}\,cm = 13.33\,cm$

Then the points (T) at which the two visual axes intersect the spectacle lenses must be found.

There are for each eye, similar triangles, with apex at C and bases at O' and ST (the distance s (SC) is assumed to be 25 mm).

Thus, $\dfrac{ST}{h_R'} = \dfrac{s}{s - l'}$ and $ST = 5 \times \dfrac{2.5}{15.0} = 0.833\,cm$

for the right eye

and $\dfrac{ST}{h_L'} = \dfrac{2.5}{35.83}$

Thus, $ST = 13.33 \times \dfrac{2.5}{35.83} = 0.930\,cm$ for the

left eye

Now, from Prentice's law (*see* p. 192), the prism effect of the right lens is $-4 \times 0.833 = 3.33\,\Delta$

base-down, and that of the left lens is $+1 \times 0.930 = 0.93\,\Delta$ base-up.

As pointed out, this gives over $4\,\Delta$ difference between the two eyes, the actual difference being $4.26\,\Delta$.

An alternative way of looking at this is to calculate the actual angles through which each eye rotates downwards, and then find the difference:

Thus, the right eye rotates downwards by an angle of

$$\tan^{-1} \frac{h_R'}{s - l'} = \tan^{-1}\left(\frac{5}{2.5 - (-12.5)}\right) = \tan^{-1}\left(\frac{5}{15}\right)$$

This is an angle of $500/15\,\Delta = 33.33\,\Delta$

The left eye rotates downwards by an angle of

$$\tan^{-1}\left(\frac{13.33}{2.5 - (-33.33)}\right) = \tan^{-1}\left(\frac{13.33}{35.83}\right)$$

This is an angle of $1333/35.83\,\Delta = 37.20\,\Delta$

The difference between the rotation required of the two eyes is thus $3.87\,\Delta$, which as expected, differs a little from the value measured in the spectacle plane, which was 4.26 Δ.

The latter method — of determining the angles through which each eye rotates — is the way in which angular values for convergence are also calculated. An object located on the midline between the two eyes (*see Figure 5.4*) is then considered as an object of height (*h*) equal to half the interpupillary distance, because this is its distance from the optical axis of the spectacle lens.

Horizontal prismatic differences are more tolerable than vertical differences. In fact, during version movements of the eyes, the anisometropic spectacle wearer learns to make allowance for the increasing prismatic difference as the visual axes intersect points at increasing distances from the optical centres. This habit of allowing for the prismatic difference shows itself as a non-comitant heterophoria which may persist for some time after contact lenses are first worn, and this can at first cause difficulty on lateral rotation of the eyes. From habit, one eye moves more than the other, and objects tend to be seen double until a new extraocular muscle balance is achieved.

Incorporation of prism

Most manufacturers of contact lenses prefer not to incorporate more than 3 Δ into a contact lens, as the thickness difference with such steeply curved surfaces makes more than this amount impracticable, although it can be done on lenses of high power.

Because the prism base always rotates downwards in corneal and soft lenses, and remains down and slightly in, it is impossible to prescribe a horizontal prism satisfactorily. Vertical prism is also limited, therefore, to one lens, and so the maximum vertical prism that may be prescribed is about 3 Δ but this may be rejected due to physical discomfort.

In scleral lenses, it is possible to prescribe horizontal and vertical prism to a maximum of 6 Δ, shared between the two eyes. This necessitates great care in fitting the scleral zone of the lens to prevent lens rotation on the eye due to the weight of the prism.

With spectacles, the difficulties of lens rotation do not arise. It is rare for more than 6 Δ to be needed in a correction, and this can easily be prescribed in spectacles.

With contact lenses some unwanted prismatic effect occurs due to movement of the lenses on the eyes. One of the aims of correct fitting is to ensure that this movement is similar for both lenses so that little prismatic difference between the two eyes is experienced.

The prism effect due to such movement is given by:

$$P = F \times c \text{ (Prentice's law)}$$

where

P is prism effect in Δ
F is back vertex power, in D, of contact-lens/liquid-lens system
c is displacement in cm

If the powers of the two lenses are the same and the movement is similar, then no prismatic difference occurs. If the two lens powers are not the same, the amount of movement enables the prismatic difference to be calculated. It is worth noting that, if a person wears a negative-powered contact lens in one eye and a positive-powered lens in the other, to counteract the prismatic effects due to vertical lens movement, the negative lens should move up (prism base-down) as the positive lens moves down (also prism base-down). With corneal lenses, because of the position of the centre of gravity and the action of the lids during blinking (*see* Chapter 10), this desirable opposite movement of positive and negative lenses frequently actually occurs.

If a lens tilts due to pressure of the upper lid on a corneal lens or to downward lag of a scleral

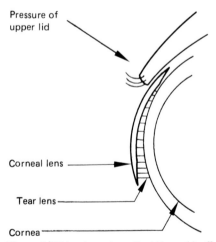

Figure 5.7 Prism base-down liquid lens: this effect is due to tilt of a corneal lens caused by pressure of the upper lid

lens, then a certain amount of extra prism base-down is introduced due to the liquid lens, as shown in *Figure 5.7*. Bennett (1985) has shown that this may be enough to counteract the prism base-up effect of a high negative scleral lens. Again, this tilt may be ignored as long as it is similar in the two eyes.

Where a contact lens has prism worked on it, then the prism power on the eye is the same as that in air. The liquid lens (unless it contains a prism element of its own due to tilt of the contact lens) has no effect on the prismatic element of the contact lens.

Cylinder effect introduced by prism, slip and tilt

The suggestion that a prism in a contact lens introduces a significant cylindrical element is incorrect. Although the refracted pencil is slightly oblique the amount of cylinder introduced is negligible. For example, taking a lens of BVP +10.00 D, BOZR 7.80 mm and centre thickness 0.40 mm, calculation shows that the cylindrical element introduced is only 0.023 D for a prism of 3 Δ. Expressed as a positive cylinder, the power is along the prism base–apex line and the axis perpendicular to it. Thus, in the example given, if the prism is base-down along 90, there will be a +0.023 D cylinder axis 180.

Lenses can also tilt by slipping on the eye. If the slipping occurs as a rotation about the centre of curvature (C_2) of the back surface then C_2 will not be displaced, but C_1, the centre of curvature of the front surface, is displaced. Thus, the chief ray is deviated and is no longer normal to the front surface. This introduces a small amount of astigmatism, as shown in the following example. Taking a lens of BVP +12.00 D, BOZR 7.80 mm and centre thickness 0.44 mm, calculation shows that if the lens slips by 2.0 mm then 0.23 D of astigmatism results. The effect increases sharply with increased slip (0.52 D astigmatism with 3.0 mm slip) but only slightly with increasing curvature. The axis of the induced positive cylinder is perpendicular to the direction of slip.

In the case of negative lenses of similar numerical power, the astigmatism induced is less.

Note that in the above examples the effect of the back surface has been neglected as the refractive index change at this surface is small.

Clearly, the induced astigmatism may be increased if the lens actually tilts on the eye as well as slipping. When the whole lens tilts through a small angle the resulting astigmatism can be found approximately by the equation:

$$\text{Cylinder} = F \tan^2 \theta$$

where θ is the angle of tilt and F is the back vertex power of the lens. The cylinder axis is perpendicular to the direction of tilt. Thus, if F = +10.00 D and θ = 5°, the induced cylinder is +0.0765 D. If the direction of tilt is vertical, i.e. about a horizontal axis, then the cylinder axis is horizontal. Such a lens tilted in the vertical about a horizontal axis, due to upper lid pressure on the top of the lens is shown in *Figure 5.7*. There is also a very small change in the spherical element given approximately by the equation:

$$\text{Sphere} = F \left(1 + \frac{1}{3} \sin^2 \theta \right)$$

Thus, in the same example the sphere is increased to +10.025 D, which is of no significance.

Sarver (1963) has studied the effect of contact lens tilt on residual astigmatism and his experimental observations confirm the above theoretical findings.

Magnification

Any correction, be it a spectacle lens or a contact lens, alters the size of the basic retinal image. (The basic retinal image is taken to be the size in the uncorrected eye assuming blur circles of zero diameter, i.e. 'pinpoint' pupils.) This change in the basic retinal image size is known as 'spectacle' magnification, even when it is the magnification due to contact lenses. In order to make a satisfactory comparison between spectacles and contact lenses, the differences in magnification given by the two forms of correction must be considered for both spherical and toric correcting lenses. This magnification is affected by the form and thickness of the lens.

Spherical lenses

Positive spectacle lenses magnify and negative lenses minify, and this magnification or minification increases with the vertex distance. Only if a corrective lens is worn in the plane of the eye's entrance pupil is unit magnification of the basic

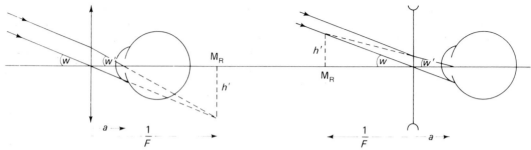

Figure 5.8 Spectacle magnification is w'/w. A distant off-axis object, subtending an angle w at the spectacle lens, is imaged by the lens of power F, in the far-point plane M_R. The image is of size h' and subtends an angle w' at the centre of the entrance pupil, which is situated at a distance of a metre from the spectacle lens. The left-hand diagram shows the situation in hypermetropia, and the right-hand diagram in myopia

retinal image achieved. Thus, a contact lens worn on the cornea approaches as nearly as possible to giving unit magnification. Only an intraocular implant can be fitted closer to the entrance pupil plane. Bennett (1985) has shown that spectacle magnification may be expressed as

$$\frac{1}{1 - aF}$$

where F is the power in dioptres of the correcting lens which is assumed to be infinitely thin, and a is the distance in metres from the correcting lens to the entrance pupil plane. *Figure 5.8* shows how this expression is derived.

The size of the retinal image is proportional to the angular subtense of the object at the entrance pupil. The angular subtense is w' when the spectacle lens is present and w when it is not.

Now, $w' = \dfrac{h'}{(1/F) - a}$ and $w = h'/(1/F)$

Thus, spectacle magnification $\dfrac{w'}{w} = \dfrac{(1/F)}{(1/F) - a} = \dfrac{1}{1 - aF}$

Note that when a spectacle lens is present, a is equal to the vertex distance plus approximately 3 mm. With a contact lens a is about 3 mm, this being the approximate distance of the entrance pupil plane from the cornea.

Thus, it can be seen that myopes who change from spectacles to contact lenses see objects larger than before, and hypermetropes see objects smaller than before. This is illustrated by the graph in *Figure 5.9*, which shows the percentage increase or decrease in retinal image size given by theoretically infinitely thin contact lenses as compared with infinitely thin spectacle lenses. More realistic values are shown for

typical aligning corneal lenses and typical scleral lenses, again compared with infinitely thin spectacle lenses. The slope for a soft lens would fall somewhere between the corneal and scleral lens slopes for positive lenses, depending on thickness and refractive index, and for negative lenses would approximate to that for

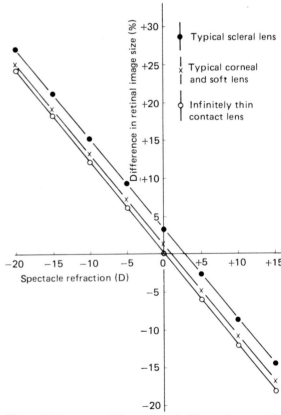

Figure 5.9 Percentage difference in retinal image size: comparison with a thin spectacle lens

corneal lenses, again depending on thickness and refractive index. (Lenses of low refractive index are normally thicker than their higher refractive index counterparts.)

Myopes can be expected to obtain increased visual acuity in contact lenses but may experience some disorientation when they are first worn owing to the apparent increase in the size of the external world.

Conversely, hypermetropes might expect to have poorer acuity with contact lenses than with spectacles; but since the difference in image size is only of real significance in the higher powers, it is only the high hypermetropes who are affected. Since most of these are aphakic, in the majority of cases they enjoy seeing objects reduced to only slightly larger than their normal size again. The disorientation experienced by an aphakic due to the magnification of his spectacles is comparable with but far worse than the disorientation felt by a high myope who transfers from spectacles to contact lenses. This is because the high positive spectacle correction causes field restriction and apparent image movement due to prismatic effects and aberrations, whereas a myope's contact lenses do not suffer from these additional defects.

The graph in *Figure 5.10* shows the different values for spectacle magnification given by four types of lenses. Theoretical values are drawn for spectacle lenses (assumed infinitely thin, and worn 12 mm from the cornea) and contact lenses (also assumed infinitely thin, and worn on the cornea, 3 mm in front of the entrance pupil) as well as more realistic values for typical polymethyl methacrylate corneal and scleral lenses, taking form and thickness into account. Again, soft lenses can be expected to fall between the two, but closer to the values for corneal lenses because of the greater similarity in thickness and lower refractive index. The latter consideration is dealt with more fully under the heading Shape factor on p. 196. The spectacle magnification of an infinitely thin contact lens should be multiplied by this factor to obtain a truer idea of the retinal image size when making comparisons with spectacles. This is borne out in *Figure 5.9*.

Toric lenses

The graph in *Figure 5.10* shows that contact lenses cause less change in size of the basic retinal image than do spectacle lenses.

A toric spectacle lens gives different magnification in different meridians, which produces distortion of the retinal image. This is particularly noticeable in oblique astigmatism, as

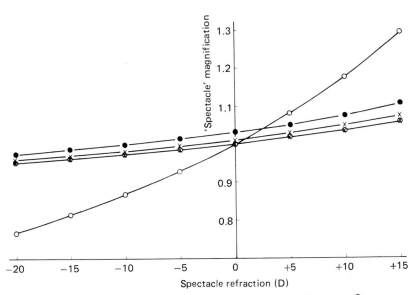

Figure 5.10 Variation of magnification with type and form of correcting lens. —●— Typical scleral lens; —×— typical corneal and soft lens; —⊗— 'thin' contact lens; —○— 'thin' spectacle lens

Bennett (1985) has pointed out. A square object seen through a toric spectacle lens may look rectangular if the principal meridians are horizontal and vertical, or diagonal like a parallelogram if the principal meridians are oblique. This distortion of shape is minimized with a contact lens because the meridional difference in magnification is reduced, as can be seen from the graph in *Figure 5.10*.

Difficulty may arise when a toric spectacle correction has been worn for many years and a perceptual allowance has been made for the distortion. On transferring to contact lenses which give a less distorted retinal image, the perceived image may appear more distorted until the processes of perception become re-adjusted to the new situation. The type of effect experienced with spectacles and contact lenses is shown in *Figure 5.11* where the spectacle lens contains a high oblique cylinder.

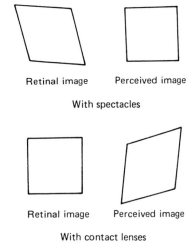

Retinal image   Perceived image

With spectacles

Retinal image   Perceived image

With contact lenses
when first worn

Figure 5.11 Perceptual compensation for retinal image distortion: this is acquired during spectacle wear and continues when contact lenses are first worn

Shape factor

The magnification of two lenses having the same back vertex power is affected by their front surface power and thickness. Shape factor is the allowance which must be made for the increase in magnification due to the form and thickness of the lens and is given as:

$$\frac{1}{1 - (tF_1/n)}$$

which is the ratio between back vertex power and equivalent power, where

n = refractive index
t = central optic thickness in metres
F_1 = front surface power in dioptres

The values for spectacle magnification for the thin lenses in *Figure 5.10* should therefore be amended to

$$\frac{1}{1 - aF} \times \frac{1}{1 - (tF_1/n)}$$

if shape factor is to be taken into account. This expression is easily applied to spectacle lenses but a contact lens system comprises a plastic lens and a tear lens in combination. The expression for the shape factor is correspondingly more involved. Bennett (1985) has derived an approximate simplified expression for shape factor of a contact lens system, based on values

which are normally known. This is:

$$1 + t(K + C) - (t_1/n_1)F_2$$

where

t = total reduced thickness in metres, of plastic lens and liquid lens = $t_1/n_1 + t_2/n_2$
K = ocular refraction in dioptres
C = keratometer reading in dioptres, where the index of calibration is assumed to equal that of the tear liquid ($= 1.336$)
t_1 = thickness of plastic contact lens in metres
n_1 = refractive index of plastic material of contact lens
F_2 = interface power in dioptres at the back optic zone surface of the contact lens

This expression was used in calculating values for the graphs in *Figures 5.9, 5.10* and *5.12*. These show that corneal and soft lenses give somewhat smaller retinal images than the corresponding scleral lens, because a scleral lens has a larger shape factor.

Figure 5.12 shows shape factor for soft, corneal and scleral lenses. Soft lenses were assumed to be 0.1 mm thick, corneal lenses 0.2 mm and scleral lenses 0.75 mm, and the liquid lens was taken to be 0.1 mm thick in the latter two cases, with zero thickness assumed behind a soft lens. This is a rather broad assumption because negative lenses, especially those of high power, are normally thinner than the values stated, while positive lenses may be considerably thicker. Also the tear lens behind a corneal lens may be less than 0.1 mm thick. However, the values assumed permit sufficient illustration of the effect of thickness on shape factor. Had more accurate thickness values been used the graphs shown would have been slightly more steeply sloped. A keratometer reading $(C)*$ of $+42\,D$ was assumed. This gives a corneal radius of 8 mm. The corneal lenses have the same back optic zone radius as the corneal radius, which is fairly typical. For comparison, values are shown for scleral lenses having the same back optic zone radius. Values are also given for scleral lenses with a back optic zone radius of 8.75 mm. (It is normal for the back optic zone of a scleral lens to be fitted about 0.50–0.75 mm flatter than the keratometer radius value.) It can be seen from the graph that this flattening has little effect on the shape factor as compared with the thickness difference between corneal and scleral lenses. Positive soft lenses are generally a little thicker than positive corneal lenses, but only slightly so, whereas negative soft lenses are often thinner than negative corneal lenses. When on the eye they fit so that the back surface of the lens almost parallels the central cornea. Because they generally have a lower refractive index than rigid corneal lenses the shape factor is slightly less than for corneal lenses.

Values used for the graph in *Figure 5.12* are:

	Soft lens	*Aligned corneal lens*	*Aligned scleral lens*	*Flat scleral lens*
n_1	1.40	1.49	1.49	1.49
n_2	1.336	1.336	1.336	1.336
t_1 (mm)	0.10	0.2	0.75	0.75
t_2 (mm)	0.00	0.1	0.1	0.1
Back optic zone radius (mm)	8.00	8.00	8.00	8.75
F_2 (interface) (D)	−8.00	−19.25	−19.25	−17.60
Corneal radius (mm)	8.00	8.00	8.00	8.00
Keratometer reading $(C)*(D)$	+42.00	+42.00	+42.00	+42.00

* Although many contact lens practitioners refer to the corneal curvature as measured by keratometry as the 'K' reading, and indeed this applies elsewhere in this book, because in visual optics the letter K is reserved for ocular refraction this chapter adopts the use of 'C' to denote the power of the cornea measured by a keratometer, where there would otherwise be confusion.

Bennett (1968, 1972) has done a considerable amount of work in calculating realistic retinal image sizes in the aphakic eye corrected by spectacle lenses and contact lenses, and in the pre-aphakic eye corrected by spectacles. He has not only taken into account the shape factor of the two types of correcting lens, but has considered the likely variations in axial length and corneal power (*Figure 5.13*). He has thereby derived some very useful values for relative spectacle magnification.

Relative spectacle magnification

This is defined as the ratio between the retinal image size in a corrected ametropic eye to that in a standard emmetropic eye. Various formulae have been given to calculate it, depending on whether the difference between the two eyes is axial or refractive. Its main use is in determining whether or not a particular type of correction is likely to improve or disrupt binocular vision, by comparing the two retinal image sizes. However, as Bennett (1985) has pointed out, such formulae, although useful, can be misleading because the human emmetropic eye does not always have the same length and power, indeed the range of values found is quite large. A much simpler approach is therefore used in this chapter, based on 'reduced eye' data and values for 'spectacle' magnification to determine retinal image sizes. This more than adequately permits an understanding of the concepts involved.

Where a person has different ocular refractions in the two eyes, the different magnification given by the two spectacles lenses (or contact lenses) may result in poor binocular vision. This is usually due to fusion difficulties resulting from unequal retinal image sizes. (Similar distribution of the retinal receptors in the two eyes is assumed although this may be a false assumption.)

It is common to think of anisometropia as being either axial or refractive. Sorsby, Leary and Richards (1962) have shown that most naturally occurring anisometropia is predominantly *axial*, but this is often accompanied by a smaller refractive difference between the two eyes.

By contrast, one obvious example of *refractive* anisometropia is unilateral aphakia. It is in such cases that contact lenses give greater similarity in retinal image sizes than do spectacle lenses.

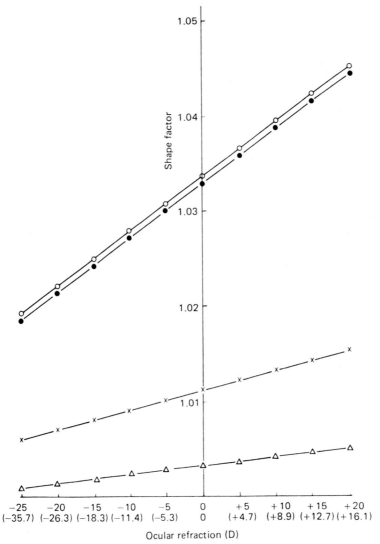

Figure 5.12 Relationship between retinal image sizes with scleral, corneal and soft lenses. The ocular refraction (D) = back vertex power of contact lens system. The values in parentheses are the spectacle refraction (D). —○— Aligned PMMA scleral lens; —●— flat PMMA scleral lens; —×— aligned PMMA corneal lens; —△— aligned soft lens ($n' = 1.4$)

As can be seen from the graphs in *Figure 5.10*, a soft or corneal lens for the aphakic eye renders the minimum amount of magnification of the basic retinal image, but in two eyes of the same length only an intraocular implant for the aphakic eye can achieve 'equality' of retinal image sizes.

The diagrams in *Figure 5.14* illustrate how two eyes of the same length and corneal power, one aphakic and the other phakic, have similar basic

retinal image sizes. Contact lenses give rise to a minimum change in this basic retinal image size, thereby permitting a good chance of binocular vision which may, however, still be difficult as study of *Figure 5.13* indicates. Retinal image size differences of as little as 1% may give rise to binocular problems in some patients.

Figure 5.15 shows how two eyes of unequal length have unequal basic retinal image sizes. In such cases, contact lenses — which scarcely

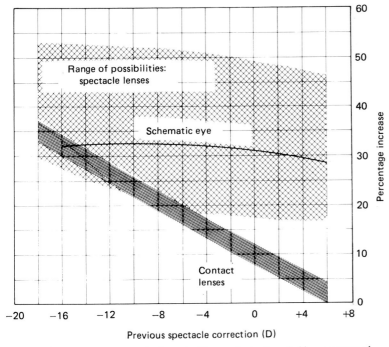

Figure 5.13 Percentage increase in the retinal image size in the aphakic eye corrected by spectacle and contact lenses. The graph indicates the possible spread of values, depending on the optical dimensions of the given eye. (Reproduced by kind permission of A. G. Bennett)

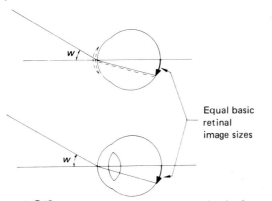

Figure 5.14 Refractive anisometropia: corneal and soft lenses cause minimum change in the basic retinal image size. w = angular subtense of distant object

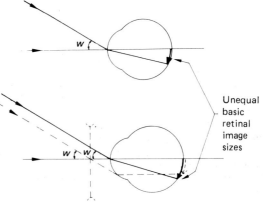

Figure 5.15 Axial anisometropia: a spectacle lens suitably placed before the ametropic eye can give equality of retinal image sizes, but this may not be desirable (*see* text). w = angular subtense of distant object

affect this basic size — are theoretically unsatisfactory if fusion is to be achieved, assuming equally spaced retinal receptors in the two eyes. A spectacle lens worn by the ametropic eye makes the retinal image in that eye closer in size to that of the other eye. Typical of such a case is unilateral myopia. However, the retinal receptor distribution may be different in the two eyes, being more widely spaced in the bigger eye. In practice it is found that axially anisometropic patients achieve better binocular fusion in contact lenses than in spectacles. This was established beyond doubt by Winn *et al.* (1986) who conducted a careful study using ultrasonography to measure axial length and other ocular component thicknesses and depths, and eikonometry to study perceived image sizes. Thus it would appear that all types of aniso-metropia and antimetropia would be better corrected by contact lenses than by spectacles, if optimum binocular vision is to be achieved.

If it becomes necessary to compare or calculate retinal image sizes, it is simplest to assume a reduced eye as shown in *Figure 5.15*. The reduced eye is assumed to have a refractive index of 4/3 and a single spherical refracting surface of radius 5.55 mm giving it a power of +60 D.

When the error (K) is known to be axial, then the power of the reduced eye (F_e') is assumed as +60 D and its length is k'.

Now, $k' = \dfrac{n'}{K'}$, where $K' = K + F_e'$

Thus, if the ocular refraction, $K = -10\,\mathrm{D}$ then

$K' = +50\,\mathrm{D}$ and $k' = \dfrac{4}{3} \times \dfrac{1000}{50} = 26.67\,\mathrm{mm}$

A standard emmetropic eye has an axial length

$f_e' = \dfrac{n'}{F_e'} = \dfrac{4}{3} \times \dfrac{1000}{60} = 22.22\,\mathrm{mm}$

When the error is known to be refractive (as in aphakia) then the power of the eye (F_e') is determined from its length (k') and its ocular refraction (K). For example, $K = +12\,\mathrm{D}$, $k' = 22.22\,\mathrm{mm}$.

Thus, $K' = \dfrac{4}{3} \times \dfrac{1000}{22.22} = +60\,\mathrm{D}$

and $F_e' = K' - K = 60 - 12 = +48\,\mathrm{D}$

As can be seen from *Figure 5.15*, the principal ray determining the basic retinal image size, undergoes refraction at the principal point of the eye according to Snell's law.

Considering this principal ray, prior to refraction the angle subtended at the eye's principal point is w, and after refraction the angle subtended by the basic retinal image is thus w/n'. (All angles are small, and the sine, tangent and angle in radians then all become equal.)

But $\dfrac{w}{n'} = \dfrac{\text{Basic retinal image size}}{k'}$

Thus, basic retinal image size $= k'w/n' = w/K'$ (in metres)

Note the principal ray may already have undergone refraction at a spectacle lens or contact lens, so that w is then equivalent to the w' of *Figure 5.8*. Thus, the spectacle magnification is taken into account in determining the angular subtense at the principal point prior to refraction by the eye. The final retinal image size then becomes

$$\frac{1}{1 - aF} \times \frac{w}{K'} \text{ (in metres)}$$

In the standard emmetropic eye the retinal image size is thus $w \times 60$ metres.

Two examples, shown in *Table 5.2*, will serve to illustrate the differences between axial and refractive anisometropia. The vertex distance is assumed as 12 mm and the distance from cornea to entrance pupil as 3 mm. Shape factor has not been taken into account.

The first example in *Table 5.2* is representative of refractive anisometropia and is a unilateral aphakic having equal basic retinal image sizes in the two eyes because the eyes are similar in length. Thus, the spectacle magnification afforded by both spectacles and contact lenses has a direct effect on the retinal image sizes. With spectacles, the difference in magnification between the two eyes is large and so, therefore, is the percentage difference between retinal image sizes. With contact lenses, it is small.

Table 5.2

Spectacle correction (D)		Ratio of basic retinal image sizes in uncorrected eyes (R:L)	With spectacle correction			With contact lenses		
			Spectacle magnification		Difference in retinal damage sizes (%)	Spectacle magnification		Difference in retinal image sizes (%)
R	L		R	L		R	L	
(1) +2	+12	60.00:60.00	1.03	1.22	18.29	1.01	1.04	3.75
(2) −1	−10	51.07:59.01	0.99	0.87	1.98	1.00	0.97	12.87

Obviously, the contact lens correction allows the greater chance for binocular vision.

The second example in *Table 5.2* is that of unilateral axial myopia in which the power of both eyes is assumed to be 60 D. Thus, the basic retinal image sizes are proportional to the axial lengths (or inversely proportional to the dioptric lengths as shown in *Table 5.2*). These basic image sizes are then affected by the spectacle magnifications; so that, with spectacles, where the difference in magnification is large there is only a small difference in the retinal image sizes. With contact lenses, the spectacle magnifications are almost the same but the retinal images are very different in size. Here, theoretically, but not in practice (as explained on p. 199), spectacles provide the better chance for binocular vision. The values found in the examples may be checked using the equations given on p. 200 for determining retinal image sizes, using standard reduced eye data, the values in *Table 5.2* being correct to two places of decimals.

It should be pointed out that where binocular vision is absolutely impossible the patient is free of any asthenopic symptoms. If binocular vision is made possible but difficult, symptoms may occur. This frequently arises with the unilateral aphakic. Because of the greater reduction in magnification afforded by corneal and soft lenses, these should allow slightly better binocular vision than sclerals. The aphakic also enjoys the other benefits of contact lenses over spectacles — but even so, the symptoms of difficult binocular vision have often caused the unilateral aphake to abandon contact lenses.

The extremes of purely refractive or purely axial anisometropia, as shown in the examples in *Table 5.2*, are rare. In most anisometropes, contact lenses afford other advantages – such as absence of differential prism – which make their effects on retinal image size worth investigating before they are ruled out entirely. In the authors' experience, the perceptual process which allows fusion of different sized images is more readily adaptable than is the extraocular musculature which has to cope with dissimilar prism effects. In spite of the fact that most anisometropia is mainly axial, contact lenses have been found to be more acceptable than spectacles to many anisometropes and as stated on p. 199, this may well be due to differences in retinal receptor spacing in the two eyes.

It is as well to note that corneal or soft lenses

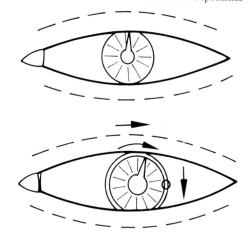

Figure 5.16 The effect of a high positive scleral lens: there is a wider lid aperture and the eye tends to rotate in the directions shown

are the better types of contact lens to use in anisometropia, as the weight difference is minimized. In scleral lenses, the weight of the high positive lens may cause hypophoria and excyclophoria of the aphakic eye (*Figure 5.16*). This is an extreme example.

Accommodation

The accommodation exerted for a given working distance varies, depending on whether spectacles or contact lenses are worn. More accommodation is required by myopes and less by hypermetropes when they transfer from spectacles to contact lenses (*Table 5.3* and the graph in *Figure 5.18*).

Table 5.3 Comparison of accommodation with spectacles and contact lenses

Spectacle refraction (D)	Ocular accommodation (D) at			
	0.33 metre from spectacle plane		0.25 metre from spectacle plane	
	Spectacles	Contact lenses	Spectacles	Contact lenses
−20	1.89	2.90	2.50	3.82
−15	2.09	2.90	2.76	3.82
−10	2.32	2.90	3.06	3.82
−5	2.58	2.90	3.40	3.82
0	2.90	2.90	3.82	3.82
+5	3.27	2.90	4.31	3.82
+10	3.72	2.90	4.89	3.82
+15	4.25	2.90	5.61	3.82

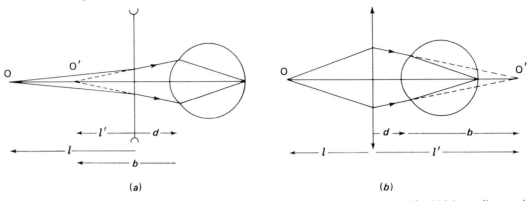

Figure 5.17 Near vision through spectacle lenses. The near object of regard, O, is imaged at O', which is at a distance, b, from the eye. The object, image and vertex distances from the spectacle lens are l, l', and d respectively. (a) Myopia; (b) hypermetropia

In order to calculate the actual amount of accommodation exerted by the eye, known as the ocular accommodation (A), it is necessary to determine the ocular refraction (K) and the distance (b) at which the near object of regard is imaged by the spectacle lens, of power F_s. For example, *Figure 5.17a* shows a myope wearing a spectacle lens of $-8\,\mathrm{D}$, who reads at a distance (l) 25 cm from the spectacle plane. Thus, the spectacle accommodation (A_s) is 4 D. Now if the spectacle lens is worn 12 mm from the eye, the ocular refraction (K) is $-7.30\,\mathrm{D}$ (*see* Appendix A and the computer program in Appendix E).

(The method of calculating ocular refraction from spectacle refraction and vertex distance, d, should be apparent from *Figure 5.19* if K is substituted for L and k for l.)

The near object, O, is imaged by the spectacle lens at O'.

Now $l = -25\,\mathrm{cm}$
Therefore, $L = -4\,\mathrm{D}$
$F_s = -8\,\mathrm{D}$
Therefore $L' = -12\,\mathrm{D}$
Thus, $l' = -8.33\,\mathrm{cm}$
But $b = l' - d = -8.33 - 1.2 = -9.53\,\mathrm{cm}$

$$B = \frac{1}{b\ (\text{in metres})}; \text{ so, } B = -10.5\,\mathrm{D}$$

But $-7.30\,\mathrm{D}$ of this corrects the ocular refraction. The remaining 2.20 D must be overcome by the use of the myope's accommodation, i.e. $A = K - B$.

This demonstrates the effectivity of the spectacle lens in permitting such a myope to use only 2.2 D of accommodation, whereas if a

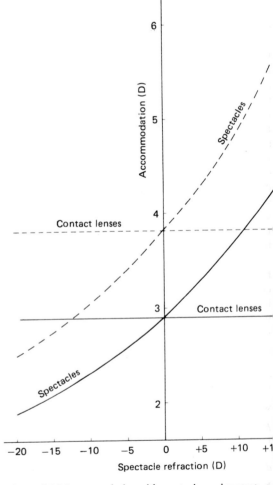

Figure 5.18 Accommodation with spectacles and contact lenses. – – – at 0.25 metre; —— at 0.33 metre. (Compare this with *Figure 5.5*)

contact lens were worn the same near object would be 26.2 cm from the eye necessitating 3.82 D of accommodation.

Figure 5.17b shows a similar situation for a hypermetrope. $F_s = +8$ D, $l = -25$ cm and $d = 12$ mm. Thus, $K = +8.85$ D (*see* Appendix A).

Now $L = -4$ D, $F_s = +8$ D
Therefore, $L' = +4$ D and $l' = +25$ cm
But $b = l' - d = +25 - 1.2 = +23.8$ cm
Therefore, $B = +4.2$ D
Since $A = K - B$, $A = +8.85 - 4.2 = +4.65$ D

This demonstrates how the ocular accommodation of a hypermetrope wearing spectacles is in excess of that required if contact lenses are worn. In this example 4.65 D of accommodation is required as compared to 3.82 D in contact lenses.

If a comparison is made of the graphs of convergence in *Figure 5.5* and the graphs of accommodation in *Figure 5.18*, it will be noted that the slopes showing convergence and accommodation with spectacles are the same. They are also the same with contact lenses. As Westheimer (1962) has already stated, this implies that the accommodation/convergence ratio (A/C ratio) is the same with contact lenses as it is with spectacles. It has also been shown by both Stone (1967) and Bennett (A. G., personal communication, 1967) that if contact lenses remain centred for all working distances and a comparison is made with spectacles centred for distance vision, the accommodation/convergence ratio remains approximately the same with both forms of correction, as shown in *Table 5.4*.

The figures for the basis of this table come from *Tables 5.1* and *5.3*. Bennett (A. G. personal communication, 1967) has derived an expression for the accommodation/convergence ratio with spectacles to that with contact lenses by using binomial approximations. This is based on a theoretical analysis and shows that:

$$\frac{\text{A/C ratio with spectacles}}{\text{A/C ratio with contact lenses}} \doteqdot 1 - F(s - 2d)$$

where

F = spectacle lens power in dioptres
s = distance from spectacle plane to centre of rotation of eye, in metres
d = vertex distance of spectacle lens in metres

Now, if $d = s/2$ it can be seen that the accommodation/convergence ratio is the same with both spectacles and contact lenses.

Table 5.4 Ratio between accommodation and convergence with spectacles and contact lenses

Spectacle refraction (D)	Ratio of accommodation (D) to convergence (Δ) at			
	0.33 metre from spectacle plane		0.25 metre from spectacle plane	
	Spectacles	Contact lenses	Spectacles	Contact lenses
−20	0.170	0.174	0.172	0.176
−15	0.173	0.174	0.174	0.176
−10	0.174	0.174	0.174	0.176
−5	0.174	0.174	0.176	0.176
0	0.174	0.174	0.176	0.176
+5	0.172	0.174	0.175	0.176
+10	0.168	0.174	0.171	0.176
+15	0.160	0.174	0.164	0.176

In *Table 5.4*, d was taken as 12 mm and s as 27 mm, which accounts for the slight discrepancies between the values found for the two forms of correction. But as d is always approximately $s/2$, the ratios are always approximately the same.

Changes in accommodation should therefore only cause difficulty in the presbyopic or pre-presbyopic myope, who may have trouble in exerting extra accommodation and convergence.

Optical considerations of contact lenses on the eye

To understand why a contact lens correction often differs considerably from a spectacle correction, the significance of the following points must be fully understood:

(1) The contribution made by the liquid (tears) lens.
(2) The effects of radius changes on back vertex power of the contact-lens/liquid lens system.
(3) The differences between total and corneal astigmatism.

This section is intended as a practical guide in determining soft and rigid corneal and scleral lens powers, and it employs the method of specifying back optic zone radii in millimetres rather than in terms of the keratometer reading in dioptres.

To correct fully an eye's refractive error, the back vertex power of the contact-lens/liquid-lens system must equal the ocular refraction (K) — not to be confused with the keratometer reading, also often denoted as 'K'.

In the following considerations, it will be assumed that surface powers are additive provided that their separations are small. This leads to some approximations. It will also be assumed that the back vertex power of a contact lens can be directly added to the vergence of the light reaching it — although this, again, is an approximation, as the following example shows.

Example

Consider a scleral lens with the following characteristics:

Back vertex power (BVP) in air	-12 D
Central optic thickness (t_c)	0.80 mm
Back optic zone radius (BOZR) = (r_2)	8.75 mm
Front optic zone radius (FOZR) = (r_1)	11.40 mm
Refractive index (n)	1.49
Refraction with this lens *in situ* (F_s)	$+8.00$ D
Vertex distance (d)	12 mm

Reference to *Figure 5.19* shows the following:

Reduced vergences   *Equivalent air distances*
$F_s' = +8.00$ D $\longrightarrow f_s' = +125$ mm
$\qquad\qquad\qquad -d = \quad 12$ mm
$L = +8.85$ D $\longleftarrow l = +113$ mm

The effective power of the spectacle lens at the front surface of the scleral lens $= L = +8.85$ D. If it is assumed that BVP of the scleral lens may be added directly to this, then the BVP of the required scleral lens

$= +8.85$ D $- 12.00$ D
$= \mathbf{-3.15\,D}$

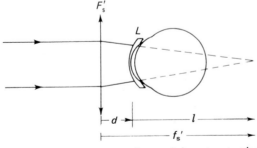

Figure 5.19 Effective power of spectacle lens at contact lens is: $L = 1/l = F_s'/(1 - dF_s')$

But this is only approximate, as more accurate calculations show:

Front surface power, $F_1 = \dfrac{(n-1)1000}{r_1}$

$\qquad = \dfrac{(1.49 - 1)1000}{11.4}$

$\qquad = +43$ D

Back surface power, $F_2 = \dfrac{(1-n)1000}{r_2}$

$\qquad = \dfrac{(1 - 1.49)1000}{8.75}$

$\qquad = -56$ D

Reduced thickness, $t/n = \dfrac{0.8}{1.49}$

$\qquad = 0.54$ mm

Reduced vergences   *Equivalent air distances*

$\quad L_1 = +\ 8.85$ D
$+F_1 = +43.00$ D
$\overline{L_1' = +51.85}$ D $\longrightarrow +19.29$ mm
$\qquad\qquad\qquad -t/n = -\ 0.54$ mm
$\quad L_2 = +53.33$ D $\longleftarrow +18.75$ mm
$+F_2 = -56.00$ D
$\overline{L_2 = -\ 2.67}$ D   This is the correct BVP of the contact lens required

It can be seen that the error due to the use of the approximate method is an over-correction of -3.15 D $- (-2.70)$ D $= -0.48$ D.

Note: Francis (1968) has compiled some very useful tables which remove most of the hard work from accurate methods of calculation. These are now incorporated into this text book and their use is dealt with later in this chapter (pp. 225–228), along with some helpful examples. The tables referred to form Appendices A–D at the end of this book.

However, the approximate method is less inaccurate: when the contact lens used for refraction purposes approximates closely to the power required, when it is thinner and when it has a lower refractive index. The example above shows why a contact lens having an entirely different back vertex power from that required should not be used for refraction.

The example above also uses a combination of positive spectacle lens and negative contact lens, which constitutes a Galilean telescope system. This should be avoided, wherever possible, since it gives a higher magnification than that obtained with the final contact lens. Hence, a false assessment of visual acuity may be made, and disappointment will follow when the final contact lens does not give the patient such a good visual acuity.

Different aspects of refraction with contact lenses will now be considered.

Ocular refraction

BVP of final contact lens in air
+ BVP of liquid lens in air (liquid lens assumed thin)
= Ocular refraction

Ocular astigmatism

Front surface corneal astigmatism
+ back surface corneal astigmatism
+ crystalline lens astigmatism (referred to the corneal plane)
= Total ocular astigmatism

Note that the front surface of the cornea usually has greater positive power near the vertical meridian, i.e. 'with-the-rule' astigmatism, whereas the other two contributors to total ocular astigmatism normally have 'against-the-rule' astigmatism, the total effect usually being 'with-the-rule', although this decreases with age.

Astigmatism of the front surface of the cornea and the effect of the liquid lens

Refractive index of tears, n_t = 1.336
Refractive index of cornea, n_c = 1.376

When a hard contact lens with spherical back surface is placed on the eye, the front surface of the liquid lens is spherical because it is formed by the back surface of the contact lens. If the front surface of the cornea is toroidal, then the back surface of the liquid lens is also toroidal, with radii (r) equal to that of the cornea, but having negative power.

The powers in air of the back surface of the liquid lens are given by $F = (1 - 1.336)1000/r$, and the powers of the front surface of the cornea are given by $F = (1.376 - 1)1000/r$. This means that the front surface astigmatism of the cornea is partly neutralized by the back surface astigmatism of the liquid lens. The amount neutralized is thus 336/376, which is almost

90%. This is of importance with toroidal corneas because it is likely that the back surface of the cornea itself will neutralize the remaining 10% of its front surface astigmatism.

Thus, with a hard, non-flexing, spherical contact lens on the eye, any residual astigmatism found is almost entirely due to the crystalline lens since practically all the corneal astigmatism is corrected, i.e.

Back surface astigmatism of liquid lens
+ front surface astigmatism of cornea
+ back surface astigmatism of cornea
= Zero (approximately)

Keratometry and corneal astigmatism

Keratometers measure front surface corneal radii but give *total* corneal power on the assumption, given above, that the back surface of the cornea has -10% of the power of the front surface.

The true refractive index of the cornea (1.376) is therefore not used to calibrate keratometers. Instead, an index of 1.3375 is usually used (n_k). This allows the instrument to read total corneal power (or approximately 90% of the front surface power).

But n_k and n_t are almost the same (1.3375 and 1.336). Indeed, some keratometers are calibrated for an index of 1.336 or even 1.332. Therefore, the astigmatism measured by the keratometer is almost the same as that corrected by the back surface of the liquid lens. In fact, the use of n_k instead of n_t gives a *power* value which is slightly too high; for a radius of 8 mm the use of n_k gives $F_k = 42.19$ D and the use of n_t gives $F_t = 42.00$ D. But astigmatism is the *difference between the two principal powers*, and the error due to the slight difference in the refractive indices is then reduced to an insignificant amount. This is illustrated in the following example of a cornea with an extreme amount of astigmatism.

Example:

Keratometry	8 mm/+42.19 D along 180
($n_k = 1.3375$)	7 mm/+48.21 D along 90
Total corneal astigmatism	+ 6.02 DC × 180
Liquid lens back surface	8 mm/−42.00 D along 180
powers ($n_t = 1.336$)	7 mm/−48.00 D along 90
Liquid lens back surface astigmatism	− 6.00 DC × 180

Even in such an extreme example it can be seen that the amount of total corneal astigmatism uncorrected by the liquid lens is an insignificant amount of $+6.02 - 6.00 = +0.02\,\mathrm{D}$. In this context, it is therefore valid to state that all the astigmatism measured by keratometry is corrected by the back surface of the liquid lens (*see* p. 204).

Residual astigmatism

Since the amount of astigmatism corrected by the back surface of the liquid lens can be measured by keratometry (as shown above), the amount of residual astigmatism with a hard spherical contact lens may be predicted in advance, although this assumes that the lens is reasonably thick and does not flex (*see* pp. 216–217). If this is so then:

Total ocular astigmatism
− astigmatism measured by keratometry
= Residual astigmatism

Care must be taken when determining the total ocular astigmatism from the spectacle refraction and vertex distance as it is incorrect to calculate the effective change in power of the cylinder alone.

The following is an example showing the correct method of calculating the effective power of a cylinder at the eye:

Spectacle refraction	$-6.00/-1.00 \times 180$
Vertex distance	$12\,\mathrm{mm}$
Spectacle refraction in crossed cylinder form	$-6.00 \times 90/-7.00 \times 180$
Ocular refraction in crossed cylinder form, after allowing for vertex distance (*see* Appendix A)	$-5.60 \times 90/-6.46 \times 180$
Ocular refraction	$-5.60/-0.86 \times 180$

This shows that the 1 D cylinder is reduced to 0.86 D due to the associated sphere power, whereas if the sphere power were ignored there would be no significant change in the power of the cylinder — which is demonstrably quite incorrect. The higher the powers of sphere and cylinder are, the greater is the effect of vertex distance.

Prediction of residual astigmatism allows the effect of this amount of astigmatism to be simulated by the use of a trial cylinder in front of the patient's usual spectacle correction. The sphere power may then be adjusted to obtain the best visual acuity. If this is inadequate, it is obvious that the contact lens must incorporate a cylinder for the correction of the residual astigmatism in order to obtain a satisfactory visual acuity. A suitable lens design may then be selected at the outset of the fitting.

With spherical soft lenses, owing to their replication of corneal astigmatism (*see* p. 214), the residual astigmatism is usually almost the same as the ocular astigmatism and if this is 1 D or more a toric soft lens or a hard PMMA lens may be necessary to obtain adequate visual acuity.

Because RGP lenses fall between the two extremes of soft and hard PMMA lenses their ability to correct corneal astigmatism is rather unpredictable and clinically, it is best to assess it with a lens, fully settled on the eye. Then, as indicated on pp. 216–217, the lens parameters or material may be changed to alter the lens flexure in order to achieve better visual acuity.

Approximate rule (1)

Generally speaking, when hard non-flexing spherical lenses are to be fitted, if the corneal astigmatism and total ocular astigmatism are both 'with-the-rule' or 'against-the-rule' and the difference between them is less than 0.75 D, this cylinder (which represents the expected residual astigmatism) may be ignored. When spherical soft or RGP lenses are to be fitted, ocular astigmatism of 0.75 D or less may usually be ignored.

Refraction with a contact lens of incorrect back optic zone radius

Fitting sets of corneal lenses, particularly at the extremes of the range, often have back optic zone radii in steps of 0.1 mm or 0.2 mm, so that the lens required to give the best fit may fall between two fitting lenses and the refraction may have to be carried out using a lens of incorrect BOZR.

A similar situation arises with scleral lenses. Not all trial scleral shells are sighted, and the refraction may have to be done with a lens of incorrect BOZR.

In this case:

Liquid lens power in air
+ trial contact lens BVP in air
+ effective power at the contact lens of the additional spectacle lens
= Ocular refraction

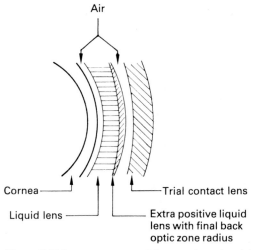

Air

Cornea

Trial contact lens

Liquid lens

Extra positive liquid
lens with final back
optic zone radius

Figure 5.20 Refraction with a trial contact lens: the trial contact lens has too flat a back optic zone radius

If the BOZR is flatter than that to be ordered, the liquid lens is more negative than it will be with the final contact lens (*Figure 5.20*). The vergence of the light reaching the front surface of the liquid lens must therefore be adjusted to allow for this. Negative power must be added to counteract the extra positive power of the final liquid lens.

When fitting soft lenses, this does not apply because they conform to the central corneal contour. Only if very big radius differences between lens and cornea are used is there any effect on the liquid lens. Even then this effect is rather unpredictable as it depends on the relationship of the back surface of the lens to the peripheral corneal contour, which varies from one eye to another. If the back surface of the lens closely parallels the entire cornea, then the liquid lens will have zero power, but if the lens touches the apex region of the cornea and clears the peripheral region there is likely to be a small negative-powered liquid lens. Soft lenses fitted with BOZR 1 mm or more flatter than the keratometer readings, may therefore possibly introduce a liquid lens of up to $-0.50\,\mathrm{D}$.

Approximate rule (2)

If when fitting hard PMMA and RGP lenses, the BOZR is flatter than that to be ordered, add $-0.25\,\mathrm{D}$ to the BVP of the contact lens for each 0.05 mm that the BOZR is too flat.

When the BOZR is steeper than that to be ordered, add $+0.25\,\mathrm{D}$ to the BVP of the contact lens for each 0.05 mm that the BOZR is too steep.

This rule can be shown to be approximately correct by checking on a Heine's scale or by using radius/power tables for a refractive index of 1.336 (*see* Appendix B, *Table B.V*).

Examples

(i)   A typical corneal lens problem
(ii) A typical scleral lens problem

		(i)	(ii)
BOZR used (mm)		8.10	8.25
BOZR ordered (mm)		8.00	8.50
Change in liquid lens power (D)	from:	+41.48	+40.73
	to:	+42.00	+39.53
	by:	+0.52	−1.20
Contact lens BVP change (D) to counteract this	Accurate method:	−0.52	+1.20
	Approximate method:	−0.50	+1.25
Error of approximate method (D)		+0.02	+0.05

These examples show that the error of the approximate method is sufficiently small to be ignored.

Back vertex power and thickness

This section applies particularly to high positive corneal and soft lenses and to scleral lenses.

The vergence of light reaching the eye must be the same with the final lens as when the refraction is done with a trial contact lens. Thus, BVP must be specified on orders for lenses. Sometimes only the front vertex power of the trial contact lens is known. When this is so the laboratory must be given the central optic thickness of the trial lens so that its BVP may be calculated.

Example

BVP of trial scleral lens	+5.62 D
t_c	0.50 mm
BOZR	8.00 mm
FVP	+5.40 D

This illustrates the difference between BVP and FVP for a typical scleral lens.

If the lens were to be ordered on the basis of

FVP without t_c being specified, it might be returned from the laboratory as:

FVP	+5.40 D
t_c	0.75 mm
BOZR	8.00 mm
BVP (instead of +5.62 D)	+5.75 D

There is thus an error in BVP of +0.12 D, and the error increases with thickness and power (*see* Appendix D). Special care should therefore be taken when ordering high positive lenses, whether corneal, soft or scleral.

Corneal lenses of PMMA and RGP materials are usually much thinner than sclerals, even in high positive powers, and the errors due to thickness differences are correspondingly much smaller. However, thickness should be specified with corneal lenses as it affects movement of the lens on the cornea as well as lid sensation and the rigidity of the lens itself (*see* Chapter 10). Soft lens thickness should also be specified for, in addition to back vertex power considerations, it affects the comfort, the rigidity and the gas transmissibility of the lens.

A program for computer calculation of harmonic and arithmetic mean thicknesses of a specified contact lens is given in Appendix E, thus enabling the potential oxygen transmission to be assessed for a material of known Dk value.

Spherical aberration becomes an important consideration when dealing with steeply curved surfaces, and with a contact lens on the eye the front surface of the lens suffers from positive spherical aberration which may seriously affect the BVP of the lens as it moves on the cornea. For example, a single vision corneal lens fitted as a distance prescription to an aphakic has been known to prove adequate in power for some close work. This occurs if the lens becomes displaced off-centre (usually upwards) relative to the pupil when the wearer looks down, and due to spherical aberration the effective power of the lens is increased. Unfortunately, not all spherical aberration effects are so beneficial, and a high positive lens which does not centre well on the cornea may therefore give poorer distance visual acuity than expected, possibly blurring to 6/18 from 6/6 if 1.00 D of positive spherical aberration is introduced.

Figure 5.21 shows that a decentration of 2.5 mm on the eye leads to an addition of +1.7 D for a lens of BVP +12.00 D, centre thickness of 0.35 mm and BOZR of 7.80 mm.

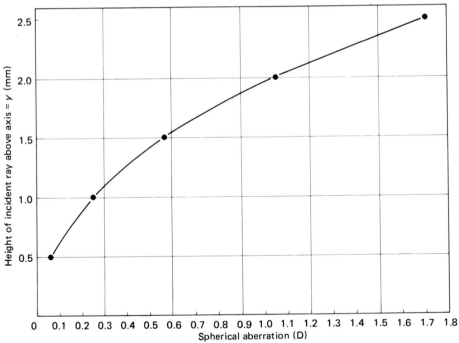

Figure 5.21 Variation of spherical aberration with aperture for a contact lens ($n = 1.490$) of +12.00 D BVP, BOZR of 7.80 mm and t_c of 0.35 mm. Parallel incident light is assumed

Aspherical front surfaces can reduce these spherical aberration effects, thereby improving visual acuity. Kerns (1974) has shown that such lenses permit improved visual acuity in patients with residual astigmatism, possibly reducing the size of the circle of least confusion, due to removal of the spherical aberration effects. The CALS and Nissel PS45 lenses for presbyopia work on this principle (*see* Chapter 16).

Power changes of soft lenses

Before being placed on an eye a soft contact lens is normally in a fully hydrated state in physiological saline solution and the refractive index is at its lowest value. The lens is also at room temperature and its curvature (i.e. its BOZR, or posterior apical radius, PAR, if the back surface is aspherical) and power should be as specified by the manufacturer.

After being placed on the eye several changes occur, all of which affect the power of the lens.

First change — flexure

The centre of the back surface takes up the same curvature as the central cornea, or almost so. This curvature change — so that the back surface of the lens takes up a different curvature on the eye from its curvature when in an unstressed and unsupported state in saline solution — is commonly referred to as flexure. The amount of the resultant power change due to flexure, be it spherical or toroidal, is small for thin lenses, but becomes significant for lenses of high positive power (Fatt and Chaston, 1981).

Various empirical methods of predicting the power change due to this flexure have been suggested, such as assuming that the front optic zone radius changes by the same amount as the back optic zone radius (Baron, 1975), or alternatively that the two surfaces change in the same ratio. Strachan (1973) termed this ratio between the pre-wear and post-wear back optic zone radii, the 'wrap-factor'. The most plausible explanation and theoretical exposition has been given by Bennett (1976), who bases his argument on the criterion that the volume of the lens remains constant even though its curvature changes. This seems a valid assumption to make. He also assumes that there is no redistribution of lens thickness, that the centre thickness remains unchanged and that the front surface of the lens remains spherical if the cornea is spherical. Bearing these factors in mind he has calculated that both positive and negative lenses change power with flexure, by the same amount as concentric lenses change power when they are bent. These changes are summarized in *Table 5.5* which is reproduced by kind permission of A. G. Bennett. He calculated the values from an equation he has derived, namely that

$$F_v' = -\frac{(n-1)}{n} \times \frac{t}{r_2^2}$$

Table 5.5 Change in power when a soft lens is moulded by the cornea to a steeper back optic zone radius, refractive index (1.43–1.44) and volume remaining the same

Thickness	Change* in power (D) for change of back optic zone radius, r_2 (mm)							
t (mm)	9.5	9.0	8.5	8.0	7.5	7.0	6.5	6.0
0.10		−0.03	−0.05	−0.05	−0.07	−0.08	−0.10	−0.12
0.15		−0.06	−0.07	−0.08	−0.09	−0.12	−0.15	−0.18
0.20		−0.07	−0.09	−0.11	−0.13	−0.15	−0.20	−0.24
0.25		−0.10	−0.11	−0.13	−0.16	−0.19	−0.24	−0.30
0.30		−0.12	−0.13	−0.16	−0.19	−0.23	−0.28	−0.36
0.35		−0.13	−0.15	−0.18	−0.22	−0.27	−0.33	−0.41
0.40		−0.14	−0.18	−0.21	−0.25	−0.30	−0.37	−0.47
0.45		−0.16	−0.19	−0.24	−0.28	−0.34	−0.41	−0.53
0.50		−0.19	−0.21	−0.26	−0.31	−0.37	−0.46	−0.58
0.55		−0.20	−0.24	−0.28	−0.33	−0.41	−0.51	−0.63
0.60		−0.21	−0.26	−0.30	−0.37	−0.44	−0.55	−0.68

* The change is invariably an addition of *minus* power and is virtually independent of the back vertex power of the original lens. For every 0.01 increase in refractive index over 1.44 the above figures should be increased by 1.5%.

The following example shows the method of use of the table: if a lens of BOZR 9.00 mm and t 0.20 mm is fitted to a cornea of radius 8.00 mm, the power change expected, if n is 1.43, is −0.09 D + (−0.11D) = −0.20 D. (The values in all columns between the two appropriate radii are added together to arrive at the power change.)

which for a value of n of 1.43 gives

$$F_v' = \frac{-300\,t}{r_2^2}$$

where F_v' is back vertex power, t is centre thickness, n is refractive index and r_2 is back optic zone radius.

Thus,

$$\Delta F_v' = -300\,t\left[\frac{1}{(r_2')^2} - \frac{1}{r_2^2}\right]$$

where r_2' is the radius to which r_2 changes after flexure. Now the refractive index of different soft lenses in their hydrated state varies between 1.36 and 1.46, but even if this variation is allowed for the values in *Table 5.5* would be altered by an insignificant amount and can safely be applied to all materials. (The greatest error introduced would be of the order of 0.10 D for a lens of centre thickness 0.60 mm and a change in r_2 from 6.5 mm to r_2' of 6.0 mm, the value for the change in power for $n = 1.36$ being −0.68 D and that for $n = 1.46$ being −0.78 D.) It is interesting that Wichterle (1967), by a completely different method, arrived at a value for $\Delta F_v'$ only 10% different from Bennett's, namely,

$$270\,t\left[\frac{1}{(r_2')^2} - \frac{1}{r_2^2}\right]$$

Had Bennett assumed a refractive index of 1.37 for soft lens materials instead of 1.43, he and Wichterle would have arrived at exactly the same expression.

Although it could be argued that Bennett's assumptions — that the centre thickness and volume of the lens remains unchanged and the front surface remains spherical if the cornea is spherical — are not absolutely correct, mathematical considerations show that errors introduced by their acceptance are of an insignificant order (Wichterle, 1967; Bennett, 1970, 1976).

Examples showing the effects of such flexure, as described by Bennett (1976), on two specific positive lenses now follow, and *Figures 5.22* and *5.23* illustrate this flexure on a positive and a negative lens respectively.

Example 1

In order to assist calculation a positive lens of knife-edge form is illustrated, but the same arguments can be applied to a lens of any specified edge thickness. A lens has BOZD 9.50 mm, TD 14.50 mm, BVP +6.00 D, $n =$ 1.44. This lens must have t_c 0.616 mm and FOZR 8.599 mm to give a knife edge (Jalie, 1974) (*Figure 5.22*).

The volume of this lens can be calculated, as explained by Bennett (1976), by subtracting the volume of the spherical cap bounded by the back surface from the volume of the spherical

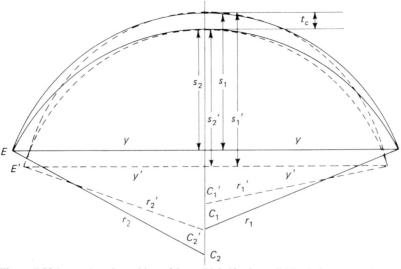

Figure 5.22 Steepening of a positive soft lens with knife edge: solid line before steepening and broken line after steepening. Before steepening: edge E, centres of curvature of front and back surfaces C_1 and C_2 with their radii of curvature r_1 and r_2 and sagitta s_1 and s_2 respectively, and semi-diameter y. After steepening these become: E', C_1', C_2', r_1', r_2', s_1', s_2' and y' respectively. Centre thickness t_c is the same before and after steepening

cap bounded by the front surface. Now, volume of spherical cap $= \pi/3(3r - s)s^2$ where $r =$ radius and $s =$ sag.

For the unstressed lens defined above, the volumes are thus:

Front spherical cap $= 361.113\,\mathrm{mm}^3$
Back spherical cap $= \underline{297.379\,\mathrm{mm}^3}$
Volume of lens, thus$=\ \ 63.734\,\mathrm{mm}^3$

If this lens is applied to a spherical cornea of radius 8.00 mm, the semi-diameter, y (7.25 mm) is reduced to some new value y' and since the BOZR is assumed to equal the corneal radius, the sag s_2' of the new back surface, can be calculated, as therefore can the volume. Because (for a knife-edge lens), $s_1' = s_2' + t_c$ and the semi-diameter y' is common to both front and back surfaces (*Figure 5.22*), the new front surface radius r_1' is readily obtainable from the general expression relating radius to sag and semi-diameter, namely,

$$r = \frac{y^2 + s^2}{2s}$$

The volume of the new front surface spherical cap can also be readily calculated.

The value of y' must be found iteratively, the correct value being the one which gives the flexed lens the same volume as the unstressed lens. In this example $y' = 6.9\,\mathrm{mm}$, $r_1' = 7.496\,\mathrm{mm}$, BVP $= +5.21\,\mathrm{D}$, showing a power change of $-0.79\,\mathrm{D}$.

After steepening the volumes become:

Front spherical cap $= 391.951\,\mathrm{mm}^3$
Back spherical cap $= \underline{328.217\,\mathrm{mm}^3}$
Flexed lens (= that of unstressed lens)$\ \ 63.734\,\mathrm{mm}^3$

From the above it can be seen that whereas the BOZR has shortened by 1.5 mm (from 9.5 to 8.0 mm) the FOZR has shortened by only 1.103 mm. If both radii had shortened by 1.5 mm the volume of the lens would have increased to:

Front spherical cap $= 460.939\,\mathrm{mm}^3$
Back spherical cap $= \underline{328.217\,\mathrm{mm}^3}$
Volume of lens, thus$=\ 167.722\,\mathrm{mm}^3$ (!)
and the centre thickness would have increased to 1.483 mm!

Clearly, if the front surface radius steepened more than the BOZR, both volume and centre thickness would increase to an even more ridiculous extent.

The differential change in radii which does

occur can be envisaged by referring to FLOM fitting (*see* Chapter 17) and thinking of the effect on sag when shortening the radius. For a given change of radius the sag is altered more when the radius is steep than when it is flat (*see* Appendix C).

Because the front surface radius of a positive contact lens is shorter than that of the back surface, the front surface radius must alter substantially less than the back optic zone radius if the volume and thickness of the lens are to remain the same.

The values used in calculating the above example and another example using a steeper cornea are listed below in case they may be of interest. Linear values are in millimetres, the volumes of the front and back spherical caps, V_1 and V_2 respectively and the volume of the lens, V, are in cubic millimetres. Back vertex powers (BVP) are used throughout. The power changes shown below agree with the findings of Bennett (1976) as shown in *Table 5.5*, which for a fractionally lower thickness value of 0.60 mm and a change of BOZR from 9.5 mm to 8.0 mm gives a power change of $(-0.21 - 0.26 - 0.30)\,\mathrm{D} = -0.77\,\mathrm{D}$.

Parameter	Unstressed	Flexed	Change
t_c	0.616	0.616	Nil
BOZR	9.50	8.00	1.50
y	7.25	6.90	0.35
BVP	+6.00	+5.21	−0.79
r_1	8.599	7.496	1.103
s_1	3.975	4.570	0.595
s_2	3.361	3.954	0.593
V_1	361.113	391.951	30.838
V_2	297.379	328.217	30.838
V	63.734	63.734	Nil

Example 2

BOZR 8.00 mm, TD 12.00 mm, BVP +10.00 D, $n = 1.44$, t_c 0.7028 mm, FOZR 6.984 mm.

Parameter	Unstressed	Flexed	Change
t_c	0.7028	0.7028	Nil
BOZR	8.00	7.00	1.00
y	6.00	5.792	0.208
BVP	+10.00	+9.059	−0.941
r_1	6.984	6.333	0.651
s_1	3.409	3.771	0.362
s_2	2.708	3.069	0.361
V_1	213.564	226.862	13.298
V_2	163.565	176.863	13.298
V	49.9989	49.9989	Nil

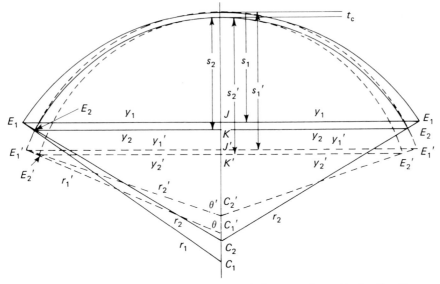

Figure 5.23 Steepening of a negative soft lens: solid line before steepening and broken line after steepening. Before steepening: front and back surface edges E_1 and E_2 with semi-diameters y_1 and y_2 intersecting the primary axis at J and K and subtending an angle θ at C_2. After steepening these become: E_1', E_2, y_1', y_2', J', K', and θ' at C_2' respectively. Other symbols are as in *Figure 5.22*

Negative lenses are treated in much the same way, except that edge thickness must be taken into account, and so it is necessary for the convenience of calculation to make one further assumption. It is assumed that the lens has a conical edge, with the apex of the cone at C_2 (*see Figure 5.23*). The edge E_1E_2 is therefore normal to the back surface and it is assumed that E_1E_2 and its relationship to the back surface remain unchanged after flexure.

The volume of the lens is the volume of the front spherical cap plus the volume of the frustum of the cone bounded by E_1E_2, minus the volume of the back spherical cap. (Volume of frustum of cone = $\pi/3 \, (y_1{}^2 \times JC_2) - (y_2{}^2 \times KC_2)$ and $\theta = \sin^{-1} y_2/r_2$ (Bennett, 1976).)

Hydrophilic lenses acquire additional positive power if they are flattened. The change of power due to flexure, $\Delta F_v' =$

$$\frac{-(n-1)}{n} t_c \left[\frac{1}{(r_2')^2} - \frac{1}{r_2{}^2} \right]$$

(n = refractive index and other symbols are as in *Figure 5.22* and as given on p. 210).

It is evident from the above formula that the change of power due to flexure is dependent on refractive index, centre thickness and the degree of bending and is independent of the original BVP (Bennett, 1976).

Unfortunately, these power changes are not always those found in practice and some of the differences are explicable as outlined in the second and third changes given below. It would appear from the work of Sarver, Ashley and Van Every (1974) and of Sarver, Harris and Polse (1975) that the spun-cast lenses of Bausch & Lomb, which have an aspherical back surface, may have a different power change due to flexure from lathe-cut lenses. Sarver and his co-workers term the change in power induced by the flexure of the lens and any liquid lens present, the 'supplemental power effect'. Most lathe-cut lenses are fitted with BOZR considerably flatter than the central cornea (*see* Chapter 11) and so flexure induces a negative increase in power or negative supplemental power effect (*Table 5.5*).

It is interesting that Sarver, Harris and Polse (1975) found a zero supplemental power effect with spun-cast lenses of PAR fitted approximately 0.50 mm flatter than the keratometer reading. Indeed, from *Table 5.5* it can be seen that for a centre thickness of less than 0.30 mm and for average PAR little change in power with flexure is to be expected for a change of 0.50 mm. However, Sarver and his co-workers remark that there is a large variation in the supplemental power effects found for a given corneal radius/PAR relationship. They state that lens thickness could be a factor contributing to the variation in supplemental power effects found. This is borne out by Bennett's work (*Table 5.5*) which shows that flexure of thicker lenses induces a greater change of lens power. They also state that peripheral corneal flattening and the shape of the back surface of the lens may be contributory factors. This seems very likely since a lens with an aspherical back surface is likely to flex differently on a given cornea from a lens whose back surface is spherical.

Voerste (1976) also considered that corneal geometry influences lens flexure. He used Hydroflex/m lenses which are lathe-cut but of similar size to Bausch & Lomb lenses, and found a preponderance of zero and low negative (mainly up to −0.50 D) supplemental power effects in a study on over 200 eyes. Only a few eyes had a positive supplemental power effect. This is good clinical evidence in support of Bennett's theoretical work (*Table 5.5*) for the Hydroflex/m lenses are fitted up to 0.4 mm flatter than the mean keratometer reading and would thus steepen on flexure. Also, the lenses used in Voerste's study were all negative lenses and therefore thin — between 0.1 mm and 0.2 mm centre thickness. Voerste also studied 30 eyes fitted with larger lathe-cut lenses (14.5–15.5 mm total diameter) and with these there was a larger negative (mainly up to −0.75 D) supplemental power effect. This again confirms Bennett's theoretical work, for the larger Hydroflex lenses are fitted up to 1.4 mm flatter than the central cornea, thereby steepening more with flexure and so inducing a greater increase in negative power, and possibly also retaining a small negative liquid lens.

Bennett also showed that on toroidal corneas the differential bending of a flatter spherical soft lens so that its back surface steepens to conform to the eye in both meridians, very slightly corrects the corneal astigmatism since there is a greater negative flexure effect along the steeper meridian. However, he showed that the amount of corneal astigmatism which can be corrected in this way is theoretically very small — from 2% to 13% dependent on centre thickness.

Second change — temperature effects

As the temperature of the cornea is 37°C and room temperature is about 20°C there is a change in temperature of the lens when it is put on the eye (Fatt and Chaston, 1980a,b, 1981) which leads to steepening with an accompanying slight increase in the negative power of the lens. (The effects on surface power of small changes in radius are shown in *Table 5.6*.)

Third change — evaporation effects

The increase in temperature and the fact that the front surface of the soft lens is exposed to the air which leads to evaporation, means that the water content of the lens decreases slightly when on the eye. This leads to a small increase in refractive index and further steepening of the lens, both of which tend to increase its negative power. (The changes in surface power due to alterations in refractive index are shown in *Table 5.7*.)

Ford (1976) terms this altered state of the lens when on the eye, 'the equilibrated state', which takes into account changes due to flexure, temperature and evaporation. He has developed tables and graphs for Sauflon material of 70% water content and for lenses of different thicknesses. These permit the changes in BVP due to equilibration and flexure to be determined from the changes in thickness and BOZR. Thereby a lens of appropriate hydrated BVP can be selected. An example is given of a Sauflon 70 lens of hydrated BVP of −9.25 D and BOZR 9.00 mm being selected 'for an eye of ocular refraction −10.00 D and keratometer reading 7.50 mm. The hydrated lens thickness of 0.21 mm would decrease to 0.204 mm on equilibration and the BOZR would alter to 8.743 mm. The effects of flexure would contribute −0.30 D, leaving the requirement of an equilibrated BVP of −9.70 D which is obtained by a hydrated BVP of −9.25 D.

Unfortunately, as Ford (1974) has also shown, the amount of change in the lens due to evaporation depends on the tear output of the wearer. Thus, greater changes occur in those lenses worn by people with *dry* eyes than in those with *normal* or *excessive* tear output. According to Ford, variations in tear output alone can contribute to differences in power of over 1 D, and he has gone so far as to suggest that in order to determine the equilibrated lens power on the eye soft lens wearers should be put into one of the above three categories according to their

Table 5.6 Rate of change of surface power in air, in terms of D/0.10 mm change in radius *r*, for surfaces of various curvatures and various refractive indices

Refractive indices	dF/dr (D/0.10 mm change) *at surface radius of curvature values* (mm) *of*						
	6.50	7.00	7.50	8.00	8.50	9.00	9.50
1.33	0.781	0.673	0.587	0.516	0.457	0.407	0.366
1.34	0.805	0.694	0.604	0.531	0.471	0.420	0.377
1.35	0.828	0.714	0.622	0.547	0.484	0.432	0.388
1.36	0.852	0.735	0.640	0.562	0.498	0.444	0.399
1.37	0.876	0.755	0.658	0.578	0.512	0.457	0.410
1.38	0.899	0.776	0.676	0.594	0.526	0.469	0.421
1.39	0.923	0.796	0.693	0.609	0.540	0.481	0.432
1.40	0.947	0.816	0.711	0.625	0.554	0.494	0.443
1.41	0.970	0.837	0.729	0.641	0.567	0.506	0.454
1.42	0.994	0.857	0.747	0.656	0.581	0.519	0.465
1.43	1.018	0.878	0.764	0.672	0.595	0.531	0.476
1.44	1.041	0.898	0.782	0.688	0.609	0.543	0.488
1.45	1.065	0.918	0.800	0.703	0.623	0.556	0.499
1.46	1.089	0.939	0.818	0.719	0.637	0.568	0.510
1.47	1.112	0.959	0.836	0.734	0.651	0.580	0.521
1.48	1.136	0.980	0.853	0.750	0.664	0.593	0.532
1.49	1.160	1.000	0.871	0.766	0.678	0.605	0.543
1.50	1.185	1.022	0.890	0.782	0.693	0.618	0.554
1.51	1.209	1.042	0.908	0.798	0.706	0.630	0.565
1.52	1.233	1.063	0.925	0.813	0.720	0.642	0.577
1.53	1.256	1.083	0.943	0.829	0.734	0.655	0.588

tear output. An allowance could then be made for evaporation based on the tear output.

Obviously, then, the determination of the required soft lens power for a given eye is rather imprecise. It depends on whether the lens is lathe-cut or spun-cast (although in general the effects of flexure are similar), on the rate of peripheral corneal flattening, on the tear output of the wearer, on the temperature and evaporation from the lens which in turn may be affected by external atmosphere and temperature as well as the lens material itself and its thickness. This section can therefore give no more than a guide as to what to expect.

The effects on astigmatism of power changes due to soft lens flexure and equilibration

Unlike the rigid hard lens, spherical soft lenses flex to match the corneal contour as already discussed on pp. 209–213. They therefore replicate the front surface corneal toricity on their own front surface. The thickness of the soft lens itself may slightly reduce the amount of toricity transferred, but as almost all soft lenses

have a refractive index higher than that of the cornea, the amount of astigmatism transferred to the soft lens front surface is usually about the same as that of the corneal front surface. Different soft lenses have different refractive indices, and the refractive index can vary with the state of hydration at which the soft lens reaches equilibrium on the eye. When fully hydrated most soft lens materials have a refractive index in the region of 1.36–1.46. Thus, the amount of astigmatism transferred to the front surface of the soft lens depends on a number of factors: the type of material and its flexibility, its thickness and its refractive index in the equilibrated state on the eye.

What is more important, is to realize that the astigmatism on the front surface of the soft lens is partly neutralized by the back surface astigmatism of the cornea as well as that at the cornea soft lens interface, and possibly by crystalline lens astigmatism also. Bennett (1976) has shown that any soft lens fitted with its back surface flatter than the cornea very slightly corrects corneal astigmatism (*see* p. 213). As it flexes to match the steeper cornea the soft lens becomes more negative in power, and this increase in negative power is greater along the steeper meridian, hence the slight correction of corneal astigmatism.

It should also be remembered that there is little, if any, liquid lens between a soft lens and the central cornea, and since the soft lens forms almost a glove fit in this region, any tear lens present is usually of zero or very low negative power.

It may be helpful at times to be able to determine the astigmatism of the front surface of a soft lens and how it may alter while *in situ* on the eye. *Table 5.6* shows the amount of astigmatism introduced by the toroidal surface of any lens (soft or hard) provided its radii of curvature and refractive index are known. It shows the change in surface power in air for a change of radius of 0.10 mm, for refractive indices between 1.33 and 1.53 in steps of 0.01. (Interpolation would permit power changes for even smaller gradations in refractive index than 0.01 to be obtained.)

Because a change of radius of 0.10 mm induces different power changes, depending on whether the curvature of the surface is steep or flat, this is allowed for by taking surface radii in 0.50 mm steps between 6.50 mm and 9.50 mm.

Thus, for example, for a large change in radius, say from 7.00 mm to 8.00 mm, and for a refractive index of 1.45, the figure in the intermediate ($r = 7.50$ mm) column should be used. So, for a lens of front surface radii 7.00 mm × 8.00 mm the power difference, or astigmatism, is 10 × 0.800 = 8.00 D, which gives an error of only 0.036 D.

If there is only a moderate radius change, as for a surface of radii 7.00 mm × 7.50 mm then (using the same refractive index of 1.45) it is best to average the figures in the two relevant columns to obtain the effect of a 0.10 mm change in radius, i.e. the average of 0.918 and 0.800 is 0.859 D, and for the 0.50 mm difference is 5 × 0.859 = 4.295 D of astigmatism. This gives an error of 0.009 D.

For small radius differences, as for a surface of radii 7.00 mm × 7.20 mm and of refractive index 1.44, then the value in the column applying to the nearest radius should be used; in this case it is 7.00 mm, and thus 0.898 D is the value for a 0.10 mm radius change. So the 0.20 mm difference in surface radii would give 2 × 0.898 = 1.796 D of astigmatism, an error of only 0.05 D.

If the front surface of a soft lens alters

Table 5.7 Rate of change of surface power in air (F) for changes in refractive index (n) of 0.01, for various radii of curvature (r)

r (mm)	dF/dn (D)	r (mm)	dF/dn (D)
6.40	1.5625	8.00	1.2500
6.50	1.5385	8.10	1.2346
6.60	1.5152	8.20	1.2195
6.70	1.4925	8.30	1.2048
6.80	1.4706	8.40	1.1905
6.90	1.4493	8.50	1.1765
7.00	1.4286	8.60	1.1628
7.10	1.4084	8.70	1.1494
7.20	1.3699	8.80	1.1236
7.30	1.3889	8.90	1.1369
7.40	1.3514	9.00	1.1111
7.50	1.3333	9.10	1.0989
7.60	1.3158	9.20	1.0870
7.70	1.2987	9.30	1.0753
7.80	1.2821	9.40	1.0638
7.90	1.2658	9.50	1.0526

curvature while it is on the eye, as for example due to temperature changes or evaporation, then there is a surface power change which may also be obtained from *Table 5.6*. Suppose the front surface of a lens steepens from 9.50 mm to 9.40 mm and the lens is assumed to have a refractive index of 1.43, then its power will change by 0.476 D, and as this is a steepening of a convex surface, the power will become more positive. Changes in toricity of a surface would lead to changes in astigmatism which can be determined from *Table 5.6* in the same way.

However, such radius changes of a soft lens occurring while it is on the eye are often accompanied by changes in refractive index, again due to equilibration factors such as temperature changes and evaporation from the lens. *Table 5.7* shows how the surface power may alter if this occurs. For example, evaporation might lead to a rise in refractive index from 1.39 to 1.40 for a surface of radius 8.50 mm. There is then a resultant power change of 1.1765 D, while a change from 1.39 to 1.41 would lead to twice this amount, i.e. 2.353 D. For a rise in refractive index, there is always an increase in power of the surface, and a drop in refractive index leads to a decrease in surface power.

Note that in *Table 5.7*, as indicated in the above paragraph, the changes in power are linear at any one radius; thus for a radius of 7.50 mm, a change of refractive index of 0.06 would give a surface power change of 6 × 1.3333

= 7.9998 D, and a change of refractive index of 0.006 would give a power change of 0.79998 D.

When these factors of radius and refractive index change with equilibration are considered, it is surprising that the power of soft lenses on the eye remain as constant as they do. Small changes in visual acuity due to alterations in power are therefore both understandable and to be expected. The effects on soft lens power of flexure, dehydration, refractive index changes, temperature and humidity changes, and thickness variations have been investigated by many researchers, among them Andrasko and Schoessler (1980), Bibby (1980), Fatt and Chaston (1980a,b, 1981), Chaston and Fatt (1981) and Port (1982), in addition to others already mentioned. Because 'water content' features largely in many of their investigations, Brennan, et al. (1986) have established definitions for hydration changes of soft hydrogel lenses, in an attempt to avoid confusion and to establish just what is meant by 'water uptake' and 'water loss'. Chapters 11 and 13 cover this aspect in further detail.

The effects of flexure on hard and rigid gas permeable lenses

In the same way that a soft lens flexes to conform to the corneal contour there is a tendency for very thin hard PMMA lenses to flex on toroidal corneas, partially replicating the corneal astigmatism. Harris and Chu (1972) found that with lens centre thicknesses of less than 0.13 mm, the thinner the lens, the more it flexes; the more corneal astigmatism present, the greater is the lens flexure. They found that thin lenses flexed in a predictable manner and induced astigmatism which affected the amount of residual astigmatism. Their results are summarized in *Figure 5.24*. As can be seen this flexure-induced astigmatism can be made use of to benefit the patient. Frequently, as explained on p. 205, if the lens does not flex, all corneal astigmatism is corrected by the liquid lens and any residual astigmatism is due to the crystalline lens. The latter is normally a small to moderate amount of against-the-rule astigmatism. If such is found, and if the cornea has

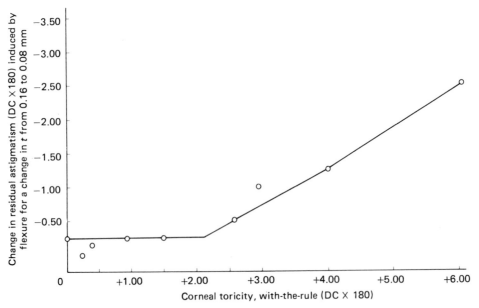

Figure 5.24 The difference in residual astigmatism between that induced by a thick PMMA lens (0.16 mm) and that induced by a thin lens (0.08 mm) for corneas of various toricities. For example, a patient has −1.25 DC × 90 residual astigmatism with a 0.16 mm thick lens, and a 4.00 D with-the-rule toroidal cornea. Changing the lens to one of 0.08 mm thickness induces −1.25 DC × 180 of astigmatism due to flexure, thereby eliminating the residual astigmatism. (Reproduced by kind permission of M. G. Harris and C. S. Chu)

with-the-rule astigmatism, then obviously by fitting a thin lens the induced with-the-rule astigmatism caused by the lens flexure can be used to partially or completely neutralize the against-the-rule residual astigmatism. The standard of visual acuity and quality may thus be improved.

Rigid gas permeable lenses also flex considerably on toroidal corneas, some materials being more flexible than others (*see* Chapter 3). Usually, the greater the oxygen permeability the greater is the flexibility of the material. This flexure can be minimized by fitting the BOZR as flat as possible (Pole, 1983; Stone and Collins, 1984) and by keeping the BOZD as small as possible (Brown, Baldwin and Pole, 1984) (*see* Chapter 10). Such flexure is similar to that of a thin PMMA lens and may be optically beneficial or, more often, prevent the lens from adequately correcting corneal astigmatism, rather like a spherical soft lens on a toroidal cornea, although the flexure is not as great with an RGP lens as with a soft lens. However, it may necessitate fitting a compensated bi-toric lens (Douthwaite, 1988).

Because flexure affects both front and back surfaces of the contact lens, thereby altering the front surface of the liquid lens, the cumulative effect on astigmatism is complex. Provided the radius changes of the lens are known — and the front surface of a lens can be measured on the eye by keratometry — then the power effects can be obtained from *Table 5.6* or from Appendix B. A computer program is presented in Appendix E, enabling the power changes due to flexure of PMMA and RGP lenses to be calculated in air and on the eye. Unfortunately the flexure effect may vary as the lens moves on the eye and, generally speaking, it is best assessed by refractive techniques (both objective and subjective) with the lens *in situ*.

Alteration of the back optic zone radius of scleral contact lenses

Sometimes a lens is supplied which has the correct BVP and is initially a good fit. After being worn for a few weeks, settling takes place and a heavy central corneal touch develops (*see* Chapters 17 and 18).

Two possibilities arise: in the first *the back optic zone may be found out using the same BOZR, thereby reducing central optic thickness*. This is usually done when the limbal clearance is also too small, as demonstrated by the fluorescein picture.

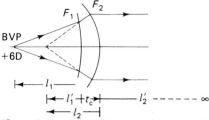

Figure 5.25 A pencil of rays traced 'backwards' through the optic zone of a scleral lens

As shown by Swaine (1956), grinding substance out of the back optic zone surface affects the vergence reaching the eye in two ways: the reduction in plastic thickness adds negative power to the BVP of the contact lens, and the increase in liquid thickness adds positive power to the tear lens. The latter may be ignored if the liquid lens is restored to its originally satisfactory thickness.

Example:

BVP of scleral lens	+6.00 D
t_c	0.60 mm
BOZR	8.50 mm
Keratometry: front corneal radius	7.75 mm

This gives central corneal touch after settling, and is ground out to:

t_c	0.40 mm
BOZR	8.50 mm
This gives liquid thickness	0.10 mm

The reduction in thickness of the contact lens adds -0.54 D to its BVP, making the BVP +5.46 D.

The increase in thickness of the liquid lens from zero to 0.10 mm changes the liquid lens power from -3.83 D to -3.72 D, an addition of +0.11 D.

Detailed calculations to obtain these BVP values are as follows. Tracing a pencil of rays 'backwards' through the scleral lens as in *Figure 5.25*, the back surface power becomes F_1 and the front surface power becomes F_2. As the BOZR = 8.5 mm

$$F_1 = \frac{(1.49 - 1)1000}{-8.5} = -57.65 \text{ D}$$

$$\begin{aligned} L_1 &= -6.00 \text{ D} \\ +F_1 &= -57.65 \text{ D} \\ \hline L_1' &= -63.65 \text{ D} \end{aligned}$$

$$l_1' = \frac{1.49 \times 1000}{L_1'} = \frac{1490}{-63.65} \text{ mm} = -23.41 \text{ mm}$$

$$t_c = 0.60 \text{ mm}$$
$$l_2 = l_1' - t_c = -23.41 - 0.60 \text{ mm} = -24.01 \text{ mm}$$

$$L_2 = \frac{1.49 \times 1000}{l_2} = \frac{1490}{-24.01} \text{ D} = -62.06 \text{ D}$$

$$L_2' = 0 \text{ D (emergent rays are parallel)}$$

$$F_2 = L_2' - L_2 = +62.06 \text{ D}$$

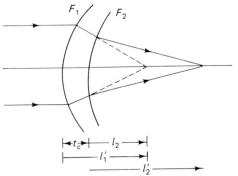

Figure 5.26 A pencil of rays traced 'forwards' through the optic zone of a scleral lens

Now that the front surface power of the lens is known, the effect of grinding out the back surface to give a new thickness, t_c, of 0.4 mm can be determined, and the new BVP ascertained.

Tracing a pencil of rays 'forwards' through the lens as in *Figure 5.26*, $F_1 = +62.06$ D (previously F_2) and $F_2 = -57.65$ D (previously F_1).

$$L_1 = 0 \text{ D (incident parallel light)}$$
$$+F_1 = +62.06 \text{ D}$$
$$\overline{L_1' = +62.06 \text{ D}}$$

$$l_1' = \frac{1.49 \times 1000}{L_1'} = \frac{1490}{+62.06} \text{ mm} = 24.01 \text{ mm}$$

$$t_c = 0.40 \text{ mm}$$
$$l_2 = l_1' - t_c = +23.61 \text{ mm}$$
$$L_2 = \frac{1.49 \times 1000}{l_2} = \frac{1490}{+23.61} \text{ D} = +63.11 \text{ D}$$

$$+F_2 = -57.65 \text{ D}$$
$$\overline{L_2' = +5.46 \text{ D}} = \text{BVP of thinner scleral lens}$$

Note that the above method of calculation, termed the 'step-along' method by W. Swaine, is an alternative to the use of reduced vergences with equivalent air distances and reduced thicknesses, as, for example, the calculations shown on p. 204.

The liquid lens power in air may be found as follows

Thus, front surface power

$$F_1 = \frac{(1.336 - 1)1000}{+8.5} = +39.53 \text{ D}$$

Its front surface radius is the BOZR of the scleral lens = +8.50 mm
Its back surface radius is the corneal radius found by keratometry = +7.75 mm

Back surface power

$$F_2 = \frac{(1 - 1.336)1000}{+7.75} = -43.36 \text{ D}$$

And for $t = 0$ mm, BVP $= F_1 + F_2 = -3.83$ D

After grinding out the back optic zone of the scleral lens, the liquid lens thickness, t, becomes 0.10 mm. The power of the liquid lens in air is then found thus.

An incident parallel beam of light is assumed, so

$$L_1 = 0$$
$$+F_1 = +39.53 \text{ D (as before)}$$
$$\overline{L_1' = +39.53 \text{ D}}$$

$$l_1' = \frac{1.336 \times 1000}{L_1'} = \frac{1336}{+39.53} \text{ mm} = +33.80 \text{ mm}$$

$$t = 0.10 \text{ mm}$$
$$l_2 = l_1' - t = +33.70 \text{ mm}$$

$$L_2 = \frac{1.336 \times 1000}{l_2} = \frac{1336}{+33.70} \text{ D} = +39.64 \text{ D}$$

$$+F_2 = -43.36 \text{ D (as before)}$$
$$\overline{L_2' = -3.72 \text{ D}} = \text{BVP}$$

These calculations may be simplified by the use of *Tables B.II, B.IV* and *B.V* of Appendix B as explained on pp. 225–227.

Approximate rule (3)

This applies to hard scleral lenses.

Reduction of 0.1 mm plastic thickness adds −0.25 D
Increase of 0.1 mm liquid thickness adds +0.12 D

In the example given above, the total effect on the vergence reaching the eye is −0.52 D + 0.11 D = −0.41 D, or if it is assumed that the original liquid thickness is restored by the grind-out, the vergence is changed by −0.52 D as the liquid lens is then unaltered (*see* Chapter 18).

For this reason, as Fletcher (1965) has stated, it is wise to order the original scleral lens a little too positive (by +0.25 D to +0.50 D, depending on the visual acuity obtainable). Even if the lens does not settle enough to require grinding out, it is bound to settle a certain amount, thereby reducing the liquid thickness and adding negative power to the liquid lens. A total settling of 0.2 mm is quite normal.

In the second possibility for alteration *the BOZR may be steepened as well as the thickness reduced*. This is usually done when the limbal clearance is more than adequate, as indicated by a large bubble in a fenestrated lens, surrounding the area of corneal touch.

The grinding out has the same effect described in the first possibility, coupled with a further increase in negative power due to the steepened BOZR. The liquid lens is made more positive, but to a lesser extent than the negative increase of the contact lens.

Example:

BVP	+6.00 D
t_c	0.60 mm
BOZR	8.50 mm

This gives heavy central corneal touch and a large limbal bubble; 0.20 mm is to be removed centrally by grinding out, and the BOZR is to be steepened at the same time to 8.25 mm. The final apical corneal clearance required is 0.10 mm.

The effect on the plastic lens is to reduce the BVP from +6.00 D to +3.74 D, which is:

−0.52 D due to the thickness reduction (*see above under* first possibility)
−1.74 D due to the radius alteration (*see* Appendix B, *Table B.II, n* = 1.49)
−2.26 D total change in BVP

This is partially offset by the increase in positive power of the liquid lens from −3.83 D to −2.52 D, which is:

+0.11 D due to the thickness increase (*see above under* first possibility)
+1.20 D due to the radius change (*see* Appendix B, *Table B.V, n* = 1.336)
+1.31 D total change in liquid lens power

The change in vergence reaching the eye is approximately −1.00 D:

−2.26 D due to the plastic lens
+1.31 D due to the liquid lens
−0.95 D total change in vergence

The BVP of the contact lens should be changed to correct this amount, i.e. from its new value of +3.74 D by +1.00 D to +4.74 D. This change must be carried out on the front surface of the lens.

Approximate rule (4)

For each 0.05 mm that the BOZR of a sighted scleral lens is steepened, +0.12 D must be added to the altered BVP of the plastic lens (by changing the front surface power) in order to keep the BVP of the plastic/liquid system unchanged.

Applying the approximate rules to the example given results in the following.

Rule (4)

BOZR steepened by 0.25 mm = 5 × 0.05 mm steepening
Compensation for negative increase at plastic/liquid interface = 5 × +0.12 D = +0.62 D to add to BVP

Rule (3)

Reduction of plastic thickness by 0.20 mm = 2 × 0.10 mm
Compensation for negative power added = 2 × +0.25 D = +0.50 D to add to BVP

Rule (3)

Increase of liquid thickness by 0.10 mm = 1 × 0.10 mm
Compensation for positive power added = 1 × −0.12 D = −0.12 D to add to BVP

Total change to be made to	+0.62 D
altered BVP by changing	+0.50 D
front surface power	−0.12 D
	+1.00 D

This yields almost the same result as that found by detailed calculation, which gave +0.95 D.

An alternative method of steepening the BOZR is to select the BOZR which will give the extra clearance required. This is done by deciding how much is to be ground out and over what diameter the BOZR is to be steepened. (This diameter is usually about 8–9 mm to allow adequate coverage of the pupil area.) Then the sagitta of the existing BOZR at this diameter may be determined (*see* Appendix C). The substance to be removed is added to this sagitta and gives the sagitta value at the same diameter for the steeper BOZR required. (Nomograms, as compiled by Clark (1970) may be used as an alternative to tables for determining sagitta values.)

Example:

BOZR	9.00 mm
Diameter	9.00 mm
Sagitta	1.206 mm
Extra clearance	= 0.20 mm
Sagitta of new BOZR	= 1.406 mm
Diameter as before	= 9.00 mm
New BOZR required	= 7.90 mm (*see* Appendix C)

This method of determining BOZR usually means that there is a considerable alteration over the central area alone which does not always result in a satisfactory fit. Central corneal clearance is achieved but touch may remain at the transition of the old and new back optic zone curves. (On the whole, it is better to steepen the BOZR by a small amount, such as 0.25 mm, after removing most of the substance required using the original BOZR.)

Toric contact lenses (*see* Chapter 14)

Both optical and fitting considerations of these lenses have been dealt with in detail by Capelli (1964), Stone (1966) and Westerhout (1969). In summary, it may be said that if the back optic surface of a contact lens is to be made toroidal, the BVP required should be found either with a lens having the correct toroidal BOZR or with a spherical lens having a BOZR equal to the flatter meridian of the toric lens to be ordered. In the latter case, which is not as straightforward as the former, some calculation is necessary in order to determine the BVP of the final toric lens to be ordered. Since the BOZR of one meridian is to be steepened by a known amount when ordering, the calculation is the same as that for a spherical lens where a refraction has been carried out with a trial lens of incorrect BOZR, as outlined on pp. 206 and 207 and summarized in Approximate rule (2). It is a simple matter of allowing for the fact that the liquid lens power in one meridian will be different with the final lens in place from the value with the spherical trial lens in place. An allowance for this difference must therefore be made on the plastic contact lens itself, as shown in the following example.

Example:

BOZR of lens to be ordered	7.50 mm along 90 8.30 mm along 180
BOZR of spherical trial lens for refraction	8.30 mm
BVP of spherical trial lens for refraction	−3.00 D
Addition spectacle lens needed	−1.00/+0.50 × 180
BVP of final contact lens along 180 is thus	−3.00 + −1.00 = −4.00
BVP of final contact lens along 90 is thus	−3.00 + −1.00 + +0.50 + allowance for radius change, of −4.00 D − see Approximate rule (2) = −7.50 D in total

(When the radius change is as large as this it is more accurate to look up the change in power of the liquid lens, remembering that this change is a change of the front surface of the liquid lens in air — see pp. 206 and 207 and see Appendix B, Table B.V, for a refractive index difference of 1.336 − 1. In this example, this gives a change of −4.32 D, i.e. 0.32 D more than the value given by Approximate rule (2). Thus, the BVP of the final contact lens along 90 should be −7.82 D.)

It can now be established whether or not a front toroidal surface will be necessary on the final lens. This depends on whether or not the cylinder power of the back surface in air is the same as the required cylinder element of the BVP of the lens in air:

Required BVP of final lens (in air)	−4.00/−3.82 × 180

For a PMMA lens back surface powers (in air) (From Appendix B, Table B.II for 1.490 − 1)	−65.33 along 90 −59.04 along 180
Back surface cylinder in air is thus	−6.29 × 180
Front surface cylinder required	−3.82 − (−6.29) × 180 = +2.47 × 180

The computer program in Appendix E may also be used to determine back surface cylinder power in air.

The above example is an obvious case where a front surface cylinder is necessary to give good visual acuity. Frequently the front surface cylinder calculated in this way is quite small and the practitioner may prefer to order a lens with a spherical front surface and risk leaving the patient with a small amount of uncorrected (but overcorrected) astigmatism. In such a case the cylinder element of the BVP of the final lens ordered must be altered by this amount, i.e. the cylinder element of the BVP is then the same as the back surface cylinder in air.

Alternatively the final lens may be ordered stating that it is to have a back toroidal surface only, and giving the back vertex power of the flattest meridian, i.e. the maximum positive or least negative power.

It often helps in considering the optical effects of contact lenses with back toroidal surfaces, to imagine the existence of a very thick tear lens, in the centre of which is sandwiched a perfectly flat layer of air. The surfaces bounding this flat layer of air are therefore of zero power in all meridians, the tears on either side forming two liquid lenses — one whose power depends on the toroidal radii of the back surface of the contact lens, and the other quite separate one whose power depends on the corneal radii. Then the optical effect of the tears on the cornea (which is to neutralize the corneal astigmatism — see p. 205) can be considered separately from the plastic/tears interface at the back of the contact lens. If appropriate the two can be added together. Thus, the rear portion of this tear lens corrects the corneal astigmatism, but further astigmatism is introduced by the front portion at the plastic/tears interface (see Chapter 14).

Compensated bi-toric lenses

These are lenses in which the front toroidal surface in air has an equal and opposite cylindrical power to the back toroidal surface in tears. It thus acts like a spherical lens on the eye, both in terms of power and in that rotation of the lens on the eye does not induce any cylindrical effect (*see* Chapter 14). Such a lens may be required for reasons of comfort or fit, or when fitting an RGP lens to replace a PMMA lens for a patient with a significantly toroidal cornea.

If, for example, a rigid spherical PMMA lens corrects the astigmatism of an eye, but for physiological (and/or fitting) reasons a gas permeable lens is to be ordered which is likely to flex, thereby inducing unwanted astigmatism, it may be desirable to fit an RGP lens with a toroidal back surface to match the corneal radii. This prevents flexure but introduces astigmatism at the interface of the lens back surface with the liquid lens front surface. The amount of this induced astigmatism is given by

$$\frac{1000 \, (n' - n)}{r_F} - \frac{1000 \, (n' - n)}{r_S}$$

where n' = refractive index of contact lens
   n = refractive index of tears = 1.336
   r_F = BOZR along flattest meridian of lens back surface
   r_S = BOZR along steepest meridian of lens back surface

To compensate for this astigmatism introduced at the back surface of the lens *in situ*, a front toroidal surface with principal meridians parallel to those of the back surface must be made which, since it is in air, will not be as toroidal as the back surface. The ratio between front and back surface toricity depends on the refractive index of the lens material and is given by

$$\frac{1/(n' - 1)}{1/(n' - 1.336)} = \frac{n' - 1.336}{n' - 1}$$

For PMMA this is

$$\frac{1.49 - 1.336}{1.49 - 1} = 0.314 \text{ or approximately } \tfrac{1}{3}$$

For an RGP material of refractive index 1.45 it is

$$\frac{1.45 - 1.336}{1.45 - 1} = 0.253 \text{ or approximately } \tfrac{1}{4}$$

Thus to provide a spherical effect on the eye, a compensated parallel bi-toric lens has a front surface cylinder which counteracts in the region of a third to a quarter of the back surface cylinder in air, depending on the refractive

index of the lens material. This information is useful when checking the lens on a focimeter. Its total cylindrical effect is thus two-thirds to three-quarters of the back surface cylinder in air — the latter being easily obtained from radiuscope readings (*see* Chapter 12) and tables for radius/power conversion (see Appendix B, *Tables B.I, B.II* and *B.III*). The computer program in Appendix E also provides this information.

If such lenses are not accurately manufactured with the principal meridians absolutely parallel on front and back surfaces, then not only is the cylinder power of the lens in air different from that expected but the lens will not provide the correct 'spherical equivalent' effect on the eye (Douthwaite, 1988). The resultant cylindrical effect can be calculated by Stokes' construction (*see* Chapter 14) or by using the computer program given in Appendix E. If the power of the cylinder on the front surface does not have the correct ratio to that of the back surface then again it will not be the equivalent of a spherical lens on the eye. This may not be problematical unless the lens rotates when the effect of the swinging cylinder may give rise to a reduction and variation in visual acuity. If the resultant refractive error is constant and the cylinder error of the lens is known, then Stokes' construction permits the misalignment of the lens on the eye to be determined (*see* the computer program in Appendix E). These erroneous effects are compounded if the front surface cylinder is both incorrect in power and not parallel to that of the back surface — which may explain the reluctance of some manufacturers to supply such lenses, as they are extremely difficult to manufacture accurately.

Bifocal contact lenses

Like bifocal spectacle lenses, contact lens bifocals are available in both solid and fused types. Chapter 16 deals with the various designs and methods of fitting. The basic principles may be understood by considering the concentric solid bifocal with distance portion in the centre and the fused bifocal with the near segment on the back surface. The latter is shown in *Figure 5.28.* An appreciation of the optical principles of these two main types should permit a general understanding of all other designs of bifocal contact lens.

Concentric solid bifocals

As *Figure 5.27* shows, these are available with the addition worked on either the front or back optic surface (and, of course, a combination of back and front surface additions could be used). When the addition is on the front surface (a plastic/air interface), the front optic zone has two radii worked on it, the steeper corresponding to the near portion of the lens. Then, provided that the lens is assumed to be infinitely thin, the near addition is equal to the difference between the two front surface powers.

For example, if the near addition to be incorporated in a PMMA lens is +3.00 D and where F_{1DP} and F_{1NP} are the front surface powers of the distance and near portions respectively, then $F_{1NP} = F_{1DP} + 3.00$. Since this is a plastic/air interface the appropriate front optic zone radii may be obtained from Appendix B, *Table B.II* (a radius/power table for polymethyl methacrylate of refractive index 1.490). If, in a particular case, F_{1DP} is calculated to be +58.00 D, the nearest value to this in the table is 57.99 giving a radius, r_{1DP}, of

$$8.45 \text{ mm} = \frac{(1.490 - 1)1000}{58.00}$$

For an addition of +3.00 D, F_{1NP} must therefore be +61.00 D and the nearest value to this in the table is 61.02, giving a radius of 8.03 mm.

If thickness is to be taken into account, reference to Appendix B, *Table B.IV* (lower figures for convergent light) should be made. In the example just given, if the centre thickness of the distance portion were 0.20 mm and that of the near portion 0.22 mm, entering the initial vergence column at 58.0 D for the distance portion, it can be seen that 0.20 mm thickness

adds 0.46 D to this power. The reduced vergence reaching the back surface is thus +58.46 D. Similarly, for the near portion, entering the initial vergence column between 60.0 D and 62.0 D, 0.22 mm thickness adds between 0.54 D and 0.57 D to the reduced vergence, say, 0.56 D. The difference between 0.46 D and 0.56 D is 0.10 D and is small enough to be ignored, but it indicates that F_{1NP} should be reduced by this amount, from +61.00 D to +60.90 D, giving r_{1NP} as 8.05 mm instead of 8.03 mm. This small radius change is not really worth making as will be shown.

In fact, most practitioners agree that there is a tendency for a small negative-powered liquid lens to collect in front of the upper and lower portions of any corneal lens due to the tears rivus along the eyelid margins. The configuration of the front surface of a solid bifocal with front surface addition (*Figure 5.27a*) is such that this tear lens may slightly reduce the front surface positive power at the periphery. If anything, then, it is wise to err on the positive side, and indeed many practitioners increase the addition they have determined, by as much as +1.00 D, to allow for this negative tear lens although its amount is rather variable depending as it does on the patient's tear output and the rate of evaporation in differing atmospheric conditions. Concern over the effect on the addition, of differences in thickness between the distance and near portions, is therefore seen to be unwarranted.

When the addition is on the back surface, no allowance for the effect of thickness need even be considered, but the major consideration here is that it is a plastic/tears interface, rather than a plastic/air interface.

In air the power of a PMMA surface depends on

$$\frac{1.490 - 1}{r}$$

whereas in tears it depends on

$$\frac{1.490 - 1.336}{r}$$

This is a factor of 0.49/0.154 or approximately 3.18 for PMMA lenses. (For RGP lenses of, for example, refractive index 1.45, this factor becomes 3.95, and for soft lenses of refractive index of 1.43 the factor becomes 4.57.) Thus, the practitioner and manufacturer must make the back surface radii such that they provide

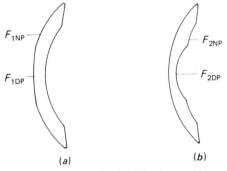

F_{1NP}

F_{1DP}

F_{2NP}

F_{2DP}

(a)   (b)

Figure 5.27 Concentric solid bifocal corneal lenses. (a) Front surface addition; (b) back surface addition

approximately three to four times the addition on the back surface (when measured in air) than is really required, due to the neutralizing effect of the tears. This point is important to remember when checking such a lens on the focimeter.

Usually this type of bifocal is fitted with a steep BCOZR (r_{2DP}) and small BCOZD, with the back peripheral optic zone radius (r_{2NP}) providing the near addition and fitted so as to align or be just flatter than the cornea. For example, if BPOZR (r_{2NP}) is 8.50 mm, reference to Appendix B, *Table B.I* for 1.490–1.336 shows F_{2NP} to be −18.118 D. (It is negative in power because the medium of higher refractive index is concave.) To give a +3.00 D addition requires that F_{2DP} be −21.118 D and thus r_{2DP}, the BCOZR, is seen by interpolation in the table, to be 7.27 mm. Now if this lens were measured in air on a focimeter, the radii of 8.50 mm and 7.27 mm would have surface powers, for 1.490–1, of −57.65 D and −67.40 D respectively (*see* Appendix B, *Table B.II*). Thus, the near addition measured in air is +9.75 D, which equals the near addition in tears × 3.18 (approximately), as stated above, depending on whether PMMA or some other material of different refractive index is used.

Fused bifocals

These are very similar to fused bifocal spectacle lenses except that most corneal lenses have the

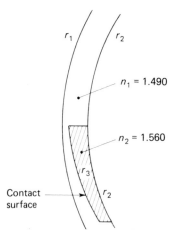

Figure 5.28 Fused bifocal corneal lens: r_1, r_2 and r_3 are the radii of the front, back and contact surfaces respectively; n_1 and n_2 are the refractive indices of the main lens and the near segment

segment on the back surface, and the refractive index of the fused segment is usually 1.56. The optical theory is easily understood if reference is made to *Figure 5.28*. Since the back surface is a negative surface and the segment has the higher refractive index, there is actually a gain in *negative* power at the back surface of

$$\frac{1.560 - 1.490}{r_2}$$

and where r_2 is in millimetres this expression becomes

$$\frac{-70}{r_2} \text{ D} = -8.75 \text{ D}$$

For example, if the BOZR (r_2) is 8.00 mm then the back surface powers in tears are:

$$F_{2DP} = \frac{(1.336 - 1.490)1000}{8.00} \text{ D} = -19.25 \text{ D}$$

(*see* Appendix B, *Table B.I*)

$$F_{2NP} = \frac{(1.336 - 1.560)1000}{8.00} \text{ D} = -28.00 \text{ D}$$

(*see* Appendix B, *Table B.X*)

The difference

$$F_{2NP} - F_{2DP} = -8.75 \text{ D} = \frac{-70}{8} \text{ D} \text{ (see above)}$$

This back surface power difference, due to the segment, may be obtained from Appendix B, *Table B.XI* for BOZR values ranging from 5.00 mm to 9.00 mm in 0.10 mm steps (and in 0.01 mm steps, by interpolation).

It should be emphasized here that the power difference due to the segment is the same whether the power is determined in air or in tears, because the BOZR (r_2), is the same throughout (as distinct from the back surface solid bifocal where $r_{2DP} < r_{2NP}$). This is easily shown using the same value for r_2 as above. The back surface powers in air are

$$F_{2DP} = \frac{(1 - 1.490)1000}{8.00} \text{ D} = -61.25 \text{ D}$$

(*see* Appendix B, *Table B.II*)

$$F_{2NP} = \frac{(1 - 1.560)1000}{8.00} \text{ D} = -70.00 \text{ D}$$

(*see* Appendix B, *Table B.IX*)

The difference, $F_{2NP} - F_{2DP} = -8.75 \text{ D} = \frac{-70}{8} \text{ D}$

This is exactly the same result as when the back surface powers were determined in tears (*see above*).

Because the back surface addition is the same measured in air as in tears, the addition read on a focimeter is the same as that on the eye.

Since the fused segment gives rise to a gain in negative power on the back surface, it must give rise to a gain in positive power at the contact surface sufficient to overcome the negative gain as well as to provide the near addition, i.e. if the power of the contact surface is F_3, then

$$F_3 = \text{Addition} - \left(-\frac{70}{r_2}\right) = \text{Addition} + \frac{70}{r_2}$$

Now F_3 (which is convex to the medium of higher refractive index)

$$= \frac{1.560 - 1.490}{r_3}D = \frac{70}{r_3}D \text{ (where } r_3 \text{ is in mm)}$$

And since $F_3 = \text{Addition} + \dfrac{70}{r_2}$

$$r_3 = \frac{70}{\text{Add.} + \dfrac{70}{r_2}}$$

(where the addition is in dioptres, and r_2 and r_3 are in millimetres).

Appendix B, *Table B.XII* gives r_3, the contact surface radius, for values of r_2, the BOZR, from 6.0 mm to 9.0 mm in 0.1 mm steps and additions from +1.00 D to +4.00 D in 0.50 D steps.

For example, if the addition were +3.00 D and the BOZR 8.00 mm,

then $F_3 = +3.00 - (-8.75) D = +11.75 D$

and $r_3 = \dfrac{(1.560 - 1.490) 1000}{11.75} \text{ mm} = 5.95 \text{ mm}$

(*see* Appendix B, *Table B.XI* used by looking up 11.75 D in the body of the table, and by interpolation, the corresponding radius is seen to be 5.95 mm).

However, r_3 is directly obtainable from Appendix B, *Table B.XII*, by reference to the BOZR (r_2) and the addition.

Optical changes of the eye caused by contact lenses

Contact lenses may bring about curvature, thickness and refractive index changes of the cornea. These effects, both with and without the contact lenses in place, are dealt with in Chapter 20.

Besides the effects mentioned in Chapter 20 it seems appropriate here to record the work of Carney (1975) who has used atmospheres of 100% oxygen tension and zero oxygen tension coupled with hard corneal lenses fitted both flat and steep to study curvature and thickness changes of the cornea induced by hard PMMA corneal lenses. A summary of his results suggests that all such lenses tend to mould the cornea to their own shape — flat lenses flattening and steep lenses steepening the central cornea. In addition, those lenses which give rise to central corneal oedema cause an unequal change in corneal thickness, it being greatest in the centre which leads to steepening of the corneal front surface. Now such steepening leads to an increase in myopia, and flattening to an increase in hypermetropia.

The resulting dioptric change in air, measurable as a change in ocular refraction, is largely masked by the wearing of the contact lens because the corneal change is neutralized by the tears. The ratio:

$$\frac{\text{Dioptric change in air}}{\text{Dioptric change with contact lens in place}}$$

$$= \frac{1.376 - 1.0}{1.376 - 1.336} = \frac{9.4}{1}$$

As can be seen it is dependent on the refractive index differences of the cornea in air relative to the cornea in tears. Thus, a person who becomes 1 D more myopic due to corneal steepening manifests less than 0.12 D of this while wearing his contact lenses.

The wearing of hard contact lenses tends to cause central corneal oedema and steepening, whilst the removal of the lenses results in central corneal thinning and flattening (Mandell and Polse, 1969; Polse, 1972). The mechanism of this change has been likened by Stone (1973) to the curvature change of a hard negative corneal lens during its hydration/dehydration cycle (Gordon, 1965). The resultant increases and decreases in myopia (and astigmatism) have been well documented by Rengstorff (*see* Chapter 20).

It is often not realized that the presence of corneal oedema alone can lead to a small increase in myopia — the lowering of the corneal refractive index due to the imbibition of water actually increases the total power of the cornea, a decrease in index of 0.01 giving rise to a power increase of approximately $+0.12\,\text{D}$. This surprising result occurs because the back surface of the cornea has no effect as a negative powered surface once the corneal refractive index drops to that of the aqueous (1.336). Therefore, as the corneal refractive index lowers during oedema, the corneal back surface has less and less neutralizing effect on the front surface power (Rengstorff and Arner, 1971). The small change in corneal thickness brought about by oedema has little effect, on its own, on corneal power. It is the lowering of refractive index and the accompanying curvature change which affects the refractive error.

With soft lens wear the cornea often suffers an increase in thickness due to oedema, but this occurs throughout the entire cornea and is not localized to the central region only as with hard PMMA corneal lens wear. The result is dependent on the degree of oedema, but the curvature change varies from very slight steepening to very slight flattening. The associated change in refractive error is also very small (Mandell, 1975). The oedema which leads to a uniform thickness increase in the cornea and therefore to a small increase in the anterior corneal radius which would decrease myopia, also leads to a drop in refractive index which would increase myopia. Thus, although soft lenses do bring about changes of the cornea, there is very little effect on refractive error and therefore very little associated 'spectacle blur'

Prescribing spectacles for contact lens wearers is a topic covered in Chapters 19 and 20. The corneal changes just described obviously influence the prescription for such spectacles.

Optical tables for contact lens work* with examples to illustrate their use

It is hoped that the tables incorporated in the appendices to this book will help to simplify and to speed up optical calculations which occur in the contact lens field. The principles involved are well covered elsewhere (Bennett, 1985), and are therefore not dealt with in detail here.

For those readers with access to a personal computer the programs which are printed and described in Appendix E should also ease the burden of more complex calculations. It will be seen that the tables printed in the other appendices at the end of

* Adapted from *Optical Tables for Contact Lens Work*, by J. L. Francis (1968). Hatton Press, London.

the book also refer to the appropriate computer program index numbers in Appendix E, and this section should be studied, bearing in mind that either the tables or the computer (or both) may be used in the resolution of optical problems.

Appendix A (program index no. 8 in Appendix E) shows the effective power of spectacle lenses at various distances from the back surface of the spectacle lens. Thus, it can be seen from the table that a lens of back vertex power $+7.00\,\text{D}$, has an effective power of $+7.76\,\text{D}$, in a plane 13 mm from the back surface of the lens, while the effective power of a $-7.00\,\text{D}$ lens at the same vertex distance is $-6.41\,\text{D}$. From this table, then, can be obtained very quickly the effective power of a trial spectacle lens at the eye. A comprehensive table of this sort can be useful in other ways, such as comparing spectacle and ocular refraction, in assessing the correction of astigmatism in near vision and in the determination of spectacle and ocular accommodation.

The contact lens

In Appendix B, *Table B.I*, the surface powers in air and for PMMA/tears (1.49–1.336) corresponding to a given radius of curvature has been plotted for various refractive indices. For the refractive index differences of (1.49–1) and (1.336–1), *see* Appendix B, *Tables B.II* and *B.V* respectively. Steps of 0.01 mm in radius have been used so that the corresponding steps in power are small enough for the table to be used in the reverse direction, i.e. the radius required to produce a given change in light vergence can be found with sufficient accuracy. To illustrate this, suppose a pencil of rays has been traced 'backwards' through a lens of index 1.49, and when incident on the front surface the divergence of the pencil is $-71.50\,\text{D}$. If the light is to emerge into air as a parallel pencil then the front surface must have a power of $+71.50\,\text{D}$. Looking down the appropriate power column of Appendix B, *Table B.II*, the nearest figure listed is 71.53 and the corresponding radius is 6.85 mm.

Table B.III (*see also* Appendix E, program index no. 1) is based in *Table B.II* but enables the change in surface power resulting from a given change of radius to be looked up directly. It applies to material in air ($n = 1.490$) and can be helpful when it is decided to fit a contact lens with a toroidal surface. For example, if the BOZR chosen for one principal meridian is 8.0 mm and that of the second principal meridian is 7.1 mm, then the difference in power between the two meridians, in air, is found from *Table B.III* to be 7.76 D. Since it is the back surface of the contact lens which is being dealt with, it is the steeper meridian which has the greater negative power.

It should also be clear that *Table B.III* can be used to give an estimate of the 'thin lens' power of a contact lens in air, i.e. the sum of the surface powers without allowance for thickness. So, if a lens has a front surface radius of 8.50 mm and a back surface radius of 7.80 mm, it can be seen from *Table B.III* that the corresponding thin lens power in air is −5.17 D, the negative sign agreeing with the fact that the back surface has the steeper radius.

Appendix B, *Table B.IV*, shows directly the change in reduced vergence due to thickness for a given initial vergence. This greatly reduces the labour involved in this type of calculation and eliminates reference to reciprocal tables and to tables of reduced thickness. This table covers initial vergences from 100.0 D to 40.0 D in 2.0 D steps for a range of thicknesses from 0.01 mm to 1.50 mm, the upper part of this range being included to cover the case of rather thick scleral lenses. In each cell of the table the lower figure gives the increase in vergence due to thickness for convergent light, while the upper figure indicates the decrease in vergence due to thickness for divergent light. The use of *Table B.IV* is best illustrated by some numerical examples. *Table B.IV* is based on the use of PMMA material of refractive index 1.49.

Example

To find the BVP in air, of a contact lens of given radii of curvature and thickness.

Take $r_1 = +7.05$ mm, $r_2 = +8.00$ mm, $t = 0.6$ mm

From Appendix B, *Table B.II*, the surface powers are found to be, $F_1 = +69.50$ D and $F_2 = -61.25$ D, so a pencil of parallel rays incident on the front surface of the lens becomes convergent after refraction to the extent of +69.50 D. Now entering the 'initial vergence' column of *Table B.IV* at the nearest figure to 69.50, i.e. at 70.00, find at this level the cell corresponding to a thickness of 0.60 mm. Since the rays are convergent use the lower figure in the cell: +2.03. This is the increase in vergence due to thickness. Thus, the rays incident on the second surface of the lens have a vergence of +69.50 + 2.03 = +71.53 D. Addition of the back surface power, with due regard to sign, gives the required back vertex power in air. Thus, BVP = +71.53 − 61.25 = +10.28 D. The process takes much longer to describe than to do. It can be conveniently set out as follows:

Sum of the surface powers	+69.50
	−61.25
	+ 8.25
Add thickness allowance	+ 2.03
BVP =	+10.28 D

It will be appreciated that some degree of approximation is involved owing to the steps used in the vergence column of Appendix B, *Table B.IV*, but errors due to this are small. In the above example, more accurate calculations give a result of +10.25 D,

so the error in the approximate result is 0.03 D, nearly 0.3%. If greater accuracy in using *Table B.IV* is desired, it is not difficult to interpolate between the rows.

Example

To find the front surface power, in air, of a contact lens of given BVP, BOZR and thickness.

Consider a PMMA lens 0.50 mm thick, of BVP = −20.00 D and BOZR = 7.80 mm

From Appendix B, *Table B.II*, the back surface power = −62.82 D

Now tracing backwards through the lens, take a pencil of rays, which initially converges towards the posterior focus of the lens, i.e. a pencil with an incident vergence of +20.00 D.

Incident vergence at back surface	+20.00
Back surface power to be added	−62.82
Vergence after refraction	−42.82 D

Entering Appendix B, *Table B.IV*, at 42.0 D the thickness allowance where $t = 0.5$ mm is 0.58 D (upper figure for divergent light), but for 44.0 D the allowance is 0.64. By interpolation therefore take 0.61 as the allowance for an initial vergence of 42.82 D. So adding 0.61 to −42.82 D gives the vergence of light reaching the front surface as −42.21 D. Clearly the front surface power required is of equal amount but opposite sign, namely, +42.21 D. From Appendix B, *Table B.II*, the corresponding radius of curvature is seen to be +11.61 mm.

This type of calculation can easily be applied to each principal meridian in turn when the lens considered has a back toroidal surface.

As a further example of the use of the tables discussed so far, consider the following. In a particular case, a choice of BOZR has been made and an afocal lens of this radius is placed on the eye. It is then found that a trial spectacle lens of +5.00 D placed 12 mm in front of the contact lens is necessary to correct the residual refractive error. The problem is: What BVP should be ordered for the finished contact lens? The liquid lens is not involved here as this is assumed to be the same in the trial set up as with the finished lens. If the BOZR chosen is 7.90 mm and the afocal lens used is 0.25 mm thick, first it is necessary to find the characteristics of the afocal lens. From Appendix B, *Table B.II*, $F_2 = 62.03$ D. Using Appendix B, *Table B.IV*, the thickness allowance for divergent light is 0.64 D so the front surface power of the afocal lens is − (−62.03 + 0.64) = +62.03 − 0.64 = +61.39 D, and *Table B.II* gives the corresponding radius as 7.98 mm. Tracing a pencil of parallel rays through the spectacle trial lens and the afocal contact lens:

Vergence after refraction at $+5.00\,D$ spectacle trial lens	$+\ 5.00$
Effective power at 12 mm (from Appendix A)	$+\ 5.32$
Front surface power of afocal contact lens to be added	$+61.39$
	$+66.71$
Allowance for thickness (from Appendix B, *Table B.IV*)	$+\ 0.76$
Incident vergence at second surface	$+67.47$
Back surface power of contact lens to be added	-62.03
Vergence in air after refraction	$+\ 5.44\,D$

The BVP to be ordered for the finished lens is thus $+5.44\,D$. Should the trial contact lens employed not be afocal, the calculation is entirely similar, the characteristics of the trial contact lens being determined as in the previous example.

The liquid lens

Tables B.V and *B.VI* are of similar type to *Tables B.II* and *B.III*, but are applicable to the liquid lens in air and are therefore based on a refractive index of 1.336. (Appendix E, program index no. 1 may be used to derive liquid lens power.) To find the power of the liquid lens in air the procedure is as follows. In a particular case let the BOZR of the contact lens be 8.00 mm, and the radius of curvature of the cornea be 7.80 mm. The surface powers of the liquid lens are obtained from *Table B.V*. These are $F_1 = +42.00\,D$ and $F_2 = -43.08\,D$, so considered as a thin lens the power of the liquid lens is the sum of these two powers $= -1.08\,D$. If the thickness of the liquid lens is 0.10 mm the effect of this can be found from *Table B.VII*. Entering this table at 42.0 D the allowance for a thickness of 0.10 mm is 0.13 D, and in this case is to be added. The BVP of the liquid lens in air thus $= +42.00 - 43.08 + 0.13 = -0.95\,D$.

The quantity which matters most in the correction of an ametropic eye is, of course, the back vertex power of the contact lens and liquid lens combined. A good approximation to this is obtained simply by adding the BVP of the contact lens to that of the liquid lens. For instance, if the contact lens in the example just quoted had a BVP in air of $-10.00\,D$, then the combination of contact lens plus liquid lens has a BVP of approximately $-10.95\,D$. If greater accuracy is required then the procedure is as follows.

With a contact lens of BVP $= -10.00\,D$ the vergence of light incident on the first surface of the liquid lens $= -10.00\,D$. Vergence after refraction at the first surface of the liquid lens $= +42.00 - 10.00 = +32.00\,D$.

Entering Appendix B, *Table B.VII* at 32.0 D, the thickness allowance for 0.10 mm $= 0.08\,D$, so the BVP of the combined contact and liquid lens is

$+32.00 - 43.08 + 0.08 = -11.00\,D$ in air. This result differs by only 0.05 D from the approximate one obtained earlier. A greater difference may arise in cases having a thicker liquid lens and a contact lens of considerable back vertex power. It should be remembered that nowadays when most cases are fitted with corneal and soft lenses, the tears thickness is so small that sufficient accuracy is obtained by ignoring any thickness allowance for the liquid lens. In these cases the power of the liquid lens is obtained by adding the two surface powers or perhaps more quickly, by using *Table B.VI* as outlined below.

Table B.VI (*see also* Appendix E, program index no. 1) gives directly the change in surface power resulting from a given change in radius for the liquid lens in air. This is probably the quickest way of estimating the liquid lens power, the effect of thickness being ignored. Thus, if the liquid lens has a front surface radius of 7.70 mm and a back surface radius of 7.60 mm, then the thin lens power is obtained directly from *Table B.VI* as $-0.57\,D$. The table may also be used when a toroidal surface is involved.

The right-hand column of *Table B.I* also gives interface powers for various radii of the back surface of the contact lens when in contact with the liquid lens (i.e. 1.49–1.336 or relative index $n_R = 0.154$), and *Table B.VIII* needs little explanation. It gives the change in power resulting from a change of radius (also for $n_R = 0.154$). Thus, a decision to alter the back optic zone radius of the contact lens from 8.00 mm (r_1 in the table) to 7.90 mm (r_2 in the table) changes the power of the contact surface by 0.24 D, and since the surface of higher refractive index is a negative surface (the back surface of the contact lens) the effect of the modification is to add $-0.24\,D$. This type of modification is often made to final sighted scleral lenses in order to improve the fit of the optic zone, and may then necessitate an alteration to the front surface power of the contact lens in order to compensate for the change in interface power and keep the combination BVP of the contact lens/liquid lens the same (*see* Chapter 18).

Fused bifocal contact lenses

Tables B.IX–B.XII relate to fused bifocal corneal lenses. The underlying theory has already been explained (*see* pp. 223–224, and *Figure 5.28*).

Table B.IX gives surface powers in air for plastic materials of refractive index 1.560, the material of which the fused segment is made. Thus, it can be used for determining the power of the back surface of the segment in air for BOZR values between 5.00 mm and 9.00 mm in 0.10 mm steps (and in 0.01 mm steps, by interpolation using the difference column). For example, if the BOZR is 8.05 mm, power F for $r = 8.00$ mm, is 70.0000 D. The difference for a 0.01 mm change in r is 0.0886 D, and therefore for a 0.05 mm change in r the difference is $5 \times 0.0886\,\text{D}$. This difference is thus $0.443\,\text{D}$ and evidently must be subtracted from $70.0000\,\text{D}$ giving $F = 69.557\,\text{D}$. This may be verified by calculating the power value midway between the powers for $r = 8.00\,\text{mm}$ and $r = 8.10\,\text{mm}$, which gives $69.568\,\text{D}$. This gives a small discrepancy of $0.01\,\text{D}$ in the second place of decimals, which is of no significance. Having determined the power value, it must be ascribed a sign, and since it is a concave surface, the power is $-69.57\,\text{D}$.

Table B.X is similar to *Table B.IX*, but gives the surface powers in tears $(1.560 - 1.336)$ and may therefore be used for determining the back surface power of the fused segment when on the eye. Again, this is a negative power since the surface is concave to the medium of higher refractive index. Used with *Tables B.II* and *B.I* for $(1.490-1)$ and $(1.490 - 1.336)$ respectively, *Tables B.IX* and *B.X* permit the power of the back surface of the segment to be compared with the back surface power of the main lens, both in air (*Tables B.IX* and *B.II*) and in tears (*Tables B.X* and *B.I*). Differences in power on the back surface between the segment and the main lens may thus be determined, but this information is directly obtainable from *Table B.XI* for $(1.560 - 1.490)$. *Table B.XI* can also be used for determining contact surface powers for radii (r_3 in *Figure 5.28*) from $5.00\,\text{mm}$ to $9.00\,\text{mm}$ in $0.10\,\text{mm}$ steps (and again by interpolation, in $0.01\,\text{mm}$ steps).

Table B.XII allows the radius, r_3, of the contact surface to be determined for various near additions and values of the BOZR. Thus for a BOZR of $8.00\,\text{mm}$ and a near addition of $+3.00\,\text{D}$, a contact surface radius, r_3, of $5.9574\,\text{mm}$, say, $5.96\,\text{mm}$ is required (compare p. 224).

Aspects of contact lens design

The main purpose of this section is to give some guidelines to those contact lens practitioners who wish to design their own lenses. It is hoped that they can then avoid the pitfall of ordering a lens of such thickness that it is impossible to manufacture. While intended primarily for the design of hard corneal lenses, the principles outlined in this section may be applied to any type of contact lens.

Readers are referred to Creighton's *Contact Lenses Fabrication Tables* (1964) for a more detailed exposition on this subject, also papers by Campbell (1987) on the calculation of tear volume between lens and cornea, and Young (1988) who gives an overview of computer-assisted contact lens design.

The computer program section of this book (Appendix E) should allow users of personal computers to carry out the following tedious iterative calculations extremely quickly. However, *Figures 5.29–5.35* and the accompanying explanatory text should provide a firm understanding of the principles involved. Although not included in Appendix E, the use of a computer permits much more complex lens forms to be considered than the multi-curve spherical design considered in the text here. It is thus possible to cope with aspherical lens surfaces in conjunction with ellipsoidal corneal surfaces of specific asphericity, and to design lenses to give a required central tear layer thickness and a specified corneal clearance at the lens edge (as also discussed in Chapter 10). Readers are recommended to study the definitive work of Bennett (1988) on the subject of aspheric and continuous curve contact lenses.

Sagitta of front and back surfaces
(*see also* Appendix E, program index nos 11 and 12)

It should be obvious from *Figure 5.29* that for both positive and negative lenses the sagitta or sag value, s, of the front surface of a lens plus the axial edge thickness, t_{ea}, must equal the primary sag (of the back surface), p, plus the centre thickness, t_c. Thus $s + t_{ea} = p + t_c$.

For a positive lens there is a danger of ordering the centre thickness too small to permit adequate edge thickness, and for a negative lens the attempt to keep the edge thickness reasonably small may result in the centre of the lens becoming excessively thin.

The values for p and s may be found as follows.

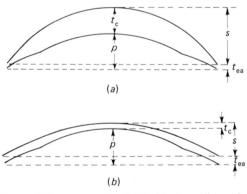

Figure 5.29 $s + t_{ea} = p + t_c$. (a) Positive lens; (b) negative lens

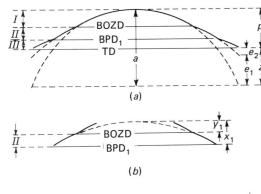

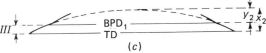

Figure 5.30 Back surface of a lens. (*a*) $p = I + II + III$; $z = a - p$; $z = e_1 + e_2$. (*b*) $II = x_1 - y_1$. (*c*) $III = x_2 - y_2$

Primary sag (p)

From *Figure 5.30* it can be seen that the primary sag of the back surface of a tri-curve corneal lens is $I + II + III$, where I is the sag of the BOZR at the BOZD. II and III may be determined by studying *Figure 5.30b, c*.

Thus, $II = x_1 - y_1$ where x_1 is the sag of BPR_1 at BPD_1 and y_1 is the sag of BPR_1 at BOZD. III is determined in exactly the same manner as II (*see Figure 5.30c*).

Thus, $III, = x_2 - y_2$ where x_2 is the sag of BPR_2 at TD (or BPD_2 if the lens has more than three back surface curves) and y_2 is the sag of BPR_2 at BPD_1.

It can be seen, then, that the primary sag of a C3 lens is given by $p = I + (x_1 - y_1) + (x_2 - y_2)$ and for a C4 lens $p = I + (x_1 - y_1) + (x_2 - y_2) + (x_3 - y_3)$.

All the individual sag values may be obtained directly or by interpolation from Appendix C (*see also* Appendix E). For example, the tri-curve corneal lens C3/8.00:7.0/9.05:7.8/10.80:8.6 has a primary sag, p, which can be calculated as follows.

I = sag of BOZR of 8.00 mm at BOZD of 7.00 mm = **0.806 mm**

$II = x_1 - y_1$

Now x_1 = sag of 9.05 mm (BPR_1) at 7.8 mm (BPD_1) = 0.884 mm (by interpolation in Appendix C).

y_1 = sag of 9.05 mm (BPR_1) at 7.0 mm (BOZD) = 0.704 mm (by interpolation in Appendix C)

Thus, II = 0.884 − 0.704 = **0.180 mm**, $III = x_2 - y_2$

Now x_2 = sag of 10.80 mm (BPR_2) at 8.6 mm (TD) = 0.893 mm

and y_2 = sag of 10.80 mm (BPR_2) at 7.8 mm (BPD_1) = 0.729 mm

So III = 0.893 − 0.729 = **0.164 mm**

And primary sag, $p = I + II + III = 0.806 + 0.180 + 0.164 = $ **1.150 mm**

Front surface sag (s)

Now suppose the lens with the above primary sag value of 1.150 mm is to be made up with BVP of +2.00 D. It is then necessary to determine the front surface radius in order to calculate the sag, s, of the front surface. To obtain the front surface radius, r_1, necessitates guessing a value for the centre thickness, t_c. In this case, suppose $t_c = 0.21$ mm. Then r_1 may be calculated as described on p. 226.

Taking a pencil of rays backwards through the lens:

Incident vergence at back surface	$= -\,2.00$ D
Power of back surface to be added	$= -61.25$ D
(*see* Appendix B, *Table B.II*)	
Vergence after refraction	$= -63.25$ D
Allowance for 0.21 mm t_c	$= +\,0.56$ D
(*see* Appendix B, *Table B.IV*)	
Vergence reaching front surface	$= -62.69$ D
Front surface power	$= +62.69$ D
Front surface radius, r_1	$=\quad 7.815$ mm
(*see* Appendix B, *Table B.II*)	
And sag, s, of r_1 at TD of 8.6 mm	$=$ **1.289 mm**
(by interpolation in Appendix C)	

Axial edge thickness (t_{ea})

When using sagitta-involved methods of designing lenses it is necessary to measure thickness values parallel to the primary axis of the lens, although this involves using axial edge and junction thicknesses, which are terms not used in International Standard ISO 8320–1986 and British Standard 3521: Part 3: 1988. The abbreviation t_{ea} has therefore been used here to denote axial edge thickness, and similarly t_{ja} to denote axial junction thickness, as compared to t_e and t_j which refer to the respective radial measurements as defined in the International and British Standards.

Continuing the above example it is known that $s + t_{ea} = p + t_c$ (*Figure 5.29*). Thus, $1.289 + t_{ea} = 1.150 + 0.21$ and $t_{ea} = \mathbf{0.071\,mm}$.

Bearing in mind that this is an edge thickness value measured parallel to the primary axis of the lens and not radial edge thickness measured perpendicular to the surface (which would give a slightly lower value), this would be too small an edge thickness to allow adequate rounding to be carried out. It may be decided, therefore, to increase the edge thickness by 0.10 to 0.171 mm. If this is done the centre thickness will obviously be altered by a similar amount to 0.31 mm. This involves recalculating the front surface radius to allow for the new centre thickness. Hence, a new value will be obtained for s, and ultimately a slightly modified value for t_{ea}. The calculation is as follows.

Incident vergence at back surface	$= -2.00$ D	
Power of back surface to be added	$= -61.25$ D	(As before)
Vergence after refraction	$= -63.25$ D	
Allowance for 0.31 mm t_c	$= +0.82$ D	
(*see* Appendix B, *Table B.IV*)		
Vergence reaching front surface	$= -62.43$ D	
Front surface power	$= +62.43$ D	
Front surface radius, r_1	$= 7.85$ mm	
(*see* Appendix B, *Table B.II*)		

With this new value for r_1 of 7.85 mm, sag, s, at 8.6 mm TD $= \mathbf{1.2825\,mm}$ (Appendix C).

Again, since $s + t_{ea} = p + t_c$
$$1.2825 + t_{ea} = 1.150 + 0.31$$
$$\text{and } t_{ea} = 0.1775 = \mathbf{0.178\,mm}$$

This edge thickness is slightly greater than that required above (0.171 mm), but is probably near enough from a clinical and manufacturing standpoint, particularly as this measurement is for a value determined parallel to the axis of the lens, and edge thicknesses are normally measured perpendicular to the surface which would result in a smaller value of, say, 0.15–0.16 mm. However, if this value for edge thickness is now greater than required further calculation could be done, reducing t_{ea} and t_c by a similar amount, recalculating s and obtaining a final value for t_{ea}.

Lenticular lenses

If, in the above example, it is felt that the t_c value of 0.31 mm is too great, but the axial edge

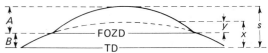

Figure 5.31 Front surface of a lenticular lens: $s = A + B$; $B = x - y$

thickness of 0.178 mm is desirable, then a lenticular front surface may be designed. Its central and peripheral radii may be determined as follows. Remembering that $s + t_{ea} = p + t_c$, suppose a t_c value of 0.21 mm is desired, then the sag of the front surface,

$$s = p + t_c - t_{ea}$$
$$= 1.15 + 0.21 - 0.178$$
$$= \mathbf{1.182\,mm}$$

If a lenticular front surface is to be made, then its total sag, s, will be composed of two portions, A and B (*Figure 5.31*), where A is the sag of the FOZR, r_1, at FOZD, and $B = x - y$, where $x =$ sag of FPR at TD and $y =$ sag of FPR at FOZD.

Now in the example being used, r_1 has already been calculated for a t_c value of 0.21 mm, and $r_1 = 7.815$ mm (*see* p. 229 under Front surface sag).

It is convenient to make the lenticular diameter the same as the back optic zone diameter, i.e. let FOZD = BOZD = 7.0 mm

Thus, $A =$ sag of r_1, 7.815 mm, at FOZD, 7.0 mm $= \mathbf{0.827\,mm}$ (by interpolation in Appendix C). But, $s = 1.182$ mm, and as $B = s - A$, then $B = \mathbf{0.355\,mm}$.

Determination of front peripheral radius

Now a front peripheral radius (FPR) must be found which gives a value for B of $\mathbf{0.355\,mm} = x - y$.

At first this value must be guessed, but some idea of where to start 'guessing' is obtained by taking a mean of the back peripheral radii, erring if anything on the flat side. In the example being used the back peripheral radii are 9.05 and 10.80 mm, the mean being 9.925 mm. Guessing the FPR as 10.00 mm gives:

$x =$ sag of 10.00 mm FPR at 8.6 mm TD $= 0.972$ mm

$y =$ sag of 10.00 mm FPR at 7.0 mm FOZD
$= 0.633$ mm

Thus, $B = x - y = \mathbf{0.339\,mm}$

Now this is slightly smaller than the value of 0.355 mm required for B. Therefore, 10.00 mm must be slightly too flat a radius to use for the

FPR. A second guess is therefore made, say 9.80 mm, the steeper radius giving a greater sag value. Using 9.80 mm for the FPR x and y are again calculated:

Thus, x = sag of 9.80 mm at 8.6 mm TD
     = 0.994 mm

and y = sag of 9.80 mm at 7.00 mm FOZD
       = 0.646 mm

so $B = x - y = \mathbf{0.348\,mm}$

This is within 0.007 mm of the required value for B.

Trying yet again and using 9.60 mm for the FPR gives:

x = sag of 9.60 mm at 8.6 mm = 1.017 mm

y = sag of 9.60 mm at 7.0 mm = 0.661 mm

Also $B = x - y = \mathbf{0.356\,mm}$ which is only 0.001 mm greater than the required value.

This is near enough to be used, and the front surface sag value, s, which equals $A + B$ is therefore 0.827 mm + 0.356 mm. Hence, s = 1.183 mm. As this is 0.001 mm greater than originally required, the axial edge thickness will be reduced by this amount from 0.178 mm to 0.177 mm. Obviously this is of no significance.

Form of the carrier zone

It is of interest here to know how the axial edge thickness, t_{ea}, compares to the axial junction thickness, t_{ja}, at the edge of the lenticular zone. The form of the carrier zone of a lenticular lens affects the position which the lens takes up on the eye. A lens is said to have a negative carrier zone when its edge thickness is greater than the junction thickness and a positive carrier zone when the reverse applies, the thickness relationship being similar to that of negative and positive lenses. Now lenses having negative and parallel surfaced carrier zones have been found to provide better attachment of the lens to the upper eyelid than positive carrier zones, which encourage the lens to drop. It is therefore desirable for the edge thickness to be equal to or greater than the junction thickness in order to provide a parallel surfaced or negative zone, respectively (see Chapter 10).

In the example already calculated, Figure 5.32 shows the central portion of the lens. Evidently $I + t_c = A + t_{ja}$.

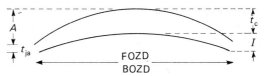

Figure 5.32 Central zone of lenticular lens: $A + t_{ja} = t_c + I$

Thus, $t_{ja} = I + t_c - A$

     = 0.806 + 0.21 - 0.827

     = **0.189 mm**

Now the axial edge thickness is 0.177 mm, and since the axial junction thickness is greater than the axial edge thickness the lens has a positive carrier zone, which, in most cases, is not desirable.

To ensure either a negative or else a parallel surfaced carrier zone, a minimum axial junction thickness of about 0.14 mm is usually desirable on positive lenticular lenses. (If thinner than this lenses of polymethyl methacrylate material are liable to crack around the edge of the lenticular zone if subjected to any accidental squeezing between the fingers.) However, in the example used, reducing the junction thickness from 0.189 mm by 0.049 mm to 0.14 mm would necessitate reducing the centre thickness from 0.21 mm, by the same amount, 0.049 mm, to 0.161 mm.

This involves recalculating the entire front surface of the lens. Therefore, let t_c now be 0.16 mm.

Tracing a pencil of rays backwards through the lens gives:

Incident vergence at back surface	= -2.00 D
Power of back surface to be added	= -61.25 D
(As before – see p. 229)	
Vergence after refraction	= -63.25 D
Allowance for 0.16 mm t_c	= $+0.43$ D
(see Appendix B, Table B. IV)	
Vergence reaching front surface	= -62.82 D
Front surface power	= $+62.82$ D
Front surface radius	= 7.80 mm
(see Appendix B, Table B.II)	
Sag A of 7.80 mm at FOZD 7.0 mm	= 0.829 mm

Now $s + t_{ea} = p + t_c$

Thus, $s + t_{ea} = 1.150 + 0.16 = 1.31$ mm

Obviously, having decided on a lenticular design any edge thickness can be chosen. If a parallel surfaced carrier zone is required, which should provide attachment to the upper lid with minimum axial edge thickness, then a t_{ea} value of 0.14 mm is indicated – the same as the axial junction thickness.

Thus, $s + 0.14 = 1.31$ and so $s = 1.17$ mm

But $s = A + B$ (*see Figure 5.31*)

Thus, $B = 1.17 - 0.829 = 0.341$ mm

Now a value for FPR must be found which yields a value for B of 0.341 mm.

Referring to previous calculations (*see* p. 230) shows that a value for FPR of 10.00 mm gives B = 0.339 mm. Evidently then, since this value for B is only 0.002 mm less than that required, a value of 10.00 mm for the FPR would be adequate and would give an axial edge thickness of 0.142 mm, resulting in a lens with a very slightly negative carrier zone.

Negative lenses

An entirely similar approach may be used for determining the front surface radii of negative lenses and if excessive edge thickness would be a problem a reduced optic design can be employed. The front peripheral radius of the carrier zone may then be determined in order to arrive at the desired edge thickness (*Figure 5.33*).

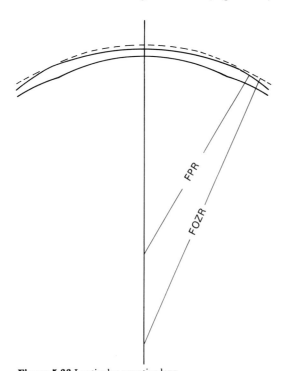

Figure 5.33 Lenticular negative lens

With negative lenses of high power, a desirable edge thickness frequently results in the lens having a positive carrier zone because the edge thickness is less than the junction thickness. This positive carrier zone encourages the lens to drop whereas it may be more desirable for the lens to attach to the upper lid. Since 'lid attachment' is more likely to be achieved with a negative or parallel surfaced carrier zone some way must be found of reducing the junction thickness of these high minus lenses. By creating a front junction radius (FJR) the junction thickness may be reduced so that it is equal to or less than the edge thickness, the carrier zone thereby becoming parallel surfaced or negative, respectively. Such an FJR is shown in *Figure 5.34*.

Occasionally, with very highly powered negative lenses a front junction radius is necessary anyway to join the FOZR to the FPR. From *Figure 5.34* it can be seen that the FJR is a shorter radius than either the FOZR or FPR.

If, for example, the FOZD and BOZD are the same (say, 7.0 mm) and the axial junction thickness at that diameter is 0.20 mm (t_{ja1}), but really a junction thickness of 0.14 mm is desired, then a radius is determined which will give this value of 0.14 mm (t_{ja2}) at a diameter of, say, 7.6 mm (FJD) as a compromise.

Reference to *Figure 5.34* shows that sag, j, of the junction radius $= b - c$, where $b =$ sag of FJR at FJD and $c =$ sag of FJR at FOZD.

Also sag, v, of BPR_1 at the width of the FJR $= x_j - y_j$, where $x_j =$ sag of BPR_1 at FJD and $y_j =$ sag of BPR_1 at FOZD. (Note that FOZD = BOZD.)

Now $t_{ja1} = u + j$ or $j = t_{ja1} - u$ and $t_{ja2} = u + v$ or $u = t_{ja2} - v$.

What is required is that $t_{ja2} = 0.14$ mm

$x_j =$ sag of 9.05 mm (BPR_1) at 7.6 mm (FJD)
  $= 0.837$ mm

$y_j =$ sag of 9.05 mm (BPR_1) at 7.0 mm (FOZD)
  $= 0.704$ mm

and $x_j - y_j = v = \mathbf{0.133\,mm}$

Since $u = t_{ja2} - v$
  $u = 0.14 - 0.133 = \mathbf{0.007\,mm}$

and since $j = t_{ja1} - u$
  $j = 0.20 - 0.007 = \mathbf{0.193\,mm}$

Thus, a radius (FJR) must be found for which $j = 0.193$ mm and, as $j = b - c$ (*Figure 5.34*),

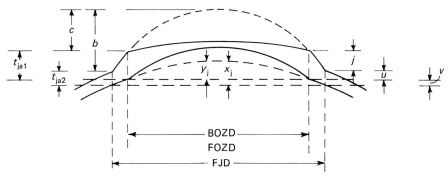

Figure 5.34 Lenticular negative lens with front junction radius: $j = b - c$; $t_{ja1} = j + u$; $t_{ja2} = u + v$; $v = x_j - y_j$

then $b - c$ also equals 0.193 mm. At first the radius must be guessed, say, FJR = 6.00 mm.

Thus, b = sag of 6.00 mm (FJR) at 7.6 mm (FJD)
       = 1.357 mm

and c = sag of 6.00 mm (FJR) at 7.0 mm (FOZD)
       = 1.127 mm

so $j = b - c = 0.230$ mm

This is too large a value for j and therefore 6.00 mm must be slightly too steep a value for FJR. A flatter value for FJR is therefore selected, say, 7.00 mm.

Again b = sag of 7.00 mm (FJR) at 7.6 mm (FJD)
        = 1.121 mm

and c = sag of 7.00 mm (FJR) at 7.0 mm (FOZD)
        = 0.938 mm

so $j = b - c = 0.183$ mm

This is now too small a value for j, which needs to be 0.193 mm, and therefore 7.00 mm is too flat a value for FJR. However, 7.00 mm is obviously much closer to the right value for FJR than was 6.00 mm (which gave a value for j of 0.230 mm). Guessing again at a value nearer 7.00 mm than 6.00 mm, 6.75 mm can be tried for FJR.

Now b = sag of 6.75 mm (FJR) at 7.6 mm (FJD)
        = 1.171 mm

and c = sag of 6.75 mm (FJR) at 7.0 mm (FOZD)
        = 0.978 mm

so $j = b - c = 0.193$ mm which is exactly the value required

Thus, a junction radius of 6.75 mm is necessary on the front surface to join FOZR to FPR and reduce the junction thickness from 0.20 mm to 0.14 mm. This then allows a suitable carrier zone to be designed.

Axial edge lift

Another aspect of lens design is to create peripheral curves which will give a desired axial edge lift (see Chapter 10 and Appendix E, program index no. 6). This may be done by calculation in the following manner.

From *Figure 5.35a* it is seen that for a tri-curve lens, the axial edge lift $z = a - p$ where p is the primary sag and equals $I + II + III$ (see *Figure 5.30a*). If the two peripheral curves are to

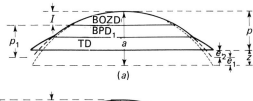

(a)

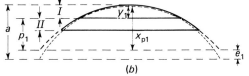

(b)

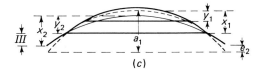

(c)

Figure 5.35 (a) Axial edge lift $z = e_1 + e_2 = a - p$.
(b) $e_1 = a - (I + p_1)$ and $p_1 = x_{p1} - y_1$.
(c) $e_2 = a_1 - x_1 - III$ and $III = x_2 - y_2$

contribute equally to the edge lift then e_1 must be equal to e_2 where $e_1 + e_2 = z$.

For example, a lens has a BOZR of 8.00 mm. The BOZD is 7.0 mm, BPD_1 is 7.8 mm and TD is 8.6 mm. An axial edge lift of 0.12 mm is required, of which 0.06 mm is to be contributed by BPR_1 and 0.06 mm by BPR_2. The values for BPR_1 and BPR_2 to give the necessary edge lift are determined as follows.

BPR₁

From *Figure 5.35b* it can be seen that the lens is treated first as if it were a bi-curve lens with BPR_1 extending out to the TD.

Then $e_1 = a - (I + p_1)$ where $p_1 = x_{p1} - y_1$

x_{p1} and y_1 are the sags of BPR_1 at TD and BOZD respectively

From above, $a = e_1 + I + p_1$ and so $p_1 = a - I - e_1$

Now a = sag of 8.00 mm (BOZR) at 8.6 mm (TD)
   = 1.254 mm

   I = sag of 8.00 mm (BOZR) at 7.0 mm (BOZD)
   = 0.806 mm

and $p_1 = a - I - e_1 = 1.254 - 0.806 - 0.06$
   = **0.388 mm**

It is now necessary to guess a value for BPR_1 which will permit x_{p1} and y_1 to be determined so as to give a value for p_1 as near to this value of 0.388 mm as possible, because $p_1 = x_{p1} - y_1$. So, let $BPR_1 = 9.00$ mm.

Then x_{p1} = sag of 9.00 mm (BPR_1) at 8.6 mm (TD)
   = 1.094 mm

   y_1 = sag of 9.00 mm (BPR_1) at 7.0 mm (BOZD)
   = 0.708 mm

giving $p_1 = x_{p1} - y_1$
   = 1.094 - 0.708
   = **0.386 mm**

This value for p_1 is close enough to the value for p_1 found above (from $a - I - e_1$) not to require further calculation. Hence, BPR_1 can be taken as 9.00 mm. Had the value for p_1 found from $x_{p1} - y_1$ been considerable different from 0.388 mm then it would have been necessary to recalculate using another value for BPR_1. A figure much smaller than 0.388 mm would have indicated that too flat a value had been selected for BPR_1 and that recalculation using a steeper value was necessary. Conversely, a value much greater than 0.388 mm would have indicated that too steep a value had been selected for

BPR_1 and that recalculation using a flatter value is necessary. As it is, the use of 9.00 mm for BPR_1 leads to a very small error of 0.002 mm in p_1 indicating that e_1 will be 0.062 mm instead of 0.060 mm (because $e_1 = a - I - p_1$). Now the remainder of the edge lift, z, is contributed by BPR_2 and is e_2. But $e_2 = z - e_1 = 0.12 - 0.062 = 0.058$ mm.

BPR₂

Thus, a value for BPR_2 must now be guessed at, which will, after calculation, yield a result of 0.058 mm for e_2.

Calculations to determine e_2 are similar to those for e_1. From *Figure 5.35c*, $e_2 = a_1 - x_1 - III$, where a_1 is the sag of BPR_1 at TD, x_1 is the sag of BPR_1 at BPD_1 and III is now $x_2 - y_2$ (*see Figure 5.35c*). x_2 is the sag of BPR_2 at TD, and y_2 is the sag of BPR_2 at BPD_2. Thus, $III = a_1 - x_1 - e_2$.

Thus, a_1 = sag of 9.00 mm (BPR_1) at 8.6 mm (TD)
   = 1.094 mm

   x_1 = sag of 9.00 mm (BPR_1) at 7.8 mm (BPD_1)
   = 0.889 mm

   e_2 is assumed to be 0.058 mm

Since $III = a_1 - x_1 - e_2$ then III
   = 1.094 - 0.889 - 0.058
   = **0.147 mm**

It is necessary to guess a value for BPR_2 which will permit x_2 and y_2 to be determined so as to give a value for III as near to this figure of 0.147 mm as possible, because $III = x_2 - y_2$. So let BPR_2 be 11.00 mm.

Then, x_2 = sag of 11.00 mm (BPR_2) at 8.6 mm (TD)
   = 0.875 mm

   y_2 = sag of 11.00 mm (BPR_2) at 7.8 mm (BDP_1)
   = 0.715 mm

giving $III = x_2 - y_2 = 0.875 - 0.715$
   = 0.160 mm

Since this value for III is bigger than 0.147 mm, then 11.00 mm must be too steep a radius for BPR_2. Therefore, another guess is made for BPR_2, say, 11.50 mm.

Again x_2 = sag of 11.50 mm (BPR_2) at 8.6 mm (TD)
   = 0.834 mm

   y_2 = sag of 11.50 mm (BPR_2) at 7.8 mm (BPD_1)
   = 0.681 mm

giving $III = x_2 - y_2 = 0.834 - 0.681$
   = 0.153 mm

This is nearer the value required, but still too large, and indicates that BPR_2 must be even flatter. Guessing yet again, let BPR_2 be 12.00 mm.

Now x_2 = sag of 12.00 mm (BPR_2) at 8.6 mm (TD)
  = 0.797 mm

  y_2 = sag of 12.00 mm (BPR_2) at 7.8 mm (BPD_1)
  = 0.651 mm

giving $III = x_2 - y_2 = 0.797 - 0.651$
  = 0.146 mm

This is near enough to 0.147 mm for it to be unnecessary to recalculate using another value for BPR_2, which may therefore be taken as **12.00 mm**. The small error of 0.001 mm in III means that e_2 is 0.059 instead of 0.058 (because $e_2 = a_1 - x_1 - III$).

The total axial edge lift, $z = e_1 + e_2 = 0.062 + 0.059 = 0.121$ mm, just 0.001 mm greater than originally required.

The value of z arrived at in the above manner may be checked by reference to *Figure 5.30* where it is seen that $z = a - (I + II + III)$.

Now a = sag of 8.00 mm (BOZR) at 8.6 mm (TD)
  = **1.254 mm**

  I = sag of 8.00 mm (BOZR) at 7.0 mm (BOZD)
  = **0.806 mm**

  II = $x_1 - y_1$

and x_1 = sag of 9.00 mm (BPR_1) at 7.8 mm (BPD_1)
  = 0.889 mm

  y_1 = sag of 9.00 mm (BPR_1) at 7.0 mm (BOZD)
  = 0.708 mm

Thus, $II = x_1 - y_1 = 0.889 - 0.708$
  = **0.181 mm**

  $III = x_2 - y_2$ and has been calculated above,
  = **0.146 mm**

and z = $1.254 - (0.806 + 0.181 + 0.146)$
  = **0.121 mm**

Any lens of known back surface specification may thus have its axial edge lift determined by this method.

Details of fitting sets with constant axial edge lift are given in Chapter 10 – *see Tables 10.1 and 10.13.*

Drawing lenses to scale

Another way to design lenses is to draw them to scale at ×40 full size as recommended by Mackie (1973), who has described the method in detail. Graph paper, 56 × 38 cm, a drawing board and beam compass (preferably 50 cm long) are essential, as well as a contact lens slide rule or tables such as those in the appendices to this book, or an electronic calculator. Some manufacturers still employ this method but computer programs such as those in Appendix E make it unnecessary, particularly if the computer can be used to do 'graphics' or diagrams of the lens which certainly assist in the understanding of lens design. Only half the lens need be drawn, as shown in *Figure 5.36* and one side of the graph paper is taken as the primary axis of the lens. It is helpful to mark up the graph paper with mm (4 cm at the chosen scale) markings both along and perpendicular to the axis, as this eases the measurement of lengths during the drawing process.

First, the BOZR is measured off and drawn as shown in *Figure 5.36* with centre, C_1, to extend from A on the axis to B representing the total diameter of the lens. Point D, indicating the limit of the BOZD can then be marked off by measurement on the graph paper. The axial or radial edge lift desired may then be measured off from B and the final edge position, E, of the lens thus located. If the lens is only to have one back surface peripheral curve, its radius is found by bisecting the line DE at right angles and finding where the perpendicular bisector intersects the axis at C_2. The BPR is then C_2D or C_2E and can be measured off with the compasses on the graph paper.

Should two peripheral curves be required then a point between B and E is marked off, say F, and a radius C_2D or C_2F is then found as above, but by locating its centre where the perpendicular bisector of DF cuts the axis. Then on the arc DF (which is now BPR_1) the limit of BPD_1 is marked where required by measurement on the graph paper. This point is denoted here as G. To obtain BPR_2, GE is now bisected perpendicularly and the centre, C_3, for the final peripheral curve is located where this perpendicular bisector of GE cuts the axis. The radius of this curve is C_3G or C_3E and can be measured with the compasses on the graph paper. Obviously any number of peripheral curves may be drawn in this fashion, contributing to the edge lift just as the lens designer wishes.

The front surface of the lens may be drawn, having first determined its radius according to

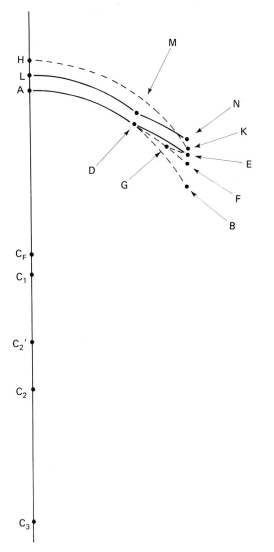

Figure 5.36 Drawing out lenses to scale (diagram not itself to scale)

the FOZR required to give the correct BVP). If necessary a lenticular lens can be designed as shown in *Figure 5.36* where the centre thickness has been reduced from AH to AL. The edge of the FOZD is marked off as required at, say, M, and a suitable curve MN (which could be parallel to DE) constructed for the FPR, so as to give a satisfactory junction thickness at MD and edge thickness at NE.

For negative lenses of high power a front junction radius similar to that shown in *Figure 5.34* can easily be constructed.

Drawing out to scale in this manner can be done for any type of lens and it has the advantage of permitting the designer to specify something which it is feasible for the manufacturer to make. It is also useful in that it allows the complete front and back surface to be specified, which encourages accurate reproduction of a lens on future occasions if duplicates are required.

Computer programs for the solution of optical problems and the related design of contact lenses

The bulk of this section forms Appendix E. The computer programs printed and explained there relate to both optical calculations and to contact lens design. Each program (or section of the whole program) is given an index no. as follows:

1   Back surface cylinder in air. This enables the astigmatic power of a surface of known radii and refractive index to be determined. The same information permits the power of an 'infinitely thin' lens of known radii and refractive index to be derived.
2   Edge lift of a known lens. Axial and radial edge lifts may be determined for lenses having up to five back surface curves.
3   Front optic zone radius. This is calculated for a known back optic zone radius, thickness and refractive index.
4   Induced cylinder. This is determined for a toroidal surface of known radii and refractive index in contact with tears.
5   Keratometer astigmatism. The corneal powers and astigmatism are provided for corneas of given radii and meridians for a refractive index of 1.3375.

the BVP required, by estimating centre thickness as described on p. 229. The centre thickness is marked off from A to point H. The centre for the front surface radius is then found by measuring off its radius from H to C_F. The FOZR (C_FH) is then drawn in from H to K, the latter point being the edge of the front surface. Thus, the edge thickness EK may be determined, and if too great or small an edge thickness results then the centre thickness can be adjusted appropriately (after checking by calculation or slide rule that this does not alter

6   Multi-curve spherical lens design. Lens back surface radii for standard or non-standard designs are obtainable for any required axial edge lift values.

7   Obliquely crossed cylinders. The resultant spherocylindrical combination is determined, allowing for any vertex distance separation of the two lenses.

8   Ocular refraction. This is obtained from spectacle refraction and vertex distance and has other similar effectivity applications.

9   Power change due to flexure. This applies to rigid contact lenses and enables the alteration in power to be obtained for lenses of known specification on a cornea of known radii.

10   Quit. This is used to exit from the program.

11   Sag of spherical surface. This gives the sagitta value for a surface of known radius and diameter.

12   Sag of multi-curve spherical lenses. The primary sagitta value is determined for multi-curve spherical lenses of up to five back surface curves.

Some of these items related to optical calculations are also listed in Appendices A–D so that new users of personal computers can cross-check, if necessary. The time-saving afforded by the use of the tables has now been extended so that practitioners and students who transfer them to their own discs will now be able to solve many complex contact lens design and optical problems literally at the touch of a few buttons. It is hoped that they will ease the burden and increase the efficiency of all serious workers in the contact lens field and eventually lead to the use of even more ambitious programs.

Examination questions and answers

The following questions have all been taken from past papers in visual optics of the Advanced Contact Lens Examination for the Diploma in Contact Lens Practice, set by the British Optical Association (now the British College of Optometrists), and are reproduced by their kind permission. The date of the questions and their answers are given in brackets after each question. Only the numerical type of questions have been included. Terminology has been brought up-to-date. It is hoped that these will be helpful to those people preparing for such examinations.

(1)   For the practitioner one of the greatest problems in verifying the characteristics of a corneal lens is that of back surface peripheral radii of curvature. Discuss methods that have been used to verify these radii and the limitations of such methods.

The following corneal lens has been ordered from a laboratory:

C2. 7.80: 6.50/8.00: 9.50/–6.00 D (refractive index 1.490).

On checking the following values were obtained:

Centre thickness	0.10 mm
Back vertex power	–6.00 D
BOZR	7.80 mm
Back vertex power of peripheral zone	–5.00 D
Thickness at centre of peripheral zone	0.20 mm

Does the peripheral radius of curvature conform to specification?
(*July, 1970; No – 7.90 mm*)

(2)   A patient with the following refractive details is to be fitted with minimum clearance scleral lenses in order to provide a satisfactory level of vision binocularly. Calculate the necessary back vertex powers of the lenses if the back optic zone radii of the contact lenses are R and L 8.30 mm.

RX   R +4.00 D/–2.00 axis 180
      Vertex distance 15 mm
      L +5.00 DS

Keratometer readings R and L
7.64 mm along 90°
8.00 mm along 180°
(*January, 1971; R + 5.78/–0.22 × 180 say +5.75 DS. L +6.93/+1.98 × 180, say +7.00 with +2.00 DC × 180 on front surface*)

(3)   A patient is fitted with an air cell underwater scleral contact lens. Calculate the radius of curvature of the front optic zone surface of the scleral component from the following details:

RE   Spectacle *Rx*
+5.00/−2.00 axis 180
Vertex distance 15 mm

7.80 mm along 90°; 8.20 mm along 180°

BOZR 8.60 mm; centre thickness 0.4 mm;
refractive index 1.490
(*July, 1971; 7.76 mm assuming contact lens BVP of +7.25 D*)

(4) Discuss the relative merits and usefulness of the following instruments for checking contact lenses: keratometer, radiuscope, focimeter and slit lamp.

A focimeter may be used to check the BOZR of a corneal lens if a lens of known characteristics is available. Given a lens of known characteristics (BOZR 8.2 mm, BVP +6.00 D) calculate the BOZR of an unknown lens given the following details:

BVP of known and unknown lens +4.00 D
BVP of known and unknown lens +3.00 D
with water (*n* = 1.336) between lenses.
Centre thickness of unknown lens 0.2 mm,
lens material refractive index 1.49

(*January, 1972; 7.68 mm*)

(5) Although spectacle/contact lens systems have been used as subnormal vision aids, they have severe limitations. If a system to be used with an emmetropic patient consists of a spectacle lens power +12.00 D vertex distance 15 mm and a contact lens, calculate the magnification produced by such a system for a distant object, and also the ocular accommodation exerted to view an object one metre from the spectacle lens (assume the system remains in normal adjustment).
(*January, 1972; × 1.22, +1.46 D*)

(6) A preformed scleral trial lens is placed on an eye and gives a satisfactory minimum clearance fit. The supplementary refraction is: +2.50 DS/+2.00 DC × 90, vertex distance 12 mm.

The trial lens has a front surface radius of 8.25 mm and refractive index of 1.49.

What will be the front surface radii of the final contact lens if it has the same rear surface construction, thickness and refractive index?

What can you deduce about the possible origins of the astigmatism if it is known that the patient normally wears spectacles

with the following correction?: −6.00 DS/ −2.00 DC × 90, vertex distance 12 mm.
(*July, 1972; 7.64 mm 180, 7.91 mm 90, crystalline lens astigmatism*)

(7) A patient with a PD of 60 mm wears a spectacle correction of −8.00 DS R and L in planoconcave form at a vertex distance of 13 mm. Subsequently a corneal lens correction is provided. Calculate the demands on accommodation and convergence when fixation is changed from a distant object to one at 32 cm from the spectacle plane using the two forms of correction.

What are the clinical implications of this calculation?
(*July, 1972; spectacles: accommodation +2.47 D, convergence 7.34 Δ each eye. Contact lenses: accommodation +3.00 D, convergence 8.70 Δ each eye*)

(8) A contact lens having a BOZR of 8 mm and a thickness of 0.15 mm has a front vertex power of −20.00 D. It is used in combination with a planoconvex spectacle lens of back vertex power +16.00 DS and 10 mm thick to provide magnification for an emmetropic eye of low visual acuity. Assume that the material of both lenses has a refractive index of 1.49. Neglect the liquid lens. Calculate:

(*a*) front surface radius of contact lens;
(*b*) lens separation for normal adjustment;
(*c*) the magnification.

(*July, 1972; (a) 11.99 mm, (b) 12.5 mm, (c) ×1.25 not allowing for shape factor*)

(9) A myope having a spectacle correction of −12 D, right and left, worn at a vertex distance of 12 mm and 25 mm from the centres of rotation of the eyes, is fitted with contact lenses. So, too, is a bilateral aphakic of spectacle refraction +12 D worn at the same vertex distance and the same distance from the eyes' centres of rotation as the myope. Each has a distance CD for the spectacles of 60 mm.

Determine in each case: (*a*) the difference in convergence required for an object 25 cm in front of the spectacle plane, when wearing spectacles and contact lenses; (*b*) the alteration in the clear field of view (assuming that, in both cases, lenticular spectacle lenses with a circular aperture of

30 mm diameter are used) between contact lens wear and spectacle lens wear.

(*January 1973; (a) myope in spectacles, 17.14 Δ; in contact lenses, 21.82 Δ. Hypermetrope in spectacles, 30.00 Δ; in contact lenses, 21.82 Δ. (b) Myope: 76° in spectacles, unlimited in contact lenses but 62° if spectacle frame present. Hypermetrope: 45.5° in spectacles, unlimited in contact lenses but 62° if spectacle frame present.*)

(10) Two solid concentric bifocal contact lenses of polymethyl methacrylate of refractive index 1.49 are made up so as to give the patient a near addition of +2.00 D. One has a front surface addition and the other a back surface addition. In each case the distance portion is in the centre and is of −2.00 D BVP and 0.20 mm centre thickness. The BOZR of the front surface addition lens is 7.60 mm, and the same radius is used on the portion of the back surface used for the near addition of the other lens. Assuming a refractive index of 1.336 for tears, calculate the two front surface radii of the front surface addition lens, and the BCOZR and FOZR for the back surface addition lens.

(*January, 1973; FCOZR, DP 7.91 mm; FPOZR, NP 7.67 mm; BCOZR 6.92 mm, FOZR 7.19 mm*)

(11) A parallel bi-toric corneal lens has a back vertex power in air of −2.00/−5.00 × 180. It is fitted so that the back optic zone surface exactly matches the with-the-rule corneal contour, and there is an afocal liquid lens. The contact lens also exactly corrects the eye's ocular refraction.

The back optic zone radii of the lens are 7.25 and 8.00 mm. What is the power and axis direction of the positive cylinder which has been worked on the front surface? (Assume an infinitely thin contact lens and, for ease of calculation, refractive indices of: lens material, 1.5; tears and cornea, 1.333.) How much of the ocular astigmatism is corneal and how much is due to the crystalline lens?

(*July, 1973; +1.47 × 180, corneal astigmatism +4.31 × 180, crystalline lens astigmatism +0.69 × 180*)

(12) A young emmetropic patient has an alternating esotropia of 15°, and uses the RE for distance and the LE for near (assumed as 25 cm from the spectacle plane). Following an accident his macular areas undergo degenerative changes and his accommodation is considerably reduced. He requires a telescopic aid for the RE and a 'microscope' aid for the LE. Corneal lenses are to be used for the eyepieces and spectacles worn at a vertex distance of 16 mm for the objectives of these aids. As his corneas are identical, two similar corneal lenses are made up, of BOZR 7.50 mm and FOZR 12.00 mm. (Assume an infinitely thin contact lens of refractive index 1.5.) If the LE continues to use the same working distance, what back vertex powers must the two spectacle lenses have and what magnification would they afford?

(*July, 1973; RE +17.86 D, ×1.40; LE +21.86 D, ×1.40*)

(13) A soft contact lens, when fully hydrated, has a back optic zone radius of 8.00 mm, a refractive index of 1.35, centre thickness of 0.30 mm and back vertex power of −3.00 D.

It is allowed to become partially dehydrated and its refractive index goes up to 1.40. Calculate the change in back vertex power on the basis of the refractive index change alone.

What other factors associated with dehydration would also contribute to a change in BVP?

(*January, 1975; −0.40 D; curvature and thickness changes*)

(14) A fused bifocal corneal lens has a segment of refractive index 1.58 in the lower part of the back optic zone and coming into contact with the tear layer of refractive index 1.336. The lens has a back optic zone radius of 7.00 mm. The main part of the lens has a refractive index of 1.49. Calculate the interface radius necessary to give the lens a near addition, on the eye, of +3.00 D. (Assume thin lens theory.)

Explain what different factors would be taken into consideration in determining the interface radius, had the segment been on the front surface.

(*January, 1975; 5.67 mm*)

(15) An aphakic eye has a spectacle refraction of +13.50 DS at a vertex distance of 12 mm. The corneal radius is 7.90 mm. Assuming a refractive index of tears of

1.333 and a keratometer, aqueous and vitreous index of 1.336, calculate:

(a) the axial length of the eye;
(b) the back vertex power of a corneal lens of BOZR 7.80 that corrects the eye;
(c) compare the spectacle magnification given by the two forms of correction, assuming also an apparent depth of anterior chamber of 3.0 mm and shape factors of 1.094 and 1.026 for the spectacle and contact lenses.

(*June, 1985; 22.78 mm; +15.57 D; ×1.372: ×1.078*)

(16) (a) Define induced astigmatism.
(b) An astigmatic eye has a spectacle refraction of –6.00/–3.75 × 170 at a vertex distance of 15 mm. The K readings are 7.95 along 180 by 7.35 along 90. A toric corneal lens of BOZR 7.90 × 7.40 is fitted and assumed to orientate along the corneal meridians. Assuming an index of 1.490 for the lens, 1.333 for tears and keratometer:
(i) what back vertex power is required in the two meridians?
(ii) what compensating cylinder has to be worked on the front surface of the lens to obtain an accurate correction (ignoring lens thickness)?

(*June, 1985; (b) Assuming corneal meridians can be treated as parallel to those of spectacle refraction: BVP of contact lens –6.10/–2.89 × 180. Front surface cylinder +1.35 × 180*)

(17) If the apparent central thickness of the optical section of the cornea produced by a slit beam is 0.42 mm, what would be its true central thickness?

Assume: refractive index of cornea = 1.376
anterior corneal surface radius = 7.8

Should the cornea become oedematous, what changes would be produced in the relationship between true and apparent thickness?

(*October, 1987; 0.566 mm; increase in true thickness with oedema, offset by reduction in refractive index, so relationship approximately the same*)

(18) (a) Define residual and induced astigmatism.
(b) A patient with refraction plano/–2.50 × 180 has K readings of 8.00 m 180 by 7.50 m 90. Using approximations, what, if any, is the remaining astigmatism when a rigid corneal lens is placed on the eye of BOZR:
(i) 7.85 spherical;
(ii) 8.00 × 7.50;
(iii) 7.90 × 7.60.
(c) If the patient in (b) is fitted with a back toroidal surface soft lens of HEMA, calculate the required radius in the steep meridian if the radius in the flat meridian is 8.5. Assume a refractive index of 1.43 in the hydrated state.
(d) A patient wearing rigid lenses of specification R BOZR 7.7 mm, BVP –6.00 D and L 7.9 mm –5.50 D respectively inserts the lenses on the wrong eyes. What is the induced error for each eye, assuming a perfect correction when worn normally?

(*December, 1986; (b) none; +1.28 × 180; +0.77 × 180; (c) 8.1 mm; (d) R –0.61 D, L +0.61 D needing lenses of equal and opposite power to correct it*)

(19) Discuss some of the possible uses of contact lenses in the management of low visual acuity.

A contact lens/spectacle combination is used to provide magnification for distance vision, in the form of a Galilean telescope. If the spectacle lens has a power of +20.00 DS, and the lens separation is 14 mm, what will be the power required for the contact lens, and what will be the magnification of the system? (Assume that the lenses are thin, neglect effects of lens form.)

(*October, 1986; –27.78 D; × 1.67*)

(20) Following cataract extraction, a previously emmetropic eye has a spectacle prescription of +11.00/+1.50 × 180 (back vertex distance 10 mm), and K readings 7.80 × 90; 8.05 × 180.

(a) Assuming that a hard contact lens were to be fitted in alignment with the flattest K, calculate accurately the FOZR for a lens with a centre thickness 0.5 mm (assume n = 1.495).

(*b*) Calculate the spectacle magnification when such a lens is worn: to what level would this improve a VA of 6/9 obtained with a spectacle magnification of unity?

(*February, 1986; (a) 6.87 mm assuming astigmatism corrected by liquid lens. In fact +0.59 DC × 180 remains uncorrected. (b) (Spectacle lens ×1.17, VA 6/7.7); contact lens ×1.04, VA 6/8.7 (assuming entrance pupil 3 mm from cornea)*)

Acknowledgements

We are indebted to the following people for help in the preparation of this chapter: Mr Roger Phillips for programming the computer and producing the figures on which Appendix D is based; Mrs Rita Watts for help in the calculations for Appendices A and B; and Mr R. G. Stone for drawing many of the diagrams.

References

ANDRASKO, G. and SCHOESSLER, J. P. (1980). The effect of humidity on the dehydration of soft contact lenses on the eye. *Int. Contact Lens Clin.* **7**, 210–212

BARON, H. (1975). Some remarks on the correction of astigmatic eyes by means of soft contact lenses. *Contacto* **19**(6), 4–8

BENNETT, A. G. (1968). The corrected aphakic eye: a study of retinal image sizes. *Optician* **155**, 106–111

BENNETT, A. G. (1970). Variable and progressive power lenses: 1. *Optician* **160**, 421–427

BENNETT, A. G. (1972). Retinal image sizes in the aphakic eye. *Contact Lens* **3**(7), 2–6; also in *Contact Lens* **4**(2), 24–28 (1973) with publisher's errors corrected

BENNETT, A. G. (1976). Power changes in soft contact lenses due to bending. *Ophthal. Optician* **16**, 939–945

BENNETT, A. G. (1985) *Optics of Contact Lenses,* 5th ed. London: Association of Dispensing Opticians

BENNETT, A.G. (1988). Aspherical and continuous curve contact lenses: Parts 1–4. *Optom. Today* **28**, 11–14. 140–142, 238–242, 433–444

BENNETT, A. G. and RABBETTS, R. B. (1984). *Clinical Visual Optics.* London: Butterworths

BENNETT, A. G. and RABBETTS, R. B. (1988). Schematic eyes – time for a change? *Optician* **196**(5169), 14–15

BIBBY, M. M. (1980). A model for lens flexure – validation and predictions. *Int. Contact Lens Clin.* **7**, 124–138

BRENNAN, N. A., EFRON, N., TRUONG, V. T. and WATKINS, R. D. (1986). Definitions for hydration changes in hydrogel lenses. *Ophthal. physiol. Optics* **6**, 333–338

BROWN, S., BALDWIN, M. and POLE, J. (1984). Effect of the optic zone diameter on lens flexure and residual astigmatism. *Int. Contact Lens Clin.* **11**, 759–766

CAMPBELL, C. (1987). A method for calculating the tear volume between the cornea and a hard contact lens with a spherical base curve. *J. Br. Contact Lens Ass.* **10**(1), 29–35

CAPELLI, Q. A. (1964). Determining final power of bitoric lenses. *Br. J. physiol. Optics* **21**, 256–263

CARNEY, L. G. (1975). The basis for corneal shape change during contact lens wear. *Am. J. Optom.* **52**, 445–454; reproduced in *Optician* **171**(4415), 11, 15–16, 20–22 (1976)

CHASTON, J. and FATT, I. (1981). The influence of temperature on the base curve of high plus soft contact lenses. *Int. Contact Lens Clin.* **8**(1), 42–50

CLARK, B. A. J. (1970). Sagitta nomograms for contact lens calculation. *Contact Lens* **2**(7), 3–6

CREIGHTON, C. P. (1964). *Contact Lenses Fabrication Tables.* New York: Creighton

DOUTHWAITE, W. A. (1987). *Contact Lens Optics,* London: Butterworths

DOUTHWAITE, W. A. (1988). Technical note: compensated toric rigid contact lenses. *J. Br. Contact Lens Ass.* **11**(2), 35–38

FATT, I and CHASTON, J. (1980a). Temperature of contact lens on the eye. *Int. Contact Lens Clin.* **7**, 195–198

FATT, I and CHASTON, J. (1980b). The effect of temperature on refractive index, water content and central thickness of hydrogel lenses. *Int. Contact Lens Clin.* **7**, 250–255

FATT, I and CHASTON, J. (1981). The response of vertex power to changes in dimensions of hydrogel contact lenses. *Int. Contact Lens Clin.* **8**(1), 22–28

FINCHAM, W. H. A. and FREEMAN, M. H. (1980). *Optics,* 9th edn. London: Butterworths

FLETCHER, R. J. (1965). Haptic lenses. In *Contact Lens Practice: Basic and Advanced,* edited by R. B. Mandell. Springfield, Ill.: Thomas

FORD, M. W. (1974). Changes in hydrophilic lenses when placed on an eye. Paper read at the joint International Congress of The Contact Lens Society and The National Eye Research Foundation, Montreux, Switzerland

FORD, M. W. (1976). Computation of the back vertex powers of hydrophilic lenses. Paper read at the Interdisciplinary Conference on Contact Lenses, Department of Ophthalmic Optics and Visual Science, The City University, London

FRANCIS, J. L. (1968). *Optical Tables for Contact Lens Work.* London: Hatton Press (these are now incorporated in the present book)

GORDON, S. (1965). Contact lens hydration: a study of the wetting-drying cycle. *Optom. Wkly* **56**, 55–62

HARRIS, M. G. and CHU, C. S. (1972). The effect of contact lens thickness and corneal toricity on flexure and residual astigmatism. *Am. J. Optom.* **49**, 304–307

JALIE, M. (1974). *The Principles of Ophthalmic Lenses,* 2nd edn, pp. 324–327. London: Association of Dispensing Opticians

KERNS, R. L. (1974). Clinical evaluation of the merits of an aspheric front surface contact lens for patients manifesting residual astigmatism. *Am. J. Optom.* **51**, 750–757

MACKIE, I. A. (1973). Design compensation in corneal lens

fitting. In *Symposium on Contact Lenses,* Transactions of the New Orleans Academy of Ophthalmology, St Louis: Mosby

MANDELL, R. B. (1975). Corneal oedema from hydrogel lenses. *Int. Contact Lens Clinic* **2**(1), 88–98

MANDELL, R. B. and POLSE, K. A. (1969). Corneal thickness changes as a contact lens fitting index – experimental results and a proposed model. *Am. J. Optom.* **46**, 479–491

OBSTFELD, H. (1982). *Optics in Vision,* 2nd edn. London: Butterworths

POLE, J. J. (1983). The effect of the base curve on the flexure of polycon lenses. *Int. Contact Lens Clin.* **10**(1), 49–52

POLSE, K. A. (1972). Changes in corneal hydration after discontinuing contact lens wear. *Am. J. Optom.* **49**, 511–516

PORT, M. (1982). Curvature changes in dehydrating soft lenses (part 1). *J. Br. Contact Lens Ass.* **5**, 42–58

RABBETTS, R. B. (1976). Large corneal lenses with constant axial edge lift. *Ophthal. Optician* **16**, 236, 239

RENGSTORFF, R. H. and ARNER, R. S. (1971). Refractive changes in the cornea: mathematical considerations. *Am. J. Optom.* **48**, 913–918

SARVER, M. D. (1963). The effect of contact lens tilt upon residual astigmatism. *Am. J. Optom.* **40**, 730–744

SARVER, M. D., ASHLEY, D. and VAN EVERY, J. (1974). Supplemental power effect of Bausch and Lomb Soflens contact lenses. *Int. Contact Lens Clinic* **1**(1), 100–109

SARVER, M. D., HARRIS, M. G. and POLSE, K. A. (1975). Corneal curvature and supplemental power effect of the Bausch and Lomb Soflens contact lenses. *Am. J. Optom.* **52**, 470–473

SORSBY, A., LEARY, G. A. and RICHARDS, M. J. (1962). The optical components in anisometropia. *Vision Res.* **3**, 43–51

STONE, J. (1959). Factors governing the back central optic diameter of a microlens. *Optician* **138**, 20–22

STONE, J. (1966). The use of contact lenses in the correction of astigmatism. *Optica Int.* **3**, 6–23

STONE, J. (1967). Near vision difficulties in non-presbyopic corneal lens wearers. *Contact Lens* **1**(2), 14–25

STONE, J. (1973). Contact lens wear in the young myope. *Br. J. physiol. Optics* **28**, 90–134

STONE, J. (1975). Corneal lenses with constant axial edge lift. *Ophthal. Optician* **15**, 818–824

STONE, J. and COLLINS, C. (1984). Flexure of gas permeable lenses on toroidal corneas. *Optician* **188**(4951), 8–10

STRACHAN, J. P. F. (1973). Some principles of the optics of hydrophilic lenses and geometrical optics applied to flexible lenses. *Aust. J. Optom.* **56**, 25–33

SWAINE, W. (1956). Optics of contact lenses and their prescription. *Br. J. physiol. Optics* **13**, 147–163

VOERSTE, K. (1976). Analysing the clinical results of fitting a type of soft contact lens. *Optician* **171**(4414), 15–18, 23

WESTERHOUT, D. (1969). Clinical observations in fitting bitoric and toric forms of corneal lenses. *Contact Lens* **2**(3), 5–21, 36

WESTHEIMER, G. (1962). The visual world of the new contact lens wearer. *J. Am. optom. Ass.* **34**, 135–140

WICHTERLE, O. (1967). Changes of refracting power of a soft lens caused by its flattening. In *Corneal and Scleral Contact Lenses,* Proceedings of the International Congress, March 1966, edited by L. J. Girard. Paper 29, pp. 247–256. St Louis: Mosby

WINN, B. ACKERLEY, R. G., BROWN, C. A., MURRAY, F. K., PRAIS, J. and ST JOHN, M. F. (1986). The superiority of contact lenses in the correction of all anisometropia. *Transactions British Contact Lens Association Conference,* 95–100

YOUNG, G. (1988). Computer-assisted contact lens design. *Optician* **196**(5171), 32–33, 37, 39

Chapter 6

Keratometry and slit lamp biomicroscopy

Michael Sheridan

A keratometer and slit lamp biomicroscope are the two major instruments used in contact lens practice. The first provides information which is helpful in deciding on the initial fitting lens and in monitoring corneal changes during the adaptation and after-care period; the second is indispensable for effective investigation of the condition of the cornea and the fit of the contact lens at every stage of fitting and after-care.

Keratometry

The main function of a keratometer is the measurement of the radius of curvature of the central portion of the front surface of the cornea, usually referred to as the optic cap (*see* Chapter 10). This result is obtained indirectly by measuring the angular size of the reflected image, formed by the cornea, of an object of known angular size. In most instruments, this is an object whose linear size is fixed or measurable at a predetermined distance from the image plane.

The technique is usually attributed to von Helmholtz, although Mandell (1960) has argued that Jesse Ramsden was, in fact, the inventor. Its subsequent development has been discussed by Emsley (1955), and the development of the allied technique of keratoscopy has been discussed by Levene (1965).

The derivation of the radius is shown in *Figure 6.1*, where B and Q represent the limits of an object of size h. The images B' and Q', formed by reflection at the front surface of the cornea, are the limits of an image of size h' formed slightly in front of the focal plane of the cornea (which intersects the axis at F, the principal focus) and at a distance d from the object plane BQ. A is the pole of the cornea and C its centre of curvature. Thus, the radius $r = AC$ and $r/2 = AF$.

Figure 6.2 illustrates the doubling principle by which the measurement of image size is made. If a prism of power P prism dioptres is interposed in half the observation aperture, an image of size h' will be seen doubled, and the doubled images will only be positioned exactly adjacent to one another at the distance a, such that $h'/a = P/100$.

In practice, the extremities of the object are represented by a pair of internally illuminated mires, the corneal images of which are observed and seen magnified through a short-focus telescope (or long-focus microscope). This incorporates a doubling device which gives rise to the four images seen in the telescope field, the two central ones being brought into contact or superimposed as shown in *Figures 6.3* and *6.4*. To obtain adjacent or superimposed images, either h' (*see Figure 6.1*) may be varied by altering the mire separation h while the power and position of the doubling device are fixed (fixed doubling), or the image size h' and mire separation h may be fixed while the power of the doubling device P or its distance a from the image plane is varied (variable doubling). In most modern instruments employing variable doubling, it is the distance a which is varied, the doubling prism travelling along the axis of the instrument between the objective and eyepiece.

In most keratometers, doubling takes place in one meridian only — along the line joining the mires. Such an instrument must be rotated about its optical axis in order to align it with each of the principal meridians of the cornea in turn and it is therefore known as a two position keratometer. A one position keratometer is an instrument in which variable doubling of mutually perpendicular pairs of mires is

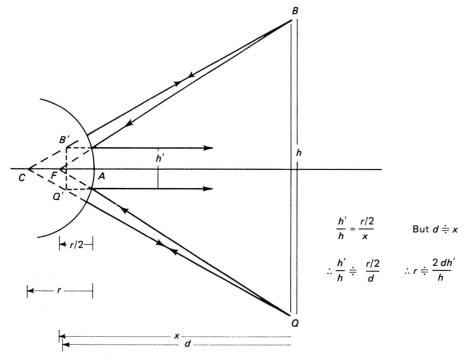

$$\frac{h'}{h} = \frac{r/2}{x} \qquad \text{But } d \doteq x$$

$$\therefore \frac{h'}{h} \doteq \frac{r/2}{d} \qquad \therefore r \doteq \frac{2\,dh'}{h}$$

Figure 6.1 Optical principle of keratometry

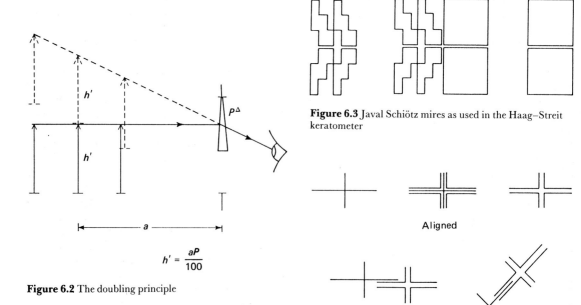

$$h' = \frac{aP}{100}$$

Figure 6.2 The doubling principle

Figure 6.3 Javal Schiötz mires as used in the Haag–Streit keratometer

Aligned

Not along principal meridian   Along principal meridian

Figure 6.4 Mires used in the Zeiss ophthalmometer

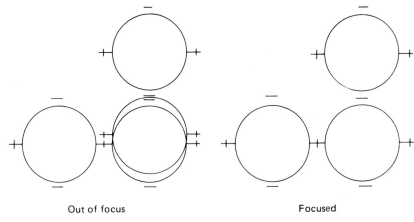

Out of focus   Focused

Figure 6.5 The Bausch & Lomb keratometer mires

produced by two doubling devices in the corresponding meridians. The instrument is rotated about its axis to align the mires with both principal meridians of the cornea (which are assumed to be at right-angles to each other) and the images in each can then be brought into contact without further rotation. A skilled observer operating both doubling devices can therefore make almost simultaneous measurements. If, however, the cornea is very toroidal, a focus adjustment must also be made as the pairs of mire reflections are formed in different planes for each meridian (Stone, 1962). The Bausch & Lomb keratometer is probably the best known instrument of this type. *Figure 6.5* shows the appearance of its mire images when out of focus and at the end-point of the measurement. Topcon produces a similar instrument. The American Optical Company's CLC Ophthalmometer is a more recent one-position design, but its mire pattern is almost identical in appearance to that of the Bausch & Lomb instrument. The American Optical Company also produces a hybrid instrument in which mire images in both principal meridians are viewed simultaneously, but a single variable doubling device is used and rotated through 90° to measure each principal meridian in turn.

Sources of error

Some of the factors which influence the accuracy of a keratometer measurement are not under the control of the observer but are functions of the design of the instrument. The relationships derived in *Figure 6.1* are based on paraxial optical theory, which has been shown by Emsley (1960, 1963) and Bennett (1966) to oversimplify the situation. The corneal areas from which the mire images are reflected are too far from the axis of the system to be considered as being in the paraxial zone of a surface with a reflecting power of about $-260\,\text{D}$. The resulting third order aberrations are too large to permit a keratometer to be calibrated by paraxial theory. Bennett (1966) has shown that the difference in the aberrations of convex and concave surfaces can account for the corrections which have to be applied when a keratometer is used to measure the back optic zone radius of a contact lens (*see* Chapter 12), whereas the paraxial formulae apply equally to concave and convex surfaces.

The second of the equations derived in *Figure 6.1* ($r = 2dh'/h$) is an approximation in which d, the separation of object and image, is assumed to be the same as x, the distance of the object from the focal point. This assumption is used in the design of most keratometers, the mires being mounted relatively close to the eye. The error thus introduced is small because of the high reflecting power of the cornea. Emsley (1955) calculates that for a cornea of 8 mm radius it amounts to 0.10 D (0.02 mm) with the Bausch & Lomb keratometer in which d is 72 mm, and that if d is increased to 150 mm the error is reduced to 0.02 D (0.003 mm). It can be completely eliminated by making the mires the targets of a collimating system. This course is adopted in the Zeiss, the Gambs and the Guilbert Routit Topographic instruments. (The latter two instruments are no longer on the market.)

Figure 6.1 also shows that the light from the

Table 6.1

Keratometer	Diameter in mm of corneal area in which each mire is reflected when the corneal radius is		
	7.00 mm	*9.00 mm*	*10.00 mm*
Bausch & Lomb	0.1	0.1	
Zeiss	0.2		0.4
Gambs	0.2		0.4
Guilbert Routit Topographic	0.5		0.8
Haag–Streit	0.4		0.3

mires is reflected, not from the keratometric pole towards which the telescope is directed, but from two small areas on either side of it. The instrument is calibrated on the assumption that these two areas are on a spherical surface and the resulting radius is attributed to the keratometric pole. If the areas from which the mire images are reflected have a curvature different from that of the pole, or from each other, the measurement will be incorrect. This error is more likely to be serious if the two reflection areas are large or widely separated, or if the keratometric pole is markedly decentred within the optic cap. It can be reduced by reducing the size and separation of the mires (Noble, 1962; Mandell, 1962a, 1965). *Figure 6.6* shows the separations of the mire reflection areas in some current instruments, and *Table 6.1* shows the diameters of the corneal reflection areas for a single mire as determined by Lehmann (1967).

The main source of error which is under the control of the observer is focusing. If the mire images formed by the objective are not accurately focused in the intended primary image plane, the radius measurement will be incorrect since

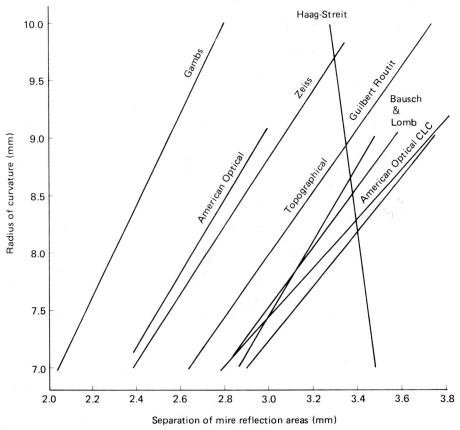

Figure 6.6 Graphs showing separation of the mire reflection areas on the corneal cap for radii of curvature from 7 to 10 mm for various keratometers. (After Mandell (1962b) and Lehmann (1967) — *see* text)

the object–image separation is then incorrect, and the out-of-focus mire images have a different separation from sharply focused ones. These out-of-focus images may not appear to be blurred if the observer accommodates. Collimated mires and a fully telecentric viewing system, as in the Zeiss or Guilbert Routit Topographic instruments, eliminate this source of error; or the observer's judgment of focus can be assisted by including a Scheiner disc in the viewing system as in the American Optical Company CLC, the Topcon and the Bausch & Lomb keratometers, where the central mire image is seen double if it is not accurately focused (*Figure 6.5*). In instruments with a fixed graticule in the primary image plane, there should be no parallax between the mire images and the graticule when the observer moves his eye from side to side; this test is valid whether or not the observer is accommodating.

The commonest cause of focusing error is proximal accommodation by the observer. The following precautions should reduce this to a minimum by avoiding unnecessary stimulation of accommodation. The observer should keep both eyes open and suppress the image in the disengaged eye. If the instrument has an adjustable eyepiece, it should be carefully focused on the graticule by turning it as far as possible in the positive direction (outwards) and then resetting it until the graticule is just clear. To ensure that convergent light emerges from the eyepiece when the instrument is out of focus, thereby encouraging the observer's accommodation to remain relaxed, the instrument should be moved as far as possible from the patient and then slowly moved forward until the mire images are just clear. By keeping errors to a minimum, readings should be repeatable to 0.02 mm, but the scales of some instruments are difficult to interpolate to this degree of accuracy (Stone, 1962).

Uses of the keratometer

A standard keratometer may be used by a contact lens practitioner for three purposes: to decide on an appropriate back optic zone radius during fitting, to monitor changes in central corneal and soft lens front surface curvature during after-care, and to check the radii of finished contact lenses.

As an aid to fitting

The value of a keratometer in fitting contact lenses depends on the fitting technique employed. If, as is usual, the specification of the prescription lens is derived by examining the fit of a number of trial lenses, the function of the keratometer is limited to indicating a starting point and providing a base record with which the measurements made in the after-care period may be compared and from which the power of the tear lens may be calculated (*see* Chapter 5). This assists in computation of the correct back vertex power. In soft lens fitting, keratometry can be carried out with the lens in place; the quality of the mire images and the stability (or instability) of the radius reading indicating whether the lens is flat or steep (*see* Chapter 11). If a keratometer is available, it is usually possible to arrive at a final specification with about half the number of trial lens insertions that would be required if it were not. This materially speeds up the fitting procedure and reduces discomfort to the patient.

In after-care

In the after-care period, comparison of keratometer readings made on successive visits provides a valuable means of detecting corneal changes produced by contact lens wear. During the adaptation period, mainly with rigid lenses, the radius of the cornea changes in an unpredictable way even with an apparently well-fitting lens. Bier (1957) suggests that a lens which is flatter than the cornea will lead to corneal flattening and vice versa, but this view has not been confirmed by subsequent investigators (Hodd, 1962; Sabell, 1962; Rengstorff, 1965a,b, 1967, 1969b; Spurrett, 1973). Regular increases or decreases in radius of up to 0.1 mm are usually tolerable during the first 6 weeks of wear, provided that spectacle blur is not persistent.

There may also be irregular changes of curvature, usually following rigid lens wear. These are revealed by distortion of the mire images, sometimes to such an extent that no satisfactory reading can be obtained. Appearances of this kind, which show that the contact lens is deforming the cornea, are common with badly fitting lenses, but slight distortion of the mire images may occur during the adaptation period even with a lens which is a good fit. It is most likely to occur with a lens whose apex clears the cornea, because the transition or peripheral zones may bear on the cornea close to the zones from which the mire images are reflected.

In order that there should be a minimum apparent variation in corneal radius due to experimental error, follow-up measurements should be made by the same observer, using the same instrument and, in view of the diurnal variations in radius reported by Reynolds (1959) and Noble and Sheridan (1962), at the same time of day.

If the front surface of a soft lens becomes coated or dirty the mire images appear indistinct, and they appear distorted if the fit is poor. Steepening of curvature indicates probable dehydration of the lens.

In the checking of contact lens radii

Since the optic radii of a contact lens are similar to those of the cornea, a keratometer may be used to check them. Keratometers are calibrated to measure convex surfaces and require re-calibration when used for concave ones. The principles of re-calibration have been investigated by Emsley (1963) and Bennett (1966), and a conversion scale for concave surfaces is available for the Bausch & Lomb, Topcon and American Optical Company CLC keratometers. The practical aspects of this use of keratometry are discussed in Chapter 12.

It sometimes happens that the surface to be measured has a radius which lies outside the range for which the keratometer is calibrated. The scleral surface of a scleral contact lens or the apex of a conical cornea are examples. The range may be extended by fitting an auxiliary lens (such as a spectacle trial case lens) in front of the objective of the keratometer to change the working distance of the instrument: a positive auxiliary lens enables shorter radii to be measured; a negative lens extends the range to allow measurement of longer radii. The instrument must be re-calibrated with the auxiliary lens in place (Sampson and Soper, 1970). Steel ball-bearings of known radii and guaranteed accuracy are ideal for this purpose. For each auxiliary lens, a graph may be drawn showing the actual radius of the balls against kerato-meter readings and, provided that the same auxiliary lenses are employed, these graphs may be used for future measurements (compare Chapter 12, p. 445).

Keratometry and keratoscopy of the peripheral cornea

Contact lenses usually extend well beyond the optic cap and, since their use became widespread, interest in the contour of the peripheral cornea has been intensified. This has resulted in the design of a number of new keratometers and the modification of existing designs to give more accurate measurements of the peripheral portion of the cornea. Mandell (1962a,b, 1965) modified a Bausch & Lomb keratometer so as to reduce the mire separation from 64 mm to 26 mm. With the addition of a series of off-axis fixation points, he was able to make measurements of the periphery of the cornea. Noble (1962) and Noble and Sheridan (1962) achieved a small mire separation by mounting small slit mires above an aperture in the telescope tube and reflecting the light along the axis of the system with a semi-silvered mirror. Bennett (1964) has described the design of a keratometer based on Drysdale's principle and intended for measurement of both central and peripheral cornea.

The system employed by Bonnet and Cochet (1960) and Bonnet (1964) and incorporated in the Guilbert Routit Topographic keratometer makes use of only one mire for the peripheral readings, which are obtained from a corneal area of only 0.5 mm in diameter. The central radius is determined by 'classic' keratometry, using two mires over a much larger chord (*Figure 6.7*). The Zeiss keratometer also provides facilities for single mire keratometry and the movable fixation point and extended radius scale which are necessary for peripheral readings.

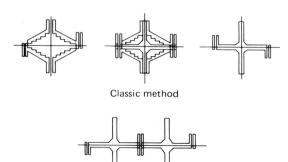

Classic method

Topographical method (one mire)

Figure 6.7 The mires used in the Guilbert Routit topographical ophthalmometer

The Rodenstock BES keratometer has been adapted by Wilms with a peripheral fixation disc designed to allow measurement of the sagittal radii of the cornea up to 30° from fixation, from which the eccentricity of the cornea can be derived and also, by measuring the change in keratometer reading as fixation is displaced along the plane of measurement, to provide an estimate for the z value of the cornea (Wilms and Rabbetts, 1977).

The Humphrey Auto Keratometer, the optical and mathematical principles of which have been fully described by Rabbetts (1985), also provides a method of specifying corneal contour. After measuring the cornea with the eye fixing centrally and also with rotations to right and left of 13.5°, the instrument computes and prints out the position of the corneal apex, the optical radii and a 'shape factor'. The most commonly used mathematical model of the corneal surface assumes it to be a conicoid which may be described by the equation $y^2 = 2r_o x - px^2$ (Bennett, 1968). Although the mathematical model used in the Humphrey Auto Keratometer is based on natural logarithms and flattens faster in the periphery than an ellipsoid, the shape factor is equivalent to $(1 - p)$, or the square of the eccentricity.

The Canon K1 Auto-Keratometer has been described by Port (1985). In this instrument a single circular mire is focused on a video monitor and a flash boosts the light output for image processing. The results displayed are radii and powers, and axes of the principal meridians, the mean radius and the degree of corneal astigmatism. These measurements may be made in any of the five fixation positions: central, nasal, temporal, superior and inferior. The peripheral fixation positions are all 10° from the central one. Port investigated the intraoperator and interoperator consistency of measurements made with this instrument and found it to be 0.03–0.04 mm which he describes as being no worse than a conventional keratometer. A similar instrument is the Nidek KM800 (Port, 1987).

The Topcon CK-1000 computerized keratometer measures central and peripheral corneal curvatures simultaneously, taking 0.5 second to do so. It prints out central corneal radii, powers and axes, as well as astigmatism and average central radius and power. It also gives eight additional radius and power readings, two each above, below, nasal and temporal to the corneal apex. For an average corneal radius of 7.7 mm these readings are obtained: centrally over a diameter of 3.3 mm and peripherally at zones separated by 4.6 mm and 5.9 mm. The instrument has a measurement range from 5.62 to 11.25 mm in 0.01 mm steps, with powers ranging from 30 D to 60 D in 0.12 D steps, and astigmatism from 0 D to 7 D in 0.12 D steps. Central readings only can be obtained in 0.1 second. The print-out includes date and time which is useful for record purposes when, for example, it is necessary to monitor the diurnal variation and changes with time following radial keratotomy.

The Topogometer (Soper, Sampson and Girard, 1962; Sampson, Soper and Girard, 1965; Sampson and Soper, 1970) is a movable fixation device designed to fit the Bausch & Lomb keratometer. As the full mire separation is used, measurement of peripheral radii is not accurate: it is used to find the position, radii and diameters of the optic cap. A similar device is available for the American Optical Company CLC ophthalmometer.

The corneal contour has also been investigated by various photokeratoscopic techniques by Reynolds (1959), Reynolds and Kratt (1959), Blair (1960), Knoll (1961), Stone (1962), Ludlam and Wittenberg (1966), Ludlam et al. (1967) and Mandell and York (1969a,b). Further information is given in Chapters 7, 8 and 10. Stereophotogrammetry — a method of stereophotography used for determining surface contour — has been employed by Bertotto (1948), Rzymkowski (1954), and Bonnet (1959, 1964). Bier (1956, 1957) used specially constructed peripheral fitting lenses and Collignon-Brach, Papritz and Prijot (1966) employed profile photography.

This activity has produced many results of scientific interest but few developments of practical clinical value, with the exception of Dunn's (1959) independent curve fitting technique — a development of Bier's method — and photoelectronic keratoscopy (PEK). All the other methods are much more time consuming than using a fitting set, and the order of accuracy obtainable with photokeratoscopy is low (Stone, 1962), although improvements have been reported by more recent workers (Cochet and Amiard, 1966, 1969; Ludlam et al., 1967; Mandell and York, 1969a). In a contact lens context, the desire to make precise measurements of the contour of an individual cornea implies that if this information were available it would be possible, without any trial fitting, to specify the back surface of a contact lens which would fit that cornea perfectly. As the fit of a contact lens depends on factors other than the relationship of its back surface to the cornea, this implication seems unlikely to be true although the PEK system attempts to take some of these factors into account in designing the lens.

An advance on the PEK system, in which the photographic record must be sent away for analysis, would appear to be the Sun PKS-1000. This has the PAL 250 supplementary system for immediate analysis of the Polaroid photograph obtained, and also provides computer-printed, three-dimensional graphics of corneal shape, as well as designing hard lenses and indicating which soft lens of a given series is most suitable for a particular cornea (Port, 1987).

At present, use of a fitting set is the most reliable way of arriving at the specification for a prescription lens, though keratometry — as already described — can play a useful auxiliary part (Guillon and Lydon, 1986).

Slit lamp biomicroscopy

The slit lamp biomicroscope is an essential tool for the contact lens practitioner. No other method permits such a detailed examination of the anterior segment of the eye or reveals possible pathological changes at such an early stage. These advantages are obtained because a slit lamp gives a stereoscopic view, at magnifications of up to ×60, of a field of view which can be illuminated in many different ways and at high intensity. Most modern slit lamps can be operated with one hand, leaving the other free to manipulate the patient's lids if necessary. The clinical aspects of the use of this instrument are discussed in Chapter 8, as part of the initial examination, and in Chapter 19 in relation to after-care. The entire anterior segment of the globe, the tear film, the canthi and the lids may be examined in detail, using suitable techniques and stains such as fluorescein and rose bengal (Norn, 1974; Pearson, 1984, 1986). With suitable attachments, the apparent thickness of the cornea and depth of the anterior chamber can be measured with great accuracy.

The illuminating system, which gives the instrument its name, is essentially a projection system of short throw, in which the slide is replaced by a slit of variable width, the image of which is focused on the patient's eye. In most instruments it is possible to use a circular aperture if desired and to vary the colour and intensity of the illumination. In some, filters may also be available in the observation system to enhance contrast when observing corneal staining. The slit image is usually vertical, but it may be arranged in any desired meridian. It is now common practice to mount the illuminating system vertically, with a narrow reflecting prism or mirror to direct the beam on to the eye. This makes it easy for the illuminating system and microscope to be arranged coaxially for gonioscopy or fundus examination (*see* Chapter 24); but in routine examination of the anterior segment, it is rare to arrange the instrument in this way or to orientate the slit image in any meridian but the vertical.

The slit lamp and binocular microscope are usually mounted on a common pivot and both are focused at a point above the centre of rotation unless deliberately uncoupled. This arrangement means that both may be focused at the same time, using a joystick control, because

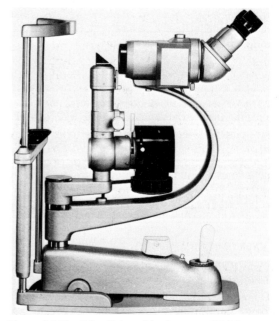

Figure 6.8 The Zeiss slit lamp biomicroscope 100/16. (Reproduced by kind permission of Carl Zeiss, Oberkochen)

the part of the eye illuminated by the slit focus will be in focus in the centre of the microscope field. The routine of focusing the slit accurately has been described by Stone (1966, 1979); if the lamp is oscillated about its pivot, the slit image will remain stationary if accurately focused. A 'with' movement shows that the focus is behind the illuminated surface and an 'against' movement shows that it is in front. *Figure 6.8* shows a typical modern slit lamp.

While the first consideration in choosing a slit lamp should be its optical performance (the slit image should be of uniform luminance, it should remain in focus while either the lamp or the microscope is swung about the pivot, its maximum length should be adequate to provide a complete optical section and its edges should be sharply defined and parallel at any slit width, while the microscope should provide a high resolution binocular view at any magnification), there are a number of features which are of particular value to the contact lens practitioner. These include the availability of attachments for measurement of corneal thickness (p. 255), the provision of a diffuser for general examination of the external eye and the inclusion of a pale-yellow filter in the viewing system, as well as a cobalt filter in the illuminating system, so that the contrast of faint fluorescein staining is enhanced (Pearson, 1984, 1986, *see*, for example, *Plates 18* and *19*). It is advisable to check that the yellow filter is not so dense as to substantially reduce the fluorescence, as well as absorbing the unwanted blue light. A green or 'red-free' filter in the illuminating system is also useful, aiding the detection and observation of neovascularization of the cornea and other vascular changes, as the blood vessels then appear black against a pale-green background as *Plate 3* shows. A magnification of at least ×40 should be available for effective examination of the endothelium. Polarizing filters in the illuminating and viewing systems permit corneal dilatation to be detected (*Plate 4*).

Types of illumination

It is conventional to describe five or six methods of illuminating the eye with a slit lamp (Doggart, 1949; Goodlaw, 1961). These are direct and indirect illumination, oscillating illumination, examination of the zone of specular reflection, retro-illumination and illumina-

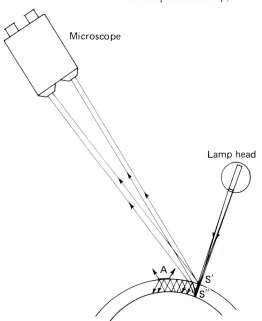

Figure 6.9 Direct and indirect illumination. The slit and microscope are focused at S′ and the section of cornea S′S″ is seen by direct illumination. Due to some light being reflected and scattered within the cornea, an irregularity at A, well outside the beam, is also seen in the microscope field by indirect illumination. *Plate 100* illustrates these methods of illumination

tion by sclerotic scatter. To this list should be added diffuse illumination, because some modern instruments now have a diffuser which can be placed in front of the reflecting mirror or prism. This is useful for general observation of the anterior eye and adnexa with low magnification. However, the first three methods mentioned are carried out simultaneously by the experienced observer, who continually varies the angle between the lamp and microscope while observing the whole of the microscope field, part of which is directly illuminated and the remainder indirectly illuminated by the slit. These methods of illumination are illustrated diagrammatically in *Figure 6.9*; they are particularly useful for general examination of the anterior segment at the first visit. Direct illumination with a narrow slit and a large angle between the lamp and microscope provides the best means of assessing the depth of an opacity or the corneal clearance of a contact lens (Marriott and Woodward, 1964). A larger width of slit allows a parallelepiped of cornea to be viewed; and by varying the depth of focus, the

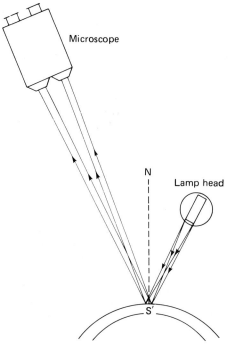

Figure 6.10 Specular reflection: the slit beam is focused at S′. NS′ is the normal to the cornea. By arranging the microscope and illuminating system at equal angles on either side of this, any irregularities of the focused surface are seen against a brilliantly lit background. *Plates 25a, 31, 64* and *65* illustrate features seen by specular reflection

front surface, intermediate area and back surface may be examined. The vertical striae at the back of the cornea, associated with corneal oedema following soft lens wear may be observed in this way (*see Plate 67*).

In contact lens practice, indirect illumination is particularly useful for the detection of epithelial microcysts (*Plate 61*) as are retro-illumination and sclerotic scatter (*see below*) both of which are forms of indirect illumination.

Examination of the zone of specular reflection requires, as shown in *Figure 6.10*, an appropriate adjustment of the angle between slit beam and microscope. It reveals minute surface defects very clearly. These appear as dark areas on a brilliant background. The discovery of corneal dimples by this method of illumination may provide the first indication that a corneal lens is damaging the surface.

Light specularly reflected from the back surface of the cornea yields an image of the endothelial cells (Vogt, 1920, 1930). Since transient changes in the endothelium as a result

of soft contact lens wear were first reported by Zantos and Holden (1977), observation of these cells has assumed increased importance, because failure of the endothelial pump leads to stromal oedema.

Unfortunately, the endothelium is difficult to see with the most commonly used clinical slit lamps which have maximum magnifications of about ×25. These may reveal the presence of the endothelial mosaic and very gross irregularities, but a view such as that shown in *Figures 6.11* and *6.12*, obtained with a Nikon photo-slit lamp adapted to specular microscopy, requires a magnification of about ×60 and high illumination from a tungsten halogen lamp. Visual observation of the endothelium requires some care and practice because the zone of specular reflection from the back surface is close to the much brighter reflex from the front.

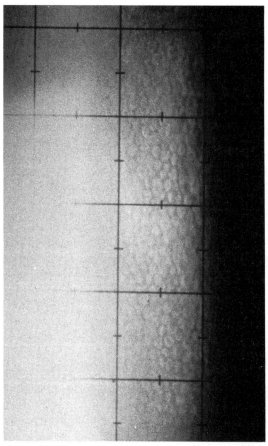

Figure 6.11 Normal corneal endothelium. (Courtesy of Dr M. Yap)

variation of size or shape and with a cell density of about 3000 cells/mm^2. With increasing age the cell density declines and there is increased variability in cell size (polymegathism) and cell shape (pleomorphism). These are illustrated in *Figure 7.79*.

The transient changes reported by Zantos and Holden were endothelial blebs; dark patches in the endothelial mosaic which appear about 10 minutes after inserting a soft lens, reach a maximum after about 30 minutes and then gradually diminish in number. They should not be confused with corneal guttata, depressions in the endothelium produced by localized thickenings in Descemet's membrane which stretch the endothelium and appear as black holes. Guttata are not transient and not specifically related to contact lens wear. *Plates 64–66* show these features.

Increased polymegathism and pleomorphism has been shown to occur in long-term contact lens wearers, although without a significant decrease in cell density (Schoessler and Woloschak, 1981).

For quantitative techniques such as cell density counts and numerical estimates of the degree of polymegathism or pleomorphism

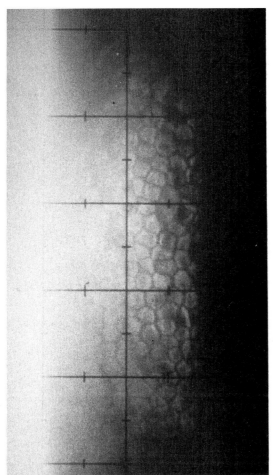

Figure 6.12 Corneal endothelium showing polymegathism and pleomorphism after cataract extraction. (Courtesy of Dr M. Yap)

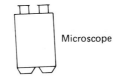

Microscope

Haag–Streit have developed a stereovariator which is fitted between the objectives and eyepieces of the binocular microscope of their slit lamp 900 BQ. This enables the angle of stereoscopic observation to be reduced from 13° to 4.5° which permits binocular, rather than monocular, observation of the corneal endothelium. This makes for easier use and enhances the appearance seen, particularly if used in conjunction with the Eisner contact lens (*see* Chapter 24). Estimation of the density of the endothelial cells is assisted by the associated use of a McIntyre eyepiece — *see Figure 24.10*. (The stereovariator has additional advantages for viewing the fundus and crystalline lens.)

The endothelium of a young person shows a uniform layer of hexagonal cells with little

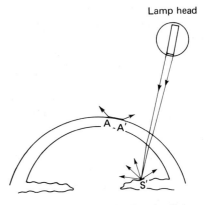

Lamp head

Figure 6.13 Retro-illumination: the slit beam and microscope may be uncoupled. An irregularity at AA′, focused in the microscope field, is seen against the light background of the iris where the slit is focused at S′. Marginal retro-illumination is shown in *Plate 53*

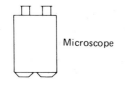

Microscope

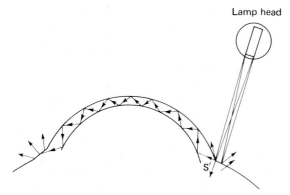

Lamp head

S'

Figure 6.14 Sclerotic scatter: the slit beam is focused at the limbus at S'. Light is totally reflected by the corneal surfaces as shown and emerges at the opposite limbus where it is scattered by the scleral tissue and shows as a glow of light as shown in *Figure 6.15*. Any corneal irregularity would similarly scatter the light which would then be seen either with or without the microscope as in *Plate 101a*

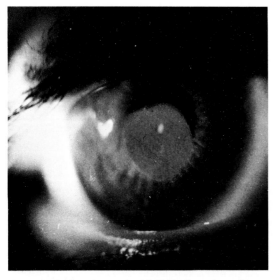

Figure 6.15 Central corneal epithelial oedema shown by scleral scatter (*see also Plate 23*)

photographic recording is ideal. The photographic techniques have been described by Holden, Zantos and Jacobs (1978) and Zantos, Holden and Pye (1980). Mayer (1984) reviews the whole field of clinical specular microscopy. The endothelial response to contact lens wear has been reviewed by Shakespeare and Yap (1984) and by Holden *et al.* (1986). Chapters 7 and 24 also deal with some of the photographic techniques. (*see Figures 7.9 and 24.1c*)

Retro-illumination and sclerotic scatter are shown in *Figures 6.13* and *6.14*. They are most easily carried out with the slit lamp and microscope uncoupled so that the microscope can be focused in front of the slit. Retro-illumination gives a particularly good view of limbal blood vessels which may be extending into the cornea. Sclerotic scatter — in which the slit is focused at the limbus and opacities or oedema revealed as luminous areas on an otherwise dark cornea — is a particularly useful technique for the contact lens practitioner, who is concerned during after-care not with gross corneal defects but with subtle signs of interference with corneal metabolism. The ease with which slight oedema of the cornea is revealed by sclerotic scatter is illustrated in *Figure 6.15*. The central circular cloudy patch, which is the manifestation of oedema following hard corneal lens wear, is most easily seen without the aid of a microscope. It is comparable to a newsprint picture, the form of which is difficult to determine if seen magnified. However, detail, such as microcysts and epithelial cell oedema, may be seen with the microscope focused on the corneal surface and uncoupled from the beam.

The slit lamp may also be used for the examination of contact lenses, both on and off the eye. Besides the estimation of corneal clearance already mentioned, the behaviour of the lens on the eye may be studied in great detail — especially its effect on the flow of tears and the behaviour of the precorneal film. The effect of a sharp transition or the edge of a fenestration hole in converting a bubble into froth can be clearly seen by this method of examination, as can the formation of dimple veil when small bubbles are pressed into the corneal surface by the lens (*see Plates 22 and 94*). Slit lamp examination also reveals the presence of unsuspected small bubbles under a corneal lens. Stone (1967) has discussed these appearances fully. With soft and rigid gas permeable lenses, the presence of deposits on the surface of the lens can be detected and their effects on wetting and tear flow over the lens can be studied. (*See* Chapter 19 and *Plates 24–26* and *31–40*.)

When the slit lamp is used as an illuminated binocular microscope for examining the surface quality and edge form of contact lenses (*see* Chapter 12), the lens is either mounted in a suitable holder and observed directly or by reflection in a mirror arranged at 45° to the axis of the illuminating system, or viewed directly by mounting in Plasticine. Surfaces, fenestrations and edges may be readily examined in this manner. However, the front surface of a contact lens is best studied when on the eye. The effects of scratches on the wettability of the surface may then be judged and the adherence to the surface of sebaceous matter from the back surface of the lids can more easily be seen in this way.

Measurement of corneal thickness

Measurement of corneal thickness (pachymetry or pachometry) has been carried out for many years as a special technique. Langham and Taylor (1956) reported that corneal thickness increased during contact lens wear, while Hedbys and Mishima (1966) demonstrated a linear relationship between stromal hydration and thickness. The popularity of the technique as a means of monitoring the fit of contact lenses has increased rapidly since Miller (1968) found corneal curvature and thickness changes to be well correlated. This finding was not confirmed by Mandell and his co-workers (Mandell and Polse, 1969, 1971; Mandell, Polse and Fatt, 1970). They did, however, find a positive association between central corneal clouding and thickness change. They also found that hard lenses which were a good fit produced an initial corneal thickening which gradually subsided during adaptation, but that poorly fitting lenses produced a persistent increase in thickness. This effect was especially marked with steep lenses. They suggest that increased thickness may be a better indicator of fit than corneal curvature changes because a central swelling may be confined to an area within the keratometer reflection points.

Polse and Mandell (1970) showed that the corneal thickness increased on reduction of the oxygen tension at the epithelial surface, and

Polse (1972) has shown that fluctuations of corneal thickness occur on discontinuing contact lens wear; these are accompanied by curvature changes similar to those described by Rengstorff (1967, 1969a) (*see* Chapter 20).

Since 1970, there has been a rapid increase in the number of soft lenses fitted and this has further increased the popularity of pachymetry as a means of monitoring lens-induced corneal changes, because a poorly fitting soft lens may produce a generalized corneal oedema which is much more difficult to detect by scleral scatter than the central oedema produced by a badly fitting hard lens (Stone, 1974).

Figure 6.16 shows the principle of pachymetry. If a narrow slit beam is directed normally at the corneal surface, the apparent thickness of the cornea can be found by measuring the width of the optical section seen through the microscope. This is now the usual technique. An alternative method in which the axis of the microscope is normal to the corneal surface was used by Donaldson (1966) and Mandell and Polse (1969). The true thickness can be found if the radius of curvature of the front surface and the refractive index of the cornea are known. For clinical purposes, measurement of the apparent thickness is sufficient, because the object is to detect changes in thickness rather than absolute values.

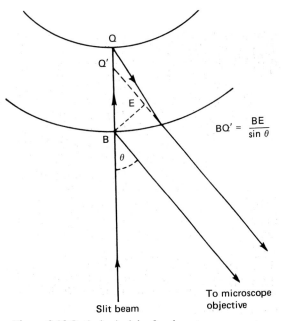

Figure 6.16 Optical principle of pachymetry

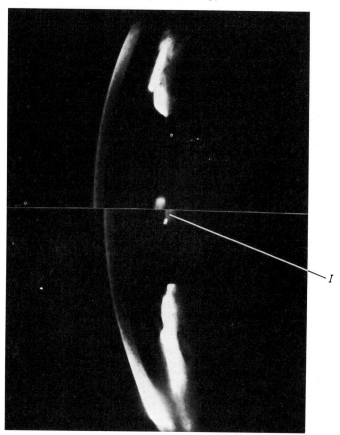

Figure 6.17 Appearance of slit section at end-point of measurement (Stone, 1974). Note vertical bisection of first Purkinje image, I, ensuring a vertically centred corneal measurement

The measurement of optical section width is made by means of a doubling device in the viewing system. The doubling is varied until (as in a keratometer) the doubled images are juxtaposed, the front surface of one image being aligned with the back surface of the other. To facilitate this adjustment, the slit lamp microscope is usually fitted with a special eyepiece so that the observer sees the top half of one image and the bottom half of the other, as shown in *Figure 6.17*. Provided the angle between the slit lamp and the microscope is kept constant, the instrument can be calibrated to read apparent depth directly.

Sources of error in pachymetry

It will be apparent from *Figure 6.16* that the measurement of apparent thickness depends on the slit beam being normal to the corneal surface. If the beam is not kept normal to the surface, an error of measurement will result.

Mishima and Hedbys (1968) used two small lights mounted at the same angle to the slit beam as the microscope, but on the opposite side of it. The images of these lights appeared on the front surface of the corneal image, one in the upper and one in the lower half of the field, only when the slit beam was normal to the cornea. A similar device, but with the lights mounted above and below the microscope objective, was used by Donaldson (1966) and Mandell and Polse (1969) to ensure that the microscope axis was normal to the corneal surface.

When measuring the thickness of the central cornea, normal incidence can be more simply maintained by asking the patient to look at the centre of the slit and checking that the reflected beam from the cornea returns to the slit aperture. A piece of translucent paper may be mounted above the slit aperture to receive the reflected beam. Vertical alignment can be checked by ensuring that the first Purkinje image of the slit, which is visible at the front surface of the crystalline lens, is bisected by the dividing line between the upper and lower halves of the field, as shown in *Figure 6.17* (Stone, 1974).

Peripheral corneal thickness measurements will be of value only if the patient's head is restrained and the slit lamp fitted with a fixation device which can be accurately and repeatably positioned so that the section measured is the same on each occasion.

It is easier to set the doubled images in coincidence if the slit beam is narrow. Norn (1974) pointed out that if a corneal parallelepiped is visible, it is possible to include the width of the slit in the corneal thickness measurement. A narrow beam, however, makes it difficult to judge the focus on the cornea and an out-of-focus image will also give an inaccurate reading. In setting up the instrument, it is essential to ensure that the slit beam and microscope are accurately focused on the corneal section. The highest magnification available should be used for this purpose. Once accurate focus has been achieved, the slit beam can be narrowed until there is just enough light to make the measurement, using the highest possible light output from the bulb.

Another possible source of error in comparative measurements arises from the fact that there is a diurnal variation in corneal thickness. Mandell and Fatt (1965) and Gerstmann (1972) found that the cornea is thicker on waking and thins, rapidly at first, then more gradually, throughout the waking day. Errors from this source can be minimized by ensuring that measurements on any particular patient are always made at the same time of day.

Kruse Hansen (1971), using the Haag–Streit instrument, found a systematic difference between the results obtained for the right eyes of his sample and those for the left, the thickness measured for the left eyes being significantly greater than those found in the right eye at the 1% level of probability. Ehlers and Kruse Hansen (1971) attribute this variation to the fact that in the Haag–Streit instrument, the microscope is always on the right side of the slit lamp during pachymetry; this means that the observation is made through a nasal portion of the cornea in the right eye and a temporal portion in the left. As the visual axis does not pass through the apex of the cornea, measurements made with the patient fixing the centre of

the slit will be made at different inclinations to the optical axis in the right and left eyes. The differences reported by Kruse Hansen are small (0.004 mm between the sample means for the right and left eyes) but in the light of these findings and those of Spurrett (1973), who found a systematic difference between right and left eyes in a group of contact lens wearers, the thickness of the right cornea apparently increasing more than that of the left, it is evident that apparent differences between the right and left eyes should be treated with caution.

References

BENNETT, A. G. (1964). A new keratometer and its application to corneal topography. *Br. J. physiol. Optics* **21**, 234–235

BENNETT, A. G. (1966). The calibration of keratometers. *Optician* **151**, 317–322

BENNETT, A. G. (1968). Aspherical contact lens surfaces. *Ophthal. Optician* **8**, 1037–1040

BERTOTTO, E. V. (1948). The stereophotogrammetric study of the anterior segment of the eye. *Am. J. Ophthal.* **31**, 573–579

BIER, N. (1956). A study of the cornea. *Br. J. physiol. Optics* **13**, 79–92

BIER, N. (1957). *Contact Lens Routine and Practice*, 2nd edn. London: Butterworths

BLAIR, W. A. (1960). Photo-electronic keratoscopy testing. *Contacto* **4**, 217–227

BONNET, R. (1959). Stéréophotogrammetrie de la cornee humaine. *Revue Opt. theor. instrum.* **38**, 447–462

BONNET, R. (1964). *La Topographic Cornéenne*. Paris: Desroches

BONNET, R. and COCHET, P. (1960). Nouvelle méthode d'ophtalmometrie topographique. *Bull. Mém. Soc. fr. Ophtal.* **73**, 687–716 (translated by E. Eagle (1962). *Am. J. Optom.* **39**, 227–251)

COCHET, P. and AMIARD, H. (1966). La photokeratoscopie, élément de biométrie cornéenne. *Bull. ds. Soc. d'ophtal. fr.* **66**, 1094–1104

COCHET, P. and AMIARD, H. (1969). Photography and contact lens fitting. *Contacto* **13**(2), 3–9

COLLIGNON-BRACH, J., PAPRITZ, F. and PRIJOT, E. (1966). Etude de l'applatissement périphérique de la cornée au moyen d'une technique photographique. *Bull. Soc. belge Ophtal.* **144**, 971–982

DOGGART, J. H. (1949). *Ocular Signs in Slit Lamp Microscopy*. London: Kimpton

DONALDSON, D. D. (1966). A new instrument for the measurement of corneal thickness. *Archs Ophthal.* **76**, 25–31

DUNN, G. M. (1959). Independent curve corneal fitting. *Optician* **138**, 501–503

EHLERS, N. and KRUSE HANSEN, F. (1971). On the optical measurement of corneal thickness. *Acta ophthal. (Kbh.)* **49**, 65–81

EMSLEY, H. H. (1955). *Visual Optics, Vol. 1*, 5th edn, pp. 301–331. London: Butterworths

EMSLEY, H. H. (1960). Revival of the keratometer. *Optician* **139**, 585–589

EMSLEY, H. H. (1963). The keratometer: measurement of concave surfaces. *Optician* **146**, 161–168

GERSTMANN, D. R. (1972). The biomicroscope and Vickers image splitting eyepiece applied to the diurnal variation in human central corneal thickness. *J. Microsc.* **96**, 385–388

GOODLAW, E. I. (1961). The use of slit lamp biomicroscopy in the fitting of contact lenses. In *Encyclopaedia of Contact Lens Practice*, Vol. 3, edited by P. R. Haynes. South Bend, Indiana: International Optics Publishing Corporation

GUILLON, M. and LYDON, D. P. M. (1986). Tear layer thickness characteristics of rigid gas permeable lenses. *Am. J. Optom. physiol. Optics* **63**, 527–535

HEDBYS, B. O. and MISHIMA, S. (1966). The thickness–hydration relationship of the cornea. *Expl Eye Res.* **5**, 221–228

HODD, F. A. B. (1962). Contact lenses in general ophthalmic practice. *Ophthal. Optician* **2**, 852–861

HOLDEN, B. A., ZANTOS, S. G. and JACOBS, K. J. (1978). The Holden–Zantos technique for endothelial and high magnification slit lamp photography. Brochure produced by Bausch & Lomb Soflens International

HOLDEN, B. A. *et al.* (1986). The endothelial response to contact lens wear. *Contact Lens Ass. J.* **12**, 150–152

KNOLL, H. A. (1961). Corneal contours in the general population as revealed by the photokeratoscope. *Am. J. Optom.* **38**, 389–397

KRUSE HANSEN, F. (1971). A clinical study of the normal human central corneal thickness. *Acta ophthal. (Kbh.)* **49**, 82–89

LANGHAM, M. E. and TAYLOR, I. S. (1956). Factors affecting the hydration of the cornea in the excised eye and in the living animal. *Br. J. Ophthal.* **40**, 321–340

LEHMANN, S. P. (1967). Corneal areas utilised in keratometry. *Optician* **154**, 261–264

LEVENE, J. R. (1965). The true inventors of the keratoscope. *Br. J. History Sci.* **2**, 324–342

LUDLAM, W. M. and WITTENBERG, S. (1966). Measurements of the ocular dioptric elements utilizing photographic methods. Part II. Cornea — theoretical considerations. *Am. J. Optom.* **43**, 249–267

LUDLAM, W. M., WITTENBERG, S., ROSENTHAL, J. and HARRIS, G. (1967). Photographic analysis of the ocular dioptric components. Part III. The acquisition, storage, retrieval and utilization of primary data in photokeratoscopy. *Am. J. Optom.* **44**, 276–293

MANDELL, R. B. (1960). Jesse Ramsden — inventor of the ophthalmometer. *Am. J. Optom.* **37**, 633–638

MANDELL, R. B. (1962a). Small mire ophthalmometry. Paper read before annual meeting of American Academy of Optometry, Miami, December, 1962

MANDELL, R. B. (1962b). Methods to measure the peripheral corneal curvature. Part 3: Ophthalmometry. *J. Am. optom. Ass.* **33**, 889–892

MANDELL, R. B. (1965). *Contact Lens Practice Basic and Advanced*. Springfield, Ill: Thomas

MANDELL, R. B. and FATT, I. (1965). Thinning of the human cornea on awakening. *Nature* **208**, 292–293

MANDELL, R. B. and POLSE, K. A. (1969). Corneal thickness changes as a contact lens fitting index. *Am. J. Optom.* **46**, 479–491

MANDELL, R. B. and POLSE, K. A. (1971). Corneal thickness and central clouding. *Am. J. Optom.* **48**, 129–132

MANDELL, R. B. and YORK, M. A. (1969a). A new calibration system for photokeratoscopy. *Am. J. Optom.* **46**, 410–417

MANDELL, R. B. and YORK, M. A. (1969b). Corneal contour from birth to five years — a cross-sectional study. Part II — corneal contour measurements. *Am. J. Optom.* **46**, 818–825

MANDELL, R. B., POLSE, K. A. and FATT, I. (1970). Corneal swelling caused by contact lens wear. *Archs Ophthal.* **83**, 3–9

MARRIOTT, P. J. and WOODWARD, E. G. (1964). A method of measuring the corneal clearance of a haptic lens. *Br. J. physiol. Optics* **21**, 61–83

MAYER, D. J. (1984). *Clinical Wide Field Specular Microscopy*. London: Baillière Tindall

MILLER, D. (1968). Contact lens induced curvature and thickness changes. *Archs Ophthal.* **80**, 430–432

MISHIMA, S. and HEDBYS, B. O. (1968). Measurement of corneal thickness with the Haag–Streit pachometer. *Archs Ophthal.* **80**, 710–713

NOBLE, D. (1962). The corneal contour and its measurement. Paper read to The Yorkshire Optical Society, Bradford, January, 1962

NOBLE, D. and SHERIDAN, M. (1962). The normal cornea, its variations and measurement. Paper read to the Contact Lens Society, Bradford, July, 1962

NORN, M. S. (1974). *External Eye, Methods of Examination*, 1st edn. Copenhagen: Scriptor

PEARSON, R. M. (1984). The mystery of the missing fluorescein. *J. Br. Contact Lens Ass.* **7**, 122–125

PEARSON, R. M. (1986). The mystery of the missing fluorescein–a postscript. *J. Br. Contact Lens Ass.* **9**, 36–37

POLSE, K. A. (1972). Changes in the corneal hydration after discontinuing contact lens wear. *Am. J. Optom.* **49**, 511–516

POLSE, K. A. and MANDELL, R. B. (1970). Critical O_2 tension at the corneal surface. *Archs Ophthal.* **84**, 505–508

PORT, M. J. A. (1985). The Canon Auto-Keratometer K1. *J. Br. Contact Lens Ass.* **8**, 79–85

PORT, M. J. A. (1987). Ophthalmic instruments: keratometry and keratoscopy. *Optician* **193**(5085), 17–24

RABBETTS, R. B. (1985). The Humphrey Auto Keratometer. *Ophthal. physiol. Optics* **5**, 451–458

RENGSTORFF, R. H. (1965a). The Fort Dix report. *Am. J. Optom.* **42**, 156–163

RENGSTORFF, R. H. (1965b). Corneal curvature and astigmatic changes subsequent to contact lens wear. *J. Am. optom. Ass.* **36**, 996–1000

RENGSTORFF, R. H. (1967). Variations in myopia measurements. *Am. J. Optom.* **44**, 149–161

RENGSTORFF, R. H. (1969a). Variations in corneal curvature measurements. *Am. J. Optom.* **46**, 45–51

RENGSTORFF, R. H. (1969b). Relationship between myopia and corneal curvature changes after wearing contact lenses. *Am. J. Optom.* **46**, 357–362

REYNOLDS, A. E. (1959). Corneal topography as found by photo-electronic keratoscopy. *Contacto* **3**, 229–233

REYNOLDS, A. E. and KRATT, H. J. (1959). The photo-electronic keratoscope. *Contacto* **3**, 53–59

RZYMKOWSKY, J. (1954). Stereophotographic and stereophotogrammetric reproduction of the cornea and sclera of the living eye. (Translated by W. P. Schumann.) *Am. J. Optom.* **31**, 416–422

SABELL, A. G. (1962). Surface distortions of the cornea from contact lenses. In *Transactions of the International Ophthalmic Optical Congress*, 1961. London: Crosby Lockwood

SAMPSON, W. G. and SOPER, J. W. (1970). Keratometry. In *Corneal Contact Lenses*, 2nd edn, edited by L. J. Girard. St Louis: Mosby

SAMPSON, W. G., SOPER, J. W. and GIRARD, L. J. (1965). Topographical keratometry and contact lenses. *Trans. Am. Acad. Ophthal. Otolaryngol.* **69**, 959–969

SCHOESSLER, J. P. and WOLOSCHAK, M. K. (1981). Corneal endothelium in veteran PMMA contact lens wearers. *Int. Contact Lens Clin.* **8**(16), 19–25

SHAKESPEARE, T. and YAP, M. (1984). Contact lens wear and the corneal endothelium. *Ophthal. Optician* **24**, 830–832

SOPER, J. W., SAMPSON, W. G. and GIRARD, L. J. (1962). Corneal topography, keratometry and contact lenses. *Archs Ophthal.* **67**, 753–760

SPURRETT, A. J. (1973). Corneal contact lens design and corneal change. *MSc Thesis*, University of Bradford

STONE, J. (1962). The validity of some existing methods of measuring corneal contour compared with suggested new methods. *Br. J. physiol. Optics* **19**, 205–230

STONE, J. (1966). The use of the slit lamp in ophthalmic practice. *Ophthal. Optician* **6**, 637–640, 645, 646

STONE, J. (1967). The use of the slit lamp in contact lens practice. *Contact Lens Practitioner*, June 1967

STONE, J. (1974). The measurement of corneal thickness. *Contact Lens J.* **5**(2), 14–19

STONE, J. (1979). The slit lamp biomicroscope in ophthalmic practice. *Ophthal. Optician* **19**, 439–455

VOGT, A. (1920). Die Sicht barkeit des lebenden Hornhordendothels. *von Graefes Arch. Ophthal.* **101**, 123

VOGT, A. (1930). *Lehrbuch und Atlas der Spaltlampen Mickroskopie des lebenden Auges*. Berlin: Springer

WILMS, K. H. and RABBETTS, R. B. (1977). Practical concepts of corneal topometry. *Optician* **174**(4502), 7, 8, 12, 13

ZANTOS, S. G. and HOLDEN, B. A. (1977). Transient endothelial changes soon after wearing soft contact lenses. *Am. J. Optom. physiol. Optics* **54**, 856–857

ZANTOS, S. G., HOLDEN, B. A. and PYE, D. C. (1980). A guide to ocular photography with the Nikon photo slit lamp. *Aust. J. Optom.* **63**, 26–32

Chapter 7

External eye photography

David Campbell-Burns

It is not intended, in a book of this nature, to attempt coverage of the whole field of ocular photography, let alone the realm of medical photography. It was also not felt to be necessary, in a book intended for such a specialized readership, to include the usual glossary of optical definitions and terms. The purpose of this chapter is to provide those basic data which will enable the practitioner to employ routine photography in his or her contact lens work. The bibliography gives references for further study. The aim must be a speedy and accurate recording of features of clinical interest, such results to be obtained with the minimum of disturbance to the practitioner's routine and the least possible inconvenience and discomfort to the patient. Apart from specialized photo-slit lamps, the hand-held camera is the preferred system, as stands, head rests, bellows and other such items can impede the swift and convenient use of the camera. Apart from the use of copy stand, bellows and transillumination stage for higher magnification photography of contact lens defects, all of the clinical work to be described here can be undertaken with the camera and flash hand held.

Many practitioners feel that their most valuable photographic record is that of the external eye, life-size, taken before fitting is commenced (*Plate 2*). Features such as lid position and conjunctival vascularization can be very clearly recorded and reference back to this photograph can be most useful. The colour plate sections of this book are a splendid illustration of the usefulness of external eye photography for record purposes in contact lens work.

The camera

By far the most suitable camera is the single lens reflex, normally referred to as an SLR (*Figure 7.1*). The particular advantage of this type is the complete absence of parallax, so important to close-up work. All except the very cheapest SLRs have automatic diaphragm control which permits framing and focusing to be done with the lens at full aperture. The diaphragm is then automatically stopped down to the chosen aperture just before the shutter releases. It is rare to find an SLR camera where the lens is not interchangeable. This facility permits the use of macro-lenses, extension tubes, bellows and lenses of different focal lengths, all of which are important in close-up photography. Examples of such accessories are shown in *Figure 7.2*.

The focusing screen fitted as standard equipment to most cameras has a circular micro-prism, surrounded by ground glass and/or a Fresnel lens to improve edge brightness. Although this arrangement is excellent for general photography, it is generally agreed that a plain ground glass or fine Fresnel screen is more satisfactory for telephoto and close-up work. Some more expensive cameras, such as the Nikon, Olympus, Minolta and Contax, feature interchangeable screens, allowing a flexible approach. Another most important, although insufficiently considered, point is that the photographer should find the camera comfortable to hold (*Figure 7.3*). This does not necessarily mean the smallest, lightest camera, as someone with large hands may find small cameras — such as the Olympus or Pentax — difficult to operate, while a woman with small hands may find it suits her perfectly. Zeiss even went to the lengths of retaining the Porsche design department to develop the body and control layout of the Contax for near perfect ergonomic efficiency. The practitioner should try holding and firing the complete equipment, i.e. the camera, the flash and the close-up equipment of choice, with one hand, as the other hand will be required for steadying oneself

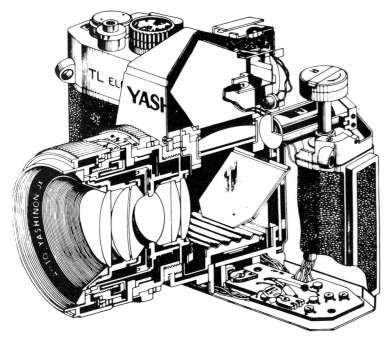

Figure 7.1 Section through a single lens reflex camera. The 45° mirror, allowing through-the-lens viewing, can be seen. This springs out of the way when the shutter is released. (Reproduced by kind permission of Yashica)

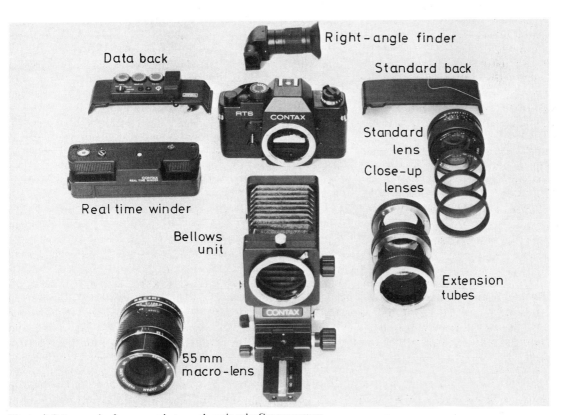

Figure 7.2 Accessories for macro-photography using the Contax system

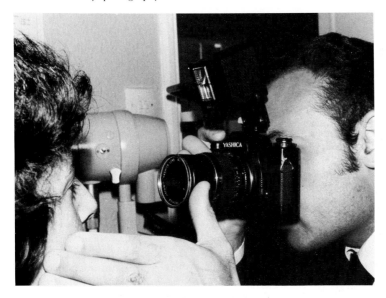

Figure 7.3 Single lens reflex system in use, showing one hand steadying the camera against the patient's face and the other hand holding the camera with forefinger ready to operate the shutter release

against the patient's brow or manipulating the lids.

Virtually all current camera systems are capable of meeting all or most of the above requirements; the smallest and lightest is probably the Olympus, the largest and heaviest the Leicaflex. Possibly the most widely used are the Pentax, Olympus, Minolta and Nikon instruments.

It is necessary to warn against the ordering of eyepiece correction lenses by direct reference to the user's spectacle prescription; most cameras do not have the viewing screen image at infinity, but have a built-in 'refractive error' of their own! The only way to ensure accurate correction is to interpose trial lenses between the eye and the viewfinder lens until the best result is found by trial and error. (The Minolta 9000 has this facility built in.) A special camera for clinical photography has been developed by Polaroid who also offer a range of user-processed instant films for 35 mm cameras.

The lens

Most SLR cameras have interchangeable lenses with automatic diaphragm control. The camera is normally supplied with a so-called 'standard' lens having a nominal focal length of 50 mm and a maximum aperture of around $f2$. This lens is likely to focus down to about 60 cm, and for closer work either supplementary lenses, bellows, extension tubes or a specially designed

macro-lens must be employed (*see Figure 7.2*). The best known macro-lenses are those from Nikon, Pentax, Minolta and Olympus, although a few are now offered by 'independent' manufacturers. These special lenses may have a longer focal length than standard lenses (for example, 55 mm), and are computed to give best results at much closer working distances than standard lenses. They allow a slightly longer working distance than bellows or extension tubes with standard lenses, thereby lessening illumination problems. They may also be used quite satisfactorily for general photography. The Micro-Nikkor macro-lens, for example, focuses from infinity down to 1:2 (half life-size) without interruption and, with the addition of an automatic extension tube, right down to 1:1.

It is preferable to use a lens of normal focal length for ocular photography up to 1:1 (life-size) because the working distance with this lens enables the photographer to steady himself against the patient's brow with the finger tips of his left hand, if normally right-handed, while the thumb is rested on the lens mount (*Figure 7.3*). A longer focal length makes lighting rather easier, but may increase the working distance too much for the above steadying technique to be employed. It must be emphasized that there is no advantage in using either longer or shorter focal length lenses in so far as depth of field is concerned, because this is a function of magnification and aperture and is independent of focal length.

A recent development is the enormous popularity of zoom lenses which feature a macro-facility. A 35–70 mm lens will not usually yield magnifications greater than 1:4, and quality would suffer with extension tubes. Longer focal lengths, or focal length ranges, are likely to be too heavy to be practicable.

Close-up (supplementary) lenses

Although these are normally sold in powers of +1, +2 or +3 D, for closer ranges very satisfactory results have been obtained with lenses of +10 or even +15 D. These lenses should, of course, be anti-reflection coated. Because it is essential in ocular photography to work at small apertures in order to yield adequate depth of field, the aberrations, which would normally preclude the use of such powerful supplementary lenses, are adequately controlled.

Extension tubes

Extension tubes are fitted between the camera lens and the camera body. As they do not contain any optical elements they do not affect the optical performance of the lens, except that the lens used may be operating in a magnification range for which it was not designed. Tubes are normally sold in sets of three and may be used either singly or in combination to give the required magnification (*Table 7.1*).

Bellows

Bellows may be regarded as continuously variable extension tubes, but, although it is possible to obtain them for some cameras with automatic diaphragm coupling, they are more unwieldy in use than tubes.

Table 7.1 Increase in magnification with extension: Macro-Takumar 50 mm f_4 lens with distance scale at 0.234 m

Magnification	Tubes used	Area to be photographed (mm)	Film-to-subject distance (mm)	Exposure factor[a]
0.50	Not used	48 × 72	234	×2.3
0.73	1 (12 mm)	33 × 49	213	×3.2
0.86	2 (19 mm)	28 × 42	209	×3.7
1.00	3 (26 mm)	24 × 36	208	×4.3

[a]Exposure factor — increase exposure by this amount.

The film

The choice of films can be broken down in two ways: are slides or prints required? Should the film be fast, for use in fluorescein photography, or slow for general external eye photography? (Colour film is assumed to be a necessity.)

Prints

Although prints may be more convenient, slides are cheaper and give much better contrast and detail. If, however, prints are preferred, suitable negative films are Kodacolor, Agfacolor or Fujicolor (ASA 100–200), although if accustomed to other brands, there are far more likely to be marked variations between the En Print type processing of one firm compared with another, than between the performances of different films. Until very recently, there has not been a freely available colour negative film which was ideal for ultraviolet illuminated work, but with the arrival of Fuji 400 and Kodacolor 400, this is now a possibility. Even faster films, up to and beyond ASA 1000, are made but the grain penalty makes them unacceptable for critical work.

The variations discussed above make the use of prints for colour matching of prosthetic lenses extremely unreliable. For best results keep to the same brand transparency film and illumination and experiment with colour temperature filtration until a satisfactory result is achieved. This technique should then be standardized. Colour compensation during processing is unlikely to be sufficiently consistent with prints.

Transparencies

For general clinical photography, Kodachrome 25 is widely considered to offer the best combination of sharpness, colour quality and processing reliability. Fujichrome, Ektachrome X, Agfacolor CT18 and Kodachrome 64 can also be recommended. Where extra film speed is called for, Ektachrome 200 is a most versatile material as it can, by varying its development times, be rated at speeds from its normal ASA 200 up to an astonishing ASA 2000! Naturally, quality suffers when the film is 'pushed' to this degree, but very acceptable results are obtained by rating it up to one and a half stops faster, i.e. up to about ASA 500.

A new, and little known, development is the service from Fuji which provides for slides and prints from one film. Any Fujichrome, or E6 compatible, slide film can be processed and returned together with 6 × 4 inch (15 × 10 cm) prints of excellent quality. This service is of great benefit to the lecturer who may wish to put the print in the patient's record and keep the slides for lectures. However, not all materials or services are available in every country.

Illumination

The modern, compact electronic flashgun combines all of the requirements for a light source in clinical photography. It is light in weight, powerful, has carefully balanced, consistent light output and is cheap to buy and run. The flash duration is very short, typically less than 1/10 000th of a second, eliminating any danger of subject movement.

The flashgun should, ideally, have a light source with a small aperture as this will produce a correspondingly small reflex when photographing subjects such as the cornea.

A few manufacturers, notably Nikon and Minolta, make special flash systems for clinical work. The Medical Nikkor is a complete lens/flash unit with variable magnification ranges while the Minolta unit is fitted to the front of the macro-lens and provides completely automatic exposure together with control of the illumination via four tiny flash tubes and a focusing light which extinguishes just before exposure.

Technique

The flashgun is best fitted to a tilting flash adaptor and both mounted on the camera accessory shoe. It must be remembered that this may render the 'hot shoe' (direct contact) feature inoperative, so that the flash unit must be connected to the camera's X synchronization contact (if present). The flashgun is then tilted downwards in order to point directly at the subject; if this angle is carefully adjusted it is possible to produce evenly illuminated photographs as close as life-size (i.e. 1:1; *Figures 7.3–7.6*). Although, in theory, the ring flash seems more suitable, in practice it produces a most inconvenient reflex right in the centre of the cornea. The light output of the smallest flash units has been found to be quite adequate even with such slow films as Kodachrome 25, producing excellent results at apertures as small as *f*16. Larger flashguns, while useful in ultraviolet photography, are of no help in normal colour work as they are too powerful and many camera lenses cannot cope with the extra

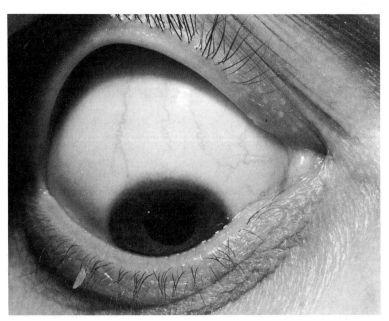

Figure 7.4 The external eye photographed at 1:1 magnification on the negative, and utilizing the technique shown in *Figure 7.3*. The photographs in *Figures 7.5* and *7.6* were also taken in the same way

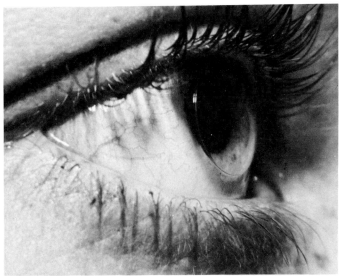

(a)

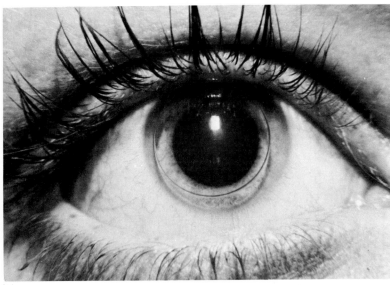

(b)

Figure 7.5 Photographs showing the position taken up by a corneal lens: (a) from the side; (b) from in front. Notable also is the low lower lid position and in (b) the shadow cast on the iris by the edge of the lens

illumination as they do not stop down further than *f*16, although most macrolenses will stop down to *f*32.

Most cameras must be set to a speed of around 1/125th of a second or slower as their focal plane shutters will otherwise produce partially exposed frames. For best results the camera handbook should be consulted. It is of no advantage to set the shutter speed at a value slower than that required for flash photography, because the result may well show blurring due to the effect of the ambient illumination, even though the flash duration is so short. The lighting used for focusing must be very carefully controlled; if it is too dim it is impossible to see properly to focus and, if too bright, particularly with ultraviolet work, the colour rendering is affected.

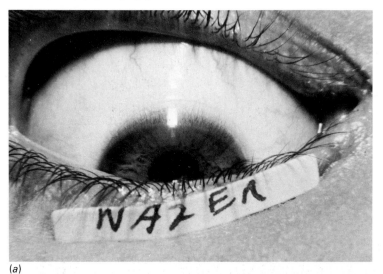

(a)

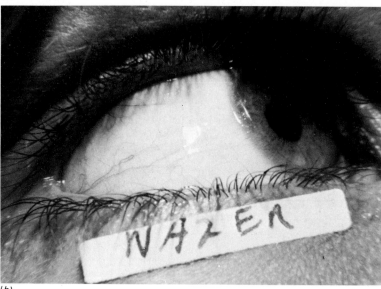

(b)

Figure 7.6 Photographs showing the positioning of a soft lens on the eye: (a) with gaze depressed and upper lid raised;   (b) looking nasally

Ultraviolet photography

The recording of corneal staining or of the fit of a hard or rigid gas permeable (RGP) contact lens requires some adaptation to the above technique (*Plates 10–20*). It is most convenient if a second camera body is available, permanently loaded with the faster film required (for example, Ektachrome 200 or 400, or Kodacolor 400). With only one camera body it is inevitable that it is loaded with the wrong film when required! A small electronic flashgun fitted with a Kodak Wratten 47B Gelatin Filter, which is blue, should be mounted, as before, on a tilting flash shoe and angled downwards. In order to increase the blue/yellow-green contrast of the photograph a pale yellow (× 2) filter must be fitted over the camera lens.

Slit lamp photography

If photographs of the external eye are all that is required, the results obtained with a conventional camera system are superior (and very much cheaper) to those obtained with a photo slit lamp. When slit section photographs are called for, such as that in *Figure 7.7*, there is no substitute for a specially designed photo slit lamp such as made by Gambs, Zeiss (West Germany), Zeiss (Jena) or Nikon (*Figure 7.8*).

The introduction by Zeiss (Oberkochen), in the mid-sixties, of a photo slit lamp with an integrated electronic flash system, marked a turning point in ophthalmic photo documentation. Together with the much improved colour emulsions then available, this instrument made possible the production of very high quality records with a minimum of operator skill. The main practical advantage was the ease with which the clinician could instantly record features of interest. Later developments include stereoscopic attachments, cine and TV/video recording. Two systems were eventually offered by Zeiss: one used a camera body mounted above, and photographing between, the microscope objectives of the slit lamp and another

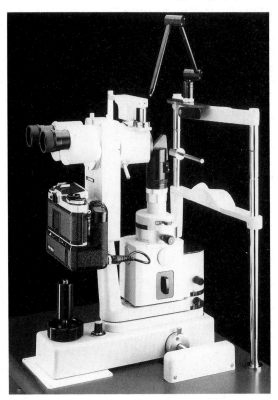

Figure 7.8 The Nikon Zoom-Photo Slit Lamp Microscope FS-2. (Reproduced by kind permission of Nikon)

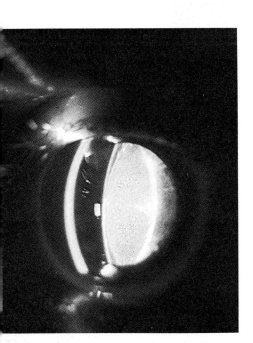

Figure 7.7 Section of cornea and crystalline lens taken with a Zeiss (Oberkochen) photo slit lamp

employed a beam-splitter between the body of the instrument and the eyepieces. The latter system achieved a true 'WYSIWYG' (what-you-see-is-what-you-get) result. The electronic flash discharge tube was neatly integrated into the lamp-housing and fired by a button on the joystick.

Later developments have included fibreoptic fill-in illumination (Gambs and Nikon), motorized film transport, simultaneous 'third-party' viewing, camera databanks and zoom lenses (Nikon). All illumination and viewing techniques employed in routine slit lamp examination may be used in biophotomicroscopy. Desirable features to look for when choosing an instrument include ease of use, one-handed operation, simplicity of exposure adjustment and the provision of fill-in illumination for external eye photography.

Suitable instruments are available from Nikon, Zeiss (Oberkochen), Zeiss (Jena), Topcon and Takagi.

Exposure

Although it is theoretically possible to calculate the correct exposure from the flash factor and the film speed, in practice the result is usually unreliable due to the very short distances involved. A much simpler method is to make an 'exposure gradient' test. The chosen film/flashgun/magnification combination is used to produce a series of test exposures from maximum to minimum aperture of the lens used. When the slides (or prints) are returned from processing they should be viewed by whichever method will subsequently be employed, i.e. projection, viewer or lightbox for slides, and the exposure of the best slide (or print) chosen. It is sometimes possible to refine this result still further by selecting an intermediate aperture, although not all lenses have 'click' settings at half stop intervals. This information should then be recorded on a label stuck to the camera or flashgun (for example, K25/1:1/ƒ16). This will, of course, have to be repeated for different film/filter combinations, although it has been found that moderate changes in magnification, for example, between 3:1 and 1:1.5, make little difference. The reason for this is that the inverse square laws relating to the increase in illumination *vs* the extra exposure required with greater extension, cancel each other out. Typical exposure data are given in *Table 7.2*.

Fundus cameras

Besides the equipment already described, fundus cameras, such as the Zeiss (Jena) model,

Table 7.2 Typical exposure data

	Film		
	K25[a]	E200[b]	E400[c]
Magnification	1:1	1:2	1:2
Lens (mm)	50	50	50
Filter (camera)	None	2 × yellow	2 × yellow
Filter (flash)	None	47B	47B
Flashgun	—	Vivitar 121	—
Aperture	ƒ16	ƒ2.8	ƒ5.6

[a]K25 is Kodachrome 25, i.e. film speed ASA 25.
[b]E200 is Ektachrome 200, i.e. film speed ASA 200.
[c]E400 is Ektachrome 400, i.e. film speed ASA 400.
All three films are made by Kodak.

may be used for external eye photography, yielding high quality transparencies. Magnification can be varied from about twice life-size (2:1) down to one-third life-size (1:3).

The Docustar Fundus Camera (Reichert) is a hand-held, Polaroid system capable of both internal and external eye photography without the need for pupil dilatation.

Photokeratoscopy

This is a technique for photographing the regularity of the corneal front surface or the front surface of a soft contact lens by means of Placido disc type rings. Examples can be seen in *Figure 11.6, 11.9* and *11.14* in Chapter 11 and *Figure 15.14* in Chapter 15. The technique is also used for measuring the corneal contour and, in one system, black and white Polaroid photographs of the corneal image are automatically scanned to give corneal curvature and eccentricity values in the two principal meridians. Corneal lenses are then designed by computer from this information (*see* Chapters 5, 6 and 10).

Photography of the corneal endothelium

Holden, Zantos and Jacobs (1978) have described a technique for endothelial and high magnification slit lamp photography where a 35 mm camera, preferably motorized, is mounted behind one of the eyepieces of a slit lamp by means of a special support. The endothelial zone is viewed through the viewfinder and the photograph (*Figure 7.9* and *see Figure 15.12*) taken by means of a cable release to avoid camera shake which could affect focus.

An entirely different approach is employed by Pocklington in the Keeler Widefield Specular Microscope. This specially designed instrument uses a contact cone together with a motorized focusing system to cover an area of 1 mm^2 and produce an image which fills the 35 mm format (36 × 24 mm). The floating cone movement of 5 mm, employs a known degree of applanation with an independent, internal mechanism adjusting the focus. In addition to the standard 35 mm camera body, a Polaroid back or video camera can be used. A normal photographic magnification would be ×30 (viewed at ×120),

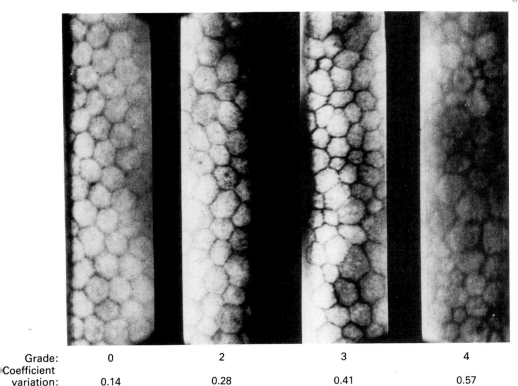

Grade:	0	2	3	4
Coefficient variation:	0.14	0.28	0.41	0.57

Figure 7.9 Corneal endothelium photographed by the Holden–Zantos technique showing normal central corneal endothelium (grade 0) on the left and various grades of endothelial polymegathism (variations in cell size) — grades 2, 3 and 4 — as indicated by the coefficient of variation given below each grade. (Reproduced by kind permission of Bausch & Lomb.) (*See also Plates 64–66*)

with variation between ×22 and ×50 being provided for.

Chapter 24 gives details of the Eisner Contact Glass used with the Haag–Streit photo slit lamp for corneal endothelial photography.

Reference

HOLDEN, B. A., ZANTOS, S. G. and JACOBS, K. J. (1978). The Holden–Zantos technique for endothelial and high magnification slit lamp photography. Brochure produced by Bausch & Lomb Soflens International, Rochester, NY, USA

Further reading

BISHOP, C. (1976). Basic aspects of ophthalmic photography. *Ophthal. Optician* **16**, 719–720, 729–731, 762–764, 769, 817–820, 845–848, 853–854

Eastman Kodak Data Book, Publication No. 3 (1972). *Clinical Photography*

Eastman Kodak Medical Publication No. 18 (1973). *Medical Photography (Clinical, Ultra-Violet and Infrared)*

HALL, J. (1973). Ophthalmic optics and the visual sciences. *Ind. comml. Photogr.* **13**, March, 84–91

HORDER, A. (1956). *The Ilford Manual of Photography*, 4th edn. Ilford, Essex: Greenwood

Kodak Information Sheet (AM-900(H)) (1977). *An Introduction to Infrared Photography*

LITTMAN, G. (1965). Slit image photography. *Zeiss Inf.* No. 56, 3–11

LANG, M. M. (1971). Fluorescence colour photography of the eye with the polaroid CU5 camera. *Aust. J. Optom.* **54**, 242–248

MAUDE, N. (1976). Developments of ophthalmic photography in the field. *Br. J. Photogr.* **123**, 298–299

PEARCE, N. (1974). Slit lamp photography of the eye. *Med. biol. Illust.* **24**, 21–27

ROSEN, E. (1976). Recent advances in retinal photography. *Med. biol. Illust.* **26**, 27–31

STEIN, H. A. and SLATT, B. J. (1971). Eye photography. In: *The Ophthalmic Assistant*, 2nd edn, Chapter 23. St Louis: C. V. Mosby

WAGSTAFF, D. F. (1970). External eye photography in ophthalmic practice. *Ophthal. Optician* **10**, 17–28

WILMOT, F. R. H. (1966). An integrated system for contact lens photography. *Ophthal. Optician* **6**, 924–926

Chapter 8

Assessment of patient suitability for contact lenses

Janet Stone

Since the first and second editions of this book were published contact lenses have become a popular form of visual correction and their fitting in private practice has become largely soft lens orientated. However, there has been a renewal of interest in corneal lens fitting with the advent of more and more gas permeable hard or rigid gas permeable (RGP) materials of increasing oxygen permeability and better wetting characteristics — many now permitting extended wear. Scleral lens fitting is now almost entirely confined to hospital departments where these lenses are used for eyes with pathological or abnormal conditions unsuited to soft or corneal lenses. The indications for this type of scleral lens are fully covered in Chapters 17, 18 and 21. Additional special uses of scleral lenses are covered in Chapter 24. Scleral lens fitting is so time consuming, and therefore costly, compared to soft and corneal lenses, that they are now rarely considered as a practical option by most contact lens practitioners.

The increasing price and complexity of spectacle lenses has led to a reduction in the cost differential between the two modes of visual correction, so that many more people are now considering contact lenses as their main form of optical correction. Also, contact lenses are often requested for specific limited use and need to be interchangeable with spectacles, so that the contact lens practitioner not only has to assess patient suitability for contact lenses in general, but also the best form of lens and material to satisfy these more sophisticated requirements. This has led to a broadening in the factors to consider when assessing patients for contact lens fitting. Limitations still exist in the types of lenses available as well as in the suitability of the prospective wearers. Careful selection benefits

both the patient and the practitioner by avoiding time wasted in attempting to fit unsuitable patients.

As far as ocular contour is concerned, it is now possible to fit any eye with a contact lens — but successful wearing depends on adequate patient motivation and absence of contra-indications. Patient selection depends on adequate recognition of these factors by the practitioner.

Certain pathological and abnormal conditions of the eye and adnexa are a definite *indication* for contact lenses.

Indications and contra-indications for contact lens wearing

These may be considered broadly under three headings: psychological influences, pathological, anatomical and physiological factors, and personal and external factors. Some overlap between the three is inevitable.

Psychological influences

A small study in 1987 by Nelson and West indicated that extroverted, well-adjusted, stable people were more likely to successfully adapt to contact lenses than anxious, introverted people. Practitioners need to keep this in mind when pointing out the following factors to their patients who should be made aware of the essential differences between the fitting and wearing of spectacles and of contact lenses. This is necessary to avoid subsequent disillusionment on the part of the patient. From the legal standpoint, it is as well to issue the patient with a printed booklet in which certain general facts about contact lenses are emphasized. This is also helpful because many patients are not fully attentive at the initial interview and may forget what is said by the practitioner, who may omit to mention or emphasize certain points.

Prior to embarking on the actual fitting of contact lenses, the practitioner should draw the patient's attention to the following special aspects of contact lens fitting and wear, so that the patient has the opportunity to reject them before being placed under any obligation.

Time taken for fitting

Since this varies from patient to patient, and depends on the skill of the practitioner and the type of lens to be fitted, it is up to each practitioner to say how long the entire fitting is likely to take. Including tuition of lens handling some 2 to 3 hours may be needed with the practitioner and/or optometric assistant. Numerous visits to the practitioner may be necessary and, if the fitting proves complicated, a longer time may be involved.

Tolerance trials add to the time spent by both patient and practitioner. Some practitioners like to arrange for a 2-week trial of contact lenses. Four hours is about the desirable minimum length for a tolerance trial. If fitting extended or continuous wear lenses, it is advisable to arrange a 24-hour tolerance trial commencing early in the day, and to see the patient again at the end of the day, as well as the following morning after the lenses have been worn all night. All this may add another hour of 'chair-side' time to the fitting, and if more than one tolerance trial is necessary the time involved with the patient during fitting may be extended and the patient involved for much longer. Tolerance trials are discussed further in Chapter 9 and in those chapters devoted to lens fitting.

Fitting children with contact lenses can be very time consuming and parents should be advised of this. The special considerations for paediatric fitting are dealt with in Chapter 21. It is especially important with children that they be dealt with in an unhurried but reassuringly firm fashion. If under the age of 12 years, ideally the child should be fitted in the presence of one of the parents, both to give the child reassurance and to demonstrate lens handling to the parent who may subsequently be required to insert and remove the lenses, particularly if the child is under the age of 7 years. At the first visit, besides the preliminary examination and measurements, it is often enough just to insert one lens and leave proper fitting for a further visit. Several hours practice are often needed for a child to perfect insertion and removal techniques, although children whose parents wear contact lenses may accomplish insertion and removal very quickly, and can be less troublesome and time consuming than adults.

Patients should also be made aware of the need for continuing clinical care involving time spent at regular after-care check-ups.

Initial discomfort — physical and visual

Patients used to wearing spectacles are sometimes totally unprepared for the initial difficulties with contact lenses and should be warned of the likelihood of corneal and lid sensation, photophobia, flare, after-wear blur with spectacles, and so on, as appropriate. These difficulties are much less noticeable with soft lenses but may still occur as may fluctuations of vision during wear due to variations in hydration, deposits on the surfaces or deformation of the surface by lid pressure and rotation of lenses during blinking and eye movements.

Gradual wearing procedure

The advisability of building up wearing time slowly, particularly with corneal lenses, is well recognized. Patients must be made fully aware of this, otherwise they may think that changing to contact lenses is as simple as changing their spectacle prescription. Only extended wear lenses do not always require a build-up time, but several visits to the contact lens practitioner are necessary in the first few weeks of wear instead.

Special storage

Owing to their effective cost, and the properties of the plastics material from which they are made, contact lenses must be handled and stored very carefully. Because of their wetting and hydration properties and the danger of transferring harmful organisms on to the eye, they must be kept in sterile conditions and certain solutions must be employed during their handling and storage. This aspect is of extreme importance (*see* Chapter 4), and patients must be informed early on which types of solution are suitable for their lenses and which ones may come into contact with the eye.

Extra hygiene

Many of the problems associated with contact lens wear result from failure to keep the lenses properly clean and/or disinfected, probably because these are time-consuming procedures. Patients who start off by carrying out these procedures adequately do not always maintain them, whereas in fact the older the lenses become the more the surfaces deteriorate with natural wear and tear, and the more likely they are to become soiled. Thus, extra cleaning procedures often become necessary as the lens material ages. By contrast spectacle wearers may spend one minute or less each day cleaning their spectacles. During handling of contact lenses the hands should be kept clean and free of grease and nicotine. Contamination of the lenses with face or eye make-up preparations must also be avoided, and special make-up creams may be necessary (Cordrey, 1972). Eye cosmetics are known to be a source of potentially serious infection (Bruch, 1973; Wilson *et al.*, 1973), and cases of conjunctival-embedded pigment from mascara and eye-liner causing long-term discomfort and excessive lacrimation have been reported by Stewart (1973). It is helpful to issue patients with a leaflet explaining the safest methods of using eye and other make-up with contact lenses, such as that issued by the Department of Optometry and Visual Science, The City University, London (1974), which is based on articles by McConnell (1967) and Gustafson (1967). Chapter 9 also deals with this aspect of eye and lens care (*see* p. 330). Patients should also examine their lenses daily to avoid wearing badly scratched, cracked or chipped lenses. These aspects add to the 'nuisance value' of the lenses and patients who are not prepared to take the necessary time and trouble to keep their lenses clean should preferably not be fitted. This is particularly so with soft lenses which are more easily contaminated than hard lenses, but gas permeable hard lenses also attract deposits and require meticulous cleaning — *see* Chapter 4. Some types of soft lens may require heat disinfection and this, unfortunately, adds to the time and the initial cost of lens maintenance,

although in the long term the use of solutions is more costly than heating, but this may be offset by slightly shorter lens life.

Stringent after-care at regular intervals

Abrasions of the cornea are easily caused by contact lenses, usually due to foreign bodies beneath them, or adherent deposits, but occasionally due to trauma from the edge of a hard lens during insertion or removal before these techniques have been mastered. Finger nails also sometimes damage the eye during these procedures. Usually the ensuing discomfort is minimal, but patients have been known to reject lens wear as a result.

Particularly as corneal sensitivity is lowered during hard contact lens wear (Boberg-Ans, 1955; Millodot, 1976), these symptoms may go unnoticed and patients should be warned in advance of the slight additional risk. Provided they understand the need for after-care and the possibility of minor emergencies arising, patients rarely forego contact lens wear for this reason. However, it is important that they realize that examination of the eyes and lenses at intervals of no greater than 1 year is advisable all the time that contact lenses are worn, so that the practitioner may detect any changes which may have taken place and advise them accordingly. This routine after-care check is, of necessity, longer and more detailed than that given to a normal spectacle wearer. Some patients require more frequent after-care checks because of recurrent symptoms or pathology. Also, if continuous or extended wear soft lenses are fitted, more frequent after-care checks should be made.

Need for and cost of insurance

Corneal lenses are easily lost, soft lenses less so, and scleral lenses hardly ever. All contact lenses are easily damaged but particularly ultrathin and high water content soft lenses. Loss or damage is most likely to occur during the initial wearing period before complete adaptation to the lenses takes place, and before facility of handling has been mastered. It is therefore essential for patients to insure lenses for their replacement value plus the estimated cost of the practitioner's fee at the time of replacement. The insurance premium may be as much as

20% of the original fee plus the cost of the lenses. This is the rate normal for soft lenses, although usually it is about 5–10% for hard lenses. Some of the lens manufacturers run insurance or replacement schemes of their own, which can be helpful to both patient and practitioner, but practitioners should be aware of the legal implications of being involved in these schemes.

Lack of protection from foreign bodies

Spectacle wearers who transfer to contact lenses always, at first, miss the protection afforded by their spectacles and should be warned of initial troubles in windy and dusty atmospheres. *Plates 12* and *59* show the effect of foreign bodies on the cornea. Soft and scleral lenses provide more protection from foreign bodies than hard corneal lenses — the degree of protection being related to the size of the lens, and the glove fit of soft lenses. Gas permeable hard lenses also have very little peripheral corneal clearance so that foreign bodies cannot easily gain entrance beneath them.

Cost of lenses, examination fees and accessories

Conscientious practitioners usually include up to 1 year of after-care in the initial fitting fee, which must therefore be adequate to cover the practitioner for the time likely to be spent with the average patient during that time. It is only fair to warn patients of other costs they are likely to incur, such as travelling expenses, and the costs of solutions and accessories. Also soft lenses may require cleaning by the practitioner from time to time (*see* Chapter 4) and hard lenses similarly may need polishing. Many practitioners run after-care or service schemes for which appropriate annual charges are made.

Fear of lenses

Another barrier that has to be overcome is the patient's fear of having anything put on the eye. Patient handling is dealt with in Chapter 9, and it is sufficient here to say that a practitioner who inspires confidence is usually able to help a patient overcome this fear very quickly. Children (and the parents who accompany them) often require a very special approach.

Apart from these possible 'psychological' disadvantages, there are many definite indications for contact lenses which have a psychological background, as will be seen from the following.

Safety

Fear of damage to the eyes from possible broken spectacle lenses in sports such as football, rugby and cricket is removed. There are many cases of contact lenses having afforded definite protection to the eyes, where otherwise a blow to the eye might have resulted in both external and internal ocular damage (Rengstorff and Black, 1974).

Security and clarity of vision

A feeling of safety is engendered by wearing contact lenses as opposed to spectacles when worn for certain sports such as horse riding, cycling (especially in the rain), shooting in rough country, skiing and bob-sleighing. The removal of the nuisance value of spectacles which steam up when playing, for example, badminton, tennis, squash and table tennis is a distinct advantage; also, spectacles become coated with spray when sailing.

Cosmetic reasons

Intense dislike of spectacles, particularly if very thick lenses are worn, has often meant that contact lenses bring about a marked cosmetic improvement. This can and does result in a beneficial personality change from introvert to extrovert. To some patients spectacles are an advertisement of a personal disability which is relieved by wearing contact lenses.

Restoration of normal appearance

Similar psychological benefits have been afforded to people (especially children) with disfigured eyes which are fitted with prosthetic lenses to give a normal appearance; for example, in albinism, aniridia, microphthalmos or an ugly eye due to injury or disease. *Plates 103–107* show such examples.

Children

Unfortunately, children who wear spectacles, still occasionally suffer taunts from their classmates. If children are of fairly placid disposition they may adapt very readily to contact lenses and thereby avoid such problems.

However, it is definitely not desirable to force children to wear contact lenses because of some whim on the part of the parents. To a child, the fitting of contact lenses can be a very traumatic experience and if it is carried out entirely against the will of the child it can lead to considerable upset and possible long-lasting psychological disturbance to the child. For this reason, if contact lenses are essential for some pathological or serious visual condition (*see* Chapter 21), it may be desirable for them to be fitted under general anaesthesia in a hospital environment, if the child is very young.

Pathological, anatomical and physiological factors

Some patients are selected for contact lens wear because no other form of visual correction is as good or even suitable. Others may be rejected due to the presence of an abnormal anatomical feature or because of the existence of a pathological condition. These aspects will now be dealt with in more detail.

Cases where contact lenses are indicated for pathological reasons

In these cases the patient is frequently referred to the contact lens practitioner by his medical adviser. If not, before fitting is undertaken, medical cooperation should be sought (*see* Chapter 9). Chapters 18 and 21 deal in detail with fitting these cases, which are briefly considered below.

Keratoconus

Early cases may be suitable for corneal lenses as may be some medium keratoconic corneas, but most medium and advanced cases are still best corrected with scleral lenses. Soft lenses with a hard corneal lens fitted steep on the front surface have been tried successfully in keratoconus (*Plate 122*). In one or two cases a soft lens has been used underneath a scleral lens as shown in *Plate 85* (Westerhout, 1973).

Corneal irregularities and scars

Unless these are small and near the limbus (when a small, carefully centred corneal lens

may be fitted), soft or scleral lenses are advisable. If the irregularity is great, flush fitting of the cornea with a scleral lens may yield best results.

Soft lenses are definitely recommended where sterile superficial corneal ulcers are present as they assist corneal healing. However, they should not be used if any infection exists, because the presence of the lens only exacerbates the condition (Leibowitz and Rosenthal, 1971). Soft lenses, either with or without the use of hypertonic saline solution every 2 hours, are also recommended for bullous keratopathy and greatly alleviate discomfort (Takahashi and Leibowitz, 1971). The results of their wear may be spectacular, sometimes obviating the need for enucleation and often giving considerable visual improvement (*see Plates 118–121*). Soft lenses are also of assistance as a form of splint to assist corneal healing following penetrating corneal wounds when they prevent leakage of aqueous and collapse of the anterior chamber (Leibowitz, 1972). Both hard and soft lenses have been put to similar use as splints following operations for cataract extraction and to hold corneal grafts in place following keratoplasty.

Protection against drying and foreign bodies

There are a number of conditions in which tear output is reduced. If these lead to drying of the eye, corneal opacification and infection may occur. An alternative to tarsorrhaphy (stitching the lids together) is the wearing of a protective scleral or soft lens with a suitable solution of artificial tears (*see* Chapter 4). A protective lens may also be required if there is lagophthalmos or marked ectropion. Trichiasis and entropion (*Plate 7*) can lead to damage of the cornea and here a protective soft or scleral lens may be indicated rather than epilation and surgery. Soft lenses are worth trying in such cases but a scleral lens affords protection to a greater area of the eye's front surface and the choice of lens must depend on the eye's actual condition.

Protection against radiation

During irradiation of malignant tumours on or near the eye, a special lead contact shell is used for protection. Opaque contact lenses have also been developed to protect the eye from harmful visible, infrared and ultraviolet radiations during operative procedures on the anterior eye involving microsurgery where the intense light source could give rise to damage to the macular area or other tissues.

The use of laser surgery has led to the development of special contact lenses which permit the laser beam to be focused accurately on the tissue involved yet shield adjacent tissues from any harmful effect.

These various lenses are described in more detail in Chapter 24.

Protection against light and ultraviolet light

Contact lenses can be tinted and can have an artificial iris portion incorporated, the latter being most effectively done in scleral lenses, the extra thickness of which permits the effect of an anterior chamber to be achieved. However, corneal and soft lenses with an iris pattern are being fitted more frequently now that manufacturing techniques have improved. More details are given in Chapter 21 and examples shown in *Plates 103–117*. Albinos are still usually helped best with scleral lenses having an opaque scleral zone to prevent scattering of light within the eye by the sclera. The resulting improvement in visual acuity may reduce the nystagmus commonly found in albinos, provided that the fitting is undertaken early in life, preferably before the age of 2 years (*see also Plate 109*). Fitting has been undertaken before the age of 1 year, but this type of fitting must be done under general anaesthesia. Patients suffering visual difficulties due to aniridia, iridectomy or polycoria experience similar advantages to the albino when fitted with a lens incorporating an artificial iris. Where an upper iridectomy has been performed during cataract extraction, it is usually covered by the upper lid and there is no need for an artificial iris.

Tints are essential where there is photophobia, such as following cataract extraction. Manufacturers can supply details of the transmission curves of tinted corneal and soft lenses. These are important for the eye is also at risk from ultraviolet radiations:

UV-A — 315–400 nm
UV-B — 280–315 nm
UV-C — 100–280 nm

(There is some overlap of wavelength between the three types of ultraviolet radiation.) According to Pitts (reported by Kerr, 1987), those people particularly at risk are: all aphakics and pseudophakics; cataract patients suffering glare due to lenticular scatter; patients taking photosensitizing drugs such as sulphonamides, tetracyclines and oral contraceptives; patients spending long hours in bright sunlight, as for example, when sunbathing, skiing or mountaineering; patients suffering from pingueculae, pterygium and macular degeneration; and finally workers in vocations which expose them to large amounts of UV-B, such as welders, electronics workers and graphic artists.

Fortunately, where required for patients at risk, contact lenses are available which absorb ultraviolet radiations below about 400 nm. All types of lens material are available — soft, gas permeable hard and PMMA (Pearson, 1984, 1985, 1986). Although these may be more expensive than their non-ultraviolet absorbing counterparts, patients needing them are well advised to be fitted. Chapter 24 includes further details of ultraviolet-absorbing contact lenses.

Cosmetic (prosthetic) contact lenses and shells

In addition to the type of eye mentioned in the preceding section, cosmetic contact shells may be fitted as prostheses where an eye has become blind or shrunken. For squinting or pronouncedly disfigured eyes — as in the case of severe burns — a sighted artificial pupil may be incorporated at an appropriate location, if useful vision can thereby be obtained. A tinted or patterned corneal or soft lens may be sufficient to mask a corneal opacity or disfigurement of the pupil or iris. However, a cosmetic corneal or soft lens incorporating an iris pattern is even better if the cornea is sufficiently regular to be fitted with one. These cosmetic lenses can be surprisingly successful, even on grossly scarred corneae. In such cases the psychological benefit to the patient is often remarkable, provided that a normal appearance is restored; but the effect may be detrimental if, for example, a squinting eye is fitted with a scleral shell having a displaced iris which then rotates! Obviously, great care in fitting must be exercised for the patient to derive maximum benefit.

Aphakia

Unilateral aphakics usually obtain some form of binocular vision, and even some stereopsis, with a contact lens for the aphakic eye. Other than an intraocular implant a corneal lens is likely to give the smallest possible retinal image size in this eye (*see* Shape factor, Chapter 5) and may therefore be optically slightly better than a scleral lens, but soft lenses are as good as corneals, for they are usually only a little thicker and are usually much more stable. An opaque shell (soft or corneal or scleral) may help if a unilateral aphakic experiences disturbing binocular diplopia, and it may be fitted to the eye with the poorer visual acuity. Of course, any patient suffering from binocular diplopia may be helped in the same way, provided that the underlying cause has been medically investigated to rule out active pathology.

Because of the reduced image size afforded by contact lenses, and their freedom from disturbing distortions as compared to aphakic spectacles, contact lenses are also regularly prescribed for bilateral aphakics. The ideal optical correction for an aphake is the intraocular lens (IOL), but certain patients, such as babies and young children, or frail elderly people unable to undergo the possible lengthy surgery or those with aphakia of traumatic origin where the eye is too damaged to take an IOL, are better fitted with contact lenses. Soft lenses, where suitable, provide the most stable and easily fitted correction, but in the presence of corneal astigmatism, unless a toric lens can be fitted (*see* Chapters 11 and 14), they may have to be used in association with spectacles to correct the astigmatism. This is rarely a hardship as the spectacles can be supplied in bifocal form to give both a good distance and near correction.

For the elderly with handling difficulties, and for babies and young children, extended wear soft lenses are ideal provided that the patients are otherwise suitable and that regular cleaning of the lenses can be arranged. Where handling is not likely to be a problem daily wear soft lenses, or lenticular corneal lenses preferably made of a good wetting gas permeable material, are excellent. The methods of fitting these lenses are covered in Chapters 10, 11 and 21, and the special considerations for lenses for extended wear are dealt with in Chapter 15. Chapter 5 discusses the optical problems involved in fitting where flexure may occur, this being a particularly serious difficulty with high positive, high water content, soft lenses.

Only in specific cases of traumatic aphakia are scleral lenses now employed, but patients do find them easy to handle compared to other types of contact lens, and their usefulness in correcting both regular and irregular corneal astigmatism still makes them useful for certain aphakes — *see Plates 75* and *83*, and Chapters 18 and 21.

High myopia

A definite improvement of visual acuity is usually obtained with contact lenses, although this may be partially offset by difficulties with convergence and accommodation (*see* Chapter 5). Here, consideration must be given to the looseness of the lids and to the state of exophthalmos. Ultrathin soft lenses, unless otherwise contra-indicated, are ideal, although there are still occasional problems of high positioning with small lenses, due to lid traction, and if a lenticular or large lens is used the upper lid may push the lens downwards due to pressure on the thick transition between the lenticular and carrier zones. Thick edges on corneal lenses make corneals difficult to tolerate by myopes with tight lids. Also, the thick edge of a high negative corneal lens is often gripped by the upper lid, and corneal lenses may therefore ride so high on the cornea as to cause drying of the lower cornea and visual disturbance due to the peripheral zone or even the edge of the lens intersecting the pupil area. However, lens constructions are available (*see* pp. 230–236 and *Figure 5.34*, Chapter 5) which overcome these difficulties (Mandell, 1974), but the problem then becomes one of manufacture rather than fitting (*see* Chapters 10 and 22).

Although theoretically the larger size and reduced peripheral clearance of gas permeable hard corneal lenses should alleviate these problems, in practice the difficulties of accurately manufacturing high minus gas permeable lenses, coupled with their flexure on the eye, makes them extremely difficult to fit in high myopia.

Microphthalmos

For this rare condition, scleral lenses yield best results both optically and cosmetically, and are easier for the patient to handle. It may be necessary to construct a specially small impression tray in order to do the fitting, as most impression trays and most preformed trial lenses are far too large — *see* Chapter 18. Corneal lenses are not ruled out, but being of high positive power are liable to drop and ride low unless made lenticular with a suitable carrier portion which will attach to the upper lid. Soft lenses are satisfactory if they can be manufactured sufficiently accurately to the high positive prescription required. The very steep front optic surface of scleral and soft lenses in particular, are apt to make the patient look keratoconic when the contact lens is *in situ* and spherical aberration is a problem if the lenses move (*see Figure 5.21*).

Non-tolerance of spectacles

Occasionally, spectacles are not tolerated owing to trauma, skin disease, allergies, nervous troubles or even absence of one or both external ears. Contact lenses may then be suitable, but some skin diseases may be made worse by their wear and appropriate medical advice should be sought if indicated. Epidermolysis bullosa, a rare inherited skin disease, in which blisters appear at sites of mechanical trauma, makes both spectacle wear and contact lens wear hazardous, but Rubinstein (1984) has reported success using high water content (extended wear) soft lenses on a daily wear basis.

People who 'cannot bear' spectacles may well not be able to put up with the trials and tribulations of getting used to contact lenses and should not be led to believe that they are essential when a lighter-weight non-allergic, spectacle frame may be all that is required. However, because soft lenses are so easy to adapt to, they may be a great help in such cases, if the patient is otherwise suitable.

Partial sight

Young people with partial sight are sometimes helped by wearing a telescopic aid to give magnification. A contact lens can form the eyepiece of such a system, with a spectacle lens as the objective (*see* Chapter 24). Generally speaking, corneal lenses perform least well because their mobility makes them a poorer eyepiece for such a system, than is afforded by a more stable soft or scleral lens. While, in theory, such systems can be used to assist any person with low visual acuity, elderly people find it extremely difficult to adapt to the contact lenses

as well as to the magnification of the telescopic-type system.

Ocular conditions needing medication

Special scleral lenses are sometimes used in hospitals for keeping medicaments in contact with the eye to promote healing and treat infection (*see* Chapter 24). Particularly for the treatment of glaucoma with miotics, soft lenses hydrated in pilocarpine which is slowly released on to the eye, have been used very satisfactorily (Hillman, 1976). Soft lenses obviously have considerable potential in the field of medication for those cases where it is desirable to keep a drug in contact with the eye for an extended period of time (*see* Chapters 21 and 24).

Pathological defects found during the examination of the eye for contact lenses

If any previously unsuspected pathological condition is found during the course of the preliminary examination, or if the history reveals the existence of a pathological condition, contact lenses should not be fitted until medical advice has been sought. Both general and ocular conditions indicating referral will be considered below.

General conditions

General debility   Tolerance of contact lenses is likely to be poor unless general health is good.

Diabetes   Unless refraction is stable, contact lenses are not practicable. The low rate of epithelial healing is an additional disadvantage. Soft lenses are therefore advised if contact lenses must be fitted, but extended wear soft lenses should be avoided if at all possible due to the increased risk of corneal neovascularization. Where the diabetes is poorly controlled there are also many other attendant risks (Rubinstein, 1987), including lowered corneal sensitivity and proneness to the development of bacterial and fungal infections.

Hyperthyroidism   The disturbed metabolism which results in exophthalmos and lack of blinking can make contact lens wear difficult as there is liable to be an insufficient tear flow to the cornea, with all its related problems.

Chronic catarrh and sinusitis The risk of ocular infection is increased if corneal abrasions from contact lenses occur. The associated mucus in the tears also causes visual problems and deposits on the lens surfaces.

In scleral lens wearers strings of mucus may collect between the back optic surface and the cornea. Frequently the nasolacrimal drainage channels become blocked, leading to epiphora which is exacerbated by contact lens wear (*see* p. 282).

Herpes simplex of the mouth There is a danger of corneal infection from 'cold sores' when contact lenses are worn. Contact lenses should not be licked. Even so, the virus may be transferred by hand from the mouth to the eye, leading to dendritic ulcers which are likely to recur if contact lens wear is not discontinued permanently. Sometimes the improvement in visual acuity provided by a contact lens following such corneal ulceration is felt to be worth the risk of this recurrence, but contact lens wear should only be resumed on medical advice.

Skin conditions and allergic reactions There is a very slight risk of some patients being hypersensitive to certain plastics (or the residual monomer therein), but a greater risk of hypersensitivity or delayed hypersensitivity to the preservatives used in some contact lens solutions, as well as to deposits which form on the lens surface during wear. Careful questioning about allergies is advisable before fitting (Larke, 1985) and the upper tarsal conjunctiva should be studied for any signs of papillary conjunctivitis likely to be of allergic origin.

Backman and Bolte (1974) have shown that desensitization treatment for chronic allergic conjunctivitis, although lengthy, is successful in most cases and useful for contact lens patients. However, the Committee on Safety of Medicines in the UK has reported (1986) a disturbing number of deaths from anaphylaxis during such treatment for allergies and it is therefore now undertaken much less frequently. If there is serious concern that a patient may react to a contact lens material or a solution preservative whose use cannot be avoided, then the patient should be referred for a patch test to be carried out. Wilson (as reported by Rengstorff, 1986) has stated that patch testing is positive where a *hypersensitivity* reaction (a gradual build-up of signs and symptoms which is slow to resolve) is likely or has previously occurred. On the other hand, patch testing is negative if there has been a *toxic* reaction where the onset and resolution of signs and symptoms are both rapid. To avoid any risk of reaction, materials of known purity should be used, such as the clinical quality (CQ) PMMA, and for soft and gas permeable hard materials only those approved for use by, for example, the Food and Drugs Administration (FDA) in the USA. Strict hygiene, to avoid the formation of deposits on the lenses, should be observed and, for soft lenses, disinfection systems which avoid the use of preservatives should be employed, and all cleaning solutions containing preservatives should be thoroughly rinsed off using sterile non-preserved saline. For hard and gas permeable lenses soaking and wetting solutions which contain the minimum number and quantity of preservatives should be selected and, if need be, rinsed off the lenses prior to their insertion on the eye. Cleaning with non-ionic surfactants is desirable to reduce the risk of any binding of preservatives to the lens surfaces, of whatever material they are made, and regular use of protein-removing systems should be initiated from the outset of wear, provided always that the protein remover is itself thoroughly cleaned and rinsed off the lenses, as patients sometimes react to the enzymes used. Chapter 4 covers these aspects in greater detail.

Where there are infections of the eye or its adnexa, soft lenses should not be fitted except under medical supervision, because the lens material is liable to become contaminated, with the risk of extending the infection.

Norn (1964), Mackie (1967) and others have shown that instillation into the conjunctival sac of one drop of 1% rose bengal will show up desquamated conjunctival and corneal epithelium and mucus, indicative of active or subclinical conditions likely to be irritated by contact lenses (*see Plate 9*). Typical of such conditions are the following, in which very special care should be taken during the fitting, with prolonged tolerance trials — despite which the contact lenses may have to be abandoned if the skin condition worsens or the eye becomes involved.

Atopic eczema This is associated with asthma and hay fever. When contact lenses are fitted, they may cause an urticarial reaction. This should be minimized with soft lenses but the lens surfaces may degrade rapidly due to excessive protein deposits. If hard lenses are fitted a low wetting angle material is desirable and this aspect may be more important than oxygen permeability. Several PMMA materials with good wetting properties have been developed — *see* Chapters 3 and 24. Moulded CAB (cellulose acetate butyrate) lenses, such as Ciba Vision's Titmus Eurocon Persecon E lenses, also have good wetting properties and encourage the minimum of deposit formation. In the high *Dk* group of materials, those containing fluorine also wet well and are helpful if oxygen supply is of paramount importance. Lid irritation from the lens edge should be avoided by fitting with minimum peripheral clearance and as large a lens as is practicable, with thin (0.12 mm radial edge thickness) and well rounded edges.

Keratoconjunctivitis sicca (Sjögren's syndrome)

This is associated with rheumatoid arthritis; there is a lack of tear secretion (*Plate 8*), and filamentary keratitis is common. Hard corneal lenses of any material should not be fitted. Soft lenses may be fitted if saline solution or artificial tear drops are instilled at regular intervals throughout the day. Even so, the lenses may dehydrate and be unwearable. Sealed scleral lenses used with a suitable artificial tear solution (*see* Chapters 4 and 18) are most likely to prove satisfactory and are a good way of protecting the cornea. Fenestrated scleral lenses may be equally good or better, and generally allow a longer wearing time, but are only satisfactory if there are sufficient tears to supplement the artificial tears which tend to evaporate or drain away because of the fenestration hole. Sometimes a channelled scleral lens provides the best compromise (*Plate 78*).

Xerophthalmia (vitamin A deficiency), congenital ichthyosis (dry skin) and sarcoidosis

These are three conditions in which scleral lenses may prove satisfactory, and possibly essential to maintain corneal integrity — *see* Chapter 18, p. 695, but corneal lenses may lead to persistent corneal abrasions. Soft lenses are best but the material is likely to deteriorate quickly.

Voke (1986) has reported a case of keratomalacia — the corneal manifestation of xerophthalmia — in a vegan (an extreme vegetarian) whose diet lacked vitamin A and carotenoids. It would therefore seem wise to question all dry-eyed patients about possible dietary causes of their symptoms (*see* Diet, p. 293). Artificial tear drops containing vitamin A are available and may be very beneficial (*see* Chapter 4 and Appendix F).

Several other skin conditions, such as the following, may flare up when contact lenses are worn.

Seborrhoeic eczema

This manifests itself as dandruff, blepharitis (*Plates 6 and 8*), and otitis externa. Only scleral or very small corneal lenses are usually tolerated as they give rise to minimal lid irritation. Soft lenses are contraindicated in the presence of blepharitis (*see* p. 284), but if this can be resolved, they can be ideal as they cause less irritation to the eye and lids than any other type of lens. However, the patient should be advised to discontinue soft lens wear during recurrences of the condition because of the risk of associated staphylococcal keratoconjunctivitis (Catania, 1987). An effective treatment for blepharitis (Mackie, 1977) is a half-dose of tetracycline, taken orally: 250 mg twice daily for 6 weeks. This must not be taken in milk, which inactivates it. It may be prescribed by arrangement with the patient's general medical practitioner, but should not be given to young children or pregnant women as it can cause side-effects such as discolouration of growing teeth.

Acne vulgaris

This occurs around the age of puberty, is not markedly aggravated by contact lens wear, but greasing and frothing of the tears may prevent satisfactory wear of any type of lens. Prolonged tolerance trials are useful to establish whether or not this is likely to occur. Wetting and soaking solutions containing polyvinyl alcohol minimize greasing of hard lenses. Corneal lenses fitted within the palpebral aperture give fairly good results because there is no massaging effect on the lids to increase the output of sebum. Soft lenses may be satisfactory but rapid deterioration of the lens surfaces is liable to occur due to contamination by sebum from the eyelids (*Plate 5*).

Acne rosacea

This is accentuated as the foreign body reaction to contact lenses increases the blood vessel dilatation of the skin of the face and conjunctiva. Punctate keratitis is associated with the condition and may be exacerbated by contact lens wear. In the absence of keratitis, soft lenses — preferably high water content, extended wear soft lenses, used on a daily wear basis — or small corneal lenses may be tolerated — otherwise, if contact lenses are essential, scleral lenses, fitted to avoid any corneal touch, may succeed.

Epidermolysis bullosa As already mentioned under Non-tolerance of spectacles (p. 277), this may necessitate the correction of any refractive error with high water content soft lenses used for daily wear. Other types of lens are likely to exacerbate the effects of the condition on the eye (Rubinstein, 1984) which include mild blepharitis and conjunctivitis to pronounced vesicle formation over the anterior eye depending on the severity of the condition.

Psoriasis This is not directly aggravated by the wearing of contact lenses, but the generally associated nervous disposition may lead to a worsening of the condition during the initial difficult period of adaptation to contact lenses. For this reason soft lenses are likely to perform best.

Other indications of general or ocular pathology These should be referred for medical advice whether or not they are specific contra-indications to contact lens wear.

Ocular conditions

A number of different techniques must be employed to examine the eyes for suitability for contact lenses. Norn (1974) has compiled an exhaustive list of techniques used in the external examination of the eye, with an excellent description of each technique. Some of these techniques are routinely used by ophthalmic opticians and optometrists in the examination of the eye. These will not be further elaborated, but those specific to contact lens fitting will be mentioned in more detail. Reference should also be made to Chapter 6 for a description of some of the equipment used. Any evidence of pathology found should indicate the need for referral.

Slit lamp examination in ocular conditions

The anterior segment of the eye and its adnexa should be examined. Magnification of ×20 is recommended for routine use, with ×40 for examination of detail. Fluorescein should be instilled and, if necessary, the excess removed by irrigation to prevent masking of small stained areas by fluorescein in the tear film. Rose bengal 1% may also usefully be instilled. The use of these stains is discussed further on p. 282.

Normal signs, using a broad beam from the side The eye should be viewed from in front, and white light, red-free illumination and blue light (cobalt filter) should be used.

Cornea and limbus Dust particles are apparent in the tear film and move with blinking. The cornea appears to have a granular structure owing to the presence of cell bodies. Several very fine nerve fibres may extend across to the centre of the cornea. Limbal blood vessel loops normally encroach into the cornea about 1 mm, but a little more than this at the upper limbus. The radial arrangement of myelinated nerve fibres around the limbus should show that the myelin ceases about 1 mm in from the limbus. Aqueous veins (usually in the horizontal meridian) may be seen. A ring or crescent of more opaque corneal tissue separated from the limbus by a narrow, normally transparent, band is frequently seen. It is normally associated with advancing age and is then known as arcus senilis, but is often seen from the early teens onwards and is usually situated near the upper and lower limbus, and consists of cholesterol deposits. In the under-35 age group, and even up to the age of 50, particularly if xanthelasma is also present, it may be indicative of the condition known as FHC (familial hyper-cholesterolaemia) associated with heart disease (Winder, 1981; Cantle, 1988). All such patients should be referred for measurement of blood cholesterol levels and medical advice.

Posterior embryotoxin may be evident as a semi-opaque, linear structure, about the width of a blood vessel, situated at the posterior corneal surface, near the limbus, and usually in the horizontal meridian where it runs parallel to the limbus (Becker, 1972). It appears to be more common than is indicated in textbooks of ophthalmology. Usually the termination of the endothelium at the anterior chamber angle is not visible except by gonioscopy when it is known as Schwalbe's line, but if tags of endothelium extend into the anterior chamber or the endothelium is raised at that point, then it becomes visible by normal direct illumination with the slit lamp. Its significance, when visible like this, is that the anterior chamber angle is likely to become blocked more easily (*see* Chapter 24); hence, care should be exercised when fitting soft or scleral lenses to avoid corneal oedema near the limbus. The rest of the endothelium should be carefully scanned to rule out the presence of any abnormalities or striate lines, which might later, subsequent to soft lens wear, be attributed to corneal oedema (*see* Chapter 19).

Bulbar conjunctiva and sclera   Conjunctival blood vessels appear to move with respect to the deeper scleral vessels during blinking and eye movements. Most conjunctival blood vessels are normally almost empty and the transparency of the conjunctiva is apparent with the slit lamp. McMonnies and Chapman-Davies (1987) have produced a reference scale for assessment of conjunctival hyperaemia due to contact lenses (*see* Chapter 19). Prior to fitting it is good practice to note the grade of hyperaemia which exists (*see*, for example, *Plate 2*). The presence of pigment, mainly near the limbus region, is normal in Asians and Negroes, but not in white-skinned races. With age, fat is deposited in the conjunctiva within the region of the palpebral aperture and appears as thickened yellow irregularities. The incidence of pinguecu-lae also increases with age, as does the irregularity of the conjunctiva and its looseness at the limbus. While these findings are normal, irregularities of the conjunctiva such as those described, may encourage xerosis of the conjunctiva during corneal and soft lens wear and contribute to limbal dessication of the corneal epithelium at the 3 and 9 o'clock positions during corneal lens wear. It is thought that these irregularities, combined with the presence of the lens, prevent the upper eyelid from massaging the mucoid layer into the surface conjunctival and corneal epithelium which normally permits these tissues to remain wetted.

Plica and semilunaris and caruncle   Fine hairs are normally visible on the caruncle. The blood vessels should not appear unduly en-gorged. Both tissues should appear smooth and not granular.

Iris and pupil   Small pigment deposits of normal chromatophores and xanthophores are frequently visible, as are pupillary remnants arising from the region of the collarette. The pupil shape and reactions may be checked.

Anterior lens surface   Epicapsular pigment stars, often associated with pupillary remnants, may be seen. The 'orange peel' effect of the anterior capsular epithelium should be visible.

Lid margins   By slightly everting the lids, their margins may be seen under magnification. Any abnormalities, such as blocking of the orifices of the meibomian glands, can be detected and appropriate action taken. Small marginal cysts, which disappear after a few days, are often visible. They give rise to discomfort when corneal lenses are worn.

Normal signs, using a narrow beam from in front   The microscope should be moved round to one side.

Cornea   When normally transparent, this shows as a slightly granular tissue in cross-section, with a brighter reflex from both the front surface (lacrimal layer and epithelium) and back surface. With age, a few pigment spots become deposited on the back surface of the cornea due to disintegration of the iris pigment epithelium. Hassall–Henle endothelial warts appear in old age.

Anterior chamber   This should appear optically empty except for normal pupillary remnants and, with age, a few pigment granules. Its depth can be assessed and the chamber angle estimated (van Herick, Shaffer and Schwartz, 1969). It is important to rule out those patients with shallow anterior chamber angles if soft lenses which may cause corneal oedema are to be fitted, for in soft lens wear the cornea is thought to swell backwards slightly, into the anterior chamber. In this connection, it is wise to refer for medical advice before fitting any patient in whom the depth of the chamber at the limbus appears to be equal to a quarter of the thickness of the cornea, or less, as seen by optical section. (The microscope should be used from directly in front of the patient with the narrow slit beam at 60° to one side.) Such narrow angles are potentially capable of closure.

Staining

Several stains may be employed to detect abnormality. Fluorescein is the most common.

Fluorescein A drop of 1 or 2% sterile sodium fluorescein solution should be instilled into the conjunctival sac or applied from a sterile impregnated paper strip moistened with sterile saline solution. The excess may be rinsed out with sterile physiological saline solution if necessary. The cornea may be examined under magnification with suitable cobalt blue filter or long wavelength ultraviolet light. (Short wavelength ultraviolet rays are dangerous.) This is then followed by slit lamp examination using × 20 magnification. Any staining of the cornea prior to contact lens fitting, except if caused by a foreign body (the prior presence of which may usually be elucidated by questioning the patient) is abnormal, although Norn (1970) states that a few punctate dots of stain, increasing in number with age, are normal in about 20% of the population. Extensive staining indicates the probable need for referral. (Following an illness or head cold, the corneal permeability is increased and the cornea absorbs some fluorescein; but this gives only a slight green haze, unlike the bright green stain of an abraded area. When the corneal permeability is grossly increased, some fluorescein may enter the anterior chamber.)

The patency of the puncta and lacrimal drainage channels may be demonstrated by asking the patient to blow his nose on to a paper tissue, which should stain green. Each side should be checked separately. It is unwise to proceed with fitting contact lenses if the nasolacrimal passages are blocked, for the conjunctival sac is less likely to be sterile. Also the presence of contact lenses, causing excess tear production, is bound to lead to epiphora in such a case. Referral is indicated for the use of decongestant eye and/or nasal drops* or, if necessary, irrigation of the nasolacrimal passages, to clear them. Blockage is common in catarrh and hay fever sufferers, and in those with dry eyes when the passages may easily get blocked with epithelial debris.

*Otrivine-Antistin (Ciba).

Rose bengal The instillation of a drop of 1% solution should not cause any marked corneal or conjunctival staining (*Plate 9*). Such staining is best sought for using red-free illumination and low magnification with the slit lamp microscope (*see Plate 3*). If found it indicates that the tear output may be reduced or an abnormal skin condition may exist and further advice should be obtained before fitting. The mucus strip along the lid margins normally stains red and thus becomes apparent. It often detaches from the lid margin during contact lens wear and if it adheres to the lens or floats in the precorneal film it may interfere with vision. (Rose bengal, which stings when instilled, particularly in dry and susceptible eyes, should be instilled after the use of fluorescein, for it may then cause the appearance of punctate staining with fluorescein. It is to be hoped that the introduction of rose bengal impregnated paper strips will reduce this stinging.)

Alcian blue and trypan blue Kemmettmüller (1962) and Norn (1964) have described the use of these dyes for the detection of abnormality. Since their action is liable to be prolonged, their use in normal contact lens practice is not appropriate.

Sensitivity

An anaesthetic cornea is an abnormal cornea. Before contact lenses are fitted to an eye with an insensitive cornea, medical advice should be obtained. Great care is needed in fitting such an eye as abrasions caused by poorly fitting lenses do not give rise to the normal discomfort symptoms. Injury to the eye and infections may occur without the wearer's realization. For this reason soft lenses are the most appropriate in such cases, provided that strict hygiene is observed. People with insensitive corneas readily accept contact lenses and it is essential to give them strict advice concerning wearing schedules and after-care, and to warn them of the dangers of ignoring this advice. Sensitivity may be quickly checked by gently holding the lids apart and touching a wisp of sterile cotton wool on to the cornea from one side, so that its approach is not seen by the patient. Touching the lashes should be avoided. A normal blink reflex response should result from both apical and limbal touch. More refined methods whereby measurements of sensitivity can be obtained are useful if there is any doubt as to whether or not sensitivity is normal. Suitable instruments are the aesthesiometer and sensitometer, and air puff methods are also available (*see* Chapter 2). Schirmer and Mellor (1961) have shown that reduced sensitivity is to be expected following cataract extraction in the sector of the cornea corresponding to the incision. Lowered sensitivity also follows interstitial keratitis and past ulceration of the cornea — as well as hard and soft contact lens wear, with recovery in both cases being rapid (Millodot, 1976).

Pachometry

The use of the slit lamp to observe the thickness of the cornea is aided by the use of a pachometer (pachymeter) or other doubling device for actual measurement of corneal thickness (*see* Chapter 6). A very thin or irregular cornea, as in keratoconus, indicates the need for referral prior to fitting. Many surgeons prefer to carry out keratoplasty while the cornea is still reasonably thick. As a thickened cornea is an indication of oedema, it is desirable to measure corneal thickness prior to contact lens fitting, as a reference for future measurements. It is also useful to know the normal values found in pachometry — the apparent central thickness of the majority of normal corneas falls between 0.50 mm and 0.60 mm.

Classic keratometry   This allows measurement of the curvature of the anterior surface of the central cornea, most radii falling within the range 7.2–8.6 mm. Radii outside this range may indicate abnormalities such as keratoconus (steep radii) and megalocornea or cornea plana (flat radii).

The amount of corneal astigmatism present is also measured. A very toric cornea may give rise to difficulties in fitting, and it is as well to anticipate these in order to warn the patient of extra time required for fitting. A big difference between ocular and corneal astigmatism should lead the practitioner to expect a large amount of residual astigmatism with a hard spherical lens, probably requiring a cylindrical correction (*see* Chapters 5 and 14). Again, this should indicate a more lengthy fitting procedure, and fair warning can be given to the patient at an early stage. Toric soft lenses are indicated where the ocular astigmatism is sufficient to require correction to achieve adequate visual acuity at both distance and near, and where rigid lenses are unsuitable. If keratometry shows that the anterior corneal surface is highly toroidal, then a soft lens with a back toroidal surface is indicated (*see* Chapter 14).

The keratometer also reveals surface irregularities of the cornea, some so small as to be invisible with the slit lamp. Any irregularity should be further investigated prior to fitting.

Peripheral keratometry   Bonnet and Cochet (1962) developed a topographical keratometer which enabled the periphery of the cornea to be measured and the rate of flattening from apex to limbus to be determined. This was of considerable help when fitting irregular corneas, where the lens design was based on the measurements found. Similar results are obtainable (some with less accuracy) using special attachments to a classic keratometer. Chapter 6 gives further details of these and other more sophisticated instruments for the determination of corneal contour. The development of surgical techniques of altering refractive error by corneal incisions (radial keratotomy — *see* Chapter 21) has led to a further need for knowledge of the entire corneal contour. Following surgery these corneas often have steeper peripheral than central curvature — the opposite of normal — which upsets the normal spherical aberration of the eye, as well as making contact lens fitting difficult. The fitting difficulty is lessened if the peripheral curvatures are known. Instruments which can measure this also permit diurnal and long-term changes in the contour of these corneas to be recorded. Because radial keratotomy operations are not always successful, the curvature details these instruments afford may be vital information in possible court actions.

Photokeratoscopy

The keratoscope, of which the most simple variety is the Placido disc, provides useful information regarding regularity and curvature of the anterior corneal surface, the amount and type of corneal astigmatism, displacement of the corneal apex and variations in the amount of peripheral flattening (or steepening, in radial keratotomy cases) from one sector of the cornea to another. Any abnormalities indicate further examination before fitting. If a photokeratoscope is used, records of unusual cases may be kept for further reference. The photographs printed by some photokeratoscopes can be scanned by an electronic computer, enabling a suitable lens design for the patient to be computed, and allowing any corneal curvature changes after contact lens wear or corneal surgery, for whatever reason, to be monitored (Bibby, 1976; *see* Chapter 6).

Tear output

Both insufficient and excessive tear output may indicate some abnormality of the lacrimal or conjunctival glands or of their nerve supply, and all diseases causing discomfort of the eye give rise to excess tears (Phelps Brown, 1987). Tear output is also affected by diet and by certain drugs (*see* pp. 291 and 293). To fit corneal lenses to a dry cornea could be harmful, whereas excessive tears would prevent a corneal lens being worn satisfactorily and, if the excess is due to a disease process, then any type of contact lens is contra-indicated until the condition has healed. In the absence of an active disease process, soft or scleral lenses could be beneficial in either case, but the abnormality should be medically investigated before fitting. It should be borne in mind that soft lenses may alter curvature considerably on dry eyes and can only be fitted if saline solution or artificial tears are repeatedly instilled.

The usual test for the measurement of tear flow is that described by Schirmer (*see* Chapter 2), but because the test papers may irritate the eye, unless they are extremely carefully applied, the test is really only adequate for the detection of gross abnormality. Nevertheless, it is very useful in revealing those very dry eyes in which even the irritation from the Schirmer test paper fails to produce any tears. It is therefore a test recommended for use before fitting any type of contact lens. Patel, Farrell and Bevan (1987) have carried out a detailed study of its reliability and intersubject variability, which confirm these comments.

Norn's test (Norn, 1965), although rarely used, is more accurate than Schirmer's test, for it involves judging the dilution of the tears in the lacrimal rivus over the central part of the lower lid exactly 5 minutes after 10 μl of a mixture of 1% rose bengal and 1% fluorescein is instilled into the lower fornix. Using the slit lamp a

comparison is made with known dilutions of the mixture in capillary tubes. Ford (1974) has interpreted Norn's work very carefully, and has predicted the amount of refractive change likely to take place due to dehydration of soft lenses on the eye, on the basis of the tear output measured by this test.

The break-up time (BUT test) of the pre-corneal film is another very useful test (*see under* Precorneal film).

General external examination of the eye

This should be carried out with a slit lamp biomicroscope (*see* pp. 280–282 and Chapter 6).

Abnormalities of the sclera and bulbar conjunctiva Abnormalities, such as pterygium or old operation scars, may make contact lenses difficult to fit and may be irritated by the presence of the lens. When large corneal lenses which bump into the limbus region are worn, any loose conjunctival tissue becomes easily injected, inviting new blood vessel growth, and it is particularly troublesome in scleral lens wear as it can block fenestration holes and channels (*see* Chapter 18).

Pingueculae are apt to be irritated by any sort of contact lens and it is only fair to warn patients of the conjunctival hyperaemia which is likely to detract from their cosmetic appearance when contact lenses are worn. With corneal lenses this is usually due to the development of '3 and 9 o'clock' drying of the cornea (*see Plates 20* and *21*, and Chapter 19). Contact lenses of any sort are contra-indicated where there is a limbal growth due to spring catarrh.

Lids The lids should be everted; and if abnormal or excessive concretions or other elevations are seen, the patient should be referred for treatment before fitting. The upper palpebral conjunctiva comes into contact with almost the entire front surface of a contact lens during blinking and lid closure, while the lower lid barely covers the lower part of a soft contact lens. Particular attention should therefore be given to the everted upper eyelid. Follicles, and papillae (when blood vessels are present in the raised area), are normal nasally and temporally and along the sulcus but not overlying the tarsal plate which should be smooth (Larke, 1985). If encountered on the tarsal plate, they are suggestive of allergy such as vernal conjunctivitis, and contact lens fitting should only proceed with great caution, and with due attention to hygiene and minimizing any possible irritants, such as surface deposits or poorly formed lens edges, or the preservatives of preserved saline solutions etc.

If ectropion, entropion or trichiasis is evident contact lenses are advisable to protect the cornea as described under Protection against drying and foreign bodies (p. 274). Incomplete lid closure (usually due to lagophthalmos following seventh nerve paralysis) again indicates the need for a protective contact lens (see p. 274).

Special scleral lenses can be fitted where there is ptosis of the upper lid (see Chapter 18).

Blepharospasm, if it is persistent, can be a nuisance to corneal lens wearers as considerable discomfort ensues. In such cases scleral lenses are advisable. Soft lenses may be satisfactory but the excessive lid pressure usually distorts the lens. In any case the cause of the blepharospasm should be investigated before fitting. It should be borne in mind that those people who are somewhat apprehensive about wearing contact lenses may exhibit an unusual amount of blepharospasm at an initial interview, simply due to nervousness, and this subsequently disappears.

Contact lenses should preferably not be fitted in the presence of blepharitis (see p. 279) as there is a risk of corneal infection. Corneal lenses also give rise to discomfort and lid soreness where blepharitis is present or where the lid margins are highly sensitive. (Lid margin sensitivity may be checked with a wisp of cotton wool or an aesthesiometer.) Recurrent styes are a contra-indication to either soft or corneal lenses, so are any lid margin growths. Where there is absence of lashes — a sign of eczema and/or alopecia — fitting should proceed with great care: the patient (and practitioner) may have difficulty in gripping the lids during insertion and removal of lenses.

Parasites may be encountered among the eyelashes. These include *Demodex folliculorum* (Coston, 1967) which breeds in the eyelash follicles, and even canine lice have been found (Londer, 1987). Removal of the former may be effected with a cotton bud soaked in alcohol applied very carefully to the lashes, and Londer reports clearing canine lice with Lacrilube (Allergan) ointment. Parasite infestation gives

the appearance of blepharitis and should similarly be cleared before contact lenses are fitted.

The depth of the fornices should be checked before fitting as past injury or surgery may restrict the limits of the conjunctival sac, making soft and scleral lenses either unsuitable or difficult to fit. Conversely, in certain inflammatory conditions such as the Stevens–Johnson syndrome and ocular pemphigus, scleral lenses may be necessary to maintain the depth of the fornices and prevent the adherence of palpebral and bulbar conjunctiva.

Palpebral aperture size and lid tightness
These may limit the size of lens fitted. A small palpebral aperture and tight lids usually make a small lens — of whatever type — necessary, whereas large palpebral apertures and loose lids make larger lenses more appropriate. This is not only true for physical reasons of fitting but physiologically also, for small lid apertures lead to a greater temperature increase behind the contact lens (Hill and Leighton, 1965). This increases the metabolic rate, which, if it cannot be met by sufficient oxygen, leads to corneal oedema. Thus, unless a highly oxygen permeable lens is fitted, the smaller the area of eye covered by the lens, the better.

If a tolerance trial with corneal lenses induces the formation of a white deposit at the canthi within half an hour of insertion, the implication is that there is an excessive temperature rise and that corneal lenses should probably be rejected unless lengthy tolerance trials with different types of lens can be arranged. Soft lenses are often more successful however, and ultrathin lenses and those of high water content are least likely to upset corneal metabolism.

The presence of foam at the outer canthus is fairly normal (Norn, 1963), but foam along the lower lid margin may be associated with instability of the tear film due to reduced meibomian secretion (Larke, 1985). Its production is increased by blinking and the presence of foreign bodies such as contact lenses. The production of excessive mucus during a tolerance trial is also a contra-indication to fitting, as is excessive meibomian activity (as shown in *Plate 5*) which may give rise to subsequent greasing problems.

Lacrimal gland This should be checked for
normality — for size, position and colour. If it is

large and prominent and scleral lenses are to be fitted, the temporal portion of the lens must be made sufficiently thin to slide under the gland without bumping it.

Precorneal film

A number of qualitative tests may be used to assess the normality of the precorneal film prior to fitting contact lenses. These have been described by McDonald (1969) and Guillon (1986a), and their relevance to contact lens fitting elaborated by Hill (1973), and by Guillon (1986a).

The wettability of the tear layer is a function of the mucoid layer, and its efficiency may be judged by observing through the biomicroscope the reflection of an ordinary movable lamp in the lacrimal rivus or prism at the lower lid margin. This prism has three zones: an upper convex one against the lower cornea, a middle concave one at the centre of the rivus, and another convex one at the limit of the tear layer on the rear of the lower lid. As the lamp is slowly moved up and down, three smoothly moving bright reflections should be seen in the prism — the upper and lower ones giving a 'with' movement and the centre an 'against' movement. It may be necessary to ask the patient to look downwards to see all three, but if all or parts of these reflections are missing, the wettability of the tears is abnormal.

The quality of the surface lipid (oily) layer which controls the rate of evaporation of the aqueous layer behind it, can be judged by looking in the same way at the corneal surface reflection of the lamp. The patient should blink normally about once every 4 seconds, and the reflection of the lamp should remain bright all the while. If streaks of interference colours appear, according to McDonald (1969) the tear layer is too thin (or there is too great an evaporation rate). If the reflection is irregular and pocked, the surface is very dry.

Guillon (1986a) has described a more refined technique for observation of the lipid layer of the preocular tear film (POTF) and the development of an instrument for use with the biomicroscope at low magnification. The instrument consists of an internally illuminated white hemispherical cup which is reflected at the tear surface as a circular white area of about 1 cm diameter, against which the lipid layer of the POTF may be viewed by low magnification.

By this means he has established that there are five basic patterns which the lipid layer forms: a *marmoreal pattern* of a grey mottled appearance occurring in about 60% of patients where the lipid layer varies between 13 and 70 nm giving rise to a marbled effect; a *contaminated marmoreal pattern* due to contamination by mucus strands or cell debris, as for example after eye rubbing, but which occurs naturally in some 10% of patients indicating an unstable tear film, and the likelihood of surface drying and deposits if contact lenses are worn; an *amorphous pattern* seen in 15% of patients where the lipid layer is between 70 and 90 nm thick and of blue-grey colour, indicating a stable POTF, and a good tolerance to contact lenses, but possibly slightly more lipid deposits on soft lenses; a wavy *flow pattern* where the lipid layer consists of different poor-mixing lipids with thickness varying from 10 to 90 nm and occurring in about 10% of patients very few of whom get problems related to their tears; and finally a *colour fringe pattern* showing different interference colours with the eyes wide open, and occurring in 5% of cases, indicating a much thicker lipid layer from 86 to 170 nm often contaminated by mucus strands. The latter appearance is often associated with excess meibomian secretion (*Plate 5a*) and chronic blepharitis (*Plate 8*), and such patients have problems with contact lenses, particularly soft ones which dry out and attract deposit formation.

Sometimes these patterns occur in combination, and a combination of amorphous and colour fringe patterns where the colours are first order yellow, brown and blue (lipid thicknesses of 90, 140 and 170 nm, respectively) is regarded by Guillon as highly favourable to contact lens wear.

A test of viscosity may be made by watching the movement of bubbles or debris in the lower tear prism. Surface particles should move more slowly than deeper ones. If the movement is simultaneous and rapid, insufficient viscosity is indicated and not enough tears will be retained on the eye. Simultaneous but slow movement indicates tears which are too viscous, and contact lenses would tend to become greasy and dirty if worn.

Other phenomena described by McDonald (1969), indicating tears which are too viscous, are the 'pleated drape' and 'rolled scum' phenomena. (These appear to correspond to

Guillon's flow and colour fringe patterns, respectively.) The former is seen by reflection of a lamp in the upper tear prism at the start of each blink, when waves, like pleats, form interference colours which close together as the lid goes up. The 'rolled scum' effect is left on the lower third of the cornea after each blink, where the two lids have parted and left an oily deposit. This is visible with a wide slit beam and is more noticeable after a high cholesterol intake. It is therefore felt that tear chemistry is related to diet (Lowther, Miller and Hill, 1970; Young and Hill, 1973).

Normal phenomena are the 'crumple' effect seen with a broad vertical slit at about 15° to the microscope axis, when the surface oil molecules undergo lateral pressure from the lids at the start of each blink and cause a diffuse (instead of uniform) reflection rather like wet silk; the epithelial drying effect, or non-invasive break-up time (NIBUT, see later) when the tear layer can be seen to evaporate after about 20 seconds without blinking which causes a reduction in acuity; and the epithelial touch effect, when a foreign body such as an eyelash or a bubble of carbon dioxide or air under a contact lens forms a furrow in the epithelium. In the latter case, after the foreign body is washed away, the furrow — visible by its oily margins — gradually widens for up to 5 minutes and then slowly narrows as the normal tear layer reforms. Such furrows retain fluorescein and, in the case of contact lens wearers, are called dimples. The speed with which the furrow disappears may well be a measure of epithelial fragility. *Plates 22, 34, 70* and *94* show dimples and furrows under a corneal lens.

Another test of the epithelial drying effect has been described by Polse (1975). He has stated that a deficiency of mucus production results in corneal dry spots which show up when the tear film is seen to break up into droplets. The test is known as the BUT (break-up-time) test. It is best seen by applying fluorescein below the cornea and observing with the slit lamp, with blue light and the largest possible circular aperture to illuminate the entire cornea. The patient is instructed to make one complete blink and then hold the eyes wide open. In normal individual dry spots, which show up as black areas within the fluorescein-covered corneal surface, usually only appear if the lids are held apart for 20 seconds or more after a complete blink, whereas they appear within 10 seconds after a complete blink in certain pathological and dry-eye conditions (*see Plate 55c*) and if there is a mucus deficiency (Lemp *et al.*, 1970, 1971; Koetting, 1976). Polse feels that the appearance of such abnormal dry spots on the cornea is a contra-indication to successful contact lens fitting, and this is confirmed by Koetting who has shown a correlation between the surface contamination/coating of hydrophilic lenses and a low tear film break-up-time, and by Andres *et al.* (1987) who found a definite relationship between reduced BUT and intolerance to contact lenses. They found 15% of 200 patients had dry eyes (BUT of 7.5 seconds or less) and 24% were borderline (BUT of 10 seconds). However, Vanley, Leopold and Gregg (1977) have cast doubts on the usefulness of the BUT test as they found considerable variation in individual eyes from one patient visit to the next. Before rejecting a patient for contact lenses on the grounds of poor tear output, several different tests should be carried out and repeated at intervals in order to get a true picture.

Guillon (1986b) has stated that instillation of fluorescein upsets the stability of the tear film and that it is preferable to observe the lipid layer using his own low magnification technique, described above, to record the non-invasive break-up time (NIBUT). Ideally this should be 20 seconds or more for successful contact lens wear and certainly not less than 10 seconds.

Most of these tests and phenomena may be observed with contact lenses in place. The tear prism at the temporal edge of the lens may be used for checking wettability and viscosity, and the lens surface for rate of evaporation, although the surface of a contact lens dries more quickly than the surface of the cornea. Guillon (1986a,b) has related the lipid layer patterns of the POTF to those of the prelens tear film (PLTF), the latter depending on the lens material and its wettability, and has discussed both in connection with the anterior surface drying time (ASDT) of various contact lenses.

Lowther, Bailey and Hill (1971) have also found that a normally wetted bulbar conjunctiva which appears smooth may become dry and irregular following corneal lens wear, due to the mechanical effect of the lids being held off the conjunctiva (especially in the 3 and 9 o'clock positions) by the lens edge, so that the conjunctiva is not properly wetted. This can occur when the tear chemistry is normal, so that the remedy is one of lens design (thinner edges and less peripheral clearance) rather than patient rejection. *Plate 20* shows 3 and 9 o'clock staining

Puncta Their presence and apposition to the globe should be checked. Abnormalities which result in poor tear drainage contra-indicate contact lens wear.

Pupil size and reactions Reactions should be normal. Large pupils create difficulties for some corneal lens wearers, particularly motorists who do a lot of night driving when considerable flare around headlights may be noticed if the optic zone is smaller than the pupil size. Also, wearers of most types of bifocal contact lenses may suffer flare and monocular diplopia if pupils are large. The deeper the anterior chamber the larger should be the optic zone of the lens for a given pupil diameter (Stone, 1959). The transition between the optic zone and the peripheral zone should be made as gradual as possible to minimize flare. Continuous curve or aspherical surfaces such as elliptical surfaces minimize these flare effects with large pupils. The maximum pupil size is readily judged by ultraviolet illumination in a dark room when the fluorescence of the crystalline lens shows up the pupil size.

Iris Normality should be established. Special lenses may be fitted if the iris is wholly or partially absent, to occlude the unwanted iris apertures. This can result in a considerable improvement in vision. Soft, corneal or scleral lenses may be used depending on the severity of the condition (*see* Chapter 21 and *Plates 106–117*).

Exophthalmos or enophthalmos Abnormalities such as Horner's syndrome should be looked for and pathological conditions ruled out. Iris-sized soft lenses or corneal lenses are cosmetically better for exophthalmos, although the latter may have to be fitted slightly steep in order to be retained on the cornea. In exophthalmos there is a risk of reduced tear flow behind the lens. For enophthalmos, sclerals look better but need to be made small to facilitate insertion and removal, which is difficult for these patients with any type of lens.

Ophthalmoscopy

This is carried out to check the media and fundi to establish absence of abnormalities. Any persistent disturbance of the normal reflex fundus glow — for example, due to lid pressure on the cornea — should be noted in case it is later mistaken for the after-effects of contact lens wear.

Visual fields

These should be checked if there are any doubts about their normality. In general, contact lenses have a beneficial effect on the visual field as compared to spectacles (*see* Chapter 5). Aphakics, in particular, benefit by losing the ring scotoma caused by high positive spectacle lenses and the surrounding frame.

Tonometry

This is usually carried out if raised intraocular tension is suspected. Cases have been encountered where a scleral lens has been thought to cause a rise of tension in an already abnormal eye. Khoo (1974) found that during the first hour of soft lens wear intraocular pressure (IOP) rises slightly, but then returns to normal. However, as stress can induce a rise in IOP (Shily, 1987) this may have been stress related, but with the thick soft lenses in use at that time it is more likely to have been due to some restriction of limbal outflow due to lid pressure over the thick lens. Because of the possible risk of contact lenses increasing intraocular tension by pressure on the anterior ciliary veins, or in the case of soft lens wear when corneal oedema could result in a narrowing of the anterior chamber angle, it is wisest to carry out tonometry both before and after fitting, whenever there is the slightest suspicion of high intraocular pressure.

If thin soft lenses are worn, accurate non-contact tonometry can be performed with the lenses in place, although a slightly high reading is obtained when positive lenses are worn, averaging 3 mmHg too high (Insler and Robbins, 1987). Polse, Haw and Fatt (1976) suggested a thin high minus soft lens be used to avoid the need for anaesthetizing the cornea, and they obtained accurate readings using the Mackay–Marg and Schiötz techniques.

Visual acuity and refraction

A consideration of the optical effects of contact lenses (*see* Chapter 5) shows that, in theory, contact lenses should give a better visual acuity than spectacles as there are no oblique aberrations or distortion with contact lenses.

Myopes   In myopes, contact lenses give bigger retinal images than spectacles, in proportion to the strength of the correction. This can lead to initial disorientation with contact lenses but should give better visual acuity. More ocular accommodation is needed, and the convergence required is greater than with spectacles, owing to the absence of the prism base-in effect. Thus, myopes tend to experience near-vision difficulties not encountered with spectacles, although the accommodation–convergence relationship should remain the same (Stone, 1967). They also have to move their eyes about more. From the point of view of others, the myope's eyes look bigger in contact lenses, as the reduced magnification of spectacles has been removed. All these effects are proportional to the power of the lenses.

Hypermetropes   In hypermetropes, the effects of contact lenses are the opposite to those for myopes. Smaller retinal images are obtained than with spectacles, and the eyes look smaller than in spectacles. Accommodation needed is less, convergence required is reduced and the eyes have to move less than with spectacles.

Astigmats   Spectacle wearers learn to compensate for the distortion of the retinal image afforded by an astigmatic spectacle correction. This compensation by the brain is continued when contact lenses are first worn, and it gives rise to a false experience of distortion which usually soon disappears. A comparison of ocular astigmatism with that measured by the keratometer allows prediction of the approximate amount of residual astigmatism with a hard spherical contact lens. A suitable lens construction may be chosen in advance if residual astigmatism is likely to cause a reduction in visual acuity. If soft lenses are being considered, any excess of ocular astigmatism over corneal astigmatism greater than 1 D suggests that a toric lens is necessary or else hard lenses capable of incorporating a cylindrical correction should be used. Where ocular astigmatism is negligible but corneal astigmatism is present, which neutralizes any crystalline lens astigmatism, soft lenses are optically ideal, provided the corneal astigmatism is not so great as to disrupt the fit.

Anisometropes   Although Sorsby, Leary and Richards (1962) have shown that most naturally occurring anisometropia is of axial origin and theoretically, in such cases, the retinal image sizes in the two eyes are more likely to be of similar size if a spectacle correction is used rather than contact lenses (*see* Chapter 5), in practice this does not necessarily work to the patient's advantage. Contrary to expectations, contact lenses often give rise to better binocular vision than spectacles (Winn *et al.*, 1986), and the binocular fusion difficulties associated with unequal retinal image sizes are not encountered. The only reasonable explanation for this is that each retina has the same number of light receptor units, and that in the longer eye these receptor units are more widely spaced than in the shorter eye, as might be expected during the growth process. Thus the bigger retinal image in the longer eye is thought to cover the same number of receptor units as the smaller retinal image in the shorter eye, which then gives rise to the ideal situation for binocular fusion.

In the over-60 age group crystalline lens changes occur which are often greater in one eye usually leading to a myopic shift of refraction and to a state of refractive anisometropia, for which contact lenses are ideal (*see* Chapter 5). Difficulties then arise, however, if the refractive error is changing fairly fast necessitating contact lens power changes every few months. Even so, this may be no more expensive for the patient than frequent changes of spectacle lens, and definitely gives far better and more comfortable binocular vision.

As a general guide, contact lenses are likely to be optically satisfactory for all young anisometropes and refractive anisometropes, but where a spectacle correction affords good binocular vision in high anisometropia and has done so for many years, then contact lenses may well be ruled out due to the aniseikonia likely to occur.

Even if the anisometropia is known to be refractive, if spectacles give satisfactory binocular vision, contact lenses may induce a state of pseudoaniseikonia owing to the relative difference between the two eyes of the change in retinal image size. An investigation of the binocular state in spectacles and in suitably powered trial contact lenses is therefore advisable before proceeding to supply final lenses. This is well worth while because a number of highly successful cases have been reported (F. A. B. Hodd, 1970, personal communication; Winn *et al.*, 1986). Where the eye with the higher refractive error is also amblyopic the author has often found that contact lens wear slowly improves the visual acuity in that eye. Part-time occlusion of the other eye, while very fine visual tasks are undertaken, has been found to help.

It may be found that non-comitant heterophorias are recorded at first with contact lenses, as the brain still continues to compensate for the ocular movements made with the anisometropic spectacle correction.

Monocular aphakia is an example in which a contact lens correction may give binocular vision where spectacles will not. However, a contact lens is worn some distance in front of the entrance pupil of the eye and it is by no means certain that contact lenses will give satisfactory binocular vision in this condition because of the residual aniseikonia. The patient may well prefer monocular vision to the asthenopic symptoms of disturbed binocularity.

Binocular vision

Heterotropias   In general, contact lenses perform as well as spectacles in the treatment and correction of squints. Very often, all that is required to correct a squint is a full spectacle correction determined with the aid of a cycloplegic. However, this may mean the patient wearing a heavy and/or unsightly pair of spectacle lenses which tend to be abandoned to the detriment of the squint. In such cases contact lenses are invaluable. The author has had some success in cases of anisometropic esotropia by fitting the more hypermetropic eye with a contact lens of power equal to the difference between the two eyes. A balanced spectacle correction is then worn in addition to the one contact lens, but it is usually easier to fit contact lenses to both eyes. However, a combination of spectacles and contact lenses permits variations in negative additions for exotropes to be made on the spectacle lenses and, where bifocals would be prescribed for either esotropia

or exotropia, contact lenses can be worn for general purposes with additional spectacles to be worn for close work. Difficulties arise where there is a residual high heterophoria requiring prismatic correction or where there is a vertical element needing prism to correct it (*see below*). As most patients requiring refractive corrections for heterotropias are children, soft lenses are particularly useful as they are quicker to adapt to and cause less discomfort in fitting. Also, if they are to be used in combination with spectacles, the latter can be used to provide any necessary cylindrical or prism correction.

High heterophorias   These are difficult to prescribe for, using contact lenses, as only about $4\,\Delta$ can be satisfactorily incorporated into a contact lens. Only with scleral lenses can the prism base be put in any direction, as long as the scleral zone is a good fit and the lens does not rotate. This allows a maximum of $8\,\Delta$ difference between the two eyes. However, with soft and corneal lenses, the base always rotates downwards, which limits any prismatic correction to $4\,\Delta$ base-down. In fact, $2\,\Delta$ is a more reasonable figure as all the prism must be put on one lens. Discomfort is likely with a very thick lower edge; also the prism base usually takes up a slightly nasal position due to lid action.

Myopes often require less prism in contact lenses than in spectacles, presumably because the bigger retinal image size with contact lenses affords a better binocular lock. However, the mobility of the retinal image, in corneal lens wear, may necessitate greater prism. There is no general rule, but the minimum prism to eliminate any fixation disparity and/or symptoms should be prescribed.

Amblyopia   Care must be taken to see that any improved visual acuity given by contact lenses does not give rise to insuperable diplopia. As visual acuity improves, orthoptic exercises may be needed to help consolidate binocular vision.

Eye movements   Pareses of extraocular muscles give rise to diplopia with contact lenses as with spectacles. As already stated, contact lenses can affect the amount of eye movement required because they remove the prismatic effects of spectacle lenses, so that both version and vergence movements may be affected.

Aniseikonia   A combination of spectacles and contact lenses can be used to create size differences to relieve symptoms due to aniseikonia. The principles are those of a Galilean telescope system, similar to the type used as an aid to the partially sighted (*see* Chapter 24).

Uniocularity   Contact lenses are a hazard — even if only a very slight one — and it may be in the best interest of a uniocular person, or one with intractable amblyopia in one eye, not to fit him with contact lenses unless this considerably improves vision as compared with spectacles, or is otherwise necessary. In any case the patient should be warned of the risk, however small. If spectacles are prescribed these should have plastics or toughened lenses.

Personal and external factors

Age and sex

Incentive, enthusiasm and handling ability are generally better in younger people, although there are remarkable exceptions. Presbyopic contact lens wearers need to use spectacles for near work unless bifocal contact lenses are fitted — and even when it is possible to fit these, they have certain limitations in use (*see* Chapter 16).

Andres *et al.* (1987) found the tear film BUT insignificantly greater (i.e. better) in men than in women, but they did find a significant reduction in BUT with age. Corneal sensitivity also reduces with age (Millodot, 1977) and in women it is affected by the menstrual cycle reducing considerably during the premenstruum and menstruation (Millodot and Lamont, 1974). However, in the latter case the possibly beneficial effect on contact lens wear from the slight loss of sensitivity may be offset by other changes (*see below*).

The eyelid tissue slackens with age making, for example, the support of a prism-ballasted bifocal corneal lens more difficult, and other tissue changes associated with ageing lead to less efficient tear drainage from the conjunctival sac. In some people these changes are beneficial to contact lens wear and in others detrimental. Each case must be assessed on an individual basis.

Women undergoing the menopause may experience difficulties with their lenses. Xerosis sometimes occurs during the menopause. Occasionally hormonal changes lead to psychological disturbances and consequent loss of motivation to wear contact lenses. Such changes are most likely to take place at the time of a pregnancy or during the menopause. Pregnancy also frequently disturbs contact lens wearing, presumably due to metabolic changes in the cornea. The change in hormone balance alters the water content of all tissues, including the cornea and lids — which may result in a corneal thickness or curvature change and a consequent alteration in lens fit. The fit of corneal lenses can become dramatically tighter, with very little peripheral clearance where plenty existed before and, if modifications are made to alleviate the ensuing discomfort, the lenses can be made wearable again until the termination of the pregnancy. Then, the cornea returns to its original state and the modified lenses become loose and uncomfortable, and must either be made smaller or replaced. In this respect soft lenses are less likely to cause problems than hard lenses, although tear output is often reduced during periods of water retention and this, coupled with corneal curvature and thickness changes, can make even soft lens wearing difficult.

Similar effects have been recorded in women taking oral contraceptives (Koetting, 1966), although improvements in these drugs have now reduced the effects to a minimal amount. Difficulties in wearing contact lenses associated with premenstrual tension have also been reported (K. Dalton, 1970, personal communication). Dalton, a gynaecologist, states:

Difficulty with contact lenses may occur before or during menstruation and I usually advise patients when first starting to use contact lenses, to practise first, after menstruation. During the premenstruum, ocular symptoms are common; non-infective conjunctivitis related to menstruation was noted as early as 1521 (Roy, 1961), and raised intraocular pressure also occurs. Landesman *et al.* (1953) studied the menstrual changes of the peripheral vascular bed of the bulbar conjunctiva and demonstrated changes during the premenstruum when the blood flow is diminished, the vessels become dilated and engorged and the arterioles constricted.

My own experience suggests that women who manage contact lenses well only have problems if they are on an unsuitable contraceptive pill and are getting other side-effects, for example, headaches, bloatedness or nausea. By changing the contraceptive pill and eliminating other side-effects, the ocular symptoms also disappear.

Similarly, women suffering from toxaemic symptoms of pregnancy (vomiting, headache, depression, lethargy) are also likely to have difficulty with contact lenses, but the ocular symptoms are eased as soon as the pregnancy symptoms are eased by treatment or the passage of time.

I have always assumed that in women with premenstrual exacerbations, or those taking the contraceptive pill, and during pregnancy, that it was the deficient progesterone and/or oestrogen excess which was responsible for their symptoms. In my experience, it is rare for women to complain of difficulty with contact lenses while on progesterone for premenstrual migraine, depression and irritability.

Farrall (1976) has shown that a reduction in tear output with associated drop in lysozyme and relative increase in globulin-type protein is to be expected when women first take the oral contraceptive pill, or change to another type, or cease to take it. The increased corneal oedema, reduced lacrimal secretion and increased mucus and lipid content of the tear film may last a few weeks but gradually subside. In a contact lens wearer, though, they may be sufficient to cause difficulty or even abandonment of contact lenses in a very few cases.

Skin, hair and eye colouring   Millodot (1975) has shown that those people with blue eyes and fair skins have more sensitive corneas than others, and most contact lens practitioners find that auburn-haired patients with fair freckled skin are particularly sensitive to hard and rigid gas permeable lenses. For these people, if appropriate, soft lenses are the contact lens of first choice.

Ability to handle lenses

Contact lenses should not be supplied unless they can be handled properly by the patient, who should be able to see both the lenses and any engraving on them. A light (neutral) tint may help. In cases such as aphakia, a spectacle frame can be supplied, glazed to a suitable prescription on one side only, the other 'eye' being left empty and the lower rim removed. The first contact lens is then inserted through the empty 'eye' of the frame, which enables the patient to see it with the other eye. The frame is then removed as the patient is able to see the second contact lens with the first in place.

People, such as the elderly, with very clumsy or shaky hands, and very young children who must wear contact lenses, are usually best fitted with extended wear lenses (soft or gas permeable hard) provided they are otherwise suitable. A relation or someone close to the patient should be taught the various insertion and removal techniques and be given all the necessary information, so that the lenses may be removed and cleaned periodically (*see* Chapters 4 and 9).

Some soft lenses are much easier to handle than others, the thin and ultrathin ones being most difficult. Ghormley (1988) has suggested that very young patients, athletes, men with large hands and others who have handling difficulties be fitted with standard thickness lenses, i.e. centre thickness 0.10 mm for negative lenses.

Working and living conditions

Contact lenses can be difficult to wear in a number of conditions: dusty and smokey atmospheres, very hot or cold temperatures, windy weather, and very dry and very humid atmospheres. An example is that of an aircraft cabin in which the humidity is usually very low, and many travellers then notice difficulty with their soft lenses due to dehydration. By contrast, hot humid conditions do not seem to affect soft lenses. People working in rarified atmospheres or at high altitudes may suffer corneal oedema due to lack of oxygen.

Soft lenses are absolutely contra-indicated for people coming into contact with any noxious fumes such as workers in the chemical industry.

If the light is poor, the pupil may dilate to a greater size than the optic zone of a corneal lens so that diplopia (ghost images) or peripheral blur is seen. Occasionally, hard lenses have been fitted with a large back optic zone diameter (BOZD), specially for night driving to avoid flare, but the advent of elliptical and other aspherical back surfaces, and of gas permeable hard lenses in which the lens design has a large BOZD, has minimized this problem.

If excessive light is likely, a tint may be necessary. Choice of tint must depend on the absorption required and the colour rendering. A neutral tint is preferable for most purposes because, as Fletcher and Nisted (1963) have shown, some tints can be dangerous if used under a monochromatic illumination the wavelength of which is not transmitted by the tint.

The effects of tints on dark adaptation should also be remembered.

Ultraviolet-absorbing lenses have already been dealt with on p. 275 and should be recommended for those patients at risk from this radiation.

Occasionally in very sensitive individuals, and particularly in the early stages of wear, certain head postures and eye movements are rather uncomfortable for wearers of hard and rigid gas permeable lenses. Looking up continually, as for example when playing snooker, and making rapid lateral eye movements, as in copy typing, may cause irritation and injection. Continually looking down, as when doing close work all day, so that the palpebral aperture size is reduced may lead to corneal oedema in certain contact lens wearers as explained on p. 285.

Patients and practitioners alike have become aware that some gas permeable hard lenses, as well as developing surface cracking (see Plate 27 and Chapter 10), at times seem to fracture spontaneously. Silk (1987, 1988) attributes this to electrical effects such as static build-up on the lenses, which may affect the polarity of the material and its surfaces. Some people are more static sensitive than others, and many man-made fibres encourage the build-up of static charges. This may in extreme cases explain epithelial damage by such lenses. Silk has found that the effects are worse in cold dry conditions rather than wet or humid ones. Thus people wearing clothing made of synthetic fibres or walking on carpets of synthetic material or even playing football on synthetic pitches, may experience more problems with their gas permeable hard lenses than at other times. These problems include greater surface deposition, proneness to fracture in the eye, surface cracking and removal of surface epithelial cells.

Drugs

Drug taking can influence metabolism, which in turn may influence contact lens wear. Tolerance trials extended over 4 weeks if necessary (as, for example, in the case of women under hormone treatment) may be advisable before prescribing contact lenses for some patients, as the corneal curvature, especially peripherally, may alter quite dramatically. The effects of oral contraceptives on tear output and corneal oedema

have been dealt with under Age and sex. Other steroid drugs may have similar effects.

Thyroxine treatment has been reported to cause intolerance to contact lenses (Marsh, 1975). Mackie, Seal and Pescod (1977) have shown that β-adrenergic blocking drugs such as practolol and labetalol, as used for certain heart conditions, may reduce tears output and lysozyme concentration, although very low doses of the latter drug may increase lysozyme concentration. Contact lenses may therefore be contra-indicated for patients on prolonged courses of these drugs.

Drugs used in the treatment of allergies, and tricyclic antidepressants have also been found to cause dry eyes (see Chapter 4).

Diet

As indicated on p. 279 under Xerophthalmia and on p. 286 under Precorneal film, diet can affect the state of the eye and in particular the quality of the tears and their output.

A high cholesterol diet, as well as obesity, have been shown to have an association with increased levels of cholesterol in the tears (Terry and Hill, 1975; Hill and Terry, 1976), while Lane (1985), who carried out hair analysis on patients with contact lens greasing problems as well as on dry-eyed patients, and compared them with a control group, showed a huge deficiency in potassium and sodium in those with coated lenses. Dietary changes to increase folic acid, ascorbic acid, vitamin B_6 and potassium and to decrease sugar intake (which otherwise reduces potassium in the body), were successful in one month in treating those with coated lenses, and many of the dry-eyed patients improved in several months.

Shreeve (1982) in a study of dry-eyed patients has discussed the role of specific prostaglandins — prostaglandin E_1 (PGE_1) being necessary for adequate tear output. The chemicals in the body necessary for the formation of PGE_1 require the availability of insulin, zinc, magnesium, ascorbic acid (vitamin C), pyridoxine (vitamin B_6) niacin (a B vitamin sometimes referred to as B_3) and the essential fatty acid cis-linoleic acid found in evening primrose oil and other vegetable oils. The formation of PGE_1 can be blocked by deficiencies of these and by excesses of trans-fatty acids, saturated fats, cholesterol, excess alcohol intake, ageing, diabetes, viruses, chemical carcinogens and ionizing radiations. Of interest may be the fact that *trans*-fatty acids are formed when *cis*-linoleic acids, found in corn, sunflower and safflower oils, are heated to a high temperature and otherwise treated to make them acceptable for cooking purposes!

There are probably many other dietary implications, as yet unknown, which may help or hinder contact lens wear and normal ocular function.

Habits

Hygiene is essential in the handling of contact lenses. People who rub their eyes a lot and who blink excessively should not be given corneal lenses unless they can cease these habits. Smoking may be a disadvantage to the wearer of contact lenses.

Hobbies

Although most gas permeable hard corneal lenses can be fitted to give minimum peripheral clearance and are therefore more difficult to dislodge as compared to PMMA hard lenses, they are still less stable than soft or scleral lenses. Soft lenses have therefore become the lens of choice for virtually all sports and have been worn satisfactorily on mountaineering expeditions at high altitude, and by swimmers in chlorinated pools (*see* Chapter 24). There is less risk of them being washed out during swimming than a corneal lens. It has been suggested that they actually protect the cornea from the swimming pool water but, because they absorb chlorinated water, they should be thoroughly rinsed in sterile saline immediately afterwards, and preferably disinfected to avoid the risk of infection by *Acanthamoeba*.

For those who need contact lenses for the stage and films, arc lights make photophobia a difficulty. Various tints are available, as are lenses having artificial iris patterns. For effect purposes, contact lenses in the form of cosmetic or prosthetic lenses can be used to alter the appearance and colour of the eyes (*see* Chapter 21).

If contact lenses are required for only occasional wear, as for social events, soft lenses are by far the best lens to fit. With hard and gas permeable corneal lenses difficulties are likely to be encountered as a satisfactory tolerance must always be built up beforehand.

Special occupations

In the UK there are certain restrictions regarding the wearing of contact lenses while driving, or piloting an aircraft, and in certain other occupations. Similar restrictions may apply in other countries and regulations regarding such use of contact lenses are normally available from the appropriate vehicle or driver/pilot licensing authority in that country or from the prospective employer. In the UK up-to-date information is published annually in their Members' Handbook by the AOP (Association of Optometrists, Bridge House, 233–234 Blackfriars Road, London, SE1 8NW). At the time of writing the following regulations apply in the UK.

Drivers

Since 1983, the wearing of contact lenses has been permissible for all classes of driver including heavy goods vehicle and public service vehicle drivers provided the other visual standards are satisfied. For motorists the minimum visual standards are: VA with corrective lenses, if needed, of at least 0.4 (6/15) in the better eye and 0.2 (6/30) in the worse eye and 0.5 (6/12) binocularly; muscle balance within 2 Δ vertically and 6 Δ horizontally; a horizontal visual field of 160° minimum; absence of diplopia.

For heavy goods and public service vehicle drivers, new applicants for licences must have a corrected VA of at least 6/9 in the better eye and 6/12 in the worse eye and an uncorrected vision of 6/60 in each eye separately. When renewing a licence first held before 1983, the corrected VA should be 6/12 in the better eye and 6/36 in the worse eye. If cataracts have been removed from one or both eyes then these drivers are only permitted a licence if intraocular lenses have been successfully implanted.

A most useful publication entitled *Medical Aspects of Fitness to Drive* has been published by the Medical Commission on Accident Prevention (35–43 Lincoln's Inn Fields, London, WC2A 3PN), the fourth edition edited by A. Raffle in 1985.

Civil pilots

The wearing of contact lenses is permitted by student and private pilots in the UK subject to certain conditions, full details of which are available from the Medical Department of the Civil Aviation Authority (CAA), but broadly the lenses must have been worn for at least 3 months and the applicant for a licence must be able to wear lenses for at least the duration of a working day. A specialist's report also has to be submitted with the application for a licence.

Professional pilots and aircrew are only permitted to use contact lenses in special circumstances. Where correction is only possible by wearing contact lenses, the Medical Department of the CAA must be informed.

Royal Air Force personnel

The Medical Board of the Royal Air Force decides on each individual's fitness and although there are no specific regulations about contact lenses, the RAF's Consultant Adviser in Ophthalmology usually makes the decision as to whether or not they may be worn in particular circumstances.

Royal Navy personnel

There is no general restriction to the wearing of contact lenses to improve visual efficiency provided that the required visual standards are met.

Merchant Navy personnel

Apart from those in the 'Deck Department' where no visual aids of any kind are permitted, contact lenses are allowed provided satisfactory visual standards are achieved and spare contact lenses or spectacles are available when on duty.

New entrants to the Merchant Navy or Fishing Industry are not allowed to wear any artificial aids to vision during the sight test and must not have had any treatment, designed to improve their form vision temporarily, undertaken shortly before the test. This would preclude the use of orthokeratological techniques to improve unaided vision.

Army personnel

The Army Medical Board judges each candidate's fitness on merit and there are no specific regulations about contact lens wear.

Police

Most but not all police forces in the UK accept contact lens wearers. Either the AOP or individual Police Authorities should be consulted about their wear and the eyesight standards required.

Prison officers

Provided the visual standards can be met, contact lenses are permitted subject to the wearer being able to defend himself and positively identify an assailant should the lenses become displaced.

Railway employees

Train drivers are not allowed to wear contact lenses, nor are workers on the running lines permitted to wear them except in special circumstances and with medical approval.

Legislative control of contact lenses and solutions

The availability of some contact lenses and solutions is limited in certain countries by government regulations. A brief outline of the current (1988) situation in the UK is appropriate here.

In the UK, since 1975, all contact lens solutions and preparations have been subject to licensing under the Medicines Act. The Department of Health and Social Security (DHSS) were approached in 1973 by the Faculty of Ophthalmologists, to bring preparations used in association with contact lenses under the control of the Medicines Act. This was because justifiable doubts had been cast on the efficacy of some solutions to kill harmful microorganisms in a suitable length of time. Also, it was felt that the toxicity of these solutions should be investigated. The DHSS, after due consideration, then set up a working party to consider guidelines which might be used in judging these preparations in the light of their mode of use. Then, in late 1975, contact lenses and associated preparations were brought under the control of the newly established Committee on Dental and Surgical Materials which was set up by Statutory Instrument to advise the Licensing Authority on various aspects of such materials.

This Committee set up a subcommittee in 1977 to advise it on 'the safety, quality and efficacy of contact lenses, contact lens blanks, contact lens fluids, such other substances or articles to which any provision of the Medicines Act 1968 is applicable and which are for administration to the human eye or which are for preventing, diagnosing, or treating adverse conditions of the human eye'. The DHSS Working Party has made recommendations to this Committee and contact lens solutions and their containers, and the sizes of the latter are now subject to statutory control. Materials and cases may be subject to regulation in due course.

In the UK, licensing of contact lens solutions became obligatory on 1st January 1980, but contact lenses and materials are still under consideration. It is understood that guidelines for their licensing have already been prepared and that such licensing will shortly come into effect.

Some idea of what is involved may be obtained from the experience of practitioners in the USA where all new contact lens materials (i.e. other than PMMA) are considered as drugs. Prior to approval by the Food and Drugs Administration (FDA) for general use they are subjected to clinical trials on rabbits and humans, and microbiological, toxicological and allergy tests are carried out with both lenses and solutions as well as tests on the associated use of their respective containers. Thus, several years may elapse between the original application to permit testing of the new lens/solution/system and its final approval. As far as extended wear contact lenses are concerned, the FDA requires the clinical trials to cover a given number of patients using the lenses for daily wear first, for a prescribed period of time. Pachometry, checks of the corneal endothelium, slit lamp examination of the upper tarsal plate, and other observations are all to be included in the clinical trials, as well as oxygen permeability studies on the lenses and their uptake of solution preservatives. If they pass these stringent daily wear trials they may then be used for similar extended wear trials.

Regulations also exist in certain European countries, but are less stringent than those of the USA. In Japan, the Ministry of Health and Welfare insists on independent testing of contact lens materials, methods of manufacture, and on contact lens solutions. University departments normally carry out the tests over a 3–5 year period which includes clinical trials. At present only a few companies are licensed to produce soft lenses. Even PMMA for hard lenses is subject to testing, and firms wishing to set up as hard lens manufacturers are rigorously controlled. As far as contact lens solutions are concerned, most mercurial compounds, such as thiomersalate (thimerosal), are banned.

Thus, in future, it may be that the practitioner's choice of lenses, solutions and containers will become much more limited, though it is to be hoped that bureaucratic intervention will not hamper genuine advances in the field of contact lenses

Sufficient has now been said about indications, contra-indications and selection of patients and contact lenses, as well as the factors to be considered in the choice of the best type of lens to fit. The reader must realize that both frustration and satisfaction are to be the lot of the contact lens practitioner at different times and with different patients.

References

ANDRES, S., HENRIQUEZ, A., GARCIA, M. L., VALERO, J. and VALLS, O. (1987). Factors of the precorneal tear film break-up time (BUT) and tolerance of contact lenses. *Int. Contact Lens Clin.* **14**, 103–107

BACKMAN, H. and BOLTE, C. (1974). Chronic allergic conjunctivitis and its effect on contact lenses. *Optom. Wkly* **65**(31), 26–30

BECKER, S. C. (1972). Clinical gonioscopy. *A Text and Stereoscopic Atlas*, pp. 165–167. St Louis: Mosby

BIBBY, M. M. (1976). Computer-assisted photokeratoscopy and contact lens design. Part 1, *Optician* **171**(4423), 37, 39, 41, 43; Part 2, *Optician* **171**(4424), 11, 14–15, 17; Part 3, *Optician* **171**(4425), 22–23; Part 4, *Optician* **171**(4426), 15, 17

BOBERG-ANS, J. (1955). Experience in clinical examination of corneal sensitivity. *Br. J. Ophthal.* **39**, 705–726

BONNET, R. and COCHET, P. (1962). New method of topographical ophthalmometry — its theoretical and clinical applications. *Am. J. Optom.* **39**, 227–251

BRUCH, C. W. (1973). Eye products: handle with care. *Optician* **166**(4297), 22, 27

CANTLE, S. (1988). Cholesterol and the eye. *Optician* **195**(5141), 29

CATANIA, L. J. (1987). Contact lenses, staphylococcus, and 'Crocodile OD'. *Int. Contact Lens Clin.* **14**, 113–115

COMMITTEE ON SAFETY OF MEDICINES (1986). Desensitising vaccines. *Br. med. J.* **293**, 948

CORDREY, P. (1972). *Cosmetics and the Eye/Contact Lens System.* London: Cordrey

COSTON, T. O. (1967). *Demodex folliculorum* blepharitis. *Trans. Am. ophthal. Soc.* **65**, 361–392

DEPARTMENT OF OPTOMETRY AND VISUAL SCIENCE, THE CITY UNIVERSITY, LONDON (1974). Eye beauty should be safe: eye make-up and contact lenses. *Optician* **168**(4355), 9, 13

FARRELL, H. (1976). Some effects of oral contraceptive steroids on the eye, related to corneal lens wear. *Optician* **171**(4423), 8–9, 13

FLETCHER, R. J. and NISTED, M. (1963). A study of coloured contact lenses and their performance. *Ophthal. Optician* **3**, 1151–1154, 1161–1163, 1203–1206, 1212–1213

FORD, M. W. (1974). Changes in hydrophilic lenses when placed on an eye. Paper read at the joint International Congress of The Contact Lens Society and The National Eye Research Foundation, Montreux, Switzerland

GHORMLEY, N. R. (1988). 'Standard' thickness soft lenses. *Int. Contact Lens Clin.* **15**, 46–48

GUILLON, J-P. (1986a). Tear film structure and contact lenses. In *The Pre-ocular Tear Film: in Health, Disease and Contact Lens Wear,* edited by F. J. Holly, Chap. 85. International Tear Film Symposium, Lubbock, Texas, November 1984. Lubbock: Dry Eye Institute

GUILLON, J-P. (1986b). Observing and photographing the pre-corneal and pre-lens tear film. *Contax* November 1986, 15–22

GUSTAFSON, J. C. (1967). Patient symptoms resulting from cosmetics and their correction. *Contacto* **11**(1), 16–19

HILL, R. M. (1973). Tears: the missing link. *Ophthal. Optician* **13**, 792–798, 800

HILL, R. M. and LEIGHTON, A. J. (1965). Temperature changes of human cornea and tears under a contact lens. Part II: Effects of intermediate lid apertures and gaze. *Am. J. Optom.* **42**, 71–77

HILL, R. M. and TERRY, J. E. (1976). Human tear cholesterol levels. *Archs Ophtal. (Paris)* **36**, 155–160

HILLMAN, J. S. (1976). The use of hydrophilic contact lenses. *Optician* **172**(4458), 9–11

INSLER, M. S. and ROBBINS, R. G. (1987). Intraocular pressure by noncontact tonometry with and without soft contact lenses. *Archs ophthal.* **105**(10), 1358

KEMMETTMÜLLER, H. (1962). Corneal lenses and keratoconus. *Contacto* **6**, 188–193

KERR, C. (1987). The UV debate. Symposium report in *Optician* **193**(5087), 14–18

KHOO, F. B. H. (1974). Paper read at National Optical Congress, University of Lancaster, September, 1974

KOETTING, R. A. (1966). The influence of oral contraceptives on contact lens wear. *Am. J. Optom.* **43**, 268–274

KOETTING, R. A. (1976). Tear film break-up time as a factor in hydrogel lens coating — a preliminary study. *Contacto* **20**(3), 20–23

LANDESMAN, R., DOUGLAS, R. G., DREISHPOON, G. and HOLZE, E. (1953). The vascular bed of the bulbar conjunctiva in the normal menstrual cycle. *Am. J. Obstet. Gynec.* **66**, 988–998

LANE, B. C. (1985). Newsbriefs: Hair it is. *Int. Contact Lens Clin.* **12**(2), 72

LARKE, J. (1985). *The Eye in Contact Lens Wear.* London: Butterworths

LEIBOWITZ, H. M. (1972). Hydrophilic contact lenses in corneal disease. IV. Penetrating corneal wounds. *Archs Ophthal.* **88**, 602–606

LEIBOWITZ, H. M. and ROSENTHAL, P. (1971). Hydrophilic contact lenses in corneal disease. I. Superficial, sterile, indolent ulcers. *Archs Ophthal.* **85**, 163–166

LEMP, M. A., DOHLMAN, C. H. and HOLLY, F. J. (1970). Corneal dessication despite normal tear volume. *Ann. Ophthal.* **2**, 258–261, 284

LEMP, M. A., DOHLMAN, C. H., KUWABARA, T., HOLLY, F. J. and CARROLL, J. M. (1971). Dry eye secondary to mucus deficiency. *Trans. Am. Acad. Ophthal. Otolaryngol.* **75**, 1223–1227

LEVEY, E. M. (1965). The sports wearer of contact lenses. *Am. J. Optom.* **42**, 21–23

LONDER, C. (1987). Canine lice in the lashes. *Optician* **193**(5094), 26

LOWTHER, G. E., BAILEY, N. J. and HILL, R. M. (1971). Conjunctival xerosis associated with contact lenses. *Am. J. Optom.* **48**, 754–758

LOWTHER, G. E., MILLER, R. B. and HILL, R. M. (1970). Tear concentrations of sodium and potassium during adaptation to contact lenses. 1. Sodium observations. *Am. J. Optom.* **47**, 266–275

McCONNELL, J. (1967). Cosmetics and contact lenses. *Contacto* **11**(1), 40–43

McDONALD, J. E. (1969). Surface phenomena of the tear film. *Am. J. Ophthal.* **67**, 56–64

MACKIE, I. A. (1967). Lesions at the corneal limbus at 3 o'clock and 9 o'clock in association with the wearing of contact lenses. pp. 66–73. In *Contact Lenses, XXth International Congress of Ophthalmology Symposium,* Munich-Feldafing, August 13th 1966, edited by O. H. Dabezies, H. Laue, A. Schlossman and G. P. Halberg. Basel and New York: Karger

MACKIE, I. A., SEAL, D. V. and PESCOD, J. M. (1977). Beta-adrenergic receptor blocking drugs: tear lysozyme and immunological screening for adverse reaction. *Br. J. Ophthal.* **61**, 354–359

McMONNIES, C. W. and CHAPMAN-DAVIES, A. (1987). Assessment of conjunctival hyperaemia in contact lens wearers. Parts I and II. *Am. J. Optom. physiol. Optics* **64**, 246–255

MANDELL, R. B. (1974). What is the gravity lens? *Int. Contact Lens Clin.* **1**(4), 29–35

MARSH, R. (1975). Thyroxine and contact lenses. In 'Points from Letters', *Br. med. J.* **2**, 689

MILLODOT, M. (1975). Do blue-eyed people have more sensitive corneas than brown-eyed people? *Nature* **255**(5504), 151–152

MILLODOT, M. (1976). Effect of the length of wear of contact lenses on corneal sensitivity. *Acta ophthal.* **54**, 721–730

MILLODOT, M. (1977). Influence of age on the sensitivity of the cornea. *Invest. Ophthal.* **16**, 240–243

MILLODOT, M. and LAMONT, A. (1974). Influence of menstruation on corneal sensitivity. *Br. J. Ophthal.* **58**, 752–756

NELSON, D. M. and WEST, L. (1987). Adapting to lenses: the personality of success and failure. *J. Br. Contact Lens Ass.* **10**, 36–37

NORN, M. S. (1963). Foam at outer palpebral canthus. *Acta ophthal.* **41**, 531–537

NORN, M. S. (1964). Vital staining in practice using a mixed stain and alcian blue. *Br. J. physiol. Optics* **21**, 293–298

NORN, M. S. (1965). Lacrimal apparatus tests: A new method (lacrimal streak dilution test) compared with previous methods. *Acta ophthal.* **43**, 557–566

NORN, M. S. (1970). Micropunctate fluorescein vital staining of the cornea. *Acta ophthal.* **48**, 108–118

NORN, M. S. (1974). *External Eye: Methods of Examination.* Copenhagen: Scriptor

PATEL, S., FARRELL, J. and BEVAN, R. (1987). Reliability and variability of the Schirmer test. *Optician* **194**(5122), 12–14

PEARSON, R. M. (1984). The mystery of the missing fluorescein. *J. Br. Contact Lens Ass.* **7**, 122–125

PEARSON, R. M. (1985). Letter to the Editor. *J. Br. Contact Lens Ass.* **8**, 43

PEARSON, R. M. (1986). The mystery of the missing fluorescein — a postscript. *J. Br. Contact Lens Ass.* **9**, 36–37

PHELPS BROWN, N. (1987). The watering eye. *Optician* **193**(5095), 47–49

POLSE, K. A. (1975). Observation of corneal dry spots. *Optom. Wkly* **66**(18), 20–21

POLSE, K., HAW, E. and FATT, I. (1976). Measurement of intraocular pressure over a gel lens. *Am. J. Optom. physiol. Optics* **53**, 3–6

RENGSTORFF, R. H. (1986). University of Maryland 2nd annual contact lens symposium, solutions cited as causing complications. *Contact Lens Forum* **11**(5), 50–51

RENGSTORFF, R. H. and BLACK, C. J. (1974). Eye protection from contact lenses. *J. Am. optom. Ass.* **45**, 270–276

ROY, A. M. (1961). Menstrual red eye. Letter in *Br. med. J.* **1**, 590

RUBINSTEIN, M. P. (1984). Epidermolysis bullosa — report of a case with contact lens implications. *J. Br. Contact Lens Ass.* **7**, 218–221

RUBINSTEIN, M. P. (1987). Diabetes, the anterior segment and contact lens wear. *Contact Lens J.* **15**, 4–11

SCHIRMER, K. E. and MELLOR, L. D. (1961). Corneal sensitivity after cataract extraction. *Am. Med. Ass. Archs Ophthal.* **65**, 433–436

SHILY, B. G. (1987). Psychophysiological stress, elevated intraocular pressure, and acute closed-angle glaucoma. *Am. J. Optom physiol. Optics* **64**, 866–870

SHREEVE, C. M. (1982). Treating the dry eye. *Ophthal. Optician* **22**, 650, 652

SILK, A. A. (1987). Puzzle of the polymers. *Transactions of the British Contact Lens Association Conference 1987*, pp. 57–61

SILK, A. A. (1988). Nissel Memorial Lecture. *J. Br. Contact Lens Ass. (Scientific Meetings)*, 18–22

SORSBY, A., LEARY, G. and RICHARDS, M. J. (1962). The optical components in anisometropia. *Vision Res.* **2**, 43–51

STEWART, C. R. (1973). Conjunctival absorption of pigment from eye make-up. *Am. J. Optom.* **50**, 571–574

STONE, J. (1959). Factors governing the back central optic diameter of a micro-lens. *Optician* **138**, 20–22

STONE, J. (1967). Near vision difficulties in non-presbyopic corneal lens wearers. *Contact Lens* **1**(2), 14–16, 24–25

TAKAHASHI, G. H. and LEIBOWITZ, H. M. (1971). Hydrophilic contact lenses in corneal disease. III. Topical hypertonic saline therapy in bullous keratopathy. *Archs Ophthal.* **86**, 133–137

TERRY, J. E. and HILL, R. M. (1975). Cholesterol: blood and tears. *J. Am. optom. Ass.* **46**, 1171–1174

VAN HERICK, W., SHAFFER, R. N. and SCHWARTZ, A. (1969). Estimation of width of angle of anterior chamber. *Am. J. Ophthal.* **68**, 626–629

VANLEY, G. T., LEOPOLD, I. H. and GREGG, T. H. (1977). Interpretation of tear film breakup. *Archs Ophthal.* **95**, 445–448

VOKE, J. (1986). A case of keratomalacia on a healthy diet. (Research review) *Optician* **192**(5075), 41

WESTERHOUT, D. (1973). The combination lens and therapeutic uses of soft lenses. *Contact Lens* **4**(5), 3–12, 16–18, 20, 22

WILSON, L. A., KUEHNE, J. W., HALL, S. W. and AHEARN, D. G. (1973). Microbial contamination in ocular cosmetics. *Optician* **166**(4298), 4, 6, 12

WINDER, A. F. (1981). Relationship between corneal arcus and hyperlipidaemia is clarified by studies in familial hypercholesterolaemia. *Br. J. Ophthal.* **67**, 789–794

WINN, B., ACKERLEY, R. G., BROWN, C. A., MURRAY, F. K., PRAIS, J. and ST JOHN, M. F. (1986). The superiority of contact lenses in the correction of all anisometropia. *Transactions of the British Contact Lens Association Conference 1986*, pp. 95–100

YOUNG, W. and HILL, R. M. (1973). Cholesterol levels of human tears: case reports. *J. Am. optom. Ass.* **45**, 424–428

Chapter 9

Patient management and instruction

K. W. Atkinson and M. J. A. Port

Some of the psychological factors likely to influence a patient have already been mentioned in Chapter 8. Many of these are worth repeating because the way in which a patient is managed is as important as pure technical ability and can make the difference between success and failure.

It is necessary for the patient to have confidence in the practitioner. This is essential in order that the patient commences to wear contact lenses, continues to wear them in spite of occasional difficulties and accurately follows any instructions given.

Simple terms should be used in explanations. Before examining a patient's eyes, it is wise to discuss the characteristics of the types of contemporary contact lenses. It is important to correct any mistaken ideas the patient has acquired. This is especially true since the advent of extended wear lenses. They have received a great deal of publicity — much of which is often over-optimistic. The practitioner should beware of making extravagant claims which may lead to loss of patient confidence or even legal proceedings if they are not met. A full explanation and discussion must cover any points on which the patient may require information.

The reason given by the patient for wanting contact lenses is important. It has a considerable effect on the successful outcome of contact lens wearing, assuming that the practitioner is fully competent to deal with any fitting difficulties. Prime motivations may be rationalized to other reasons on enquiry by the practitioner, but cosmetic results are the usual consideration in general practice. Intelligence, dexterity, environment, motivation and the needs of the patient all have a bearing on the type of lens selected.

A demonstration of hard and soft lenses may be useful. Even though contact lenses are in wide usage many are still unsure of size and flexibility, for example. The practitioner might consider a demonstration on his own eyes before using the patient's eyes.

If lens insertion and removal can be shown to be smooth, simple and painless procedures, confidence in the practitioner is enhanced and at the same time the patient's apprehension is reduced regarding his own ability to tolerate a contact lens.

Discussion tends to relax patients. They are normally tense and worried at the first visit. This discussion should include the advantages and disadvantages of contact lenses together with a brief résumé of adaptive difficulties. Reasons for using different types of contact lens can be given. It is important to anticipate a particular patient's visual expectations wherever possible, especially if the practitioner is considering fitting soft lenses.

Hydrogel lenses may give a reduced visual *quality* even though Snellen acuity is good (Applegate and Masof, 1975). Visual degradation may be caused by surface drying, surface distortion and surface deposits. The use of contrast sensitivity tests or low contrast charts may give more information than just the Snellen acuity (Woodhouse, 1987).

The practitioner should explain how much time is involved in fitting and what this entails. At this stage, the cost of the lenses and professional fees may be mentioned. The patient should be informed of the annual cost of wearing contact lenses; this normally consists of a fee for an after-care examination, an insurance premium to cover accidental loss of lenses, and the cost of maintaining the prescribed hygiene regimen. On a per annum basis, most patients are unaware of the relatively high cost of solutions and enzyme tablets. If patients do become aware of the costs this may lead to poor hygiene regimen compliance. Collins and

Carney (1986) found that only 25% of patients within their sample were truly compliant with practitioner instructions. They further found that a worsening ocular response to contact lenses was correlated to non-compliance with hygiene regimens.

Most patients wish to know how long their lenses are going to last them. With careful handling, cleaning and storage, PMMA lenses might last from 5 to 15 years but their usage is diminishing. Gas permeable hard (RGP) lenses are generally more brittle, less strong and more inclined to scratch. However, these characteristics are improving compared to the earliest RGP lenses and a typical life of 2–3 years may be expected. The polymers used tend to degrade with time and this may adversely affect strength, comfort, performance and optical quality. Two years for a PHEMA soft lens is probably about the longest useful life. Some manufacturers operate frequent replacement schemes, the idea being that soft lenses renewed on a regular basis cut down on chair time, lens cleaning costs and patient problems. However, taking loss or breakage of a lens into account, there may well be little difference between the average life of a hard and a soft lens.

The practitioner must lay great emphasis on the need for regular after-care visits after the initial supervised period. These may be carried out at 9- or 12-month intervals, more frequently for extended wear lenses. After the first year of wear a fee is normally charged.

Routine examination

Routine examination helps to determine the limitations that the patient himself may impose on the possibility of successful contact lens wear. It also helps to determine which type of lens will be most suitable. The patient's history is most important and should cover all the contra-indications mentioned in Chapter 8, with particular reference to general systemic conditions, systemic medication, previous ocular pathology and general ocular history (squint, amblyopia, eye operations and diseases).

The refractive condition of the patient should be considered as follows.

(1) Degree and type of ametropia, and whether or not corrected. Differences between the corneal astigmatism and the spectacle astigmatism are worth noting (see Chapters 5 and 14).

(2) Length of time spectacles have been worn. The patient may feel incomplete without spectacles if these have been worn for a considerable number of years. Conversely, the ability to see clearly without spectacles may be a strong motive.

(3) Whether the prescription is worn continually or only intermittently. A patient who wears a spectacle correction intermittently may not have sufficient motivation to persevere with contact lenses.

(4) The best visual acuity with the spectacle correction worn, the best visual acuity obtainable and whether or not the patient has been fully corrected previously.

(5) Correction required for vocation or leisure activity. It may well be, for example, that a gardener or rugby player will not need the good acuity of a graphic designer.

(6) The need of a correction for near vision. Motivation may be lessened when the patient realizes that a near correction is still necessary with contact lenses, be this in the form of bifocal contact lenses (see Chapter 16) or supplementary reading spectacles. Myopes invariably find that presbyopia appears a few years earlier if they are wearing contact lenses rather than spectacles.

(7) Tints — rigid and soft lenses are available in a wide range of tints. The purpose may be to aid location of the lens, to counteract photophobia, to change the colour of the iris, or to provide protection. The last case is particularly important for aphakic eyes. Without a crystalline lens, the retina receives a much higher level of ultraviolet light and adverse effects of this have been reported (Wittenberg, 1986). A contact lens for aphakia should therefore incorporate some tint that absorbs ultraviolet wavelengths (see Chapter 8). Soft lenses normally have their tinted portion the same size as the iris. The tinted portion may surround a clear pupil area if it is needed purely for cosmetic reasons. Reproducibility of soft lens tints is not always accurate. Scleral lenses can be supplied with a tinted optic portion.

If the patient knows other contact lens

wearers, their success or failure may affect his attitude and it may be worth while to mention individual variations in contact lens tolerance; for example, hours worn, degree of adaptation, lens comfort.

General ocular examination

Some parts of this examination assume added importance in contact lens work, but the following is a guide to the necessary tests (Chapter 8 gives an expansion of this information).

(1) External examination.
(2) Motility.
(3) Measurement of heterophorias at distance and at near. (Vertical prism can be included in soft, corneal and scleral lenses but horizontal prisms can only be incorporated in scleral lenses and then only up to 3 Δ in each lens.) Cover test for squint; speed of recovery of heterophoria; measurement of near point of convergence; fixation disparity tests.
(4) Visual acuity with spectacles.
(5) Ophthalmoscopy.
(6) Retinoscopy: a swirling movement may be indicative of keratoconus, but is also seen just after removal of PMMA lenses in some patients.
(7) Refraction — if the best acuity obtainable with trial lenses, of one or both eyes, is worse than 6/6, the practitioner should endeavour to find a reason for this. Checking with a pinhole disc may be useful.

External ocular characteristics related to contact lenses

General considerations

(1) Vertical and horizontal measurement of palpebral apertures.
(2) Vertical and horizontal visible iris diameters.
(3) Pupil diameters in average illumination and the maximum diameter in low illumination. It is most convenient to do this with a hand-held ultraviolet lamp. The fluorescence of the crystalline lens seen with this makes comparison with a pupil gauge very easy.

(4) Any irregularity of the pupil shape and any difference in size between the two.
(5) The profile of the cornea should be observed against the lower lid margin for Munson's sign (this is visible in keratoconus when the ectatic cornea distorts the outline of the lower lid margin). The anterior chamber depth, the central corneal radius and the nature of the limbal junction may be estimated at the same time.
(6) The size of the globes should be noted, i.e. large or small, and the general shape of the sclera.
(7) Lid tension, texture and thickness.
(8) Conjunctival texture, thickness and vascularity. Abnormalities are recorded; for example, pingueculae, limbal injection, blebs.

It is important to examine the upper and lower lids using a slit lamp. Lid margins and palpebral conjunctivas should be examined for signs of meibomitis and meibomian gland dysfunction (see Plate 5). The palpebral conjunctival surfaces should be examined for colour (hyperaemia) and surface texture. The position, size, density and type of surface elevations should be noted (see Plate 71). As with other aspects of the slit lamp examination (limbus, oedema, vascularization, staining, bulbar injection etc.), it is very worth while using a ranking (grading) system. For example, palpebral conjunctival colour:

0 = normal
1 = mild hyperaemia
2 = moderate hyperaemia
3 = severe hyperaemia

The patient record might show 1/3, indicating grade 1 on a scale of 0 to 3.

Other considerations

(1) It is useful to make a drawing of the upper and lower lid positions relative to the cornea. The importance of this together with other lid characteristics should not be underestimated when the centration and performance of lenses is being considered.
(2) Active corneal and conjunctival conditions can be detected by instilling staining agents (Norn, 1972).
(3) Corneal sensitivity can be established gross-

ly with a wisp of tissue. Correct use of a corneal aesthesiometer will give more accurate information. An instrument designed by Cochet and Bonnet (1961) or Draeger (1984) is the technique usually employed.

(4) Keratometry (*see* Chapter 6).

(5) A thorough slit lamp examination (*see* Chapters 6, 7, 8 and 19). Where possible this should include pachometry, to measure at least the central corneal thickness (Stone, 1974). The pachometer should be properly calibrated and a mean of 10 readings is more useful than single readings. The practitioner should be aware of the effect of menstrual and diurnal variations in corneal thickness (Fujita, 1980).

(6) A Placido disc, Klein keratoscope or photo-electric keratoscope (PEK) should be used if prior examination has led the practitioner to suspect the presence of keratoconus or corneal irregularity. Keratometry, slit lamp examination, refraction, visual acuity and pachometry also give clues.

(7) Assessment of tear output and volume. Significant departures from the norm can be detected using a thread test (Hamano *et al.*, 1982) or with Schirmer paper strips. The figures given by Zappia (1972) are fairly typical but variation is wide (Schapiro and Merin, 1979).

A new generation of paper strips with transparent covers helps minimize evaporation from the strip and they are therefore more efficient than the original design.

A large percentage of the tear volume is held in the tear rivus which interfaces the lid margins and globe. Careful inspection of this rivus gives an indication of tear volume.

(8) Tear film integrity — using a slit lamp, fluorescein and blue light, the break-up time (BUT) is assessed when dry spots appear in the tear film (*Plate 55*). The patient is asked not to blink during the test. Lemp *et al.* (1970) found that a BUT of less than 10 seconds was critical. It has been argued (Mengher *et al.*, 1985) that the use of fluorescein produces an abnormal tear film. Thus, non-invasive break-up time (NIBUT) without the dye can be employed *see* Chapter 8, pp. 286 and 287.

(9) Photography of the external eye with both white light and ultraviolet light (*see* Chapter 7).

Not all the above tests are necessary for every patient. Tests 6, 7, 8 and 9 may be carried out at the discretion of the practitioner, although it may be valuable to do them for every patient.

If the history or ocular examination yields evidence that an active pathological process is present, then in the UK it is necessary by statute to refer the patient to his or her doctor. If the patient is receiving treatment for a general condition it is prudent to contact the general medical practitioner concerned to discuss the advisability of fitting contact lenses. Those who refuse to consult a medical person should be asked to provide a letter stating their reasons for refusal, and careful records should be kept.

The practitioner must be very careful to examine the eyes for active or passive pathological conditions before proceeding to place a contact lens on the eye. As stated above, with any active condition, referral is imperative before fitting is started. In the case of a passive condition, careful notes and diagrams should be entered on the patient's record card. Such conditions may not prevent successful contact lens wear, but the patient should be made aware of their presence.

If, for example, an early case of endothelial dystrophy had been discovered and it is decided not to proceed with fitting, it would be wise to inform the patient and provide him with a covering note to this effect. The practitioner should obviously keep a copy for his or her own protection. This same patient might well consult someone else with a view to having contact lenses fitted. Such a subtle condition could well be overlooked and contact lenses might be supplied to the detriment of the patient's cornea, unless the patient has already been told why he was rejected for contact lenses. Where conditions exist that are 'abnormal' but may not fit precisely into an 'active' or 'passive' category, the opinion of an ophthalmologist should be sought, who may also be able to give opinions as to whether such conditions would be aggravated by the wearing of contact lenses.

Changes in the condition of the eyes in subsequent years may be blamed on contact lenses. These changes may be old or may have arisen concurrently with contact lens wear. Accurate records monitoring the condition of the eyes over the years are therefore of paramount importance.

At this stage it is necessary to decide whether

to proceed with fitting, bearing in mind the contra-indications which might have been discovered. Some conditions may impose restrictions on the performance of contact lenses and the patient should be made aware of these limitations.

If the practitioner decides to proceed with the fitting, he must also decide whether to fit hard or soft lenses, taking all considerations into account.

Insertion of the first lens

The methods of lens insertion and removal by the practitioner and by the patient are very similar — although, of course, the patient may occupy a different position, either sitting or reclining backwards when the lens is being inserted by the practitioner, and leaning over some flat surface or over a mirror when doing it himself. The methods described in detail are only some of those which can be used, and variations can be left to the ingenuity of the individual.

It is better to use finger methods as these are much less likely to cause trauma and, when it comes to handling lenses, confidence is more easily achieved when a minimum of artificial aids is necessary.

The patient who has lost his suction holder and is dependent on it to remove his lenses can be in a real dilemma. For this reason suction holders should only be supplied for removing lenses from the cornea as a last resort after all other methods have been tried in vain, and when used a spare should always be supplied.

Patients with enophthalmic eyes and loose lids may have to rely on a suction holder for lens removal. The safe and hygienic keeping of the suction holder must be emphasized to users. Recommending spare suction holders to be kept safely at work and at home is expedient.

Insertion and removal of hard and rigid gas permeable corneal lenses

Insertion is more easily managed by working from the same side as the eye on to which the lens is to be placed, so that the facial contours do not interfere with lens manipulation.

Finger method of insertion

The lens is placed on the forefinger of one hand. The second finger of this hand is used to hold the bottom lid down and also to steady the inserting hand. The other hand is used to hold up the top lid and, while some fixation point is regarded with the other eye, the lens is gently placed on to the cornea. If the lids are held apart for a moment after the lens has been placed on the cornea, then the lens is less likely to be dislodged on the first strong blink. The patient should then look down. Best lid control is obtained if the lids are held near to but not actually over the lashes (*Figure 9.1*).

By the practitioner

Standing beside the patient, ideally the practitioner should work on the same side as the eye being fitted, for best lens control. It needs a little practice to become equally adept with either hand, but the ease of doing it this way makes the practice worth while.

The patient's head should be upright with the back of the head against the headrest of the chair.

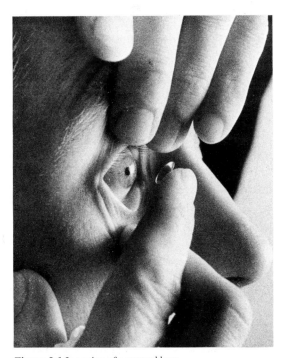

Figure 9.1 Insertion of a corneal lens

The patient is instructed to look at a suitable object so that the line of sight is depressed, and the lens is gently placed on to the upper part of the cornea and allowed to move into place before the lids are released.

The patient's head should remain in the same position after the lids have been released. Looking up and around tend to be initially uncomfortable.

By the patient

This may be done over a horizontally placed mirror. Fixation is maintained by the eye which is not receiving the lens. This reduces the avoidance reflex causing eye deviation if the lens is watched as it approaches the cornea. When the lens insertion technique has been mastered efficiently with the mirror the patient should try to insert the lens without the mirror. The eye receiving the lens has to fixate the lens or, better still, looks at some object directly ahead so that the cornea remains centred within the palpebral aperture. Many patients prefer to learn this way as they find it upsetting to watch themselves in a mirror.

Some patients prefer to use a vertical mirror. They should be warned that the lens is more likely to slip off the finger and get lost with this method.

The patient learning to insert corneal lenses has to remember a number of points and they are not always coordinated immediately. Three main points are worth underlining when instructing the patient: keep a very firm grip on the lid margins; only let the lids go when the lens is definitely felt to have settled on the cornea; keep fixation stationary until both lids have been gently released.

Insertion by the suction holder method

Instead of being placed on the forefinger, the lens is lightly pressed on to the end of a moistened suction holder and transferred from this to the eye by the technique set out above. This is a less satisfactory method than placing the lens on the forefinger as it is more likely to cause damage when inexpertly used and generally causes a larger avoidance eye movement. It also relies on the patient always having a suction holder to hand.

Variations of the suction holder technique are sometimes employed and usually incorporate a fixation target such as a light seen through the hollow suction holder handle. High hyperopes, presbyopes, and aphakics may have to resort to such methods of lens insertion if they cannot see to manipulate the lens at short distances. They may also find it useful to have a spectacle frame, glazed on one side only with a prescription for near work. The lower part of the front on the other side is removed from the frame and the first contact lens is inserted through the empty half of the frame. It should then be possible to see to insert the other lens.

One-handed insertion

This method is occasionally necessary when a patient has only one hand which can be used. In this case, the lids are held apart with the first and third fingers while the second finger is used to place the lens on the eye. Some patients can inhibit the blink reflex so well that they only need hold the bottom lid down with the middle finger and place the lens on the cornea with the forefinger.

Insertion technique variations

Patients often develop ingenious and sometimes awkward-looking methods for inserting and removing contact lenses. As long as the method is unlikely to damage their eyes or lenses there is no reason for change.

Removal by both the practitioner and the patient

With the cornea central in the palpebral aperture, the lids are opened as wide as possible. To keep the lids taut the patient should be told to keep his eyebrows raised and stare wide all the time until the lens is expelled. The forefinger, middle finger or thumb is placed at the outer canthus. The lids are then pulled outwards in the direction of the top of the ear so that both lids are tensioned equally at the top and bottom of the lens. An extra pull with the finger or a strong blink will then lift the lens off the eye as shown in *Figure 9.2*. Some patients find that a slight head turn to position the cornea just in the nasal part of the aperture is a useful posture to adopt prior to starting the removal technique. As the lens comes off the

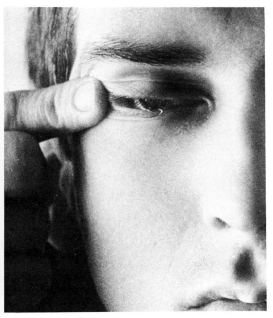

Figure 9.2 Lid removal of a corneal lens using one finger

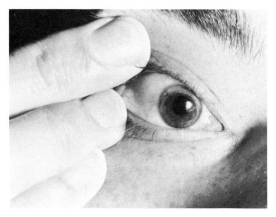

Figure 9.3 Lid removal of a corneal lens using two fingers

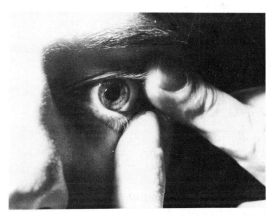

Figure 9.4 Lid removal of a corneal lens using one finger of each hand

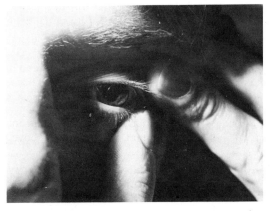

Figure 9.5 Later stage of removal — the lens is just coming away from the cornea. Temporal movement of the lens is almost inevitable

cornea it may drop, in which case it may be caught with a free hand. Alternatively it may stick on the lashes. In this case the patient closes his eyes and then the lens is removed with the fingers.

'Scissors' method of removal

Using one hand

The cornea is again positioned centrally or slightly nasally in the palpebral aperture. The middle finger is placed on the upper lid margin and the third finger on the lower lid margin as shown in *Figure 9.3*. The two fingers can control the upper and lower lids independently. It is important that the margins are in contact with the globe; an 'ectropion' lid posture cannot result in successful lens removal. When correctly positioned, the lids are pulled towards the ear as described above.

If this method is used by the practitioner, it is useful for the patient to fixate one of the practitioner's fingers — about 25 cm in front of the eye. When the practitioner sees that the lids are taut and are on the top and bottom edges of the lens, he should move the fixation finger laterally — in the direction of the patient's nose. At the same time as the fixation finger is moving nasally, the lids should be pulled temporally. This is a very effective technique unless the eyes are very enophthalmic.

Using two hands

The forefingers of each hand are positioned on the top and bottom lids as shown in *Figures 9.4* and *9.5*. The method is essentially the same as in using one hand only.

The scissors method is normally used when the conventional method is inadequate, the usual reason for failure being the top lid descending over the lens while the pulling action occurs. Before trying the scissors method it may be worth positioning the single finger more on the top lid rather than exactly at the outer canthus.

A variation of this method is to place the fingers on the lid margins just above and below the highest and lowest parts of the lens. The lid margins are then used to lift off either the superior or inferior edge of the lens. A practitioner should be careful not to use too much force and cause discomfort.

Suction holder removal of lens

The lids are held apart in the same way as that used for inserting a lens. With the top lid held up by the free hand and the lower lid held down by the hand using the moistened suction holder, the thumb and forefinger hold the suction holder bulb, which is squeezed before the flat end is pressed gently against the lens. When the thumb and forefinger are eased apart, the lens is sucked on to the holder and can be removed from the eye. Sometimes a small twist as the lens comes off the cornea helps to break the suction between lens and cornea (*Figure 9.6*). This method is often useful when dealing with a tense patient.

A large amount of suction is not required in most cases. A common fault is not getting the cup end of the suction holder central and parallel to the lens. Patients having to use this method as a last resort usually have narrow apertures and/or enophthalmic eyes.

Before any repeated attempts are made at lens removal by this method, the patient should be instructed to check that the lens is still on the cornea in order to prevent possible corneal insult by the suction holder.

The normal way is to ask the patient to close or cover the other eye. If the vision is still normal then the contact lens is still in place.

With all the above methods of lens removal, the practitioner must be willing and able to help the patient by demonstrating on himself. It is also useful for him to remove a lens from the patient's eye to demonstrate a particular aspect; for example, the force used by the fingers when pulling the lids. When using the fingers in conjunction with a mirror the practitioner must emphasize that pulling on the lids after the top lid has passed over the lens edge can have no effect except to keep the lens in and make the eye sore. Similarly, it is difficult to remove a corneal lens if there is excessive lacrimation. Tears should be allowed to subside before attempting removal. The lid margins can then grip and pass under the lens edges more effectively.

Lens on the bulbar conjunctiva

Some corneal lens wearers habitually place the lens on to the conjunctiva and then centre it. Occasionally, the practitioner may place the lens on to the conjunctiva of a nervous patient and then move it carefully on to the cornea.

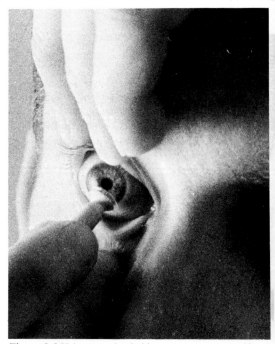

Figure 9.6 Using a suction holder to remove a corneal lens

More frequently a corneal lens locates itself on the conjunctiva from faulty insertion or removal technique. The patient must be able to find the lens if this happens, and it must be emphasized that the lens cannot get lost behind the eye. The position of the lens can usually be located because it can be felt as the eye moves, except when in the upper fornix. To expose the lens maximally, it is usually easier to use a vertical mirror. The patient can expose various sections of the bulbar conjunctiva by appropriate head movements; for example, tilting the head down and looking up, if the lens is displaced downwards. Pulling the lids away from the globe can also help in the search for a misplaced lens. Having found the lens it can be removed with a suction holder or recentred on to the cornea.

The lens can be centred by using the lid margin to push the lens into the required position or back on to the cornea. *Figure 9.7* shows a lens being moved from the lower conjunctival sac towards the cornea. The lid is pulled down as necessary, so that the margin is beyond the furthest edge of the lens. Then, using two fingers to prevent the lens moving sideways, the lid margin is used to push the lens back on to the cornea. It is useful to press down gently on the edge of the lens furthest from the cornea.

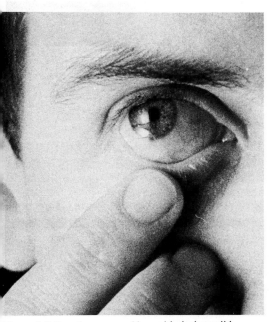

Figure 9.7 Centring a corneal lens with the lower lid

This will lift the lens edge closest to the cornea and minimize the risk of abrasion when the lens is centred. From the patient's point of view the lens is most easily centred when it is on the upper or lower sectors of the conjunctiva. It is often simpler to move the lens into one of these areas before attempting to centre it. Again, the lid margin can be used to move the lens across the conjunctiva to the desired area. When using the lower lid to manipulate the lens, it is best to tell the patient to hold the upper eyelid up, out of the way, and vice versa.

Alternatively, the lens can sometimes be located by closing the eye and feeling through the lids with one or two fingers. The lens may be centred by forming the fingertips of one hand into a circle and, with the eye still closed, massaging through the lids to centralize the lens. This is a haphazard approach and is often unsuccessful. It can be useful if the lens has moved into the superior fornix where it may be occluded by the orbital margin.

Insertion and removal of scleral lenses

Insertion

The insertion methods are the same whether done by the practitioner or by the patient. The lens is best inserted into the superior fornix. With the eye looking down, the upper lid is lifted by the opposite hand. The lens is grasped at or slightly below its horizontal meridian on each side by the thumb and second finger (*Figure 9.8*). If the lens is fenestrated, then the fenestration should be orientated before the lens is inserted on to the eye. The first finger is positioned against the lower front optic zone and serves to support the lens. The top edge of the lens is gently touched on to the superior portion of the bulbar conjunctiva and allowed to follow the contour of the eye into the superior fornix. While it is held in this position by the fingers, the forefinger of the other hand is used to manipulate the top lid down over the lens, which holds the lens in position. The patient then looks up and the lower lid is simultaneously pulled down so that the lower portion of the lens moves on to the inferior bulbar conjunctiva and the lens is then in position. During this procedure, blinking or closing the eyes must be resisted as a really hard blink may trap the lower lid under the

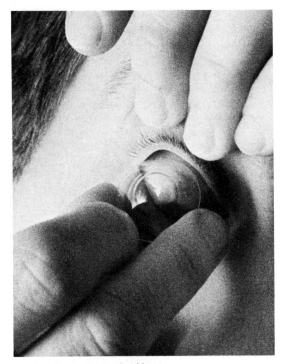

Figure 9.8 Inserting a scleral lens

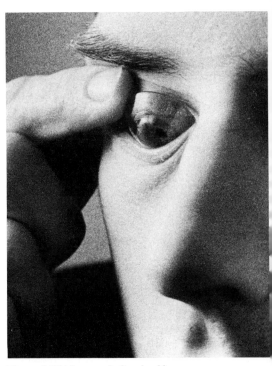

Figure 9.9 Lid removal of a scleral lens

lower edge of the lens and it is then necessary to pull the lid free so that it moves comfortably over the lens.

Many scleral lens wearers prefer to insert the lens with the optic zone filled with saline. This is feasible with all scleral lens types. In this instance the lens is held and inserted horizontally.

Removal

Removal is accomplished by looking downwards, which exposes the upper edge of the lens when the upper lid is raised. The tip of the forefinger is used to hold the top lid at its nasal margin close against the eye above the lens, and pulling it taut up across the superior aspect of the eye causes the lid margin to move under the top edge of the lens and lever it away from the eye. By looking upwards and pulling the lower lid away from the eye, the lens is finally expelled (*Figure 9.9*).

Alternatively, a small suction holder placed on to the superior scleral zone of the lens may be used to pull the top of the lens away from the eye, if the lid method is not successful. A slight twist of the suction holder helps to break any suction between lens and eye.

Care should be taken to supervise patients habitually using the lid removal method to make sure that a fingernail is not used to lever the top of the lens from the eye as this could lead to trauma and, possibly, infection.

Insertion and removal of hydrophilic lenses

Insertion

Often a soft lens can be inserted exactly as described above for the insertion of hard corneal lenses, i.e. by placing directly onto the cornea either at the superior aspect with the patient looking down or centrally with the patient looking straight ahead (*Figures 9.10, 9.11 and 9.12*). Because of its greater size and flexibility, the interpalpebral gap must be larger than the lens diameter and the lids must be gripped at the edges and held well apart to make insertion easy. When the initial lenses are being inserted, patient comfort can be enhanced by having the patient look away and placing the lens onto the

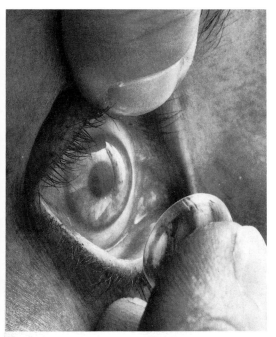

Figure 9.10 Inserting a hydrophilic lens

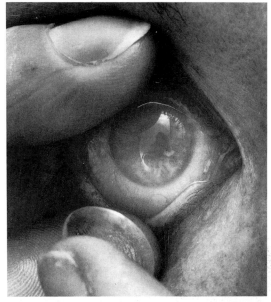

Figure 9.12 Holding the lids apart with the same hand and inserting a hydrophilic lens

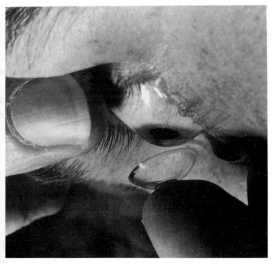

Figure 9.11 Inserting a lens with the head horizontal

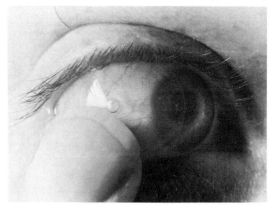

Figure 9.13 A hydrophilic lens being moved from the temporal conjunctiva to the cornea

temporal side of the cornea or pressing it onto the temporal conjunctiva. The lens can be centred by having the patient look into it or by pushing the lens gently on centre either with the lids or with a finger as shown in *Figure 9.13*. Transfer from the finger onto the eye is easy if the lens has dried out a little and excess moisture is removed, either by transferring it

from one forefinger to the other or by dabbing the moisture pool at the base of the lens with a tissue. Care should be taken not to introduce foreign material onto the lens in the process of drying it. A slightly dry thin lens will actually be taken up from the finger to the eye by the attraction of the tears on the eye's surface, so that the lens need only be touched gently against the eye — the tear layer completing the transfer. If a lens is placed onto the eye inside out it will move excessively and give poor vision and discomfort. *Figures 9.14* and *9.15* show a lens the

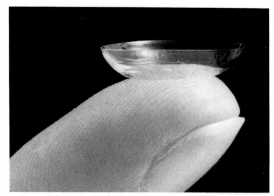

Figure 9.14 A hydrophilic lens correct side uppermost

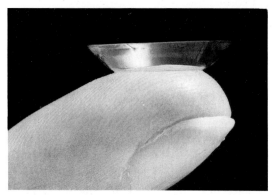

Figure 9.15 The same lens inside out

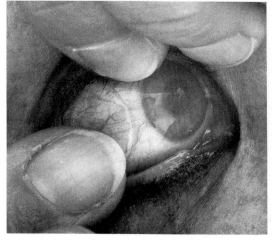

Figure 9.16 A hydrophilic lens pulled onto the conjunctiva to remove a foreign body

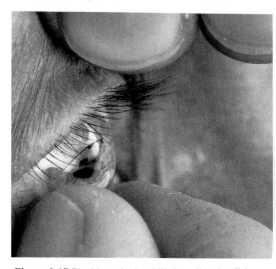

Figure 9.17 Pinching a hydrophilic lens directly off the cornea

correct way round, and the same lens inside out. With very thin lenses the difference is not so obvious. A further check can be made by folding the lens inwards gently between thumb and forefinger. If the edges move inwards the lens is the right way round, if they bend outwards it is inside out. Discomfort can also be caused by a foreign body being trapped between the lens and the eye. Using the tip of one finger to slide the lens either temporally or inferiorly off the cornea and onto the bulbar conjunctiva and then back on centre will often remove the source of irritation (*Figure 9.16*).

Removal

The method chosen to remove the soft lens will depend on dexterity, lid and palpebral characteristics as well as factors such as the size of lens, lens thickness and lens material. It is worth while consulting the manufacturer's literature regarding lens removal.

The pinch method is easiest especially with a nervous patient. The lens is pinched off either from the central position as shown in *Figure 9.17* or pulled either inferiorly (*Figure 9.18*) or temporally with the tip of the forefinger and then pinched between the fleshy parts of forefinger and thumb.

The scissors method can be carried out by placing the fingers directly at the lid margins above and below the lens and pulling the lids first apart then pushing them tightly onto the eye and then together to squeeze the lens out through the lid gap. *Figure 9.19* shows this sequence.

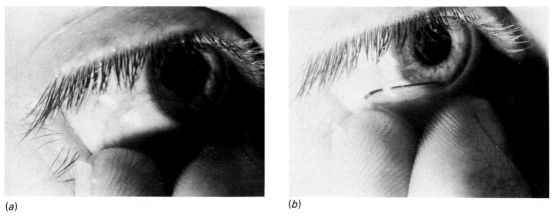

(a)   (b)

Figure 9.18 Pinching a hydrophilic lens between finger and thumb of one hand to remove the lens from the lower fornix

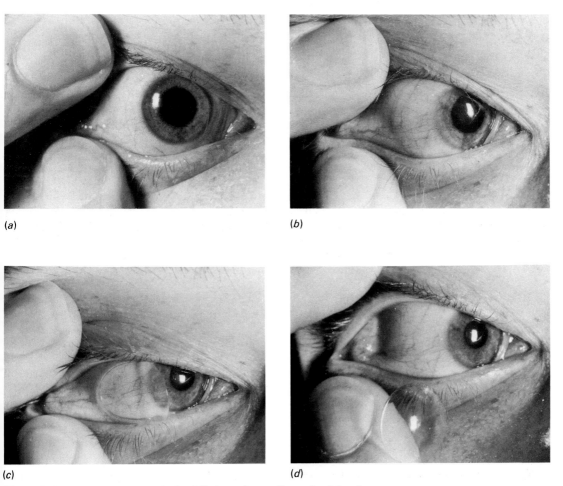

(a)   (b)

(c)   (d)

Figure 9.19 Removal sequence of a hydrophilic lens using one finger of each hand

Artificial aids such as suction holders are not recommended but if used at all should first be modified so that in fact no suction can be exerted. The suction holder is used as a wedge, being forced under the lens edge and then away from the eye to break the lens cohesion to the eye.

On removal, a thin or spun-cast lens can become rolled or stuck together. Care needs to be taken to prevent lens damage when separating the lens. The pinch method of removal is more likely to cause the edges of a lens to become stuck together on removal. Instillation of saline into the eye prior to removal or wetting the fingers with saline prior to pinching can help. A rolled or stuck lens can sometimes be separated by gently rolling it between the fingers as shown in *Figure 9.20* or on the palm of the hand having wetted it with saline or cleaning solution which is more viscous. Soaking in warm saline or heating in saline or distilled water is sometimes needed for a lens that is difficult to separate.

Reactions to the first lens

Cleanliness is vital in all aspects of contact lens practice. The patient should be made aware of this both by modelling behaviour on the practitioner's own example, as well as by instruction and demonstration.

The patient must be prepared physically and psychologically for the insertion of the first lens.

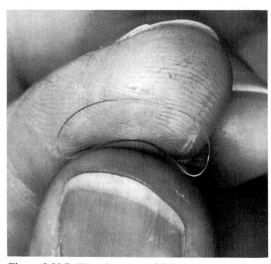

Figure 9.20 Rolling a lens to unstick it

It should be stated that some initial discomfort (use of the word 'pain' is deprecated) and lacrimation is quite normal. It is explained that these initial symptoms usually subside quickly and the lens becomes more tolerable. Most patients admit that the first lens feels much better than expected and there is no harm telling a new patient this before the lens is inserted.

Patient management

There may well be some irritation for the first minute or two. The new patient has no experience in deciding what may be the cause of this irritation. The practitioner should bear in mind such factors as pH and tonicity of solutions, and foreign bodies. A small piece of dust or fluff behind the lens can be very irritating. Removing the lens, cleaning it appropriately and re-inserting it can often give a dramatic improvement. With a soft lens it is often sufficient to move the lens on to the conjunctiva for a few seconds and then centre it back on the cornea (*Figure 9.16*).

Patients should always sit comfortably with head supported, and be given a tissue to wipe away any overflow of tears.

Both soft and hard lenses need to be cleaned with an appropriate surfactant and then thoroughly rinsed in sterile saline (or cold water for hard lenses). A really clean lens is more comfortable and settles more quickly as well as giving better visual results when refraction is done through the contact lens. It also makes it easy to assess the fit once the initial adaptive response has subsided.

A soothing explanation of what is taking place helps to calm the patient. It should be treated as a matter of course if the lens should fall before being inserted, or if the first attempt is not successful. It is essential not to panic at any stage.

Excess lacrimation, blepharospasm, engorgement of conjunctival vessels or extreme sensitivity may contra-indicate the use of contact lenses, if these symptoms do not subside in a reasonable time. These symptoms may also indicate a foreign body or a dirty, damaged or poorly fitting lens and these possibilities need to be examined.

Unless a scleral lens is fitting very poorly, the patient does not experience much discomfort relative to that felt with a hard corneal lens. If the lens is too large there may be localized sensation at the edges. It is often reported that the eye feels full and hot.

With a hard corneal lens most of the sensation comes from the top lid moving over the lens edge, because the lid margins are very sensitive. The lids being somewhat tense will cause some pressure effects on the lens. These points can easily be demonstrated by the practitioner moving the lids well away from the lens; the patient then admits that the sensation virtually disappears completely.

Assuming no foreign bodies and a reasonable fit, the symptoms from a corneal lens soon pass. Patient relaxation and reduction in corneal sensitivity obviously assist this process. The patient can be told this will occur.

Most people react very favourably to hydrophilic lenses. There is often significantly less reaction than with a hard lens and, although the reaction of a patient is of consequence, the practitioner must not choose a lens type only on this basis. Other significant factors must be taken into account before this very important decision is taken.

A patient who sweats profusely, sways about in the chair, complains of a 'stuffy atmosphere', or turns pale, may be in the first stages of fainting or vomiting. It is useful to be prepared for this after the insertion of the first lens. If in doubt, the patient should be asked if he feels well, and if necessary his head may be held down. The patient should not be left alone in this state as he may fall from the chair and injure himself. The contact lens should be removed as soon as it is practicable to do so and the patient given adequate time to recover. It is usually of no use to continue the fitting as the patient may faint again if another lens is inserted. It is useful to be able to obtain assistance easily in any emergency so that a glass of water or smelling salts can be handed to the patient. The presence of another person is desirable for the practitioner's own protection and will be reassuring to the patient.

An initial settling period of at least 10 minutes, and sometimes 20 minutes, is necessary so that lacrimation and blink rate become more normal before an assessment of the fit is made. After assessing all aspects of the fit of the first lens, it is then removed. Excess lacrimation and renewed tension at this prospect often make removal difficult. It is essential, therefore, that the practitioner is proficient at this. He or she should have several methods at his or her disposal, and should be able to vary them according to the circumstances so that the lens is quickly removed with minimum discomfort.

The basic fitting methods for hard corneal lenses, hydrophilic lenses, and scleral lenses are dealt with in Chapters 10, 11, 17 and 18.

Refraction with contact lenses

Hard lenses

Excess lacrimation can make patient observations difficult. A satisfactory end-point in subjective refraction is not always easy. If the lens does not centre well or the patient blinks at a high rate, then refraction is variable. The duochrome chart may help. The maximum positive power acceptable should be given and the Humphriss balancing technique is useful in helping to keep accommodation relaxed.

Although in most cases only a spherical correction is necessary, the astigmatism with a contact lens in place should still be measured. This may be done most easily with a retinoscope — but if good acuity is not obtainable with a spherical correction, or if the patient is hypercritical, a subjective measurement should be made. The methods and criteria for correcting residual astigmatism are set out in Chapter 14.

It is generally found that up to 0.75 D of astigmatism may be left uncorrected without reducing visual acuity, although individual acceptance varies.

It is important to check for any vertical heterophoria when the patient has a lens in each eye. The spectacle correction gives a clue as to whether correcting prism may have to be incorporated.

It is often useful to order the power of the lens +0.25 D more than the power deduced from the refraction. The excess lacrimation with the trial lens provides a temporary increase in negative power and the discomfort of a contact lens can cause the patient to accommodate slightly.

If power changes are necessary, they can be carried out once the patient is fully adapted when it is easier for the patient to concentrate and make accurate judgements in subjective testing. For this reason, binocular balancing is best left until this time.

Hydrophilic lenses

Many of the points mentioned above in relationship to hard lenses still apply to soft lenses. It is important to remember that neither the practitioner nor the soft lens laboratory can satisfactorily modify the power of finished lenses.

Refining the refractive end-point can be done at the first after-care check by exchanging the lenses using a lens from the practitioner's own inventory or one of the variety of exchange plans that can be arranged with the laboratory. To ensure accurate refraction with hydrophilic lenses a stable lens fit is required.

A trial lens with power and other parameters as close as possible to the patient's intended prescription is helpful, as well as behaving more nearly like the final lens.

Most corneal astigmatism is transmitted by a soft lens. Residual astigmatism is sometimes less and sometimes more than expected (*see* Chapters 5 and 14). It should be measured, recorded and its effects anticipated in every case.

Lenses should be well settled before a refraction is performed. It is preferable, and convenient, to do this after a tolerance trial, but 20 minutes wear would be a minimum before a final assessment is made. If vision checks are performed during fitting a shorter time for the lens to settle has to be allowed even though this is not ideal.

Vision which cannot be stabilized to a satisfactory level is a contra-indication for fitting soft lenses. If it is stable and the quality is poor, the practitioner should think of alternative lens designs (soft and hard). The quality of vision may be judged by asking the patient to look at a small spotlight in the dark. If it does not appear round and well defined, but instead looks distorted or streaky, then the quality of vision is poor. The use of toric hydrophilic lenses may be helpful if poor quality is related to residual astigmatism that is quantitatively consistent (*see* Chapter 14).

Contrast sensitivity tests or reduced contrast letter charts may be used to assess quality of vision.

Tolerance trials

Tolerance trials should be carried out routinely. Whether this is a short-term trial of half an hour to a couple of hours, or a longer trial of all day or several days or weeks, or a combination of these, depends on the practitioner and the individual patient and the lenses being used.

There are very good reasons for doing tolerance trials both for the patient and for the practitioner. They provide the patient with experience and confidence about their ability to wear contact lenses and will demonstrate or eliminate those without the necessary confidence. Patients will find lens handling and practising insertion and removal easier if they have worn lenses prior to doing this, and the practitioner gains insight to possible adverse ocular responses that may occur with long-term wear, and which could be modified with alternative fittings, lens materials, shorter wearing times or appropriate care and storage systems for the lenses. More immediately the practitioner is provided with extra information as to the accuracy of the initial fitting and refractive findings, as the performance of the lenses can be reassessed once the initial responses have diminished and more normal tearing and blink rates have been established.

Short-term tolerance trials can be done with fitting or trial lenses either close to the patient's refraction, or with low power lenses and the patient's spectacle correction worn over that. While this is an adjustment period for the patient, for the practitioner it provides the settling down time needed to get a stable acuity and to judge the fit of the lenses and physiological response of the eye.

Responses after tolerance trials

Following tolerance trials, an abbreviated after-care examination should be carried out. The advantages of doing a tolerance trial are to be able to anticipate and eliminate causes of difficulty which, if occurring later, could interrupt the smooth passage of easy adaptation to the contact lenses and, more damagingly, affect the patient's confidence about wearing contact lenses. Sometimes it is obvious that a change in lens design or lens materials is needed and this is best done before issue to the patient. Sometimes patients decide that, having worn contact lenses for a tolerance trial, that is as far as they want to proceed and it is easier to stop at this stage rather than later, when a greater investment of money and time has been made.

The routine after-care examination is similar for soft and hard lenses and can be considered under the following headings:

(1) Patient responses:
confidence and ease of wearing;
comfort, lens awareness;
perceptual adjustment to a new prescription.
(2) Practitioner observations:
is the fit still satisfactory?
does the lens still centre and provide adequate pupil or corneal cover?
ascertain correct lens power and relate visual acuity to that with spectacles.
(3) Lens responses — as comfort increases alterations in tear flow and blinking may alter how a lens performs.
(4) Physiological responses:
corneal epithelial and endothelial changes, stromal swelling with striae and folding in Descemet's membrane;
changes in the tears with alterations in volume and tear composition;
changes in the lid margins or palpebral conjunctiva;
alterations in limbal vasculature and conjunctival vessels.

Some of these changes will be adaptive and will diminish with time while others may be sufficiently severe to be signals for a different lens design or a different lens material. Some problems or limitations may be insoluble and patients should be told of these possibilities so that their expectations of how the lens is likely to perform remain realistic.

Post-wear changes are discussed in more detail in Chapter 19.

Lens insertion and removal by the patient

During the initial examination, some practitioners like to give patients some experience in inserting and removing lenses themselves. This can help the patient's confidence in his or her ability to wear and handle lenses. Whether this is done depends on the time available, but it is useful to have some idea of the patient's ability to handle lenses before proceeding further. Inability to insert and remove lenses is as important a contra-indication to contact lens

wear as any of the others. However, with a very tense patient, further instruction may solve any difficulty of lens handling, and the use of an eyebath between consultations may aid relaxation. It has been found very useful with those having difficulty, to instruct them to spend 5 or 10 minutes daily practising the techniques of lens placement and removal. They should do this in front of a mirror and are told to get a drop of water on the insertion finger and imagine it is the lens. This not only helps them to relax, but it also gives them confidence in handling their eyes and lids, so that by the time they collect their lenses they are usually adept at controlling their eyelids and eye movements.

Ordering

The practitioner has now amassed the information needed to decide if the lenses are to be ordered and, if so, the necessary specification. He must be sure that the patient stands a reasonable chance of successfully adapting to contact lenses and wishes to continue. If the patient is likely to have any particular difficulty, then he should be told of this before the practitioner continues. If the patient still desires lenses and there are no disqualifying contra-indications, then an appointment is made to collect the finished lenses.

If lenses of the correct power and fit have been ordered for the tolerance trial then these lenses may be issued to the patient. If the practitioner's own trial lenses have been used for the tolerance trial as well as for the fitting, then the desired lenses can be ordered from this information.

Before the patient leaves, a careful examination of the cornea is essential. An antimicrobial eye drop may be administered if any abrasions are present. If the conjunctiva is injected, a vasoconstrictor may be instilled for cosmetic reasons.

Delivery of contact lenses

The lenses should be checked for accuracy and rejected, or modified if necessary (*see* Chapters 12, 13 and 23). Delivery is the time of transfer of some responsibility for the contact lenses and their effects from the practitioner to the patient. With this transfer comes a need for confidence on the part of the patients that they have been told everything they need to know: that they have been thoroughly instructed in the handling and cleaning of the lenses and can do it with some confidence but that complete confidence will take a little longer to achieve; that they have an appropriate and complete care system for the lenses; that they have written instructions to reinforce what they have been told; that they know how to contact their practitioner if they need more advice and if things are obviously not going properly; and that they know that their progress will be supervised and difficulties dealt with at subsequent appointments. The time spent instructing a patient is vital, and crucial to the preparation for handling lenses when alone. Competent lens handling and understanding of all aspects of lens wear is an encouragement to success. The areas to be covered need to include:

(1) Handling.
(2) Insertion.
(3) Recentring.
(4) Removal.
(5) Disposing of a foreign body.
(6) Dealing with inverted or rolled lenses; right and left discrimination.
(7) Use of the solutions.
(8) Use of the container.
(9) Wearing schedules.
(10) Some warning of adaptive difficulties.
(11) The need for after-care and arranging of the next appointment.

Handling, insertion and removal, recentring, lens inversion, right and left discrimination and dealing with a foreign body can probably be considered together and make up an area where care and time must be taken to make sure the prospective contact lens wearer is competent to deal with these situations. The practitioner needs to be familiar with a variety of methods and, while preferring one particular method, must also be flexible and able to change from one method to another to find a technique that the patient finds easy and successful.

A great deal of information is imparted on this occasion and it is very useful to have a printed sheet, covering the main points, which can be given to the patient for future reference. Addenda I and II, pp. 321 and 325 gives examples of information sheets for wearers of hard and soft lenses, respectively. This is reassuring from the patient's point of view, as it provides an available source of information and guidance. It is also a source of protection for practitioners if they should forget to mention anything, and it is desirable from a legal standpoint.

Handling

Most of the handling techniques used by the patient are similar to those used by the practitioner and already described in pp. 303–312. However, some methods are slightly different and a description of the important aspects is pertinent here. Insertion and removal usually need to be done using a mirror at first. The critical factors are the holding the lids and the position of the eye in the interpalpebral aperture.

The two-handed method may be used where the lens is placed either on centre or on the bulbar conjunctiva. One hand holds the top lid up, the other hand holds the bottom lid down and also places the lens onto the eye using either the first or second finger. Alternatively the one-handed method may be taught, where one hand holds the lids apart and the other hand puts the lens in.

The lids should be held at the margins for greater control and the interpalpebral aperture made larger than the lens diameter especially with soft lenses. The eye should be in the primary position. Having touched the lens onto the eye the patient should wait a second and then blink gently to give the lens time to settle. Once each lens has been inserted, the other eye should be covered and vision checked to see that it is correctly on centre.

Recentring and dealing with a foreign body

Soft lenses can be pushed over with a forefinger if off-centre or if put in off-centre. If the lens is on-centre and uncomfortable, something may be trapped between the lens and the eye. The contact lens is pulled down onto the bulbar conjunctiva and then pushed on-centre again to eject the foreign body. Hard lenses are more difficult to locate and recentre. They can be more easily dealt with from the inferior ocular position (*see Figure 9.7*) with the head tilted to expose the area of attention. Two fingers at the lid edge are used to control the lens from slipping sideways and the lid edge (*not* a finger) is used to push from the far side of the lens and cause the lens edge closest to the limbus to ride up and over the cornea. If the lens is displaced nasally, then looking away and turning the head will expose the nasal conjunctiva and, with the bottom lid held away, the top lid can be manipulated to push the lens inferiorly from where it can be recentred more easily. Hard lenses displaced superiorly are harder to locate as the superior fornix is deeper and the superior orbital margin protrudes more. It may not be possible to see the lens (unless the top lid is everted) and it may be necessary to look down and massage the lens down, having felt it through the lid. Displaced lenses are also easily dealt with by the patient using a suction holder or by having some other person, for example a family member, use the suction holder. A twist once the suction holder is on the lens helps to break the suction. To ensure ease of use only a good quality suction holder should be employed.

Removal

Removal methods are different for hard and soft lenses.

Soft lens removal

Pinch method

The pinch method is easier to learn and more successful for a beginner but has more risk of lens or eye damage. The lids may be held apart as for insertion, the forefinger pulls the lens down onto the inferior sclera as the patient looks up (see Figure 9.18), and it is then gently pinched between the pads of the forefinger and thumb. Those with long fingernails need to shorten them in the early stages. Alternatively, but with more risk of corneal trauma, the lens is gently pinched across its greatest diameter (see Figure 9.17) with the patient looking straight ahead in the mirror or fixing on a spot on the mirror.

Scissors method

This is harder to learn but safer as the fingers are off the lens and away from the cornea. With the eye in the primary position, the forefingers of each hand are placed vertically one centrally at the very edge of the top lid and one centrally at the very edge of the bottom lid. The lids are

pulled apart to just greater than the lens diameter, then pressed firmly onto the eye and then moved together. If the lid edges are tight enough, instead of passing over the lens, the lens edges are pushed together and the buckled lens is squeezed out through the lid gap and onto the lid or lashes (see Figure 9.19). This is safer for a nervous person and less likely to cause lens or eye damage for someone who is rough with himself.

Suction holder removal

A suction holder can be used for soft lens removal and works better with thicker lenses. A suction holder which has been modified by having a hole either through the flange or through the centre so that it cannot exert suction is eased under the edge of the lens and swept across the eye to break the cohesion of the lens on the eye and lift it out. Because of the strong cohesion of the soft lens on the eye and the risk of removing corneal epithelium as well, a soft lens cannot be grasped directly by a suction holder to remove it as would be done with a hard lens.

Hard lens removal

Stare–pull–blink method

Hard lens removal is most commonly done by the stare–pull–blink method (as in Figure 9.2). This requires forefinger stretching at the outer canthus to stretch the lids sufficiently to grip the lens, and a blink action to pop the lens out and away from the eye. To be successful it needs to be done in the order of its name and deliberately. The cornea needs to be placed centrally or slightly nasally in the interpalpebral aperture to make sure the lids are well stretched around the cornea and lens. The lid aperture must be greater than the lens diameter (i.e. with the patient staring), the forefinger placed in the centre of the outer canthus and a gentle pull made in the direction of the top of the ear, so that a similar stretch is made to top and bottom lids to stop the lens slipping under the loose lids. Finally a deliberate blink is made to eject the lens. Once proficiency is attained then the opposite hand is cupped over the eye to catch the lens. The suction holder can be used as for removal of a decentred lens but with the lens still on the cornea. The lids are held apart as for insertion and the previously moistened suction holder is placed on the lens and removed with a small twirl to help break the cohesion. Note that after an unsuccessful attempt the patient should check that the lens is still on-centre before making another attempt or the suction holder could be unintentionally attached to the cornea from which it is difficult to remove without removing epithelium at the same time. However, should this happen the suction holder may be gently rotated and slipped across the cornea and over the limbus onto the conjunctiva before attempting its removal.

The scissors method can be used as for soft lens removal.

Cleaning contact lenses on removal

Hygiene is vital and should be modelled on practitioner behaviour. Hand washing before handling the lenses or eyelids both for insertion and removal, and when cleaning the lenses is essential. Not only can bacteria, for example, be transferred, but a variety of other hand contaminants can also be damaging to contact lenses, for example hand-lotions and make-up. Care and cleaning of the contact lens container is also necessary. All contact lenses need to be cleaned with a surfactant cleaner on removal. Hard lenses are cleaned by rubbing with the fingers using the surfactant, and soft lenses either being rubbed in a circular motion in the palm of the hand (*Figure 9.21*) while supported on the

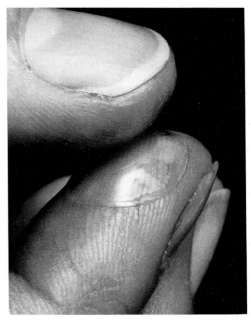

Figure 9.22 Rubbing a hydrophilic lens with thumb and forefinger to clean it

forefinger of the other hand, or else supported on the end of the forefinger or thumb (*Figure 9.22*), and rubbed with surfactant using the other hand. If the fingers or hand are rough, a smooth finger (usually the little one) may be used to rub the lens on a sponge pad.

Surfactants should be well rinsed off as the residue can be irritating to the eye or damaging to the lens surfaces. A saline rinse must be used for soft lenses. In areas where tap water is drinkable, then this may be of sufficient quality to rinse hard and gas permeable lenses and a thorough rinse, with the plug in the basin of course, will ensure a clean, surfactant-free lens. Sterile saline solution can also be used, but this is more expensive and less effective unless used in adequate quantities. Prior to removal and cleaning, the lens container should have been prepared, opened and filled with the appropriate solution. The cleaned and rinsed lens is then transferred to the container, taking care that it is completely in the body of the container and in the appropriate solution. The container is then closed.

A soft lens which has become folded or stuck together may be separated by gently rolling between thumb and forefinger or on the palm of the hand having been wetted with saline. More

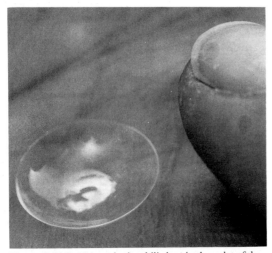

Figure 9.21 Rubbing a hydrophilic lens in the palm of the hand to clean it

stubborn cases can be separated by heating in saline or distilled water. This is best done by the practitioner. Sticking on removal can be avoided by moistening the fingers prior to pinch removal or by using the scissors method of removal. Sticking is more likely with new lenses, low power lenses and lenses with very thin edges. Note that too much force can tear or damage a lens.

Having dealt with lens handling and insertion and removal, the solutions used and the use of the container should be discussed and demonstrated. Care systems are discussed in Chapter 4.

Wearing schedules

Adaptation to contact lenses is usually necessary and the daily wearing time is therefore gradually increased. Wearing schedules can be variable and the schedule should provide for the fastest passage possible through to maximum daily wear, provided that the patient is physically and visually reasonably comfortable in the process. There is no advantage in slow adaptation if proper safeguards are met. With the advent of soft lenses, comfort problems are reduced and a start of 4–6 hours per day with an increase of 1–2 hours daily is typical. Sensitive eyes and lenses with thicker edges, for example prism ballasted torics, may need a slower schedule. RGP lens wearers could be started at 4 or 6 hours depending on lid sensitivity and confidence, and add 1 hour extra daily. Schedules should all be given with the proviso that wearing time can be held at the same level for some days, or built up more slowly if there are problems, or the lenses not worn at all if things are obviously wrong.

Early difficulties

Many early problems are possible; some are adaptive and will diminish with time, some may relate to lens or solution problems which may need appropriate changes or changes in use, while some problems may be impossible to solve if, for example, an incorrect decision on patient suitability has been made. Naive contact lens wearers need reassurance that their problems are normal and under the control of the

practitioner, and will either resolve with time or else be dealt with by the practitioner at subsequent after-care visits. Those people who are not confident or who are poorly motivated will find numerous problems, which, as soon as they are solved are replaced by new ones. Sources of difficulty are often in the areas covered at delivery and provide some feedback as to the effectiveness of the methods used and the quality of instruction. Early problems can include:

(1) Difficulties getting lenses in and out.
(2) Lenses off-centre.
(3) Lost lenses.
(4) Soft lenses stuck together.
(5) Soft lenses inside out or difficulty in the detection of lenses inside out.
(6) Difficulties distinguishing right and left.
(7) Handling and cleaning difficulties.
(8) Poor vision.
(9) Variable vision.
(10) Perceptual — adaptive problems.
(11) Discomfort on insertion.
(12) Variable discomfort depending on the environment.
(13) Discomfort after lenses are removed.
(14) Sensitivity to solutions.
(15) Unsatisfactory or incompatible cleaning and care systems.
(16) Glare.
(17) Self-consciousness.

Some problems go with time; others need to be dealt with speedily to maintain patient confidence. Some patients present problems which need simple reassurance that everything is normal, and gentle pressure to resume their wearing schedule.

What should be done at delivery?

The lenses should have been checked and cleaned prior to the delivery appointment as described in Chapters 12 and 13, a care system selected, and solutions and container collected together. An instruction sheet or booklet should be provided (see pp. 321–330) and this should be gone through with the patient at the delivery appointment. Audiovisual aids can be used at this time and a variety of good video films are available to assist with patient instruction.

Delivery time is too late to start making fitting

and lens power changes. If the fitting process was accurate and lenses supplied as ordered, then the lenses should only need to be briefly checked in the eye to make sure that the original decisions were correct. A quick look at the fit and a check on the acuities provides patient confidence. As long as the lens is safe on the eye and the vision adequate, re-fitting decisions are best left to the first after-care appointment when adaptive problems have hopefully been overcome. This of course needs to be balanced by the patient's welfare.

The patient should start with hand washing. Lens handling and instruction on insertion and removal are taught initially followed by patient practice, until reasonable competence is attained. Patients must be able to remove the lenses satisfactorily before they can take the lenses home. Recentring of displaced lenses should be shown and, for soft lens wearers, the means of identifying that a lens is inside out either by inspection or by demonstration of reduced comfort and vision. The use of the container and the methods of cleaning the lenses and using the solutions supplied should follow. The wearing schedule should be discussed, early problems mentioned and the patient advised that some difficulties may arise but that these will go with time and adaptation. The instruction booklet should be gone through and the necessary items on use of solutions and wearing schedules completed. The next after-care appointment is the final thing to arrange and the patients should go on to wear the lenses on their own and to achieve the confidence and competence that is needed to succeed as a contact lens wearer in the long term.

Fitting children's contact lenses

There is nothing particularly unusual about children's eyes. Teenagers are usually very good patients if they are well motivated. Maturing earlier, girls usually have a more responsible attitude towards contact lenses than boys of the same age. If the parents are paying for the lenses good communication and cooperation with them is essential, and a financial contribution from the individual involved also assists in their care.

Fitting children under the age of 10 years is a specialized area and thus requires a specialized approach. Chapter 21 provides information on paediatric contact lenses.

Written instructions

Every patient should receive written instructions to reinforce the verbal instructions and demonstrations given at the time of issuing their contact lenses. A great deal of information is given at issue and written instructions and information provides a novice contact lens wearer with reassurance as to their accuracy of recall. It also provides more information should this be necessary, and useful items such as contact telephone numbers. These written instructions also provide the practitioner with reassurance that the patient will be able to perform as they were instructed.

They provide an important link between patient and practitioner at a time when contact lens skills are being established.

Ideally, the instructions should be able to be varied for the system and varieties of solutions used and terminology kept simple for easy understanding. The instructions should include information on hygiene and lens handling, insertion and removal method with illustrative diagrams and pictures, care of the eyes, normal adaptive symptoms and a wearing programme advised. The need for after-care and the intervals advised for this is useful.

Patient procedure for contact lens emergencies, especially for use with extended wear lenses, should also be included.

Addendum I for RGP lenses and Addendum II for soft lenses are examples based on those used by one of the co-editors (A. J. Phillips) in his practice.

Addendum I

Instructions to patients wearing hard and rigid gas permeable contact lenses

Rigid gas permeable (RGP) lenses represent one of the latest generation of contact lens materials. Considered simply, they represent an attempt to provide lenses which combine the optical advantages of hard lenses and the physiological advantages of soft lenses. Although RGP lenses are superficially the same as conventional hard lenses, you *must* adhere to the following instructions or permanent damage to the lens may result.

Basic instructions for handling RGP lenses

(1) Hands should be thoroughly washed and all traces of soap rinsed off before handling lenses and the eyes and lids. Avoid contamination with face and hand-creams, nicotine and perfumes. When using hair lacquer and aerosol sprays, keep the eyes closed for a moment until the air has cleared.

(2) While handling the lenses work over a smooth soft surface such as a paper towel or paper handkerchief. This simplifies finding a dropped lens and avoids scratching or loosing a dropped lens.

(3) If a lens is dropped, do no more until the lens is located. Lift the dropped lens by wetting the finger tips or suction holder and gently touching the surface.

(4) Never wipe your lenses with a handkerchief. If wiping is necessary use only the softest of paper tissues. To avoid damaging the lenses, handle them gently and avoid holding the lenses by the edges. Avoid leaving the lenses in a hot place as they may distort.

(5) Finger nails should be clean and reasonably short to avoid scratching the eyes and the contact lenses.

Hygiene and lens storage

Absolute cleanliness is essential in the handling and storage of contact lenses. In order to prevent dirt or any harmful organisms being transferred to the eye, the following rules must be observed:

(1) The lenses should be stored in the container provided in a solution suitable for the storage of RGP lenses. As a general guide, any soft contact lens storage and disinfecting solution may be used and the large majority of hard lens storage solutions, although caution should always be exercised when changing to a new solution. 'Combination' soaking and wetting solutions such as Soaclens, Combisol and Total, generally appear effective with RGP lenses. Wearers prescribed the Menicon O_2 lenses *must* use the O_2 Solution while the Boston Solution made for Boston RGP lens wearers is not absolutely essential.

(2) The level of soaking solution should be maintained in the container so that each lens is completely immersed in the solution. At least once a week the container should be emptied out and cleaned by being filled with Savlon (ICI). This is left for a period of at least half an hour (for instance, while the lenses are being worn) and then rinsed out with running tap water (or, ideally, boiled water that has been allowed to cool). The container is then refilled with fresh solution (never use bleach or other antiseptic solutions as they may be absorbed by the plastic of the container and then contaminate the lenses). Savlon must *not* be used for the overnight storage or cleaning of RGP lenses as it may cause severe subsequent discomfort on lens wear. Certain other proprietary antiseptics may also permanently damage the lens and should not be used.

(3) The lenses must *never* be stored dry as this allows the growth of bacteria and affects the curvature of the lens and the wetting ability of its surface.

(4) Before inserting your lenses, rinse off the soaking solution with cold water and apply one drop of recommended wetting solution to each lens, spreading it on to both surfaces of the lens with the fingers. The wetting solution maintains lens sterility, helps the surface wet more easily, and forms a protective cushion in the event of a lens

being inserted too quickly. However, in the case of Menicon O_2 lenses, the O_2 Solution should be rinsed from the lens prior to insertion. Wetting solutions should not be used with this lens.

(5) On removal of your lenses clean with the recommended cleaner, e.g. Polyclens, LC65, Lobob, Cleaner No. 4 etc., and rinse off with fresh, cold, tap water before replacing the lenses in their container. Be sure to put the plug in the hand basin before rinsing lenses under running cold tap water.

(6) Never lick your lenses as harmful organisms can be transferred from the mouth to the eye.

(7) Keep hair clean and free of dandruff as this may lead to eye discomfort with contact lenses.

(8) Examine the lenses regularly for scratches and chips and to ensure that each lens is being worn in the correct eye. One or both lenses may be engraved with dots or R and L to identify them. Some RGP lenses may also be marked with a code to identify the lens material, e.g. 'ALB' for Alberta material.

(9) For some wearers an additional cleaning technique is sometimes necessary (*see* Enzyme cleaning).

Insertion of lenses

Place the wetted lens on the tip of the forefinger of one hand, where it will be retained. Look downwards and, using two fingers of the other hand, hold the upper lid and eyelashes well up clear of the cornea. Now use the middle finger of the hand holding the lens to pull down the lower lid by the very edge. Keep the head and eye pointing in the same direction and place the lens gently on the cornea. Remove the forefinger, release the lower lid and finally the upper lid. The whole procedure is reversed for the other eye. The very tip of the second finger may be used as an alternative, with the third finger holding down the lower lid, if any difficulty is experienced using the forefinger. Check that the lens is on-centre by covering the other eye and making sure that you can see well.

If the lens slips on to the white of the eye, it may be replaced by lifting one lid beyond the lens and pushing it back on to the cornea with the lid margin, using a finger on either side of the lens as a guide. A mirror will aid lens location, and this should be held so that the eye is looking in the opposite direction from where the lens is positioned. Alternatively, a suction holder may be used, if one is available, either by yourself or someone else.

If you cannot remove it from the white of the eye — *do not panic* — it is quite safe to leave it there overnight if necessary, until you can obtain assistance. It cannot disappear behind the back of the eye as a fold of tissue prevents this. Nevertheless, in the case of an apparently missing lens, remember to check that it has not moved well under the lids.

Removal

Although the first method below is the simplest and most commonly used, you are strongly advised to practise all three techniques so that should one not work, an alternative method may be used:

(1) Again, work over a table or hold the free hand cupped to catch the lens. Bend the head slightly and tilt it so that the eye is turned slightly towards the nose. Open the eyes as wide as possible, so that both lids are beyond the edges of the lens. Stare straight in front of you and place a finger at the outer corner of the eye, separating the lids slightly. Pull the lids towards the direction of the top of the ear and give a single blink, then the lens should be ejected from the eye. At first it may often stick to the lashes, from where it is easily removed. A quick glance in the opposite direction to the pull of the fingers at the same time as the blink may aid lens ejection.

(2) The second method is to place the forefinger of each hand on the very edge of the upper and lower lid at the inner corner of the eye. Each lid is then slowly stretched around the lens and then together. Working over a mirror may be helpful at first, although this should be discarded as soon as possible as such artificial aids may not be available in an emergency. This also applies to the use of a suction holder as suggested in the third method of removal described below and a suction holder should not be used except

where there is any initial difficulty with either of the above methods.

(3) The free hand should hold the upper lid away from the lens. Squeeze the bulb of the moistened suction holder firmly and place the end gently against the dome of the lens. Release the pressure on the bulb and slowly withdraw both holder and lens, twisting them slightly to relieve the cohesion between lens and eye.

Care of the eyes

(1) Insert and remove the lenses gently and slowly to avoid scratching the eyes.
(2) In the event of a foreign body becoming trapped behind the lens, the following procedure should be carried out: if initial blinking does not move the particle, look downwards and hold the upper lid away from the eye for a few seconds. Repeat several times if necessary. If the particle is still present, remove the lens, clean and replace. The lens must *not* be left on the eye if there is a foreign body beneath it. If there is any discomfort when the lens is removed, the lens should not be re-inserted until the following day. If the discomfort persists until the following day, report to your practitioner for examination.
(3) Always seek advice if:
   (a) your eyes remain red or painful during or after wear;
   (b) you continually see coloured haloes around lights or if your vision becomes misty;
   (c) you notice white spots on the cornea which do not move on blinking. If in doubt leave the lenses *out* and seek professional advice immediately.
(4) Always report for an examination of your eyes and lenses when advised and at least once a year after the first 12 months of wear.
(5) Do not wear your lenses if you are ill or have a bad cold, or at least reduce your daily wearing time. Female patients may occasionally experience slight lens discomfort during the menstrual period, and possibly in the first month or two of taking the contraceptive pill or in the latter stages of pregnancy. Advice should be requested where necessary.

Enzyme cleaning

As RGP lenses are porous, certain people are susceptible to deposits from their tears 'binding' to the lens surface. Such deposits are sometimes very tenacious and not completely removed by daily cleaning. Over a period of weeks or months these deposits build up and reduce both comfort and vision slightly during lens wear. All wearers should carefully dry the lenses with a soft paper tissue every 2–4 weeks when any deposits can be seen as a milky haze on the lens, or part of the lens, when viewed against a bright light. If such deposits become visible the following procedure should be carried out *in addition* to the daily cleaning routine and you may well be advised to do it monthly or fortnightly in any case as a preventive measure. Your practitioner will advise you on the need for this type of cleaning:

(1) A starter kit of enzyme (or protein-removing) tablets should be purchased, e.g. Soflens Cleaning Tablets, Allergan Cleaning Tablets, Alcon Enzymatic Cleaner or Amiclair Tablets.
(2) One tablet is sufficient to clean two RGP lenses. Make up the solution according to the manufacturer's instructions by placing a tablet in one of the vials provided and filling the vial to the fill-line with either saline, or purified or distilled water as appropriate. Once the tablet has dissolved transfer half the solution to the other vial. A container is now available for RGP lenses which permits one tablet to clean both lenses simultaneously.
(3) The lenses should now be removed from the eyes, carefully cleaned with the daily cleaner in the usual way, and rinsed thoroughly. They are then placed in their respective vials and left overnight.
(4) The following morning, the lenses should be removed from the vials, cleaned very thoroughly to remove the enzyme by-products, rinsed and inserted as usual.
(5) Refill packs of enzyme tablets provide the most economic long-term method of enzyme cleaning.

Normal symptoms

Some symptoms, such as the following, are normal during the adaption period and should not cause anxiety.

(1) Excessive blinking and watering of the eyes.
(2) Discomfort in bright lights, high winds and dusty atmospheres. Avoid these where possible in the first few weeks during lens wear.
(3) Discomfort when reading and in a stuffy atmosphere. Avoid both where possible in the first few weeks during lens wear.
(4) Comfort is greater out of doors than in-doors.
(5) Moments of blurred vision and temporary double vision.
(6) Slight blurred vision with spectacles after wearing contact lenses. This should last a few minutes only and may not be noticeable. Report anything more noticeable than this and particularly any obvious difference between the two eyes (allow for a possibility of an outdated spectacle prescription).
(7) Displacement of lenses on the eye — usually due to poor insertion or removal.
(8) Annoying reflections from lights due to the increased lens movement present over the first few weeks.
(9) Headaches and tension in the face and forehead — often found where the wearer is not relaxing the muscles in the brow.

If you are in any doubt about symptoms, please ask for advice.

Wearing programme

The speed of adaption varies greatly from individual to individual. The following gives a good guide, although it may be necessary to adapt slightly more slowly or quickly depending on individual tolerance.

(1) On the first day, wear the lenses for from 2 to 4 hours depending upon comfort. Increase by 1 hour every day for 3 days, 1½ hours for the next 3 days, and 2 hours per day thereafter until maximum tolerance is achieved.
(2) Wear your lenses every day. This is very important during the adaption period.
(3) *Never* wear your lenses longer than the recommended period no matter how comfortable they may be. Severe discomfort may be experienced several hours after lens removal if there has been gross over-wear. If the lenses have been left out for several days, for example, due to illness, re-adapt over several days. In cases of prolonged illness, special advice should be requested.

(4) Slight discomfort of both lenses towards the end of the wearing schedule may be ignored, but the lenses should be removed if there is any marked discomfort of one or both lenses. If any discomfort occurs every day, mention this to the practitioner as occasionally a small modification to the lens becomes necessary as it settles on the eye.
(5) *Never* leave the lenses in all night unless your practitioner has fitted you with special extended wear lenses. You may rub the eyes during sleep and have sore eyes on waking. Also the presence of most types of lens deprives the cornea of its oxygen supply during sleep.
(6) *Do not drive* with contact lenses in until you are fully adapted to them and have comfortable vision. This is particularly so at night when you may notice haloes or streamers around lights. Remember to keep a pair of spectacles in the car in case emergency removal of your contact lenses is necessary; for example, you may lose a lens or get something in your eye. These spectacles should provide good vision — do not rely on an old pair. Cyclists and motor cyclists should wear protective goggles or glasses. In the daytime, sunglasses can give protection from both light and dust, but *never* wear tinted glasses at night or at dusk although glare from headlights may be troublesome with contact lenses, for the tint could then cause you to miss seeing poorly lit cars and pedestrians.
(7) Where possible, wear your lenses outdoors at first and try to do something which will take your mind off your lenses. For instance, do not sit watching television or reading a book.
(8) Make a note in your diary that in the event of an accident your contact lenses should be removed.
(9) When you report for your first examination, usually after 1–2 weeks, *you must be wearing your lenses* and have been wearing them for the maximum period of tolerance that you have achieved, i.e. if you have achieved a wearing time of 6½ hours, then you must have been wearing your lenses for this time when you come for your appointment. Bring your most up-to-date spectacles with you as they may be needed at the time of each after-care examination.

Addendum II

Instructions for the care and handling of soft contact lenses

Hydrophilic 'soft' lenses are designed to cover the entire cornea and overlap onto the white of the eye. As the lenses are made of a resilient porous material, it is essential that they are handled with great care. Further, as the lenses contain a percentage of fluid, daily disinfection and cleaning of the lenses is most important. Lenses which are not cleaned regularly may cause eye infections and discomfort.

(1) Hands should be thoroughly washed and all traces of soap rinsed off before handling lenses and the eyes and lids. Avoid contamination with face and hand-creams and nicotine and perfumes. When using hair lacquer and aerosol sprays keep the eyes closed for a moment until the air has cleared.
(2) While handling the lenses work over a smooth surface such as a paper towel or paper handkerchief. This simplifies finding a dropped lens and avoids scratching or losing a dropped lens.
(3) If a lens is dropped, do not move until the lens is located. Lift a dropped lens by gripping it with special soft-tipped tweezers or the finger tips, not the fingernails. If the lens has dried it may be necessary to wet it with sterile saline and leave it to soften for several minutes before attempting to lift it.
(4) Never wipe your lenses with a handkerchief. If wiping is necessary use only the softest of paper tissues. To avoid damaging the lenses, handle them gently and don't pinch them with your finger nails.
(5) Finger nails should be clean and reasonably short to avoid scratching the eyes and the contact lenses.

Lens disinfection

Lens disinfection may be carried out by one of the following three methods. You will be advised if any method is particularly suitable or unsuitable for your own lens material.

Chemical disinfection

Solutions such as Hydrocare, Hydrosoak, Flexcare, Sterisoft etc., have been developed exclusively for the disinfection of soft contact lenses. As soft lenses have the effect of concentrating some antiseptics on the lens surfaces (and hence causing eye irritation), it is of vital importance that all solutions specifically state that they are for use with hydrophilic or soft lenses. Under *no* circumstances should the lenses be stored in tap water, purified, distilled or rain water or contact lens solutions designed for hard lenses, or solutions of household disinfectants.

Before removing the lenses at night, the contact lens container should be empty of all used solution and filled with fresh solution direct from the bottle. It is important that this is done daily as the low antiseptic concentration in the solution (to prevent eye irritation) may not maintain sterility beyond 24 hours when the lenses are in use.

Patients with high water content lenses (who will be advised of this) or a history of storage solution allergy problems may be advised to use specific disinfection solutions, such as Sterisoft, Sensitive Eyes Saline, Sorbisal etc. solutions described below. Alternative systems such as hydrogen peroxide methods, heat disinfection, Softabs or Aerotabs may also be prescribed.

Boiling the lenses

Because the tears contain a proportion of salt, it is important for comfort that the lenses are stored in a physiological saline solution. This is obtainable:

(1) As preserved saline manufactured especially for this purpose such as Bausch & Lomb Saline for Sensitive Eyes, Alcon saline, Allergan saline.
(2) Unpreserved sterile saline is available in clear plastic single dose sachets such as Scanlens rinse, the Allergan or Barnes–Hind plastic containers or in aerosol dispensers.
(3) Unpreserved sterile saline solution is available in a transparent flexible container

(normally half or one litre) possibly used as intravenous saline in hospitals. Once opened it should be stored in a refrigerator and discarded after 1 month.

(4) It can be made up from salt tablets by following the instructions with them.

Boiling is ideally carried out in an aseptor unit made especially for this purpose. These provide thoroughness, convenience of operation and can give several years of trouble-free use. If the aseptor is not working or if you are away from home, then simply place the lens container (with the lenses inside) into a saucepan of boiling water to simmer for 15 minutes, taking care that all the water in the saucepan does not evaporate.

Pasteurizing the lenses

The lenses are stored in saline as above. The lens container (with the lenses inside) is gently slid into a full vacuum flask of boiling water. Lightly cap the flask and leave overnight or for at least half an hour. Ensure that the container has cooled before removing the lenses and inserting them. This may be speeded up if necessary by holding the lens container under running cold tap water.

Disinfection by boiling or pasteurizing must be done regularly to avoid risk of lens contamination. Ensure that the lens container screw tops are fully tightened to prevent solution loss during heating. However, if the solution has escaped from the container and the lens has stuck to the container, fill the container full with saline (or storage solution), replace the cap, tighten and shake. Let the lens soak for 1 or 2 hours more and, if possible, reboil or pasteurize before wear.

Softab and Aerotab systems

These methods use a low level chlorine release system to disinfect the lenses. They have the advantages of being simple to use, inexpensive and, because the chlorine has evaporated from the solution by the next morning, there are no preservatives introduced into the eye which can occasionally cause sensitivity problems on lens insertion. The lenses should be cleaned in the normal way (*see below*) and rinsed with saline. Each lens should then be placed separately on the dome at each end of the container taking

care to ensure that the correct lens is placed on each side and that when the lens case is snapped shut it will not damage the lens.

The container is then filled to the fill-line with fresh sterile *unpreserved* saline and one disinfecting tablet added. This is then left overnight. The lenses are simply removed from the container the next morning and inserted.

The Softab and Aerotab containers can be used to allow one enzyme tablet to clean both lenses at the same time (prior to Softab overnight disinfection).

Hydrogen peroxide methods

Several methods using hydrogen peroxide are now available. These are becoming increasingly popular because the method aids in lens cleaning as well as disinfection. The disadvantage of these systems is that a specific neutralizing step is usually involved and this must be adhered to.

Barnes–Hind method

The lenses are cleaned in the normal way to remove loose debris etc. and then soaked for *five* minutes in the hydrogen peroxide. The lenses are then thoroughly rinsed in preserved saline and stored overnight, again in a preserved saline. This technique is quick and effective in killing most 'germs', but has very little cleaning effect. In this short contact time no hydrogen peroxide is absorbed into the lens and no specific neutralization step is required. However, some people do notice stinging on insertion and neutralizing tablets and a solution are now available, if needed.

American Optical methods

The lenses are stored for 15–30 minutes in container number one with hydrogen peroxide (Lensept). The container top and lens basket is removed and rinsed with saline before being placed in container number two in preserved saline (e.g. Lensrins) overnight or at least for 4 hours. Container number two contains a platinum compound, catalyst disc in the base which breaks down the hydrogen peroxide. The catalyst should be replaced ever 100 times it is used or approximately every 3 months. An alternative system, 'AOSept', allows disinfection and neutralization in one step as an overnight procedure.

Allergan, Mirasept and Bausch & Lomb methods

The lenses in the container lid baskets are placed in hydrogen peroxide (Oxysept 1 Disinfection solution, Mirasept 1, or HP1) for 20 minutes or overnight. The container lid and lens basket are removed and the hydrogen peroxide emptied out. The container and lenses are rinsed with Oxysept 2 Rinse and Neutralizer, Mirasept 2 or HP2 solution and the container half-filled with the same solution. The lens basket is replaced and left for a minimum of 10 minutes (or preferably overnight). Oxysept 2, Mirasept 2 and HP2 contain a catalyst or other ingredients to break down the hydrogen peroxide.

Enzyme cleaning is still usually necessary for additional lens cleaning but may not be needed so frequently. Please discuss this with your practitioner.

Daily lens cleaning

Unless lenses are thoroughly cleaned prior to soaking or boiling, proteins and other tear contaminants will accumulate on the lens. The soaking or boiling then alters the state of the protein so that it adheres to the lens and can irritate the eye. You may then notice any or all of the following symptoms:

(1) A drop in the standard of vision.
(2) Loss in comfort.
(3) Lens discolouration.
(4) A red eye.
(5) Distorted or wrinkled lenses.

The importance of thorough daily cleaning cannot be over-emphasized. Deposits on soft lenses represent the major cause of patient symptoms and are the main reason for lens replacement.

Several proprietary cleaners such as Polyclens, Cleaner No. 4, Pliagel, Miraflow, Preflex, Amiclean, LC65 etc., are available. The lenses are removed from the eye, placed in the palm of the hand concave side upwards, and a drop of cleaning fluid dropped onto the lens. The lens is then massaged around the palm of the hand using a smooth finger of the other hand for at least 30 seconds. Alternatively, the lens may be placed concave side downwards on the first or second fingers and massaged with the thumb. In either case, the cleaning solution should be rinsed from the lens with storage solution prior to being placed in the container. In the case of patients with particularly severe deposit problems, the lenses may be cleaned and rinsed a second time prior to insertion in the eye. Sponge pads also assist lens cleaning for people whose hands have rough skin likely to damage lenses.

Enzyme cleaning

In spite of daily cleaning, the porous nature of the lens material still allows deposits to build up on the surface. This is similar to the build-up of dental plaque on teeth which occurs in spite of regular cleaning, although, as with soft contact lenses, the problem can be reduced or delayed by regular daily cleaning. Research has shown that the longer deposits remain on soft lenses the more difficult they are to remove. The following method should therefore be carried out at least once a week or once a fortnight in addition to the use of the daily cleaner to minimize deposits building up on the lens surface.

(1) A starter kit of enzyme or protein removing tablets should be obtained.
(2) One tablet is placed in each plastic vial and the vial filled to the fill-line with distilled or purified water or unpreserved saline depending on the tablets.
(3) The lenses are now removed from the eyes, carefully cleaned with the daily cleaner in the usual way and thoroughly rinsed. They are then placed in their respective vials and left for the appropriate period recommended for the enzyme cleaner being used.
(4) At the end of this period the lenses should be removed from the vials, cleaned very thoroughly with the surfactant cleaner again and rinsed.
(5) As the enzyme has no disinfecting action, the lenses should then be taken through a full disinfection cycle. Generally, it is most convenient to remove the lenses and enzyme clean during the evening so that the lenses can then be disinfected in the normal way overnight.
(6) In summary, once weekly the routine should be: remove, clean and rinse, enzyme clean, clean and rinse, disinfect.

(7) Some enzymes are now available for use in hydrogen peroxide which eliminates the need for separate enzyme cleaning prior to this method of disinfection.

Lens insertion

To prevent the right and left lenses being interchanged accidently, they should be removed from their storage container and inserted one at a time. The following procedure is carried out for the right eye (and repeated for the left eye) after ensuring that the lens is not inside out.

(1) Support the lens on the ball of the forefinger (or middle finger of the right hand), work over a large smooth surface if possible. A mirror is often helpful at first. Allow ultrathin lenses to dry out for about 30 seconds.
(2) Bring the left hand down over the forehead, look right down and grasp the upper right lid firmly with the middle or forefinger. Now look straight ahead (at your eye in the mirror).
(3) Pull down the lower lid with the middle finger or next finger of the right hand, keeping the lens away from the eye.
(4) Bend the head well forward over the mirror or flat surface and, holding the lids well apart, gently place the lens on the cornea. Obviously the distance between the lids must be greater than the lens diameter; the lashes must be kept well out of the way.
(5) Slowly release both lids.

There may be very slight irritation for the first minute or so. In the case of marked irritation, a particle of dust or fluff may have become trapped behind the lens; it should be removed, rinsed with sterile saline or storage solution and re-inserted. Sometimes a small foreign body behind the lens can be removed by moving the lens onto the white of the eye (the side nearest the ear is often convenient), and then sliding it back onto the cornea.

Rather than insert the lens directly onto the cornea some patients may prefer to look in the mirror, turn their head to the right, and place the lens on the white of the eye then use a finger on the lens to gently move it onto the cornea. Or, without a mirror, you can look up, pull the lower lid well down, and place the lens below the cornea. Looking slowly down will then centre it before letting go of the lower lid. When inserting the left lens the head is turned to the left or you can look up and place it below the cornea.

Before placing the lens on the eye always check that it has not accidently become turned inside out. There are two simple methods of checking that this is not the case.

(1) Place the lens on the tip of the forefinger concave side upwards, and hold it up to a light or a window. Look at the shape of the lens from the side in silhouette. If the lens is the correct way round the edges will point up almost vertically. If the lens is inside out the edges will turn slightly outwards.
(2) Balance the lens on the tips of the thumb and forefinger, concave side upwards. Gently fold the lens inwards slightly. If the edges bend inwards then the lens is the right way round and, if they bend outwards, it is not.

Lens removal
Method 1

(1) Hold the upper and lower lids apart as described in insertion above. This time the mirror may be used in either a vertical or horizontal position.
(2) Turn the head so that you are looking across your nose into the mirror, i.e. for the right eye turn your head to the right so that you are looking to the left to see in the mirror.
(3) Using the index finger slide the lens off the cornea towards the ear onto the white of the eye.
(4) Keep hold of the upper lid but take away the right hand and turn it so that the side of the thumb and forefinger are facing the eye.
(5) Keeping the head position constant, hold the lids at the corner of the eye apart with the side of the thumb and forefinger and gently pinch the lens off the eye with the thumb and forefinger.

Method 2

Bend the chin in to the neck so that you look upwards to see the eye straight ahead in a mirror. Pull the lower lid down and slide the lens below the cornea. Pinch the lens off using the thumb and forefinger (or middle finger as before). If you have long fingernails, deepset eyes or a smaller than average distance between the lids, Methods 1 and 2 may prove difficult.

Method 3

(1) Raise the eyebrows and keep staring wide.
(2) Use one finger of each hand. Put one fingertip at the edge of the top lid and the other at the edge of the bottom lid. Both lids should be held about half-way along.
(3) Pull the lids towards the ear keeping the edges of the lids in close contact with the white of the eye.
(4) Look towards your nose almost at the same time as (3); the lens should be expelled from the eye.
(5) Alternatively push the lid edges tightly together across the surface of the eye to expel the lens.

Method 4

Proceed as in Methods 1 and 2 but instead of pinching the lens off the white of the eye between forefinger and thumb use a suction holder inserted under the edge of the lens to lever the lens off the eye.

Wearing schedules

Unless otherwise advised, start at 4 hours on the first day and increase by 1 or 2 hours each day if it is comfortable to do so. Endeavour to wear your lenses every day during the adaptation period. An alternative wearing schedule may be advised as follows:

First day .... Fourth day .... Seventh day ......
Second day ... Fifth day .... Eighth day ....
Third day ..... Sixth day ......

General notes

(1) Always wash your hands thoroughly before handling soft lenses to ensure they are free from all traces of creams, make-up, nicotine etc. Dry them on a lint-free well washed towel.
(2) If your lenses accidently dry out (becoming smaller and losing their flexibility), handle them with extreme care. Preferably drop saline solution onto them and let them soften for about half an hour before touching them. Then place them gently in the container and soak in saline or storage solution for at least 2 hours. Ideally, they should be disinfected by your usual method before wearing. Never put a partly dry lens on the eye.
(3) As lenses are not generally marked right and left care must be taken not to get them confused.
(4) There is very little chance of dust getting beneath the lens during wear. (*See under* Lens insertion in case this happens.) If discomfort persists consult your contact lens practitioner.
(5) There is little risk of lens loss from the eye, except when swimming, although they may be displaced onto the white of the eye if the eyes are rubbed. Swimming goggles may of course be worn.
(6) Take care to keep the eyes closed when using aerosols and other sprays. Remember that the droplets may persist in the room for several minutes. Such chemicals may cause subsequent irritation and could ruin the lenses permanently.
(7) If the lens is irritating your eye and you suspect that it may be contaminated with make-up etc., clean the lens very carefully. Boil the lens for at least an hour in distilled water and return the lens to physiological saline or storage solution for at least one additional hour. If this procedure is ineffective go through the recommended routine with an enzyme cleaner. If discomfort persists, stop wearing the lens and get in touch with your contact lens practitioner.
(8) Unless your lenses are designed for continuous or extended wear, never sleep in your lenses for more than very short periods of time. If you should forget, however, check immediately on waking to see if the lenses will move on the eyes. If they do not move readily, do not attempt to move them. Place several drops of saline solution in the eyes every few minutes and try moving them again. If after several applications, the lenses will still not move, you must consult your contact lens practitioner.
(9) If after placing the lens on the eye you do not see clearly through it, massage the closed lid gently to centre the lens and smooth out any wrinkles in it. If the vision is

still not clear check if you have put in the wrong lens or if the lens is inside out.

(10) You may wish to insure your lenses.

(11) The lenses should not be worn if using eye drops unless your contact lens practitioner has approved or suggested using an 'in eye wetting solution' and named one as suitable.

(12) Make a note in your diary that you are a soft contact lens wearer and that in the event of an accident the lenses should be removed within a few hours.

(13) After-care check-ups will be advised at periodic intervals until complete integrity of the eyes has been ascertained. Further appointments but at longer intervals and about once every 12 months are essential to ensure that no abnormal corneal changes are taking place, as often such changes do not cause symptoms. If you are in doubt about the state of your eyes or lenses always seek advice.

(14) Always bring your spectacles, contact lenses and case to after-care appointments.

Cosmetics and the contact lens wearer

During the first month when your eyes are adapting to lenses, it is best to keep eye make-up to a minimum and if the eyes water excessively, then they are best avoided for a time. Remember eye make-up should be applied after the lenses have been inserted because you can then see what you are doing and there is less risk of smearing the lenses or smudging the make-up. The best cosmetics to use are those which are non-greasy and water soluble and less likely to irritate the eyes and the delicate surrounding skin. Hypoallergenic unperfumed beauty products are the best choice for contact lens wearers but even with these, skin reactions can occasionally occur. Lenses should also be removed before removing make-up. This is not applicable of course to wearers of extended wear lenses who should be particularly careful in their choice and application of eye cosmetics. Eye make-up should be removed before general facial make-up as it is generally thicker and may get rubbed in to the surrounding skin pores. Removing facial make-up afterwards should therefore prevent this. If make-up gets in the eye it is best removed using a saline eye bath.

Eye pencils and eye liners

Eye pencils and eye liners should be used outside the line of the lashes. This not only provides extra emphasis but prevents particles falling off the delicate inner edge of the eye lid onto the eye and causing irritation. Using eye liners on the inner lid margins can occasionally cause infections. Avoid the twin extremes of too hard pencils which may score the lid or easily dislodge the lens and too soft or kohl-type crayon that can become greasy in hot weather.

Mascaras

A water resistant, i.e. non-waterproof, type is better than a waterproof one. Waterproof mascaras are difficult to remove from the lids and undue rubbing may be necessary to remove at night thereby aggravating the lid area.

Lash-building mascaras

Lash-building mascaras containing tiny filaments are not to be recommended to lens wearers as the fibres often drop into the eye with painful results. In the case of those with light-coloured lashes an alternative is to have the lashes dyed. Lenses should be removed during this procedure.

Products to remove eye cosmetics

It is preferable to use a non-greasy preparation with a pH (acid–alkali level) matched to that of the tears so that if any runs into the eye it will not sting. This will be found by experience. Moisturizing and removal creams are preferable to lotions which can more easily get into the eye area.

Acknowledgements

The authors are indebted to Roger Taylor for *Figures 9.1, 9.2* and *9.6–9.9*, Geoff Woodward for *Figures 9.3–9.5, 9.11, 9.20, 9.21* and to Godfrey Boehnke for *Figures 9.10,* and *9.12–9.19.* They are also indebted to Maureen Colyer and Judith Palliser of the Department of Optometry, University of Auckland, New Zealand for the typing.

References

APPLEGATE, R. A. and MASOF, R. W. (1975). Changes in the contrast sensitivity function induced by contact lens wear. *Am. J. Optom. physiol. Opt.* **52**, 840–846

COCHET, P. and BONNET, R. (1961). L'estesiometrie corneenne. Realisation et interet pratique. *Bull. Soc. Ophtal Fr.* **7**, 541–550

COLLINS, M. J. and CARNEY, L. G. (1986). Patient compliance and its influence on contact lens wearing problems. *Am. J. Optom. physiol. Opt.* **63**, 952–956

DRAEGER, J. (1984). Corneal sensitivity — measurement and clinical importance. Vienna: Springer-Verlag

FUJITA, S. (1980). Diurnal variation in human corneal thickness. *Jap. J. Ophthal.* **24**, 444–456

HAMANO, H., HORI, M., MITSUNAGA, S., KOJIMA, S. and MAESHIMA, J. (1982). Tear secretion test (Preliminary report). *J. Jap. Contact Lens Soc.* **24**, 103–107

KIELY, A. M., CARNEY, L. B. and SMITH, B. (1983). Menstrual cycle variation of corneal topography and thickness. *Am. J. Optom. physiol. Opt.* **60**, 822–829

LEMP, M. A., DOHLMAN, C. H. and HOLLY, F. J. (1970). Corneal dessication despite normal tear volume. *Ann. Ophthal.* **2.**, 258–261, 284

LEMP, M. A., HOLLY, F. J., IWATA, S. and DOHLMAN, C. H. (1970). The pre-corneal tear film. *Archs Ophthal.* **83**, 89–94

LOWTHER, G. E. and HILL, R. M. (1968). Sensitivity threshold of the lower lid margin in the course of adaptation to contact lenses. *Am. J. Optom.* **45**, 587–594

MENGHER, L. S., BRON, A. J., TONGE, S. R. and GILBERT, D. J. (1985). A non-invasive instrument for clinical assessment of the pre-corneal tear film stability. *Current Eye Res.* **4**, 1–7

NORN, M. S. (1972). Vital staining of cornea and conjunctiva: fluorescein and rose bengal mixture and tetrazolium–alcian blue mixture. *Acta ophthal.* (suppl.) **113**, 3–66

PHILLIPS, A. J. (1969). Alterations in curvature of the finished corneal lens. *Ophthal. Optician* **9**, 980–986, 1043–1054, 1100–1110

SCHAPIRO, A. and MERIN, S. (1979). Schirmer test and break up time of tear film in normal subjects. *Am. J. Ophthal.* **88**, 752–757

STONE, J. (1974). The measurement of corneal thickness. *Contact Lens J.* **5**(2), 14–19

WILSON, M. S. (1970). Instruction of contact lens patients with particular reference to hospital practice. Paper read at the summer Clinical Conference of The Contact Lens Society, Bradford, 1970

WITTENBERG, S. (1986). Solar radiation and the eye: A review of knowledge relevant to eye care. *Am. J. Optom. physiol. Opt.* **63**, 676–689

WOODHOUSE, J. M. (1987). Contrast sensitivity measurement in optometric practice. *Optician* **193**(5079), 19–20

ZAPPIA, R. J. (1972). Fluorescein dye disappearance test. *Am. J. Ophthal.* **74**, 160–162

Further reading

BAILEY, I. L. and CARNEY, L. G. (1973). Corneal changes from hydrophilic contact lenses. *Am. J. Optom.* **50**, 299–304

BARRADELL, M. J. (1975). Future requirements of soft lenses. *Optician* **169**(4363), 14–16

BERMAN, M. R. (1972). Central corneal curvature and wearing time during contact lens adaptation. *Optom. Wkly* **63**, 132–135

BIER, N. (1957). *Contact Lens Routine and Practice*, 2nd edn. London: Butterworths

BLACK, C. J. (1972). Experiences with soft lenses. *Contacto* **16**(1), 57–58

BRUNDGARDT, T. F. and POTTER, C. E. (1972). Adaptation to corneal lenses: profile of clinical tests. *Am. J. Optom.* **49**, 41–49

ENOCH, J. M. (1972). The fitting of hydrophilic (soft) contact lenses to infants and young children. *Cont. Lens med. Bull.* **5**(3–4), 41–49

FILDERMAN, I. P. and WHITE, P. F. (1968). *Contact Lens Practice and Management*. Philadelphia: Chilton

FINNEMORE, V. (1973). Common factors in contact lens failure. *Am. J. Optom.* **50**, 50–55

FLETCHER, R. J. (1961). Routine and records in contact lens practice. *Ophthal. Optician* **1**, 429–431

FLETCHER, R. J. and NISTED, M. (1963). A study of coloured contact lenses and their performance. *Ophthal. Optician* **3**, 1203–1213, 1259–1262, 1269

GROSVENOR, T. (1963). *Contact Lens Theory and Practice*. Chicago: Professional Press

GROSVENOR, T. (1972). Visual acuity, astigmatism, and soft contact lenses. *Am. J. Optom.* **49**, 407–412

GROSVENOR, T. (1972). Soft lens patient selection and criteria for success. *J. Am. optom. Ass.* **43**, 330–333

HARRIS, M. G. (1972). Identifying potentially unsuccessful contact lens patients. *Contacto* **16**(3), 50–58

HARRIS, M. G. and SARVER, M. D. (1971). Health history and failure in wearing contact lenses. *J. Am. optom. Ass.* **42**, 550–553

HARRIS, M. G. and SARVER, M. D. (1972). The prefitting eye examination and failure in wearing contact lenses. *Am. J. Optom.* **49**, 565–568

HARRIS, M. G. and MESSINGER, J. H. (1973). Personality traits and failures in wearing contact lenses. *Am. J. Optom.* **50**, 641–646

HARRIS, M. G., BLEVINS, R. J. and HEIDEN, S. (1973). Evaluation of procedures for the management of spectacle blur. *Am. J. Optom.* **50**, 293–298

HILL, J. (1973). Tear analysis for successful contact lens wear. *Optom. Wkly* **64**, 943–946

HILL, J. (1973). Physical and physiological differences in fitting soft contact lenses. *Optom. Wkly* **64**, 621–623

HILL, J. (1975). A comparison of refractive and keratometric changes during adaptation to flexible and non-flexible contact lenses. *J. Am. optom. Ass.* **46**, 290–294

HILL, R. M. (1970). Comments on contact lens adaptation: osmotic pressure of the tears. *Contact Lens Soc. Am. J.* **4**(4), 36–39

HILL, R. M. (1971). Apertures and contact lens control. *J. Am. optom. Ass.* **42**, 749–750

HOLDEN, B. (1973). The present and future of contact lenses. *Aust. J. Optom.* **56**, 429–442

KOETTING, R. A. (1973). Keratometric reflexes on flexible lens surfaces. *Am. J. Optom.* **50**, 722–726

KOETTING, R. A. and MUELLER, R. C. (1961). A routine for examination of contact lens patients. *Am. J. Optom.* **38**, 211–220

LARKE, J. R. and SABELL, A. G. (1971). A comparative study of the ocular response of two forms of contact lens. *Optician* **162**(4187), 8–12 (Part 1); **162**(4188), 10–14 (Part 2)

LEMP, M. A. and HAMILL, J. R.(1973). Factors affecting tear break-up time in normal eyes. *Archs Ophthal.* **89**, 103

MACKIE, I. A. (1970). Blinking mechanisms in relation to 3 o'clock and 9 o'clock limbal lesions associated with contact lens wear. *Cont. Lens med. Bull.* **3**(2), 16–20

MANDELL, R. B. (1971). Contact lens adaptation. *J. Am. optom. Ass.* **42**, 45–50

MANDELL, R. B. (1974). Lathe cut hydrogel lenses. *Int. Contact Lens Clin.* **1**(1), 54–62

MANDELL, R. B. (1974). *Contact Lens Practice: Hard and Flexible Lenses*, 2nd edn. Springfield, Ill: Thomas

MANDELL, R. B. (1974). New thoughts on gel lenses. Why don't we find keratometer changes and spectacle blur in gel lens wearers? *Int. Contact Lens Clin.* **1**(1), 34–35

McMONNIES, C. W. (1972). Predicting residual astigmatism with flexible hydrophilic contact lenses. *Aust. J. Optom.* **55**, 106–111

MORRISON, R. J. (1973). Comparative studies in visual acuity with spectacles and flexible lenses: ophthalmometer readings with and without flexible lenses. *Am. J. Optom.* **50**, 807–809

MOSS, H. L. and POLISHUK, A. (1972). Oral contraceptives and contact lenses. *J. Am. optom. Ass.* **43**, 654–656

PHILLIPS, A. J. (1969). Contact lens plastics, solutions and storage — some implications. *Ophthal. Optician* **8**, 1058, 1075–1076, 1134–1136, 1143, 1190–1192, 1203–1205, 1234–1238, 1312–1315, 1405–1408; **9**, 19–20, 25–27, 65–66, 75–79

POLSE, K. A. and MANDELL, R. B. (1971). Contact lens adaptation. *J. Am. optom. Ass.* **42**, 45–50

RACUSEN, F. R., CORRALL, E. and McGEE, T. F. (1964). An explanatory investigation of factors associated with success or failure in contact lens wearing. *Am. J. Optom.* **41**, 232–240

ROCHER, P. (1972). Optical and metabolic problems with hydrophilic contact lenses. *Optician* **162**(4209), 6–8

SABELL, A. G. (1970). Oral contraceptives and the contact lens wearer. *Br. J. physiol. Optics* **25**, 127–137

SARVER, M. D. (1972). Vision with hydrophilic contact lenses. *J. Am. optom. Ass.* **43**, 330–333

SCHOESSLER, J. P. and LOWTHER, G. E. (1971). Slit lamp observations of corneal oedema. *Am. J. Optom.* **48**, 666–671

SCHMIDT, P. P., SCHOESSLER, J. P. and HILL, R. M. (1974). Adaptation: 'hard' vs 'soft' contact lenses. *J. Am. optom. Ass.* **45**, 282–284

STEIN, H. A. and SLATT, B. J. (1973). Clinical impressions of hydrophilic contact lenses. *Can. J. Ophthal.* **8**, 83–91

STEWART, C. R. (1968). Functional blinking and contact lenses. *Am. J. Optom.* **45**, 687–691

STEVENS, A. V. (1972). A simple device for the removal of contact lenses. *Br. J. Ophthal.* **56**, 442

TABAK, S. (1972). A short Schirmer test. *Contacto* **16**(2), 38–42

WATTS, G. (1973). Soft lens wearers: how are they doing? *Optician* **165**(4282), 25–26, 30

WILSON, M. S. (1970). Corneal oedema from contact lens wear, its causes and treatment. *Trans. UK Soc. Ophthal.* **90**, 31–45

YORK, M., ONG, J. and ROBBINS, J. C. (1971). Variation in blink rate associated with contact lens wear and task difficulty. *Am. J. Optom.* **48**, 461–467

Chapter 10

Rigid gas permeable and hard corneal lens fitting

A. J. Phillips

Basic requirements

The student new to contact lens practice is often confused by the multitude of different lens materials and fitting techniques available, each claiming its own special advantages. The basic requirements of a good fitting contact lens are often forgotten and should be stressed from the outset. These are simply:

(1) Maintenance of corneal integrity (including integrity of the related ocular and extra-ocular tissues).
(2) Maintenance of normal tear flow behind and over the lens.
(3) Adequate vision.
(4) Patient comfort.
(5) Invisibility.

It follows, therefore, that the best fitting technique or lens construction to use in any one particular instance is the one which most readily satisfies these criteria. For many patients, several different techniques may all perform adequately; in others, the use of a specific technique may give improved results.

The ideal corneal lens material should have a high degree of the following properties:

(1) Oxygen permeability.
(2) Surface wettability.
(3) Low surface reactivity.
(4) Dimensional stability.
(5) Flexure resistance and recovery.
(6) Surface hardness.
(7) Machining and polishing capability.
(8) Fracture resistance.
(9) Material and quality control, i.e. different batches of the material should have the same chemical and physical characteristics

and should behave in an identical manner during the lens fabrication process.
(10) Wide range of tints and depths of tint.

With the exception of oxygen permeability, polymethyl methacrylate (PMMA) satisfies all these requirements to a good or acceptable degree. Indeed the manufacturers of rigid gas permeable (RGP) materials have been forced to sacrifice several of the other material considerations in order to gain oxygen permeability. Because PMMA lenses are still fitted to a reasonable extent, particularly in certain parts of the world, and because the advent of new materials may lead to the development of less flexible materials which may simulate the properties of PMMA, the fitting of both PMMA and RGP materials will be dealt with in this chapter. Both sections should be read and understood since the development of modern RGP lenses has historically followed from many years of clinical experience with PMMA lenses.

Corneal contour

In the fitting of corneal lenses, a knowledge of corneal contours is essential. To review the enormous volume of research on this single topic would be impossible in this chapter. Nevertheless, for fitting purposes, a basic knowledge will suffice.

In the late 1940s and early 1950s, the main instrument available for measurement of corneal curvature was the keratometer. This gave an accurate value for the central corneal curvature, but a single curve lens made to this curvature and a total diameter of 9.0–10.0 mm showed a fluorescein picture (*see* p. 338) of central and

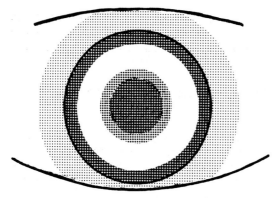

Figure 10.1 Fluorescein picture obtained when fitting a mono-curve corneal lens of approximately the same curvature as the central cornea. Shading within the lens circumference indicates corneal bearing and the unshaded ring indicates corneal clearance

peripheral touch with intermediate corneal clearance (*Figure 10.1*).

Observations such as this led Bier (1956) to conceive the idea of a triple zone cornea (*Figure 10.2*). Bier believed there to be a central, regular and positively curved zone; outside this a less curved or *relatively* negative zone; and beyond this a further zone of steeper curvature. From this general idea arose the concept of a 'corneal cap'. This commonly used term in contact lens practice was meant to indicate the central, regular corneal area. Bier stated that in the average case the corneal cap was decentred 0.2–0.6 mm nasally and 0.2 mm superiorly.

Modifications to the keratometer confirmed the peripheral flattening of the cornea but

representations of this flattening were often incorrectly shown, as in *Figure 10.3*. The centre of curvature for the central region lies at C_1 and at C_2 for the peripheral portion. The construction so produced supported the concept of a central corneal cap, a secondary negative zone and tertiary positive zone.

The introduction of more accurate methods of assessing corneal contour — such as single mire keratometry, photokeratoscopy and other photographic methods — have shown that the cornea has a constantly varying radius of curvature; also the centre of curvature is constantly changing to a new position, the centres of curvature forming a locus of points which extends from the centre of curvature of the central point to an off-axis position. The locus of centres of curvature for a constantly varying curve is known as an *evolute*. The general appearance of a corneal evolute is shown in *Figure 10.4*.

It is now possible to see why the original single curve lens made to the same curvature as the central keratometer reading gave the fluorescein picture shown in *Figure 10.1*, and how this led to the concept of a triple zone corneal configuration as described by Bier. However, although the concept of a 'corneal cap' is not strictly correct, for clinical purposes it is often convenient to assume that one does exist, for the following reasons.

(1) The flattening close to the centre of the cornea is so small that the central region may be assumed close to spherical, in each principal meridian, for clinical purposes.

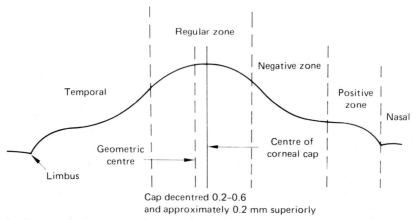

Figure 10.2 Diagrammatic representation of the corneal contour. (After Bier, 1956)

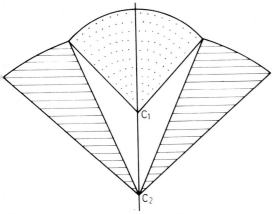

Figure 10.3 Incorrect representation of peripheral corneal flattening as measured by a keratometer

(2) The keratometer reading obtained for fitting purposes is not the curvature value at the geometric centre of the cornea but of two points some 1.2–1.8 mm each side of the centre (*see* Chapter 6). For a typical back optic zone diameter (BOZD, *see* p. 350) of 6.00–7.00 mm, the keratometer reading is therefore approximately the mean value of the curvature at the geometric centre* and that at the edge of the back optic zone. A curvature value is therefore obtained which should closely approach the cornea over this diameter.

(3) Where it is attempted to align too large a central area of the cornea with one single curve of a lens, the peripheral corneal flattening shows a circle of non-alignment of the fluorescein pattern in the midperiphery of the curve, similar to that shown in *Figure 10.1*. Earlier writers on corneal lens fitting claimed that this was because the back optic zone diameter was larger than the corneal cap, and they recommended that a smaller BOZD be used. While it has been shown that the corneal cap is a misconception, the clinical remedy of improving the area of

alignment by reduction of the BOZD still holds good as an attempt to align a spherical contact lens with a non-spherical cornea.

Mathematical models of corneal curvature

The use of computers has enabled the design, in recent years, of sophisticated lenses which more accurately reflect the true shape of the cornea. For their design, mathematical models of the corneal curvature are necessary for the appropriate calculations to be made.

Conic sections, i.e. the curves exposed when sections are taken through a cone, produce a suitable clinical model for the cornea (Bibby, 1976). The notation given by Bennett (1966) is generally accepted and is shown in *Figure 10.5*.

The oblate curve represents the flattening and the prolate the steepening parts of the ellipse.

Bennett, taking the origin of the coordinates at the apex of the cornea, gives the relationship between the x and y values for any point on the curve as:

$$y^2 = 2r_o x - p x^2$$

where r_o is the radius of curvature at the apex of the cone and p is the 'shape' factor†. The 'shape'

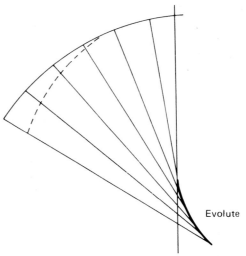

Figure 10.4 General appearance of a corneal evolute

*Arias (1960) has pointed out that, since the visual and geometric centres of the cornea do not normally coincide, when the patient fixates the keratometer target, he is looking along the visual axis and a slightly flat value of central curvature is obtained. The curvature at the geometric centre may be 0.02–0.05 mm steeper than the keratometer reading. This has been confirmed for emmetropes by Sheridan (1970) although in myopes the visual axis appears to pass through the steepest part of the cornea.

† Not to be confused with the usual optometrically accepted meaning for the term 'shape' factor which is one of the components of spectacle magnification, and this also applies to contact lenses (*see* Chapter 5).

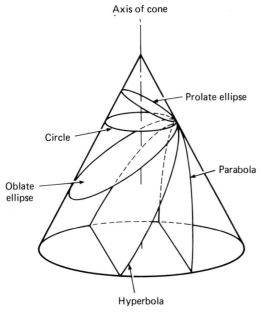

Figure 10.5 Mathematical representation and notation for conic sections. Circle, $p = 1$; ellipse, $0 < p < 1$ and $p > 1$; parabola, $p = 0$; hyperbola, $p < 0$

factor indicates the level of asphericity, i.e. the departure of the actual curve from the apical radius, and takes the following values:

Hyperbola, $p < 0$
Parabola, $p = 0$
Oblate (flattening) ellipse $\quad 0 < p < 1$
Sphere $\qquad\qquad\qquad\quad p = 1$
Prolate (steepening) ellipse $\quad p > 1$

Another term often used to define the corneal asphericity is the eccentricity (e). It is applicable to all the conic sections and there is a relationship between 'shape' factor and eccentricity:

$$p = 1 - e^2$$

Guillon, Lydon and Wilson (1986) have shown that the majority of corneas approximate to an oblate ellipse with a typical 'shape' factor of 0.85 ($e = 0.39$). However, a large variation was found even within the normal population with some corneas remaining unchanged in curvature towards the periphery whilst a small number even steepened at the periphery (range 0.21–1.20). A high correlation was found between 'shape' factors of the flat and steep meridians of individual patients indicating that, for the majority of eyes, the central and peripheral astigmatism is similar. Again, large individual variations were sometimes found

confirming the clinical impression when, in occasional cases, the astigmatic fluorescein patterns (*see below*) observed under the lens are different at the centre and periphery. Such factors need to be borne in mind in the designing of fitting sets and serve to stress the fact that each patient must be treated as an individual.

Barr (1984) gives an average corneal shape factor of 0.75 ($e = 0.50$), Brungardt (1984) of 0.77 ($e = 0.48$), and Guillon, Lydon and Sammons (1983) of 0.83 ($e = 0.41$), with extremes of 0.70 and 0.88.

According to Burek (1977), Wesley–Jessen refer to e^2 as 'shape' factor or SF (*see Figure 10.14*). Thus

$$SF = 1 - f$$

Because the term 'shape' factor may therefore be misunderstood, it seems best to adopt Bennet's (1988) suggestion of referring to the general term 'asphericity' and denoting it by p, e or e^2.

Terms relating to corneal lenses

Detailed terminology relating to cornea lenses is summarized in the Glossary of terms at the beginning of the book. For ease of reference, the major terms are summarized in *Figure 10.6*. The reader is strongly advised to obtain a full copy of ISO standard 8320 – 1986.

Forces affecting the lens on the eye

For a correctly fitting lens, a balance is necessary between those forces acting to hold the lens against the cornea and those acting to move the lens or eject it from the eye. The most important of these forces are reviewed as follows.

Capillary attraction

The force of attraction between the lens and the cornea varies inversely with the distance between the two surfaces (Wray, 1963). In other words, the more nearly a lens surface matches the corneal contour the greater is the force of attraction. If the lens curvature is made slightly flatter than that of the cornea, the capillary attraction is lessened and the lens moves more easily. Because the cornea is not spherical, it should be impossible to achieve exact alignment with a spherical corneal lens. However, because the cornea is compressible, lenses which closely

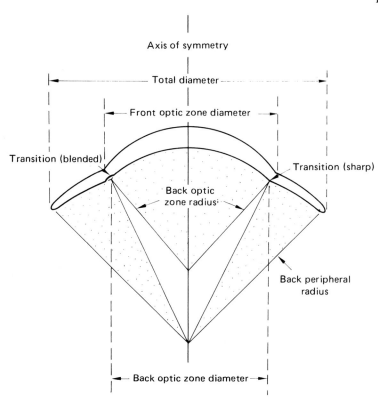

Axis of symmetry

Total diameter

Front optic zone diameter

Transition (blended)

Transition (sharp)

Back optic
zone radius

Back peripheral
radius

Back optic zone diameter

Figure 10.6 Diagrammatic representation of corneal lens dimensions as recommended by the International Standards Organisation (1986)

approximate the corneal curvature can 'mould' the cornea to the shape of the lens and appear as a good alignment fitting. With lenses fitted steeper than the corneal curvature, although capillary attraction is lessened, the compressibility of the cornea allows the edge of the lens to press into the cornea during blinking, and lens movement is reduced by reason of the suction effect so produced.

In practice, while it is desirable to achieve a reasonable area of corneal alignment with the lens to prevent corneal insult, a lens which *exactly* conforms to the corneal contour over the *whole* of its surface cannot be comfortably tolerated. In this instance the capillary attraction would be so great that lens movement would be minimal and adequate tear circulation beneath the lens would be prevented.

Gravity

The effects of gravity on the lens are most easily envisaged by the use of the concept of the centre of gravity. This has the property that the object acts as though all of its weight were concen-

trated at that one point. For a corneal lens, the position of the centre of gravity is near the back surface or actually behind the lens. The further the centre of gravity moves behind the lens the greater the area of support above the centre of gravity. As the centre of gravity moves towards the front surface of the lens, there is less support for the lens and it tends to drop or 'lag' more readily under the effect of gravity.

The position of the centre of gravity is affected by the lens total diameter, back vertex power, thickness and BOZR (*Figure 10.7*). Thus, the effect of gravity is less for a negative lens, minimal centre thickness and steep corneal curvature.

Related to and affected by gravity is the lens mass or weight. Augsburger and Hill (1971) have published the five following 'rules of thumb' for relating alterations in the parameters of negative corneal lenses to changes in their mass.

(1) A change of 0.01 mm in t_c can change lens mass by 3–12%.
(2) A change of 0.1 mm in TD can change lens mass by as much as 4% for a −5.00 D lens

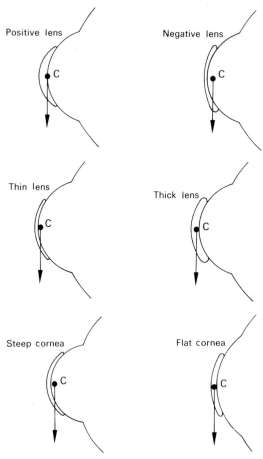

Figure 10.7 Diagrammatic representations of the centre of gravity (C) with lenses of differing power, thickness and BOZR

of TD 8.00 mm, or as little as 2% for a −1.00 D lens of TD 10.00 mm.

(3) A change of 1.00 D in BVP can change lens mass by 2–6%.

(4) A change of 0.1 in the BOZD/TD ratio can change lens mass by 3–4.5% over the BVP range −1.00 to −5.00 D.

(5) A change of 0.1 mm in BOZR changes lens mass by only 0.3–1.5%.

It is thus apparent that changes in lens thickness, total diameter and power are those parameter changes most likely to affect lens position on the eye.

Tear meniscus

The existence of a tear meniscus under the edge of a corneal lens is essential for its centration

(Mackie, Mason and Perry, 1970; Mackie, 1973). For any given lens, the greater the circumference of the meniscus, the better the lens centration. Fenestration holes which permit the formation of a tear meniscus between lens and cornea, also therefore aid in lens centration, as they add to the effective 'length' of the tear meniscus between lens and cornea.

Lid force and position

Many corneal lenses ride in such a position that the upper lid covers a small portion of the lens. The lens is thus held between the cornea and lid. This force contributes to but is not necessary for holding the lens on the eye.

In many cases, the lower lid is sufficiently high for the lens to rest on it between blinking.

Frictional forces

A corneal lens tends to remain stationary on the eye because of frictional forces. This is largely due to the viscosity of the precorneal film. If the precorneal layer is thin, friction may also occur directly between the surface of the lens and the corneal epithelium.

Variations in the viscosity of the precorneal film affect the frictional forces and so affect the position of the lens on the cornea. Thus, the foreign body reaction produced by a lens when first worn, or by a lens with a misshapen or damaged edge, causes an increase in lacrimal production. This serous liquid is less viscous than the normal precorneal liquid and lowers its frictional effect, allowing greater lens movement. Since the precorneal film thickness is also increased, the capillary attraction is lessened and, again, lens movement is increased.

Fluorescein patterns

Fluorescein patterns (*see Plates 10–18*) are the pictures obtained when one drop of 2% sodium fluorescein is instilled into the lower fornix or on to the bulbar conjunctiva above the lens in order to give colour to the tears. The lens fit is then viewed under ultraviolet light, which renders the tears fluorescent. A different pattern is obtained as the lens moves upwards and downwards following each blink and as the fluorescein gradually drains from behind the lens. It is thus a dynamic picture and not easily represented pictorially. The following diagrams and cross-sectional representations can only serve as a useful guide and must be complementary to clinical study (*Figure 10.8*).

Fitting techniques for hard (PMMA) lenses

In the following review, the student should not forget that the fitting technique is but a means to the end of achieving the desiderata listed at the beginning of this chapter. The fitting technique selected should be that which most easily allows the fulfilment of these desiderata. However, while considering the following techniques the reader should bear in mind the accumulated experience of many contact lens practitioners over the last four decades. This is that the fitting technique least likely to upset corneal integrity is the so-called 'alignment' technique, whereby the back optic zone of the corneal lens follows as closely as possible the central corneal contour. It is obviously difficult to align a toroidal cornea with the spherical back surface of a lens, but *Table 10.3* on p. 350 gives an idea of the BOZR likely to give the best possible approximation to alignment in such cases, as well as indicating when a lens with a toroidal back surface should be considered. Although a spherical lens fitted to a markedly toroidal cornea is often optically satisfactory and encourages tear flow beneath the lens, it may mould the cornea so much as to cause a considerable alteration in the spectacle refraction with a resultant severe drop in VA, if the original spectacle prescription is worn. Thus, alignment fitting using a toroidal surface becomes necessary provided that adequate tear flow can be maintained. A careful balance must always be achieved between the need for tear flow and minimizing the moulding effect on the cornea. As a general guide when fitting a spherical BOZR to a toroidal cornea, the BOZR chosen should be slightly steeper than the flattest corneal meridian by approximately one-third of the astigmatic difference of the cornea. In all cases the fit should be checked with fluorescein to confirm its adequacy. With spherical and almost spherical corneas it may be necessary at times to choose a BOZR slightly flatter (up to 0.10 mm) than the keratometer

reading, especially if a large BOZD (7.00–8.00 mm) is chosen. This is because the cornea flattens beyond the region measured by the keratometer and, in order to achieve an overall alignment, it is necessary to fit flatter than the flattest radius measured by keratometry.

Many techniques and lens constructions are available, some being very similar, but each claiming its own especial advantages. They may be divided into two main groups: extrapalpebral and intrapalpebral aperture fitting techniques.

Extrapalpebral aperture fitting techniques

This group of techniques uses lenses larger than the vertical interpalpebral aperture (though smaller than the vertical visible iris diameter). Three main examples follow.

Contour technique

This technique was one of the first which attempted to follow more closely the contour of the cornea, from which it derived its name. It arose from the observations of Bier (1957), who attempted to improve on the fitting of the mono-curve 'microlens'. As it had proved impossible to align a single curve lens with the cornea over the whole of its surface when made to the same curvature as the keratometer reading, the microlens was generally fitted about 0.3 mm flatter than the central corneal curvature (Dickinson, 1954). This resulted in heavy central bearing, excessive lens movement, alteration in corneal curvature, and usually eventual corneal insult and lens rejection.

Bier suggested a back optic zone diameter of around 7.00 mm over which it should be possible to align closely to the cornea. The peripheral curve is fitted flatter than the cornea in order to prevent the lens edge from pressing into the cornea. The clearance given must also be sufficient to prevent the edge from digging in on lens movement to the flatter corneal periphery. The fluorescein picture is that shown in *Figure 10.8a*, so that a reservoir of tears collects beneath the peripheral zone. As the lens is moved up and down by the action of the lids, the tears pass under the back optic zone, thereby maintaining normal corneal metabolism.

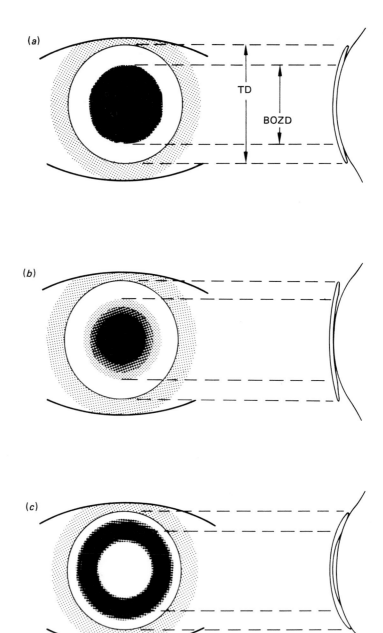

Figure 10.8 Typical fluorescein patterns of corneal lenses with the lens centred and lids slightly separated. The cross-section of the lens fit is shown on the right-hand side. Shading within the lens circumference indicates corneal bearing and the unshaded area indicates corneal clearance. (*a*) Alignment of the back optic zone and clearance of the peripheral zone (a 'contour' fit). The fluorescein pattern appears as a dark area of alignment over the BOZD and a bright fluorescein band beyond (compare *Plate 12*). (*b*) Flat back optic zone and peripheral zone. The fluorescein pattern appears as a dark area of contact towards the centre of the back optic zone and shows increasing fluorescence towards the lens periphery (compare *Plates 11* and *18g, h*). (*c*) A lens with BOZR steeper than the cornea showing central clearance and bearing on the transition between the back optic zone and peripheral curves (an example of a 'tight' lens fit). The fluorescein pattern appears as a central trace of fluorescein, the amount depending on the relative steepness of the lens, a dark ring of bearing in the transition region, and a bright ring of fluorescein towards the lens edge where the lens is flatter than the cornea (compare *Plate 18a–d*).

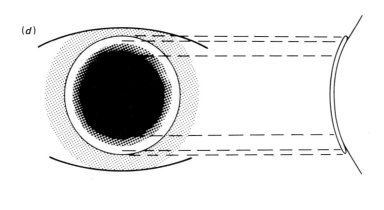

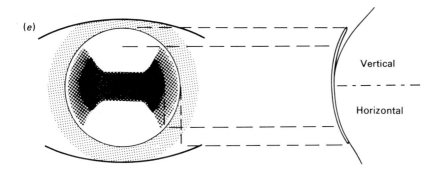

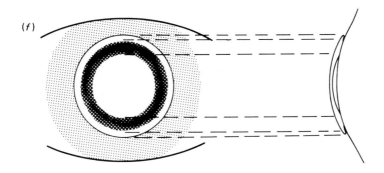

Figure 10.8 (*cont.*) (*d*) Alignment or slight clearance of the back optic zone, near alignment of the first peripheral curve moving towards shallow clearance, and complete clearance of the narrow second peripheral curve (a 'modified contour' fit) (compare *Plate 17*). The fluorescein pattern appears as a dark area of central alignment gradually merging into a bright ring of fluorescein towards the lens edge. (A similar appearance is given by the correct fitting of a 'tapered' and an 'all-aspheric' continuous curve lens — compare *Plates 12* and *16*.) (*e*) A 'contour' lens on a 'with-the-rule' astigmatic cornea. In the horizontal meridian the lens shows alignment of the back optic zone curve and has been fitted with near alignment of the peripheral curve in this meridian to reduce excessive edge clearance in the vertical meridian (*see* split cross-sectional diagram) (compare *Plate 13*). (*f*) A small lens showing central clearance, alignment of the first peripheral curve and clearance of the narrow second peripheral curve ('Bayshore' technique, *Plate 14*). The fluorescein pattern appears as a bright circle of fluorescein over the back optic zone, a dark area of alignment over the first peripheral curve and a bright ring of fluorescein over the second peripheral curve

In cases of corneal astigmatism, the lens is fitted to align with the flattest corneal meridian or may be fitted slightly steeper than this meridian since the flatter meridian often becomes steeper with lens wear (*see* p. 350).

Further details of this technique are discussed under Fitting routine, p. 349.

Advantages

(1) The back surface of the lens parallels the cornea closely enough to distribute the lens weight evenly and yet differs enough from the true corneal curvature to allow tear circulation beneath the lens.
(2) The even distribution of the lens weight gives rise to a minimum of spectacle blur (*see* Chapter 19) or corneal distortion.
(3) The success of this method is shown by the fact that it was the most commonly used fitting technique for many years, and that all modern fitting methods are extensions of the same technique.

Disadvantages

(1) Occasional poor centring. Once the lens moves to the peripheral cornea, it often stays there due to alignment of the peripheral zone with the cornea.
(2) Lenses often 'ride high', due to the top of the lens being held by the upper lid.
(3) Moderately large lens movement. This very commonly shows as a ring or part ring of indentation around the limbus, which collects fluorescein where the lens edge has indented the bulbar conjunctiva in this region.
(4) A small amount of corneal steepening (for example, due to oedema) or slight lens flattening gives rise to a flat fitting lens with the accompanying disadvantages mentioned above.
(5) Nearly all possible modifications to the lens effectively make the fit flatter (*see* Effect of variations in the BOZD).

Summary of typical specfications

BOZR $= K_F \pm 0.10$ mm*
BPR $=$ BOZR $+ (0.40 \rightarrow 0.80)$ mm
BOZD $= 6.50 \rightarrow 7.50$ mm
TD $= 8.50 \rightarrow 10.00$ mm

*$K_F =$ flattest corneal meridian in millimetres as measured by the keratometer.

Modified contour technique

This technique is similar to the contour technique but attempts to eliminate some of the disadvantages associated with that method. The first peripheral curve is made to approach the cornea most closely and there is usually a small, flat, second peripheral curve at the very edge to act as a tear reservoir and to prevent the edge digging in on lens movement (*Figure 10.8d*). The junction between the BOZR and BPR₁ must be well blended since both curves are close to corneal alignment. The BOZR may be fitted slightly steeper than the flattest corneal meridian to aid lens centration in certain cases (*see* pp. 345 and 350). The aim is for a fluorescein pattern similar to that in *Plate 16*.

Advantages over contour technique

(1) Better centration and less lens movement.
(2) High-riding lenses are less common because the lens adheres more to the cornea than the upper lid, due to the greater area of corneal alignment with this technique.
(3) The lens is more amenable to modification and there is less likelihood of a flat fit.
(4) There is less edge sensation because the edge lies closer to the cornea.

Disadvantages

(1) Greater accuracy is required in fitting, especially of the first peripheral curve.
(2) Many laboratories have difficulty in manufacturing an accurate first peripheral curve, which greatly affects the efficacy of this method.
(3) Following from (1) and (2) above, it is relatively easy to obtain a 'tight lens, i.e. a fitting where the lens weight is concentrated on to a narrow band, usually at a transition or near the lens edge, causing a restriction in tear flow under the lens.

Summary of typical specfications

BOZR $= (K_F - 0.05) \pm 0.05$ mm
BPR₁ $=$ BOZR $+ (0.30 \rightarrow 1.00)$ mm
BPR₂ $= 9.50 \rightarrow 12.50$ mm, $0.20 \rightarrow 0.40$ mm wide
BOZD $= 6.00 \rightarrow 7.50$ mm
TD $= 8.50 \rightarrow 9.50$ mm

Multi-curve or tapered lenses

A further attempt to match the corneal contour more closely and to eliminate some of the disadvantages associated with the two foregoing techniques is the multi-curve lens (Hodd, 1958) (*see Plates 12* and 17). Typically, these lenses have four or five back surface curves, usually well blended with a similar number of curves. The edge clearance is not as excessive as may be imagined (*see* discussion and table of examples of edge lifts on p. 349), and there is less likelihood of edge or transition indentation. The main disadvantage is the difficulty of checking the narrow peripheral curves (*see* Chapter 12). Either the central alignment or minimal apical clearance methods of fitting may be used and the peripheral flattening varied to allow adequate tear flow and prevent indentation by this zone on lens movement.

Summary of three typical specifications

$$BOZR = (K_F - 0.05) \pm 0.05 \, mm$$

Three possible variations of the peripheral zone curves follow

(1) BPR_1 = BOZR + 0.50 mm
     BPR_2 = BOZR + 1.00 mm
     BPR_3 = BOZR + 1.50 mm
     BPR_4 = 12.25 mm

(2) BPR_1 = BOZR + 0.50 mm
     BPR_2 = BOZR + 1.25 mm
     BPR_3 = BOZR + 2.25 mm
     BPR_4 = 12.25 mm

(3) BPR_1 = BOZR + 0.50 mm
     BPR_2 = BOZR + 1.50 mm
     BPR_3 = BOZR + 2.70 mm
     BPR_4 = 12.25 mm

     BOZD   = 7.00 mm
     BPD_1 = 7.60 mm
     BPD_2 = 8.20 mm
     BPD_3 = 8.80 mm
     TD   = 9.20 mm

The range for BOZD and TD, which has been omitted to avoid over-complication, is the same as for the modified contour technique.

Constant axial edge lift lenses

Stone (1975) and Rabbetts (1976) have designed multi-curve lenses of various total diameters so that throughout each fitting set the lenses all have the same axial edge lift (*see* p. 349 and Chapter 5, pp. 233–236). These lenses are a much more logical approach to fitting, because

if the axial edge lift (AEL) is constant throughout the set, all lenses are equally likely to have similar peripheral clearances on the eyes to which they are fitted, whereas with a standard flattening in radius of the first and second peripheral curves throughout the fitting set, the flat lenses have a much smaller edge lift than the steep lenses (*see Table 10.2*, p. 349). The flat lenses therefore give less peripheral clearance to the eyes on which they are fitted, than do the steep lenses.

Lenses with constant edge lift are fitted by the modified contour technique. Some typical fitting set specifications are given in *Table 10.1* (AEL 0.15 mm at TD 9.00 mm) and *Table 10.13* (AEL 0.12 mm at TDs 9.80 and 9.50 mm).

Other types of lens having constant edge lift are dealt with later (*see* p. 348). Chapter 5 refers to a computer program (given in Appendix E) for determining lens specifications to give a desired edge lift and another to determine the edge lift if the back surface parameters are known.

Lens–lid attachment (parallel-surfaced peripheral zone lenses)

Corneal lens intolerance has been related, among other reasons, to the development of corneal oedema under the lens and corneal dessication in areas that the lens does not cover. Oedema can be avoided (assuming the lens is fitted correctly) provided a smaller area of cornea is covered or, alternatively, the movement of the lens on the cornea is increased. The small lens, which satisfies both these criteria, has the disadvantage of sometimes inducing abnormal blinking because it is often unstable after each blink. According to Korb and Korb (1974), the ideal contact lens should simulate the actions and movements of the tear layer in order to prevent this oedema occurring.

Because almost all precorneal film movement is the result of upper lid action, and because the precorneal film may in effect be considered as attached to the upper lid, Korb and Korb argue that the ideal contact lens should therefore be effectively attached to the upper lid. This concept of lens performance, in which the lens remains immobile without upper lid action or eye version movements, but moves during blinking as if the corneal lens were attached to

Table 10.1 Fitting set designed by J. Stone with a constant axial edge lift of 0.15 mm at the TD of 9.00 mm

								Edge lift				Ratio
								Axial (AEL)			Radial (REL)	REL/ AEL
BOZR	BOZD	BPR$_1$	BPD$_1$	BPR$_2$	BPD$_2$	BPR$_3$	TD	at 7.8	at 8.6	at 9.0	at 9.0	at 9.0
7.00	7.0	7.40	7.8	8.40	8.6	10.00	9.00	0.018	0.083	0.147	0.113	0.77
7.10	7.0	7.55	7.8	8.60	8.6	10.20	9.00	0.019	0.085	0.148	0.115	0.78
7.20	7.0	7.70	7.8	8.80	8.6	10.40	9.00	0.020	0.086	0.148	0.116	0.78
7.30	7.0	7.85	7.8	9.10	8.6	10.40	9.00	0.021	0.091	0.149	0.118	0.79
7.40	7.0	8.10	7.8	9.30	8.6	10.50	9.00	0.025	0.095	0.150	0.120	0.80
7.50	7.0	8.30	7.8	9.50	8.6	10.60	9.00	0.028	0.097	0.150	0.121	0.80
7.60	7.0	8.40	7.8	9.70	8.6	10.80	9.00	0.027	0.097	0.150	0.122	0.81
7.70	7.0	8.55	7.8	9.90	8.6	11.00	9.00	0.028	0.098	0.149	0.121	0.81
7.75	7.0	8.65	7.8	10.00	8.6	11.10	9.00	0.029	0.098	0.150	0.123	0.82
7.80	7.0	8.75	7.8	10.10	8.6	11.30	9.00	0.029	0.098	0.150	0.123	0.82
7.85	7.0	8.80	7.8	10.20	8.6	11.40	9.00	0.029	0.098	0.150	0.123	0.82
7.90	7.0	8.85	7.8	10.40	8.6	11.50	9.00	0.028	0.099	0.150	0.124	0.82
8.00	7.0	9.00	7.8	10.60	8.6	11.70	9.00	0.028	0.100	0.151	0.125	0.83
8.10	7.0	9.20	7.8	10.80	8.6	11.90	9.00	0.030	0.101	0.150	0.125	0.83
8.20	7.0	9.30	7.8	11.00	8.6	12.10	9.00	0.030	0.101	0.150	0.126	0.84
8.30	7.0	9.45	7.8	11.30	8.6	12.40	9.00	0.029	0.101	0.150	0.126	0.84
8.40	7.0	9.60	7.8	11.60	8.6	12.60	9.00	0.029	0.102	0.150	0.127	0.85
8.50	7.0	9.80	7.8	11.70	8.6	12.90	9.00	0.031	0.101	0.150	0.128	0.85
8.60	7.0	10.00	7.8	11.90	8.6	13.10	9.00	0.032	0.102	0.150	0.128	0.86
8.70	7.0	10.40	7.8	12.00	8.6	13.20	9.00	0.036	0.104	0.150	0.129	0.86

the upper lid, facilitates the movement of tears during the acts of blinking and eye movement, and permits the successful training of blinking.

The main technique of 'lid attachment' is achieved by arranging that 0.75–1.00 mm of the most peripheral portion of the lens has parallel front and back surfaces or is even slightly negative in cross-section (i.e. slightly thicker at the very edge). This may be done by simply requesting it from the laboratory, by tables (Korb and Korb, 1974), by drawing to ×40 magnification (Mackie, 1973), or by calculation (J. Stone, 1975, personal communication). The latter two methods are dealt with in Chapter 5, pp. 233–236.

Unlike all other techniques, Korb and Korb recommend that the lens is fitted flatter than the central cornea to give an approximate alignment fit when riding superiorly on the cornea and actually moving some 3 mm onto the inferior sclera during blinking. The lens edge is made more blunt and rounded than normal to increase the tear meniscus. This is acceptable because the upper lid does not have to pass over the lens edge. Lens mass is kept to an absolute minimum.

Summary of typical specifications

BOZR = $K_F + (0.40 \rightarrow 0.50)$ mm
BPR = fitted to give satisfactory clearance with the lens in the superior position
FPR = arranged to be parallel with the back surface over $0.75 \rightarrow 1.00$ mm. A lenticulated lens is usually necessary
BOZD = typically 7.00 mm
TD = $8.20 \rightarrow 9.40$ mm, typically 9.00 mm
t_c = minimum possible to allow lens manufacture and to keep edge thickness to around 0.06 mm for plano lenses, with a range of $0.05 \rightarrow 0.12$ mm

In spite of the Korbs' recommendation to fit flat, Stone (J., 1975, personal communication) has found the technique of using parallel-surfaced peripheral zones very successful using a standard modified contour technique with BOZR = $(K_F - 0.05) \pm 0.05$ mm and an AEL of approximately 0.15 mm. Lenses are drawn out to scale or calculated to give edge thickness of approximately 0.15 mm and are made lenticular with the FOZD equal to the BOZD. This technique is particularly successful for making positive lenses and low-power negative lenses (up to −2.0 D) ride high. For lenses of −7.0 D

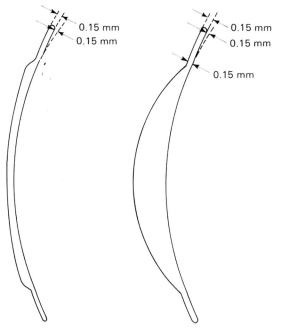

Figure 10.9 Cross-sections of parallel-surfaced peripheral zone lenses: negative (left) and positive (right). The carrier zone is held by the upper lid

and upwards, the technique is also helpful as it minimizes edge thickness. For very high-power negative lenses, an extra front surface junction curve must be worked on and the appearance then is similar to the gravity lens described by Mandell (1974) (*Figure 10.9* and *see Figure 5.34*).

Whereas Stone uses peripheral thicknesses of 0.15 mm and axial edge lifts of 0.15 mm, Mackie uses peripheral thicknesses of 0.10 mm and radial edge lifts of 0.10 mm. Both report considerable success with this modification of Korb's technique.

For drawing out lenses to scale at ×40 magnification, large sheets of graph paper, a drawing board and a beam compass are required. The drawing itself is simple and is done by normal geometrical principles.

If lens curvatures are determined by calculation, sag tables (*see App*endix C) and an electronic calculator or computer are ideal (J. Stone, 1975, personal communication) — *see* Aspects of lens design, Chapter 5, pp. 228–236 and Appendix E, program index nos 10 and 11.

Another technique for assisting the upper eyelid to hold up a corneal lens has been described by Hersh (1974). This involves making a groove, some 0.05 mm deep and

0.08 mm in width, in the front peripheral portion of the lens, about 0.4–0.8 mm in from the edge depending on lens total diameter. The inner margin of the upper eyelid aligns and penetrates the groove at the upper part of the lens thereby holding it up. It is essential that the groove is well polished, otherwise the patient suffers considerable lid sensation.

Interpalpebral aperture fitting techniques

This group of techniques uses lenses smaller than the vertical interpalpebral aperture. Lester and Braff (1963) list the following conditions as particularly suitable for these small lenses.

(1) When the lid aperture is narrow.
(2) When the lids are more sensitive than average.
(3) When large lenses do not centre.
(4) When the peripheral cornea is highly irregular.
(5) When the cornea abrades easily.
(6) When the lenses are worn in hot or humid climates.
(7) When very large lenses of high positive power would otherwise be necessary.
(8) When the patient has a backward head tilt with conventional lenses.

To which may be added

(9) In cases of moderate corneal astigmatism where the fitting of a small lens may obviate the need for a lens with a toroidal back surface.
(10) When the wearer spends most of his time doing close work.
(11) When the lower lid margin is situated below the lower limbus.
(12) Some cases of 3 and 9 o'clock staining (although often a larger lens works better).
(13) Persistent corneal oedema.

Small bi-curve and tri-curve lenses

The fitting technique is basically that of the contour or modified contour philosophy except that the total diameter of the lens is made smaller than the interpalpebral aperture but should be at least 2.00 mm larger than the maximum pupillary diameter. Jessen (1961) suggests total diameters in the range of 7.50–8.40 mm, Morrison (1967) an average of 7.80 mm, Davis (1964) from 7.30 to 8.20 mm, and Moore (1974) from 8.00 to 8.30 mm.

The BOZR necessary to give an alignment fitting may be slightly steeper than the keratometer reading because the cornea steepens towards its apex, and this becomes more apparent with the generally smaller BOZD (*see p. 350*). The central thickness of the smaller lenses is often less than that of the extrapalpebral aperture lenses. Various other modifications to small lens fitting have been suggested. Morrison (1967), for example, utilizes a narrow peripheral zone width of 0.30–0.40 mm and a relatively large BOZD.

Summary of typical specifications

BOZR $= K_F - (0 \to 0.15)$ mm
BPR $=$ BOZR $+ (0.30 \to 1.00)$ mm
BOZD $= 5.00 \to 6.50$ mm
TD $= 7.30 \to 8.40$ mm

Bayshore technique

Probably the most well known of the interpalpebral aperture fitting techniques (although not now fitted so frequently), this method (*see Plate 14*) reverses the bearing surfaces of the contour technique to give central clearance, first peripheral curve alignment and a small, flat second peripheral curve (*see Figure 10.8f*). The total diameter is normally determined by the vertical lid aperture less 0.20 mm, with a minimum of 7.00 mm and a maximum of 8.80 mm (Bayshore, 1963).

The main advantage of this method is the excellent lens centration. This arises from the fact that it is possible to achieve much better alignment of the non-spherical cornea with a narrow first peripheral curve than with the wider back optic zone. Thus, the cornea is steeper on one side of the bearing surface and flatter on the other, giving the lens a strong tendency to move to the position of first peripheral curve alignment. It is therefore important to stress the accuracy with which this curve must be fitted. The disadvantages of this method are mainly those that apply to the modified contour technique, and also the corneal oedema and surface irregularity which often arise unless fitted extremely carefully.

The Bayshore technique may also be applied as an extrapalpebral technique in certain cases, although some of the advantages of the smaller lens may be lost. In this instance, the recommendation of subtracting 0.30 mm from the radius of the flattest corneal meridian to give the

BOZR (Bayshore, 1962, 1963) would give rise to excessive central clearance from the cornea with the use of a wider BOZD. Approximately half this amount gives the same central clearance as the smaller lens.

Summary of typical specifications

BOZR	$= K_F - 0.30$ mm
BPR$_1$	$=$ generally $1.00 \to 1.50$ mm flatter than BOZR to give alignment
BPR$_2$	$= 17.00$ mm radius*, $0.10 \to 0.30$ mm wide
BOZD	$= 5.60 \to 6.60$ mm, generally governed by subtraction of the first peripheral curve width (ideally $0.80 \to 0.90$ mm) and second peripheral curve width, from the total diameter
TD	$= 7.00 \to 8.80$ mm (interpalpebral aperture less 0.20 mm)
Fenestration	a central fenestration, $0.20 \to 0.25$ mm in diameter is recommended if a restriction of lacrimal interchange should cause objective symptoms or subjective signs of oedema.

Lester and Braff (1963) list some of the disadvantages of interpalpebral fitting lenses as follows.

(1) They are more difficult to handle and are more easily lost.
(2) The lens edges need more precise finishing.
(3) There is less variation possible for a good fit.
(4) If the corneal apex is decentred, the small lens is usually decentred.
(5) There is often a problem with flare.
(6) Modification of small lenses usually requires greater care.
(7) They tend to lose their dimensional stability more than larger lenses.

Continuous curve lenses

These more recent types of lens construction (*see Plate 16*) may be used for either interpalpebral or extrapalpebral aperture fitting techniques. As their name would suggest, these types of lens

---

*In practice, if this curve is polished using a soft felt tool which tends to take up the shape of the lens, it is unlikely that the curve will remain as flat as this after polishing. The author would not recommend such a flat curve if harder tools (for example, those made of wax or hard felt) are to be used.

eliminate transitions, so that the back surface of the lens is apparently of one continuous curve. In practice, the back surface may be made with a single aspherical curve or the peripheral zone may follow on from the edge of the back optic zone without a sharp junction. The accurate use of terminology used to describe them is therefore most important. The advantages claimed for this lens type are as follows:

(1) It is possible to align more accurately the gradually flattening cornea with a non-spherical lens construction
(2) There is no risk of corneal abrasion from a transitional area.
(3) There is less likelihood of flare.
(4) The precise lens construction is, in theory, easier to reproduce.
(5) Due to fewer parameters, they are generally simpler to fit.

The main disadvantage is that the practitioner is at the mercy of the laboratory in as much as it is impossible at the present time to check accurately all such peripheral zone constructions. Stone (1975), however, has described methods of checking radial and axial edge lifts.

There are three basic types of lens construction, as follows.

Offset peripheral curve lenses

The back peripheral curve is cut on a conventional lathe but the centre of curvature is offset so that its radius passes through the centre of curvature of the back optic zone at the transition between the two curves (*Figure 10.10*). This eliminates a sharp transition between the two curves which, at that point, both have a common tangent. As the centre of the peripheral curve is offset to the opposite side of the centre of curvature of the central portion, as in *Figure 10.10*, it is known as a 'contralateral offset continuous curve' lens. Bennett (1968) has termed this type of lens construction a 'continuous bi-curve' lens.

The amount of flattening is usually specified by the distance, at the lens edge, between the back optic zone curve (extrapolated to this point) and the peripheral curve(s). The distance, in millimetres, is normally measured along a line parallel to the axis of symmetry (*Figure 10.10*) and is known as the axial edge lift

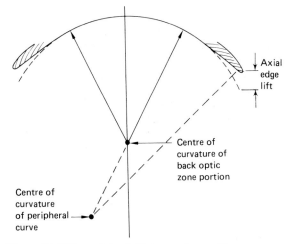

Figure 10.10 Contralateral offset or continuous bi-curve lens

(AEL) — previously known as the 'flattening factor' or 'Z value' (Bennett, 1968). Some writers prefer to measure the radial edge lift (REL) along the radius of curvature of the back peripheral zone at the lens edge — previously known as the 'Z factor' (Hodd, 1966; Ruben, 1966). When comparing peripheral lens flattening, it is important to check if axial or radial edge lifts are being referred to.

The centre of curvature of the peripheral curve may also be displaced to some homolateral point, although this does not give a 'continuous curve' lens when a flatter peripheral curve is used.

Conical peripheral zone lenses

With this type of lens, it can be readily appreciated that for each BOZR at a certain BOZD there is one tangent to the lens at this point. A tangent rotated around the axis of symmetry gives a conical peripheral zone with no visible transition. The cone angle is expressed in degrees as the included (apical) angle of the conical surface (*Figure 10.11*) although ISO standard 8320–1986 defines it as half this value.

In the 'Conoid'* type of construction (Thomas, 1967), the lens rests on the conical peripheral region and shows central optic clearance. Centration is extremely good with

*Conoid — Focus Laboratories Ltd under licence from Corneal Lens Corporation Pty Ltd, Australia.

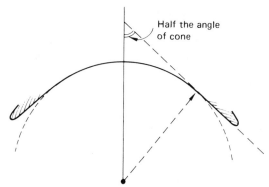

Figure 10.11 Conical periphery continuous curve lens. (Note: since the introduction of these lenses ISO 8320–1986 has recommended that cone angle be defined as the angle between the generating line and its axis of resolution – *see* p. 347)

this type of fitting, as with the Bayshore technique, and the same degree of central steepness of BOZR is recommended for both techniques ($K_F - 0.30$ mm). It is argued that the gradually increasing and decreasing bearing across the contact band in the conical periphery gives rise to less corneal discomfort and distortion than that of the conventional spherical lens on the aspherical cornea. In the optimum fitting of this technique, there is a bright glow of fluorescein over the central area, surrounded by a dark band of contact which should circle the apical clearance. The apical pool may be circular or elliptical in shape, depending on the degree of corneal astigmatism present. Around the edge of the lens there should be a band of fluorescein 0.30 mm wide at the narrowest part of the band. A 0.25 mm diameter fenestration, 2.00 mm in from the lens edge (with a lens of total diameter 9.00 mm), aids lacrimal interchange. Comparison with the fenestration diameter during fitting aids selection of the cone angle to give the correct width of peripheral clearance. Toroidal back optic zones with elliptical conoidal peripheries are available where the corneal astigmatism does not permit a complete ring of corneal bearing with a standard lens. Conoid lenses are generated with a lathe working on the pantograph system and the cone angles are claimed to be accurate to within 0.1°.

In the 'Conic'* construction (Stek, 1975), the back optic zone is fitted to align the cornea,

*Conic — Optimedic Ltd.

while the conical peripheral zone is adjusted (normally by the laboratory) to give a constant radial edge lift of 0.10 mm (considered to be the ideal). Where there is excessive peripheral corneal flattening this may be increased. The cone angle is always within 2° of being an exact tangent so that, while it may not be a true 'continuous curve' lens, the transition is virtually eliminated. It is argued by the originators of the technique that the constant radial edge lift in conjunction with almost complete lack of transition permits a more normal corneal metabolism and causes less corneal distortion than with other lens designs. Conic lenses appear to be suitable in cases of up to 3.00 D of corneal astigmatism and conic peripheries in conjunction with toroidal back optic zones are available for use where the corneal astigmatism is in excess of this value.

Complete aspheric (or conicoid) lenses

The third type of lens construction has a complete single aspherical back surface curve from lens centre to edge and may therefore be correctly termed a 'continuous curve' lens. Over a central 1.00 mm diameter area, the curvature is extremely close to spherical and this serves as the nominal central curvature of the lens.

Nissel (Steele, 1969) has produced three aspheric fitting sets, each set having the same axial edge lifts for every lens. Thus:

Set 1 — known as the 12/18 set has an axial lift of 0.12 mm at a diameter of 8.00 mm and of 0.18 mm at a diameter of 9.50 mm

Set 2 — known as the 7/11 set has an axial lift of 0.07 mm at a diameter of 8.00 mm and of 0.11 mm at a diameter of 9.50 mm

Set 3 — known as the 5/8 set has an axial lift of 0.05 mm at a diameter of 8.00 mm and of 0.08 mm at a diameter of 9.50 mm

Each set can be made with any desired total diameter. The addition of a small, flat 0.50 mm wide well-blended curve at the lens margin has been found to prevent indentation of the lens edge at the corneal periphery (Gegg, 1969).

In the fitting of this type of lens, the aim is to match the aspherical surface of the cornea with the continuous aspherical back surface of the lens. Because the keratometer gives the corneal

Table 10.2 Back surface specifications and edge lift values of comparable corneal lenses

	Axial edge lift (mm)
Bi-curve lenses	
C2/7.20:7.00/7.70:9.00	= 0.06
C2/7.80:7.00/8.30:9.00	= 0.05
C2/8.40:7.00/8.90:9.00	= 0.04
Tri-curve lenses	
C3/7.20:7.00/7.70:8.40/10.00:9.00	= 0.12
C3/7.80:7.00/8.30:8.40/10.00:9.00	= 0.09
C3/8.40:7.00/8.90:8.40/10.00:9.00	= 0.06
Multi-curve lenses	
C4/7.20:7.00/7.70:7.80/8.20:8.60/10.50:9.00	= 0.13
C4/7.80:7.00/8.30:7.80/8.80:8.60/11.00:9.00	= 0.10
C4/8.40:7.00/8.90:7.80/9.40:8.60/12.00:9.00	= 0.09

Conoid lenses
Not applicable since these lenses are fitted with apical clearance and use the peripheral curve as the bearing surface

Conic lenses	
Constant for every BOZR and TD (BOZD = 6.80 mm) at:	0.10

Kelvin Continuous Curve lenses
Impression moulded lenses with a spherical back optic zone surrounded by an annulus whose curvature constantly changes from the edge of the back optic zone. Toroidal continuous curve lenses are also available. Various radial edge lifts are possible and each is held constant for every BOZR. Thus lenses with a *constant radial edge lift* of 0.10 mm at 9.00 mm TD will give the following axial edge lifts (AEL) for:

	BOZR = 7.20, AEL	= 0.14
BOZD = 7.00 mm	BOZR = 7.80, AEL	= 0.13
	BOZR = 8.40, AEL	= 0.12

Nissel Continuous Offset lenses

Set 1 (Ref. 3/4/2).

	BOZR = 7.40 mm	= 0.09
BOZD = 6.50 mm	BOZR = 7.80 mm	= 0.08
TD = 9.50 mm	BOZR = 8.40 mm	= 0.06

Set 2 (Ref. 146/0914).

	BOZR = 7.30 mm	= 0.15
BOZD = 6.50 mm	BOZR = 7.80 mm	= 0.12
TD = 9.50 mm	BOZR = 8.35 mm	= 0.09

Set 3 (Ref. 5/2/51/2).

	BOZR = 7.20 mm	= 0.19
BOZD = 6.50 mm	BOZR = 7.80 mm	= 0.16
TD = 9.50 mm	BOZR = 8.40 mm	= 0.12

Nissel Aspheric (Conicoid) lenses

Set 1 (Ref. 12/18).

All nominal BOZR	At 8.00 mm diam.	= 0.12
	At 9.50 mm diam.	= 0.18

Set 2 (Ref. 7/11).

All nomimal BOZR	At 8.00 mm diam.	= 0.07
	At 9.50 mm diam.	= 0.11

Set 3 (Ref. 5/8).

All nominal BOZR	At 8.00 mm diam.	= 0.05
	At 9.50 mm diam.	= 0.08

curvature approximately 1.5 mm each side of the geometric centre, the correctly fitting lens is generally some 0.10 mm steeper than this value as the nominal lens curvature is taken at the lens centre (Steele, 1969). This may be varied by individual practitioners, however, according to their own fitting philosophy.

A similarly constructed lens has been produced by Focus Contact Lens Laboratory Ltd, and is known as the 'Uni A' lens.

Examples of axial edge lifts

It is of interest to compare edge lifts for various types of lens construction (*Table 10.2*). It should be emphasized that the values given are axial edge lifts (measured along a line parallel to the axis of symmetry) and not radial edge lifts (measured along a line normal to the lens edge).

The significance of the edge lift must be considered in relation to the different types of lens construction and the ways in which these bear upon the cornea. Thus, two lenses having the same edge lift and the same TD may give different edge clearances from the cornea as well as different widths of peripheral corneal clearance.

Fitting routine

The following are required before fitting commences:

(1) General discussion with the patient on advantages and disadvantages of contact lenses, patient suitability etc., as discussed in Chapters 8 and 9.
(2) Corneal, as well as lid and limbal, integrity should be established with a slit lamp (*see* Chapters 6 and 8).
(3) Accurate keratometer readings. These govern the choice of the BOZR of the first trial lens (*see* Chapters 5 and 6).
(4) Horizontal and vertical visible iris diameters (which approximately equal the corneal diameters). These partly govern the choice of total diameter.
(5) Interpalpebral aperture size. Again, this partly governs the choice of total diameter.
(6) Pupil size in average and low illuminations. This largely governs the choice of BOZD.
(7) Accurate spectacle refraction and calculation of ocular refraction. This enables a

subsequent check on the liquid lens power to be made, which should be zero in a true alignment fit.

(8) Decision of lens type to be used — corneal, hydrophilic or scleral.

Selection of the first trial lens

For simplicity it will be assumed that the fitting of a bi-curve contour lens is being carried out. The basic routine varies only with the lens dimensions, as discussed under the different fitting techniques.

BOZR

It is best to approach alignment from the steep side rather than the flat side as a central fluorescein pool is easier to see than fluorescein just inside the transition. For this reason, lenses as much as 0.20 mm flatter than correct alignment may *appear* to give an alignment picture. The student new to contact lens practice is well advised to select a BOZR approximately 0.15 mm steeper than the flatter keratometer reading for the first trial lens so that a definite central fluorescein pool is obtained. The BOZR may then be flattened in steps of 0.05 mm until central alignment is obtained.

The majority of contact lens patients have some degree of corneal astigmatism. Keratometry indicates the corneal radii and amount of corneal astigmatism. *Table 10.3* indicates the optimum value of BOZR found from clinical experience in the majority of cases.

Table 10.3

Astigmatism (by keratometer)	Approximate BOZR
Under 0.75 D	Flattest keratometer reading to 0.05 mm steeper
0.50–1.00 D	0.05–0.10 mm steeper than the flattest keratometer reading
1.00–2.00 D	Steeper than the flattest keratometer reading by approximately one-third of the difference between the principal meridians (consider a toroidal back optic zone)
Over 2.00 D	As above, but a toroidal back optic zone is recommended (*see* Chapter 14)

BOZD

This should be at least 1.00 mm bigger than the pupil diameter in average room illumination, and larger if the lenses are to be used in the dark (for example, for night-driving).

It has been found from clinical experience that if a given BOZR over a certain BOZD gives a satisfactory central alignment, then 0.05 mm should be added to the BOZR for each 0.50 mm increase in BOZD in order to maintain a satisfactory fit (*see* p. 354).

BPR

To give adequate peripheral clearance, this must be approximately 0.50 mm flatter than the BOZR, more for flat corneas (8.20 mm and above) and less for steep corneas (7.60 mm and below). Toroidal peripheral curves may be considered for corneal astigmatism of about 3.00 D and over (*see* Chapter 14).

In assessing the fit of the peripheral curve, it must be ensured that this curve shows adequate clearance when centred on the cornea but not such excessive clearance that the lens can pass over the limbal region. Conversely, if inadequate clearance is given, the lens may dig into the peripheral cornea on lens movement, necessitating a flatter peripheral curve or the addition of an even flatter second peripheral curve. In general, several peripheral curves are preferable to one, in order to give the desired peripheral clearance.

TD

This should be at least 1.40 mm smaller than the largest visible iris diameter, and often 2.00 mm smaller. If the lids are tight, or if there is a narrow vertical palpebral aperture or a lot of corneal astigmatism, a smaller total diameter may be selected.

Assessment of the fit

At least 5 minutes should be allowed after insertion of the first lens for lacrimation to subside. This is not normally necessary with subsequent lenses. Patients usually comment that the lens is more comfortable than expected and the practitioner should maintain conversation to reassure patients and to take their minds off any irritation produced by the lens. While adapting to the lens, the patient should be instructed to look downwards (where the lids are at their most relaxed) and blink normally.

White light assessment

(1) Lids in the normal position: as the eye moves, the lens should remain within the limbal area.
(2) Lids separated: the lens should drop slowly when pushed to the top of the cornea. A flat fitting lens falls more quickly and often drops in a curved path as it pivots around the apex of the cornea. A steep fitting lens falls more slowly and often remains at the corneal apex.

Ultraviolet light assessment

One drop of 2% fluorescein is applied from a wetted impregnated paper strip, or with a sterile glass rod, on to the conjunctiva above the cornea with the patient looking down and the lids retracted. The series of fluorescein patterns depicted in *Plate 18* should be studied here.

Lens centred

Table 10.4 supplements the fluorescein patterns represented pictorially in *Figure 10.8* and *Plate 18*.

Table 10.4

Fit		Fluorescein picture
Central	Peripheral	
Ideal alignment	—	Even dark blue over BOZD with a 0.5–1.0 mm wide green band at edge of lens. A central trace of fluorescein is acceptable
—	Flat	Bright green under the entire peripheral zone
Flat	—	Green encroaching under periphery of back optic zone
—	Steep	Narrow blue touch band at extreme edge, green within this. Possible blue transition touch with wide peripheral curves
Steep	—	Blue transition with green under back optic zone and bubble if very steep

Lens displaced upwards

Fluorescein should disappear from under the upper periphery of the lens, except at the extreme edge, and should collect under the lower periphery and lower part of the back optic zone. Care should be taken to ensure that the extreme edge of the lens does not indent the peripheral cornea.

Movement

With fluorescein present, the movement of the lens is observed with the lids in the normal position, during blinking and normal eye rotations (*Table 10.5*). The BOZD is checked relative to the pupil size as the lens moves. The lens should centre itself after each blink and eye movement. Whenever a lens consistently takes up an incorrect position, areas where the transition or edge may be bearing on the cornea should be looked for and blended.

Table 10.5

Lens position	Possible cause*
Continually high, not dropping after blinks	Flat peripheral zone; too large a lens; too wide a peripheral zone; lens too thin; thick edges; (lens slightly steep, occasionally;) lens too light in weight due to small total diameter, or too thin, or both; negative lens
Continually low, with rapid dropping after blinks	Too small a lens; too thick a lens; (prism) ballasted lens; too heavy a lens due to large total diameter or thickness, or both; positive lens
Continually to one side	Apex of cornea displaced; lens too small or too flat; spherical lens on an 'against-the-rule' cornea
Hardly any movement from the centre	Lens too steep
Lens moving about too much and beyond limbus	Profuse lacrimation due to foreign body or poor lens edge; lens too flat, allowing excessive movement; lens too flat or too steep, causing irritation and lacrimation; spherical lens on a toroidal cornea

*Reference should also be made to *Figure 10.7* for the effects of centre of gravity on lens position.

Fitting astigmatic corneas

When fitting a spherical lens to an astigmatic cornea, a compromise fit is called for as dealt with in under BOZR on p. 350. If a 'with-the-rule' astigmatic cornea is assumed fitted with a lens showing central alignment of the flattest meridian and a peripheral zone also showing near alignment in this meridian, then the fluorescein picture should show:

(1) *Centrally* — an elongated H or dumb-bell-shaped blue touch area as wide as the BOZD (*see Plate 13*).
(2) *Peripherally* — blue touch in the horizontal meridian and green stand-off in the vertical. The peripheral alignment should not occupy more than one-third of the lens circumference. Vertical stand-off is liable to cause discomfort when blinking. This can be minimized by making the lens as small as possible and the peripheral zone narrow (*see Plates 13 and 15*).

Refraction

This should be performed with the patient wearing the lens whose BOZR is the nearest to the correct fitting. The contact lens refraction is a means of checking the fit, as with exact alignment the liquid lens power should be zero and the contact lens refraction (plus any power of the trial contact lens) equal to the ocular refraction. If the contact lens refraction shows less negative or more positive power than the ocular refraction, then a slightly flat fitting should be suspected. A steep fitting (positive liquid lens) gives a more negative or less positive contact lens refraction.

Tolerance trials

Once the desired fitting information has been obtained, the practitioner should order the lenses in the manner described later. Following an instruction session (*see* Chapter 9) and once the practitioner is satisfied with the patients' ability to handle the lenses, they are then issued for a tolerance trial of usually 1–2 weeks. Because of the curvature change with hydration, lenses should ideally be soaked for 24 hours before being worn (*Figure 10.12*). It should be explained to patients that they are being *loaned* lenses for an assessment period. It should also

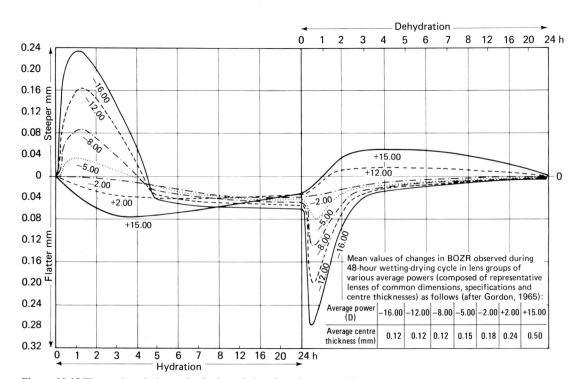

Figure 10.12 The wetting–drying cycle of polymethyl methacrylate corneal lenses

be stressed that patients are free to consult the practitioner should any problems arise or if they should decide not to have contact lenses (when an appropriate fee will be charged). Similarly, the practitioner must reserve the right to reject any patient considered as being unsuitable for corneal lenses.

At the end of the tolerance trial, the fitting of the lenses is noted (and any necessary modifications carried out), the patient's objective and subjective reactions noted, and the corneas examined for oedema or any abrasion which may indicate epithelial fragility. Tolerance trials are discussed fully in Chapter 9.

Fitting sets

Ideally, a large number of trial sets of varying dimensions and powers is desirable. In most average-sized practices this is unrealistic, although a small but growing number of practitioners are now fitting from (a large) stock covering the most commonly used parameters. The student may begin with one or two sets and aim at extending these as soon as possible.

A tri-curve back surface and a fairly sharp transition between the three curves allows an accurate assessment of the fit of both back optic and peripheral zones. Further transitional or peripheral curves may then be ordered on the final lens if found to be needed. Trial lenses may be ordered with slightly greater central thickness than prescription lenses to aid maintenance of lens curvature with handling. Because most contact lens patients are myopic, many trial sets are made with low to moderate negative power. Lenses which are approximately afocal have the advantage that, in many cases, the patient may wear his spectacle correction over the contact lenses during a short tolerance trial but the effect of the correct lens power on lens position and movement is thereby sacrificed.

Table 10.6 gives the minimum requirements for an initial fitting set. Those in lighter type show additional lenses which may be obtained later. Additional fitting sets are shown in *Tables 10.7* and *10.8*.

Further fitting sets may be acquired as practitioners develop their own techniques. Sets of high positive and negative lenses are useful for fitting aphakics and high myopes. The thickness variations cause such lenses to behave different-

Table 10.6 Initial 19 lens fitting set (heavy type) extending to 27 lenses

BOZR	BOZR	BOZR	
7.20	**7.70**	8.15	
7.30	**7.75**	8.20	
7.35	7.80	8.25	BOZD 7.00 mm
7.40	**7.85**	**8.30**	
7.45	**7.90**	8.35	BVP approximately afocal
7.50	**7.95**	**8.40**	
7.55	**8.00**	8.45	BPR 0.50 mm flatter than
7.60	**8.05**	**8.50**	BOZR, 0.70 mm after
7.65	**8.10**	8.60	BOZR 8.00 mm
			t_c 0.23–0.25 mm
			TD 9.00 mm

Table 10.7 Second fitting set

Specifications as for the initial set but with:

BOZD 6.50 mm and TD 8.50 mm
BVP −3.00 D t_c 0.19–0.22 mm

Table 10.8 Third fitting set

Specifications as for the initial set but with:

BOZD 7.25 mm and TD 9.50

ly on the eye from low-powered lenses of otherwise similar specifications, although when made in lenticular form, as is usual, high positive lenses with parallel-surfaced or negative carrier zones, behave like low-powered negative lenses. Even when high-powered negative lenses are made lenticular it is difficult to stop them from riding high on the cornea, due to upper lid traction, but the 'gravity lens' type of construction (*see* p. 345) helps, particularly if the edge is made like that of a positive lens.

Becoming increasingly popular are fitting sets with a constant axial edge lift as discussed earlier (*see* pp. 343 and 349).

All trial lens specifications should be checked at frequent intervals as these may alter with age, handling etc. All curvatures should be noted to the nearest 0.01 mm and each lens engraved with some suitable identification engraving. Lenses may be lightly tinted in some colour sequence to help prevent confusion of the lenses in the fitting set.

Ordering

During the fitting routine, it is unlikely that a single lens will be available which will be correct in all its specifications. It may be necessary to combine specifications from several lenses or to extrapolate a dimension from the nearest available trial lens. The following notes indicate those allowances necessary.

BOZR

Effect of variations in the BOZD

As mentioned earlier, since the cornea flattens towards its periphery, as the BOZD is increased, the BOZR must be flattened to maintain the nearest to an alignment fit. The opposite applies on reducing the BOZD. It has been found from clinical experience that for every 0.50 mm increase in BOZD the BOZR must be flattened by approximately 0.05 mm, and vice versa.

Effect of hydration

Due to plastic expansion, all lenses flatten with hydration. Thus, since lenses flatten during storage and wear, an allowance should be made for this at the time of ordering (Phillips, 1969). A table of average hydration flattening has been given by Gordon (1965) and is reproduced in *Table 10.9*. Generally, as the lens is made thinner so the flattening with hydration is increased.

Figure 10.12 shows the effects of hydration and dehydration on the BOZR of PMMA lenses of different powers. Lenses made of other materials, such as cellulose acetate butyrate (CAB), show fairly similar hydration and dehydration changes. CAB, however, is generally less stable than PMMA and the changes are much more marked (Stone, 1978).

BPR

The same allowances apply as for the BOZR, both for alterations in the total diameter and hydration flattening (usually taken to the nearest 0.05 mm owing to the difficulty of accurately manufacturing and checking peripheral curves).

BOZD and TD

See notes under BOZR and BPR.

BVP

Comparison of spectacle and contact lens correction

The initial spectacle refraction is best written in negative cylinder form because the tear lens acts as a negative cylinder in a lens aligning the flattest corneal meridian and corrects most of the corneal astigmatism (*see* Chapter 5). Thus, the power of these two negative cylinders can be compared and, where the spectacle astigmatism

Table 10.9 Flattening of back optic zone radius with maximum hydration of PMMA lenses

Range of powers of lenses (D)	Lens centre thickness (mm)	Flattening at maximum hydration	
		Group flattening range (mm)	Mean value of lens flattening (mm)
+10.00 to +20.00	0.40 to 0.60	0.020 to 0.035	0.028
+5.00 to +9.00	0.25 to 0.40	0.020 to 0.035	0.030
+1.00 to +3.00	0.20 to 0.28	0.025 to 0.040	0.033
−1.00 to −3.00	0.12 to 0.22	0.030 to 0.045	0.038
−4.00 to −6.00	0.10 to 0.20	0.030 to 0.050	0.042
−7.00 to −9.00	0.08 to 0.18	0.035 to 0.060	0.047
−10.00 to −13.00	0.08 to 0.17	0.035 to 0.065	0.052
−14.00 to −18.00	0.08 to 0.16	0.040 to 0.070	0.058
−19.00 to −22.00	0.07 to 0.15	0.045 to 0.080	0.065

As measured by Gordon (1965). Each group contained 20 lenses and 90% of the findings fell within the group flattening range.

and keratometer astigmatism are approximately the same, the astigmatism should be corrected by the tear lens and then the cylinder in the spectacle correction may be ignored. The spherical component of the spectacle refraction referred to the corneal plane should then equal the liquid lens power along the flattest corneal meridian, plus the BVP of the contact lens. If there is more than 0.50–0.75 D difference between spectacle and keratometer astigmatism, depending on individual patient acuity and tolerance, it may be necessary to incorporate a front surface cylindrical correction. To maintain lens orientation in these cases, a prism-ballasted lens or double truncation may be used where the cornea is close to spherical; alternatively a toroidal back surface lens may be fitted where possible (*see* Chapter 14).

Vertex distance

A refraction is carried out with the trial contact lens in place, and provided adequate visual acuity is achieved the 'best sphere' power is used.

The BVP of the trial contact lens is then added to the power of the spectacle addition, having made due allowance for the vertex distance, to give the BVP of the lens to be ordered.

A table of vertex distance allowances is given in Appendix A, or the ocular refraction may be determined from the computer program in Appendix E, index no. 8. It can be seen that for spectacle corrections of less than 4.00 D the effects of vertex distance may generally be ignored, provided that the latter lies within normal limits.

Effect of variations in the BOZR

It may be necessary to carry out the refraction with a trial contact lens whose BOZR is not the same as that to be ordered on the final lens. As any alteration of the BOZR alters the power of the tear liquid lens, an allowance must be made to the BVP of the lens to be ordered. It can be calculated that, for small amounts and for corneas of average curvature, an alteration of 0.05 mm in the BOZR requires an alteration in BVP of 0.25 D.

Thus, if the trial lens used is of BOZR 8.00 mm and BVP −3.00 D, and the lens

ordered has a BOZR of 8.05 mm, then the liquid lens becomes more negative powered and the BVP of the lens must be ordered as −2.75 D to compensate for this.

No alteration to the BVP should be made where the BOZR is altered to compensate for flattening with hydration. This allowance normally disappears when the lens becomes fully hydrated.

Centre thickness

Although the centre thickness of a lens is normally specified, the edge thickness is just as important clinically. An edge which is either too thick or too thin gives rise to lid irritation. An edge thickness of around 0.14–0.18 mm appears to be the ideal. A lens which is too thin flattens excessively with hydration and often becomes distorted or damaged if handled incorrectly. Conversely, a lens which is too thick is relatively heavy and constantly positions low on the cornea.

A list of suggested centre thicknesses for variations in BVP and TD is given in *Table 10.10*.

It is suggested that the higher powers are made in lenticular form because this provides a great reduction in lens weight, thereby aiding lens centration and giving easier control of edge thickness. When a lens is ordered in lenticular form, it is necessary to specify a front optic zone diameter (FOZD), and the desired final edge thickness. The FOZD is generally around 0.50 mm larger than the BOZD. Junction thickness may also be specified (*see* pp. 231–233, Chapter 5).

Transitions

These may be left sharp or blended lightly, moderately or heavily. Although a heavily blended transition lessens any risk of corneal abrasion caused by this area, there are two possible disadvantages. First, it is difficult to check if the BOZD has been made correctly; if incorrect, it effectively alters the fit of the back optic zone. Secondly, the transition, if polished well into the BOZD, reduces its effective diameter, often causing flare under conditions of low illumination. Ideally, the transition should be ordered lightly blended and the blending increased later by the practitioner as necessary.

If blending is carried out, a tool should be

Table 10.10 Corneal lens thickness chart

Negative powered lenses

BVP (D)	Total diameter (mm)					
	8.50 to 8.80	8.90 to 9.20	9.30 to 9.60	9.70 to 10.00	10.10 to 10.30	10.40 and over
Afocal to −0.50	0.215	0.210	0.210	0.210	0.200	0.180
−0.75 to −1.00	0.215	0.210	0.200	0.190	0.190	0.170
−1.25 to −1.50	0.210	0.200	0.190	0.190	0.175	0.160
−1.75 to −2.00	0.200	0.200	0.190	0.180	0.165	0.155
−2.25 to −2.75	0.190	0.190	0.175	0.170	0.155	0.150
−3.00 to −3.25	0.180	0.180	0.160	0.155	0.150	0.145
−3.50 to −4.25	0.170	0.160	0.150	0.145	0.140	0.130
−4.50 to −5.00	0.160	0.155	0.140	0.135	0.125	0.115
−5.25 to −5.50	0.150	0.145	0.130	0.120	0.110	0.105
−5.75 to −6.00	0.140	0.135	0.120	0.105	0.100	0.100
−6.25 to −7.00	0.130	0.120	0.110	0.105	0.100	0.100
−7.00 and over	0.100	0.100	Make in lenticular form			

Positive powered lenses

BVP (D)	Total diameter (mm)					
	8.40 to 8.70	8.80 to 9.20	9.30 to 9.70	9.80 to 10.00	10.50 (approx.)	11.00 (approx.)
Afocal to +1.00	0.210	0.220	0.230	0.235	0.240	0.245
+1.25 to +2.00	0.230	0.240	0.250	0.255	0.265	0.270
+2.25 to +3.00	0.260	0.270	0.280	0.290	0.310	0.330
+3.25 to +4.00	0.280	0.295	0.310	0.325	0.350	0.370
+4.25 to +5.00	0.305	0.315	0.330	0.360	0.395	0.450
+5.25 to +6.00	0.330	0.345	0.365	0.385	0.420	0.470
+6.25 to +7.00	0.350	0.370	0.395	0.440	0.470	0.520
+7.00 and over			Make in lenticular form			

The figures given above for centre thickness (mm) are the average for the power and total diameter groups and generally give an edge thickness of about 0.14–0.18 mm for an average tri-curve lens (P. Bryant, 1975, personal communication). Lens thicknesses should be ordered to two decimal places only.

Note: Lenses with a BVP of about ±5.00 D may be made in lenticular form. Lenses with a BVP of ±7.00 D or more should be made in lenticular form. To reduce the incidence of corneal oedema, centre thickness of greater than 0.40 mm should be avoided where possible by the use of lenticulation. Some practitioners advocate lenticular construction for all positive lenses to minimize centre thickness but give adequate edge thickness and similarly for very low minus lenses, up to −2.00 D.

chosen whose radius lies one-third to mid-way between the BPR and BOZR so that most of the lens substance is removed from the peripheral curve.

Distinguishing marks for right and left lenses

Right and left lenses should be distinguished by the letters R and L or by small dots — one for the right lens and two for the left (British Standard, BS 5562:1978, awaiting re-publication in revised form in 1989). Although used mainly for scleral lenses, if dots are used for identification marks, often only the right lens is so marked because the drilling of two small holes into the lens surface may weaken the lens. A hole filled with black pigment shows less against the iris background, in most cases. A dot is more easily visible to presbyopes even without their near correction. All marks are positioned near the lens edge so that there is no risk of visual interference and, ideally, both lenses should be engraved. A disadvantage of lens engraving marks is that they are sometimes inadvertently removed when power alterations are carried out. Also, like scratches, they may encourage deposits (*Plate 24*).

Lens tint

The use of tinted plastic material enables the contact lens practitioner to prescribe a tinted lens for his patient either for photophobia or to alter or enhance the iris colour within certain limits. Surface-dyed lenses are no longer used since the tint is not permanent and it has been suggested that certain of the pigments used in the dyeing process may be carcinogenic.

The arguments used by Giles (1960) to deprecate the over-prescribing of tinted spectacle lenses also apply to tinted contact lenses. However, the use of very light neutral tints in contact lenses, for example, code numbers 911 (very light grey) and 912 (light grey), is often beneficial in practice for two reasons. First, location of a clear lens on the sclera or in a bowl of water is extremely difficult, whereas even a lightly tinted lens can be easily observed. Secondly, the contact lens wearer is often more light sensitive than when wearing spectacles and the use of a lightly tinted lens may help to relieve this. The reasons for this photophobia have been suggested as three in number (Phillips, 1968), as follows:

(1) The increased light transmission of the contact lens since there is only one air–lens surface, which causes the greatest light loss by reflection. (However, the wearing of plano spectacle lenses over the contact lenses does not relieve the photophobia —Bergevin and Millodot, 1967.)
(2) The small amount of corneal oedema usually present in new wearers while adapting to their lenses, which causes increased scattering of light.
(3) The foreign-body sensation of the lens edges, again present in new wearers, which probably causes reflex iris blood vessel dilatation, iris congestion and pain on sphincter constriction.

Because both (2) and (3) above are normally temporary in nature, the temptation to prescribe a deeper tint should be avoided. However, in the case of a badly fitting lens causing increased corneal oedema, or a poor lens edge exaggerating the foreign-body reflex, the photophobia may well be excessive and prolonged. In these instances, the answer lies in improving the lens design or construction and not in prescribing a deeper tint.

Tinted lenses are discussed further in Chapter 24. Where available, the use of CQ (clinical quality) material is recommended.

A list of tints available in PMMA material is given in Chapter 22, *Table 22.1*. Only 9042 and 9043 are CQ tints.

Fenestration

While some practitioners utilize fenestrations initially in every case the majority of practitioners fenestrate lenses only as a subsequent modification, usually to eliminate corneal oedema or staining due to inadequate tear flow under the lens. Fenestrations should only be used in those central areas which are definitely clear of the cornea, otherwise an additional tear meniscus is formed between lens and cornea which tends to reduce lens movement. In addition there is a greater risk of epithelial trauma from the edge of the fenestration.

Atkinson and Phillips (1971) have listed the proposed advantages of fenestrations in PMMA corneal lenses:

(1) To relieve oedema and corneal staining not alleviated by other methods (Friedberg, 1961; Korb, 1961, 1962a,b; Sellers, 1964; Boyd, 1965) (*Plates 23* and *93*).
(2) To allow larger than normal lenses or back optic zone diameters to be fitted, for example, in the case of large pupils or high-riding lenses, where the large lens would otherwise cause oedema (Haynes, 1960; Korb and Filderman, 1961; Korb, 1962a,b; Boyd, 1965; Neill, 1967).
(3) For non-blinkers, where there is constant oedema (Boyd, 1965).
(4) To remove small bubbles under the lenses not removed by other modifications (Korb and Filderman, 1961; Boyd, 1965).
(5) For patients who have difficulties in hot, stuffy atmospheres (Korb, 1961, 1962a,b; de Carle, 1965, 1967).
(6) To reduce or remove photophobia caused by an interference with normal corneal physiology (Korb, 1962a,b).
(7) To allow normal tear flow with lenses that have to be fitted steeper than the flattest corneal meridian and/or with less than normal lens movement (Sellers, 1960, 1964; Korb and Filderman, 1961; Bayshore, 1962; Korb, 1962a,b; Neill, 1967).

(8) To lighten heavy hyperopic lenses by making eight to ten fenestrations (Boyd, 1965).

(9) In high plus corrections where the thickness of the lens induces physiological problems (Korb and Filderman, 1961; Korb, 1962a,b).

(10) To improve tear circulation in toroidal back surface and truncated lenses which do not rotate and therefore have a poor tear flow beneath them (Friedberg, 1961; Korb, 1961, 1962b).

(11) To allow quicker lens settling and to improve the patient's speed and regularity of adaptation (Sellers, 1960, 1964).

(12) To prevent 'corneal exhaustion' where this has arisen by a minimal but prolonged interference with normal corneal metabolism (Korb, 1961, 1962b).

(13) To aid in reducing spectacle blur in certain lenses (Friedberg, 1961).

(14) To improve normal corneal physiology in high-riding lenses with superior pooling (Friedberg, 1961).

The suggested size of fenestrations fall into three main groups: around 0.10 mm diameter, often positioned centrally; the most commonly suggested group, around 0.25 mm diameter, and positioned near the edge of the back optic zone; and a larger fenestration of around 0.50 mm.

Hill and Uniacke (1968) have shown that there is little oxygen movement (via the tears) through the fenestration itself but that any physiological improvement is more likely to be due to the prevention of negative pressure under the lens.

Methods of lens fenestration by the practitioner are described in Chapters 22 and 23. Lenses fenestrated by a laser beam permit multiple well-finished fenestration holes of 0.10 mm diameter. These are reported by Brucker (1975) to be very successful. *Figure 1.10* (p. 26) shows such a lens.

The written prescription

The form of the written prescription has been recommended by British Standard BS 3521: 1979, now withdrawn. (A new Standard awaits publication in 1989.)

The radius of each zone is given in turn from the centre outwards, immediately followed by its external diameter. Dimensions are invariably to be given in the following order:

(*i*) The letter C followed by the figure *1* for single curve, *2* for a double curve, *3* for a triple curve lens etc.

(*ii*) Radius of the back optic zone surface followed by its diameter or the total diameter, whichever applies.

(*iii*) Radius of each surrounding back surface followed by its external diameter or the total diameter, whichever applies.

(*iv*) Displacement of the optic (where applicable).

Examples

(1) Please supply one corneal lens

R.C3/7.70:6.50/8.15:8.00/10.00:8.80/D1
   (*i*)   (*ii*)   (*iii*)   (*iii*)   (*iv*)

BVP − 6.00 D

t_c 0.14 mm

Transitions left sharp

Mark one dot (black)

Clear tint

(2) Please supply one pair corneal lenses

R. C2/8.00:7.00/8.50:9.30

BVP − 3.25 D

t_c 0.17 mm

L. C2/8.05:7.00/8.55:9.30

BVP − 1.00 D

t_c 0.20 mm

Transitions lightly blended

Engrave R & L

9043 tint

(3) Please supply one corneal lens

R. C3/8.15:7.00/8.70:8.20/9.50:9.40

BVP − 7.00 D

Front surface lenticular, FOZD 8.00 mm, to give edge $t = 0.20 \pm 0.02$ mm

Transitions moderately well blended

Engrave R

911 tint

Other examples

The following example indicates the importance of knowing the accurate parameters of the fitting lenses in use and the final lens to be fitted. At the same time it illustrates the importance of the various allowances discussed earlier.

Supposing a
trial lens is
engraved as: 7.80 mm BOZR and 7.00 mm BOZD
but actually
measures: 7.77 mm BOZR and 7.20 mm BOZD

A lens is
ordered to the
same para-
meters as the
trial lens but
comes as   7.82 mm BOZR and 6.80 mm BOZD

i.e. net
effect on the   _____   _____
lens fit is   ≡ 0.05 mm flat   ≡ 0.04 mm flat

Now the lens is also a $-10.00\,D$ and the flattening with hydration has been ignored. This will average 0.06 mm

The total effect of the fit will therefore be

≡ 0.05 + 0.04 + 0.06 mm flat

≡ 0.15 mm flat.

The lens will therefore appear grossly flat in this instance.

While the use of trial lenses, over-refraction etc., is considered essential by most authorities it may be instructive to consider the following example of 'theoretical' fitting:

Keratometry, right eye 7.80 at 180, 7.71 at 90
Spectacle R_x $-6.00/-0.75 \times 180$
Horizontal corneal diameter: 11 mm
Maximum pupil size   :   6 mm

First, applying the rule-of-thumb that 0.05 mm change in radius ≡ 0.25 D change in power, we can see by comparing the K readings that there is approximately 0.50 D corneal astigmatism, i.e. 0.25 D less than the spectacle astigmatism, indicating that theoretically there should be approximately 0.25 D of residual astigmatism.

The lens ordered may be typically:

C4/7.73:7.00/8.25:8.00/10.00:8.40/12.25:8.80

BVP $-5.75\,D$

t_c 0.10 mm
t_e 0.16–0.18 mm

Transitions moderately blended

912 tint

Engrave R

The BOZR is derived from a compromise of the K readings, as explained earlier, of 7.77 mm + $(-0.04\,\text{mm})$ hydration allowance for this BVP.

The BVP is derived from $-5.50\,D$ (after allowing 0.50 D for the vertex distance) + $(-0.25\,D)$ to compensate for the positive powered liquid lens which will be introduced as the BOZR is 0.04 mm steeper than the flattest K reading, i.e. 7.81–7.77 mm (the hydration allowance can be ignored, as explained earlier).

Rigid gas permeable corneal lenses

Although PMMA corneal lenses have been fitted in large numbers over a period of 30 years, certain disadvantages have become apparent in a significant proportion of patients. These are:

(1) Corneal oedema (as central corneal clouding or disc oedema, and hypoxic intracellular epithelial oedema — see Plates 23 and 93).
(2) Induced refractive and corneal curvature changes (see Chapters 5 and 20).

(3) Corneal staining.
(4) Prolonged adaptation period for many individuals.
(5) Flare in low levels of illumination.
(6) Discomfort in dusty surroundings.
(7) Poor tolerance in adverse environments.
(8) Ease of lens loss.

Although some of these problems were solved with the advent of hydrogel lenses, these also suffered from their own specific disadvantages (*see* Chapter 11):

(1) Poor or difficult correction of astigmatism.
(2) Tendency to deposit formation on the lens surfaces.
(3) Complex and expensive maintenance.
(4) Relatively short lens life.
(5) Corneal vascularization in some cases.
(6) Reactions to solutions and cleaners.
(7) Palpebral lid reactions, e.g. giant papillary conjunctivitis (GPC).

For these reasons, over the last 15 years the development has taken place of gas transmissible hard lenses. These are commonly referred to as 'gas permeable hard' (GP or GPH) lenses, or 'rigid gas permeable' (RGP) lenses. Although the material is not rigid (*see below*) this latter term is sometimes used to avoid patient confusion with 'hard' PMMA lenses that may have given problems in the past.

Using a material which is transmissible to oxygen and carbon dioxide may be expected to provide the following specific advantages over other types of lens.

Advantages over hard (PMMA) lenses

(1) Fewer physiological problems such as central corneal clouding (oedema).
(2) Quicker adaptation.
(3) Few over-wear syndromes.
(4) Less spectacle blur/post-wear refractive changes.
(5) Lenses may be fitted larger because anoxia due to corneal coverage by the lens is no longer of great significance. This will generally provide greater comfort because the lens edge can be fitted to locate under the upper lid and, secondly, a larger back optic zone will normally reduce night-time flare problems due to dilated pupils.
(6) Extended wear becomes possible as transmissibility increases.
(7) Alternation of daily and extended wear becomes feasible.
(8) Less likelihood of lens loss because RGP lenses can be fitted with minimal edge clearance (*see below*).

Advantages over soft (hydrogel) lenses

(1) Good visual stability and better correction of astigmatism.
(2) Less deposit problems and easier lens maintenance.
(3) Less solution allergy or toxicity problems.
(4) Excellent tear interchange and lack of debris build-up behind the lens.
(5) Ability to be modified or repolished in most cases.
(6) Interchange between daily and extended wear without the fragility problems associated with extended wear soft lenses.
(7) Less likelihood of GPC.

In fitting patients with RGP lenses the points made for fitting PMMA lenses in general still apply. The following additional points should be taken into account.

Selection of lens material

There is now a multitude of RGP materials for the practitioner to choose from (*Table 10.11* and *see Table 3.5*, p. 117). While there has been a general trend towards meeting all the desirable criteria listed at the beginning of this chapter, often the gain of one material property, e.g. oxygen permeability, means a trade-off against another, e.g. increased flexibility. The majority of currently available materials can be grouped into the following general headings below. By understanding the advantages and disadvantages of each group, practitioners can make a more logical selection of the material most appropriate for each individual patient.

Cellulose acetate butyrate (CAB)

This was one of the first gas permeable materials available in the early 1970s (Stahl, Reich and Ivani, 1974). Made from natural substances, it was originally developed by Eastman Kodak in 1938 for photographic purposes. The three major constituents are cellulose, derived from wood and cotton, acetic acid from vinegar, and butyric acid from natural gas. The initial prime attraction of the material as a plastic was that it was not flammable. As well as being slightly permeable to oxygen the material dissipates heat and wets much better than PMMA. This

Table 10.11 Some of the gas permeable materials currently available with PMMA and modified PMMA for comparison

Brand name[a]	Material	Water content (%)	Specific gravity	Oxygen permeability[b] or Dk at 35°C $10^{-11} \times$ (cm ml O_2)/ (cm^2 s mmHg)
PMMA	PMMA	0.2–2.0	1.19	0.001
BP Flex	PMMA cross-linked	1.6–2.4	1.21	1–2.2
Airlens	Styrene		0.99	22–25
Alberta II (XL 30) (GP IV) (Sil-O_2-Flex)	Silicone–acrylate	1.9	1.13	22
Boston Equalens	Fluorosilicone–acrylate	1.0	1.18	71
Boston II (Kelvin GP) (Hydron GP)	Silicone–acrylate	0.9	1.14	14–15
CAB (Cabcurve) (Persecon) (Paracab) (GP II) (Meso)	CAB	1.8	1.20	4.5–10
Calgary (XL 20) (GP III)	50% PMMA+ 40% CAB+ 10% silicone	3.2		5
Conflex	CAB + ethyl vinyl acetate	2.5	1.21	8
EW Flex	Silicone–acrylate			56
Fluoropolymer (Fluorofocon A)	Perfluorether NVP/MMA			90–94
Fluoroperm	Fluorosilicone–acrylate		1.11	92
GP 26 (Boston IV) (Boston EW)	MMA/dimethyl itaconate/siloxane	1.75		26–27
Hyperm	MMA/siloxanylamyl-methacrylate	1.0	1.12	18.5
Menicon O_2	Silicone–acrylate + MMA	1.4	1.11	10.5
Menicon SP	Fluoromethacrylate/ siloxanyl methacrylate/ methyl methacrylate		1.187	32
Menicon EX	Fluoromethacrylate/ siloxanyl methacrylate/ methyl methacrylate			
Optacryl 60	Silicone–acrylate	1.61	1.12	10–12
Optacryl K	Silicone–acrylate		1.11	20
Oxyflow	Silicone–acrylate	5.4	1.08	28
Paraperm O_2	Silicone–acrylate	1.1	1.12	12–18
Paraperm O_2 Plus	Silicone–acrylate	1.0	1.09	38–39
Paraperm EW	Siloxymethacrylate copolymer	1.0	1.07	57
Polycon II	Polysiloxanyl alkyl acrylic/ester copolymer 30% silicone	0.7	1.13	9–12
Polycon HDk	Siloxymethacrylate copolymer	1.0	1.08	50
Silcon	Silicon	0.02	1.15	16–17
Silflex	Silicon/silicic acid	10.2	1.10	79.8

[a]Alternative names are shown in brackets.　[b]Manufacturers' claimed values.　*See also Table 3.5.*

latter property should improve retro-lens tear flow and may help patients with marginally dry eyes. Several CAB materials are suitable for contact lens fabrication, all with slightly varying properties.

Advantages

(1) First RGP material available (*Dk* up to 8–10*).
(2) Good wettability.
(3) Not prone to protein deposition.
(4) Greater heat conductivity than PMMA reduces corneal oxygen demand by not increasing corneal metabolism.

Disadvantages

(1) Low modulus of elasticity, or poor shape retention. The material does not retain its shape when flexed or stressed. Clinically this leads to warpage of the lens from handling during cleaning procedures. The material tends to be distorted by the lathing bit and, unless great care is exerted during manufacture, the softness and heat sensitivity of the material will result in inaccurate or warped peripheral curves. Because of the small area used by a radiuscope, a blurred reading will sometimes be obtained. A more accurate reading of the BOZR will be obtained if a keratometer is used because of the larger lens surface area used.

In order to minimize manufacturing problems some laboratories, in recent years, have manufactured CAB lenses by moulding techniques. Such lenses are claimed to be less liable to distortion or warpage.
(2) Because of (1), lenses are normally made thicker than equivalent PMMA and silicone–acrylate (*see below*) lenses. This may produce greater lens awareness and decreases oxygen transmissibility (*Dk/t*) (*see* Chapter 3).
(3) Ammonia-based compounds, such as Silvo, will hydrolyse the lens material and turn it yellow. Alcohol and petroleum products also cause opacification of the material. Lens cleaners, such as Miraflow (Cooper) which contain alcohol, will not cause lens damage if used correctly for their purpose,

i.e. lens cleaning, but may cause surface damage if inadvertently used as an overnight storage solution.
(4) The softness of the material leaves it vulnerable to scratches and chips.
(5) Large hydration–dehydration changes. These may be similar to or greater than those discussed for PMMA lenses earlier (Pearson, 1978; Smith, 1979). Slow longer-term changes have also been reported and the BOZR should be rechecked on lenses where unexpected fitting changes have occurred. Where checking is carried out, the lenses should be blotted dry and quickly measured before curvature changes begin to take place.
(6) The material appears prone to lipid deposition (*see Plate 26*).

Silicone–acrylate (or siloxanyl–acrylate)

Although highly permeable to oxygen, pure silicone polymers are soft and hydrophobic. They are therefore normally combined with PMMA to enhance the hardness and stability of the material. To ensure adequate wettability, hydrophilic monomers such as methacrylic acid are also incorporated into the polymer. Surface treatment or special solutions are not therefore usually necessary to maintain adequate wettability and this allows subsequent laboratory and practitioner modification or repolishing of the lens. Different additives such as dimethacrylate may be used to enhance tensile strength and resistance to deformation.

The ratio of PMMA to silicone is generally 65% PMMA to 35% silicone. The greater the proportion of silicone the higher the oxygen permeability, but the poorer the wettability, stability and strength. Similarly, the greater the proportion of wetting agent, the greater the surface wettability but the poorer dimensional stability and the greater the affinity for surface deposition because of increased surface reactivity. Thus the range of *Dk* values between the materials commonly available is fairly limited (generally 9–16 units*), although some laboratories have achieved higher values by incorporation of proprietary compounds without excess sacrifice of other desirable properties.

As with all RGP materials, great care should be exerted during lens fabrication although there is less susceptibility to distortion than with

---

*Oxygen permeability units or *Dk* units are expressed as units of 10^{-11} (cm ml O_2)/(cm^2 s mmHg).

CAB materials. Warpage often indicates excessive over-heating during the button blocking or lathing procedures (*see* Chapter 22). Ammoniated polishes are best avoided and alcohols, esters, ketones and aromatic hydrocarbons will damage the material.

Advantages

(1) PMMA acts as a thermal insulator. Not only does the lack of oxygen permeability create corneal hypoxia but, by insulating the cornea, it raises the basal metabolic rate and increases the oxygen demand of the corneal epithelium. However, silicones, either in the pure form or polymerized with PMMA, are thermal conductors which remove the heat of metabolism away from the corneal surface thereby decreasing oxygen requirements. The silicone–acrylates are approximately twice as good thermal conductors as PMMA and CAB and this becomes extremely useful for patients living or working in warm or hot environments.
(2) The oxygen permeability of the silicone–acrylate group ranges from fifty to several hundred per cent greater than CAB.
(3) The material is less susceptible to warpage and hydration–dehydration changes than CAB.

Disadvantages

(1) The silicone–acrylate group of materials are still softer and more flexible than PMMA. Thus, lenses will still scratch more easily than PMMA lenses and flex on astigmatic corneas (*see below*). Most RGP lenses are also more easily broken than PMMA lenses.
(2) The hydrophobic nature of silicone allows the attachment of both lipid and protein deposits to the lens surface.
(3) As a rough guide there is a manufacturing trade-off with increasing oxygen permeability. Thus increased permeability is often traded for poor optical quality, poor wettability etc. Manufacturers have attempted to incorporate proprietary ingredients to counteract these problems. Certain high *Dk* value silicone–acrylate materials also appear prone to surface cracking (*see below*).

Silicone

The use of pure silicone as a contact lens material dates back to the late 1950s when Dow Corning in the USA began their research with this material. Dow Corning now market a rigid silicone lens under the tradename 'Silcon', and a rubber-like lens under the tradename 'Silsoft'.

The advantages of pure silicone are much the same as for the silicone–acrylate group. In addition, because silicone resin material has an excellent shape retention, if a patient warps the lens the original curvature may be restored by heating in saline. Two or three cycles through a soft lens thermal unit are sometimes necessary.

Because of the natural hydrophobicity of silicone, the finished lens must be surface treated to render the surface wettable. This in turn means that lenses cannot be modified or repolished.

To maintain surface wettability, lenses should always be wet stored. If a lens is stored dry the wettability of the surface will be considerably reduced. Stronger cleaners, such as Bausch & Lomb's 'Intensive Cleaner' which contain 'friction enhancing agents', should not be used since these can remove or damage the surface coating (Barr and Hettler, 1984).

Fitting is usefully done by using PMMA lenses of the same parameters so that wet storage of the trial set is not essential, although the effect of lens flexure on astigmatic corneas will not be apparent (*see below*). Lenses are normally shipped to the practitioner in sealed glass vials in sterile water. Fitting from practitioner inventory removes the need for parameter modification in most instances. At the time of writing this material is only available in the USA.

Styrene

The Airlens was developed by Wesley–Jessen in the USA and consists of a three-dimensional network of cross-linked alkylstyrene copolymer chains.

Advantages

(1) Good oxygen permeability. The *Dk* value is better than most silicone–acrylate materials.
(2) More resistant to flexure than silicone–acrylates.

(3) Low specific gravity. This material is unique in that its specific gravity is less than 1.0, i.e. it will float on water. This property should help patients with high prescriptions whose lenses would normally lag low. The higher Dk value of this material is also helpful in these invariably thicker lenses.

Disadvantages

(1) The low specific gravity necessitates the use of a container that forcibly retains the lens below the surface of the disinfecting solution.
(2) Solutions preserved with chlorhexidine should not be used with this material as the surface wettability is reduced.

Fluorosilicone–acrylate

As stated earlier, attempts to increase the oxygen permeability of silicone–acrylate polymers, particularly for extended wear, resulted in compromises in dimensional stability, flexure resistance and/or lens surface interaction with tear components.

Polymer Technology attempted to avoid these problems in the 'Boston Equalens' by using a polymer incorporating a fluorinated monomer and combining it with a silicone–acrylate moiety. The fluorinated component enhances the material's capability of resisting mucus adhesion and deposit formation while promoting its affinity for tear mucin and soluble proteins for superior lens wettability *in vivo*. The high oxygen permeability (*see Table 10.11*) is provided by the siloxanyl groups while the itaconate backbone* of the molecule aids in maintaining the integrity of the optical surface of the lens for correcting corneal astigmatism.

An ultraviolet absorber has been integrated within the Equalens polymer matrix in response to growing concern over the potential cataractogenic and retinal toxic effects of ultraviolet light.

Other fluorosilicone–acrylates are now available (*see Tables 10.11 and 3.5*).

*The itaconate backbone is a patented monomer used in the Polymer Technology range of gas permeable hard materials to add rigidity to the polymer, i.e. to increase flexure resistance.

Advantages

(1) High oxygen permeability.
(2) Resistance to mucus and deposit formation.
(3) Dimensional stability equal to silicone–acrylate materials.
(4) Clinically acceptable flexure, scratch and fracture characteristics.
(5) Effective ultraviolet light filtration (in some lenses — *see* Chapter 24).
(6) Suitability for daily or extended wear, or intermittent extended wear.

Disadvantages

(1) The incorporation of an ultraviolet absorber in some materials means that conventional hand ultraviolet lamps cannot be used for assessing fluorescein patterns. A white light with blue filter or the blue light of a slit lamp must be used.†

Care must be taken in ascertaining if a new patient being seen for after-care is wearing a lens of this material or a misjudgement of lens fitting may be made and inadequate edge clearance may be incorrectly assumed.
(2) Lenses are less resistant to breakage than silicone–acrylate lenses.
(3) The lens material is more vulnerable to flexure and is slower to recover from flexure. Hardness is also poorer so that lenses are very vulnerable to abrasion.
(4) Although lenses are capable of being modified in both fitting and power the response of the material is quicker than that of silicone–acrylate materials and should therefore only be done by skilled technicians. Polishing compounds that contain ammonia, alcohol or organic solvents should not be used.

Fluoropolymer

Fluorocarbon gases have been widely used since the early 1900s as a form of refrigerant (e.g. Freon), and gaseous propellant for aerosol

†A Burton Lamp with a Kodak Wratten Filter Blue No.47 placed over *white* illuminating fluorescent tubes and a Wratten Filter No.12 placed over the viewing lens are ideal for viewing the fitting of these lenses. Alternatively, the cobalt blue light of a slit lamp may be used with the viewing system set at a low magnification.

sprays. Fluoroplastics include high temperature cable insulation, heat resistant plastics for piping and gaskets, low friction and anti-stick applications for non-lubricated bearings and coating of cooking utensils (e.g. Teflon). Recently, more elaborate uses of fluorine-based compounds have been investigated. Researchers have discovered that liquid fluorochemicals are highly efficient carriers of oxygen and carbon dioxide. These properties have led to the use of fluorochemicals in physiological salt solution as a form of artificial blood. The newly created 'blood' supplies oxygen to the body tissues while carrying away waste products such as carbon dioxide.

Early reference to fluoroplastics for contact lenses appeared in patents by the Dupont Corporation in 1970 and Gaylord in 1974. These early contact lens materials never reached the commercial stage of development partly due to the poor wetting characteristics, softness, high specific gravity (1.60) and low index of refraction (1.388) (Caroline and Ellis, 1986). Recent research has aimed to modify or overcome these problems.

The fluoropolymer developed by 3M has a high fluorine content pendant to the backbone of the polymer chain. Present in small amounts are *N*-vinyl pyrrolidone, which contributes to the inherent wetting, and methyl methacrylate, which controls the mechanical strength and influences flexibility. The aim has been to provide a material to satisfy both daily and extended wear physiological requirements with a low tendency to accumulate deposits and good mechanical strength.

Advantages

(1) Extremely high oxygen permeability.
(2) Minimal tendency to deposit formation.

Disadvantages

(1) Lenses are currently only available as spun-cast or cast-moulded although lathe-cut versions are in the development stages. This means that laboratory designed lenses only can be fitted. Lenses can be modified or repolished but not by conventional methods.
(2) There is moderate lens flexure on astigmatic corneas.

(3) Lenses are made relatively thick (0.18–0.22 mm centre thickness) to minimize the on-eye flexure (*see below*). Even in this thickness, however, the oxygen transmissibility of the lenses is superior to all other RGP lenses currently available.

Fitting techniques applicable to RGP materials

The following represents a generalized summary for most currently available materials. With the further development of new materials, the guidelines given may change. Laboratory manuals and current literature should constantly be reviewed.

In many respects the same general philosophies follow as for PMMA discussed earlier. The following adaptations follow because of the materials' oxygen permeability and flexibility.

Fitting philosophy

Five techniques are commonly used with RGP lenses

Modified contour technique

This is as described under PMMA lenses above. Extrapalpebral or interpalpebral diameters may be used and with the lenses fitted slightly flatter than PMMA equivalents (*see below*) retro-lens tear flow to provide corneal oxygen becomes less important, so that minimal edge clearance can be used to reduce lid awareness of the lens edge. Generally speaking, larger diameter lenses are used with gas permeable materials. A typical fitting set is illustrated in *Table 10.12*.

Lid attachment technique

As described under PMMA lenses, during primary gaze, upward gaze and between blinks, the upper edge of the lens should be retained

Table 10.12 Four representative lenses from the 10.50 mm total diameter lens fitting set designed by J. Mountford

7.50:9.00/8.20:9.50/8.50:10.00/11.50:10.50	−3.00
7.80:9.00/8.50:9.50/8.80:10.00/11.50:10.50	−3.00
8.10:9.00/8.80:9.50/9.10:10.00/11.50:10.50	−3.00
8.40:9.00/9.10:9.50/9.40:10.00/11.50:10.50	−3.00

under the upper lid. The bottom edge of the lens should be above the lower lid but below the inferior pupillary margin in order to prevent flare. During primary gaze, the lens should not intrude upon the temporal or nasal limbus. The lens should move with the upper lid during blinking. To achieve this a lens BOZR approximately 0.1–0.3 flatter than the flatter K reading is usually necessary associated with a larger BOZD than used with PMMA lenses.

Constant axial edge lift

It was obvious to clinicians even as early as the 1950s (Bier, 1957) that while the simple fitting set concept of providing a secondary curve of, say, 0.5 mm flatter than the BOZR worked well for average keratometer readings, at the extremes of corneal curvature, the edge clearance became excessively great at the steep end of the range and too little at the flat end.

Work by Stone (1975) and others considerably improved fitting by the design of fitting sets of lenses having constant axial edge lift. Lenses were computed to provide the same axial edge lift at each of the peripheral curves over the whole range (*see Figure 10.10*). Many fitting sets of these designs are still in current use and provide a more uniform approach to the fitting of all corneas, from steep to flat, than the earlier sets mentioned above.

Typical fitting sets are shown in *Table 10.13*.

Tear lens thickness and axial edge clearance techniques

Careful observation of lenses fitted using the constant axial edge lift approach still frequently showed lenses on steep corneas that were often too steep at the centre and too flat at the periphery, and vice versa for flat corneas. To further improve the match of lens to corneal contour, the concepts of tear lens thickness (TLT) and edge clearance (EC) were developed by Bibby (1979), Guillon (Guillon, Lydon and Sammons, 1983; Guillon, Lydon and Wilson, 1986), Atkinson (1984, 1985), and others (*Figure 10.13*). The underlying principles and assumptions should first be stated.

(1) Because the cornea is aspherical in shape, a small amount of tear liquid must exist between the cornea and spherical back optic zone of the lens. This volume will increase

Table 10.13 Constant axial edge lift fitting sets designed by J. Stone

BOZR:BOZD	BPR₁:BPD₁	BPR₂:BPD₂	BPR₃:TD
(a) 9.80 mm total diameter set with 0.12 mm AEL			
7.00:8.00	7.30:8.80	7.75:9.40	8.90:9.80
7.10:8.00	7.45:8.80	7.90:9.40	9.15:9.80
7.20:8.00	7.55:8.80	8.05:9.40	9.40:9.80
7.30:8.00	7.70:8.80	8.25:9.40	9.65:9.80
7.40:8.00	7.80:8.80	8.40:9.40	9.95:9.80
7.50:8.00	7.90:8.80	8.55:9.40	10.20:9.80
7.60:8.00	8.05:8.80	8.70:9.40	10.50:9.80
7.70:8.00	8.15:8.80	8.85:9.40	10.80:9.80
7.80:8.00	8.25:8.80	9.00:9.40	11.10:9.80
7.90:8.00	8.40:8.80	9.15:9.40	11.40:9.80
8.00:8.00	8.50:8.80	9.35:9.40	11.70:9.80
8.10:8.00	8.65:8.80	9.50:9.40	12.00:9.80
8.20:8.00	8.75:8.80	9.65:9.40	12.35:9.80
8.30:8.00	8.90:8.80	9.85:9.40	12.70:9.80
8.40:8.00	9.00:8.80	10.00:9.40	13.05:9.80
8.50:8.00	9.15:8.80	10.15:9.40	13.40:9.80
8.60:8.00	9.25:8.80	10.35:9.40	13.75:9.80
8.70:8.00	9.35:8.80	10.50:9.40	14.10:9.80
8.80:8.00	9.50:8.80	10.70:9.40	14.50:9.80
(b) 9.50 mm total diameter set with 0.12 mm AEL			
7.00:7.50	7.45:8.20	7.90:9.00	8.15:9.50
7.10:7.50	7.60:8.20	8.05:9.00	8.35:9.50
7.20:7.50	7.70:8.20	8.20:9.00	8.50:9.50
7.30:7.50	7.85:8.20	8.35:9.00	8.70:9.50
7.40:7.50	7.95:8.20	8.50:9.00	8.90:9.50
7.50:7.50	8.10:8.20	8.65:9.00	9.10:9.50
7.60:7.50	8.20:8.20	8.80:9.00	9.30:9.50
7.70:7.50	8.35:8.20	9.00:9.00	9.45:9.50
7.80:7.50	8.45:8.20	9.15:9.00	9.65:9.50
7.85:7.50	8.55:8.20	9.20:9.00	9.75:9.50
7.90:7.50	8.60:8.20	9.30:9.00	9.85:9.50
8.00:7.50	8.75:8.20	9.45:9.00	10.10:9.50
8.10:7.50	8.85:8.20	9.65:9.00	10.30:9.50
8.20:7.50	9.00:8.20	9.80:9.00	10.50:9.50
8.30:7.50	9.10:8.20	9.95:9.00	10.70:9.50
8.40:7.50	9.25:8.20	10.15:9.00	10.90:9.50
8.50:7.50	9.40:8.20	10.30:9.00	11.15:9.50
8.60:7.50	9.50:8.20	10.50:9.00	11.35:9.50
8.70:7.50	9.65:8.20	10.65:9.00	11.60:9.50
8.80:7.50	9.80:8.20	10.80:9.00	11.90:9.50

or tend to increase when the lens is decentred and thereby serves to re-centre the lens on lens movement by the negative pressure thus induced. In the case of an aspheric lens, negative pressure can only be induced if the lens creates a positive tear layer between the lens centre and point of contact with the cornea.

(2) Although in practical terms the back surface of the lens will approximate the corneal

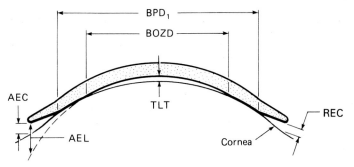

Figure 10.13 Diagrammatic representation of the tear layer trapped between the back optic zone of the lens and cornea. The central clearance (which may not exist in practice) between lens and cornea is known as the *tear layer thickness*. Also shown is the axial and radial edge clearance from the cornea and axial edge lift between the lens edge and extended BOZR (dotted). TLT = tear layer thickness; AEC = axial edge clearance; AEL = axial edge lift; REC = radial edge clearance; BOZD = back optic zone diameter; BPD₁ = first back peripheral curve diameter

shape, for calculation purposes there can be assumed to be a tear layer of finite thickness known as the tear lens (or layer) thickness (TLT) as shown in *Figure 10.13* trapped between the back of the lens and the cornea. Thus the TLT = sag of the BOZR − sag of the cornea at the BOZD where the sag of the contact lens = $r - \sqrt{r^2 - y^2}$ (r = BOZR and y = BOZD/2) and the sag (x) of the cornea (assumed elliptical) can be determined from

$$y^2 = 2r_o x - px^2$$

where y = BOZD/2, r_o = apical corneal radius and p = asphericity ('shape' factor). Also $r_o = b^2/a$ and $p = b^2/a^2$ where a and b are the semi-major and semi-minor axes of the corneal ellipse (Baker, 1943; Bennett, 1988).

r_o can be determined by assuming the K

Table 10.14 BOZD values giving fixed TLT of 0.02 mm for various asphericities (all BOZRs fitted 0.05 mm steeper than K)

Asphericity p	BOZR (mm)		
	7.20	7.80	8.40
0.70	6.70	7.20	7.60
0.75	7.00	7.40	7.90
0.79	7.20	7.70	8.20
0.83	7.50	7.90	8.40
0.88	7.90	8.40	8.90

reading to represent a spherical reading of a 3 mm chord and from this sag it is possible to work back to r_o for any given corneal asphericity (p).

(3) The axial edge clearance (AEC) represents the axial distance of the lens edge from the cornea and is therefore a more relevant term in the clinical context than axial edge lift (AEL) which relates to the lens and not the eye (*Figure 10.13*). The axial edge clearance can be calculated from:

AEC = AEL − (sag of BOZR at lens TD − TLT − sag of cornea at lens TD)

If intermediate values are to be calculated, i.e. from the point of touch of the BOZR at the BOZD outwards, it is only necessary to obtain the axial lift at that point and the sags of the BOZR and cornea at the same required diameter. From this information it is possible to draw up a profile of the tear layer thickness across the whole lens.

(4) At the beginning of this chapter the variations in corneal shape were stressed. *Table 10.14* sets out the BOZD values for steep (7.25 mm), average (7.85 mm), and flat (8.45 mm) keratometer readings, asphericities (p) of 0.70–0.88 and lenses fitted 0.05 mm steeper than K to give a TLT of 0.02 mm*. This value is considered

*For thinner lenses greater lens flexure will occur and lenses should be fitted flatter as discussed below.

optimal by Atkinson (1985) from clinical experience. Eliminating the more extreme values the majority of corneal shapes can therefore be covered by typical BOZDs of 7.20, 7.70 and 8.30 mm.

(5) The choice of peripheral curve diameters and total lens diameter is deduced as follows. As stated earlier, the functions of the peripheral and edge curves are four-fold:

  (a) to allow proper circulation of tears beneath the lens during lens movement in order to maintain the correct metabolism of the cornea;

  (b) to prevent the edge digging into the corneal surface on lens movement;

  (c) to support a tear meniscus at the edge of the lens to provide forces that cause the lens to centre (following eyelid movement and lag of the lens when looking laterally);

  (d) to allow the lens to be removed.

  Functions (a) and (b) are partially contradictory to (c). The first two require increasingly flatter radii whereas (c) improves with a steeper radius and close edge alignment. With gas permeable lenses the edge clearance can be reduced from that required for PMMA lenses because tear flow under the lens is not so vital for normal metabolism due to the material's gas permeability. This in turn reduces edge sensation. An intermediate curve allows more accurate following of the corneal contour and reduces the sudden change in curvature from BOZR to edge curve.

  Bibby (1979) has shown that the ideal width of peripheral curves is approximately 0.50–0.60 mm. For smaller widths of peripheral curve, a large change in radius is necessary to change the edge clearance significantly but a small error in the diameter during manufacture would change the edge clearance significantly. Similarly, at large peripheral curve widths, a small error in radius would be significant but a large error in diameter less significant.

  From clinical experience total diameters of 8.70, 9.20 and 9.80 mm would cover the majority of cases normally encountered. For the BOZDs previously selected and the discussions above, the edge curve selected is 0.5 mm wide with the intermediate band width therefore 0.25 mm.

(6) Choice of intermediate peripheral radii: if the profile of a lens is assessed when the BOZR is 7.85 mm and the BOZD is 7.70 mm, with a first peripheral curve 0.25 mm wide and 0.50 mm flatter than the BOZR, we obtain a corneal clearance of 0.005 mm at the edge of the band. A curve 0.80 mm flatter than the BOZR will give 0.011 mm clearance, and 1.10 mm flatter will give 0.017 mm. From clinical experience, a clearance of 0.005 mm leaves too little clearance and 0.017 mm too much. By going 0.80 mm flatter than the BOZR throughout the range, we tend to flatten the periphery at the steep end of the range and steepen it at the flat end which is as desired from the earlier discussion above.

(7) The final peripheral curve, and edge clearance: Bibby (1979) suggested an average radial edge clearance for PMMA lenses of 0.08 mm. In axial terms this is approximately 0.093 mm. As mentioned above, this figure is now considered unnecessarily great for RGP lenses and Atkinson and Kerr (1987) consider a figure of 0.08 mm as being adequate. However, with the introduction of flatter BOZRs and the tendency to fit on alignment it is now considered possible that the edge clearance can be reduced to the order of 0.06 mm although this has not been clinically proven as yet.

Thus for a lens on a spherical cornea of 7.90 mm radius and fitted 0.05 mm steep, the final specification would be:

7.85:7.70/8.65:8.20/9.75:9.20

TLT   0.020 mm
AEL   0.101 mm
AEC   0.080 mm

For steeper corneas also fitted 0.05 mm steeper than K of, say, a 7.30 mm cornea, the lens will have the following specification:

7.25:7.70/8.05:8.20/8.75:9.20

The TLT now, however, will be slightly too great at 0.025 mm and the lens will effectively fit more tightly. Fitting the next lens flatter, i.e. specification:

7.30:7.70/8.10:8.20/8.85:9.20

would reduce the TLT to 0.017 mm which is significant, but the edge clearance would change only from 0.080 mm to 0.086 mm which is not so

Table 10.15 A partly illustrated fitting set giving a tear layer thickness of 0.020 mm and axial edge clearance of 0.08 mm on corneas of average asphericities

7.25:7.10/7.75:7.60/ 9.15:8.60
7.45:7.30/8.05:7.80/ 9.35:8.80
7.65:7.50/8.35:8.00/ 9.55:9.00
7.85:7.70/8.65:8.20/ 9.75:9.20
8.05:7.90/8.95:8.40/10.00:9.40
8.25:8.10/9.25:8.60/10.25:9.60
8.45:8.30/9.55:8.80/10.50:9.80

All lenses fitted 0.05 mm steeper than K on a cornea with p 0.79.
After Atkinson, 1985.

Table 10.16 Partly illustrated three fitting set approach incorporating the tear layer thickness and edge clearance technique

Set		TLT	AEC	AEL
1	7.25:7.20/7.75:7.70/ 9.15:8.70	0.020	0.081	0.105
	7.85:7.20/8.35:7.70/10.25:8.70	0.015	0.080	0.098
	8.45:7.20/8.95:7.70/11.50:8.70	0.012	0.081	0.095
2	7.25:7.70/8.05:8.20/ 8.75:9.20	0.025	0.079	0.111
	7.85:7.70/8.65:8.20/ 9.75:9.20	0.020	0.080	0.101
	8.45:7.70/9.25:8.20/10.95:9.20	0.016	0.080	0.098
3	7.25:8.30/8.05:8.80/ 8.60:9.80	0.033	0.080	0.123
	7.85:8.30/8.65:8.80/ 9.60:9.80	0.025	0.080	0.111
	8.45:8.30/9.25:8.80/10.60:9.80	0.020	0.079	0.102

After Atkinson, 1985.

significant. For flatter corneas the opposite effect would occur.

A further option would be to reduce the BOZD of the lens for the steeper radii and vice versa. By keeping the same TLT, edge clearance and peripheral curve width, this gives smaller lenses at the steep end and larger lenses at the flat end of the range. This is a logical approach as steep corneas are usually smaller than flat ones. A fitting set on these lines has been designed by Atkinson (1985) and is partly shown in *Table 10.15*.

However, because of the variety of asphericities found for the human cornea as discussed at the beginning of this chapter, at least three different BOZDs and TDs are ideally required and fitting sets based on all the foregoing are now shown in *Table 10.16*.

As we acquire greater understanding of the corneal topography, tear volume under the lens, tear mixing, and tear film formation over and under the lens, more sophisticated lens designs will undoubtedly continue to emerge.

Photoelectric keratoscopy (PEK)

It can be seen from the foregoing that improved fitting techniques have evolved with greater understanding of corneal contour and lens design. The difference in individual corneal asphericities has also been stressed. Generally these differences have to be assessed by fluorescein pattern observation using trial sets. This arises because the keratometer measures radius of curvature by determining the chord length between two reflection areas approximately 3 mm apart. Thus the information is simply the corneal curvature 1.5 mm each side of the visual axis. One attempt to overcome this has been the use of photoelectric keratoscopy where a photograph is taken of a Placido disc-type target reflected from the anterior corneal surface. Several systems are now available, the most well known of which is probably the Wesley–Jessen System 2000.

Practitioners use the PEK to take a polaroid keratograph picture of the cornea. Trial lens fitting is not considered necessary. The photograph is enlarged ×50 and the cornea three-dimensionally mapped by computer analysis.

Information supplied by the practitioner is used in conjunction with the analysis of the cornea to calculate the BOZR, intermediate and peripheral curves. These curves are designed to provide controlled tear layer thickness, parallel bearing surface and controlled lens thickness at the edge of the lens. The computer also calculates the front curve necessary to achieve the required power and any peripheral front curve that may be required to reduce the edge thickness to comfortable proportions.

The system provides for the use and design of both spherical and aspherical back curves. It also designs toroidal back curves to fit toroidal corneas when the corneal toricity exceeds a predetermined amount, and for bi-toric lenses when a toroidal back surface leaves unacceptable residual astigmatism (Bibby, 1976).

The results of the computer analysis are printed on the form shown in *Figure 10.14*. A copy of this is returned to the practitioner along with the patient's lenses.

The advantages of the system are as follows:

(1) Reduction of chair-side time
(2) Common problems occurring from faulty lens design are eliminated because of the computer program.

SYSTEM 2000
CORNEAL ANALYSIS
HAMBLIN CONTACT LENSES LTD. (COMPUTER ANALYSIS)

PATIENT	L E	DATE	29 10 87
PRACTITIONER	/LIVERPOOL	ORDER No.	O/N:000

INPUT DATA

	SPHERE	CYLINDER	AXIS	DIAM	TEAR LAYER THICKNESS	CYCON LIMIT	TRIAL LENS BCOR	BACK VERTEX POWER	DIAM
R	1 - 3.50	3 - 0.50	5 180	9.00	0.005	0.5	10	12 + 0.00	14
L	2 - 3.75	4 - 0.75	6 10	7 9.00	8 0.005	9 0.5	11	13 + 0.00	15

VERTEX DISTANCE	COLOUR	MATERIAL	MARKING	
13.00	GY	XL20		
16 13.00	17 GY	18 XL20	19	20

CONTACT LENSES

	BASE	INTER	PERIPH	THICK	DIAM	BACK VERT PWR	RESID ASTIG	V.I.D.
R	21 8.01	23 8.6	25 11.1	27 0.13	29 9.0	31 - 3.12	33 -0.14	0.0
L	22 8.01	24 8.6	26 10.8	28 0.13	30 9.0	32 - 3.25	34 -0.15	35 0.0

OTHER DATA

BCOR	RH	RV	LH	LV	
	36 8.01	37 7.93	38 8.01	39 7.90	40

NOTES

SOFT 38:   R   9.00/ -3.75/13.5;   L   9.00/ -4.00/13.5

41

APEX 42   RE   mm at   LE   mm at
0.   10   0.   135

	REFERENCE	CORNEA		REFERENCE	CORNEA		REFERENCE	CORNEA		REFERENCE	CORNEA
CENT CURVE 43	7.97	7.97		7.86	7.86		7.96	7.96		7.81	7.81
SHAPE FACTOR 44	.25	0.21	R	.25	0.28	R	.25	0.24	L	.25	0.36
45											
READ ANGLE 46	5			—			180			—	

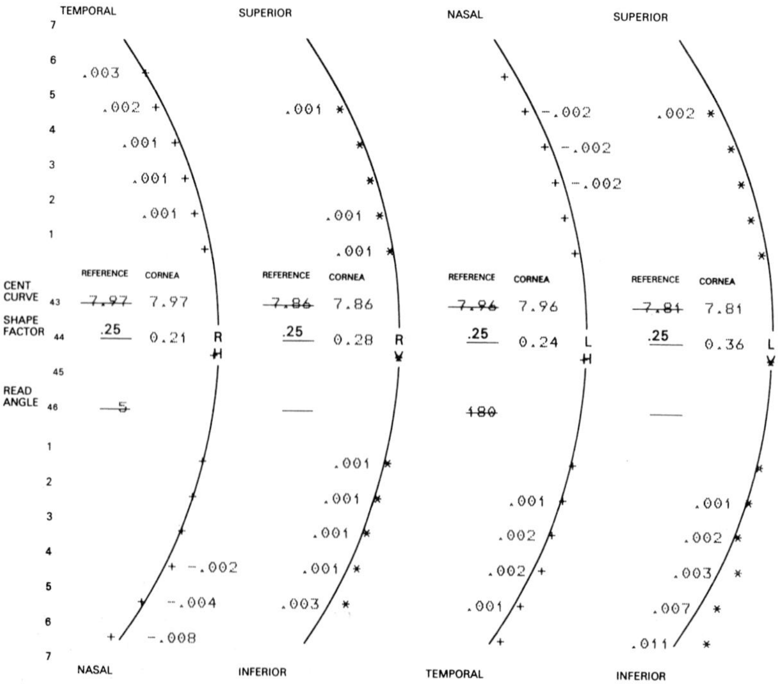

Figure 10.14 Typical Wesley–Jessen System 2000 Computer Analysis Sheet

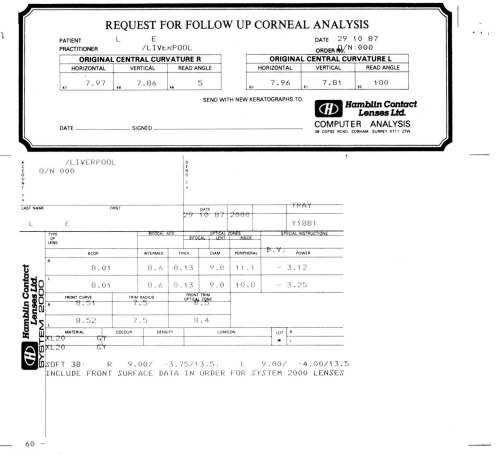

Figure 10.14 (*cont.*)

(3) A high rate of 'first-fit' success and minimal subsequent modification is claimed.

(4) From (3), replacement of lost lenses is straighforward.

(5) Minimal practitioner skill at fitting and lens design is required.

The disadvantages are as follows:

(1) The system is dependent on the accuracy and clarity of the keratograph. Errors in the photograph or measurements taken from it will result in an inaccurate lens.

(2) Factors such as lid hypersensitivity, lid tightness, hyperlacrimation etc., only become apparent if a trial lens is placed on the eye.

(3) Assessment of fluorescein patterns is still essential for proper after-care and deduction of problems so that this skill is still necessary.

(4) No system is any better than the laboratory that actually fabricates the lenses. The system necessitates the use of the laboratory that markets the system with no freedom of practitioner choice.

(5) The PEK typically measures only a 9.00 mm diameter across the cornea. Thus, larger lenses cannot accurately be fitted by the system.

(6) If used for the fitting of soft lenses, no information of the limbal topography is obtained from the keratograph that would be visible by assessment of a trial fitting.

(7) Photokeratoscopy can only be used for normal corneas and does not allow fitting of such cases as keratoconus, postkeratoplasty etc.

(8) The PEK must be purchased as a specific fitting tool.

Total diameter

The oxygen permeability and greater thermal conductivity of most RGP materials allows practitioners to fit larger lenses. This provides three specific advantages:

(1) A larger lens is generally more comfortable because the top edge lies beneath the upper lid. This will apply whether the lens is fitted by the modified contour or lid attachment techniques (*see* earlier).
(2) A larger lens fitted with minimal edge clearance moves less so that there is again less visual or physical awareness of the lens edge.
(3) A larger BOZD is possible which considerably reduces post-blink and night-time flare from refracted light through the peripheral curves. This also allows a flatter BOZR to be used which is ideal to minimize flexure on toroidal corneas (*see below*).

Lens–cornea relationship and lens flexibility

Four factors should be taken into account:

(1) Because the keratometer measures corneal curvature approximately 1.5 mm each side of the visual axis, it will not give the average curvature required for lens alignment with the large BOZDs commonly employed with RGP lenses. The same allowances must be made as under PMMA lenses discussed earlier although the full 0.05 mm flattening for each 0.5 mm increase in BOZD is not applicable as the rate of corneal flattening slows down as one moves away from the corneal apex. Thus a K reading of 7.90 may require a 7.90 mm BOZR lens to give correct alignment over a 7.00 mm BOZD. For an 8.50 mm BOZD this figure would typically only increase to an 8.00 mm BOZR. Ideally trial lenses should always be used to verify the fitting.
(2) When the eyelid moves over the cornea during blinking it presses the eye back about 1.25 mm (Holden, 1984). Clearly the front surface of the contact lens is subjected to considerable force. With PMMA, this results in distortion of the shape of the cornea over years of wear. In the case of the flexible RGP materials, the eyelid succeeds

in distorting the shape of the lens itself. The lens does not then return to its original shape but stays flexed because the surface tension in the tear meniscus around the contact lens edge is sufficient to hold it in place. For PMMA, the critical centre thickness at which flexure on the eye can be observed is about 0.12 mm. For many RGP lenses flexure is still obvious at 0.15 mm (greater for CAB materials).

One would expect to find that, if an RGP lens is placed on a with-the-rule astigmatic cornea, then with-the-rule flexure of the lens on the eye would occur. In practice, not only will the degree of flexure depend upon the rigidity and thickness of the lens being used, but it will also depend upon the lens–cornea relationship. Stone and Collins (1984), Herman (1984) and others have shown that in the case of with-the-rule astigmatic corneas, as the BOZR becomes flatter than the flattest keratometer (K_F) reading, the lens flexes in an *against-the-rule* fashion. Conversely, as the lens BOZR becomes steeper than K_F, the lens flexes in a with-the-rule direction.

The explanation for this is as follows (Herman, 1984): as the lens is fitted flatter, corneal adhesion is minimized while the influence of the upper lid is maximized. The pressure exerted by the upper lid will then be largely against the flat front periphery of the horizontal meridian of the lens (since the lens will have rocked to align the upper half of the corneal vertical meridian). This will cause the horizontal meridian of the lens to steepen which will then be accompanied by a corresponding flattening of the vertical meridian, i.e. the lens will flex against-the-rule. Correspondingly, as a lens is fitted steeper, corneal adhesion is maximized and the influence of the upper lid minimized. Tear film adhesion will obviously cause the lens to flex in the same direction as the corneal toricity, i.e. with-the-rule on a with-the-rule cornea. Herman found mathematically that at approximately 0.14 mm flatter than K, zero flexure (± 0.25 D) was observed, i.e. lid compression and tear film adhesion cancel or negate each other allowing lens rigidity to dominate.

Thus, if a lens is actually required to flex with-the-rule (and sometimes this may be desirable to neutralize internal astigmatism), it might be preferable to fit the lens slightly steep. This should allow the lens to centre so that it is not totally affected by the upper lid and is therefore allowed to flex somewhat with-the-rule. If, after the relationship of the K reading and refractive spectacle correction has been examined, it seems more desirable to minimize or create an against-the-rule effect, then the lens should be fitted flatter, allowing it to ride high, behind the upper lid, maximizing lid compression to minimize with-the-rule flexure.

The numerical BOZR/K reading relationship, however, must only be used as a guideline. Fluorescein patterns must be observed for individual cases. Such factors as peripheral corneal flattening and corneal diameter can make a significant difference. Thus the fluorescein pattern must be coordinated with the measured flexure (by keratometry over the lens) and over-refraction to produce both an optimal fit and visual result. It should be emphasized that, although the lens BOZR may be nominally flatter than K, a large BOZD is commonly used and the fluorescein picture may still be that of corneal alignment.

The foregoing explanation applies only to with-the-rule corneas. In the case of against-the-rule corneas both the tear film adhesion factor and the upper lid forces are additive, both acting in an against-the-rule direction, causing significant flexure in the against-the-rule direction of almost any BOZR placed on the eye. In such cases toric fitting lenses are preferable. The only possible exception is the higher values of hyperopic astigmatism where lens thickness may prevent flexure on the eye.

(3) The increased flexibility of most of the higher Dk RGP lenses reduces their capability of resisting the compression forces created during reflex blinking. If the lens is fitted even slightly on the steep side of alignment, blink-induced compression may create a temporary seal between the periphery of the lens and the underlying cornea. As the lens decompresses during the opening phase of each blink cycle, the resulting hydrodynamic forces can create a transient negative pressure at the corneal surface that will cause increasing lens awareness as well as unstable vision. The fitting of lenses should always therefore be slightly on the flat side of alignment (see also Lens adhesion phenomenon below).

(4) The amount of lens flexure may be influenced not only by peripheral corneal flattening, lid pressure and capillary attraction of the tears, but also by the back surface geometry of the lens and its cross-sectional thickness distribution which themselves have an influence on lid pressure and the tear meniscus. For example, an elliptical back surface lens may flex slightly differently from one with a multi-spherical curve back surface, and a lenticular construction may differ from a non-lenticular construction.

Astigmatism

It can now be appreciated that a different approach to dealing with astigmatism is needed with RGP lenses than for PMMA lenses. Ideally a short tolerance trial should be carried out with lenses of the same material, thickness and diameter as the final lens and practitioners are well advised to stockpile old or non-prescribed lenses for this purpose.

Generally the lower the Dk value of the material and the greater the centre thickness the more similar is the fitting to that of PMMA (see earlier guidelines, p. 350). As the Dk value increases and the centre thickness decreases, the fitting of the BOZR should approach the flatter K reading to slightly flatter than K_F in cases of with-the-rule astigmatism. In the case of against-the-rule astigmatism, the practitioner will fairly quickly require a toroidal back surface lens, if available.

Sevigny and Bennett (1984) advise increasing the centre thickness by 0.02 mm/D of corneal astigmatism or decreasing the BOZD by 0.2–0.4 mm to minimize flexure in cases of with-the-rule astigmatism. It should be remembered, however, that increasing the lens centre thickness will reduce its oxygen transmissibility.

The approach becomes different again as the higher Dk value materials are used and flexibility increases. The Boston Equalens Manual gives the guide to the choice of initial BOZR shown in *Table 10.17*.

Table 10.17 Choice of the initial BOZR as recommended by the Boston Equalens fitting manual

Corneal astigmatism	BOZR (mm) compared to K_F for lens total diameters of		
(D)	8.70 mm	9.20 mm	9.70 mm
0.0–0.50	0.10 flatter	0.10 flatter	0.15 flatter
0.75–1.25	On flat K	0.05 flatter	0.10 flatter
1.50–2.00	0.10 steeper	On flat K	0.05 flatter
2.25–2.75	0.15 steeper	0.05 steeper	On flat K
3.00–3.50	0.20 steeper	0.10 steeper	0.05 steeper

Fitting sets

Various fitting sets have been suggested in *Tables 10.12–10.16*. These are commonly still made from PMMA material as this is less expensive and more resistant to distortion with handling. The variation in flexure with the final lens should be borne in mind as discussed above. Most practitioners will accumulate lenses of different materials rejected for one reason or another and short wearing trials with lenses approximating to the patient's prescription and selected lens material usually prove very helpful.

The use of computers and pocket calculators plus modern instruments allowing the asphericity of the cornea to be determined has led to elegant mathematical approaches to lens design as discussed earlier (*see* Chapters 5 and 6). This trend will undoubtedly continue.

Logically it might be expected that lenses will gradually become single-cut aspherical curves on the back surface. The advantages are largely those of no flare from the peripheral curves and no indentation from transition junctions and hence improved comfort. However, clinical experience at the present time appears to show few advantages for aspherical designs and Forst (cited by Lloyd, 1986) has shown poorer centration with aspheric lenses due to loss of the central tear 'pool', i.e. the small tear lens volume trapped between the spherical back optic zone and aspherical cornea. The negative pressure created in this area when lenses are decentred by lid action or eye movement normally tending to re-centre the lens. For this reason aspheric lenses need to be fitted steeper or larger than spherical designs. Nevertheless, it remains likely

that aspherical designs and fitting sets will become increasingly available over the next few years.

Lens adhesion phenomenon

The intermittent adhesion of the flexible high *Dk* value lenses to the cornea during sleep is a phenomenon almost unique to the overnight wearing of these lenses. Such lenses are found fixed to the underlying cornea, partially overlapping the limbus and with the patient usually asymptomatic. In most instances, the lens adhesion disappears spontaneously shortly after awakening leaving a compression ring that resolves after a few hours (*see Plate 19*). This ring is identified by the instillation of fluorescein which collects in the circular groove. Too steep a fit or poor blending of the peripheral curves should be suspected if the base of the compression groove stains with fluorescein and causes discomfort. Some patients are more susceptible to this phenomenon than others and should be advised to check that the lenses move freely on waking. Patients experiencing occasional adhesion should be instructed to free the lens by compressing the lid margin just above or below the lens to release the suction. Additionally the centre thickness of the lens may be increased by at least 0.03 mm to reduce lens flexure, the BOZR flattened by 0.05–0.15 mm, or the edge clearance increased slightly if the problem persists. However, some patients seem prone to lens binding and overnight wear should be discouraged if this problem resists all corrective measures (*see* Chapter 15).

Swarbrick (1987) has shown that fenestrating RGP lenses has little effect on lens binding indicating that lens flexure or tight fitting is not necessarily the causative factor. Sodium fluorescein also penetrates only very slowly under bound lens, spreading in a fern-like pattern. From these observations, Swarbrick postulates that the lens preferentially expresses the aqueous layer of the tear film overnight leaving the mucous layer to act as an adhesive between lens and cornea.

Three and nine o'clock staining

Although 3 and 9 o'clock staining of the exposed peripheral cornea is often seen in PMMA lens wearers (*see* Chapter 19 and *Plate 20*), it is more commonly observed in RGP lens wearers for the following reasons:

(1) The reduced edge clearance techniques used minimize lens movement.
(2) The larger lens TDs increase edge thickness for negative-powered lenses.
(3) Many gas permeable materials themselves, because of their tendency to attract deposits, cause reduced surface wettability and hence disruption to the tear film.

The effect of these is to create an inadequate tear film in the exposed 3 and 9 o'clock areas which leads to corneal dessication. While minor 3 and 9 o'clock staining may be acceptable, persistant or marked conditions may lead to dellen (thinning of the epithelium), erosions and possible eventual local neovascularization or ulceration. Where necessary, the following action should be taken:

(1) Thin the edges if considered thick.
(2) Check the lens has not been fitted too steeply.
(3) Give blink exercises and lateral eye movement exercises.
(4) Flatten peripheral curves to create more lens movement.
(5) Increase lens TD if considered small or decrease TD if considered too large.
(6) Steepen the peripheral curves if considered excessively flat.
(7) Flatten the fitting to utilize the lid attachment technique, i.e. create more lens movement.
(8) Try a better wetting material.
(9) Use in-eye lubricant drops.

Changes in BOZR

As discussed earlier, the changes occurring with PMMA lenses during hydration and dehydration are well known. The plethora of new RGP materials has discouraged the accumulation of similar data which would be of clinical value to the contact lens practitioner.

CAB materials are known to be at least, if not more, sensitive to hydration–dehydration changes as PMMA. Pearson (1977, 1978) and Smith (1979) found flattening of 0.05–0.10 mm in BOZR with hydration, with the degree of flattening increasing as the lens centre thickness decreased and high minus lenses being quite unstable.

The incorporation of wetting agents, such as methacrylic acid, into a silicone–acrylate polymer can be responsible for the BOZR flattening observed when this group of lens materials is hydrated. If this change is modest, consistent and limited to the higher minus powers, it is acceptable. Because of the lower water uptake than either PMMA and CAB, the silicone–acrylate group generally undergoes smaller hydration changes than these other two groups of materials. Significant and unpredictable fluctuation in BOZR measurements that occur after hydration are undesirable and may reflect a weakness in the design or polymerization of the material. Because of its potential to alter the anticipated fit and visual correction of the lens, the dimensional stability of all new products should ideally be evaluated by measuring the BOZR of a series of negative-powered lenses before and after 24 hours of hydration.

Occasionally flattening of lens BOZR will be observed that cannot be explained by normal hydration changes, e.g. 0.05–0.20 mm flattening on low-powered lenses. The common cause would appear to be stress put on the lens during the lathe-cutting process in the form of heat transfer (Schwartz, 1986). If the laboratory technician runs the cutting lathe too fast, makes the cuts too fast or too deep, polishes the lens too long or does not use enough coolant, then stress is induced into the lens which will cause the subsequent lens flattening. This stress may be cumulative and is also more likely if the practitioner orders a lens too thin for a particular material. Finally, stress-induced flattening is more likely in larger diameter and higher minus-powered lenses due to the difference in thickness between lens edge and centre. To minimize this effect, front surface lenticulation should be ordered from around lens BVPs of −3.0 D and +1.0 D upwards as opposed to the ±5.0 D upwards of PMMA lenses.

Walker (1987) has reported BOZR flattening with hydration of the order of 0.10 mm for −7.50 D and 0.25 mm for −15.00 D lenses made from Paraperm EW and 0.17 mm for −15.00 D lenses made from Boston IV and Equalens. Unlike PMMA, high positive-powered lenses (+15.00 D) are steepened by 0.05 mm for Paraperm EW and Equalens and 0.03 mm for

Boston IV material. Interestingly by using photokeratograms Walker has shown that these curvature changes are largely restricted to the central 3–4 mm so that the effect on fitting (but not vision) may not be as great as may be expected. Ideally all RGP materials, especially CAB, should be hydrated before being dispensed, and the BOZR periodically monitored.

Surface crazing and cracking phenomenon

Over a period of time, many patients show deposit build-up on lens surfaces. In some patients this appears as plaques or areas of deposit, while in others it may appear as surface lines or patterns. In this situation of surface crazing, the answer lies in improving the patient's cleaning regimen and including the addition of extra or more frequent use of proteolytic enzymes. Surface crazing is also amenable to repolishing by the laboratory.

More serious is the appearance of surface cracking. These are deep fissures within the lens surface (*Figure 10.15* and *Plate 27*) and, at the time of writing, appear largely in the higher *Dk* silicone–acrylate group of materials. Early research by the author does not appear to show causative factors as either ultraviolet or preservative exposure. It may possibly originate from either surface stress introduced during lens manufacture and ultimately show as cracking from repeated flexure during blinking on the eye or from constant hydration–dehydration changes.

Surface cracking is often not visible to the patient, but symptoms of slight loss of comfort and visual deterioration are presented, especially if the cracking is central. Only rarely does it show on the lens back surface (Grohe, Caroline and Norman, 1987). Cracking is visible to the practitioner either by slit lamp examination or hand-held magnifier. It cannot be removed by repolishing and, in view of the subjective symptoms and potential for a bacterial nidus or base for foreign bodies or deposits, lens replacement is the only answer.

Lens care and maintenance

The solutions used with RGP lenses have been discussed in Chapter 4. Patients who have been previous PMMA wearers must be warned of the greater fragility of RGP materials, their greater vulnerability to scratching and distortion, and the greater emphasis on cleaning necessary. Specifically, patients should be advised to:

(1) Exercise care when retrieving lenses from the storage case, especially if the lens has been inadvertently placed in its compartment convex side up.
(2) Minimize lens compression during cleaning and handling.
(3) Clean the lenses in the palm of the hand as with a soft lens rather than between the thumb and fingers.
(4) Avoid handling the lenses by the opposing edges.
(5) Avoid dropping the lenses on hard surfaces and exercise care when retrieving a dropped lens.
(6) Be sure that the lens is centred in the storage compartment before it is closed to avoid edge breakage during closing.
(7) Use only solutions advised by the practitioner as being suitable for the lens material prescribed.
(8) Regularly check the lens for deposit build-up after drying and observing against a good light (*see Plate 25*). Most patients will benefit by the intermittent use (typically monthly) of an enzymatic cleaner.

Re-fitting the former PMMA wearer

Although RGP lenses are rapidly becoming the material of first choice for all patients requiring a rigid lens, moderate numbers of former PMMA wearers require re-fitting with RGP lenses. The change of material is often helpful for patients with marked spectacle blur, persistent corneal staining or decreased wearing time.

Methods of re-fitting long-term PMMA wearers include reducing wearing time, or immediate re-fitting. The advantages of immediate re-fitting with RGP lenses are that patients are not inconvenienced, because they can continue full-time wear with rigid lenses and, in most cases, experience no significant drop in visual acuity or inhibition of corneal recovery with the new lenses. However, the decision as to the optimum method of re-fitting depends upon the state of the patient's corneas.

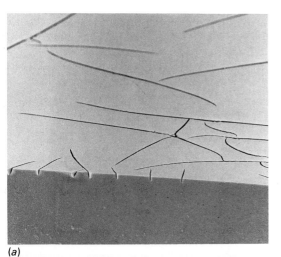

(a)

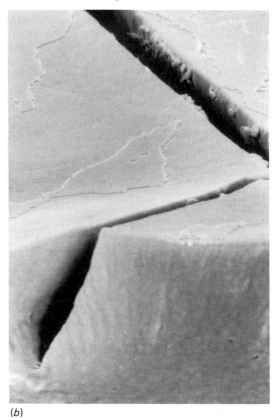

(b)

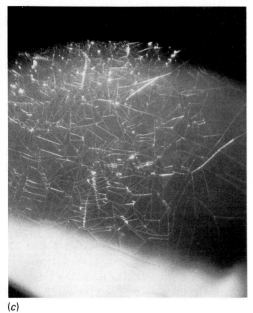

(c)

Figure 10.15 Surface cracking of an RGP lens. (*a*) Low magnification in cross-section showing both the surface pattern and depth of crack. (*b*) High magnification showing debris accumulating in the crack. Surface protein deposits are also visible. (*c*) Slit lamp appearance of surface cracking on the eye (*see also Plate 27*)

To make an adequate assessment of corneal physiology (staining, oedema etc.) and post-wear spectacle refraction and acuity, a preliminary evaluation of the patient's PMMA lenses should be scheduled after a minimum of 4 hours of lens wear. If the induced changes are minimal, the patient can be re-fitted at that time. If excessive corneal staining, oedema, significant spectacle refractive or acuity changes, or keratometric mire distortion is present, a more feasible option would be to gradually decrease the patient's lens wear, possibly one eye at a time if that is helpful, to the minimum number of hours possible. Spectacles,

if available, usually fail to provide adequate visual acuity so that a decrease to 8–12 hours of lens wear is the minimum schedule most patients will adhere to.

The patient should then maintain a limited wearing schedule until the dispensing visit of the re-fitted RGP lenses. Although the patient's progress should be closely monitored, immediate full-day wear or rapid re-adaptation can be instructed. Spectacles can also be prescribed once the patient's refraction has stabilized although this may be 3–12 weeks after dispensing, depending on the severity of the corneal changes. In the case of heavily distorted corneas, patients should be warned that further re-fitting is sometimes necessary as corneal regularity and curvature stabilize following the first re-fitting. A return to the original pre-PMMA-fitting keratometer readings often indicates when stability has been reached. If these are not available a request to the patient's original practitioner will often provide the necessary information.

Patients re-fitted with RGP lenses may initially complain of lens awareness even though the lens fitting may be excellent and corneal physiology improved. This 'initial transfer irritability' occurs because corneal sensation usually improves when a gas permeable lens is worn. Thus a PMMA lens-wearing patient who tolerates corneal oedema, erosions or epithelial infiltrates because of corneal hypaesthesia may be quite irritable with new lenses that are gas permeable even though the corneal state is much improved. The symptoms of increased sensation usually last 2–4 weeks and the patient *must* be warned in advance to accept this.

Ordering RGP lenses

RGP lenses are ordered in the same manner as that for PMMA lenses described earlier but with the following variations:

(1) *Material* — this should be clearly stated, e.g.

   Polycon II, Paraperm EW etc.

(2) *Thickness* — manufacturers literature should be studied for each material but in general the centre thicknesses should be 0.02–0.04 thicker than those shown in *Table 10.10*.

(3) *Engraving* — where possible a suitably obvious code for the lens material should be ordered in addition to the normal R, L or dots, e.g.

   'BOS' for Boston material, 'ALB' for Alberta material etc.

Identification of RGP materials

From time to time, every practitioner is confronted by a patient wearing corneal lenses who has a complication, such as oedema, corneal staining or spectacle blur, of an unacceptable degree. If the lenses were fitted elsewhere, the practitioner must first establish the material from which the lenses are made. If the nature of the material can be discovered, correct management of the problem is facilitated. In some cases, this will constitute re-fitting with a RGP material or an alternative RGP material of high oxygen permeability.

There are several ways of identifying the material:

(1) *Ask the patient* — often the patient is aware of the fact that he or she is wearing RGP lenses if not the specific material. Specific solutions or cleaning techniques may give useful clues. Some patients are issued with lens prescriptions or identification cards. The patient's former practitioner, if available, will usually be able to supply relevant clinical information.

(2) *Check the lens* — some practitioners engrave a code to identify the lens material as mentioned earlier.

(3) *Spectroscopy* — in theory, lens materials may be identified by spectroscopy, principally in the infrared region (Pearson, 1986). While materials may be identified in terms of their general groups, e.g. silicone–acrylate, batch variations of materials and even variation along rods of materials, make specific identification difficult.

(4) *Specific gravity* — Refojo and Leong (1984) used a series of 21 solutions of calcium chloride with concentrations ranging from 18% to 38%. Specific gravity was established by noting the solution in which the lens neither floated nor sank upon immersion. Materials of higher oxygen permeability were associated with lower values of specific gravity.

A simplified specific gravity test has been devised for use by the contact lens practitioner or manufacturer (Whitford, 1984). The lens, or button, is placed in a solution the specific gravity of which is probably about 1.17. Lenses or buttons which float are deemed to be gas permeable while samples which sink are either PMMA or CAB. Practitioner kits available for material identification include the Opti-Mis (Optacryl) and Clik Kit (Paragon). Specific gravities of various materials are shown in *Table 10.11*.

Disadvantages of RGP lenses

The advantages of RGP lenses over PMMA and hydrogel lenses were listed at the beginning of this section. It is now possible to list their disadvantages.

(1) Patients experience the typical hard lens initial discomfort, although this is often less than with PMMA lenses if larger total diameters are used. Foreign bodies under the lens are still experienced.
(2) There is still some potential for corneal distortion.
(3) Greater incidence of 3 and 9 o'clock staining.
(4) Problems due to lens flexure.
(5) Distort and scratch more easily than PMMA lenses.
(6) Shorter life and more expensive than PMMA lenses.
(7) Because of flexure and larger total diameters, toric lenses are more frequently necessary than smaller, PMMA lenses.
(8) More prone to deposits than PMMA. Greater care and cost of upkeep is therefore necessary, although this is less than for hydrogel lenses.
(9) Reduced range and depth of tints compared to both PMMA and hydrogels.

Summary

In spite of the disadvantages of gas permeable lenses just discussed, there is no doubt that these materials will displace all but a small proportion of PMMA lenses fitted over the next few years. Competition between material manufacturers is such that materials of higher oxygen permeability, better wettability, reduced deposit tendency, greater rigidity etc., are increasingly likely to become available. Gas permeable lenses have found increasing favour with practitioners and are becoming the lenses of first choice in a growing number of cases.

The final lens

Whatever the lens material, the final lens is first checked as described in Chapter 12. Ideally, the transitions are blended to facilitate tear flow under the lens and prevent bubble entrapment and corneal abrasion. The lenses are fully hydrated before being checked on the eye — carried out in the same manner as in the fitting routine. A gradual transition across the lens from touch to clearance is the ideal for most fitting philosophies. If any hard blue arcuate bearing areas (possibly indicative of a relatively sharp transition or too steep a peripheral curve) are apparent, either with the lens centred or as it moves on the cornea, these should be blended.

The patient is instructed in the wear and handling of his lenses, as described in Chapter 9 and the period of after-care then begins.

Acknowledgements

The author wishes to acknowledge the help and constructive comments made in the preparation of this chapter by Janet Stone, Terry Atkinson and Chris Kerr.

References

ARIAS, C. M. (1960). Are we measuring the true apex of the cornea with the keratometer? *Contacto* **4,** 195–198

ATKINSON, K. W. and PHILLIPS, A. J. (1971). Fenestrations in corneal lenses. *Br. J. physiol. Optics* **26**, 1–14

ATKINSON, T. C. O. (1984). A re-appraisal of the concept of fitting rigid hard lenses by the tear layer and edge clearance technique. *J. Br. Contact Lens Ass.* **7**, 106–110

ATKINSON, T. C. O. (1985). A computer assisted and clinical assessment of current trends in gas permeable design. *Optician* **189** (4976), 16–22

ATKINSON, T. C. O. and KERR, C. (1987). The Kelvin equalens design. *Optician* **193** (5078), 20–29

AUGSBURGER, A. R. and HILL, R. M. (1971). Contact lens mass: the most elusive feature. *J. Am. optom. Ass.* **42**, 78–82

BAKER, T. Y. (1943). Ray tracing through non-spherical surfaces. *Proc. phys. Soc.* **55**, 361–364

BARR, J. T. (1984) Contact lens materials. Aspheric hard corneal contact lenses are better? *Int. Contact Lens Clin.* **11**, 204

BARR, J. T. and HETTLER, D. H. (1984). Effects of emulsion cleaners on Silcon lenses. *Contact Lens Forum* **9**(11), 45–49

BAYSHORE, C. A. (1962). Report on 276 patients fitted with micro-corneal lenses, apical clearance and central ventilation. *Am. J. Optom.* **39**, 552–553

BAYSHORE, C. A. (1963). Report on 600 cases of micro-corneal lenses fitted with apical clearance. *Am. J. Optom.* **40**, 351–353

BENNETT, A. G. (1966). The calibration of keratometers. *Optician* **151**, 317–322

BENNETT, A. G. (1968). Aspherical contact lens surfaces. *Ophthal. Optician* **8**, 1037–1040, 1297–1300, 1311; **9**, 222–230

BENNETT, A. G. (1988). Aspherical and continuous curve contact lenses. *Optom. Today* **28**, 11–14, 140–142, 238–242, 433–444

BERGEVIN, J. and MILLODOT, M. (1967). Glare with ophthalmic and corneal lenses. *Am. J. Optom.* **44**, 213–221

BIBBY, M. M. (1976). Computer assisted photokeratoscopy and contact lens design. *Optician* **171**(4423), 37–44; **171**(4424), 11–17; **171**(4426), 15–17

BIBBY, M. M. (1979). Factors affecting peripheral curve design. Part II. *Am. J. Optom.* **56**, 618–627

BIER, N. (1956). A study of the cornea in relation to contact lens practice. *Am. J. Optom.* **33**, 291–304

BIER, N. (1957). The Contour lens. *J. Am. optom. Ass.* **28**, 394–396

BIER, N. (1957). *Contact Lens Routine and Practice*, 2nd rev. edn, pp. 194–195. London: Butterworths

BOYD, H. H. (1965). Perforation of contact lenses. *Am. J. Ophthal.* **60**, 726–728

BRITISH STANDARD 5562 (1978). *Specification for Contact Lenses*. London: British Standards Institution

BRITISH STANDARD 3521 (1979). *Glossary of Terms Relating to Ophthalmic Lenses and Spectacle Framess — BS 3521: 1979. Part 3. Glossary of Terms Relating to Contact Lenses*. London: British Standards Institution

BRUCKER, D. (1975). Laser fenestrated lenses. Chapter 20 in *Micro-Corneal and Soft Contact Lenses* by S. K. Dastoor. Bombay: Popular Prakashan

BRUNGARDT, T. F. (1984). Eccentricity of the corneal topography. *Int. Contact Lens Clin.* **11**, 214–218

BUREK, H. (1987). Conics, corneae and keratometry. *Optician* **194** (5122), 18–33

CAROLINE, P. J. and ELLIS, E. J. (1986). Review of the mechanisms of oxygen transport through rigid gas permeable lenses. *Int. Eyecare* **2**(4), 210–213

DAVIS, H. E. (1964). Why the small contact lens? *Br. J. physiol. Optics* **21**. 215–218

DE CARLE, J. (1965). A comparison of materials used in the manufacture of contact lenses. *Contact Lens Practnr* **6**, 29–32

DE CARLE, J. (1967). Small lenses. *Contact Lens Practnr.* **8**, 9–11

DICKINSON, F. (1954). Report on a new corneal lens. *Optician* **128**(3303), 3–6

FRIEDBERG, M. A. (1961). Contact lens apertures and toric curve designs. *J. Am. optom Ass.* **32**, 642–644

GEGG, B. R. (1969). Aspherical contact lenses — development and doubts. *Contact Lens* **2**(5), 20–24, 31

GILES, G. H. (1960). *The Principles and Practice of Refraction*. London: Hammond & Hammond

GORDON, S. (1965). Contact lens hydration: a study of the wetting-drying cycle. *Optom. Wkly* **56**, 55–62

GROHE, R. M., CAROLINE, P. J. and NORMAN, C. (1987). Rigid gas permeable surface cracking. *Contact Lens Spectrum* May, 37–45

GUILLON, M., LYDON, D. P. M. and SAMMONS, W. A. (1983). Designing rigid gas permeable contact lenses using the edge clearance technique. *J. Br. Contact Lens Ass.* **6**, 19–26

GUILLON, M., LYDON, D. P. M. and WILSON, C. (1986). Corneal topography: a clinical model. *Ophthal. physiol. Opt.* **6**, 47–56

HAYNES, P. R. (1960). Aperture venting techniques in corneal contact lenses. In *Encyclopedia of Contact Lens Practice*, edited by P. R. Haynes, South Bend, Indiana: International Optics Publishing Corporation

HERMAN, J. P. (1984). Lens flexure: clinical rules. *J. Am. optom. Ass.* **55**, 169–171

HERSH, D. (1974). The Hersh palpebral traction lens. *Int. Contact Lens Clin.* **1**(4), 65–71

HILL, R. M. and UNIACKE, N. P. (1968). Lacrimal fluid and lens design. *Contacto* **12**, 59–61

HODD, F. A. B. (1958). Clinical experience in fitting microlenses. *Br. J. physiol. Optics* **15**, 205–226

HODD, F. A. B. (1966). A design study of the back surface of corneal contact lenses. *Ophthal. Optician* **6**, 1175–1178, 1187–1190, 1203, 1229–1232, 1235–1238; **7**, 14–16, 19–21, 39

HOLDEN, B. A. (1984). Predicting contact lens flexure from in-vitro tests. *J. Am. optom. Ass.* **55**, 171

JESSEN, G. N. (1961). New bifocal technique results in more comfortable single vision lenses. *Contacto* **5**, 237–243

KORB, D. R. (1961). Contact lens news and views: application of multiple micro-holes. *J. Am. optom. Ass.* **32**, 11, 891–892

KORB, D. R. (1962a). The evolution of fenestrated corneal lenses. *Pennsylvania Optom.* **22**(3), 23–28

KORB, D. R. (1962b). Recent advances in corneal lens fenestration. In *Encyclopedia of Contact Lens Practice*. Vol. **3**, Suppl. 14, pp. 58–66, edited by P. R. Haynes. Sound Bend, Indiana: International Optics Publishing Corporation

KORB, D. R. and FILDERMAN, I. P. (1961). A new approach to contact lens ventilation. *Optom. Wkly* **52**, 2375

KORB, D. R. and KORB, J. E. (1974). Fitting to achieve a normal blinking and lid action. *Int. Contact Lens Clin.* **1**(3), 57–70

LESTER, R. and BRAFF, S. (1963). The management of small corneal contact lenses. Calcon Comment, El Monte, California. Cited by R. B. Mandell in *Contact Lens Practice, Basic and Advanced*. Springfield, Ill.: Thomas

LLOYD, M. (1986). Is there a future for rigid aspherics? *Optician* **191** (5032), 21

MACKIE, I. A. (1973). Design compensation in corneal lens fitting. In *Symposium on Contact Lenses: Transactions of the New Orleans Academy of Ophthalmology*. St Louis: Mosby

MACKIE, I. A., MASON, D. and PERRY, B. J. (1970). Factors influencing corneal contact lens centration. *Br. J. physiol. Optics* **25**, 87–103

MANDELL, R. B. (1974). What is the gravity lens? *Int. Contact Lens Clin.* **1**(4), 29–35

MOORE, C. (1974). A new concept for fitting ultrathin lenses. *Int. Contact Lens Clin.* **1**(3), 47–54

MORRISON, R. J. (1967). Minalens technique. *Refractionist* January/March, 35–44

NEILL, J. C. (1967). Electronic venting of corneal contact lenses. *Contacto* **11**, 9–11

PEARSON, R. M. (1977). Dimensional stability of several hard contact lens materials. *Am. J. Optom. physiol. Optics* **54**, 826–833

PEARSON, R. M. (1978). Dimensional stability of lathe-cut CAB lenses. *J. Am. optom. Ass.* **49**, 927–929

PEARSON, R. M. (1986). The clinical performance of hard gas-permeable lenses. *Clin. Exp. Optom.* **69**, 98–102

PHILLIPS, A. J. (1968). Filters used by drivers at night. *Ophthal. Optician* **8**, 707–713, 756–763

PHILLIPS, A. J. (1969). Alterations in curvature of the finished corneal lens. *Ophthal. Optician* **9**, 980–986, 1043–1054, 1100–1110 ·

RABBETTS, R. B. (1976). Large corneal lenses with constant axial edge lift. *Ophthal. Optician* **16**, 236, 239

REFOJO, M. F. and LEONG, F. L. (1984). Identification of hard contact lenses by their specific gravity. *Int. Contact Lens Clin.* **11**, 79–82

RUBEN, M. (1966). Use of conoidal curves in corneal contact lenses. *Br. J. Ophthal.* **50**, 642–645

SCHWARTZ, C. A. (1986). Radical flattening and RGP lenses. *Contact Lens Forum* **11**(8), 49–53

SELLERS, F. J. E. (1960). The adjustment of multi-curved corneal lenses. *Contact Lens Practnr* **1**, 26–32

SELLERS, F. J. E. (1964). Fenestrations first — not last. *Contacto* **8**(2), 17–30

SEVIGNY, J. and BENNETT, E. (1984). Trouble shooting with silicone acrylate lenses. *Rev. Optom.* **122**(12), 24–30

SHERIDAN, M. (1970). The investigation of corneal form. *Ophthal. Optician* **10**, 892–894

SMITH, H. C. (1979). A study of the stability of lenses fabricated from cellulose acetate butyrate. *Int. Contact Lens Clin.* **16** (4), 190–193

STAHL, N., REICH, L. and IVANI, M. S. (1974). Report on laboratory studies and preliminary clinical application of a gas-permeable plastic contact lens. *J. Am. optom. Ass.* **45**, 302–307

STEELE, E. (1969). The fitting of aspheric contact lenses. *Contacto* **4**, 55–58

STEK, A. W. (1975). Conic contact lens — design and fitting technique. *Optician* **169**(4378), 30–35

STONE, J. (1975). Corneal lenses with constant axial edge lift. *Ophthal. Optician* **15**, 818–824

STONE, J. (1978). Changes in curvature of cellulose acetate butyrate lenses during hydration and dehydration. *J. Br. Contact Lens Ass.* **1**, 22–35

STONE, J. and COLLINS, C. (1984). Flexure of gas-permeable lenses on toroidal corneas. *Optician* **188**(4951), 8–10

SWARBRICK, H. (1987). Paper read to the Sixth International Australian Contact Lens Congress, Surfers Paradise, Queensland

THOMAS, P. F. (1967). *Conoid Contact Lenses*. Australia: Corneal Lens Corporation

WALKER, J. (1987). Poster presentation. British Contact Lens Association, Clinical Conference, Windsor, UK

WHITFORD, M. J. (1984). More about those Bostons. *Ophthal. Optician* **24**, 90

WRAY, L. (1963). An elementary analysis of the forces retaining a corneal contact lens on the eye. *Optician* **146**, 239–241, 373–376

Chapter 11

Soft (hydrogel) lens fitting

Andrew Gasson

During the last 15 years, hydrophilic lenses have remained one of the fastest developing aspects of a constantly evolving contact lens technology. This has been due to improvements and changes in polymers and materials, techniques of manufacture, cleaning and disinfection procedures and methods of fitting. Within this timespan the status of soft lenses has changed from occasional experimental use in difficult cases to a routine and indispensable part of contact lens practice.

Terminology

Since their introduction, in addition to brand names, the new lenses have become known by a variety of descriptions, such as soft, hydrophilic, hydrogel, gel, flexible, and pliable, in order to distinguish them from both corneal lenses, which are now described as hard, PMMA, stable, rigid or firm, and gas permeables (GPs). 'Soft' (defined as yielding to pressure), with the advantage of simplicity, has become the most acceptable and widely used term. Hydrophilic (water loving), although applicable to most lenses mentioned in this chapter, is not a strictly accurate description, since it is more properly used to define the surface characteristics of a material in relation to the angle of contact, or wetting angle (*see* Chapter 3). It is a term which can also be applied to hard lenses and rigid gas permeable lenses, so that a hydrophobic hard lens may be coated to become hydrophilic. Similarly, a flexible silicone lens is extremely hydrophobic unless the surface is treated to become hydrophilic. The term 'hydrogel' signifies a material made from a hydrogel polymer, which absorbs and binds water into its molecular structure. It usefully describes those lenses mentioned as having a percentage water content, although not all hydrogels need necessarily be soft. Before hydration these hydrogels are

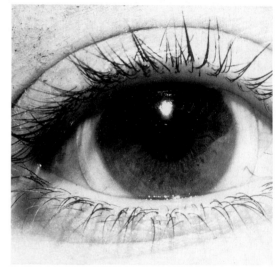

(a)

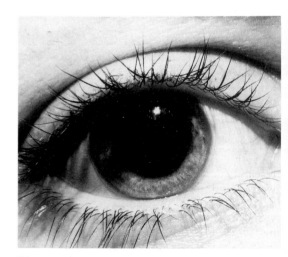

(b)

Figure 11.1 (*a*) Large diameter, high water content semi-scleral lens. (*b*) Corneal diameter soft lens

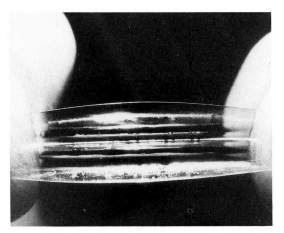

Figure 11.2 The elastic property of a low water content hydrophilic lens being stretched

referred to as zerogels. Within the category of hydrogels there are a great many individual polymers, some of which, such as hydroxyethyl methacrylate (HEMA), have themselves become generic. *Figure 11.1a, b* shows, respectively, a high water content semi-scleral lens, and a corneal diameter lens which cosmetically is almost invisible on the eye. *Figure 11.2* shows the considerable elasticity of a typical soft lens.

Historical background

The first soft lenses were produced in Czechoslovakia by Wichterle and Lim, two polymer chemists from the Prague Institute of Macro-Molecular Physics. Having worked in association with Dreifus, they reported that certain hydrogels developed for biological application could successfully be used for the manufacture of contact lenses (Wichterle and Lim, 1960). The early lenses, known as Geltact or Spofa, were made by spin-casting HEMA. They were successful in a country which had no hard lens industry, but when compared by foreign researchers with their own corneal lenses, they were found to be difficult to fit and to give unsatisfactory vision. The material was of variable quality and the lifespan short. They nevertheless represent an important milestone in the history of contact lenses, for they provided the impetus to the rest of the world for the vast programmes of research and development undertaken since that time into new materials

and lens forms. This has resulted in soft lenses being routinely fitted in practice as an acceptable form of visual correction and, indeed, they are now the lenses of first choice for a high proportion of patients.

The rights to the Czechoslovakian lens were acquired in 1965 by the American company, National Patent Development Corporation, who in turn, during 1966, licensed Bausch & Lomb in the USA to continue its manufacture by the spin-casting process. At the same time production of lenses was started in various other countries around the world by the more usual method of lathing or 'lathe-cutting' under the name of Hydron, as well as using the same HEMA material for many other applications such as biological implants. Bausch & Lomb spent 5 years in improving and developing all aspects of the spun-cast lenses, and eventually gained approval from the US Food and Drugs Administration (FDA) in March 1971.

In the mid-1960s a great many non-HEMA materials were investigated and the Bionite lens appeared in 1969, together with the then new method of semi-scleral fitting.

In the UK, Sauflon material was investigated from 1968, and fitted to patients in 1970, at about the same time as early Permalenses were first fitted (de Carle, 1972). Bionite was first prescribed in 1971, Hydron early in 1972, and the Bausch & Lomb Soflens in July of the same year. Since then there has been a huge proliferation of new materials and lenses, mostly HEMA based and for daily use. The majority of early high water content soft lenses, despite the recognition of their physiological advantages for problem solving, did not gain widespread acceptance because of repeated difficulty with fragility, reproducibility and discolouration.

By the mid-1970s, when it was realized that the HEMA lenses then used could cause problems such as oedema, vascularization, arcuate staining and giant papillary conjunctivitis (alternatively referred to as contact lens-induced papillary conjunctivitis), soft lenses evolved into smaller and thinner designs of the same low water content material because of the, by then, predictable problems with high water content lenses. Indeed, 'thin' HEMA maintained its almost universal position and continued to work very well for daily use despite the introduction of medium to high water content lenses, such as Hydrocurve II and Duragel, with

Table 11.1 Properties of commonly available soft lenses

Lens	Laboratory	H_2O^a	Dk^b	T(°C)	Polymer	Fit	Remarks	Daily/extended wear (D/EW)
Hydron Mini	Allergan Hydron	38.6	8.0	21	HEMA	C		D
Hydron Zero 6/Z Plus		38.6	8.0	21	HEMA	SD		D
Hydron Z4		38.6	8.6	21	HEMA	SD	Cast-moulded	D/EW
Hydron HX		65	26 / 30	23 / 34	HEMA + MA	SD		D/EW
Soflens/ Sofspin	Bausch & Lomb	38.6	{9.2/ 8.0/	35/ 21	HEMA	C+S/S	Spun-cast	D/EW
Optima 38		38.6	{9.2/ 8.0/	35/ 21	HEMA	SD	Spun-cast and lathed	D
B & L 70		70	23.4	35	NVP + HMA + AMA + EGDMA	SD		D/EW
CW 79		79	46.5	21	Copolymer of NVP + MMA + AMA + EGDMA	SD	For aphakia	EW
Hydrothin/Hydrolens	Cantor & Silver	38	8.0	21	HEMA	C+S/S		D
Hydrofit		38	8.0	21	HEMA	SF		D
Hydrolens E		72.4	33	35	HEMA-based	C		EW
Hydrofit HP55		35	17	55	Terpolymer of MMA + G-MEMA	C+S/S		D/EW
Weicon 38E/38EX	CIBA Vision (Titmus)	38.6	{8.5/ 7.3	35/ 21	HEMA	C	Aspheric	D/EW
Weicon CE60		60	28	35	Copolymer of MMA + VP	C+S/S	Aspheric	D/EW
CIBA Soft		38	{8.5/ 7.3	35/ 21	HEMA	SD		D
Scanlens 75		71	36	35	Terpolymer of NVP + acrylic monomers	C+S/S		D/EW
Sauflon 70	CLM	70	39	35	Copolymer of NVP + MMA	C+S/S		D
Sauflon 77		77	50	35	Copolymer of NVP + MMA	C+S/S		D/EW
Sauflon PW		70	57.4	35	Copolymer of NVP + MMA	C+S/S		EW
Permalens	CooperVision	71	34.3 42.0	20 36	Terpolymer of HEMA + NVP + MA	C+S/S		EW
Permaflex		74	34.0 43.0	25 36	Copolymer of MMA + VP + MMA + other methacrylates	SD	Cast-moulded	D/EW
Cooperthin		38	8.5	25	HEMA	SF	Cast-moulded	D
Lunelle ES70	Essilor	70	35	25	Copolymer of PMMA + PVP	C		D/EW
Hoya Soft	Hoya	35	7	30	HEMA copolymer	C		D

Lens	Manufacturer	Water content (%)[a]	Oxygen permeability[b]		Polymer	Fit	Features	Wear
Igel CD	Igel International	38.6	7.0	20	HEMA	SD		D
			13	35				
Igel 67		67.5	17	21	Terpolymer of VP + hydrophobic monomers	SD		D/EW
			29	35				
Igel 77		76.5	33	21	Terpolymer of VP + hydrophobic monomers	SD	Cast-moulded	D/EW
			46	35				
Incanto 78	Nissel	78	64	37	Copolymer of PMMA + PVP	C+S/S		D/EW
Hyperthin 45 (ICL)		45	22.2	35	HEMA + EGDMA + PMMA + PVP	SD		D
CSI/CSIT	Pilkington Barnes–Hind	38.5	12	34.5	GMA + MMA	C+S/S	Non-HEMA low water content	D/EW
Hydrocurve II 55		55	19.2	36	Copolymer of HEMA + Acrylamide + MA	S/S		D/EW
Softmate II		55	19.2	36	Acrylate VP	S/S		D/EW
Polysoft 70		67.5	39.5	35				D/EW
Alges	University Optical Products	45	11.3	35	Copolymer of HEMA + NVP	SD	Bifocal	D
Vistamarc	Vistakon (Johnson & Johnson)	58	20	35	Random copolymer of HEMA + MA + EGDMA + TPT	SF	Toric	D/EW
Vistakon UV Bloc		58	20	35		C+S/S		D/EW
Acuvue		58	20	35		C+S/S	Disposable lens	D/EW
Hydroflex/mini/SD	Wöhlk–Contact–Linsen (Zeiss)	38.6	7.3	21	HEMA	C		D
Geaflex 70		69	43.1	21	Copolymer of MMA + VP	C+S/S		D
Weflex 55		55	23.1	21	Copolymer of polyalkyl methacrylate + VP	C+S/S		D

Many other good quality comparable soft lenses are available from laboratories not mentioned in this table.

[a] Water content (%).

[b] Oxygen permeability, $\times 10^{-11}$ (cm ml O_2)/(cm^2 s mmHg).

Abbreviations used are:

Fit
C corneal
S/S semi-scleral
SD single diameter (i.e. choice of radius)
SF single fitting (i.e. no choice of radius or diameter)

Polymer
HEMA 2-hydroxyethyl methacrylate
MA methacrylic acid
EGDMA ethylene glycol dimethacrylate
AMA alkyl methacrylate
NVP N-vinyl-2-pyrrolidone
PVP polyvinyl pyrrolidone
MMA methyl methacrylate
GMA glyceryl methacrylate
TPT trimethylol propane trimethacrylate
G-MEMA glyceryl methoxy-methacrylate

such descriptions as 'extended wear capability'. Since 1984, a whole new generation of high water content materials has appeared from many of the major laboratories. These include, among others, Geaflex 70, Incanto 78, Lunelle and Permaflex. Most of the new lenses have significant advantages and can also claim suitability for extended wear to a greater or lesser degree. Nevertheless, they are not without problems (*see* p. 427) and HEMA is still widely used. The new lenses and materials have been accompanied by the development of such allied technologies as lens disinfection, storage and cleaning, while many of the earlier lens forms have already disappeared because of their unsatisfactory clinical performance.

Table 11.1 provides brief details for many of the lenses available in the UK at the present time (1989). This list is by no means exhaustive but it illustrates the range of polymers, water contents, *Dk* (oxygen permeability) values and fitting methods currently in use. These will undoubtedly be supplemented by the arrival of future lens forms.

Permeability, transmissibility and equivalent oxygen performance

Oxygen permeability is an inherent property of a material and is independent of thickness. It is frequently expressed as the *Dk* value where *D* represents the diffusion coefficient and *k* the solubility of oxygen (Fatt, 1977). The oxygen tension at the lens–cornea interface is less than that at the front surface of the lens, the drop in oxygen tension being a function of the oxygen permeability for that material. There is a further relationship between oxygen flow and lens thickness (Larke and Sabell, 1971; Fatt, 1977), so that the transmissibility for a particular lens is thickness-related and given by the expression *Dk/t*, where *t* refers to the thickness.

The normal values for oxygen tension at the corneal surface are 155 mmHg and 55 mmHg, respectively, for open- and closed-eye conditions (Fatt and Bieber, 1968) and it is to this latter figure that many considerations for extended wear are related (*see* Chapter 15). In practical terms, Rocher (1977) has suggested that for a 40% water content HEMA lens, the cornea's oxygen requirements are met for open- and closed-eye conditions if the maximum lens

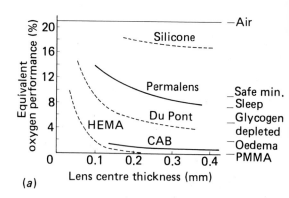

(a)

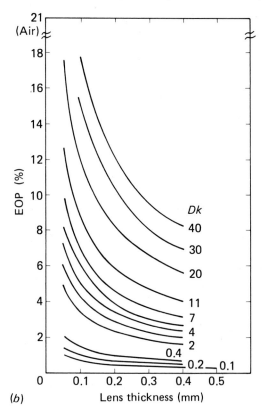

(b)

Figure 11.3 (*a*) A comparison of the equivalent oxygen performances of several general classes of hard and soft contact lens material. Performances vary within a given class depending on differences in the particular material and lens fabrication techniques used by each manufacturing laboratory. No account has been taken of any mechanical 'pump' effect under the lens. (By 'equivalent oxygen performance' is meant that the cornea responds as if it were in an atmosphere containing that particular percentage of oxygen; after Hill, R. M., 1977.) (*b*) The calculated curves of equivalent oxygen performance (EOP) responses anticipated for materials with various permeability constants (*Dk*) measured at 23°C in units × 10^{-11} (cm ml O$_2$)/(cm^2 s mmHg), over the range of lens thicknesses shown. (After Loshaek and Hill, 1977)

thicknesses are 0.14 mm and 0.04 mm, respectively. With 70% water content lenses, the equivalent values for maximum lens thickness are 0.47 mm and 0.13 mm, respectively.

Equivalent oxygen performance (EOP) means that the cornea responds as if it were in an atmosphere containing a particular percentage of oxygen (Hill, 1977). *Figure 11.3a* shows the relationship between equivalent oxygen performance and lens thickness for a variety of contact lens materials (*see* Chapter 15, p. 564). *Figure 11.3b* shows the relationship deduced by Loshaek and Hill (1977) between EOP and oxygen permeability over a range of lens thicknesses. The correlation between EOP and *Dk* was further explored by Fatt and Chaston (1982).

Holden and Mertz (1984) have shown that the mean oxygen requirement to avoid oedema on a daily wear basis is an EOP of 10% with individual variations from only 4% to atmospheric 21%.

Oedema, of course, is not only caused by anoxia, but may also be regarded as the cornea's response to a variety of disturbances. One of the most significant of these is osmotic imbalance which can cause epithelial oedema by the flow of water across the tears/cell membrane barrier (Hill and Uniacke, 1969). In addition, Hill and Terry (1978) have described the diurnal variations in the tears and have concluded that some patients are naturally so near their oedema threshold that they cannot be successfully managed as contact lens patients.

Mandell (1975) pointed out that there are many substances in the tears necessary for corneal health, and Hamano *et al.* (1980), over a long period, have advocated that the exchange of tears is as important as oxygen supply.

Methods of soft lens manufacture

Lenses may be manufactured by either moulding or lathing ('lathe-cutting').

Moulding obviously lends itself to mass production of lenses and various methods are in use. The Bausch & Lomb Soflens, following the principle of the original Czechoslovakian production method, is manufactured by the spincasting process. Now that the original patents have expired, other laboratories are also employing this method. Certain lenses, such as the Bausch & Lomb Optima, are hybrid in character, being lathe-cut after initial spincasting. Other lenses, such as the Hydron Z4, Permaflex, Permalens-XL and Cooperthin, are produced by the cast-moulding method. Silicone lenses, on the other hand, are compression moulded in the same way as some hard lenses.

The majority of laboratories, however, still manufacture by lathing. This technique is ideally suited to the production of individual lenses and specialized designs, but with modern automatic lathes, it is also successfully used for mass production.

Clinically, the different flexibility and surface characteristics of a moulded lens mean that it may centre less well than the equivalent lathe-cut lens, even if manufactured to the identical specification (*see Figure 11.19* and p. 413).

Advantages of soft contact lenses

There are numerous advantages which soft lenses of all types possess in common; they are as follows.

Greater comfort

Hydrophilic lenses are in nearly all cases significantly more comfortable than hard lenses, patients frequently stating that they can scarcely feel the presence of the lens even from the first moment of insertion. With all types of contact lens, there are two different adaptation processes involved. The first is that of the lids to the sensation caused by the presence of a foreign body on the eye; the second is that of the cornea to changes in its normal metabolism. It is the reduction, or even complete absence, of lid sensation which allows a hydrophilic lens to be immediately comfortable. The softness of the lens material is certainly concerned with this initial comfort, but just as important is the hydrophilic nature of the lens surface, so that the lid is in contact with a smooth, moist surface which gives a very similar sensation to that of the cornea itself. Soft lenses of smaller than corneal size tend to be unstable in fitting and, because of their excessive movement, can be as irritating as hard lenses. They have, therefore, evolved in their design to be the same size as the cornea or slightly larger. Stability, currently achieved through this relatively large total diameter, is a very important requirement for comfort, for exactly the same reason that a scleral lens is usually quite comfortable on initial insertion — because there is no differential sensation of the lid making and breaking contact with the edge of the lens. Manufacturing considerations are also important, and the lens edge must be thin and well formed.

Ease of adaptation

Soft lens wearers are normally able to adapt to their lenses within a very few days. This is due to the physical and chemical properties of the hydrogel material, and to the already mentioned absence of lid sensation. There is no disincentive to proper blinking, and tear exchange occurs readily with the pumping action of the lids on a well-fitting lens where this is not too thin (thinner lenses 'drape' the cornea more effectively and therefore move less). The cornea thus receives an adequate supply of oxygen with a minimum of disturbance to its normal metabolism.

Normal head posture and facial expression

Abnormal head posture and unnatural facial expressions are commonly seen with both hard and rigid gas permeable lens wearers in the early stages of adaptation. Because of the initial comfort, soft lens wearers generally look perfectly natural from the beginning of their wearing schedule.

Longer wearing time

Hydrophilic lenses can frequently be worn for longer periods of time than corneal lenses. This is especially true of those patients who have achieved only limited success with hard or rigid gas permeable lenses.

Lower incidence of corneal oedema

Corneal oedema is seen less frequently with soft lens wearers and, even if present, it is usually only of a mild degree and difficult to detect.

Rare occurrence of the 'over-wear syndrome'

Because oedema is so much less of a problem with a well-fitting lens, patients who wear soft

lenses for excessively long periods are unlikely to suffer acute epithelial necrosis often referred to as the 'over-wear syndrome'. Moderate stinging and burning with conjunctival injection is sometimes encountered, but this usually disappears rapidly when the lenses are removed. Over-wear is normally self-limiting with soft lenses, because discomfort usually occurs before they have caused any severe epithelial damage.

Absence of spectacle blur

It is uncommon for spectacle blur to occur with hydrophilic lenses because, under normal circumstances, they do not produce significant changes in corneal curvature as established by keratometer readings. Even if oedema is present with an increase in corneal thickness, it is uniform and extends from limbus to limbus. There is little or no localized change in radius or physical distortion of corneal curvature as occurs with hard corneal lenses. Even when small changes of corneal curvature do occur, these are not permanent (Hill, J. F., 1975, 1976).

The absence of noticeable spectacle blur means that patients can change from soft lenses to spectacles whenever they wish, and that the long-term clinical management of their spectacle refraction is straightforward. This can be undertaken at any convenient time, without requiring lenses to be removed for a specified number of hours or days (see Chapter 20).

Maintenance of corneal sensitivity

The wearing of hard lenses can cause a temporary but significant loss of corneal sensitivity. This potentially dangerous situation does not occur with soft lenses to anything like the same extent; the sensitivity loss is only half that with hard lenses (Millodot, 1971, 1974, 1976; see Chapter 2).

Lower incidence of corneal staining

Because hydrophilic lenses are soft, large and stable, corneal insult of the sort inherent in the use of a hard lens, such as apical, arcuate or 3 and 9 o'clock staining is not commonly encountered. However, the use of high water content soft lenses sometimes gives rise to midperipheral drying stains.

Occasional wear

The ease of adaptation and the absence of spectacle blur mean that soft lenses are ideal for patients who wish to wear contact lenses irregularly for sporting or social occasions.

Absence of photophobia and lacrimation

The typically adaptive photophobia and lacrimation found with corneal lenses is almost invariably absent with hydrophilic lenses.

Lower incidence of flare

Because of their large optic zone diameter, patients rarely complain of flare or peripheral reflections when wearing soft lenses.

Less difficulty with dust and foreign bodies

Because the lenses are of corneal diameter, or greater, they effectively protect the eye against dust and wind. Except on insertion — for it is quite easy to inadvertently place a lens on the eye with a speck of dust — patients wearing soft lenses are rarely troubled by foreign bodies.

Lower risk of loss

Well-fitting soft lenses do not generally fall out except in cases of extreme dehydration. They are not easily ejected from the eye by rubbing or lid tension and are not normally dislodged onto the sclera. Where loss occurs, it is almost always a result of careless handling.

Therapeutic uses

Hydrophilic lenses have proved effective in treating several pathological conditions. These include bullous keratopathy, the dry-eye syndromes, corneal burns and sterile indolent ulcers. Apart from their use as a corneal bandage, they are also employed as a drug release mechanism (Hillman, 1976; *see* Chapter 21).

The successful re-fitting of hard lens failures

Perhaps the major advantage of soft lenses is that it is now possible to re-fit, with some degree of success, the majority of patients who have previously failed with hard or rigid gas permeable lenses. The instant comfort of soft lenses by comparison with the earlier discomfort of their hard lenses proves a reassuring factor in the decision of many patients to recommence contact lens wear.

Disadvantages of soft contact lenses

Despite their many advantages, soft lenses have several drawbacks which must be carefully evaluated for each patient.

Distance vision

Visual acuity is often not as good as that obtained with hard lenses. Poor vision generally relates to uncorrected astigmatism, but may also result from limitations imposed by lens geometry or the inherently more variable nature of soft lens acuity. The materials are softer than the cornea and so are more readily deformed by eyelid pressure.

Near vision

It is quite common for patients to complain of poor near vision, while distance acuity is perfectly satisfactory (*see* p. 395).

Variable vision

Visual acuity can vary with hydrophilic lenses as a result of fluctuations with blinking and in the tear film or because of environmental factors affecting the level of hydration and fitting characteristics (*see* p. 392).

Breakage and tearing

Soft lenses can suffer from tearing, breakage and edge nicks. The frequency of replacement depends on the tensile strength and water content of the lens, as well as the handling ability of the patient.

Lens ageing and surface degradation

Hydrophilic lenses deteriorate with age. They discolour and the surfaces become deposited with mucoprotein, calcium and lipids. Lenses

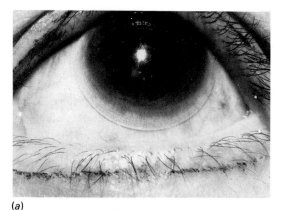

(a)

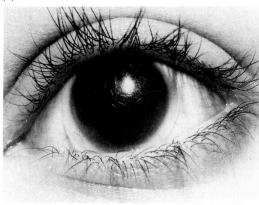

(b)

Figure 11.4 (a) An old worn lens exhibiting surface deposits and discolouration. (b) Surface scratching of an old, loosely fitting, low water content soft lens

eventually become uncomfortable, their fitting characteristics alter, and visual acuity may be reduced. Lenses showing surface deposits and scratches are shown in *Figure 11.4a,b* and *Plates 30–40*.

Difficulty of cleaning

The various cleaning processes which have been introduced must be applied by the patient with painstaking regularity if they are to be effective. They are frequently expensive and time consuming.

The need for lens disinfection

Hydrophilic lenses must be disinfected daily to avoid the risk of contamination by microorganisms. Many patients find boiling an unacceptable procedure, while others develop an adverse reaction to solutions. The efficacy of both methods has been criticized on microbiological grounds, while certain of the newer peroxide systems have proven too complicated (Bernstein and Maddox, 1973; Bernstein, Stow and Maddox, 1973; Norton *et al.*, 1974; *see* Chapter 4).

Unknown but limited lifespan

It is not possible to predict with certainty the lifespan of any given soft lens, but it is almost invariably less than that of a hard lens. High water content lenses, in particular, frequently last only a few months (Haig-Brown, 1985).

The inability to modify soft lenses

It is not generally feasible to modify either the power or the fitting parameters of soft lenses. If the patient's refractive error should alter, it is necessary to supply a new lens. The limited modifications possible are discussed in Chapter 23.

Difficulty of lens checking and verification

Methods for checking and verifying soft lenses are not as straightforward for speedy use in the consulting room as those for hard lenses. In addition, such factors as temperature and storage solution details must be taken into account. Chapter 13 covers these aspects in detail.

Vascularization and other pathological complications

Long-term wear of hydrophilic lenses has produced limbal vascularization and nodules in a small number of patients. Other complications are secondary vernal conjunctivitis causing papillae of the upper palpebral conjunctiva (giant papillary conjunctivitis), general conjunctival injection, stromal and endothelial disturbances of the cornea with rare cases of apparent endothelial detachment and nummular keratitis (Allansmith *et al.*, 1977; Mackie, 1977). *Plates 46–71* show some of these conditions.

Chemical contamination

It is possible for hydrophilic lenses to absorb chemicals into their naturally porous structure, for example if worn in a polluted environment or used for swimming in chlorinated water, when these chemicals may be retained and become a future source of ocular irritation. It is also preferable not to use eye drops while wearing soft lenses, because the preservatives may be similarly absorbed.

Cost factors

Apart from the initial fitting fees, it is also important to consider the greatly increased ongoing cost of solutions if soft lenses are to be correctly cleaned and disinfected throughout their lifespan.

Patient selection for soft lenses

With so many advantages and disadvantages, careful discussion is required with patients at the first consultation to determine their full history and discover their reasons for wanting to wear contact lenses. These aspects are fully covered in Chapters 8 and 9.

Generally, if patients have not already tried hard or rigid gas permeable lenses and are willing to persevere with the normal range of adaptive symptoms, rigid gas permeable or PMMA lenses may well be the first choice. If patients have already failed with a hard lens form, or their tolerance looks unpromising at the initial consultation, then soft lenses can be tried straight away. There are, in fact, many instances where a soft lens is the obvious choice with which to commence fitting. The various factors in evaluating this decision of hard or soft may be considered briefly under the headings of ocular factors and other factors, but it should always be remembered that any influence which tends to cause or exacerbate dry eyes is more likely to contra-indicate specifically the use of soft lenses.

Ocular factors

Considerations here are the type and degree of astigmatism, the standard of vision likely to be obtained with a soft lens and, just as important, the standard of vision actually required by the patient. There is little point in insisting that a patient should obtain 6/5 acuity with a hard lens, when 6/9+ with an immediately comfortable soft lens is perhaps perfectly adequate for

his or her needs. Corneal and lid sensitivity, accounting for the majority of hard lens failures, are equally important factors. A soft lens may well prove the answer in the type of case where a small corneal lens gives flare, but where a corneal lens of larger total diameter causes oedema which cannot be resolved by improvements to the fit or even by the use of a rigid gas permeable material. The same has applied where fenestrations were ineffective or when the fenestrations themselves were the cause of visual disturbance. Hydrophilic lenses should be considered for hypermetropes and low myopes who may be unhappy with a corneal lens because of the relative thickness and weight, which in turn give rise to excessive lens mobility on blinking. Pupil size is important because flare with hard lenses is nearly always avoided with the larger optic zone diameter of a soft lens. Patients with awkward anatomical features for corneal lenses, such as proptosed eyes, a low lower lid position or a decentred corneal apex, may prove much more successful with a hydrophilic lens.

The presence of any abnormal ocular condition, dry eyes and poor tear flow must also be considered.

Other factors

It is essential to determine from patients the reasons for wanting contact lenses, and the regularity of wearing schedule which they intend to adopt. The irregular or intermittent wearer is ideally suited to soft lenses, particularly if sporting requirements demand a stable fitting. Economic factors must be taken into account, not only the fees for initial fitting, but also the long-term costs of future lens replacements, accessory solutions and cleaning agents. The availability of these various solutions, geographical locations and working environments are important; whether they are hot or cold, humid or dry, dusty or clean, and whether they are likely to contain noxious fumes or chemicals.

The prolonged use of computer screens in difficult office environments particularly causes dryness and blinking problems with soft lenses and may contra-indicate their use (Gasson, 1983).

Airline crews have noted difficulty in the low humidity and pressurized atmosphere of aircraft cabins. Arias (1968, 1973) mentioned problems encountered in the high altitude of Mexico. This is not surprising for Hill (R. M., 1976) has shown that, in Mexico City, the percentage of oxygen in the atmosphere is only 16% compared to 21% at sea level. On the summit of Mount Everest it is only 7%. Clarke (1976) has reported the successful use of Permalenses at up to 24 000 feet, some 5000 feet below the summit. In Australia something over 75% of contact lenses fitted have been hydrophilic because of their greater comfort in the dust and heat (Gilford, 1975).

Psychological factors should be considered for those patients who need the sense of security of a stable fitting lens which it is almost impossible to dislodge from the eye by accident, or for those who are temperamentally unsuited to undergo the slower or more difficult adaptation process required by hard or rigid gas permeable lenses. Many patients find the insertion and removal of soft lenses rather easier than hard lenses.

Visual considerations

The refractive result obtained with soft lenses, as opposed to hard lenses or spectacles, is neither fixed nor absolute. It may be of extreme variability, changing from moment to moment, or from day to day, depending on external environment and lens fitting and performance. The visual standard is very much a subjective interpretation by the patient, and does not necessarily correlate with the Snellen acuity on the letter chart. Applegate and Massof (1975), for example, found marked changes in contrast sensitivity although the visual acuity remained the same, stressing that acuity is only one aspect of visual performance. Similar conclusions were reached by Rosenblum and Leach (1975) with Bausch & Lomb Soflens patients.

Guillon, Lydon and Wilson (1983) confirmed with larger groups of patients that contrast sensitivity is capable of pinpointing the exact nature of any reduction in visual performance and whether this occurs for distance or near, or for high or low spatial frequencies. They found specifically that soft lenses showed a poorer performance for high frequencies at near and that soft lenses (in common with rigid gas permeables) showed a decrease in contrast sensitivity for mid-frequencies under high illumination.

The defining of visual acuity therefore represents something of a problem, because the quality of vision is just as important as the precise number of lines read on the test chart. In some circumstances, a good 6/9 may be more acceptable than a poor 6/6, so that Snellen acuity is not always a reliable guide to a patient's potential visual success with soft lenses. Practitioners are obliged to place more than usual reliance on the patient's subjective impression of whether vision is good enough for his needs. This is especially true of near vision, and this factor must always be considered in relation to the patient's work and visual requirements. Variations of vision with hydrophilic lenses can be due to several different causes, as follows.

Environmental factors

The power of a lens depends upon its basic lens dimensions of back and front optic zone radii, thickness, refractive index and total diameter, which can all vary with environmental factors. These include such ocular effects as temperature and the pH, tonicity and volume of the tears. Some of these are, in turn, influenced by external factors such as ambient temperature, humidity, atmospheric pressure or the state of the lens when placed on the eye.

Generally, lenses manufactured from HEMA-based polymers undergo smaller variations than those made from high water content materials, as, for example, with the effect of temperature. Tonicity was investigated by Poster and Skolnik (1974), who demonstrated a 1.6% decrease in size when a Bausch & Lomb Soflens was taken from distilled water and placed in isotonic saline solution. A further decrease of 2.8% occurred when the lens was transferred to hypertonic, 1.8% saline solution. Eriksen, Randeri and Ster (1972) also showed changes of size with PHEMA (polyHEMA) lenses, but signficantly greater changes with the high water content Bionite lenses. They also found that pH had little effect on the dimensions of PHEMA lenses, but gave a measurable decrease in size for Bionite in acidic solution. Harris and Mock (1974) were able to demonstrate changes in both power and light transmission according to the tonicity of lens storage solutions. Ford (1974) showed how the degree of lens hydration, and all of these other influences, can summate to give a significant error of power when a lens has fully settled on the cornea.

Lens flexure and optical considerations
(*see also* Chapter 5)

A second possible cause of power change is the effect of lens flexure. This has been argued for all types of lenses, whether corneal or semi-scleral, and occurs when a flexible lens fitted either flatter or steeper than 'K' bends to conform to the corneal curvature. Wichterle (1967) gave a mathematical analysis of this effect and, in 1967, Vincent (Blackstone, 1968) reported that in practice the original Czechoslovakian lenses increased their effective negative power when allowed to steepen, and vice versa. Sarver, Ashley and Van Every (1974) described how a thin corneal-sized soft lens with back and front surface radii of 8.00 mm and 8.50 mm, respectively, increased its power from $-3.25\,\mathrm{D}$ to $-4.00\,\mathrm{D}$ when allowed to steepen by 1.00 mm, and proposed the term 'supplemental power effect'. This represents the total change in power, due first to lens flexure and secondly to a liquid lens, if the posterior surface of the contact lens fails to conform to the front surface of the cornea. In practice, any supplemental power effect is likely to be created by a combination of these two causes, with the greater proportion resulting from flexure. In the case of a modern, 'thin', soft lens which completely drapes over the cornea, it can be assumed that there is virtually no liquid lens power.

Strachan (1973) suggested that both positive and negative lenses increase their power on steepening, in direct proportion to the degree of flexure and to the power of the original lens. A different mathematical analysis by Bennett (1976), assuming only that the volume of the lens remains constant, showed that refractive changes due to flexure are independent of power and invariably add negative power. This closely agrees with the earlier analysis of Wichterle, as well as with Sarver's clinical findings.

Another variable factor which can affect the power of a hydrophilic lens is refractive index (*see Tables 5.6* and *5.7*, Chapter 5). Strachan (1973) evaluated a hypothetical case of a 60% water content lens, with a refractive index (n) of 1.52 in the dry state. When fully hydrated this lens becomes a mixture of 40% polymer ($n = 1.52$) and 60% water ($n = 1.333$), with a resultant refractive index of 1.40. If the lens is in a state of partial dehydration on the eye, the refractive index increases, with a consequent change of power. In Strachan's example, a $-3.00\,\mathrm{D}$ lens becomes $-3.12\,\mathrm{D}$ and $-3.37\,\mathrm{D}$, when the refractive index changes from 1.40 to 1.42 and 1.46, respectively, and conversely a $+3.00\,\mathrm{D}$ lens alters its power to $+3.18\,\mathrm{D}$ and $+3.55\,\mathrm{D}$, respectively. Ford (1976) demonstrated a typical water loss of 8.79% when a 70% water content soft lens reached a state of equilibration on the eye, with the refractive index changing from 1.4300 to 1.4397.

When a soft lens is placed on a toroidal cornea, the final refractive result depends on the way in which the lens moulds itself to the corneal topography. If a lens partially dehydrates within the palpebral aperture, there can be an astigmatic power change due to alteration in the refractive index, and to the lens becoming less flexible meridionally, with differential power changes because of the resulting flexure. These effects tend to become very complicated, but they can sometimes partially neutralize corneal astigmatism, reducing it to a level suitable for spherical soft lens fitting.

Ageing effects

Changes in visual acuity also occur with time and use. Discoloured lenses (*Plate 35*), and those affected by mucoprotein or calcium deposits from the tears, are commonly seen (*Figure 11.5*

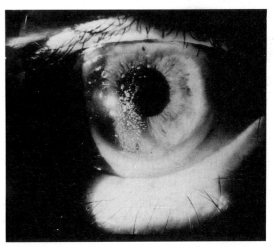

Figure 11.5 White spots (calcium) on a high water content soft lens

and *Plates 31* and *32*). Such deposits and discolouration may sometimes cause a serious reduction in visual acuity. At the same time, older lenses have a greater tendency to dehydrate on the eye so that noticeable alterations in fitting characteristics are frequently observed. Apparent refractive changes of −0.50 D are quite common and marked differences have been shown in the light transmission curves between new and old lenses (Gasson, 1975).

Over-refractions*

The various factors already mentioned — environment, flexure, degree of hydration, ageing and dimensional changes — all combine to give a refractive result at a particular time for a particular set of conditions. It cannot be assumed that this refraction will remain constant, and it does frequently change by small amounts. If, for example, a patient should move from indoors to outdoors, temperature and humidity will alter, and the lenses must reach a new state of equilibration on the eye. Usually, no very great concern is caused, although there may be complaints of visual fluctuation, especially in the early days of wear when the tear flow has still not returned to normal.

If the over-refractions are carefully monitored, these changes can be easily demonstrated. Also, cylinder power and axis can both vary widely and apparently at random. There does not seem to be any correlation with 'K' readings (Larke and Sabell, 1971), and Gasson (1975) has shown the same type of variation with a series of different lens types on the same eye, and also with the same lens on the same eye examined on different occasions. It was originally held that thicker lenses (over 0.2 mm centre thickness) would more effectively mask corneal astigmatism, transferring less cylinder through to the anterior surface of the soft lens, but this idea was rejected by Morrison (1973) who found, in a study of three HEMA-based materials, that neither thickness, diameter, power, water content nor method of manufacture seemed to have an appreciable effect on the the amount of astigmatism transferred to the front surface of the lens. Generally, lenses with a standard thickness of approximately

0.10–0.14 mm are likely to give the best visual result. Thicker lenses should be avoided for physiological, visual, and cosmetic reasons and ultrathin lenses of 0.07 mm or less often do not give as good a quality of vision on toroidal corneas as their standard thickness counterparts or modern high water content semi-scleral lenses. When a soft lens is placed on the eye the spherical anterior surface may become an aspherical or irregular curve with different optical qualities. Such effects are not predictable, so that the prescription and quality of vision must be determined empirically by placing lenses on the cornea. Even if the same over-refraction can be demonstrated with quite different designs of lens, it may be only one type of fitting which gives an acceptable visual result to the patient. Stability of vision is important, and semi-scleral lenses are often preferred by patients with corneal astigmatism. It can be demonstrated that the addition of a quite small cylinder, perhaps only −0.50 D, can give a very significant improvement in acuity, eliminating ghosting and distortion. The typically small degree of residual astigmatism, which can be easily ignored by both patient and practitioner when prescribing hard lenses, cannot always be so readily discounted with soft lenses. It is also found that the binocular visual acuity is frequently better out of all proportion to the monocular results so that R and L 6/9−, may well give 6/6+ binocularly. For this reason, essentially monocular patients are likely to be rather less happy with their soft lens visual acuity, particularly if they are wearing a toric or bifocal soft lens where variations in vision are more common.

Corneal and residual astigmatism

Two basic assumptions should be made when assessing the potential success of astigmatic patients being fitted with spherical soft lenses:

(1) Total ocular astigmatism = corneal astigmatism + lenticular astigmatism.
(2) All corneal astigmatism is transferred through the lens to its anterior surface.

Patients may therefore be divided into the following four groups at their initial examination by reference to spectacle correction and 'K' readings.

---

*A refraction carried out when a contact lens is being worn is termed an 'over-refraction'.

'Spherical cornea' with spherical refraction

Rx: −3.00 DS
'K': 7.85 mm along 180° (43.00 D);
       7.85 mm along 90° (43.00 D).

This is the ideal optical situation for contact lens fitting. Vision should be equally good with either hard or soft lenses.

'Spherical' cornea with astigmatic refraction

Rx: −2.00/−1.75 × 90
'K': 7.85 mm along 180° (43.00 D);
       7.90 mm along 90° (42.75 D).

The astigmatism is almost entirely lenticular, so that the visual result is the same with either a hard or soft lens. In either case, a front surface toric lens is required to correct the 1.50 D of residual astigmatism.

Astigmatic cornea with astigmatic refraction

Rx: −2.00/−1.75 × 180
'K': 7.80 mm along 180° (43.25 D);
       7.50 mm along 90° (45.00 D)

All of the astigmatism is corneal, so that a spherical hard or suitable rigid gas permeable lens, or a toric soft lens should be fitted.

Astigmatic cornea with spherical refraction

Rx: −3.00 DS
'K': 7.80 mm along 180° (43.25 D);
       7.50 mm along 90° (45.00 D).

In this example, there is 1.75 D of with-the-rule corneal astigmatism together with an equivalent degree of against-the-rule lenticular astigmatism, to give a resultant spherical refraction. A spherical hard lens form would leave a residual cylinder of −1.75 D × 90. A soft lens, *because* it transfers all of the corneal astigmatism through to its front surface without optically neutralizing it, is the lens of choice.

These theoretical considerations should be confirmed by clinical observation with a soft lens placed on the eye. The arbitrary figure of 1.50 D ocular astigmatism is frequently given as the upper limit for which good visual acuity can be obtained with a spherical hydrophilic lens. In practice, this limit can be as low as 0.50 D or 0.75 D for patients who are critical observers, accustomed to good vision and required by their occupation to undertake exacting visual tasks. Conversely, satisfactory acuity has occasionally been obtained with cylinders as high as 4.00 D for less critical and strongly motivated patients. In these cases, the distance visual acuity is usually more acceptable than that for near. With such a high degree of astigmatism, success is unlikely and patients should not be unduly encouraged. Nevertheless, it is worth while trying a spherical lens, especially with those for whom all other considerations, including perhaps hard or rigid gas permeable lens failure, indicate a soft lens, and where time and expense rule out a toric soft lens fitting. Such a procedure, in any case, demonstrates to the patient the visual limitations of a spherical soft lens. In order to make a proper assessment, trial lenses should be as close as possible to the expected prescription. Because lenses are fitted flatter than flattest 'K', the most satisfactory vision is usually obtained for myopic patients with the least myopic focal line on the retina, rather than with the predicted best vision sphere. For example, spectacle *Rx* −3.50/−1.00 × 180; the likely back vertex power (BVP) of soft lens is −3.50 DS. In borderline cases, plano-cylindrical spectacles can be worn for critical vision and driving, and cylinders may be incorporated into a normal presbyopic correction.

Near vision problems

When prescribing soft lenses, near vision should be carefully assessed as a separate function from distance acuity. Frequently, patients who can wear soft lenses comfortably and see well for distance, find their near vision completely unsatisfactory. Clinical results show that the deciding factor for soft lens success or failure can often be the quality of near vision, especially if it interferes with work or study. There are many causes of near vision difficulty. Stone (1967), in an assessment of this problem with hard lenses, suggested four main reasons, as follows:

(1) Alteration in the accommodation–convergence relationship.
(2) Reduced size of palpebral aperture.
(3) Reduced evaporation of tears.
(4) Alteration in corneal curvature during convergence.

From their very nature, the last three of these effects are likely to be of greater significance with hydrophilic lenses, but there are several other possible causes, any or all of which could produce problems.

(1) Borderline acuity for distance.
(2) Lid pressure, causing irregular buckling or flexure of the lens with the eyes in the near vision position.
(3) Irregular astigmatism at near.
(4) Reduced blink rate, causing drying of the lens surface.
(5) Changes in scleral topography during convergence.
(6) A decentred lens.
(7) A poor fitting.

Visual advantages of soft lenses

Despite all the visual problems which can arise, the majority of patients do achieve a good and worthwhile standard of soft lens vision. Indeed, many claim that their quality of vision and field of view are better with soft lenses than with either hard lenses or spectacles. The size and stability of fitting ensure that hydrophilic lenses have certain natural advantages over corneal lenses. There is a significant reduction in the incidence of flare and peripheral reflections, especially at night or in dim illumination when the pupils are enlarged. Patients adapting to soft lenses, which have relatively large optic zone diameters, rarely complain of the flare so commonly observed with hard lenses. For those with naturally large pupils and where corneal lenses cannot be made to give satisfactory centration, a hydrophilic lens may be the only means of eliminating intolerable visual disturbance. Many patients wearing conventionally fitted hard or rigid gas permeable lenses of positive or low negative power find the constantly altering vision, which is unstable after blinking, quite unacceptable. A soft lens with its very limited vertical movement nearly always provides a satisfactory solution.

Water content and polymers

In this context the following definitions are used:

$$\text{Percentage water content} = \frac{\text{Weight of fully hydrated lens} - \text{Weight of fully dehydrated lens}}{\text{Weight of fully hydrated lens}} \times 100\%$$

British Standards recommends that this should apply to lenses under equilibrium conditions with physiological (normal) saline solution at a temperature of $20 \pm 0.5°C$.

$$\text{Percentage water uptake} = \frac{\text{Weight of fully hydrated lens} - \text{Weight of fully dehydrated lens}}{\text{Weight of fully dehydrated lens}} \times 100\%$$

Thus, lenses with a water content of 38% have a water uptake of approximately 61%. Care must be exercised when interpreting brand names which include a numerical suffix, because these do not always accurately reflect the water content.

In the context of soft lens materials, the suffix '-filcon' is used for polymer names in the USA. This is a requirement of the FDA who also divide polymers into four groups:

(1) Low water content, non-ionic polymers, e.g. Crofilcon (C.S.I., 38.5%).
(2) High water content, non-ionic polymers, e.g. Lidifilcon A (Sauflon, 70%).
(3) Low water content, ionic polymers, e.g. Bufilcon A (Hydrocurve II, 45%).
(4) High water content, ionic polymers, e.g. Etafilcon A (Vistamarc, 58%).

Lenses have been produced with water contents from 3 to 85%, with the wide range of polymers indicated in *Table 11.1*. However, a great many of the lenses currently being used are still HEMA-based with water contents in the 35–45% region.

Low water content lenses have been predominantly fitted because of their greater tensile strength and longer lifespan. They have the further advantage that they can be made thinner, because of their smaller swell factor during hydration. In addition, the various cleaning and rejuvenating agents have, in the main, been developed for HEMA-based lenses.

High water content soft lenses

Advantages

High water content lenses however have significant advantages which are listed below.

High Dk values

Most of the materials have *Dk* values between three and six times that of HEMA. The very good oxygen permeability of these lenses means that they are suitable in this respect for almost all new patients. In addition, the lenses have two other obvious applications:

(1) For cases of early vascularization – although a modern rigid gas permeable or flexible silicone lens is often more effective in allowing vessels to empty or recede.
(2) Cases of oedema with low water content materials, especially with hypermetropic patients where lens thickness is considerably greater.

Better comfort

Because these new materials are much softer, often matching the water content of the cornea, they are frequently more comfortable with less lid sensation, over and above any advantage given by their high *Dk* value.

Longer wearing time

As a result of the first two advantages, patients often achieve a much longer wearing time.

Faster adaptation

The majority of patients can build up their wearing time more rapidly with higher water content lenses.

Extended wear

The ultimate example of this rapid adaptation is given by the true extended wear lenses where both all day and all night wear can often be achieved from the beginning.

Easier to handle

Most high water content lenses are thicker than their low water content 'thin' counterparts. Particularly in the lower negative powers, they are much easier to handle. The additional thickness of plus and very high minus lenses, however, can be a disadvantage in removal because of their reduced flexibility in these power ranges.

Better vision

For the same reason of increased thickness, some patients with borderline acuity with moderate astigmatism (−0.75 D to −1.25 D) may achieve a much better visual result than with thinner low water content lenses.

Better for intermittent wear

Longer periods of intermittent wear for social and sporting use are much easier with high water content lenses.

Ease of fitting

Because some types of these lenses have only one predominent fitting, lens selection is rapid and simple.

Disadvantages

Despite the foregoing, it is also necessary to consider a number of disadvantages, as given below.

Environmental sensitivity

High water content lenses are more sensitive to environmental factors. Chief among these is temperature which may have a significant effect on dimensional stability, lens hydration and *Dk* value.

Greater fragility

Although modern high water content lenses are far superior to many of the earlier examples of this type, breakage can still represent a major problem.

White spots

White spots have previously been associated rather more with extended wear than with daily wear lenses. Some of the newer high water content materials seem particularly prone to this problem even when worn purely on a daily basis. Patients are less concerned with whether the origin is lipid or calcium than with the fact that a new lens – often within a few weeks of fitting – has developed irreversible deposits and needs replacement. The main, common factor appears to be dryness. The origin may be ocular, because of minimal, tear flow, wide palpebral aperture or poor blinking, or environmental because of factors such as air conditioning or central heating, or occupational, for example with the use of visual display unit (VDU) screens (*see* p. 391).

In addition, within the same make of lens there often seem to be variations in material, because one lens may exhibit severe white spots (*see Figure 11.5*) within a very short time while its successor may prove to be altogether free of this particular problem.

Discolouration

The majority of high water content lenses appear in use to suffer from rapid brown discolouration (*Plate 35*). Indeed, many new lenses appear marginally discoloured on removal from their laboratory sealed vials. In addition, they seem more prone to pink or blue discolouration which possibly emanates either from disinfection solutions or the use of systemic medicines (*see* Chapter 4).

Disinfection

Because discolouration is greatly exacerbated by heat disinfection, this is rarely the method of first choice with high water content lenses. In addition, because these highly absorptive materials are more likely to retain chemical preservatives within their structure, there is an increased possibility of either stinging or a serious solutions reaction. The preferred method, which also conveniently bleaches away some of the discolouration, is therefore peroxide. However, many of the patients who are scarcely willing to disinfect their lenses properly with a simple one-stage preserved system are completely unwilling to employ a more complex and lengthy, usually two-stage system.

Poor reproducibility

Once again, the modern lenses are a vast improvement over their historical counterparts.

Nevertheless, problems with reproducibility are still encountered in practice, even with some of the moulded lenses.

More variable vision

In some cases, particularly with thinner lenses, visual acuity may be more variable and therefore less satisfactory than with standard thickness HEMA lenses.

Longer fitting time

It takes much longer for high water content lenses to reach proper equilibration on the eye before the fitting can be reliably judged, and significant power changes can occur while settling. The fitting characteristics of these lenses, particularly where smaller diameters in the region of 13.50 mm are used, mean that it is not always possible to achieve ideal centration and movement.

Dryness problems

The main problem with high water content lenses has been an increase in dryness-related symptoms. Even patients with apparently normal tear flow may complain of extreme discomfort and reduced wearing times of no greater than 3 or 4 hours, often despite having previously worn HEMA lenses without difficulty.

In some of these cases of failure, slit lamp examination reveals no corneal insult, but the patients complain of varying degrees of dryness and discomfort. In many instances, however, there is very evident arcuate staining. This proves more common towards the upper limbus, but also occurs in various other midperipheral areas of the cornea (*see Plates 49* and *58*). Some eyes produce the same type of stain in different regions of the cornea with a succession of different makes of lens, whereas others will only be affected by certain makes of lens.

It is particularly interesting that this sort of stain is very similar in appearance to that seen with old-fashioned, thick, semi-scleral lenses made from HEMA, and rarely observed since the use of 'thin' HEMA lenses. Its reappearance with modern high water content lenses, which are frequently fitted in a semi-scleral fashion, suggests a strong correlation with their relatively greater thickness and fitting technique. The staining now, as then, seems to be due to a combination of: indirect mechanical pressure from the upper lid through the portion of the lens near its lenticular junction, and increased dehydration of the material on the eye (*see also* Chapter 15).

Dehydration of soft lenses

One of the major reasons for the clinical success or failure of a particular lens on the eye relates to its dehydration characteristics. The literature on this complex subject is sometimes contradictory and is not always consistent with actual clinical experience.

Dehydration of a lens on the eye causes a reduction in the *Dk* value, changes in lens parameters and, therefore, its fitting characteristics, increased deposition, and generally reduced comfort. In addition, with high water loss it is unlikely that a good tear film can be maintained, remembering also that, even under normal conditions, the tear film break-up time (BUT) is reduced during contact lens wear.

Frankland (1980) considered the water content contained within the polymer matrix to consist of 'bound' water, which is directly attached to the hydrophilic sites by van der Waals forces, and 'free' water which is readily lost from the lens by evaporation. Notionally, the higher the 'bound' water, the less any particular material will dehydrate on the eye and cause clinical problems.

Andrasko and Schoessler (1980) described how the amount and speed of evaporation depend upon ocular factors, such as volume and quality of tears, blink habits, osmolarity and palpebral aperture, and environmental factors which will include temperature, relative humidity and wind velocity. Young and Mandell (1983) stressed that the success of a contact lens for extended wear depends upon the transport of water molecules through the material and that water loss is proportional to water content. This relationship was quantified for certain conditions by Kohler and Flanagan (1985) who proposed that dehydration can increase by approximately 1% for each 4% increase in water content. He also concluded that temperature is a highly significant factor in lens dehydration.

On a practical level, except when a lens is in its vial, it is rarely at its full, stated hydration level. Indeed, Wechsler, Johnson and Businger (1983) suggested that the main water loss occurs within the first 5 minutes on the eye. Andrasko (1983) found that high and low water content lenses lose, respectively, 14.8% and 10.4% after 30 minutes. Other investigators have quantified water loss for different materials and found that, under adverse environmental conditions of very low relative humidity, a lens might lose nearly 20% of its water content (Hill, 1982).

More specifically, Bilton and Guillon (1984) found that Permalenses took 30 minutes to equilibrate on the eye and lost 15% water to achieve a final water content of 56%. Hydron HX lenses, by comparison, took 15 minutes to equilibrate and lost only 4% to end with a water content of 61%. Standard and 'thin' HEMA lenses lost, respectively, 4% and 8%. They also proposed a water gradient across the thickness of the lens. More recently, however, Fatt and DiMartino (1985) concluded that both the front and the back surface of a lens on the eye maintain the same water content, and that the tear film beneath a soft lens contains only non-aqueous mucin and lipid components.

Bilton and Guillon also recognized the importance of the tear film and refer to J. P. Guillon's work in relation to different lens materials and thicknesses with normal eyes. Thick HEMA lenses give the most stable tear film. The prelens tear film for Permalens proves thin but stable, whereas those for Duragel, Hydron HX and Sauflon are all thin and unstable. Very thin HEMA lenses, such as the Bausch & Lomb 'O' series, have a thin aqueous tear film with no lipid content.

These last results are very much in accord with clinical experience, where drying problems are frequently encountered with very 'thin' HEMA, and such lenses are almost unwearable by even normal eyes in hot, dry climates. They also explain why patients who are perfectly comfortable with HEMA lenses are sometimes unable to wear the theoretically superior high water content lenses with which they have just been re-fitted.

The rehydration characteristics of the lens should also be considered. Hill (1983) suggests that it can take nearly 1 hour for a lens to stabilize at a higher hydration level, when changing from an adverse to a favourable environment. Young and Mandell (1983) suggested that the ratio of water loss to gain is different for each lens and that, in some cases, the hydrated level on the eye is governed by evaporation but in others by rehydration.

Dry eyes

Soft lenses may well be contra-indicated for patients working in an unsuitably dry atmosphere or where there is a serious deficiency in tear flow. In the case of the marginally dry eye, it is necessary to evaluate whether it is likely to benefit from the greater volume of fluid contained within a lens of higher water content and which will remain greater than a lower water content material even after partial dehydration, or whether a lower water content lens will prove better because relatively reduced dehydration will cause less disturbance to an already minimal tear film.

In most cases, it seems preferable to avoid higher water content and thinner lenses in favour of lower water content and thicker. The ultimate example of this would be the successful use on even seriously dry eyes of flexible silicone lenses which have virtually no water content.

Success with high water content lenses depends upon many factors. The lens must have a high enough water content to offer a worthwhile advantage over HEMA, but not so high that it will dehydrate too rapidly or too much on the eye. It must be fitted thick enough to maintain a stable tear film and take advantage of good vision, but not so thick that it can cause arcuate staining. It must be thin enough to be comfortable and give proper fitting characteristics, but not so thin that it will upset tear film stability, or cause visual problems.

These several factors explain why different makes of high water content lens give completely different clinical results and why sometimes they may all perform significantly worse than HEMA. There is no certain way of predicting how well a particular high water content lens will perform on a particular eye even with a normal tear film, until it has been worn by the patient in his or her normal environment.

Lens thickness and 'thin' lenses

The typical centre thickness for a 'standard thickness' corneal diameter HEMA lens of power $-3.00\,\text{D}$ is in the region of 0.10–0.15 mm

(e.g. Hydroflex mini = 0.10 mm; Hydron = 0.12 mm). Lenses below 0.10 mm may be regarded as 'ultrathin' and represent a very satisfactory way of increasing transmissibility (Dk/t) and improving physiological performance. On the basis of centre thickness, a reduction from 0.11 mm to 0.07 mm is likely to give an improvement in transmissibility of nearly 40% and an increase of about 60% in the estimated oxygen tension at the anterior surface of the cornea for a HEMA lens; Wilson, Rafferty and Lewerenz (1978) found a four-fold increase in the oxygen diffusion rate for a thin compared with standard thickness Hydrocurve lens.

It is important to remember that the oxygen performance for a lens cannot be judged solely in relation to its specified centre thickness but must be considered for the entire lens. Edwards (1985) analysed the zonal oxygen transmission (EOP) profiles for hyperthin HEMA lenses (i.e. lenses of centre thickness less than 0.05 mm) of various powers across the whole lens. These showed that over about $-4.00\,\text{D}$ the increased peripheral thickness would be unlikely to meet Holden's 10% criterion for oedema-free daily wear. Sammons (1980, 1981) showed the mathematical complexities of analysing the harmonic or mean lens thickness and that taking an inappropriate average thickness (*see* Appendix E) could result in a 30% error in the predicted oxygen flux. Low plus and aphakic lenses cannot truly be considered as 'thin' because of their necessarily greater centre thickness. Nevertheless, positive lenses such as the Hydron Z Plus and Hydroflex SD are significantly thinner than their standard counterparts and often resolve cases of oedema. A centre thickness of 0.05 mm or less is theoretically necessary to sustain extended wear in closed eye conditions with a 38% HEMA lens (Fatt, 1977). However, many patients have been known to sleep wearing lenses of even normal thickness for varying periods of time. In these cases ultra- and hyperthin lenses much more closely approach the theoretically required figure and possess an inherent safety factor.

Theoretical considerations are well confirmed by good clinical results in practice (Haig-Brown, 1978; Solomon, 1978), and by Fanti and Vollmer (1979) who found a much reduced increase in corneal thickness after 9 hours of wear compared to that measured with standard thickness wear. The fitting characteristics of thin and standard lenses differ even if otherwise having the same specification. Generally, ultrathin lenses tend to completely drape the cornea and may become almost immobile. The thickness of the lens may therefore be regarded as an additional fitting variable.

Advantages of thin soft lenses

The advantage of thin lenses may be summarized as follows:

(1) Lower incidence of corneal oedema because of the improved transmissibility.
(2) Reduced lid sensation because of the much thinner lens edge. This is especially beneficial for sensitive patients at their initial fitting.
(3) Reduced limbal irritation for the same reason and because lenses are fitted slightly larger.
(4) The different fitting characteristics often permit better centration compared with standard thickness lenses.
(5) They are an easier lens to fit because their increased flexibility means that fewer fitting radii are necessary.
(6) They are a safer lens should patients doze while wearing them.

These important factors mean that thin lenses are frequently the first choice, but there are certain disadvantages which should also be taken into account.

Disadvantages of thin soft lenses

(1) Handling is more difficult, particularly in the low minus powers below about −2.00 D.
(2) The breakage rate is somewhat greater than with standard thickness lenses, although by no means the problem experienced with high water content soft lenses.
(3) The lifespan of thin lenses is shorter particularly when heat disinfection is used. With current thinking towards more frequent replacements, this may be regarded as beneficial.
(4) For patients with toroidal corneas, visual acuity may be less satisfactory than with standard thickness lenses (*see* p. 397).
(5) Thin lenses have a greater tendency to dehydrate on the eye and may disturb the precorneal tear film (*see* p. 399).

Additional techniques in soft lens fitting

Certain techniques additional to those routinely used with hard lenses are sometimes used in soft lens fitting.

Slit lamp techniques

Pachometry (*see* Chapter 6)

If increased corneal thickness is to be used as a potential indicator of oedema, a pachometer attachment to the slit lamp is required (Stone, 1974).

Photography (*see* Chapter 7)

The use of clinical photography permits a permanent record to be maintained of the eye, particularly its vascular state prior to fitting (*Plate 2*).

Graticules

A calibrated graticule in the slit lamp eyepiece can be used to assess both the corneal diameter and the total diameter of a soft lens in wear. It can also be used to estimate the rotation of a marked toric lens.

Placido disc and Klein keratoscope

These simple devices permit a qualitative assessment to be made of the regularity of the anterior surface of a soft lens while it is being worn. Any noticeable distortion of image quality suggests a poor fitting, and is likely to be accompanied by poor subjective acuity (*Figure 11.6a,b*).

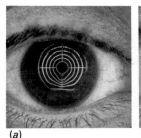 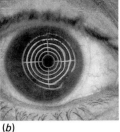

(a)   (b)

Figure 11.6 Photokeratoscopy showing distortion from the front surfaces of steeply fitted soft lenses during wear. (*a*) A high water content 'extended' wear lens of corneal size; (*b*) a low water content semi-scleral lens

Aesthesiometry

If it is desired to monitor corneal sensitivity, aesthesiometry should be carried out prior to fitting (*see* Chapters 2 and 8).

Lens verification and inspection

The instruments for this purpose are fully described in Chapter 13 but essentially the practitioner needs to verify with reasonable speed the radius, by means of the spherometer principle or ultrasound, the power, by a focimeter method, and the diameter — for this last measurement, those instruments most valuable for consulting room use include the facility for projection magnification. They provide an easy method of assessing lens condition and also demonstrating to the patient any flaws which might have developed in the surface or edge (*see Figure 13.20*). Also useful are a dark-field analyser for demonstrating surface deposits; and a refractometer for providing an assessment of water content.

Consulting room procedures and equipment

A constant supply of physiological saline is required in the consulting room for rinsing and cleaning lenses prior to insertion and for their subsequent disinfection after use. Ideal for this purpose is one of the proprietary aerosol salines, either buffered or unbuffered. These contain no preservatives and employ sterile air as the propellant.

Lenses are most easily extracted from their vials by means of soft-ended plastic tweezers or a glass rod. For the more fragile high water content lenses, the complete contents of the vial should be tipped into a small dish. This has the additional advantage of making sure that the storage solution is changed on each occasion that the lens is used, and is therefore a good procedure to adopt with any type of lens. Additional 5 ml or 10 ml lens vials are useful for storing patients' lenses when they are removed during an after-care examination, or if lenses are retained for cleaning and rejuvenation. For the latter purpose a small hotplate or magnetic stirrer is required, together with an autoclave or large heat sterilizer for disinfecting several trial lenses at the same time. The smaller pharmaceutical vials require a crimping device for re-sealing their metal caps. Because many soft lenses are not marked and are therefore unidentifiable without time-consuming measurement, small self-adhesive labels are extremely useful for the identification of lenses temporarily stored in otherwise plain bottles. A selection of lens vials is shown in *Figure 11.7*.

Hygienic procedures are extremely important in practice to avoid cross-infection within the consulting room (Sheridan, 1987).

Assessment of tear flow

It is important to be able to recognize dry-eyed patients with inadequate tear flow, as they are very likely to develop into problem cases. Schirmer's test (*Figure 11.8a,b*) is the most commonly cited method of measuring tear output and is described in Chapters 2, 8 and 21. However, it is not always a reliable method unless very carefully carried out and other tests are often preferable. Ordinary fluorescein can be used as a simple diagnostic test by observing the

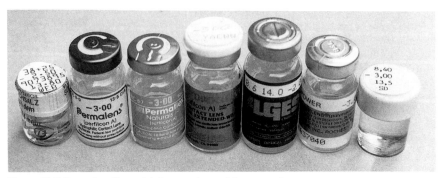

Figure 11.7 Examples of lens vials from various soft lens manufacturers

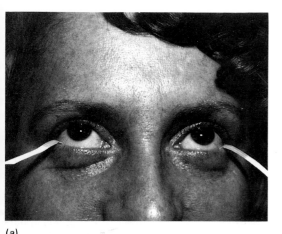

(a)

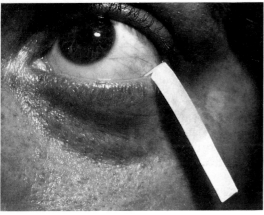

(b)

Figure 11.8 Schirmer's test showing how the tear fluid wets the paper strips: (a) being carried out on both eyes at once; (b) close-up of one eye. This is best carried out on one eye at a time with the patient looking up and in, as shown in (b). The normal output for a young adult is 15 mm of the paper strip wetted in 5 minutes or 10 mm wetted in 3 minutes. Measurement is made from the notch at the lid margin

break-up time (BUT) of the precorneal film which is normally about 10–12 μm thick (Rengstorff, 1974). A small drop of fluorescein is instilled into the lower fornix, and the patient instructed to blink several times, and then to stare straight ahead. Observation is made with the slit lamp at about × 15 magnification, using a blue filter. Break-up of the precorneal film is easily seen by the presence of dark areas against the otherwise bright green background as shown in *Plate 55* on a compromised cornea. A break-up time of 10–60 seconds is considered normal. If it occurs in less than 10 seconds, a deficiency of either the volume or wetting properties of the tears is indicated or may suggest the presence of meibomian gland dysfunction (Larke, 1985a).

Norn (1974) has described a more elaborate, quantitative procedure whereby fluorescein is mixed with 1% rose bengal. The colour of the composite stain is evaluated according to a time-scale related to the dilution effect of tear flow on a single 10-μl drop instilled into the conjunctival sac (*Table 11.2*). Observation with the slit lamp is made on the lacrimal rivus in the central portion of the lower lid after exactly 5 minutes. Ford (1974) has further extended this technique to give the predicted water loss from a hydrophilic lens during wear thereby enabling him to calculate the probable change of power caused by lens dehydration.

Tear pH

Norn (1974) has also discussed the use of bromothymol blue as a pH indicator for the tears in the range 6.8–7.6, as shown in *Table 11.3*. The colour is assessed after exactly 5 seconds, before carbon dioxide from the tears renders the lacrimal rivus more alkaline.

Table 11.2 Tear dilution test

Group	Colour	Dilution	Indicated tear flow per hour (ml)*	Water loss (from 70% water content lens) (%)
1	Intense red	Insignificant	<0.18 (3)	
2	Pale red	4–1	0.36 (6)	13–23
3	Intense orange	16–1	1.8 (30.6)	5–12
4	Weak orange	64–1	7.6 (128)	<5
5	Yellow	256–1	30.6 (520)	

After Norn (1974) and Ford (1976).
*The values in parentheses are the number of drops.

Table 11.3 Bromothymol blue as a pH indicator for tears

pH	Colour of tears
≤6.8	Yellow
7.0	Yellowish-green
7.2	Green
7.4	Greenish-blue
≥7.6	Blue

From Norn (1974).

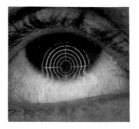

Figure 11.9 Limbal photography as shown by reflection from an A.I.M. photokeratoscope. The patient is looking up at the fourth ring from the centre

Assessment of limbal topography

Chapters 10, 17 and 18 on corneal and scleral lens fitting have stressed the respective importance of corneal and scleral topography. In the fitting of soft lenses these factors are no less important, but practitioners are also concerned with those aspects of global topography which it is least easy to quantify and measure. These are the diameter of the cornea, the rate of flattening of the corneal periphery and the configuration of the corneoscleral junction, all of which can only be assessed by observation rather than by direct measurement. They can often account for the unusual behaviour of a soft lens, and explain why two eyes with the same refractive error and keratometer readings may require soft lenses with completely different specifications in order to establish a satisfactory fit.

Corneal diameter is usually measured as the horizontal visible iris diameter (HVID) and varies from 10 to 14 mm, with an average of about 12 mm. Direct measurement with, for example, a graticule in the slit lamp eyepiece, only gives an assessment of the dimensions concerned, because it is not truly possible to ascertain exactly where the cornea finishes and the sclera begins. The horizontal axis is normally longer than the vertical by about 0.5–1.0 mm. The effective corneal diameter is perhaps best evaluated by placing a corneal soft lens of known total diameter on the eye and examining it *in situ*.

Peripheral flattening of the cornea can be studied with the topographic keratometer (Sampson and Soper, 1970), but this can be time consuming to undertake routinely. Alternatively, the Photo-Electric Keratoscope (PEK) may be used (Bibby, 1976). Limbal topography can also be assessed by observing the continuity of a slit beam as it crosses the corneoscleral

junction, and is most easily seen with a vertical slit at the lower limbus with the patient looking upwards. The reflection of a Placido disc at the limbus is also helpful in assessing its contour as shown in *Figure 11.9* in which the patient's gaze is directed slightly upwards. A corneal diameter lens on an eye with a shallow corneoscleral junction typically decentres and lags more easily than on an eye with a well-defined junction.

The use of fluorescein in fitting

Ordinary fluorescein cannot be used with hydrophilic lenses because it will be absorbed into the porous structure of the material. Except for high water content polymers, from which the colour may gradually fade, the lenses can be permanently stained (*Plate 81*). Because the fluorescein, in any case, rapidly spreads behind, in front and within the lens, it would be of little use. There have now appeared various forms of high-molecular-weight fluorescein, such as Fluoflex and Fluorexon, whose molecular size is sufficiently great to prevent immediate penetration into the soft lens materials (*Plate 28*). Fluorexon was introduced in 1972 by Refojo and others (Refojo, Korb and Silverman, 1972; Refojo, Miller and Fiore, 1972). It has a molecular weight approximately double that of fluorescein and the full chemical name is bis[N,N-bis(carboxymethyl)aminoethyl]fluorescein tetrasodium (Refojo, Miller and Fiore, 1972; Mossé and Scott, 1976). The degree of fluorescence, however, is much less than with standard fluorescein, and the fitting pattern difficult to observe and of doubtful value with a standard ultraviolet light. Poster (1977) found much better clinical results using a Kodak Wratten filter No. 47. Nevertheless, such dyes have been used in practice to demonstrate tear flow (Rocher, 1977). One or two drops are instilled into the lower fornix and the eye observed after a few blinks. If fluorescein can then be seen beneath the lens, it confirms that an interchange of tears occurs on blinking. If no fluorescein is observed, it suggests that the fitting is too tight, and the lens periphery is creating a seal where the edge of the lens presses against the bulbar conjunctiva.

Clinical routine

The complete clinical routine consists of the following steps:

(1) The taking of general and optical history.
(2) A complete routine refractive examination, including all the usual procedures such as ophthalmoscopy and tests of binocular function.
(3) Keratometry.
(4) Preliminary external eye examination, including slit lamp examination, lid eversion, tear film assessment and other techniques as outlined on p. 401 onwards.
(5) Discussion with the patient about lens types, and the decision to fit soft rather than other types of contact lens.
(6) The decision as to which variety of soft lens should be fitted or tried initially.
(7) Insertion of lenses.
(8) Initial assessment of fitting, vision and over-refraction.
(9) Tolerance trial with sufficient time for lens settling and equilibration.
(10) Re-assessment of vision, over-refraction, fitting and lens type.
(11) Re-examination with slit lamp, and other instruments as required.
(12) Ordering of lenses.
(13) Dispensing of lenses and patient instruction.
(14) After-care examinations.

Preliminary examination

The first steps are refraction, recording of monocular and binocular acuities and keratometry. These are all especially important with soft lens fitting, because an early assessment of visual suitability has to be made with respect to corneal and refractive astigmatism. A detailed slit lamp examination should then be made,

paying particular attention to the limbus and perilimbal blood vessels. If it is intended to insert soft lenses shortly afterwards, fluorescein and rose bengal cannot be used at this stage. However, they should be employed where the possibility of some prevailing corneal or conjunctival condition is suggested, warranting a more definite diagnosis before fitting can be safely commenced. In cases where these dyes are used, to prevent their absorption into the lens the conjunctival sac should be irrigated with saline solution afterwards and fitting delayed. External eye examination should always include eversion of the upper lid to confirm the normality of the palpebral conjunctiva (Allansmith *et al.*, 1977), and an assessment of the patient's tear flow, either by Schirmer's test or, better, by direct observation of the precorneal film (McDonald, 1969). An estimate of the horizontal corneal diameter is made and, if part of the normal routine, clinical photography and pachometry are carried out prior to fitting (*see* p. 401).

Lenses may be inserted by the practitioner in a variety of ways. Those of corneal size may be handled in much the same way as a hard lens, and placed directly onto the cornea. Thin lenses, however, are particularly unstable at the moment of insertion if an air bubble should be trapped behind and they may be expelled by an involuntary blink. The risk of this occurring is reduced if patients are requested to look down with gentle eye closure after insertion. Allowing the lens to dry for half a minute on the practitioner's finger prior to insertion encourages its transfer to the eye as the patient's tear film attracts it onto the eye from the finger, and prevents a thin lens from folding back on itself.

A second method is for the patient to look upwards at some suitable fixation target, and then to place the lens onto the inferior sclera, from which it will position itself correctly on the cornea when the eye turns to the primary position. A further method is to have the patient look down and nasally, while the lens is placed on the temporal sclera. It may then be slid across quite easily into the correct position. A right-handed practitioner may well find it simpler with a tight-lidded patient to approach the left eye first. In some cases, where the palpebral aperture is small, it may be necessary to partially fold a standard thickness lens between finger and thumb effectively to reduce its total diameter during insertion. Alternatively, it is sometimes helpful to balance the lens between the first and second fingers, particularly if it is a high positive lens, and unstable on only one finger because of its weight and the steep curvature of the lenticular portion of the front surface.

Certain of the proprietary solutions for storing hydrophilic lenses may cause some degree of stinging with sensitive eyes so that lenses should be cleaned and rinsed with sterile, non-preserved physiological saline prior to insertion. This also removes any particles which may be present on the lens surface. Care should be taken to avoid touching the back surface of the lens after it has been rinsed. Once the lens has assumed its correctly centred position on the cornea, the patient should be no more than slightly aware of its presence. Any significant level of discomfort is likely to be due to a foreign body trapped behind the lens. This may have been a speck of dust or make-up carried in, for example, from the eyelashes, or it may have been already present in the tear film and subsequently trapped by the lens. If discomfort is only mild, and patients sometimes describe this foreign body sensation as stinging, the lens should be slid onto the temporal sclera with a circular motion and allowed to recentre. This wiping action is usually sufficient to eliminate the cause of the discomfort, but if it persists the lens should be removed from the eye, cleaned and re-inserted.

Removal can sometimes be effected by the hard lens method of applying lid pressure, but a much simpler technique is to slide the lens onto either the temporal or inferior sclera from where it is pinched directly out of the eye. Although not ideal, suction holders can be used as described in Chapter 9.

Initial assessment of fitting and vision

When a hydrophilic lens is removed from its vial, it is fully hydrated with the maximum water uptake permitted by its particular storage medium. The lens, in settling on the eye, loses water by evaporation from its anterior surface and by the squeezing action of the eyelids. Some part, but not all, of this water loss is replenished by normal tear flow, until a state of equilibrium has been achieved for the environmental conditions prevailing in the consulting room. At the same time, the lens is adjusting to the temperature of the cornea, and to the pH and tonicity of the tears. The movement of the lens and therefore its fitting characteristics, unless grossly loose or tight, cannot be reliably judged for at least 20 minutes, until this state of equilibration on the cornea has been reached. The vision, on the other hand, if it is going to prove satisfactory, usually settles within the first 5 minutes, although the refractive result is not necessarily accurate after so short a time. If the visual acuity is initially poor it is unlikely to improve and the lens should be changed.

In some instances, particularly with ultrathin lenses, false fitting results can occur. A lens sometimes settles within its storage vial so as to adhere to the base, neck or lid. It therefore has a temporarily distorted shape, unrelated to its true fitting parameters, and its behaviour on the eye may be very different from that of the same lens in an unstressed state. Similarly, if a lens has been disinfected by heating and not allowed sufficient time to cool and revert to its proper dimensions, it may well appear to fit too tightly. The same effect can be produced by a lens stored in hypotonic saline solution, which may sometimes even give a temporary osmotic adhesion to the cornea. Eventually, the patient's natural tear flow restores the osmotic balance and allows the lens to move but the process is assisted by the liberal application of physiological saline. This situation is illustrated in *Figure 11.10*. In practical terms, this means that if a lens is completely immobile just after insertion, it is more likely to be a tonicity rather than a fitting problem.

Methods of observing the fit

Lens movement and position are most easily observed by using the slit lamp with low magnification and white light. The action of the lens edge on blinking can be judged in relation to the position of the limbal vessels. In some eyes with rather loose conjunctival tissue, however, the appearance can be misleading. Movement of possibly even a tight fitting may be attributed to the lens when it is, in fact, motion of the bulbar conjunctiva. A further indication of fit may be obtained by using $\times 35$ or $\times 40$ magnification and observing the passage of blood through the limbal vessels beneath the lens edge, to ensure that there is no obstruction

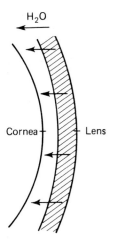

Figure 11.10 A soft lens stored in hypotonic saline solution adhering to the cornea due to the osmotic pressure difference which encourages water to enter the cornea from the lens. The application of physiological saline solution eventually restores the osmotic balance permitting the lens to be removed

to its normal steady flow. Without a slit lamp, lens movement is best seen by directing the beam from a hand-held pen torch, not necessarily from in front, but from the side or below so that the junction of the lenticular portion of the lens casts an easily observed annular light pattern and shadow onto the iris background (*Plate 29*). The movement of this is more easily discernible than that of the lens itself. A further simple test for semi-scleral lenses is to slide the lens gently onto the temporal sclera, two-thirds of the way off the cornea, and to observe the way in which it recentres. A correctly fitting lens has a quick recovery movement, whereas that of a flat fitting is considerably more sluggish. A steep lens, although recentring sharply, may be difficult to slide off the cornea.

Because most fitting criteria relate to lens movement and quality of vision, the slit lamp, keratometer and retinoscope have become important fitting instruments.

Tolerance trials

Once the initial fitting characteristics have been confirmed as satisfactory, ideally the next stage of the clinical routine is a long tolerance of about 2–4 hours, using, where possible, lenses of the correct power and fitting. Patients can then wear lenses in their normal daily environment,

carrying out their usual visual tasks. In this way a fairly reliable assessment is possible of their potential success, and latent problems such as dry eyes or near vision difficulty may be discovered. When a lengthy trial is not practicable, it still remains essential to leave lenses for enough time to settle fully. A minimum of 20–30 minutes is recommended. A long tolerance trial, however, is especially important for previous hard or rigid gas permeable lens failures so that, on the one hand, the practitioner can be more certain of a satisfactory result and, on the other, the patient may be reassured with regard to contact lenses in the light of earlier failure (*see also* Chapter 19).

After the trial, fitting and refraction are carefully reassessed. Any marked deterioration in visual acuity other than that due to uncorrected astigmatism suggests the fitting is steep. This occurs when tear flow has returned to normal, lens mobility decreases and an initially acceptable fit has become tight. Examination of the eye itself should confirm the absence of corneal oedema and striae, punctate epithelial staining with fluorescein, limbal and conjunctival irritation, and scleral indentation. If any elevations of the upper palpebral conjunctiva had been previously noted, the lids should be everted to make sure that there is no irritation or staining of these areas with fluorescein.

At this stage, the clinical decision can usually be made as to whether the patient is suitable for hydrophilic lenses. In cases of doubt, either visual or physiological, the tolerance trial should be repeated on another occasion. If possible, patients are loaned lenses of optimum fitting and power for several days, in order to extend the trial period. This procedure is straightforward if lenses are fitted from stock, or if the manufacturer concerned operates a lens exchange system.

Patients frequently confuse right and left lenses and it can be particularly difficult to identify two unmarked lenses of only 0.25 D power difference. When feasible, it is much easier to avoid this problem by ordering the final powers to be the same for both eyes. The alternative is to make the two lenses as different as possible so that the patient is more likely to realize if they have been inadvertently switched, or else to have a dot engraved on one lens (*see* Chapter 23).

Table 11.4 Fitting characteristics of soft lenses

Observation	Good fit	Steep fit	Flat fit
Comfort	Good	Good, initially	Poor
Centration	Good, with complete corneal coverage	Usually good, may be decentred, no recovery on blinking	Poor
Movement on blinking	Up to 1.0 mm	Less than 0.5 mm	Excessive, over 2.0 mm
Movement on upwards gaze	Up to 1.5 mm	Little or none	Excessive, over 3.0 mm
Movement on lateral gaze	Up to 1.5 mm	Little or none	Excessive, over 3.0 mm
Vision	Good	Poor and variable, momentary improvement on blinking	Variable, may improve on staring after blinking
Over-refraction	Precise end-point, power correlates with BVP of spectacle *Rx*	Poorly defined end-point, positive liquid lens	Variable, negative liquid lens
Retinoscopy reflex	Clear reflex, before and after blinking	Poor and distorted, central shadow, momentarily improved on blinking	Variable, may be clear centrally with peripheral distortion
Slit lamp after settling	No limbal injection or scleral indentation	Conjunctival or limbal injection, scleral indentation	Localized limbal injection, possible edge stand-off
Keratometer mires	Sharp, stable before and after blinking	Irregular, momentary improvement on blinking	Variable and eccentric, changing on blinking
Placido disc	Regular image	Irregular image anywhere but at the edge of the lens	Irregular image, more often peripheral only but occasionally central as well

Fitting characteristics for soft lenses

The general fitting characteristics for soft lenses are summarized in *Table 11.4*.

Characteristics of a good fitting

A lens which is fitting well is comfortable in all directions of gaze, gives complete corneal coverage and appears properly centred. Normal blinking results in about 1 mm of vertical movement when the eye is in the primary position. The lens lags by up to 1.5 mm on upwards gaze or lateral movements of the eye. Vision is good, remaining stable on blinking. Refraction gives a precise end-point, correlating with the BVP of the spectacles. The retinoscopy reflex is crisp and sharp both before and after a blink. Keratometry of the front surface of the lens on the eye shows the mires to be stable and undistorted. The slit lamp shows no irritation of the limbal vessels or compression of the conjunctiva.

Characteristics of a steep fitting

A lens fitting too steeply gives little or no movement either on blinking or as the eye changes fixation. Initially, a tight fitting is quite comfortable, sometimes more so than a correct fit, because a completely immobile lens produces the minimum of lid sensation. Centration is usually good, although a corneal-sized lens may sometimes assume a decentred position. This is easily differentiated from a decentred flat fitting because of the lack of movement. The slit lamp may show irritation of the conjunctival or limbal vessels and, with very tight semi-scleral

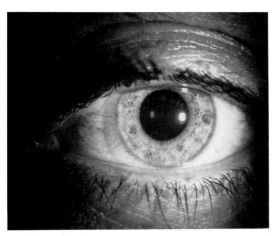

Figure 11.11 Nasal scleral indentation following the wearing of a tight semi-scleral lens

lenses, an annular ring of conjunctival compression may be seen, which is often visible even after the lens has been removed (*Figure 11.11*).

A steep fitting soft lens vaults the corneal apex, but is momentarily pressed onto the eye on blinking. Vision is, therefore, unstable and of poor quality, although showing some transient improvement after a blink. Subjective refraction is difficult, with no clearly defined end-point, and more negative power than predicted may be required because of a positive liquid lens and flexure. Retinoscopy reflex and keratometer mires both show irregular distortions such as those indicated by photokeratoscopy in *Figure 11.6a,b*. They may also improve momentarily on blinking.

Characteristics of a flat fitting

A flat fitting is more easily diagnosed because of the absence of proper centration, greater lens mobility on blinking, and excessive lag on lateral eye movements as shown in *Figure 11.12*. Such a fit is often very uncomfortable, especially on looking upwards, when the lens may slide down 3 mm or more, and catch against the upper lid on blinking. In the primary position, lower lid sensation is experienced if the lens sags, and discomfort is accentuated if the lens is so flat that the periphery buckles to give edge stand-off (*Figure 11.13* and *Plate 29*). Vision and over-refraction are variable, but nevertheless may still give a satisfactory result. The retinoscopy reflex may be clear centrally but with peripheral distortion. Keratometry mires change according to lens movement, showing an eccentric shape on blinking. *Figure 11.14* shows the photokeratoscope image from a flat lens, the

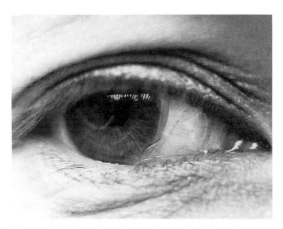

Figure 11.13 Very loose fitting showing buckling of lens edge

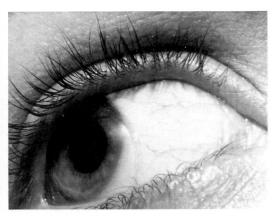

Figure 11.12 A flat-fitting spun-cast lens of corneal size showing excessive lag on temporal excursion of the eye. The edge of the lens is clearly visible

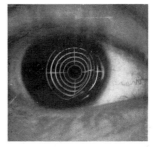

Figure 11.14 An eye wearing a flat-fitting low water content lens of corneal size. The photokeratoscope shows up the peripheral distortion

peripheral distortion being most marked. Occasionally a flat fitting lens may appear to fit well but in a decentred position.

Fitting philosophies and soft lens selection

Selecting the most appropriate soft lens is not always a straightforward procedure because of the very wide range of lens forms now available. Several factors must be taken into account including: size (corneal or semi-scleral), water content (high or low), thickness (standard or 'thin'), geometric and optic design (spherical or aspheric) and manufacturing method (lathed or moulded). All have some influence on vision, comfort and fitting characteristics. Frequently, however, it is the total diameter which determines the method of fitting.

Although there is some degree of overlap with certain of the single-diameter lenses, the two main fitting philosophies into which soft lenses may be divided are semi-scleral and corneal. (In theory there is a third, in which lenses are fitted smaller than the corneal diameter, but in practice such lenses have not proven successful with the present range of materials.)

Semi-scleral lenses

Semi-scleral lenses are fitted significantly larger than the visible iris diameter to give deliberate apical touch with further support beyond the limbus where they overlap onto the sclera (*Figure 11.15*). They vary in size from 13.50 mm to 16.00 mm with the majority in the range 14.00–15.00 mm. Lathed semi-scleral lenses almost always have a greater thickness than

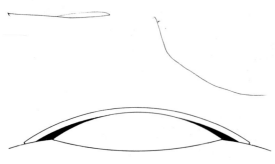

Figure 11.15 A semi-scleral soft lens giving apical and scleral touch but bridging the limbus region

corneal lenses so that, although it is easily possible to manufacture them from the entire range of materials, for physiological reasons, nearly all such lenses are now of medium to high water content. Semi-scleral lenses frequently give greater stability of vision and fitting than corneal lenses and may well prove much more successful for patients with sensitive lids or limbus.

The high water content varieties give very good initial comfort and their high Dk values mean that they can be recommended for the majority of cases including moderate degrees of astigmatism and patients prone to corneal oedema. For this last reason they are very often the preferred choice for hypermetropes where they also achieve better centration.

Cosmetically, semi-scleral lenses are more noticeable on the eye and in practice many of the varieties must be contra-indicated for the usual reasons associated with high water content, of breakage, shorter lifespan, dryness and dehydration, and environmental factors (*see* p. 392).

Fitting technique

Most of the early forms of hydrophilic lens made the same size as, or smaller than, the cornea proved to be very unstable because of their relative thickness; they gave poor vision and were very uncomfortable because of lid sensation. It is for this reason that the 'semi-scleral' method of fitting evolved, in order to give stability of fitting and vision.

The intention of the fitting philosophy is to give definite apical touch, with further support for the lens edge being provided beyond the limbus by a much flatter peripheral curve resting on the sclera. It is essential that the total diameter of the lens is large enough not to interfere with the blood vessels in the limbal region.

Initial lens selection is determined by two factors: the keratometer readings, and the horizontal corneal diameter.

HEMA lenses are usually fitted between 0.7 mm and 1.3 mm flatter than the flattest 'K'. High water content materials may be fitted more steeply than this. Where a choice is available, the total diameter is selected to be 2–3 mm larger than the horizontal visible iris diameter (HVID).

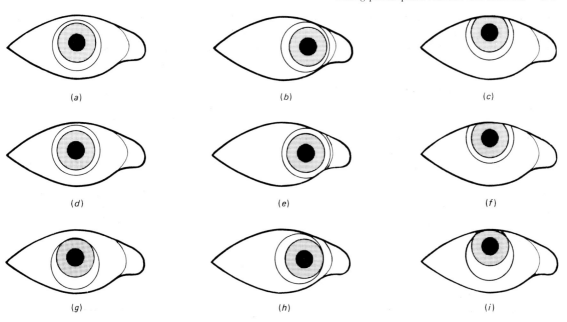

Figure 11.16 Semi-scleral lenses shown with the eye in the primary position, on the left-hand side, looking laterally in the centre column and looking upwards on the right-hand side. The upper three diagrams, (*a*), (*b*) and (*c*), show a correctly fitting lens; the centre three diagrams, (*d*), (*e*) and (*f*), show a tightly fitting lens; the lower three diagrams, (*g*), (*h*) and (*i*), show a loose fitting lens

The fitting characteristics of correct, steep and flat lenses are as described on pp. 408–410 and summarized in *Table 11.4*. *Figure 11.16a–c* shows diagrammatically the limits of acceptable lens movement and position for semi-scleral lenses with the eye in the primary position and in lateral and upward gaze respectively. *Figure 11.16d–f* shows the lack of movement with a tight lens. *Figure 11.16g–i* shows the excessive mobility of a loose fitting lens as also shown in *Figure 11.17*.

Because of liquid lens or flexure effects, the power of a correctly fitting lens shows approximately 0.25 D to 0.50 D less minus than the spectacle *Rx*, allowing for any vertex distance considerations.

Primary sagitta

The choice of action required to correct an unsatisfactory semi-scleral fitting was related by Brailsford (1972), Rocher and Schwegler (1974) and Hodd (1976) to the primary sag or sagittal height of the lens in the same way as described for FLOM lenses (fenestrated lenses for optic measurements) in Chapter 17. In this way, a steep lens is corrected by decreasing the sag (flatter radius or smaller total diameter), and a flat lens by increasing the sag (steeper radius or larger total diameter).

The principle of clinical equivalents therefore also applies as it does to FLOM lenses, so that two lenses of different but related specification may behave in the same way on the same eye. For many semi-scleral lenses a change of radius of 0.3 mm is approximately equivalent to altering the total diameter by 0.5 mm.

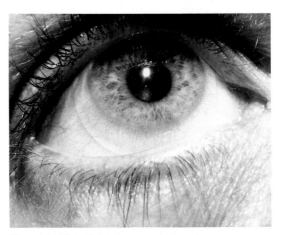

Figure 11.17 A slightly loose semi-scleral lens

Clinical equivalents do not, in fact, have the same primary sag because of their different diameters, and Cooke (G. E., 1976, personal communication) suggested that the ratio between primary sag and total diameter is more meaningful. Thus, 8.40:14.0, 8.70:14.5, and 9.00:15.0, which may be considered clinically equivalent in terms of their fitting characteristics, have almost the same sag to total diameter ratios.

A steep fitting may, therefore, be corrected in two ways, either by selecting a lens with a flatter radius, or by employing a smaller total diameter. If the initial lens has proved very tight, it may be necessary to combine both of these fitting changes. For example, if a lens of specification 8.7:14.5 is too steep, it may be progressively loosened by the following lenses: 8.7:14.0, 9.0:14.5, and 9.0:14.0. Generally, altering the radius has a greater effect on the fitting than changing the total diameter.

Conversely, a flat fitting may be corrected by choosing a steeper radius, or a larger total diameter, or possibly both. Thus, 8.70:14.0 may be progressively steepened by the lenses: 8.70:14.5, 8.40:14.0, and 8.40:14.5.

Corneal diameter soft lenses

The majority of corneal diameter soft lenses are still manufactured from low to medium water content materials to give reproducible lenses of good durability. The thinner varieties, in particular, give a minimum of interference with normal corneal metabolism and they have an excellent cosmetic appearance. They can be recommended for the majority of straightforward cases, patients with poor handling ability, particularly those with small palpebral apertures, and most of those cases prone to oedema with hard or rigid gas permeable lenses. They may be contra-indicated for some patients with tight lids and shallow corneoscleral junctions if these cause lens decentration and consequent visual problems, or peripheral arcuate staining. Patients with sensitive lids may find adaptation difficult because of the sensation experienced each time the lid margin crosses the edge of the lens on blinking.

Fitting technique

A correctly fitting corneal diameter soft lens gives complete corneal coverage with proper centration. It should be the same size as or slightly larger than the horizontal visible iris diameter extending beyond the limbus by up to 0.5–0.75 mm. Lenses vary in size from 11.5 mm to 14.50 mm with the majority in the range 12.50–13.50 mm. The thin varieties, as well as high water content, and high positive and negative lenses, are fitted approximately 0.5 mm larger than those of standard thickness in order to ensure stability on the cornea.

The radius for standard HEMA lenses is usually between 0.3 mm and 0.6 mm flatter than flattest 'K'. High water content lenses are fitted closer to alignment whereas the more rigid lower water content materials may require radii 0.7 mm or more flatter than flattest 'K'.

Most corneal diameter soft lenses have a mono-curve back surface and the two principal parameters of radius and diameter frequently have fitting steps of 0.2 mm and 0.5 mm, respectively.

Fitting characteristics are mainly as outlined in *Table 11.4*. Corneal diameter lenses require careful observation of centration and movement since they can be significantly influenced by such factors as corneal and limbal topography, lid pressure and size and position of the palpebral aperture.

Figure 11.18a–d shows the four common ways in which a lens may position on the cornea with the eye in the primary position. In *Figure 11.18a* an optimum fitting is shown. The lens is perfectly centred and there should be 0.5–1.0 mm of vertical movement on blinking. In *Figure 11.18b*, the lens is riding slightly high, influenced, for example, by a tight upper lid. This may prove acceptable provided the decentration is no more than about 0.5 mm, but an attempt should be made to improve the fitting by selecting a larger diameter.

In *Figure 11.18c*, the lens is shown riding in a low position. It generally represents an unsatisfactory fitting which is too small or too flat and the patient is likely to complain of unacceptable lid sensation. It can also result from the downwards pressure of a relatively heavy upper lid creating a fitting which is too tight, although initially quite comfortable. There is the possibility of arcuate staining at the superior limbus after several hours of wear together with oedema because of insufficient tear exchange.

In *Figure 11.18d*, the lens is eccentrically located. This may also be due to a fitting which

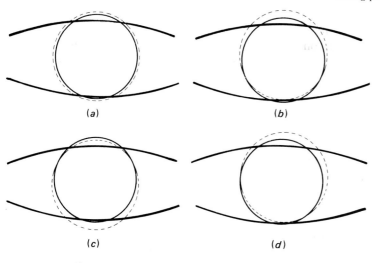

(a)

(b)

(c)

(d)

Figure 11.18 The four common positions taken up by soft lenses of corneal size (shown with dashed outline), on an eye in the primary position. (*a*) Correctly centred: (*b*) slightly high; (*c*) slightly low; (*d*) laterally decentred

is too small or too flat, or because of lid pressure combined with a shallow corneoscleral junction. It represents a rather unsatisfactory fitting although it may sometimes prove acceptable if the decentration is limited to 0.5 mm. A larger total diameter should be tried.

Lenses must give complete corneal coverage to avoid the risk of epithelial dehydration and arcuate staining of any exposed area. An attempt should always be made to improve the fitting characteristics of a decentred lens by selecting a larger diameter. Where this fails, it may be necessary to consider a semi-scleral lens. The principle of clinical equivalents frequently applies so that a change in diameter of 0.5 mm ≃ a change of radius of 0.2 mm.

Thus, 7.90:12.50 is approximately clinically equivalent to 8.10:13.00, and 8.30:13.00 is approximately clinically equivalent to 8.50:13.50.

A loose fitting may be improved by choosing either a larger total diameter or a steeper radius, but it is usually preferable to achieve a more stable fitting by increasing the total diameter. Maintaining a flatter radius is likely to give better visual acuity by keeping the lens in alignment with the cornea.

A tight fitting may be improved by selecting a flatter radius or a smaller total diameter. It is important to avoid fitting too tightly — either too steep or too large — because of the risk of oedema. This can occur even with thin or high water content lenses with high *Dk* values, particularly for thicker lenses of positive power. It is also essential to ensure adequate lens mobility to allow proper tear flow for removal of debris from beneath the lens.

General fitting points

With all soft lens fitting, if there is a possible choice between two radii when selecting a lens, it is much better to commence with the flatter. There are three main reasons for this. First, it is much easier to see the movement of a lens which is too loose and therefore excessively mobile rather than the relative lack of movement of a steep fitting; secondly, a sharper end-point can be obtained with over-refraction; thirdly, soft lenses become tighter after settling.

Steep corneas require lens selection to be relatively much flatter than flat corneas where the optimum fitting is likely to be significantly closer to flattest 'K'. This applies to both corneal and semi-scleral lenses. Thus, a radius of 8.10 mm may be necessary for a 13.00 mm lens on a 7.40 mm cornea, whereas an 8.40 mm cornea might well require a radius of 8.70 mm or even 8.50 mm.

Lens flexibility

A further important influence on the fitting characteristics is the flexibility of the material. This accounts for two lenses of apparently the same specification and material behaving in entirely different ways on the cornea. *Figure 11.19* illustrates the difference in flexibility of several soft lens materials (Burgess *et al.*, 1985). It explains why Permalens, which is very flexible, often requires to be fitted steeper than

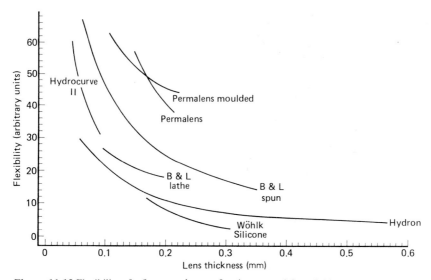

Figure 11.19 Flexibility of soft contact lenses of various materials and thicknesses

'K' compared with other more rigid materials where the more usual flatter than 'K' approach is correct. Similarly, thin spun-cast and moulded lenses with their overall thin cross-section and inherently greater flexibility than their lathed counterparts, lend themselves better to a 'one-fit' fitting philosophy which relies on draping the cornea.

Examples of lens types

It is not possible in a chapter of this nature to include a detailed description of the fitting procedures for each and every soft lens currently available. Existing lens designs are constantly being improved upon while new varieties are continually being introduced. The lenses described here, although relating to an individual laboratory, have been chosen as typical examples of the same general type. It should therefore be possible to deduce the fitting method for any soft lens not specifically mentioned* by reference to the general fitting principles described.

A selected list of commonly available lenses is given in *Table 11.1*, which is intended to give an idea of the range of polymers, water contents and oxygen permeabilities currently in use.

Hydron Mini

A standard thickness, corneal diameter lens manufactured from HEMA.

*Omission of some of these excellent laboratories is not intended as a reflection on the quality of their work.

Manufactured by: Allergan Hydron Limited.

Material properties

Chemical nature	HEMA cross-linked polymer
Water content	38.6% at 20°C
Oxygen permeability*	8.0×10^{-11} at 20°C and 10×10^{-11} at 35°C
Refractive index	1.513 (dry), 1.43 (wet)
Swell factor (not linear)	1.19
Optical transmission	95%
Density	1.17 g/ml
Tensile strength	8 kg/cm^2
Tear strength (initiation)	3 (approximately) g/mm^2
Water permeability	$\sim 10 \times 10^{15}$ cm^4/dyn (10^{16} cm^4/μN)

Manufacturing method

Lenses are lathe-cut according to the tolerances shown in *Table 11.5*.

Table 11.5 Tolerances of Hydron soft lenses

Parameter	Dry	Hydrated
Back optic radius (mm)	±0.04	±0.05
Thickness (mm)	±0.02	±0.024
Total diameter (mm)	±0.05	±0.06
Power (D)	±0.12	±0.14

*In this section all oxygen permeabilities (*Dk* values) are in units ($\times 10^{-11}$) of (cm ml O$_2$)/(cm^2 s mmHg).

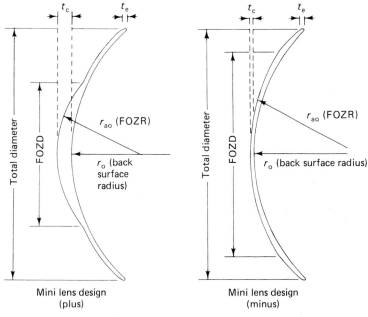

Figure 11.20 Hydron Mini lens design

Lens geometry

The Mini design is shown in *Figure 11.20*. Lenses are lenticulated to give the centre thicknesses and front optic zone diameters (FOZDs) shown in *Table 11.6*.

Table 11.6 FOZD and centre thickness for Hydron Mini lenses

Back vertex power (D)	FOZD (mm)	Centre thickness (mm)
−20.00	8.4	0.12
−10.00	8.4	0.12
−5.00	10.0	0.12
−2.00	11.4	0.12
Plano	11.4	0.14
+2.00	9.0	0.21
+5.00	7.8	0.30
+10.00	7.2	0.38
+20.00	7.2	0.56

Parameters available

These are given in *Table 11.7*.

Table 11.7 Parameters available for Hydron Mini lenses

Back surface radius (mm)	7.90–8.90 in 0.20 steps	8.10–9.30 in 0.20 steps
Total diameter (mm)	12.50	13.00
Back vertex Power (D)	±10.00 in 0.25 steps ±10.50 to ±30.00 in 0.50 steps	

Fitting set

This is given in *Table 11.8*.

Table 11.8 Recommended fitting set for Hydron Mini lenses

Back surface radius (mm)	Total diameter (mm)
8.10	13.00
8.30	13.00
8.50	13.00
8.70	13.00
8.90	13.00
9.10	13.00
	Power −3.00 D

Fitting technique

The total diameter should be at least 1 mm larger than the HVID total. Lenses of diameter 13.00 mm are therefore used in approximately 90% of cases. The initial back surface radius is selected to be about 0.7 mm flatter than flattest 'K'. Fitting characteristics are as described for most corneal diameter soft lenses (p. 412–413) and in *Table 11.4*. A flat fitting lens is shown in *Figure 11.21*

Typical lens specification

A typical lens specification is 8.70:13.00 −3.00 D.

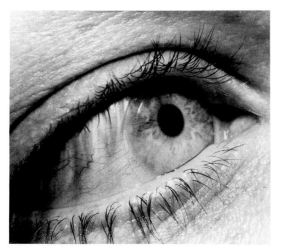

Figure 11.21 Flat fitting corneal diameter soft lens, showing excessive lag on nasal rotation of the eye

Lunelle ES 70

A high water content corneal diameter lens for daily or extended wear.
Manufactured by: Essilor.

Material properties

Chemical nature	Copolymer of PMMA and polyvinyl pyrrolidone
Water content	70%
Oxygen permeability	35×10^{-11} at 25°C
Refractive index	1.38
Linear swell factor	1.5
Optical transmission	98.6%
Modulus of elasticity	15.00 kgf/cm^2 (147 N/cm^2)
Tensile strength	18 ± 2 kgf/cm^2 (176 $\pm$ 20 N/cm^2)

Manufacturing method

Lathe-cutting.

Lens geometry

Lenses have a spherical back surface with an average thickness of 0.15 mm. The relative stiffness of the material gives an advantage in correcting low-to-medium degrees of astigmatism (0.75–1.25 D).

Parameters available

These are given in *Table 11.9*.

Table 11.9 Parameters available for Lunelle ES 70 lenses

Back surface radius (mm)	7.70–8.30 in 0.30 steps	8.00–9.20 in 0.30 steps
Total diameter (mm)	13.00	14.00
Back vertex power (D)	Plano to −12.00	±20.00

Fitting set

This is given in *Table 11.10*.

Table 11.10 Recommended fitting set for Lunelle ES 70 lenses

Back surface radius (mm)	*Total diameter* (mm)	
7.70	13.00	
8.00	13.00	
8.30		14.00
8.60		14.00
8.90		14.00
Back vertex power (D)	−3.00	±3.00

Aphakic trial lenses are also available.

Fitting technique

A total diameter of 13.00 mm is the initial selection for corneas of diameter 11.25 mm or less; for larger corneas 14.00 mm lenses are used. The manufacturers recommend fitting 0.30 mm and 0.60 mm flatter than flattest 'K' for 13.00 mm and 14.00 mm lenses, respectively. Both Atkinson (1986) and Fanti (1986), however, achieved better clinical results with back surface radii flatter still. Lens movement should be 1.00–1.50 mm on blinking. The most common fittings are, therefore, 8.60 and 8.90 mm back surface radii with the 14.00 mm total diameter.

Typical lens specification

A typical lens specification is 8.90:14.00 −3.00 D.

Additional comments

A low rate of lens dehydration is claimed which is useful either to avoid or assist dry eye problems. Fanti (1986), however, deduced from refractive results that there was some degree of reduced water content on the eye, requiring over-correction in the higher power ranges.

The Lunelle ES 70 provides the basis for fitting other Lunelle lenses:

(1) Two toroidal front surface designs.

(2) The Solaire, which includes a sun-filter and an ultraviolet inhibitor.

(3) The Aphakic UV, which contains an ultraviolet inhibitor.

Hydroflex SD

A thin HEMA corneal diameter lens.

The Hydroflex SD is the thin version of the standard thickness Hydroflex/m (SD derives from the German 'super dünn' or 'super thin').

Manufactured by: Wöhlk–Contact–Linsen, a subsidiary of Zeiss.

Material properties

Chemical nature	HEMA
Water content	38.6%
Oxygen permeability	7.3×10^{-11} at 21°C
Refractive index	1.448 (at 23°C)
Swell factor (wet length/dry length)	1.69
Softening temperature	109°C
Elasticity	11.3 mm elastic deformation
Penetration strength	4.81 N
Hardness (at 20°C)	85.6 Shore-D-units
Ash content (3 g ashed at 550°C)	<0.1%

Manufacturing method

All lenses are lathe-cut.

Lens geometry

All minus lenses have a centre thickness of 0.08 mm and an edge thickness of 0.05 mm. The FOZD is constant at 7.80 mm for both positive and negative lenses.

Parameters available

These are shown in *Table 11.11.*

Table 11.11 Parameters available for Hydroflex SD lenses

	Low powers	Aphakic powers
Back surface radius (mm)	7.60, 8.00 8.40, 8.80	8.40, 8.80 9.20
Total diameter (mm)	13.00, 13.50	14.50
Back vertex power (D)	±10.00 in 0.25 D steps	+14.00 to +20.00 in 0.25 D steps

Fitting set

This is shown in *Table 11.12.*

Table 11.12 Recommended fitting set for Hydroflex SD lenses

Back surface radius (mm)	Total diameter (mm)		
7.60	13.00		
8.00	13.00	13.50	
8.40		13.50	14.50
8.80		13.50	14.50
9.20			14.50
Back vertex powers (D)		±3.00 D	+14.00 D

Fitting techniques

Fitting characteristics of thin lenses differ from their standard counterparts. It is, therefore, not possible to assess the fitting on the basis of a standard mini trial set. The greater degree of flexibility means that, in most cases, fitting can be satisfactorily accomplished with larger back surface radius intervals of 0.4 mm.

The most commonly used total diameter is 13.50 mm, but 13.00 mm lenses are useful for smaller corneas or where the larger size causes irritation of the lower lid. Initial back surface radius is selected to be approximately 0.3–0.5 mm flatter than flattest 'K'.

Fitting characteristics are mainly as described on pp. 412–413 and in *Table 11.4*, except that a smaller degree of movement on blinking may be permitted because of the superior *Dk/t* value.

Typical lens specification

A typical lens specification is: 8.40:13.50 −3.00 D.

Additional comments

Thin lenses may be contra-indicated for poor lens handlers and where they give a less satisfactory visual acuity.

Weicon 38 Elliptical (W38E)

An aspheric corneal diameter soft lens.
Manufactured by: CIBA Vision (previously Titmus-Eurocon).

Material properties

Chemical nature	HEMA
Water content	37.5% ± 1%
Oxygen permeability	8.5×10^{-11} at 35°C
Refractive index	1.43
Linear swelling	18.0% ± 1%
Ball pressure hardness (60 s)	$18 \pm 1\,kgf/mm^2$ ($176 \pm 10\,N/mm^2$)
Contact angle (captive bubble method)	19° ± 1°

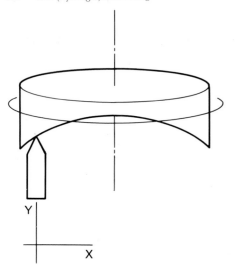

Figure 11.22 Schematic representation of computer numeric controlled (CNC) lathe, where X and Y coordinates are controlled by a microprocessor

Manufacturing method

All lenses are manufactured on computer numeric controlled (CNC) lathes. This is represented schematically in *Figure 11.22* where the X and Y coordinates of the diamond tool are controlled by a microprocessor.

Lens geometry

All lenses have an elliptical back surface. *Figure 11.23* shows this diagrammatically, together with a typical

CIBA Vision-style engraving. Lenses do not have a true back surface radius, but have a choice of two 'fitting values' which are designated either 'flat' (FL) or 'steep' (ST). Both vertex radius and eccentricity are varied to give a consistent performance throughout the power range. Lenses also feature the 'tangential bevel' shown in *Figure 11.24*, which gives a continuous transition from the back surface to the lens edge where it permits a 'ski' effect.

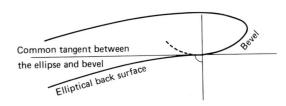

Figure 11.24 'Tangential bevel' of the Weicon 38E which allows a continuous transition from the elliptical back surface to the lens edge

Parameters available

These are shown in *Table 11.13*.

Table 11.13 Parameters available for Weicon 38 Elliptical lenses

Fitting value	Flat (FL) or steep (ST)
Total diameter (mm)	13.00, 13.80, 14.60
Back vertex power (D)	±20.00

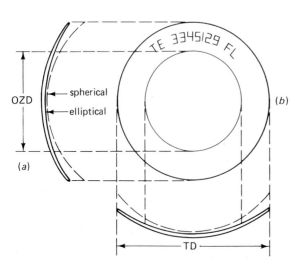

Figure 11.23 Diagram of a typical Weicon 38E lens showing (*a*) how the elliptical back surface geometry differs from that of a spherical lens, and (*b*) a CIBA Vision-style engraving for lens identification

Fitting set

This is shown in *Table 11.14*.

Table 11.14 Recommended fitting set for Weicon 38 Elliptical lenses

Total diameter (mm)	Back surface power (D) and fitting value
13.00	−3.00(FL), −1.50(ST)
13.80	−1.50(FL), −3.00(FL), −3.00(ST)
14.60	−4.00(FL)

Low plus and aphakic sets are also available.

Fitting technique

The initial trial lens is generally selected to have a 13.80 mm total diameter with the flat fitting value. Because of the aspherical back surface, changing the total diameter does not necessarily alter the fitting characteristics. The steeper fitting value is tried only if the lens is obviously mobile after complete settling.

A correctly fitting lens will behave in the main as indicated in *Table 11.4*, but lens mobility of between 0.5 mm and 2 mm is acceptable. Although the elliptical design is suitable for a wide range of patients, there are nevertheless some corneal geometries for which a satisfactory fitting cannot be achieved. These require a more traditional lens design with a spherical back surface.

Typical specification

A typical specification is FL 13.80 −3.00 D

Additional comments

The Weicon elliptical design is the basis for the fitting of other CIBA Vision soft lenses.

Weicon 38EX   This is an ultrathin lens with a centre thickness of 0.035 mm. It is available with only the flat fitting value, total diameters of 13.00 mm and 13.80 mm and power range plano to −7.00 D. The lens is recommended to achieve greater comfort or for weekly extended wear.

Weicon CE 60%   This has a 60% water content with a *Dk* of 28. It may be used for either daily or extended wear.

Weicon 38E Bifocal   This is a concentric bifocal with a central distance portion.

Weicon 38E Ellipticolour   Four colours are available each in 10% and 20% light absorption, i.e. transmission of 90% and 80%.

Permaflex

A high water content semi-scleral lens for daily or extended wear.
Manufactured by: CooperVision, in the UK.

Material properties

Chemical nature	A hydrophilic cross-linked copolymer of methyl methacrylate, vinyl pyrrolidone, and other methacrylates
Water content	73.5%
Oxygen permeability	34×10^{-11} at 25°C
	43×10^{-11} at 36°C
Refractive index	1.385
Linear swell factor	1.600 at 21°C
Tensile strength	$7.6 \, kg/cm^2$
Elongation at break	315%

Manufacturing method

Lenses are cast-moulded.

Lens geometry

A typical lens of power −3.00 D is shown in *Figure 11.25*. Centre thickness varies from 0.08 mm to 0.22 mm for negative powers with a minimum FOZD of 7.50 mm.

Parameters available

These are shown in *Table 11.15*.

Table 11.15 Parameters available for Permaflex lenses

BOZR (mm)	8.70, 8.90
TD (mm)	14.40
BVP (D)	−10.00 to +6.00

Fitting set

Lenses are provided in a range of powers for the two radii. The preferred method of fitting is from a lens stock.

Fitting technique

The spherical 8.70 mm BOZR fits a high percentage of patients and except for very flat corneas is the parameter selected initially. Because of the high water content, sufficient time must be allowed for lens settling or an apparently correct fitting may subsequently become tight. It should be noted that lenses of 8.90 mm BOZR fit significantly flatter than those of

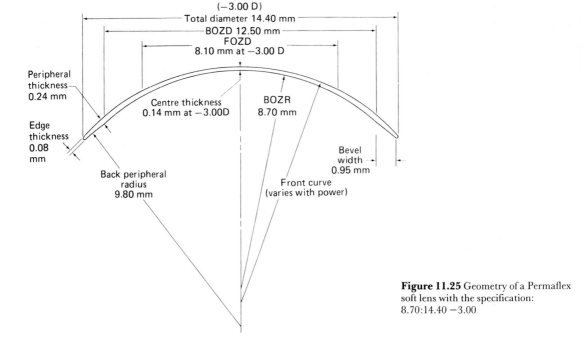

Figure 11.25 Geometry of a Permaflex soft lens with the specification: 8.70:14.40 −3.00

8.70 mm, rather more than would be anticipated, because the posterior surface is, in fact, an aspherical curve *equivalent* to 8.90 mm.

Typical specification

A typical specification is: 8.70:14.40 −3.00 D.

Additional comments

Permaflex lenses in negative powers and the 8.70 mm BOZR are also available with an ultraviolet inhibitor or in a range of five tints.

Hydrocurve II 55

A medium water content, semi-scleral lens for daily or extended wear.
Manufactured by: Pilkington Barnes–Hind.

Material properties

Chemical nature	A copolymer of HEMA, *N*-(1,1-dimethyl-3-oxobutylacrylamide) and methacrylic acid
Water content	55% (or 45% — *see below*)
Oxygen permeability	14.2×10^{-11} at 21°C
Refractive index	1.41
Light transmission	90%
Specific gravity	1.15

Manufacturing method

Lathe-cutting, although spherical lenses have a moulded back surface radius.

Lens geometry

The posterior surface is of mono-curve construction. Centre thickness is 0.05 mm for a lens of power −3.00 D.

Parameters available

The parameters available (mm) are 8.50:14.00 and 8.80:14.50 in powers from +20.00 D to −12.00 D.

Fitting set

Lenses are provided in a range of powers for the two available fittings. The preferred method of fitting is from a lens stock.

Fitting technique

The flatter fitting, 8.80:14.50, is used in the majority of cases. It is, therefore, the initial choice of lens unless the cornea is obviously very small. The total diameter should be 1.50–2.00 mm larger than the horizontal visible iris diameter. A lens which is too flat tends to buckle at the edge and gives unacceptable lid sensation (*see Figure 11.13*).

Typical specification

A typical specification is: 8.80:14.50 −3.00 D.

Additional comments

Hydrocurve II lenses are available in a variety of other forms:

(1) With a lower water content of 45%. Fitting parameters are: 8.30:13.50, 8.60:13.50 and 8.90:14.50, all in the same power range of +20.00 D to −12.00 D.
(2) A toroidal back surface design.
(3) A concentric bifocal consisting of a central distance portion surrounded by a variable focus near portion.
(4) A range of four tints (using the name 'Softmate 1').
(5) The 'Elite', with deposit-resistant properties.

Hydron Zero 6 and Z Plus

Thin HEMA semi-scleral lenses.
Manufactured by: Allergan-Hydron Ltd.

Material properties

HEMA — as for the Hydron Mini (p. 414)
Water content   38.6%

Manufacturing method

Lathing.

Lens geometry

The Zero 6 geometry and edge design are shown in *Figure 11.26*. Negative lenses with powers of −3.00 D

and greater, all have a centre thickness of 0.06 mm. Lenses are designed to give a deliberately thickened midperiphery to assist with handling. This is particularly useful for low negative powers. *Table 11.16* shows the centre thickness and FOZD for the remainder of the power range. The BOZD and peripheral curve width are constant at, respectively, 13.28 mm and 0.36 mm for all powers.

Table 11.16 FOZD and centre thickness for Hydron Zero 6 and Z Plus lenses

BVP (D)	FOZD (mm)	Centre thickness (mm)
−20.00	6.7	0.06
−10.00	6.7	0.06
−5.00	9.0	0.06
−3.00	11.0	0.06
−1.25	13.4	0.08
Plano	10.8	0.12
+2.00	9.6	0.16*
+6.00	9.0	0.25*
+10.00	8.3	0.31*

*Average thickness = 0.10 mm.

Parameters available

The parameters available in the UK are shown in *Table 11.17*.

Table 11.17 Parameters available for Hydron Zero 6 and Z Plus lenses in the UK

BOZR (mm)	8.10, 8.40, 8.70, 9.00, 9.30
TD (mm)	14.00
BVP (D)	+20.00 to −20.00

NB A wider range of parameters is available in other countries, e.g. Australia.

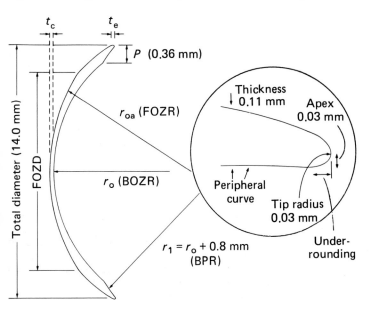

Figure 11.26 Geometry and edge design for Hydron Zero 6

Fitting set

The fitting set is shown in *Table 11.18*.

Table 11.18 Recommended fitting set for Hydron Zero 6 and Z Plus lenses

BOZR (mm)	TD (mm)	
	Zero 6	Z Plus
8.40	14.00	
8.70	14.00	14.00
9.00	14.00	14.00
9.30		14.00
	−3.00 D	+3.00 D

Fitting technique

There is no very firm relationship between flattest 'K' and BOZR because of the greater lens flexibility. Approximately 70% of negative and positive prescriptions are successfully fitted with respective BOZRs of 8.70 mm and 9.00 mm. Fitting criteria are as noted in *Table 11.4* and *Figure 11.16*.

Because diameter is available, Zero 6 and Z Plus lenses may prove unsuitable where the cornea is either very small or very large.

Typical specification

A typical specification is: 8.70:14.00 −3.00 D.

Additional comments

The Zero 6 and Z Plus designs are the basis for fitting other, related lenses: a range of tinted lenses and the Zero 6 front toroidal surface design.

Hydrofit

A single-fitting, thin HEMA semi-scleral lens. Manufactured by: Cantor and Silver Limited.

Material properties

Chemical nature	HEMA
Water content	38%

(For additional properties *see* p. 414)

Manufacturing method

Lenses are produced on computer-controlled automatic lathes.

Lens geometry

All lenses have a constant BOZR and TD. The posterior surface is of bi-curve construction, the peripheral radius being 10.75 mm. Centre thickness for minus lenses varies between 0.05 mm and 0.07 mm. Edge and junction thickness are, respectively, 0.15 mm and 0.20 mm.

Parameters available

The parameters available are shown in *Table 11.19*.

Table 11.19 Parameters available for Hydrofit lenses

BOZR (mm)	8.80
TD (mm)	14.50
BVP(D)	±20.00

Fitting set

The preferred method of fitting is from a lens stock. However, a 10 lens trial set is available, consisting of lens pairs in powers of −2.00 D, −3.00 D, −4.00 D, −5.00 D and +3.00 D.

Fitting technique

Fitting is assessed with lenses as near as possible to the correct power. Thin semi-scleral, 'one-fit' lenses can give a satisfactory result in a high percentage of cases because of their flexibility and large total diameter. Because no modification is possible, it is important to recognize early those cases for whom the fitting characteristics fail to meet the criteria given on pp. 408–410 and in *Table 11.4*. Particular care must be taken with corneas which are very small, large, steep or flat.

Typical specification

A typical specification is: 8.80:14.50 −3.00 D.

Additional comments

The semi-scleral Hydrofit is also the basis for the Hydrofit Mini, a single-fitting corneal diameter lens with parameters of 8.40:13.75 mm.

Spun-cast lenses

Bausch & Lomb Soflens

The Bausch & Lomb Soflens is manufactured by the spin-casting process, which is the same in principle as the centrifugal technique employed for the original gel lenses from Czechoslovakia. Bausch & Lomb extensively refined the basic spinning process from 1966 onwards. They redesigned the lens geometry and introduced elaborate techniques to ensure quality control and reproducibility.

Bausch & Lomb was the first contact lens manufacturer to receive FDA approval on March 18th, 1971, not specifically for the lens, but for the entire system. It therefore included such items as the carrying case, heat disinfection unit and storage vials.

Material properties

Chemical nature	HEMA cross-linked polymer
Water content by weight	
Equilibrated in water	41.7%
Equilibrated in 0.9% saline solution	38.6%
Oxygen permeability	8.0×10^{-11} at 20°C
Refractive index	1.43 (wet)
Linear swell factor	18%
Softening point	120°C
Visible light transmission	> 97%

Manufacturing method

The manufacturing process has been described by Watts (1971) and Wycoff (1972). The monomer mixture and the solvent, glycerol, are introduced into ground and highly polished female moulds, which are mounted on a central spindle to permit rotation at speed. Polymerization takes place while the mould is spinning about its central axis. Water is then pumped in to replace the glycerol and to hydrate the lens, which is afterwards removed manually from the mould for edging. The lenses are extracted for 22 hours in circulating distilled water at 87°C to remove any remaining unreacted monomers, catalyst or water-soluble polymer. After checking, the lenses are finally sealed in 5-ml pharmaceutical vials for autoclaving. The process is different from the cast-moulding or pressing techniques employed by other manufacturers for two reasons. First, the mould is open and, secondly, it is spinning during polymerization.

Lens geometry

The spherical curvature of the mould itself determines the anterior surface of the lens which is designated the 'base curve' or 'Series'. The posterior lens surface, which governs the power, is aspherical, due to centrifugal force distributing liquid polymer away from the apex of the mould according to its speed of rotation. A faster speed gives a higher minus lens, and vice versa. The exact shape of the back surface depends on a number of other factors, including the volume of polymer used, surface

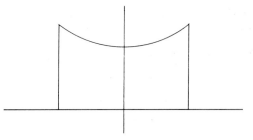

Figure 11.27 Female mould used for spin-casting

tension, rate of polymerization and the duration of the polymerization process. The following formula, associated with *Figure 11.27*, has been applied (Wichterle and Wichterle, 1970; Coombs, 1981).

$$Z = \frac{W^2 X^2}{2g} + K$$

where
Z	= distance on vertical axis
X	= distance on horizontal axis
W	= speed of rotation
g	= gravity constant
K	= a function of surface tension

The aspherical posterior surface of the lens was related by Poster (1975) to the mathematical form of an ellipse. Within a particular Series, the surface shape gradually changes from oblate to prolate as the power is increased as indicated in *Figure 11.28*.

The back surface cannot therefore be defined as having a BOZR since only the central 2–3 mm is in fact spherical. Thus, the term 'posterior apical radius' (PAR) has been used.

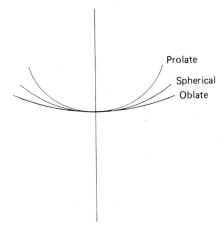

Figure 11.28 Aspherical back surfaces of spun-cast lenses: the steepest curve, associated with the highest negative power, is in the form of the prolate portion of an ellipse, while the flattest curve is that of the oblate portion of an ellipse, the intermediate curve being spherical

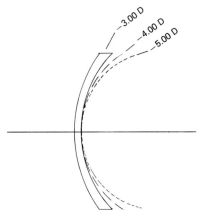

Figure 11.29 Bausch & Lomb Soflenses. The front surface radius is constant. Variation in power is achieved by altering the posterior apical radius (PAR); the steeper it is , the higher the negative power

Figure 11.29 shows how progressively higher powers are obtained by using steeper posterior apical radii in conjunction with a constant sag and fixed radius for the front surface. It illustrates the way in which a spun-cast lens differs fundamentally from any other type of lens, either hard or soft. First, the 'base curve' or series is always the anterior surface of the lens; this is the opposite of lathe-cut lenses where the BOZR, sometimes referred to as the 'base curve', is always the posterior surface. Secondly, the power for any given series is determined by the back surface, also the opposite of all other lenses.

The spin-casting process has certain advantages. It is possible to design and manufacture lenses with better surface quality and edge shape. It is a mass production process so that reproducibility and consistency of manufacture are more easily maintained (Hanks, 1976). On the other hand, the method imposes limitations on the variety of back surface

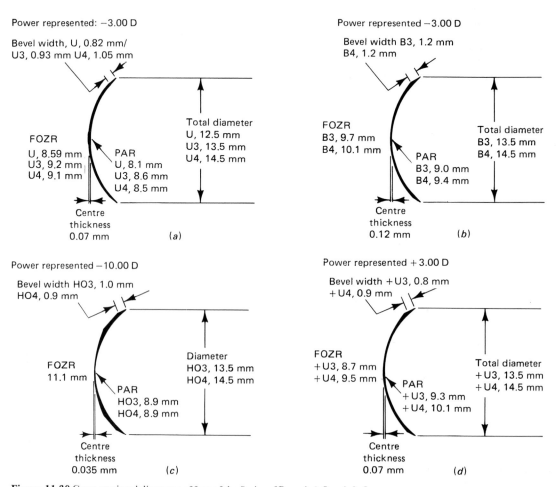

Figure 11.30 Cross-sectional diagrams of four of the Series of Bausch & Lomb Soflens

forms which may be conveniently obtained and the entire range of powers is not produced for every anterior surface radius.

Figure 11.30 shows cross-sectional diagrams of some of the spun-cast Bausch & Lomb lenses.

Parameters available

The parameters available are shown in *Table 11.20*.

Fitting set

The preferred method of fitting is from a comprehensive lens stock. However, six lens trial sets are available for most series.

Fitting technique

The range of Bausch & Lomb HEMA lenses currently available are shown in *Table 11.20*. All are spun-cast with the exception of the Optima 38 which is hybrid in character. It has a spun-cast front and lathed posterior surface. Most of the lenses for myopia have a constant centre thickness and, since the lenses for a given series are produced from identical moulds, the sag of all lenses in that series is constant.

Spun-cast lenses possess greater flexibility than their lathed counterparts (Burgess *et al.*, 1985). Lenses therefore drape more effectively over the cornea. This factor and the constant sag means that, for any given series, a 'one-fit' approach is more feasible, despite variations in the PARs. (A change in power of 0.25 D is approximately equivalent to a change in PAR of 0.05 mm.) Fitting therefore depends mainly upon lens thickness and total diameter, and the specification is expressed as a letter and a number. The letter for a series not only defines the front surface curvature, but also the centre thickness. The number refers to the total diameter. Thus the suffix '4' denotes a 14.50 mm diameter; the suffix '3' a 13.50 mm diameter; and where there is no numerical suffix as for the U and original F Series, a 12.50 mm diameter.

The recommended fitting method is to select lenses on the following basis:

(1) Power according to spectacle *Rx* and vertex distance.
(2) Diameter on the basis of horizontal corneal diameter: 13.50 mm lenses are used where the visible iris diameter is less than 11.75 mm, and 14.50 mm lenses where this is greater.
(3) Series and thickness according to physiological and handling considerations.

Table 11.20 Parameters available for Bausch & Lomb Soflenses

Lens series	BVP (D)	TD (mm)	Centre thickness (mm)	Sag (mm)
Sofspin	−0.25 to −12.00	14.00	0.05 to 0.09	
U	−0.25 to −9.00	12.50	0.07	2.89
U3	−9.00 to +6.00	13.50	0.07 to 0.18	3.09
U4	−9.00 to +6.00	14.50	0.07 to 0.18	4.05
L3	−0.25 to −3.00	13.50	0.06	3.09
L4	−0.25 to −3.00	14.50	0.06	3.65
B3	−20.00 to +6.00	13.50	0.12 to 0.30	3.10 (3.20*)
B4	−9.00 to +6.00	14.50	0.12 to 0.30	3.59
O3	−1.00 to −9.00	13.50	0.035	3.18 (3.12†)
O4	−1.00 to −9.00	14.50	0.035	4.10 (3.68‡)
F§	−0.25 to −9.50	12.50	0.18	2.84
M3	+3.00 to +14.00	13.50	0.23 to 0.44	3.41–3.61
M4	+3.00 to +14.00	14.50	0.23 to 0.44	3.66–3.86
N (non-lenticulated)§	+0.25 to +6.00	12.50	0.18 to 0.36	3.86–4.02
N§	+6.50 to +18.50	13.50	0.40 to 0.75	
H3	+10.00 to +20.00	13.50	0.48 to 0.61	3.40–3.47
H4	+10.00 to +20.00	14.50	0.48 to 0.61	3.69–3.80
HO3	−8.00 to −20.00	13.50	0.035	3.61
HO4	−8.00 to −20.00	14.50	0.035	3.67
Optima 38	−0.25 to −6.00	14.00	0.06	3.60/3.82

Sag values are those shown but the values in parentheses apply to the following denoted BVP ranges (D):

*−12.50 to −20.00;   †−1.00 to −1.25;   ‡−1.00 to −1.75.

§Discontinued in 1989 but may still be available.

U3 and U4 Series   The U3 and U4 Series with a centre thickness of 0.07 mm are the most commonly used and generally provide very good comfort. The other minus Series are used in the following circumstances:

O Series (centre thickness = 0.035 mm)   Where greater oxygen transmissibility is required or for extended wear. However, these lenses are extremely difficult to handle and have a tendency to dehydrate more readily on the eye (*see* Chapter 15).

B3 Series (centre thickness = 0.12 mm)   For easier handling and to provide an extension to the power range.

L3 and L4 Series (centre thickness = 0.06 mm) For low minus powers, up to −3.00 D. The lens is designed to be ultrathin in the centre with a relatively thicker peripheral geometry to permit easier handling than either O or U Series, for the same total diameter.

HO3 and HO4 Series (centre thickness = 0.035 mm)   For high minus powers. The large front optic zone, despite lenticulation, means that the periphery remains relatively thick. These lenses are, therefore, not always ideal in cases prone to corneal vascularization.

F Series (centre thickness = 0.18 mm)   For very small corneas where handling difficulties are encountered with the 12.50 mm U Series.

Optima 38 (centre thickness = 0.06 mm)   Where a choice of two sags is required combined with a lathed posterior surface to provide greater rigidity and easier handling. 'Sag I' (3.60 mm) gives greater movement and is for flatter corneas; 'Sag II' (3.82 mm) gives better centration and is for steeper corneas.

Sofspin (centre thickness = 0.05–0.09 mm)   Where a variable centre thickness may be required with a single total diameter (14.00 mm) for ease of fitting.

Fitting characteristics for Bausch & Lomb lenses are mainly as described in *Table 11.4*, except that movement on blinking is only about 0.5 mm, a little less than other types of soft lens. It is particularly important to achieve proper centration with complete corneal coverage. A decentred lens, because of its aspheric optic, can give poor visual acuity. It can also result in arcuate staining at the limbus where the lens edge produces a combination of corneal drying and abrasion. This would typically occur on the nasal side of the cornea of the eye as in *Figure 11.31* which shows a lens decentred slightly temporally. Lens decentration might occur with either a loose or a tight fitting,

but in the latter case there is no recovery movement on blinking.

If adequate centration cannot be obtained with the initial total diameter, the next larger lens in the same 'letter' Series, should be tried, for example if a U3 lens is too small, try a U4.

Plus lenses are selected according to similar principles, although centre thickness varies with power. It should also be noted that the power range is divided into three overlapping groups, each with a different sag.

Typical specification

A typical specification is: −3.00 U4.

Additional comments

The U3, U4 and B3 Series are produced in a range of four tints. Bausch & Lomb also have available a toric and an extended wear version of the optima lens (the Optima 38 EW only being available in some parts of the world) as well as high water content extended wear lenses, the Bausch & Lomb 70 and CW79.

Since the expiry of the Bausch & Lomb patent, other companies such as American Hydron have begun to produce spun-cast lenses of different design. The fitting principles, however, are similar.

Extended wear lenses

Extended wear is covered in detail in Chapter 15, but it may be noted here that soft lenses have been routinely fitted for this purpose since the early 1970s with the introduction of Permalens

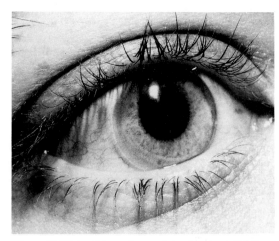

Figure 11.31 A soft lens of corneal size decentred slightly temporally. This can give rise to nasal corneolimbal drying and abrasion

by de Carle (1972) and Sauflon PW by C.L.M. Group Ltd.

Since this time, improvements have occurred not only in lens designs and materials, but also in the understanding of the physiological requirements of the cornea to achieve extended wear with relative safety.

An essential requirement is for lenses to provide an adequate supply of oxygen to the cornea even under closed eye conditions. Soft lenses attempt to achieve this in one of two ways:

(1) By means of a high water content, e.g. Permaflex (74%) and Incanto (78%). Lenses have high Dk values, but the potential problems with this approach are lens fragility, deposits and discolouration, and a greater likelihood of solution reaction.
(2) By making lower water content lenses extremely thin, e.g. Bausch & Lomb O series (thickness = 0.035 mm) and CSI T (thickness = 0.035 mm). These rely on their Dk/t values, but there can be problems with handling and less efficient tear exchange on blinking to remove debris from beneath the lens.

With both types of approach, problems may arise with lens dehydration and corneal desiccation, oedematous responses such as striae or microcysts, giant papillary conjunctivitis, long-term vascularization, and the ever-present risk of infection. Extreme care is, therefore, required by both patient and practitioner in fitting extended wear lenses. The patient must be made aware of the potential hazards and given careful instructions, preferably in writing, about:

(1) How and when to remove lenses.
(2) The need for regular lens replacements.
(3) Proper lens cleaning and disinfection, peroxide and enzyme tablets being the preferred method in most cases (Kotow, Grant and Holden, 1986).

When used for purely cosmetic reasons, the clinical need must be carefully balanced against the possible risks. However, there are many patients for whom extended wear lenses are the most suitable if not the only possible form of visual correction:

(1) Aphakics, where handling difficulties preclude daily wear.

(2) Other poor lens handlers.
(3) Therapeutic cases where the lens is used as a corneal bandage for conditions such as bullous keratopathy, recurrent erosions and burns (*see* Chapter 21).
(4) Young children, where daily handling is not feasible.
(5) For certain occupations or vocational uses where good acuity is required immediately on wakening.
(6) Where soft lens patients have no facility for lens disinfection.
(7) As one component of a low vision aid system, where poor acuity precludes regular lens handling.

In addition, there are obvious advantages in wearing on a mainly daily basis lenses which are suitable for extended wear because of their excellent physiological properties. Although lenses are removed nearly every evening, most patients may be permitted the flexibility of using them on an occasional overnight basis with little or no chance of adverse ocular response.

Toric soft lenses

Full details of toric lenses are given in Chapter 14, but the following practical considerations should be taken into account during fitting:

(1) Unlike most hard lenses for astigmatism, toric soft lenses are prescribed, not to improve the physical fitting, but to provide good visual acuity where spherical lenses are unable to achieve this.
(2) Several different designs have now evolved so that toric soft lenses may be of corneal or semi-scleral diameter, with the toroidal curve on either the back or front surface, and of either low or high water content.
(3) The main influences acting on a soft lens have been described as gravity, hydrostatic forces, lens elasticity and lid pressure (Grant, 1986).
(4) In cases of with-the-rule astigmatism, the thickest portions of the correcting toric lens lie at the top and bottom. The normal action of the lids is to rotate the lens 90° off-axis to bring the thickest part of the lens into the horizontal meridian. To prevent rotation, and to maintain correct orientation of the lens with respect to the cylinder

axis, soft lenses must be stabilized on the eye. Various methods have been used for this purpose, either on their own or in combination: prism ballast, truncation, 'dynamic stabilization', back surface toricity, shapes other than circular.

Toroidal back surface soft lenses

Toroidal back surfaces have evolved logically from the fact that most of the astigmatism encountered in practice is predominantly corneal. It is measurable with the keratometer and a comparison with the spectacle refraction gives an immediate prediction of the likelihood of visual success. Because the back surface of the lens is essentially designed to neutralize the toroidal cornea, by replacing it with the spherical front refracting surface of the lens, lenticular astigmatism is not theoretically correctable with such a lens. Clinically, however, reasonable results can sometimes be obtained. Despite the complexity of the actual lens design, fitting procedures are straightforward and the toric calculations relatively simple. Cylinders as high as 6.00 D can be corrected.

The toric difference between the radii of the principal meridians, representing the cylinder to be corrected in minus form, may be determined from a radius to surface power conversion chart such as Appendix B, *Table B.I*. Additional considerations relating to induced astigmatism are discussed in Chapters 5 and 14.

Because least distortion occurs when it is correctly aligned, the elasticity of the lens ensures that the back surface has a natural stabilizing effect when placed in apposition to an equivalently toroidal cornea (Grant, 1986). However, stabilization is markedly assisted either by prism ballast (e.g. Hydroflex/m-T, Hydrocurve II) or by truncation (e.g. Hydroflex TS).

Toroidal front surface soft lenses

Toroidal front surfaces are capable of correcting both corneal and lenticular astigmatism, although constraints of lens thickness and geometry generally put an upper limit of about 4.50 D on the cylinder to be corrected. Several designs of lens are possible, the methods of stabilization being prism ballast (e.g. Bausch & Lomb), truncation (e.g. Durasoft) or dynamic

stabilization (e.g. Weicon). The back surface may be either spherical (e.g. Vistamarc) or aspherical (e.g. Hydron).

Truncation may be either single or double (e.g. Sauflon). Sometimes it is sufficient to achieve stabilization on its own, but single-truncated lenses are usually more effective when incorporating about $1\,\Delta$ base-down. Dynamic stabilization was a term first used by Fanti (1975) with the introduction of the Weicon-T design. The method consists of chamfering the top and bottom portions of the front of the lens in order to reduce the thickness where the stabilization zones fit beneath the eyelids. The optic zone is a central 8 mm band which lies within the palpebral aperture.

For either toroidal back or front surfaces, a further refinement of lens design is to incorporate the stabilizing prism only in the peripheral areas of the lens (e.g. Hydron Zero 6 Toric). A prism-free optic allows lenses to be made thinner. It has the additional advantage that, where only one eye requires toric correction, there is no likelihood of introducing vertical imbalance. Toric lenses should ideally be made from high *Dk* value materials to compensate for their necessarily greater thickness. However, physiological requirements must be balanced against greater difficulty in manufacture and shorter lifespan. With all types of toric soft lens, there is a much greater tendency for deposition at the thicker base of the lens or along the edge of the truncation. Patients must therefore be advised to pay particular attention to surface cleaning in this area of the lens.

Toric lenses may be either individually prescribed and calculated or selected from a simplified range predetermined by the laboratory.

The former method permits the fitting of most prescriptions which it is technically feasible to manufacture, with a comprehensive range of lens parameters, water contents, spherical and cylinder powers, and axis positions. The main disadvantages are the length of time required to obtain lenses and additional costs.

The latter, simplified method enables rapid fitting from either the practitioner's or laboratory's stock of lenses. However, for this to be feasible, fitting parameters are usually very restricted. Cylinder powers may be limited to 0.50 D or 0.75 D steps with an upper limit of about 2.50 D, because this will be sufficient for all but about 10% of patients (Holden, 1975). Oblique cylinders, which are generally more difficult to fit, are frequently omitted, axes being limited to about 20° either side of horizontal and vertical.

Fitting routine

(1) Decide on whether a toroidal back or front surface is required with respect to corneal or lenticular astigmatism and cylinder power.
(2) Decide on method of stabilization. A truncated lens placed on one eye and a circular lens on the other usually determines both a preference in comfort by the patient and whether prism or truncation is likely to give better stabilization.
(3) Determine the best fitting trial lens.
(4) Determine the lens orientation on the eye from the angle at which the truncation settles or from the lens markings present on most non-truncated trial lenses. These are usually a dot or radial engravings at the base of the lens, or in the 3 and 9 o'clock position. Trial lenses establish at the fitting stage whether compensation is required for the cylinder axis. The most common result is a 5° nasal rotation of the lens base. Success is unlikely if the rotation is more than about 20°, even if consistent, and it is usually better to try a different fitting or lens type.
(5) Over-refract with a fully settled spherical trial lens of power as near as possible to the spectacle *Rx*. Apart from any vertex distance considerations, this is always worth while to ensure that the results correlate, particularly in respect of cylinder power and axis. If there is any discrepancy, the procedure should be repeated with a different trial lens.
(6) If axis compensation has been incorporated because of lens rotation at the initial fitting, the prescription lens should also settle with exactly the same degree of rotation.
(7) The nature of the over-refraction may be used as a guide with the prescription lens. If cylinder is present at the original axis or at 90° to this, under- or over-correction is suggested. If it takes the form of a plus sphere with a minus cylinder of twice the power (e.g. $+0.50\,\mathrm{D}/-1.00\,\mathrm{DC}$) at an oblique axis, it is likely to be caused by mislocation of the cylinder axis (*see Table 14.2*).
(8) Particular care should be taken with fitting essentially uniocular patients. They are much more disturbed by any instability of vision caused by lens rotation on blinking.

Bifocal soft lenses

Bifocal soft lenses, like torics, may be either individually designed by the practitioner or selected from predetermined laboratory systems.

Various designs are now available (*see* Chapter 16), although most of the more successful current types are concentric and based on the principle of simultaneous vision. The majority of these have a central distance portion surrounded by an annulus containing the reading addition (e.g. Hydrocurve, Soflens PA1, Weicon 38E). The reverse approach is also possible (e.g. Alges), with the reading area at the geometric centre of the lens surrounded by the distance portion. There are also segment bifocals and those based on the principles of diffraction, and asphericity.

Where a successful result cannot be achieved with a bifocal, the so-called 'monovision' technique of incorporating the near prescription in the correction of the non-dominant eye can work very well because of the greater stability of vision.

Silicone lenses

Silicone rubber has been investigated as a material for contact lens use since 1962. It is chemically and physiologically inert (Breger, 1971; Elze, 1976), and its very high permeability to oxygen and carbon dioxide, together with its negligible effects on corneal physiology have been demonstrated respectively by Fatt (1969), Hill (1966, 1977), Hill and Schoessler (1967), Fatt and St Helen (1971) and by Burns, Roberts and Rich (1971). Roth *et al.* (1980), however, have reported on a variety of clinical complications found with these lenses.

Silicone lenses differ from PMMA hard lenses in several ways. They can be flexed, stretched and turned inside out; they have excellent elastic properties, partly conform to the shape of the cornea in wear, and have an oxygen permeability several times greater than either HEMA or most rigid gas permeable lenses. They are also unlike hydrophilic lenses because they are extremely tough, and their natural state is dry. Since they do not absorb water to any significant extent, fluorescein can be used in their fitting, and they do not need disinfecting in the same way as soft lenses. Silicone should therefore be regarded as a completely different category of flexible lens which lies somewhere between 'hard' and 'soft'.

Because of the amorphous nature of the silicone rubber raw materials, lenses are produced by a moulding and vulcanization technique, which also assists in maintaining good reproducibility. The main difficulty with silicone is that its natural surface is extremely hydrophobic, and it has been necessary to devise a method of rendering the surface permanently hydrophilic without interfering with any of its optical or physical properties. The final stage of manufacture is therefore surface treatment by ion bombardment.

The first silicone lenses were fitted with a total diameter of 10.50 mm, but, because of their relatively great centre thickness of 0.30 mm, they tended to be low riding (Black, 1972; Long, 1972). Subsequent lenses have been made either thinner or larger in order to achieve better centration. Silicone lens fittings are illustrated in *Plates 41–43*.

Advantages of silicone lenses

(1) Very high oxygen permeability.
(2) Better and more stable visual acuity than many soft lenses.
(3) Less variation in comfort or fitting with environmental factors.
(4) Little likelihood of loss or damage.

Disadvantages of silicone lenses

(1) They are difficult to fit, requiring as much or greater precision than hard lenses and a longer time to settle.
(2) A negative pressure effect, particularly if not fitted correctly, so that some lenses have a tendency to stick to the cornea (Fatt, 1979).
(3) Short lifespan because of breakdown in surface coating and build-up of deposits (*see Plates 44* and *45*).
(4) Difficulties with surface wetting.

(5) Difficulties with foreign bodies, especially with loose fittings.

Because of the disadvantages, silicone has remained very much a minority lens with the following types of limited application:

(1) Dry eyes and other therapeutic cases (Woodward, 1984).
(2) Fitting corneas where vascularization has occurred with other lens forms.
(3) Extended wear for very young children who would lose or break soft lenses.

Special features

Lens identification

Several makes of lens have some form of identification at the periphery. This may represent:

(1) A code, serial or lot number.
(2) Details of partial or complete lens specification.
(3) Location of cylinder axis or prism base.
(4) Position of segment to assist bifocal fitting.

The earlier problems with mechanical engravings, which could either develop fractures or attract deposits, have largely been eliminated by modern laser techniques. Other laboratories imprint the information onto the lens by photographic means; and this same method can be used by the practitioner to mark prescription lenses with 'R', 'L' or dots (*see* Chapters 22 and 23). In general, lens markings prove extremely useful because they assist both patient and practitioner with lens identification.

Hard–soft combination lenses

The use of a hard–soft combination lens for keratoconus was first described by Little in 1971. The soft lens achieves comfort with an otherwise sensitive cornea and the hard lens, fitted to match its anterior surface, provides a good visual result (*Plates 121* and *122*). Combination lenses have also been used in fitting pathological cases (Westerhout, 1973; Chapter 21), and astigmatic patients (Mavani, 1976a,b; Harwood, 1977). McKay Taylor (1976) has suggested that the hydrophilic-base lens may be fenestrated, channelled or toric edged in order to promote tear flow. De Carle (1985) described how a rigid corneal lens could be inset into the front surface of a carrier lens and sandwiched by a further soft lens.

The ideal combination lens consists of a rigid gas permeable optic zone permanently bonded during manufacture to a soft periphery. Saturn II lenses of this type have been produced, but their fitting has so far found only limited application due to limited parameters and breakage at the soft–hard interface. Astin (1985) has reported on their use for therapeutic cases.

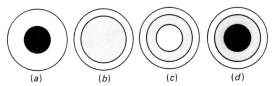

(a)   (b)   (c)   (d)

Figure 11.32 Variations possible with soft lens tints. (a) A black (opaque) pupil on a clear lens; (b) a tinted iris with clear peripheral annulus; (c) a tinted iris with clear peripheral annulus and clear pupil; (d) a tinted iris with clear peripheral annulus and black (opaque) pupil

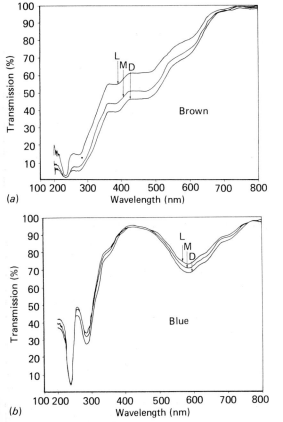

(a)

(b)

Figure 11.33 (a) Light transmission curves for brown-tinted soft lenses (light, medium and dark) with 37% water content. (b) Light transmission curves for blue-tinted soft lenses (light, medium and dark) with 37% water content

Tinted and cosmetic soft lenses

The need for tinted soft lenses is much less than with hard lenses because of the low incidence of adaptive photophobia. Several laboratories, however, offer a range of tinted lenses, mainly for cosmetic reasons. Tints may be translucent, to enhance the colour of the patient's own iris pattern, or opaque and semi-opaque to provide a more radical change of appearance. Solid tints may be either printed or photographically produced. Lenses usually have an iris diameter of about 11.50 mm, surrounded by a clear annulus to give a natural appearance on the eye. It is also possible to provide clear or black pupils (*Figure 11.32a–d, Plates 106–117* and Chapter 21).

Figure 11.33 shows the transmission curves for brown and blue lenses of 37% water content. Brown tints are generally more effective at reducing light transmission than blues or greens both in the visible and ultraviolet parts of the spectrum. Soft lenses have also been produced with inhibitors, specifically to eliminate the ultraviolet part of the spectrum and with a 'sun' filter.

A further application of tinting is with the dark red X-Chrom lens. The monocular use of this is intended to enhance colour discrimination in patients having a red–green deficiency (*see* Chapter 24).

Instructions to patients

Patients should be given clear instructions, both verbally and in writing. Lens handling is fully described in Chapter 9, but the most important points to be discussed may be listed as follows:

(1) Any identification marks on the lenses.
(2) The wearing schedule. This should be uncomplicated, and a typical example is 3–4 hours on the first day for low water content lenses, increasing by 1 hour extra each day. Positive lenses may well require a slower rate of adaptation.
(3) Lens comfort should be no worse than that already experienced on a tolerance trial, and the eyes should not become unduly red or sore.
(4) The method of lens disinfection.
(5) The solution in the lens case should be changed every day.

(6) The importance of cleaning lenses, and the distinction between cleaning and disinfection.

(7) Spectacle blur should not be experienced.

(8) Hard lens solutions should never be used.

(9) Soft lenses should not be worn while eye drops or ointment are being used for any reason.

(10) Environments containing fumes, chemicals, or sprays should be avoided.

(11) The importance of always removing any trace of noxious chemicals from the hands.

(12) Extreme environments in terms of temperature or humidity may temporarily affect both comfort and vision.

(13) If a patient falls asleep or enters certain extreme environments, lenses may give a temporary adhesion to the cornea. This can be released by the application of physiological saline solution.

(14) The lens case should be carried at all times, containing the appropriate storage solution.

(15) Lenses are not necessarily spoiled if they dry out, because they recover their normal shape after rehydration, but they are very fragile when dry.

(16) Patients should bring with them for their first after-care examination both their lens case and their spectacles. They should arrive having worn the lenses for as long as possible on that particular day.

Disinfection of soft lenses

A continuing concern with soft lenses is the risk of contamination by harmful microorganisms. It can also be argued, however, that worse problems have been created by the disinfection procedures themselves; by accelerated lens ageing with boiling on the one hand, and hypersensitivity reactions to solutions and patient error on the other. Nevertheless, it is essential that all patients are properly advised with respect to the appropriate disinfection and cleaning procedures for their particular type of lens. It is also extremely important that they understand the distinction between cleaning and disinfection, because a sterile but 'dirty' lens produces as many problems as a clean contaminated one. Full details of the methods currently employed for lens disinfection are described in Chapter 4 but the two basic approaches are heat and chemical.

Heat

Heat disinfection is best carried out by using a thermostatic or time-controlled heating unit designed for this purpose. Alternatively, a suitable storage case containing the lenses in unpreserved physiological saline may be placed in boiling water for approximately 15 minutes or in a vacuum flask containing water which has just been boiled. These procedures are not truly sterilization, because they fall short of the absolute efficacy of autoclaving, and are better described as disinfection — sometimes referred to as pasteurization or ascepticizing (see Chapter 4).

Chemical

Hard lens solutions, which contain such preservatives as benzalkonium chloride or chlorbutanol, should under no circumstances be used with soft lenses because of their propensity to concentrate on and within the hydrophilic material.

Chemical disinfection is carried out by using a variety of proprietary soft lens solutions commonly based on chlorhexidine and thiomersalate (thiomersal or thimerosal), which are effective against bacteria and fungi, respectively. Unfortunately, chlorhexidine also tends to concentrate within hydrogel materials to a certain extent and bind to deposits on the lens surface.

Allergic responses, sometimes extremely severe, are also quite common with thiomersal. Nevertheless the chlorhexidine–thiomersal combination is an effective antimicrobial system and is still used successfully by many millions of contact lens wearers throughout the world.

Oxidizing systems, such as those based on 3% hydrogen peroxide or chlorine, have emerged as the preferred method of lens disinfection for many patients, because when properly used, allergy problems are rare. Peroxide, in particular, apart from being a very efficient disinfecting agent, has cleaning properties which enhance the lifespan of the lenses. It is especially suitable for high water content lenses. In addition, other disinfectants are increasingly becoming available (see Chapter 4).

After-care

After-care for patients fitted with soft lenses, particularly at their early visits, is very much an extension of the fitting procedure. This is frequently the case with those patients for whom lenses have been fitted and dispensed on the first visit, where a lens may require to be changed for a different fitting or power. The examination is more than usually directed at the lenses while still being worn. A comprehensive treatment of all aspects of after-care is to be found in Chapter 19, but the clinical routine should contain the following steps: discussion with the patient; over-refraction; examination of the lenses *in situ*, with and without magnification; slit lamp examination and staining, with lenses removed; change of lens fitting or lens type, if necessary; reappraisal of wearing schedule.

The initial discussion with the patient establishes the wearing time which has been achieved, together with the wearer's subjective appraisal of comfort, distance vision and near vision. The monocular and binocular visual acuities are then recorded, and over-refraction carried out to determine any residual error. The usual importance is given to the quality of the retinoscopy reflex. Lenses may then be examined *in situ*, with the keratometer, Placido disc, and slit lamp. The latter is especially important because not only can the fitting best be judged with low-to-medium magnification, but so also can the general condition of the lens surface. Embedded foreign particles can easily be seen, as can possible deposits from the tears, or contamination from make-up. The integrity of the lens edge is also studied in this manner, as well as its possible effect on the limbal or conjunctival blood vessels. Lenses engraved with identification marks are easily confirmed as being worn both the right way round, and in the correct eye.

Lenses are then removed, cleaned and placed in the patient's carrying case. It is sometimes necessary at this stage to consider a change of fitting, power, or even lens type. By the time of the first after-care examination, lenses will have been worn for 1 or 2 weeks, tear flow will be back to normal, and the fitting may have significantly altered. Usually lenses become tighter rather than looser, so that a reduction in visual acuity, or scleral indentation, may have occurred. For physiological reasons it may be necessary to change the type of lens, so that a higher water content material may be indicated. If there is some doubt about the comfort given by a particular lens, it is often instructive deliberately to switch right and left lenses into the opposite eyes. If the discomfort follows the lens into the alternate eye, then it must be suspected as being faulty and replaced. Assuming that no other lenses are to be tried on this occasion, ordinary fluorescein is used and the slit lamp examination continued to confirm the absence of corneal insult.

It is sometimes necessary to change the wearing schedule at this stage. Finally, patients are instructed that the lenses may be worn again after a gap of 2 hours, by which time, virtually all traces of fluorescein will have disappeared from the eye.

Severe problems do not arise frequently with hydrophilic lenses, but it should not be assumed that, because they are so soft and flexible, ocular changes do not occur, and practitioners must expect that at least some small percentage of their patients will one day present themselves with, for example, a suddenly contracted red eye. Punctate staining of an adaptive nature is sometimes observed centrally or peripherally. Crescentic areas of stain have been observed in the midperiphery, and arcuate stains are seen at the limbus with some types of corneal-sized lens; this is due to a combination of corneal drying by the lens edge, and physical abrasion. Corneal desiccation may be seen with some ultrathin or high water content lenses (*see Plate 58*). Patients who are hypersensitive to disinfection or cleaning solutions show diffuse punctate erosions in the superficial epithelium (*Plates 55, 56* and *58*); they may or may not exhibit discomfort, photophobia and lacrimation. Striae (*Plate 67*) may be seen as folds in Descemet's membrane (Wechsler, 1974; Katz, 1976). These occur if corneal swelling exceeds 7% (Polse, Mandell and Olsen, 1975). Limbal injection (*Plates 53* and *56*) may be observed either in association with these foregoing conditions, or on its own. Long-term soft lens wearers have produced true neovascularization spreading from the limbal arcades (*Plate 54*); arcuate staining near the superior limbus has also occurred accompanied by vascularization caused by the downward pressure of a tight upper lid (*Plates 48–52*). Greyish infiltrates have been seen in the corneal stroma (*Plate 57*) and cases of disciform (nummular) keratitis and superficial punctate keratitis have been diagnosed.

Corneal oedema is sometimes present, but compared to that found with hard lenses it is difficult to observe. It is an overall effect, extending from limbus to limbus with no clearly defined edge to be seen against the background of the pupil area. There is usually very little or no change in either refraction or 'K' readings, which accounts for the absence of spectacle blur. Carney (1975) found that epithelial anoxia gives both central and peripheral thickness changes, so that there is no actual change in the corneal topography. Mandell (1975) described a linear relationship between corneal thickness increase and corneal oedema. For these reasons, pachometry is probably the only sure way of diagnosing the low levels of oedema encountered with soft lenses. Compared with hard lenses, Hamano *et al.* (1975) found less morphological changes in the cornea, and a smaller reduction in glycogen levels.

Chapter 19 gives details of the procedures to be adopted in dealing with the problems which arise during contact lens after-care.

Lens ageing

Hydrophilic lenses stored in sealed vials continue to remain in good condition for several years, but once they are worn regularly lens deterioration occurs in a variety of ways. Unlike hard lenses, ageing effects are as common a cause of lens replacement as either loss or damage. The degree to which any particular lens is affected depends on several factors:

(1) The polymer from which the lens is manufactured. HEMA lenses age differently from those of higher water content.
(2) The wearing schedule. Extended wear lenses are more badly affected than daily wear lenses, and these are, in turn, more badly affected than those worn only occasionally.
(3) The nature of the tear chemistry (Larke, 1985b). Some patients' lenses last only a few months, whereas others remain in good condition for several years.
(4) Method of disinfection. Lenses generally have a shorter lifespan when sterilized by heat as opposed to solutions. Hydrogen

peroxide, in particular, is beneficial in maintaining optimum lens condition.
(5) The regularity and method of cleaning.
(6) The environment in which the lenses are worn. Dry atmospheres are especially harmful.

Types of ageing effect

Protein deposition

Most lenses suffer from mucoprotein deposits, although HEMA lenses are more badly affected. Cumming (1973) considered that there is a chemical bonding between the proteins of the tears and the hydroxyl groups of the polymer. Some degree of deposition is therefore inevitable, but heat disinfection compounds the problem by denaturing protein on the lens surface which has not been removed by proper cleaning. In the early stages a blue-grey film is seen when the lens is observed by oblique illumination against a dark background, or if the patient refrains from blinking and the lens is allowed to dry on the eye during slit lamp examination (*Plate 31*). Eventually large areas of deposit are clearly visible, even without magnification. Spring (1974) has described the allergic response of some patients to the protein deposits on their lenses.

Discolouration

High water content lenses very commonly suffer from brown discolouration, even when not disinfected by heat. HEMA lenses can also be affected. Gasson (1975) and Ganju and Cordrey (1976) demonstrated a reduction in light transmission of such discoloured lenses. The brown colour may be due to adrenaline compounds in the tears, or, if the lenses fluoresce under ultraviolet light, it may be due to chlorhexidine bound to surface deposits (*Plate 35*). High water content lenses have also been observed with pink and blue discolouration (*see* Chapters 4 and 13).

White spots

These are usually considered to be largely lipid in content, often containing some calcium. They rarely occur with daily wear corneal-sized lenses, and spun-cast lenses are especially good in this respect. High water content lenses are much more often affected, particularly with dry-eyed patients who are poor blinkers. White spots always occur on the front surface of the lens. They may sometimes be observed as a cloud of fine punctate dots, but are more usually seen as quite noticeable discrete white spots scattered irregularly over the lens surface in the area of the exposed palpebral aperture. In severe cases, particularly with extended wear lenses, they can be extremely large and uncomfortable. These larger deposits are sometimes referred to as 'mulberries' (inorganic) or 'jelly-bumps' (organic) as shown in *Plate 32*.

Rust spots

Rust spots affect all types of hydrophilic lens. They are mainly due to atmospheric pollution, but have occasionally been found as a manufacturing fault. Loran (1973) has shown them to be a form of ferrous contamination, and they are more often observed in patients who live or work in industrial areas (*see also* Chapter 13 and *Plate 40*).

Surface and edge deterioration

Lathe-cut HEMA lenses can develop fissures relating to manufacturing lathe marks (Barradell, 1973), and they gradually suffer from surface scratching. The integrity of the edge, with age, can break down to produce small chips and imperfections; and engraving marks can sometimes become encrusted with deposits (*see Figure 13.31*, Chapter 13). Lenses affected by protein tend to dry more easily on the eye and, if this occurs unevenly at the periphery, the edge may become crenellated.

Fitting changes

Lenses with deposits, scratches, or other surface irregularities, are more influenced by the mechanical pressure of the upper lid, so that significant changes in fitting characteristics can occur. Usually they become looser, and corneal diameter lenses may become badly decentred because the lens surface tends to adhere to the upper lid. High-riding lenses are frequently associated with giant papillary conjunctivitis, because the papillae 'grip' the lens and displace it superiorly. As a secondary effect, apical or peripheral corneal staining is sometimes observed.

Refractive changes

Old lenses frequently give a reduced standard of vision, not only because of surface deposits, but also as a result of spurious changes in the over-refraction of as much as 1.00 D. If the patient is subsequently checked with a new lens, the refractive change is often found to be either smaller or unnecessary. This may be due to refractive index and flexure changes (*see* Chapter 5).

Patients sometimes produce a severe ocular response to the wearing of contaminated lenses. This may be either corneal, or conjunctival of an allergic follicular nature (Allansmith *et al.*, 1977).

The majority of the foregoing difficulties are resolved by thorough lens cleaning. It is not possible to predict with any degree of certainty the lifespan for a soft lens. Although the various cleaning and rejuvenation procedures now available could make 2–3 years feasible, there are considerable clinical benefits from regular lens replacement, for example, the Johnson & Johnson Acuvue lens. Patients should be supplied from the beginning with the appropriate solutions. Ideally, they should use daily a surface acting cleaner effective against mucoprotein, combined with a periodic enzymatic or other cleaning process.

General comments on soft lens practice

There are now a great many types of hydrophilic lens available to the practitioner. They differ in water content, chemical composition, size, geometric construction, method of manufacture and technique of fitting so that they may have little in common, except for the fact that they are described by the adjective 'soft'. They are best regarded as complementary rather than competitive systems, for the question: 'Which is the best soft lens?' does not necessarily have an answer unless it relates to a particular patient, or perhaps even to a particular eye. If it is intended to fit as many patients as possible, it is essential to have available more than one variety of lens. Thin lenses of corneal size are preferable in many cases; but semi-scleral or thicker lenses are still necessary in some others, as are materials of different water contents or *Dk* values. It is not possible to prescribe lenses of one type based on the fitting set of another. A comprehensive range of lenses for one preferred fitting philosophy should therefore be supplemented by at least a minimum set of an alternative method. It is not possible to prescribe only one sort of hard lens and nor is this feasible with soft lenses.

In choosing a soft lens system it is desirable to fit and prescribe those lenses and materials produced by the major soft lens manufacturers, who have carried out the necessary preclinical studies to ensure the safety of their lenses, and who continue with research and development into new materials and improved lens designs. It is advantageous to use a lens which is part of a complete system, backed by an easily workable warranty, exchange and replacement scheme. This enables the practitioner to maintain an efficient fitting service, and the patient to have at least some idea of what the future costs might be as a soft lens wearer. Such a system should not be too rigid, for the things which happen to soft lenses can sometimes defy classification.

The material from which lenses are made must be durable and avoid rapid deterioration, and it must withstand patient handling in order that a reasonable lifespan may be expected. Good reproducibility is essential and lenses should be capable of being autoclaved, so that any method of disinfection may be used.

The preferred way of prescribing soft lenses, of any variety, is from a substantial lens stock. This facilitates lengthy tolerance trials when necessary and the clinical evaluation of lenses close to the patient's fitting and power. If, however, a start is made with a limited trial set, it should be possible to extend this by the subsequent addition of further fitting units. Because positive and negative lenses can behave very differently on the eye, both should be included in even a basic fitting set. Lenses with standardized parameters and recommended fitting procedures are preferred in most cases, but any soft lens system should ideally be sufficiently versatile to provide non-standard lenses when clinically necessary.

Acknowledgements

The author would like to acknowledge all those contact lens companies which kindly made available detailed information concerning their lenses and to the following for their permission to reproduce diagrams and photographs: Bausch & Lomb (*Figure 11.30*), CIBA Vision (*Figures 11.22, 11.23, 11.24*) CLM (*Figure 11.5*), CooperVision (*Figure 11.25*), Hydron Europe (*Figures 11.20, 11.21, 11.26a,b*), Igel International (*Figures 11.32a–d, 11.33*). My thanks are also due to Bausch & Lomb for arranging the art-work for *Figure 11.19*, and to Miss Robyn Edlington for typing the manuscript.

References

ALLANSMITH, M. R., KORB, D. R., GREINER, J. V., HENRIQUEZ, A. S., SIMON, M. A. and FINNEMORE, V. M. (1977). Giant papillary conjunctivitis in contact lens wearers. *Am. J. Ophthal.* **83**, 697–708

ANDRASKO, G. (1983). Hydrogel dehydration in various environments. *Int. Contact Lens Clin.* **10**, 22–28

ANDRASKO, G. and SCHOESSLER, J. P. (1980). The effect of humidity on the dehydration of soft contact lenses on the eye. *Int. Contact Lens Clin.* **7**, 210–212

APPLEGATE, R. A. and MASSOF, R. W. (1975). Changes in the contrast sensitivity function induced by contact lens wear. *Am. J. Optom.* **52**, 840–846

ARIAS, M. C. (1968). Contact lens fitting in high altitudes and/or dry climates. *Contacto* **12**(3), 10–13

ARIAS, M. C. (1973). Paper read at Conference of International Society of Contact Lens Specialists, Chateau d'Artigny, Montbazon, France, and reported in *Optician* **166**(4291), 18–19, 23–24

ASTIN, C. (1985). The use of Saturn II lenses following penetrating keratoplasty. *Transactions of the British Contact Lens Association Conference*, pp. 2–5

ATKINSON, T. C. O. (1986). The Lunelle ES 70. A preliminary report. *Optician* **191**(5032), 31–33

BARRADELL, M. J. (1973). Soft lenses compared. *Optician* **166**(4304), 39, 43–44

BENNETT, A. G. (1976). Power changes in soft lenses due to bending. *Ophthal. Optician* **16**, 939–945

BERNSTEIN, H. N. and MADDOX, Y. (1973). Evaluation of the 'asepticization' procedure for the Soflens hydrophilic contact lens. *Contact Lens* **4**(3), 3

BERNSTEIN, H. N., STOW, M. N. and MADDOX, Y. (1973). Evaluation of the asepticization procedure for the Soflens hydrophilic contact lens. *Can. J. Ophthal.* **8**, 575–576

BIBBY, M. M. (1976). Computer-assisted photokeratoscopy and contact lens design. *Optician* **171**, Part 1, (4423), 37, 39, 41, 43; Part 2, (4424), 11, 14–15, 17; Part 3, (4425), 22–23; Part 4, (4426), 15, 17

BILTON, S. and GUILLON, M, (1984). *In vivo* hydrogel lens dehydration. Paper presented to a meeting of the North East Contact Lens Society

BLACK, C. J. (1972). Silicone lens. In *Soft Contact Lens*, edited by A. R. Gassett and H. E. Kaufman, Chap. 14, pp. 126–138. St Louis: C. V. Mosby

BLACKSTONE, M. R. (1968). Hydrophilic contact lenses: 1967, 1968 and onwards. *Optician* **155**, 156–159

BRAILSFORD, M. I. D. (1972). The importance of sag heights when fitting Bionite lenses. *Ophthal. Optician* **12**, 1047–1048

BREGER, J. L. (1971). The silicone rubber lens. *Optician* **162**(4189), 12–14

BRITISH STANDARD 5562. (1978). *Specification for Contact Lenses — BS 5562:1978*. London: British Standards Institution

BURGESS, C. J., CAMBRIDGE, J. J., HOLDEN, B. A., MARTIN, D. K. and SWEENEY, D. (1985). Flexibility of soft contact lenses of various materials and thicknesses. Unpublished work from the Cornea and Contact Lens Research Unit, Sydney

BURNS, R. P., ROBERTS, H. and RICH, L. F. (1971). Effects of silicone contact lenses on corneal epithelial metabolism. *Am. J. Ophthal.* **71**, 486–489

DE CARLE, J. (1972). Developing hydrophilic lenses for constant wearing. *Aust. J. Optom.* **55**, 343–346

DE CARLE, J. (1985). Paper presented to the International Society of Contact Lens Specialists, Venice, Sept.

CARNEY, L. G. (1975). Effect of hypoxia on central and peripheral corneal thickness and corneal topography. *Aust. J. Optom.* **58**, 61–65

CLARKE, C. (1976). Contact lenses at high altitude. *Br. J. Ophthal.* **60**, 470–480

COOMBS, W. F. (1981). Spin casting of Hema lenses. Paper presented at the October 1981 meeting of the Contact Lens Manufacturers Association in New Orleans

CUMMING, J. S. (1973). The future of soft contact lenses. *Mfg Optics Int.* **26**(6), 309–312

DECKER, M., POLSE, K. and FATT, I. (1978). Oxygen flux into the human cornea when coverd by a soft contact lens. *Am J. Optom.* **55,** 285–301

EDWARDS, K. (1986). The gasman cometh. *J. Br. Contact Lens Ass.* (Scientific meetings), pp. 2–13

ELZE, K. L. (1976). Toxicity of soft contact lens material. *Contact Intraoc. Lens med. J.* **2**(1), 57–61

ERIKSEN, S., RANDERI, K. and STER, J. (1972). Behaviour of hydrophilic soft contact lenses under stress conditions of pH and tonicities. In *Symposium on the Flexible Lens*, edited by J. L. Bitonte and R. H. Keates, pp. 213–217. St Louis: C. V. Mosby

FANTI, P. (1975). The fitting of a soft toroidal contact lens. *Optician* **169**(4376), 8–9, 13, 15–16

FANTI, P. (1986). Practical results with the Lunelle 70. *Optician* **191**(5027), 16–24

FANTI, P. and VOLLMER, W. (1979). Sind dünne HEMA-linsen verträgliche? *Dtsch. Optikerztg.* **4**, 139–147

FATT, I. (1969). A pre-clinical study of gas permeable contact lens material. *Contact Lens* **2**(4), 3–5

FATT, I. (1977). A rational method for the design of gas-permeable soft contact lenses. *Optician* **173**(4470), 12, 13, 15

FATT, I. (1979). Negative pressure under silicone rubber contact lenses. *Contacto* **23**, 6–8

FATT, I. and BIEBER, M. T. (1968). The steady-state distribution of oxygen and carbon dioxide in the *in vivo* cornea. I: The open eye in air and the closed eye. *Expl Eye Res.* **7**, 103–112

FATT, I. and CHASTON, J. (1982). Relationship of oxygen transmissibility to oxygen tension or E.O.P. under the lens. *Int. Contact Lens Clin.* **9**, 119–120

FATT, I. and DiMARTINO, R. B. (1985). Water content of a hydrogel lens on the eye. *Optician* **190**(5011), 19–22

FATT, I. and ST HELEN, R. (1971). Oxygen tension under an oxygen-permeable contact lens. *Am. J. Optom.* **48**, 545–555

FORD, M. W. (1974). Changes in hydrophilic lenses when placed on an eye. Paper read at the joint International Congress of The Contact Lens Society and The National Eye Research Foundation, Montreux, Switzerland

FORD, M. W. (1976). Computation of the back vertex powers of hydrophilic lenses. Paper read at the Interdisciplinary Conference on Contact Lenses, Department of Ophthalmic Optics and Visual Science, The City University, London

FRANKLAND, J. (1980). Advances in contact lens polymer application. *Optician* **179**(14), 13–21

GANJU, S. N. and CORDREY, P. (1976). Removal of adsorbed preservative in soft contact lenses. *Optician* **171**(4423), 16, 18, 20–21

GASSON, A. P. (1975). Visual considerations with hydrophilic lenses. *Ophthal. Optician* **15**, 439–448

GASSON, A. (1983). VDUs and contact lenses. *Contact Lens J.* **11**, 13–16

GILFORD, S. J. W. (1975). How atmosphere affects soft lens wearers. (Letter) *Optician* **169**(4375), 30

GRANT, R. (1986). Mechanics of toric soft lens stabilisation. *Transactions of the British Contact Lens Association Conference*, pp. 44–47

GUILLON, M., LYDON, D. P. M. and WILSON, C. (1983). Variations in contrast sensitivity function with spectacles and contact lenses. *J. Br. Contact Lens Ass.* **6**, 120–124

HAIG-BROWN, G. (1978). The use of ultra-thin soft contact lenses especially in problem cases. *Optician* **176**(4543), 20–22

HAIG-BROWN, G. (1985). A clinical study of high water content contact lenses in the daily wear regime. *Transactions of the British Contact Lens Association Conference*, pp. 12–15

HAMANO, H., HORI, M., HIRAYAMA, K., KAWABE, H. and MITSUNAGA, S. (1975). Influence of soft and hard contact lenses on the cornea. *Aust. J. Optom.* **58**, 326–336

HAMANO, H., HORI, M., KAWABE, H., MIKAMI, M. and MITSUNAGA, S. (1980). Changes of oxygen tension in corneal stroma with various kinds of contact lenses. *Contacto* **24** (1), 9–16

HANKS, A. J. (1976). A study of the reproducibility of spin cast hydrophilic lenses. *Aust. J. Optom.* **59**, 341–347

HARRIS, M. G. and MOCK, L. G. (1974). The effect of saline solutions of various compositions on hydrogel lens dimensions. *Am. J. Optom.* **51**, 457–464

HARWOOD, L. W. (1977). Combination Soflens contact lenses/hard lenses — use on high-toric corneas. In *Proceedings of the Second National Research Symposium on Soft Contact Lenses*, pp. 131–137. Chicago, Illinois, August

16–17, 1975. Amsterdam: Excerpta Medica

HILL, J. F. (1975). A comparison of refractive and keratometric changes during adaptation to flexible and non-flexible contact lenses. *J. Am. optom. Ass.* **46**, 290–294

HILL, J. F. (1976). Changes in corneal curvature and refractive error upon refitting with flatter hydrophilic contact lenses. *J. Am. optom. Ass.* **47**, 1214–1216

HILL, R. M. (1966). Effects of a silicone rubber contact lens on corneal respiration. *J. Am. optom. Ass.* **37**, 1119–1121

HILL, R. M. (1976). Perils of the pump. *Int. Contact Lens Clin.* **3**(3), 48–49

HILL, R. M. (1977). Oxygen permeable contact lenses: how convinced is the cornea? *Int. Contact Lens Clin.* **4**(2), 34–36

HILL, R. M. (1982). Lenses in ambience. *Int. Contact Lens Clin.* **9**, 94–96

HILL, R. M. (1983). Dehydration deficits. *Int. Contact Lens Clin.* **10**, 364–365

HILL, R. M. and SCHOESSLER, J. (1967). Optical membranes of silicone rubber. *J. Am. optom. Ass.* **38**, 480–483

HILL, R. M. and TERRY, J. E. (1978). Predestined edema. *Contact Lens Forum* **3**(4), 41–43

HILL, R. M. and UNIACKE, N. P. (1969). Tear chemistry of a new contact lens wearer. *J. Am. optom. Ass.* **40**, 3

HILLMAN, J. S. (1976). The use of hydrophilic contact lenses. *Optician* **172**(4458), 9–11

HODD, N. F. B. (1976). How to fit soft lenses — No. 6: Vergo group AO: Aoflex. *Optician* **172**(4449), 15, 17, 20

HOLDEN B. A. (1975). Principles and practice of correcting astigmatism with soft contact lenses. *Aust. J. Optom.* **58**, 279–299

HOLDEN, B. A. and MERTZ, G. W. (1984). Critical oxygen levels to avoid corneal oedema for daily and extended wear contact lenses. *Invest. Ophthal. Vis. Sci.* **25**, 1161–1167

HOLLY, F. J. and REFOJO, M. F. (1972). Oxygen permeability of hydrogel contact lenses. *J. Am. optom. Ass.* **43**, 1173–1180

KATZ, H. H. (1976). A hypothesis for the formation of vertical corneal striae as observed in the wearing of Soflens contact lenses and in keratoconus. *Am. J. Optom.* **53**, 420–421

KOHLER, J. E. and FLANAGAN, G. W. (1985). Clinical dehydration of extended-wear lenses. *Int. Contact Lens Clin.* **12**, 152–160

KOTOW, M., GRANT, T. and HOLDEN, B. A. (1986). Evaluation of current care and maintenance systems for hydrogel extended wear. *Transactions of the British Contact Lens Association Conference*, pp. 66–67

LARKE, J. R. (1985a). *The Eye in Contact Lens Wear*, pp. 5–6. London: Butterworths

LARKE, J. R. (1985b). *The Eye in Contact Lens Wear*, p. 44. London: Butterworths

LARKE, J. R. and SABELL, A. G. (1971). Some basic design concepts of hydrophilic gel contact lenses. *Br. J. physiol. Optics* **26**, 49–60

LITTLE, I. (1971). Soft lenses in keratoconus. (Letter) *Optician* **162**(4204), 26

LONG, W. E. (1972). Silicone rubber corneal contact lens. In *Symposium on the Flexible Lens*, edited by J. L. Bitonte and R.

H. Keates, pp. 73–79. St Louis: C. V. Mosby

LORAN, D. F. C. (1973). Surface corrosion of hydrogel contact lenses. *Contact Lens* **4**(4), 3–6, 8, 10

LOSHAEK, S. and HILL, R. M. (1977). Oxygen permeability measurements: correlation between living-eye and electrode-chamber measurements. *Int. Contact Lens Clin.* **4**(6), 26–29

McDONALD, J. E. (1969). Surface phenomena of the tear film. *Am. J. Ophthal.* **67**, 56–64

McKAY TAYLOR, C. (1976). Combining hard and soft lenses with applied fitting techniques. *Ophthal. Optician* **16**, 356–364

MACKIE, I. A. (1977). Complications of soft lenses. Paper read at Summer Clinical Conference of the British Contact Lens Association, April 1977, Torquay, Devon

MANDELL, R. B. (1975a). Corneal edema and curvature changes from gel lenses. *Int. Contact Lens Clin.* **2**, 88–98

MANDELL, R. B. (1975b). Is oxygen our only problem? *Int. Contact Lens Clin.* **2**, 1

MAVANI, M. R. (1976a). The correction of high astigmatism. *Optician*, **172**(4453), 34

MAVANI, M. R. (1976b). The concept of the correction of high astigmatism with a combination of hard and soft lenses. *Contacto* **20**(6), 31–33

MILLODOT, M. (1971). Corneal sensitivity and contact lenses. *Optician* **162**(4210), 23–24

MILLODOT, M. (1974). Effect of soft lenses on corneal sensitivity. *Acta ophthal.* **52**, 603–608

MILLODOT, M. (1976). Effect of the length of wear of contact lenses on corneal sensitivity. *Acta ophthal.* **54**, 721–730

MORRISON, R. J. (1973). Comparative studies: visual acuity with spectacles and flexible lenses, ophthalmometer readings with and without flexible lenses. *Am. J. Optom.* **50**, 807–809

MOSSÉ, P. and SCOTT, V. (1976). What use is large molecular fluorescein in contact lens fitting? *Optician Special Supplement*, January, 1976, **171**(4414), 15–19

NORN, M. S. (1974). *External Eye, Methods of Examination*, p. 121. Copenhagen: Scriptor

NORTON, D. A., DAVIES, D. J. G., RICHARDSON, N. E., MEAKIN, B. J. and KEALL, A. (1974). The antimicrobial efficiencies of contact lens solutions. *J. pharm. Pharmac.* **26**, 841–846. Also reproduced in *Optician* **168**(4360), 14–16

POLSE, K. A. and MANDELL, R. B. (1970). Critical oxygen tension at the corneal surface. *Archs Ophthal.* **84**, 505–508

POLSE, K. A., MANDELL, R. B. and OLSEN, M. (1975). Origin of striate corneal lines. *Int. Contact Lens Clin.* **3**(3), 85–88

POSTER, M. G. (1975). A rationale for fitting the Bausch & Lomb Soflens. *J. Am. optom. Ass.* **46**, 223–227

POSTER, M. G. (1977). Lens/eye relationships of hydrogel lenses using fluorescein analysis. Paper read at National Research Symposium on Soft Contact Lenses, August, 1977, Rochester, New York

POSTER, M. G. and SKOLNIK, A. (1974). The effects of pH and tonicity change on some parameters of the Soflens. *J. Am. optom. Ass.* **45**, 311–314

REFOJO, M. F., KORB, D. and SILVERMAN, H. (1972). Clinical evaluation of a new fluorescent dye for hydrogel lenses. *J.*

Am. optom. Ass. **43**, 321–326

REFOJO, M. F., MILLER, D. and FIORE, A. S. (1972). A new fluorescent stain for soft hydrophilic lens fitting. *Archs Ophthal.* **87**, 275–277

RENGSTORFF, R. H. (1974). The precorneal tear film; break-up time and location in normal subjects. *Am. J. Optom.* **51**, 765–769

ROCHER, P. (1977). Hydrogel lenses and oxygen permeability. *Optician* **174**(4493), 7–8, 10–11, 13

ROCHER, P. and SCHWEGLER, Y. (1974). A fitting method for soft hydrophilic lenses based on sagittal height differences. Paper read at Annual Meeting of American Academy of Optometry, Miami, Florida, December, 1974

ROSENBLUM, W. M. and LEACH, N. E. (1975). The subjective quality (SQF) of Bausch & Lomb Soflens. *Am. J. Optom.* **52**, 658–662

ROTH, H. W., IWASAKI, W., TAKAYAMA, M. and WADA, C. (1980). Complication caused by silicon elastomer lenses in West Germany and Japan. *Contacto* **24**(3), 28–36

SAMMONS, W. A. (1980). Contact lens thickness and all that. *Optician* **180**(4667), 11–18

SAMMONS, W. A. (1981). Thin lens design and average thickness. *J. Br. Contact Lens Ass.* **4**, 90–97

SAMPSON, W. G. and SOPER, J. W. (1970). Keratometry. In *Corneal Contact Lenses*, Chapter 6, pp. 65–92, 2nd edn, edited by L. J. Girard. St Louis: C. V. Mosby

SARVER, M. D., ASHLEY, D. and VAN EVERY, J. (1974). Supplemental power effect of Bausch & Lomb Soflens contact lenses. *Int. Contact Lens Clin.* **1**(1), 100–109

SHERIDAN, M. (1987). AIDS virus in tears. *Optician* **193**(5083), 15

SOLOMON, J. (1978). An investigation of the ultra-thin Soflens contact lens. *Int. Contact Lens Clinic* **5**, 2

SPRING, T. F. (1974). Reaction to hydrophilic lenses. *Med. J. Aust.* **1**, 449–450

STONE, J. (1967). Near vision difficulties in non-presbyopic corneal lens wearers. *Contact Lens J.* **1**(2), 14–16, 24–25

STONE, J. (1974). The measurement of corneal thickness. *Contact Lens J.* **5**(2), 14–19

STRACHAN, J. P. F. (1973). Some principles of the optics of hydrophilic lenses and geometrical optics applied to flexible lenses. *Aust. J. Optom.* **56**, 25–33

WATTS, G. K. (1971). Hydrophilic contact lenses — a review. *Optician* **161**(4174), 10–13

WECHSLER, S. (1974). Striate corneal lines. *Am. J. Optom.* **51**, 852–856

WECHSLER, S., JOHNSON, M. and BUSINGER, U. (1983). *In vivo* hydration of hydrogel lenses — the first hour. *Int. contact Lens Clin.* **10**, 349–352

WESTERHOUT, D. (1973). The 'combination lens' and therapeutic uses of soft lenses. *Contact Lens J.* **4**(5), 3–10, 12, 16–18, 20, 22

WICHTERLE, O. (1967). Changes of refracting power of a soft lens caused by its flattening. In *Corneal and Scleral Contact Lenses*, The Proceedings of the International Congress, paper 29, pp. 247–256, March 1966, edited by L. J. Girard. St Louis: C. V. Mosby

WICHTERLE, O. and LIM, D. (1960). Hydrophilic gels for biological use. *Nature* **185**, 117–118

WICHTERLE, K. and WICHTERLE, O. (1970). Surface shapes of fluids in rotating vessels. *Appl. Sci. Res.* **22**, 150–158

WILSON, G., RAFFERTY, W. B. and LEWERENZ, D. C. (1978). The relative oxygen permeability of soft contact lenses. *Int. Contact Lens Clin.* **5**, 61–65

WOODWARD, E. G. (1984). Therapeutic silicone rubber lenses. *J. Br. Contact Lens Ass.* **7**, 39–40

WYCOFF, P. (1972). Hydrophilic contact lenses. *Contact Lens Soc. Am. J.* **6**(3), 12–21

YOUNG, W. and MANDELL, R. (1983). A study of water loss and imbibition of some contact lenses. *Contacto* **27**(6), 15–21

Chapter 12

Hard lens verification procedures

Rita Watts

Contact lenses should be checked for quality and physical characteristics whether they are for prescription use, contact lens fitting sets or research purposes. Contact lens manufacturers are not bound by any statutory regulations, but many laboratories publish details of the accuracy to which their lenses are made, and the British Standards Institution has issued guidance on tolerances for use by practitioner and laboratory (*see* Addenda I and II, pp. 460 and 461).

This chapter is divided into the following sections: parameters to be checked and verification procedures.

Parameters to be checked

Table 12.1 shows the various parameters which may need checking in each group for corneal and scleral lenses, they are: radii; diameters and linear parameters; thickness; the optic; quality, tint etc.

A pair of lenses should match for tint, transition and edge forms. Diameters and zone widths should not differ by more than a certain tolerance. The maximum difference in thickness for a pair of lenses of relatively equal power should not exceed a specified tolerance unless this is specifically requested to facilitate lens checking.

Verification procedures

Radii

Various methods are available for verifying contact lens radii.

Radiuscopes

There are several instruments available (*Figure 12.1* and *see Figures 12.3* and *22.10*) which differ in construction, but all use Drysdale's method for the measurement of small radii (Drysdale, 1900). This method is based on the principle that for a curved mirror an image is formed in the same plane as the object when the object is at the centre of curvature of the surface. This is because the reflected light returns along its incident path. An image may also be formed on the surface, and thus the distance between the two images — which is equal to the radius of the surface — may be measured (*Figure 12.2*).

A radiuscope consists essentially of a microscope with a dial gauge attached (calibrated to 0.01 mm) to read the position of the microscope body or microscope stage. Light from an illuminated target (consisting of a ring of dots or radial lines) attached to the microscope is imaged by the microscope objective after being reflected through a right-angle by a semi-transparent mirror.

Some radiuscopes (*Figure 12.3*) have dispensed with the external dial gauge shown in *Figures 12.1* and *22.10*, and the radius reading is shown on a scale at one side of the field of view in the microscope. The knurled knob on the left-hand side of the instrument in *Figure 12.3*, just above its nameplate, is used to set a pointer to zero on this scale when the surface image of a concave surface is in focus. To focus the centre of curvature image, the coarse and fine focusing wheels at the lower back of the instrument are used to raise the microscope objective and, at the same time, this movement is recorded by the pointer on the scale — so giving the radius reading directly. The use of instruments with dial gauges is outlined below.

Table 12.1 Contact lens parameters which may need verifying

Group	Corneal lenses	Scleral lenses
Radii (spherical and/or toroidal)	Back optic zone radius Back central optic zone radius Back peripheral optic zone radius/radii* Back peripheral zone radius/radii* Front optic zone radius Front central optic zone radius Front peripheral optic zone radius/radii* Front peripheral zone radius/radii*	As for corneal lenses
	Effective or equivalent back optic zone radius	Back scleral zone radius/radii* Back transition zone radius/radii*
Diameters and linear parameters (maximum and minimum dimensions if not circular)	Back optic zone diameter Back central optic zone diameter Back peripheral optic zone diameter(s)* Back peripheral zone diameter(s)* Front optic zone diameter Front central optic zone diameter Front peripheral optic zone diameter(s)* Front peripheral zone diameter(s)* Total diameter Displacement of optic Bifocal segment size and position	As for corneal lenses
	Back diffractive zone diameter Axial and/or radial edge lift	Primary optic diameter Back scleral size Transition width(s)
Thickness	Central (optic and/or geometric) Edge Lenticular junction At any other specified point	Central optic Average scleral Edge Transition At any other specified point
Optic — lens prescription	Back vertex power Front vertex power Near addition Prism and base direction Cylinder power and axis Aberration	As for corneal lenses
Quality etc.	Finish and quality Polish Edge form Transitions Tint Material	As for corneal lenses

* Where there is more than one such zone.

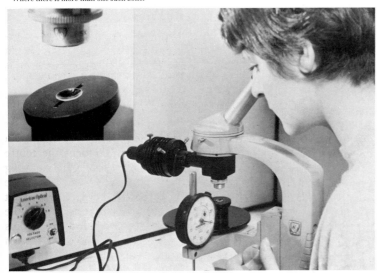

Figure 12.1 American Optical Company Monocular Radiuscope with corneal lens in place for measurement of back optic zone radius. Inset: close-up of lens in place, holder tilted to measure back peripheral radius

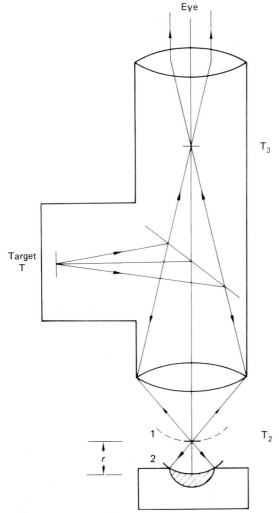

Figure 12.2 Diagram to show Drysdale's principle. (1) First position of lens, image focused on lens surface; (2) second position of lens, image is now at centre of curvature of surface. r = lens radius

Procedure for using a radiuscope, concave surfaces

(1) A suitable lens holder is filled with water.
(2) The clean lens is placed centrally on the holder, convex surface in complete contact with the water. The water minimizes reflections from the front surface of the lens because its refractive index is very similar to that of the lens material. (Without the water present, the images formed by reflection at the front surface are as bright as the images formed by the back surface, and it then becomes difficult to tell quickly which image

is required.) Only a small quantity of water should be used, otherwise the lens floats and may move during measurements.
(3) The holder is placed on the microscope stage and centred.
(4) The microscope eyepiece is correctly adjusted and then, by observation through the microscope, the target is imaged on the surface of the lens by moving either the microscope and target or the microscope stage, depending on the type of instrument used.
(5) The dial gauge reading is recorded (or the dial gauge is set to zero).
(6) A second focus, at the centre of curvature of the surface, is obtained by racking the microscope up or the stage down.
(7) The second reading is recorded.
(8) The difference between the two dial gauge readings gives the radius of curvature of the surface.
(9) This procedure should be repeated twice and the average of the three readings taken. To minimize user errors, the fine focusing drum should be racked in the same direction when making each setting. The radius should also be measured at different points on the lens as it may vary (Tannehill and Sampson, 1966).

The focused target must be central. Usually, it is possible to move the microscope stage horizontally to centralize the image. A diaphragm and/or rheostat is incorporated in most instruments to reduce brightness.

The target image will appear distorted if the surface is irregular. If any water is left on the surface being measured, it can result in distorted surface images. On toroidal surfaces, two measurements for the principal radii must be made. When a radial line target is being used, the lens must be rotated so that its principal meridians coincide with one pair of perpendicular radial lines.

On some instruments it is necessary to use a special holder (*Figure 12.4*) when measuring back scleral radius. By using the holder, the travel of the microscope is increased to cope with the larger radii encountered.

Measurement of back peripheral radii

A similar procedure is followed but the lens holder is tilted and the microscope stage moved

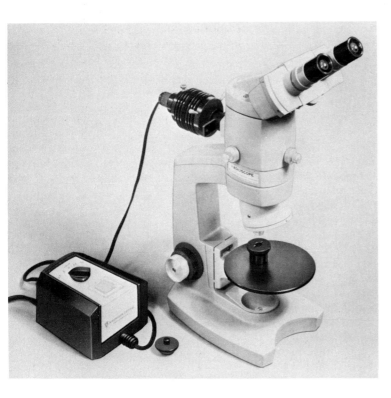

Figure 12.3 American Optical Company Binocular Radiuscope with internal scale. (Photograph kindly provided by British American Optical Company)

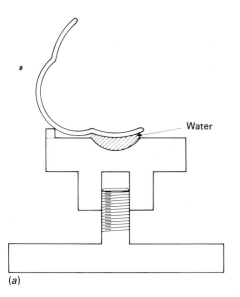

Water

(a)

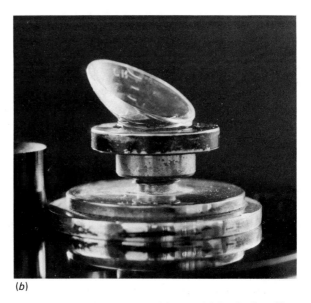

(b)

Figure 12.4 Scleral lens holder for use with Drysdale's method. (*a*) Diagram of section through holder with lens in place. Note screw section by means of which a greater distance may be obtained between the lens surface and microscope objective. (*b*) Holder in use, back scleral radius being measured

across so that the target is focused in the peripheral band of the lens. Care is needed to centre the surface image in this band. Provided that the band is 1 mm wide and light incidence is still normal to the surface being measured, it is possible to measure its radius. It is therefore possible to measure any intermediate radii on the lens which occur over a wide enough band. Where each peripheral curve is too narrow, the centre of curvature image is similar to that of a toroidal surface. A line image (formed by the surface along the band) can be focused and is parallel to the direction of the tilt. This is closest to the correct radius. The image formed by the surface across the width of the band is longer than the correct radius because it is influenced by the areas of surface to either side of the band being measured.

Attempts have been made (Brungardt, 1962) to measure back peripheral radii using a focimeter. Because of the change in back surface radius between the centre and the periphery, it may be possible to obtain two power readings on the focimeter. Provided that the front surface is one single curve, the difference between the two power readings is due to the radius difference on the back surface. If the back optic zone radius is known, its corresponding negative surface power may be obtained from radius/power tables* and the back peripheral surface power found by adding the difference in focimeter readings (the periphery has the less negative value). By further using radius/power tables, the back peripheral radius may be determined. This method is inaccurate with multi-curve lenses. The thickness difference between centre and periphery contributes to the inaccuracy for all lenses.

Measurement of convex surfaces

The concave surface is mounted on water, if possible, or blacked out with a soft grease pencil or felt-tip pen. The convex surface is placed uppermost on a special holder (*Figure 12.5*) on a radiuscope. A similar procedure to that outlined above for concave surfaces is followed, but the surface and centre of curvature images are reversed.

*Tables for radius to power conversion — *see* Appendix B, *Table B.II.*

Keratometers

The keratometer is used with a special contact lens holder (*Figure 12.6*) which utilizes a front surface silvered mirror and a lens support. The lens rests on water in a small depression on a horizontal support. The mirror is set at 45° to the optical axis of the instrument and reflects light from the instrument on to the surface to be measured.

Another type of holder (*Figure 12.7*) requires that the lens be attached to a depression, which lies in a vertical plane, by some adhesive substance such as Plasticine or double-sided sticky tape. There is a possibility that the lens may be distorted using this procedure.

The keratometer can be used to measure optic zone radii of corneal lenses and optic radii of scleral lenses. Because an area of approximately 3 mm in diameter is needed to check a particular radius using conventional keratometers (Lehmann, 1967), it is not possible to measure intermediate and peripheral radii on corneal lenses by this method. Using a single mire of the topographical ophthalmometer (*see* Chapter 6), which utilizes a very small area of reflecting surface, such readings may be possible, however.

Because the keratometer mires are reflected from regions of the surface outside the paraxial zone, an allowance is made during calibration for the aberrations thus introduced. As keratometers are calibrated for convex surfaces and, when used to measure back optic radii of contact

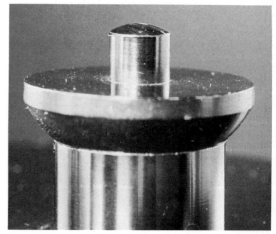

Figure 12.5 Holder for measuring convex surfaces on the radiuscope. The lens has been displaced slightly in order to make it visible

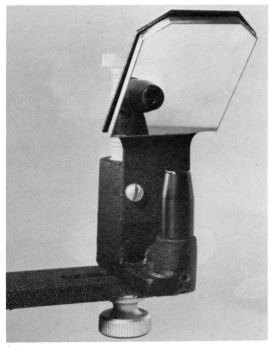

(a)

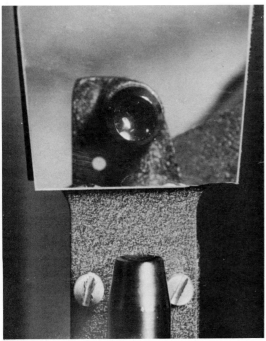

(b)

Figure 12.6 Mirror-type contact lens holder for use with a keratometer. (*a*) On the keratometer; (*b*) close-up. The lens, which is resting on the concave depression of the support, can be seen reflected in the mirror

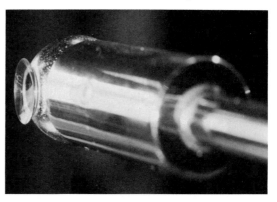

Figure 12.7 Contact lens holder for use with keratometer. The holder is screwed to the head-rest arm, and the lens is held in the depression by an adhesive substance

lenses, concave surfaces are involved, an error is introduced. This is because the aberrations produced by a concave surface are different from those produced by a convex surface. As stated in Chapter 6, p. 248, Bausch & Lomb and other keratometer manufacturers have produced conversion tables for converting convex to concave radii and these show the error to range from 0.02 mm for steep radii (of the order of 6.50 mm) up to 0.04 mm for flat radii (of about 9.50 mm). In all cases, the radii for concave surfaces are greater than for convex surfaces. Thus, for most of the back optic zone radii encountered in contact lens work, it is sufficient to add 0.03 mm to the radius reading given by the keratometer.

To measure back scleral radii the range of the keratometer needs extending. This may be done by recalibrating the keratometer using a $-1.00\,\mathrm{D}$ or $-2.00\,\mathrm{D}$ trial case lens taped in front of the objective as mentioned on p. 248. Three steel balls are used for recalibration having accurately known radii of, say, 9.00 mm, 12.00 mm and 15.00 mm. A graph is then drawn of measured radius (ordinate) against actual radius (abscissa). Provided the same trial case lens is always employed, the same graph may then be used for determining longer radii than the keratometer was designed to measure. Steep radii may be determined similarly, by taping a positive trial case lens, of about $+1.50\,\mathrm{D}$, in front of the keratometer objective and recalibrating with steep steel balls and drawing another graph. (This is useful for measuring the radii of keratoconic corneas, if sufficiently undistorted readings can be obtained.)

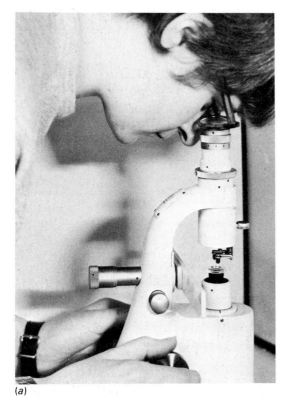

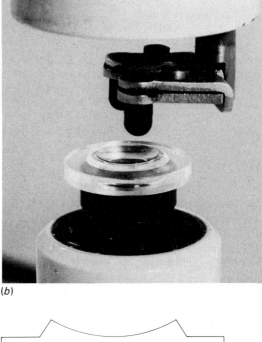

(b)

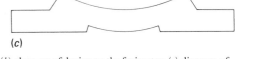

(a)   (c)

Figure 12.8 The radius checking device. (a) On the focimeter; (b) close-up of device on the focimeter; (c) diagram of cross-section of device. Note design of the convex side. The outer flat section rests on the focimeter stop, and the apex of the convex portion is in the same plane

The radius checking device

This device (*Figure 12.8*), developed by Sarver and Kerr (1964), is used in conjunction with a focimeter. The device is made of plastics, refractive index 1.49, and has a depression on one surface which is flatter than the front surface radius of most corneal contact lenses. The other surface has a convex portion, radius 8.87 mm, designed to rest in the plane of the focimeter stop. A small amount of liquid of refractive index 1.49 is placed in the depression and the lens to be measured is placed with its convex surface in contact with the liquid. The device with lens in place can be considered as a thick lens since all the components — device, liquid and lens — have the same refractive index.

Thus if,

Front surface of device $= F_1$ D $= +55.24$ D
Thickness of device $= t_1$ mm
Thickness of contact lens $= t_2$ mm

Back surface power of
  contact lens $= F_2$ D
Back surface radius of
  contact lens $= r_2$ mm
Front vertex power of the
  system $= F_v$ D

then from the formula for front vertex power:

$$F_v = \frac{F_2}{1 - \left(\frac{t_1 + t_2}{1000n}\right)F_2} + F_1$$

From the above

$$r_2 = \frac{(1 - n)1000}{F_v - F_1} + \frac{(t_1 + t_2)(1 - n)}{n}$$

(a)   (b)

The front vertex power of the system is found using the focimeter. The thickness of the liquid between lens and device is negligible. The thickness of the contact lens is determined by a suitable method. Tables have been prepared and published (Dickins, 1968) for use with the device. Thus, once F_v and $(t_1 + t_2)$ have been determined, two figures are obtained from the appropriate tables for the two parts of the formula (*a*) and (*b*). This device can only be used to measure the back optic zone radius of a corneal lens. It is possible that a separate device could be designed for use with scleral lenses.

Templates

Plastics rings of various radii, with chamfered edges, have been used to measure back scleral radii (Stone, 1964).

Other methods

There are various other methods for measuring contact lens radii which are in the main only laboratory techniques. It is possible that other instrumentation may be developed using these techniques.

Interference patterns

Interference patterns, which may be parallel fringes or rings, can be produced in a number of ways. Interference fringes are the basis of many lens testing techniques. Moiré fringes were utilized in the Toposcope (*Figure 12.9*). It was used for measuring radii and diameters of corneal lenses. The target, which consisted of a series of straight lines, was viewed through a screen with similar lines. The shape and

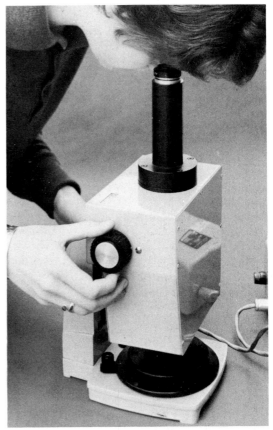

Figure 12.9 The Toposcope

orientation of the fringes formed were a function of the relationship between the two sets of lines. Straight parallel fringes indicate a spherical surface, curved fringes indicate an elliptical surface (*Figure 12.10*). Any warpage or dimples

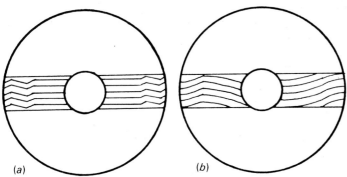

(*a*)   (*b*)

Figure 12.10 Fringes as seen with the Toposcope. (*a*) Straight parallel fringes indicate spherical curves; central fringes correspond to the back optic zone radius, peripheral fringes the back peripheral radius. A transition zone and edge bevel are apparent. (*b*) Curved fringes indicating an elliptical surface

in the surface was indicated by irregularly shaped fringes.

Methods of measuring radii using fringes may be needed more in the future with the developments in aspheric and continuous curve lenses, because it is not possible to measure these surfaces accurately with the other methods discussed.

Garner (1970) undertook an investigation concerning the measurement of contact lens radii using Newton's rings. Although his apparatus was too complicated to form the basis for an instrument for use by practitioners, it made use of test plates and was accurate to 0.003 mm in radius determination. With it he showed that hydration of hard lenses maintains the spherical nature of their surfaces (if spherical to start with), and that surface polishing with wax tools can lead to flattening of the periphery of a spherical surface with effective steepening at the centre due to distortion.

Pneumatic gauging

This method uses an air jet as part of a direct reading spherometer (Smith, 1966), the pressure from a small air jet being proportional to the sagitta of surfaces to which it is applied.

Focimeter and trial lenses

Linnell Fearn (1970) suggested taking a focimeter reading with the front surface of a trial lens resting on the back surface of a test lens of unknown dimensions. A second reading is taken with water between the contact surfaces. The difference between the readings gives the liquid lens power. Knowing the front surface radius of the trial lens, and assuming a negligible liquid lens thickness and refractive index of 1.336, the back optic zone radius (BOZR) of the test lens can be determined. The fluid lens power must be kept to a minimum. This requires the use of about three trial lenses with different known front surface radii depending on the BOZR of the lens to be tested.

Accuracy of methods

Of the methods described for determining contact lens radii, the radiuscope appears to be the most accurate and versatile (Dickins and Fletcher, 1964). The keratometer is limited because a large area is usually needed on which to take measurements. Most keratometers are not calibrated with a sufficiently small scale to measure to 0.01 mm positively. Because a keratometer utilizes reflections from outside the paraxial zone, it is calibrated to allow for the aberrations introduced by convex surfaces. When used for measuring concave surfaces the radius is slightly underestimated by approximately 0.02–0.04 mm (Bennett, 1966) (see p. 445).

The accuracy of the radius checking device has been investigated (Dickins, 1966a,b) and found to be reasonable. Measurements can be made to an accuracy of 0.02 mm provided that the constants of the device are accurately known.

Templates provide only an approximate value for the back scleral radius. Sources of error are the pliability of the lens and the difficulty of rotating the template about the axis of symmetry of the lens.

In an investigation into the accuracy of the Toposcope, Storey (1969) found it to be poor, particularly for peripheral radii, and most errors were negative. However, a more recent study by Janoff (1977) had shown that, with an experienced observer, the Toposcope proved quicker to use and gave less variable readings than the radiuscope. Also the Toposcope utilized fringes formed over the whole back optic zone and was capable of detecting and measuring aspherical surfaces to a limited degree of accuracy.

For most instruments, the precision (repeatability) of measurements is high, but the accuracy may not be high. The quality of the image obtained may vary according to the material used for the contact lens.

It should be remembered when checking contact lens radii that finished corneal lenses alter in curvature with hydration and with release of any stresses in the lens material (Phillips, 1969).

Diameters and linear parameters

Several devices are available for measuring the different linear parameters. With some methods, the problem of parallax occurs as the measuring scale is not in the same plane as the parameter being measured.

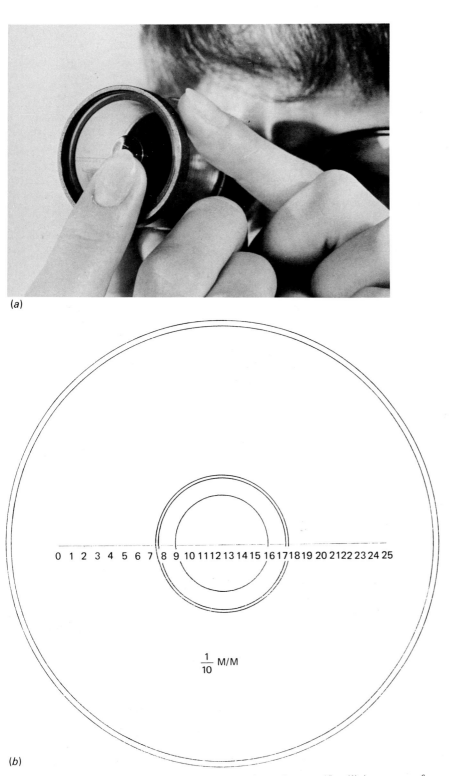

(a)

(b)

$\frac{1}{10}$ M/M

0 1 2 3 4 5 6 7 8 9 10 11 12 13 14 15 16 17 18 19 20 21 22 23 24 25

Figure 12.11 (*a*) Lens being positioned against scale of measuring magnifier. (*b*) Appearance of zones of corneal lens as seen through a measuring magnifier

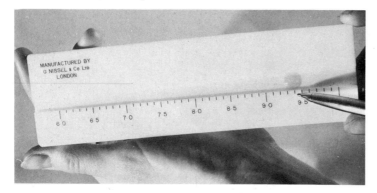

Figure 12.12 V gauge in use. Pen indicates position, to read lens total diameter of 9.40 mm to nearest 0.10 mm

Measuring magnifier

The measuring magnifier (*Figure 12.11* and *see Figure 22.12*) has an adjustable eyepiece through which an engraved scale is viewed. The lens is held with the concave surface towards the scale. The total diameter of the lens may be checked with this device. The back optic zone diameter and any intermediate optic diameters may also be checked in this way provided that the transitions are reasonably sharp. The lens should be rotated and several readings taken to check overall and optic zone roundness. Any displacement of the optic may be checked with this instrument. Because the scale is usually only 20 mm long, the device is only used with corneal lenses.

V gauge

V gauges (*Figure 12.12*) are made of metal or plastics and have a V-shaped channel cut into the material. The channel may vary in width from 6.00 to 12.50 mm. The corneal lens to be measured is placed at the widest end of the channel, concave side downwards, and then allowed to slide down under gravity until it is stopped by the sides of the gauge. The total diameter is then read from a scale beside the

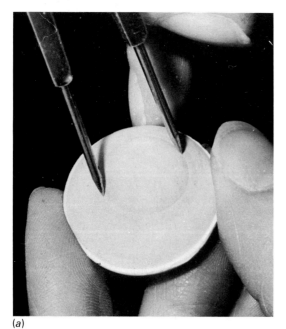

(a)

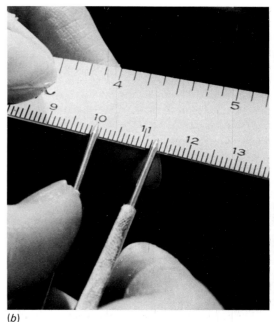

(b)

Figure 12.13 (a) Cast of scleral lens with dividers placed to measure back optic zone diameter. (b) Dividers placed against scale giving measurement of 13.0 mm

channel. The lens must be clean and dry or it will not slide freely. The lens must not be forced along the channel as this can result in compression and even breakage.

Other methods

Various contact lens viewers are available for determination of linear parameters as shown, for example, in *Figures 13.17* and *22.43*. These usually incorporate a screen and use projection magnification. The principle on which they are based is that of the microfiche viewer.

Alternative, a reticule within the eyepiece of any viewing instrument can be used for linear measurements.

Cast, dividers, transparent rule

Most scleral lens parameters are measured on a cast of the lens (*Figure 12.13*). The cast is made from dental stone mixed with a small amount of water to a smooth paste. The lens is supported horizontally on Plasticine. After ensuring that all air bubbles have escaped from the dental stone by tapping the sides of the mixing bowl, the dental stone is poured into the lens until it is completely full. Care must be taken that an excess of dental stone does not drip over the sides of the lens and so cause difficulty in the removal of the cast. When the dental stone is set, the cast is removed from the lens, using a fingernail. The cast has all the lens features clearly marked on it. The transition width, back optic zone diameter and optic displacement can be measured from the cast by placing the dividers at the appropriate points and measuring the distance apart of the dividers with a rule. The primary optic diameter of a preformed scleral lens may be deduced by adding the transition width to the back optic zone diameter, measured on a cast at the point where the transition curve intersects the optic curve. Displacement of optic is found by measuring on the cast, the major and minor scleral chords (usually on the temporal and nasal sides, respectively) and taking half the difference between the two. A scleral chord is measured from the outer edge of the transition to the edge of the cast.

The total diameter and back scleral size of a scleral lens are determined by direct measurement with a transparent rule.

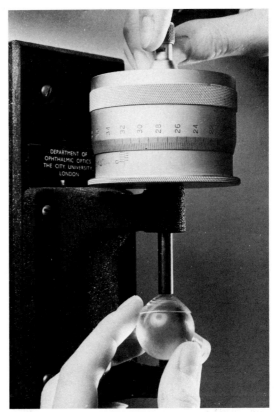

Figure 12.14 Micrometer method of measuring primary optic diameter. The lens is placed on a sphere. When the vertical plunger is in contact with the front surface of the lens the scale reading gives the distance x (*see Figure 12.15*)

Micrometer and spheres

A special problem arises in checking the primary optic diameter of a scleral lens because the sharp demarcation between back optic zone and scleral surfaces is usually removed by the transition. It is possible to measure this diameter by finding the difference between optic and scleral zone sags (Stone, 1964).

A sphere with radius equal to the back scleral radius of the lens to be measured is placed on the base plate of a vertical micrometer (*Figure 12.14*) with the lens on top. The maximum measurement x (*Figure 12.15*) is determined. From this is subtracted the thickness of the optic, t, and $2h$, the diameter of the sphere, to find the difference between the sags, a.

The value a is found in the appropriate table* indicated by the back scleral radius and back

---

*Tables used when measuring primary optic diameter with a micrometer (Stone, 1964).

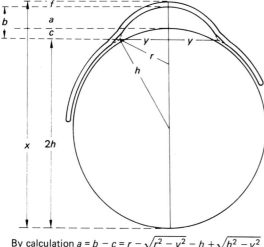

By calculation $a = b - c = r - \sqrt{r^2 - y^2} - h + \sqrt{h^2 - y^2}$
By measurement $a = x - t - 2h$

Figure 12.15 Principle of micrometer method of measuring primary optic diameter. h = back scleral radius; r = back optic zone radius; $2y$ = primary optic diameter; b and c are determined from the exact sag formula

optic zone radius, and the primary optic diameter can then be read off. Values of a have been computed for back optic zone radii from 7.00 to 10.50 mm in 0.125 mm steps, back scleral radii from 11.50 to 15.50 mm in 0.25 mm steps, and primary optic diameters from 12.00 to 15.50 mm in 0.125 mm steps.

Axial edge lift measurement

Stone (1975) has described two methods, as follows.

Method 1

The lens is placed on the radiuscope holder in the usual manner, and a microscope cover slide placed on top (*Figure 12.16*). Central readings are taken successively on the underside of the

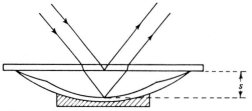

Figure 12.16 Axial edge lift measurement. A cover slide on the lens (which is placed in the radiuscope holder) permits s to be measured

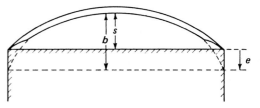

Figure 12.17 Axial edge lift $e = b - s$. Here the lens is placed on a holder having a stem diameter equal to its total diameter. Other stem diameters may be used

cover slide and then the back surface of the lens. The difference between these readings gives the lens primary sag. From sag tables (*see* Appendix C) the sag b, corresponding to the back optic zone radius of the lens under test at a diameter corresponding to the total diameter of the lens, is found. The axial edge lift $e = b - s$ (*Figure 12.17*). This does not allow for edge rounding.

Method 2

The radiuscope is first focused on the flat uppermost surface of a holder or stem of known diameter such as that shown in *Figure 12.17*. The test lens is then placed on this, convex surface upwards, and the radiuscope is re-focused at the apex of the convex surface. The difference between these readings gives the sag s plus the lens thickness. From sag tables (*see* Appendix C), the sag b corresponding to the back optic zone radius of the lens under test at a diameter equal to that of the stem is found. The axial 'edge' lift $e = b - s$. This gives the true axial edge lift at the known diameter of the stem.

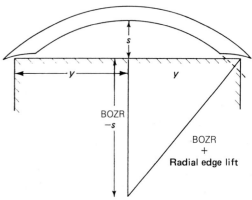

Figure 12.18 Determination of radial edge lift. (After Newlove, 1974)

Radial edge lift

As described by Newlove (1974) and Stone (1975), and shown in *Figure 12.18*, the radial edge lift also may be found by placing the lens concave surface down on a holder of known diameter. It can be seen from the right-angled triangle in *Figure 12.18*, that by Pythagoras' theorem:

$$(\text{Radial edge lift} + \text{BOZR})^2$$
$$= \left(\frac{\text{Stem diameter}}{2}\right)^2 + (\text{BOZR} - \text{sag})^2$$

If stem diameter = $2y$ and sag = s, then

$$\text{Radial edge lift} = \sqrt{y^2 + (\text{BOZR} - s)^2} - \text{BOZR}$$

s is found as described above, by focusing the radiuscope first on the upper flat surface of the stem and then at the apex of the front surface of the lens, and subtracting the centre thickness of the lens from the measurement obtained.

Note. If the stem diameter is the same as the total diameter of the lens, the sag value, s, obtained is that of the primary sag of the lens.

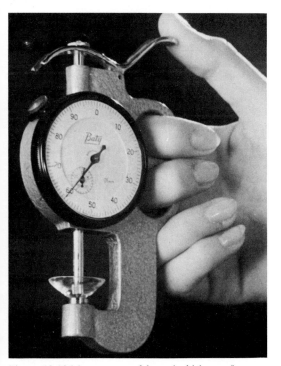

Figure 12.19 Measurement of the optic thickness of a scleral lens. Scale reading 0.60 mm

Thickness

The thickness of the centre and edge, or any other part of a corneal lens, as well as the optic and scleral zones of a scleral lens, may be determined with a suitable thickness gauge. Thickness gauges usually incorporate a dial gauge calibrated to 0.01 mm (*Figures 12.19, 12.20* and *see Figure 22.40*). *Radial thickness* is measured perpendicular to the front surface of a lens (although in practice, when the two surfaces are not parallel, the actual measurement may be made along an axis which is the nearest compromise to being perpendicular to both surfaces — *see Figure 12.20b*). *Axial thickness* is measured parallel to the primary axis of the lens. For most lenses the centre thickness is measured at a common geometric and optical centre, and at that point radial and axial thickness are the same. For points away from the optical centre, while radial thickness is easy to measure, axial thickness is not; but from the manufacturer's point of view it is axial thickness which is the easier value to calculate from the sagitta values of the lens surfaces — *see* Chapter 5. This may mean that practitioner and manufacturer have a different understanding of 'edge thickness' for example. Pearson (1986) has discussed in detail the calculation and measurement of both radial and axial thickness as well as the relationship between them, and he has derived approximate conversion formulae. He also gives equations for deriving average thickness which is of significance when considering the oxygen transmission of a lens.

Guillon, Crosbie-Walsh and Byrnes (1986) have described the use of a modified digital pachometer for the measurement of axial edge thickness of hard lenses, giving an accuracy for single measurements of $\pm 20\,\mu m$, but the technique has not been marketed.

A modified thickness gauge (*Figure 12.20*) permitting radial edge thickness measurement at a precisely determined distance in from the very edge of the lens, has been evaluated by Port (1987), who found it excellent. It also permits accurately positioned centre thickness measurement and determination of the base–apex line of prismatic lenses. Supplied with a pre-programmed computer, it can be used to compare theoretical values of axial and radial thickness of rigid lenses of known geometry with the actual thickness at any realistic distance from the lens edge.

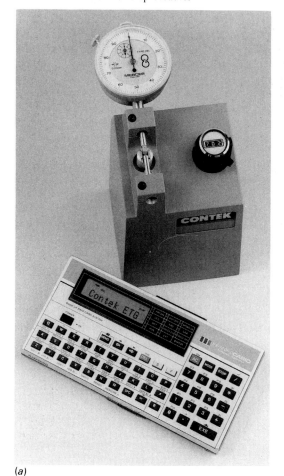

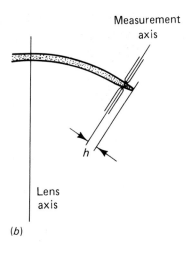

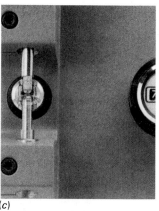

(a)

(b)

(c)

Figure 12.20 (a) The Contek edge thickness gauge and computer; (b) the radial thickness measurement it makes at a precise distance, h, in from the edge; (c) close-up of lens in place during edge thickness measurement. (Reproduced by kind permission of Contek Ltd)

A spectacle lens measure may be used for thickness measurement if the lens is placed convex side down on a flat surface. The two outer legs of the lens measure should contact the flat surface outside the lens, and the centre leg be located on the concave surface of the lens where the thickness measurement is needed. The sag value obtained is then equal to the thickness of the lens. (Note: this method should not be attempted if the legs of the lens measure have sharp points; it is only safe if the legs have rounded tips.)

Another method is to use the radiuscope. Water is not used in the lens holder when the thickness of a lens is being determined. The target is focused on each lens surface in turn. The distance between the two foci multiplied by the refractive index of the material gives the lens

thickness. Or a flat plate may be put on the radiuscope holder, on which surface the radiuscope is first focused and set at zero. The lens is then placed, convex side down, on the plate and the radiuscope focused at the centre of its back surface. This gives a direct reading of the lens centre thickness.

Optic — lens prescription

The back vertex power of a contact lens may be measured using a focimeter. If the focimeter is mounted vertically, the lens can rest freely on the stop. A corneal lens, if held against the stop, may be distorted by the pressure of the fingers. Unless its construction permits angling to a vertical position, it is possible to arrange for a focimeter to be mounted vertically by means of a

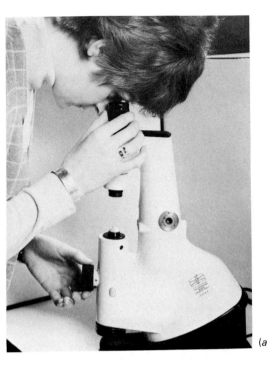

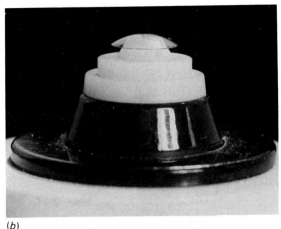

(b)

(a)

Figure 12.21 (*a*) Measurement of back vertex power on a focimeter; (*b*) close-up of lens in place against stop. It can be seen that the back vertex of the lens is not in the plane of the stop

special stage (*Figure 12.21*). The focimeter is used in the normal way to determine the prescription. Care is needed in centring the lens to determine any prism.

One problem in determining the back vertex power of a contact lens is that the back surface of the lens may not be in the plane of the focimeter stop. This is because contact lenses have highly curved surfaces. With scleral lenses, the scleral zone may prevent the back surface of the lens from lying in the correct plane. The back vertex power may therefore be recorded as being a greater positive or smaller negative value than it actually is. This is because the back vertex focal length of a lens is measured from the plane of the stop to the target position (*Figure 12.22*). Because the back surface of the lens is not in the plane of the stop, the true back vertex focal length is actually greater. This error can be minimized either by using a smaller stop or removing the stop collar, if possible, so that the back surface of the lens is in approximately the correct position.

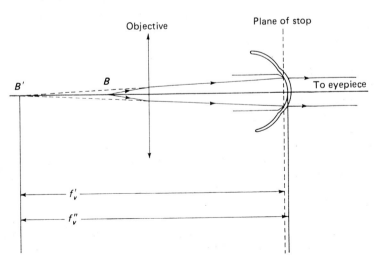

Figure 12.22 Error in measuring back vertex power. f_v' = back vertex focal length of lens under test as measured on the instrument; f_v'' = true back vertex focal length; B = target; B' = image of target formed by objective

456

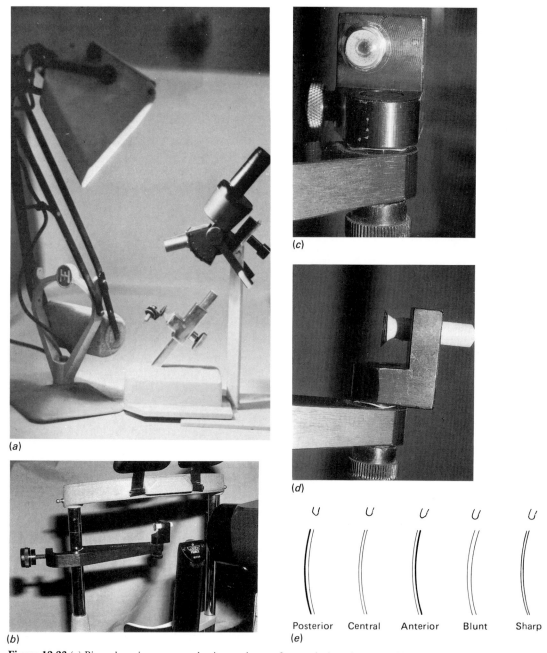

(a)

(b)

(c)

(d)

(e)

Posterior   Central   Anterior   Blunt   Sharp

Figure 12.23 (*a*) Binocular microscope used to inspect lens surfaces and edges. An external light source is used. The lens is held on the suction holder which can be rotated about its own axis and about the plane of the lens, the rotating holder being movable along its angled support to permit accurate focusing. The rotating holder and support were built by Ronald B. Rabbetts (Rabbetts, 1978) for The London Refraction Hospital (LRH, now the Institute of Optometry), and were the prototype for (*b*) The LRH — Nissel Edge Checking Device. (*b*) This is shown fixed to the head rest of a Gambs slit lamp. The binocular microscope is used to study the edge shape and finish, with illumination provided by the slit beam. A similar lens-holding device is the Krieger Contact Lens Holder available in the USA from Ocular Instruments Inc. (*c*) Close-up of the lens surface which is seen to be dirty. (*d*) Lens edge. When seen through the microscope the width of the central bright reflection, at the very edge nearest the observer, can be used to judge the edge shape as in (*e*). (*e*) The position and width of the bright edge reflection — shown as the gap between the lines — from several corneal lens edges whose profiles are shown above, and with the position of the peak of the edge given below. [(*a*) and (*e*) reproduced by kind permission of R. B. Rabbetts]

Special contact lens holders are available for many focimeters. (Rodenstock make a special attachment to their focimeter, for measuring corneal lenses. The stop may be screwed up or down depending on the BOZR of the lens which is indicated on a scale.)

Alternatively, instead of back vertex power, front vertex power may be measured by resting the front surface of the contact lens on an optical flat placed in the focimeter's stop. The former may then be determined by calculation or from tables (Appendix D) if the central optic thickness and back optic zone radius are known.

Surface quality and polish, edge form, material tint

A binocular microscope (*Figure 12.23*), radiuscope, contact lens viewer or measuring magnifier may be used to examine the surface of a contact lens. Alternatively, the lens is observed against a uniformly illuminated background with or without magnification. The blending of the transition may be observed at the same time. For the back transitional curve, the horizontal image produced from an elongated light source such as a fluorescent tube can be observed with a × 10 loupe or hand magnifier (*see Figures 19.1* and *19.2*; Bailey, 1959; McMonnies, 1986). Lenses should be free from material defects and surface imperfections.

Any distortion of the optic or unwanted cylinder may be found using a cross-line chart and the lateral and rotational tests, or by using a focimeter, radiuscope or Toposcope.

The shape of the edge of a contact lens may be examined by observation with a binocular microscope with the lens mounted on a suitable rotating holder as shown in *Figure 12.23*, or by projecting a shadow of the edge onto a screen. Casting the edge in dental stone or impression materials, or pressing the lens edge into Plasticine may be utilized and in each case the impression left on the material is examined under magnification with a binocular microscope, for example, on a slit lamp. The edge is cast by inserting the edge of the lens into a small pool of dental stone on top of a rubber band on a square of plastics material (*Figure 12.24*). The lens is placed at right-angles to the rubber band. When the dental stone is just set, the lens is gently removed and the dental stone is pulled off the rubber band. The dental stone is scored on

the back by the rubber band so that it is easy to break in half and the edge cast can be examined in cross-section. With more fragile rigid gas permeable lenses, it is better to use impression material which sets quickly and can be cut with a razor blade to reveal the contour of the lens edge in cross-section. However, because impression material dehydrates and shrinks, the cast is only accurate for a short time, compared to the permanent record provided by a dental stone cast.

Plasticine provides a quick and easy means to examine the edge, but the cast tends to lose shape. If the lens is left. in the Plasticine, the edge shape can be seen in profile against the Plasticine when examined with the binocular or slit lamp microscope.

McMonnies (1986) advocates the use of a × 20 hand magnifier to inspect the outer edge

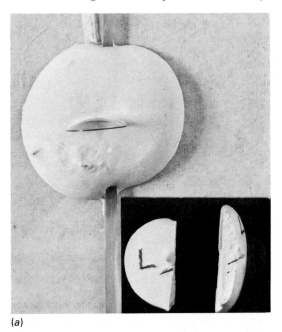

(a)

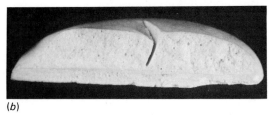

(b)

Figure 12.24 (*a*) Lens edge being cast in dental stone. Inset — cast broken in half. (*b*) Magnified view of section through cast. A square-shaped edge is seen. Provided that it is not distorted, impression material is quicker and safer to use

profile, the lens being held in a horizontal plane, concave surface down, between index finger and thumb, with the magnifier being held in the other hand in the same way. The thumbs can be kept in contact with each other to minimize movement. The illumination from a single fluorescent tube reflected in a bench-mounted mirror obviates the need to raise the hands above the head.

The edge should be examined at a number of different points by one of the above methods.

The entire circumference of the lens edge should also be rotated before a binocular microscope to check for any localized distortions (*see Figure 12.23*).

The colour of a contact lens may be observed against a white background.

A specific gravity test may be used to establish the basic type of material (*see* Chapter 10, p. 378). Some rigid gas permeable lenses are engraved with a material identification mark by the manufacturer.

Stress

Stress may be checked by placing the lens between crossed polarized filters. If stress is present a strain pattern is seen, otherwise the appearance is devoid of any pattern.

Surface and undersurface stresses can lead to subsequent flaking of the surface layers, in final lens working, polishing or in later use (Cordrey, 1973).

Stress and electrical charges such as static and piezo-electric effects are thought to be responsible for the spontaneous fracture and surface crazing of many rigid gas permeable (RGP) lenses. A surface-crazed lens is shown in *Figure 10.15* and *Plate 27*). The whole subject of stress in polymers is a very complex one. Silk (1987) has discussed the matter in some detail indicating all the factors to be taken into consideration to avoid problems for wearers of PMMA and RGP lenses (*see also* Chapter 8).

Toric lenses

When a radiuscope is used to check toroidal surfaces, the target image formed on the lens surface appears uniformly focused as seen through the microscope, but, as a toroidal surface has two centres of curvature correspond-

ing to the two principal meridians, there is not a uniformly focused target image formed at the two centre of curvature positions. Instead, only one of the target lines will appear sharply focused and the lens must be rotated so that each principal meridian coincides with one of the target lines. Then the centre of curvature of each principal meridian is located by focusing the two perpendicular target lines in turn. If the target consists of a ring of dots there is no need to rotate the lens to locate the principal meridians.

If a keratometer is used, the procedure is the same as for carrying out keratometry on a toroidal cornea, the usual small allowances being made for the measurement of a concave surface instead of a convex one.

The back optic zone diameter of a corneal lens may be oval, depending on the method of manufacture, so maximum and minimum values should be found.

For checking the power of toric lenses *see* Chapter 14.

Aspheric lenses

DeFazio and Lowther (1979) investigated two methods of clinically inspecting and verifying aspherical back surfaces of hard contact lenses. In the first method a radiuscope was modified with a tilting table. By measuring radii at off-axis points, the eccentricity was calculated for each aspherical surface tested. The conformity of the surface to a true conicoid could then be evaluated.

More recently, Garner (1981) has described a method of assessing the back surface of hard contact lenses using a modified low-power stereomicroscope to view the interference fringes formed between the contact lens and a test plate. He outlined how the instrument could be used to measure the radius of curvature of the optical zone and the periphery of aspheric contact lenses, and to assess the quality of the back surface of the lens.

The ability to reproduce aspherical back surface designs to nominal specifications is important. Garner (1981) and DeFazio and Lowther (1979) produced results that suggested some variation between the nominal specifications of the lens surfaces and the measured values.

Table 12.2 Determination of the effective BOZR of Pilkington Diffrax bifocal lenses from the measured radius (using a radiuscope) and near addition

Near addition (D)	+1.00	+1.50	+2.00	+2.50	+3.00
Effective BOZR (mm)	Radiuscope measured radii (mm)				
7.10	7.283	7.380	7.480	7.582	7.687
7.20	7.389	7.488	7.591	7.696	7.804
7.30	7.494	7.597	7.702	7.810	7.922
7.40	7.600	7.705	7.813	7.925	8.040
7.50	7.705	7.814	7.925	8.040	8.158
7.60	7.811	7.922	8.037	8.155	8.277
7.70	7.917	8.031	8.149	8.271	8.396
7.80	8.023	8.140	8.261	8.386	8.515
7.90	8.128	8.249	8.374	8.502	8.634
8.00	8.234	8.358	8.486	8.618	8.754
8.10	8.340	8.467	8.598	8.734	8.874
8.20	8.447	8.577	8.712	8.851	8.993
8.30	8.553	8.686	8.825	8.967	9.114
8.40	8.659	8.796	8.937	9.084	9.235
8.50	8.765	8.906	9.051	9.201	9.356
8.60	8.872	9.016	9.165	9.318	9.477

Bifocal lenses

The near addition may be checked using a focimeter. For solid PMMA bifocals, where the addition is on the back surface, its value in air is 3.18 times that on the eye (*see* Chapter 5, p. 222). The diameter and position of the near vision zone may be checked using a measuring magnifier.

Diffractive bifocal lenses

At the time of writing, the only lens of this type available is the Pilkington Diffrax rigid gas permeable lens — *see* Chapter 16. Its various diameters and thicknesses are measured in the conventional way used for hard lenses as described on pp. 448–454.

Table 12.3 Near addition power corresponding to number of diffractive zones or visible rings of the Pilkington Diffrax bifocal RGP lens

Near addition (D)	No. of diffractive zones
+1.00	6
+1.50	8
+2.00	11
+2.50	14
+3.00	17

The effective BOZR is a non-existent curve. A radiuscope measurement of the diffractive surface is easily obtained, but its value is not that of the effective BOZR. The radius measured depends on both the dioptric value of the near addition and the effective BOZR (*Table 12.2*). Thus, for example, a lens having a near addition of +2.00 D and an effective BOZR of 7.5 mm would give a radiuscope reading of 7.925 mm. Thus the near addition of the lens must be known and checked in order to ascertain the effective BOZR.

Verification of the near addition is simple as it is directly related to the number of diffractive zones — which appear as rings — on the back optic zone surface, as shown in *Figure 16.27*. *Table 12.3* shows the number of diffractive zone for each of the available near addition powers. The number of rings is most easily counted by placing the lens with its back surface against the scale of a scale magnifier, as in *Figure 12.11*, then slowly moving the rings across one of the graduation marks on the scale, counting them as the lens is moved. With experience it is possible to judge how many rings are present from the appearance of the lens.

Another method of determining the near addition is to put a drop of water on the diffractive surface and place on this a single vision lens whose front surface curvature is approximately the same as that of the effective BOZR. This 'thick' lens is then placed on the focimeter and the difference between the two power readings obtained is the near addition (*see* Chapter 16).

The distance back vertex power (BVP) of the lens cannot be determined directly from the focimeter reading in air — which yields a multiplicity of images, some of them coloured. The maximum positive green reading should be used (best found by placing a green filter in the optical system between the lens and the observer) and from this value twice the near addition is deducted to obtain the distance BVP. For example, a Diffrax lens has a maximum positive power reading of +2.00 D and has eight diffractive zones (+1.50 D near addition). Its true distance BVP is therefore +2.00 − (+1.50 × 2) = −1.00 D.

General

Wehking (1981) makes the point that instrumentation should be checked for working efficiency, and periodically against test standards for precision.

Addendum I Dimensional tolerances for hard contact lenses (all dimensions in millimetres)

	Corneal	Scleral	Method of test
Back (central) optic zone radius	±0.02	±0.05	(1) Keratometer (calibrated for concave surfaces) (2) Radiuscope (3) Interferometry techniques
Back (central) optic zone diameter	±0.20	±0.20	× 10 measuring magnifier
Back scleral zone radius (of preformed lenses)	—	±0.10	(1) Keratometer (calibrated for concave surfaces) (2) Radiuscope (3) Interferometry techniques
Basic or primary optic diameter	—	±0.10	Sagitta method
Back peripheral (optic) radius	±0.10	±0.10	(1) Keratometer (calibrated for concave surfaces) (2) Radiuscope (3) Interferometry techniques
Back peripheral (optic) diameter	±0.20	±0.20 (for preformed lenses)	× 10 measuring magnifier
Axial edge lift	±0.02	For all lenses	(1) Radiuscope (2) Sagitta method*
Radial edge lift	±0.02	For all lenses	(1) Radiuscope (2) Sagitta method*
Total diameter	±0.10	±0.25	(1) V-channel gauge (2) × 10 measuring magnifier (3) Projection magnifier with scale
Front (central and/or peripheral) optic zone diameter	±0.20	±0.20	× 10 measuring magnifier
Bifocal segment height	±0.10	—	× 10 measuring magnifier
Centre thickness	±0.02	±0.03	(1) Measuring dial gauge† (2) Radiuscope (3) Projection magnifier with scale
Edge thickness	±0.02	—	Measuring dial gauge†
Vertex clearance (from cast)	—	±0.02	Measuring dial gauge†
Fenestration Truncation Displacement Scleral zone thickness	10% allowance on specification		

*Sagitta method — *see* Stone, J. (1975). Corneal lenses with constant axial edge lift. *Ophthal. Optician* **15**, 818–824.
†Measuring dial gauge calibrated in units of 0.01 mm in accordance with BS 2795: Part 1.
(Formerly reproduced by kind permission of the British Standards Institution from *BS 5562/1978 Specification for Contact Lenses*.) This Standard has now been withdrawn pending the publication of a new Standard. An International Standard is also in the process of preparation.

Addendum II Optical tolerances for hard contact lenses

	Corneal	Scleral	Method of test
Back vertex power (in the weaker meridian):			
+10.00 D to −10.00 D	±0.12 D	±0.12 D	Focimeter with an aperture of not
Over ±10.00 D	±0.25 D	±0.25 D	less than 4 mm
Prism (measured at geometrical centre of optic portion)	±0.50 Δ	±0.50 Δ	Focimeter with an aperture of not less than 4 mm
Optical centration (maximum error)	0.50 mm	0.50 mm	Focimeter with an aperture of not less than 4 mm
Cylinder power:			
Up to 2.00 D	±0.25 D	±0.25 D	Focimeter with an aperture of not
2.00 D to 4.00 D	±0.37 D	±0.37 D	less than 4 mm
Over 4.00 D	±0.50 D	±0.50 D	
Cylinder axis	±5°	±5°	For a prism ballast front surface toric lens, the resultant cylinder axis is measured with the prism base down, i.e. the base–apex line at 90°. For a bi-toric lens the resultant cylinder axis is measured with respect to the orientation of the flattest meridian of the back toroidal surface

(Formerly reproduced by kind permission of the British Standards Institution from *BS 5562:1978 Specification for Contact Lenses*.) This Standard has now been withdrawn pending the publication of a new standard. An International Standard is also in the process of preparation.

Acknowledgements

The author is indebted to Mr C. Wilson, formerly of the Department of Optometry and Visual Science, The City University, London, and later at Bath University, for preparing photographs for all the figures; and to Mr G. Nissel for the loan of the Toposcope for photography.

References

BAILEY, N. J. (1959). The examination and verification of a contact lens. *J. Am. optom. Ass.* **30**, 557–560

BENNETT, A. G. (1966). The calibration of keratometers. *Optician* **151**, 317–322

BRUNGARDT, T. F. (1962). A fast, accurate and practical measurement of the secondary curve radius. *J. Am. optom. Ass.* **34**, 131–134

CORDREY, P. (1973). Technical and economic effects of contact lens production methods. *Ophthal. Optician* **13**, 230–236

DeFAZIO, A. J. and LOWTHER, G. E. (1979). Inspection of back surface aspheric contact lenses. *Am. J. Optom. physiol. Optics* **56**, 471–479

DICKINS, R. (1966a). An investigation into the accuracy of the radius checking device. *Optician* **151**, 265–269

DICKINS, R. (1966b). Further results using the radius checking device. *Optician* **152**, 135–137

DICKINS, R. (1968). Tables for use with the radius checking device. *Optician* **155**, 292–294

DICKINS, R. and FLETCHER, R. J. (1964). Contact lens measurement, a comparison of several devices. *Br. J. physiol. Optics.* **21**, 107–115

DRYSDALE, C. V. (1900). On a simple direct method of measuring the curvature of small lenses. *Trans. opt. Soc.* **2**, 1–12

GARNER, L. (1970). The design and measurement of the back surface of contact lenses. *PhD Thesis*, The City University, London

GARNER, L. F. (1981). A simple interferometer for hard contact lenses. *Am. J. Optom. physiol. Optics* **58**, 944–950

GUILLON, M., CROSBIE-WALSH, J. and BYRNES, D. (1986). Application of pachometry to the measurement of hard contact lens edge profile. *Transactions of the British Contact Lens Association Conference*, pp. 56–59

JANOFF, L. E. (1977). A pilot study of the comparison of validity and reliability between the radiuscope and toposcope. *Int. Contact Lens Clin.* **4**(2), 68–73

LEHMANN, S. (1967). Corneal areas utilised in keratometry. *Optician* **154**, 261–264

LINNELL FEARN, W. W. (1970). The use of the focimeter for measuring the central radii of contact lenses. *Contact Lens* **2**(6), 20–22

McMONNIES, C. W. (1986). Assessment of hard lens edges. *Int. Eyecare* **2**, 532–538

NEWLOVE, D. B. (1974). Development of a new hard lens material. *Optician* **169**(4368), 16–23

PEARSON, R. M. (1986). How thick is a contact lens? *Transactions of the British Contact Lens Association Conference*, pp. 82–86

PHILLIPS, A. J. (1969). Alterations in curvature of the finished corneal lens. *Ophthal. Optician* **9**, 980–982, 985, 986, 1043–1046, 1051–1054, 1100–1104, 1109, 1110

PORT, M. J. A. (1987). A new method of edge thickness measurement for rigid lenses. *J. Br. Contact Lens Ass.* **10**, 16–20

RABBETTS, R. B. (1978). Corneal lens edge checking device. *Ophthal. Optician* **18**, 202

SARVER, M. D. and KERR, K. (1964). A radius of curvature measuring device for contact lenses. *Am. J. Optom.* **41**, 481–489

SILK, A. A. (1987). Puzzle of the polymers. *Transactions of the British Contact Lens Association Conference 1987*, No. 4, pp. 57–61

SMITH, I. C. P. (1966). Pneumatic gauging applied to contact lenses. *Br. J. physiol. Optics* **23**, 161–167

STONE, J. (1964). Checking preformed contact lenses. *Br. J. physiol. Optics* **21**, 264–286

STONE, J. (1975). Corneal lenses with constant axial edge lift. *Ophthal. Optician* **15**, 818–824

STOREY, S. (1969). An assessment of the O.M.I. Toposcope. *Student project*, The City University, London

TANNEHILL, J. C. and SAMPSON, W. G. (1966). Extended use of the radiuscope in contact lens inspection. *Am. J. Ophthal.* **62**, 538–540

WEHKING, K. (1981). Contact lens inspection. *Contacto* **25**, 9–12

Further reading

ANON (1963). What's new — B.A.O. Radiuscope. *Ophthal. Optician* **3**, 76

BENNETT, A. G. (1958). On accuracy in contact lens manufacture. *Optician* **135**, 357–358

BENNETT, A. G. (1966). *Optics of Contact Lenses*, 4th edn. London: Association of Dispensing Opticians

BENNETT, A. G. (1968). Aspherical contact lens surfaces. *Ophthal. Optician* **8**, 1037–1040

BENNETT, A. G. (1968). Aspherical contact lens surfaces, part two. *Ophthal. Optician* **8**, 1297–1311

BENNETT, A. G. (1969). Aspherical contact lens surfaces, part three. *Ophthal. Optician* **9**, 222–224, 229–230

BLACKSTONE, D. (1961). A new instrument. *Ophthal. Optician* **1**, 614–615

BLACKSTONE, M. (1966). The toposcope examined. *Optician* **152**, 38–39

CHARMAN, W. N. (1972). Diffraction and the precision of measurement of corneal and other small radii. *Am. J. Optom.* **49**, 672–680

EMSLEY, H. H. (1963). The keratometer — measurement of concave surfaces. *Optician* **146**, 161–168

FLETCHER, R. J. and NISTED, M. (1961). The accuracy of corneal contact lenses. *Ophthal. Optician* **1**, 217–219

FORST, G. (1971). Optical homogeneity and contour of contact lenses and tests. *Ophthal. Optician* **11**, 739–744

FREEMAN, M. H. (1965). The measurement of contact lens curvature. *Am. J. Optom.* **42**, 693–701

GOLDBERG, J. B. (1961). Lens evaluation inadequacies. *Contacto* **5**, 357–358

HAYNES, P. R. (1960). Quality control and inspection of contact lenses. In *Encyclopaedia of Contact Lens Practice*, **1**, Ch. 23, 8–63. South Bend, Indiana: International Optics

LAYCOCK, D. E. (1957). A microlens measuring aid. *Am. J. Optom.* **34**, 538–539

MANDELL, R. B. (1965). *Contact Lens Practice: Basic and Advanced*. Springfield, Illinois: Thomas

NISSEL, G. (1962). Measuring instruments used in the manufacture and checking of contact lenses. *Optician* **144**, 58–64

PORT, M. (1986). A spherical lens measurement exercise. Part 1. Rigid lenses. *J. Br. Contact Lens Ass.* **9**, 26–35

SARVER, M. D. (1963). Verification of contact lens power. *J. Am. optom. Ass.* **34**, 1304–1306

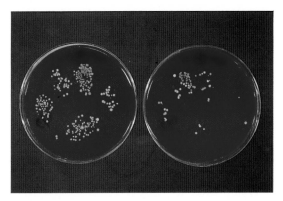

Plate 1 Hygiene and hand-washing. Two agar plates are shown with a practitioner's fingers and thumbprint before (left) and after (right) hand-washing. The reduction but not complete elimination of bacterial colonies is clearly visible. (Courtesy of C. Copley)

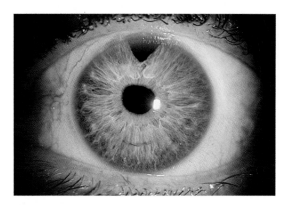

Plate 2 General record of external eye prior to fitting. Special features such as the nasal pinguecula, degree of bulbar conjunctival injection, pupil shape and upper peripheral iridectomy can be used for comparison with the appearance of the eye after fitting. (Courtesy of A. P. Gasson)

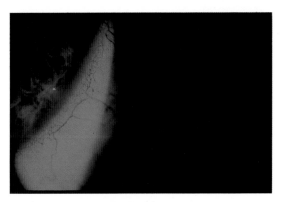

Plate 3 Limbal blood vessel engorgement shown up by red-free illumination – the blood vessels appearing black. (Courtesy of Bausch & Lomb)

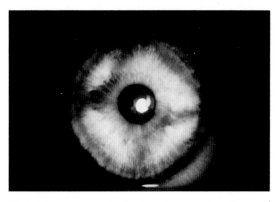

Plate 4 Stress patterns in the normal cornea viewed by polarized biomicroscopy. The pattern will alter in certain disease conditions, e.g. keratoconus, and after surgical procedures such as keratoplasty. (Courtesy of J. Mountford)

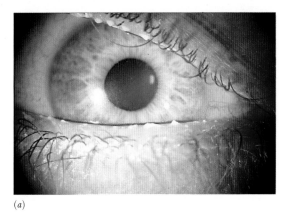

(a)

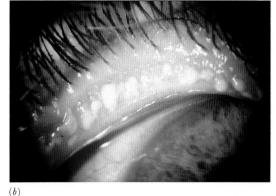

(b)

Plate 5 Severe meibomian hypersecretion. (a) The secretion can be seen along the lid margins and the oiliness of the precorneal tear film is visible; (b) upper lid margin shown in more detail. (Courtesy of A. J. Phillips)

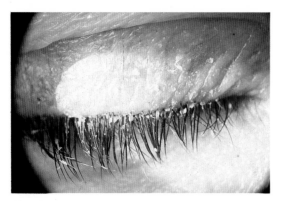

Plate 6 Blepharitis indicating the need for treatment and sustained lid hygiene to improve the chances of good contact lens tolerance. Dead epithelial tissue accumulates around the base of the lashes. This material is a nidus for infection and is irritating in the tear film. (Courtesy of C. McMonnies)

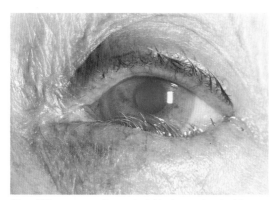

Plate 7 Severe entropion and trichiasis associated with blepharitis. The use of a bandage soft lens allowed regeneration of damaged corneal epithelium and prevented further disturbance prior to surgery. (Courtesy of D. Westerhout)

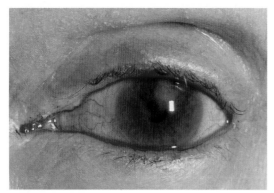

Plate 8 Keratoconjunctivitis sicca associated with chronic blepharitis where both aqueous and lipid layers of the precorneal tear film are affected. (Courtesy of D. Westerhout)

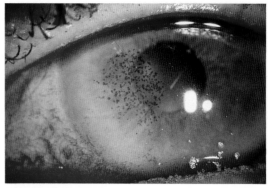

(a)

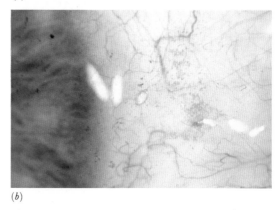

(b)

Plate 9 Rose bengal staining of a dry eye: *(a)* corneal; *(b)* conjunctival. ((*a*) Courtesy of A. J. Phillips and (*b*) courtesy of C. McMonnies)

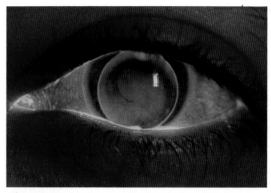

Plate 10 The tri-curve lens C3/7.80:7.00/8.30:8.80/ 12.25:9.20 on an eye with keratometer readings of 7.91 mm along 180, 7.81 mm along 90. The fluorescein pattern shows slight apical corneal clearance and very little peripheral clearance. Such a lens in PMMA material would probably cause central corneal oedema with steepening of the corneal apex giving rise subsequently to the appearance of apical corneal touch as in *Plate 11*. In an RGP material this might be an ideal fit, the minimum peripheral clearance avoiding flare and lid sensation. (Courtesy of M. Wilson)

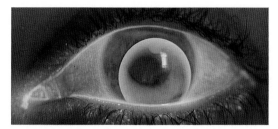

Plate 11 The tetra-curve corneal lens C5/8.10:7.00/ 8.60:7.60/9.60:8.20/10.80:8.80/12.25:9.20 on the same eye as in *Plate 10*. The fluorescein pattern shows the central flat fit with bearing on the apex of the cornea and a slight epithelial abrasion as a result. The lens is riding lower temporally. The lens periphery also appears to have excessive clearance, partially due to the central flat fit. (Courtesy of M. Wilson)

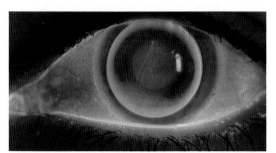

Plate 12 A penta-curve 'tapered' corneal lens C5/7.85:7.00/ 8.35:7.60/9.10:8.20/10.10:8.80/12.25:9.20 on the same eye as in *Plate 10*. The lens is fitted with the back optic zone in alignment with the cornea and with gradually increasing peripheral clearance which would be unnecessarily great for an RGP lens. A foreign body track is also present as shown up by the fluorescein staining of the damaged epithelium. (Courtesy of M. Wilson)

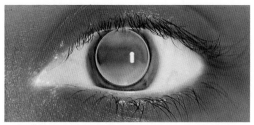

Plate 13 An interpalpebral spherical corneal lens with the back optic zone in alignment with the horizontal meridian of a toroidal cornea having 'with-the-rule' astigmatism. (Courtesy of M. Wilson)

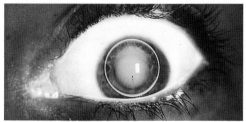

Plate 14 A 'Bayshore' type interpalpebral corneal lens fitted slightly too steep. It shows excessive central clearance with a small entrapped bubble, alignment of the first peripheral curve and a narrow band of clearance at the lens edge due to the flat second peripheral curve. (Courtesy of M. Wilson)

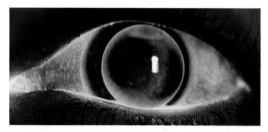

Plate 15 A spherical lens fitted with a slight apical clearance to a 'with-the-rule' toroidal cornea, the steepest corneal meridian being 70°. The peripheral zone has been fitted slightly steep to prevent too much edge clearance at the top and bottom, in order to minimize discomfort when blinking. There are two crescentic bands of corneal touch on either side of the 160° meridian, and fluorescein shows on the front surface of the top of the lens. Slight central clearance can just be seen along the 70° meridian. (Courtesy of M. Wilson)

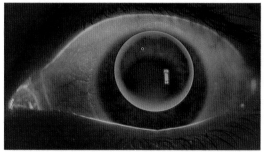

Plate 16 A 'continuous curve' lens with a single 0.25 mm diameter fenestration hole fitted with very slight central clearance. There is gradually increasing clearance at the periphery, more noticeable at the bottom of the lens which is situated over the central cornea following a blink. In RGP material the fenestration would not be necessary. (Courtesy of M. Wilson)

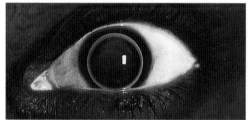

Plate 17 A spherical tetra-curve lens on a cornea with spherical keratometer reading. The optic zone and the first peripheral curves give an almost matching fit, and the second and third peripheral curves give gradually increasing clearance. If it were necessary to assist tear flow behind the lens the junction between the first and second peripheral curves could be blended to widen slightly the band of peripheral clearance. (Courtesy of M. Wilson)

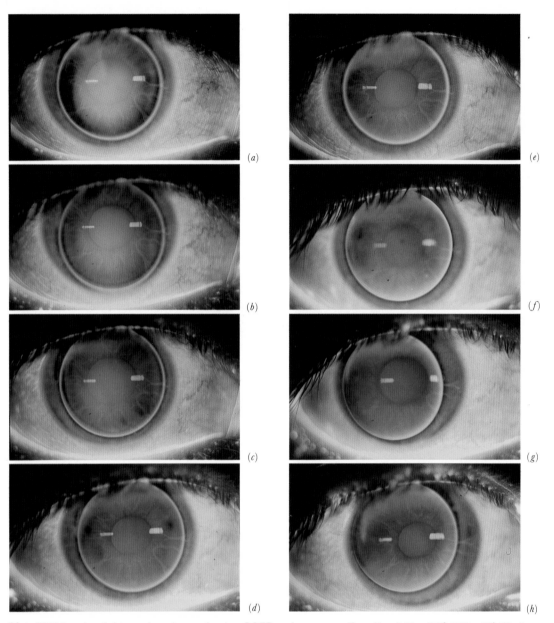

Plate 18 This series of pictures shows lenses of various BOZR on the same eye, K readings 7.90 at 180°, 7.70 at 90°. The lens TD is 9.60 mm, and BOZD 7.5 mm. The horizontal visible iris diameter is 11.50 mm. (Courtesy of The Cornea and Contact Lens Research Unit, Sydney). (*a*) BOZR 7.65 mm: the central fit is grossly steep with accumulation of fluorescein under the whole back optic zone. (*b, c*) BOZRs 7.70 and 7.75 mm, respectively: the steep central fit is still obvious with the depth and intensity of fluorescence reducing as the fitting approaches corneal alignment. (*d*) BOZR 7.80 mm: the BOZR is still slightly steeper than the flattest horizontal corneal meridian and the slight fluorescence centrally can just be seen. There is more peripheral clearance in the vertical meridian. (*e*) BOZR 7.85 mm: the BOZR is now in good compromise alignment over most of its area. Lack of fluorescence from the tear film over the back optic zone is apparent. (*f*) BOZR 7.90 mm: by assessment of the fluorescein pattern the lens still appears in good alignment with the cornea. A BOZR of 7.85 and 7.90 mm may indeed give a good fit but it is extremely difficult to judge a very slightly flat fit that could possibly result from the 7.90 mm BOZR, although the peripheral clearance is now greater. (*g*) BOZR 8.00 mm: a slightly flat fitting lens is now apparent. The lens cannot balance on the corneal apex and so tilts to (in this instance) the temporal cornea so that central and temporal contact become apparent. (*h*) BOZR 8.05 mm: a definite flat fitting lens can now be seen rocking from the apex to the temporal corneal zone

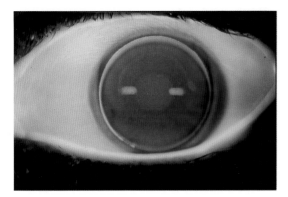

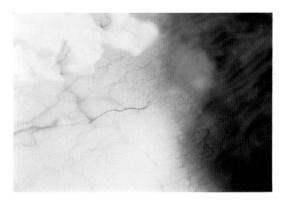

Plate 19 Lens binding occurs with extended wear RGP lenses after overnight wear. The lens fails to move with normal blinking for 1–5 hours in 10–50% of wearers. On lens removal the epithelium typically displays some central punctate staining and often a prominent indentation or compression ring corresponding to the lens edge shown above. The compression ring may itself stain with fluorescein although more typically there is pooling rather than true staining. (From Swarbrick and Holden (1987), *Am. J. Optom. Physiol. Optics*, **64**, 815, with kind permission. © The American Academy of Optometry, 1987)

Plate 21 A case of pseudopterygium in an RGP lens wearer. This is the sequel to chronic nine o'clock epithelial dessication, staining and erosion. (Courtesy of C. McMonnies)

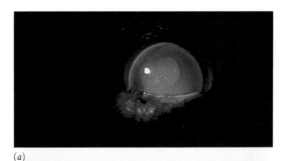

(a)

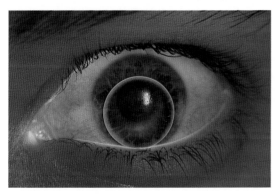

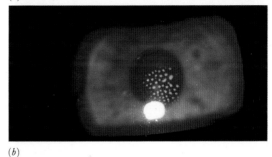

(b)

Plate 20 Three and nine o'clock corneal staining here shown associated with a dry and lipid-coated rigid lens. It can often be attributed to peripheral corneal dessication resulting from inappropriate lens design and fitting, and can occur with both hard (PMMA) and RGP lenses. It is most commonly due to too thick a lens edge and/or excessive edge clearance of the lens which creates a pool of tears under the lens edge drawing tears from adjacent areas. A bridging effect is also caused where the lid is lifted away from the adjacent cornea as it passes over the lens. Thus the eyelid cannot properly resurface the cornea with mucin adjacent to the lens edge or rewet the peripheral cornea, leading to localized drying and dessication. Thus this type of staining only occurs in those areas exposed to the atmosphere between blinks. If the lower lid is very low then similar staining may also occur in the six o'clock position. (Courtesy of D. Westerhout)

Plate 22 (*a*) Small bubbles trapped under a corneal lens have caused furrows and dimples in the epithelium during lens movement; (*b*) fluorescein has collected in these furrows and dimples. The resultant deterioration in vision is known as 'dimple veil' (*see also Plates 34, 70 and 94*). (Courtesy of A. J. Phillips)

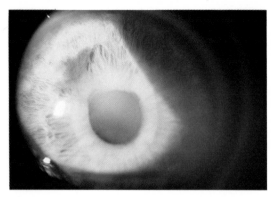

Plate 23 Central corneal clouding or oedema such as that seen following the wear of a tight fitting PMMA corneal lens. This gives rise to hazy or smoky vision known as veiling or Sattler's veil, Fick's phenomenon or simple veil (*see also Plate 93*). (Courtesy of B. Czigler)

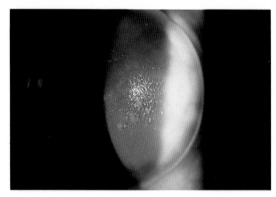

Plate 26 The effect on an RGP lens of a modern hand cream. The appearance is that of a totally non-wetting lens. A similar but less exaggerated appearance is seen in lenses coated with lipid secretion or in surface-treated lenses when the coating has worn off or been inadvertently removed, e.g. by polishing. (Courtesy of A. J. Phillips)

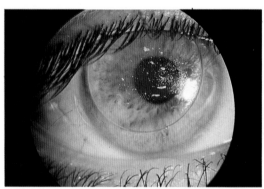

Plate 24 Grease and mucus on the scratched front surface of a corneal lens. (Courtesy of A. P. Gasson)

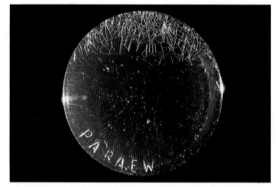

Plate 27 Surface crazing and cracking of high oxygen permeable silicone–acrylate lenses is often seen as the lenses age. Symptoms can range from slight loss of vision if occurring centrally, to some loss of comfort. Removal of the cracks is not possible and lens replacement is the only answer, but in the early stages of surface crazing it may be possible to repolish the surface. (Courtesy of A. J. Phillips)

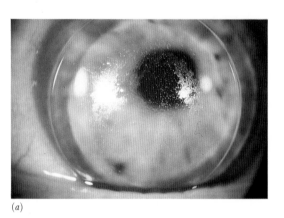

(a)

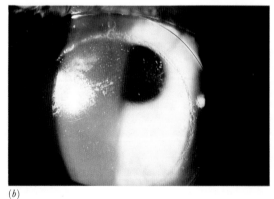

(b)

Plate 25 (a) Protein deposition can occur on both soft (*Plates 31* and *32*) and RGP lenses. Here deposits on an RGP lens can be seen by direct, indirect and specular reflection illumination with the slit lamp. (b) Deposits occurring in the lenticular junction shown by indirect illumination. These build up because of the lack of the normal sweep action of the lid into this area combined with a similar effect in lens cleaning. Slight loss of lens tolerance eventually occurs. Regular use of a proteolytic enzyme cleaner is indicated. (Courtesy of A. J. Phillips)

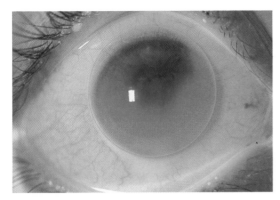

Plate 28 Fluorexon (high-molecular-weight fluorescein) stain used to show the flat fit of an upper temporally displaced soft lens. (Courtesy of B. Czigler)

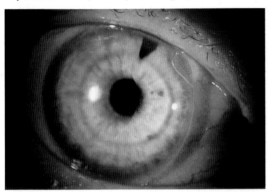

Plate 29 Grossly flat fitting high positive soft lens. The lens is shown at low magnification to be decentring badly with edge standoff under the upper lid. A similar effect can sometimes occur with a heavily coated lens causing relative dehydration of the front lens surface, or in giant papillary conjunctivitis when the swollen upper lid drags an otherwise correctly fitting soft lens upwards. The dark shadow of the lenticular junction is clearly visible on the iris. This can aid observation of lens movement. (With negative lenses, the shadow is a light ring.) (Courtesy of A. J. Phillips)

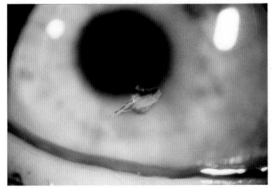

Plate 30 Damaged soft lens, with central nick possibly caused by a foreign body or finger nail, or due to folding a partially dehydrated lens. (Courtesy of A. J. Phillips)

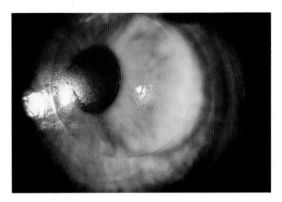

Plate 31 Deposits on a lenticulated soft lens are shown here largely by specular reflection. As the surface dries out between blinks the deposits are more readily visible. Deposits may be seen by direct, indirect or specular reflection methods of slit-lamp illumination and all three methods should normally be employed. (Courtesy of A. J. Phillips)

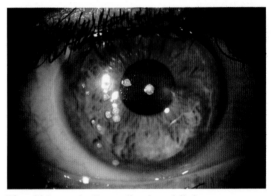

Plate 32 Lens calculi or mulberries or jelly bumps represent localized areas of lipid build-up with calcium salts sometimes also present. The calculi build up around the edge of dry spots on the lens surface until they eventually break through the tear film. Because of their interaction with the lid on blinking the lens is often rotated until the majority of calculi lie in the lower half of the lens when on the eye, severely affecting vision. (Courtesy of A. J. Phillips)

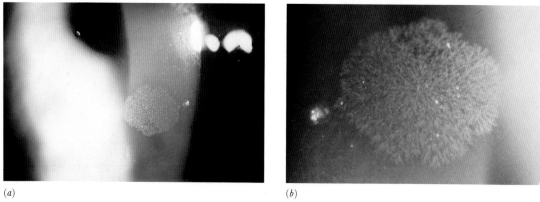

(a)   (b)

Plate 33 Fungal growths can occasionally be seen in inadequately disinfected soft lenses. Few symptoms are reported by the patient unless the growth is central when vision may be affected. The fungal hyphae can be detected (*a*) at low magnification and are clearly visible (*b*) at high magnification. (Courtesy of A. J. Phillips)

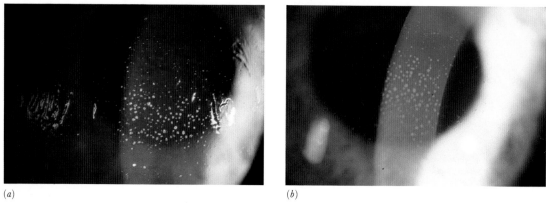

(a)   (b)

Plate 34 Dimple staining can occur with both hard (*Plate 22*) and soft lenses. (*a*) Here lipid droplets are shown beneath a soft lens. With hard lenses the dimples are more often caused by the break-up of a bubble into froth. On immediate removal fluorescein collects in the dimples or hollows left where lid pressure through the lens has compressed the droplets or bubbles into the epithelium shown in (*b*). Dimple staining can be recognized by its bright staining and sharply defined edges. Staining lasts no more than a few minutes as normal tear action (or irrigation) will remove the fluorescein from the hollow since true staining has not occurred. Even with no staining the dimples may be seen by indirect slit-lamp illumination both against the dark pupil and the light iris background (retroillumination). If severe enough, they may produce blurring of vision known as 'dimple veiling'. (Courtesy of A. J. Phillips)

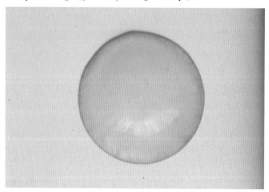

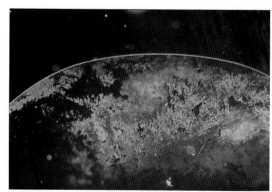

Plate 35 Discoloured soft lens. (Courtesy of A. P. Gasson)

Plate 36 One of the best methods of viewing deposits on contact lenses is by dark field microscopy. Shown above are protein deposits with superimposed calcium deposits centrally and lower right. (Courtesy of R. Payor)

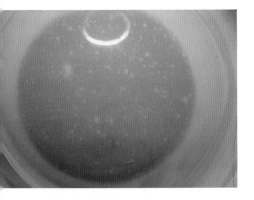

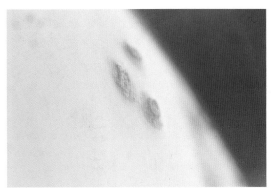

37 Many creams for acne vulgaris contain benzyl
...de. These and other oxidizing agents, if brought into
...ct with tinted soft lenses may cause the patchy
...ing shown above. Information should be sought from
...dual manufacturers as to the stability of their
...ular tinting process. (Courtesy of R. Payor)

Plate 38 Calculi stained for lipid with Oil-Red-O showing
the crater or doughnut effect as they build up around the
edge of dry spots. (Courtesy of A. J. Phillips)

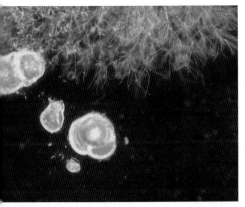

39 The doughnut nature of many soft lens calculi is
...y shown here by dark field microscopy. Fungal growth
... visible at the top of the picture. (Courtesy of A. J.
...ps)

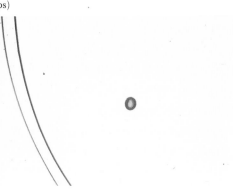

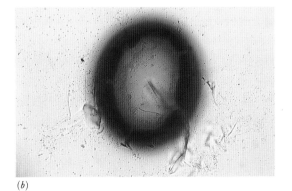

(b)

40 (*a*) Small pin-point red dots seen in hydrogel lenses are usually rusting metallic particles. Careful differential
...osis from small fungal growths should be made. Most rust spots create no subjective or objective problems. (*b*) Under
...magnification the split in the lens surface where the foreign body entered can easily be seen. The rust stain from the centre
...particle has diffused out through this split. (Courtesy of A. J. Phillips)

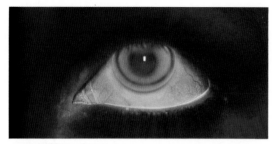

Plate 41 Ideal fluorescein pattern of correctly fitting Silflex (silicone) lens. (Courtesy of D. C. Campbell-Burns)

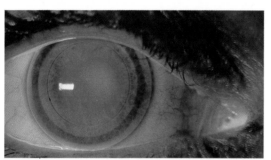

Plate 42 Silicone rubber lens (Silflex 2) fitted too steeply. (Courtesy of D. Westerhout)

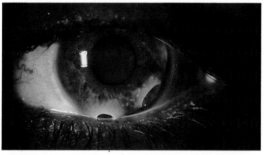

Plate 43 Silicone rubber lens (Silflex 2) fitted far too flat with bubbles under the edge. (Courtesy of D. Westerhout)

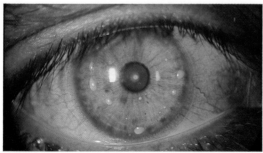

Plate 44 Silicone rubber lens with hydrophobic surface caused by excessively vigorous surfactant cleaning for 4 months which damaged the hydrophilic lens coating. (Courtesy of D. Westerhout)

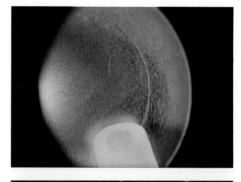

(a)

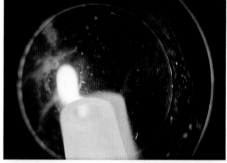

(b)

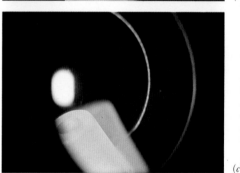

(c)

Plate 45 Silicone rubber contact lens. (a) Heavily protein contaminated after only 3 months use. (b) The same lens after cleaning with 5% sodium hypochlorite and rinsing saline. (c) The same lens after a further rinse with distilled water now showing a clean surface. (Courtesy of D. Westerhout)

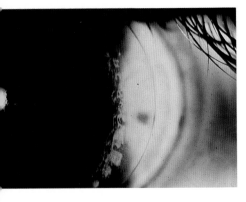
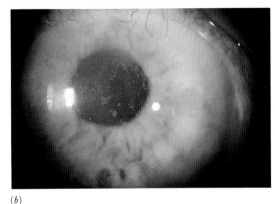

(b)

46 One cause for concern with any extended wear lens binding to the cornea is that while the lens is adherent there is no ~ation of tears behind the lens. Consequently corneal deswelling after overnight hypoxic stress may be impeded although ~ay not cause significant problems with lenses of high oxygen transmission. More importantly, however, tear debris and ~s remain trapped behind the lens typically (a) collecting in a ring behind the mid-periphery of an RGP lens and (b) ~lly under a soft lens. This trapped debris has the potential to provoke an acute red eye reaction. Some upper ~larization can be seen in (b). ((a) Courtesy of B. Holden and D. Sweeney and (b) courtesy of A. J. Phillips)

47 A severe complication associated mainly with ~ded wear hydrogel and silicone soft lenses is the acute ~e reaction shown here with a string of mucus detached ~the upper lid margin on the left hand side. This is ~y present on waking with signs and symptoms which ~nclude epithelial decompensation and erosion, limbal ~onjunctival hyperaemia, ciliary injection, aqueous ~stromal infiltrates, epithelial microvesicles, endothelial ~wing, photophobia and pain. The causative mechanism ~ fully understood and suggestions have included ~rvative sensitivity, tight fitting lenses, overnight ~dration causing tightening of fit, post-lens debris ~sing inflammatory stimuli, lowering of tear pH by ~nic and lactic acids causing water loss from the lens ~ightening of fit, viral infections, and bacterial toxins. ~rtesy of A. J. Phillips)

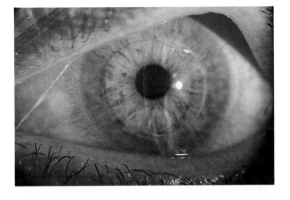

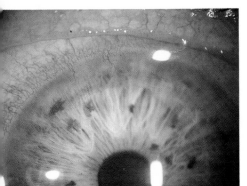
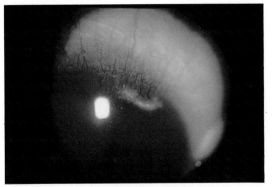

48 Contact lens-induced superior limbic keratitis ~s hyperaemia of the superior limbus and adjacent ~nctiva, stromal infiltrates, a fibrovascular ~opannus, epithelial haziness and corneal and ~nctival staining to fluorescein (*Plates 49* and *50*). Exact ~logy is uncertain but may include prolonged hypoxia, ~anical irritation from the lens edge, an immunological ~nse from protein deposits on the back lens surface, or ~ion preservatives. (Courtesy of A. J. Phillips)

Plate 49 Superior limbal epithelial splitting and hypertrophy stained with fluorescein and showing vascularization. (Courtesy of A. P. Gasson)

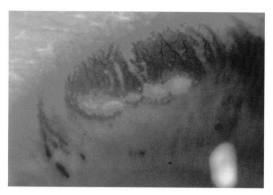

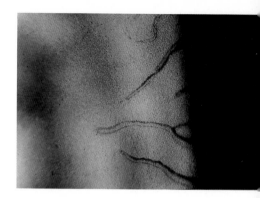

Plate 50 Superior limbal epithelial split found in a hydrogel lens wearer. Dense staining and diffusion of the stain into the underlying stroma occurs, with increased vascularization as compared to *Plate 49*. (Courtesy of C. McMonnies)

Plate 53 Increased limbal vessel proliferation and hyperaemia are normal, if undesirable, findings in association with extended hydrogel lens wear and certai other conditions. New corneal vessels may be distinguis from normal limbal vessels by locating the translucent limbal transition zone using marginal retroillumination the slit lamp. Vessels extending beyond this zone should viewed with concern. (Courtesy of B. Holden and D. Sweeney)

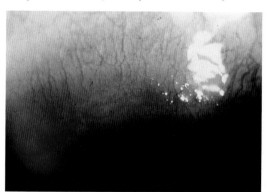

Plate 51 The same type of contact lens-induced superior limbal keratitis as in *Plates 48, 49* and *50*, showing rose bengal staining of the damaged epithelium. This should be differentiated from that in *Plate 52*. (Courtesy of A. J. Phillips)

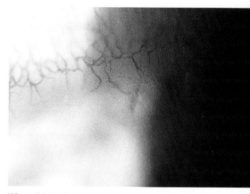

Plate 54 Active stage of new limbal vessel growth showi new spike projecting from an existing arcade and surrounded by exudate. (Courtesy of C. McMonnies)

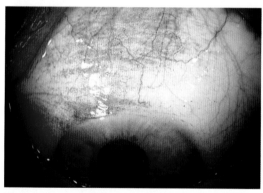

Plate 52 Superior limbic keratitis (SLK) occurs when there is abnormal frictional force between lid and globe. The condition is commonly associated with thyrotoxicosis. Epithelial staining to rose bengal can be seen in the area above the globe and a fold of loose or stretched conjunctiva hangs over the upper limbal area. The condition often responds well to the use of an extended wear bandage lens, ocular lubricants and, of course, the treatment of any underlying condition. True SLK should be differentiated from contact lens-induced SLK (*see Plates 48–51*) which also stains similarly with rose bengal. (Courtesy of A. J. Phillips)

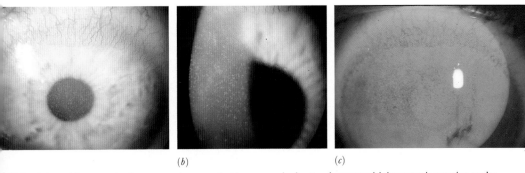

(b)   (c)

55 Toxic keratitis may arise from several sources but is commonly due to a hypersensitivity or toxic reaction to the
~~rvative~~ in a lens storage solution which leaches onto the cornea when the lens is inserted. The pattern is that of a diffuse to
~~y~~ punctate keratitis over a large area or the whole area of the cornea. The limbal area is also commonly injected.
~~Low~~ and high magnification white light photographs respectively; (c) low magnification blue light photograph showing
~~term~~ thimerosal toxicity with diffuse fluorescein staining of the epithelium and a pronounced dark dry spot. (Courtesy of
~~rant~~)

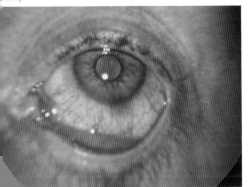

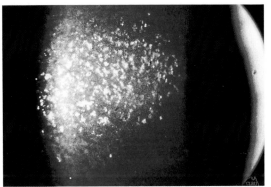

56 Conjunctival hyperaemia due to the sensitivity
~~nse~~ to preservatives in a soft lens storage solution
~~h~~ frequently adhere to mucus deposits on the lens
~~ce.~~ (Courtesy of G. Haig-Brown)

Plate 58 Epithelial erosions may occur when soft lenses
dehydrate on the eye, such as this case of multiple confluent
erosions following short-term wear of a very thin high water
content hydrogel lens. It is postulated that small areas of
epithelial tissue become attached to the lens and are torn
away when the lens is removed. They may also occur when
mild degrees of punctate stain remain untreated for long
periods or in cases of sterile ulceration, also when debris
builds up under a lens or adheres to its back surface. (From
Holden, Sweeney and Seger (1986), *Clin. expl Optom.*, **69**,
103, with kind permission).

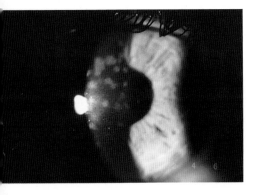

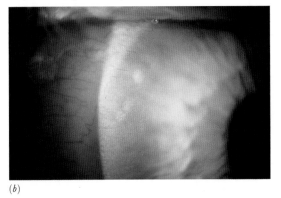

(b)

57 Stromal infiltrates may occur in association with a variety of adverse reactions to lens wear, such as the acute red eye
~~ion,~~ contact lens-induced superior limbic keratoconjunctivitis, stromal vascularization and corneal ulceration. Infiltrates
~~ar~~ as hazy, grey areas which (a) may be focal, or (b) diffuse. They typically occur near the limbus and the adjacent
~~nctiva~~ is often hyperaemic. Infiltrates are most probably leucocytes or monocytes lying between collagen fibres in the
~~na.~~ ((a) Courtesy of B. Holden and H. Swarbrick, (b) courtesy of A. J. Phillips)

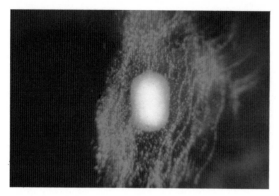

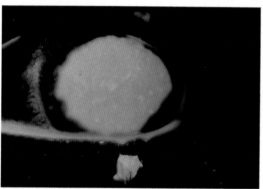

Plate 59 Multitrack foreign body corneal abrasion and staining seen under high magnification. (Courtesy of C. McMonnies)

Plate 60 Prolonged soft contact lens-induced hypoxia can significantly reduce epithelial adhesion. This may provide an explanation for the SLACH syndrome (soft lens associated corneal hypoxia syndrome) where there is spontaneous loss of up to 40% of the epithelial surface during lens wear. (Courtesy of B. Holden and D. Sweeney)

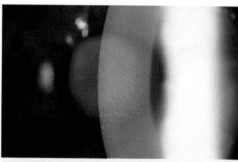

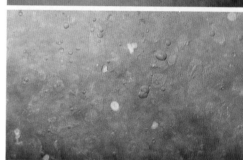

Plate 62 In localized epithelial oedema vacuoles of fluid form throughout the epithelial layer. These move toward the surface where they rupture. The general appearance (*a*) is similar to superficial punctate keratitis. However, by high magnification the small ruptured and non-ruptu vacuoles or cysts can be seen thereby exhibiting what is known as 'microcystic oedema'. (*c*) Empty (clear) and fil microcysts can be seen by using an endothelial camera b focusing in the epithelium area. (Courtesy of A. J. Philli

Plate 61 Epithelial microcysts are the small inclusions displaying reversal illumination, i.e. the distribution of light within the inclusion (darker on the left side) is opposite to that of the background (darker on the right side). Microcysts are seen best by indirect illumination at the highest magnification possible. Inclusions displaying unreversed illumination, i.e. the light distribution within is the same as the background, are fluid vacuoles. (Courtesy of B. Holden and H. Swarbrick)

Plate 63 Endothelial bedew observed in the region of the inferior pupil margin 3 days after the intense oedema fro an over-wear episode had cleared. Bedewing is though represent inflammatory cell adhering to the endothelium (compare with *Plate 61* – epithelial microcysts). (Courtesy of C. McMonnies

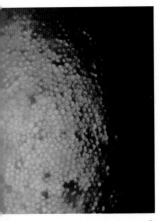

64 Blebs appear as black, non-reflecting areas of the ?helium using the highest slit-lamp magnification and ?ng to one side of the specularly reflected light source. ?occur within minutes of inserting a contact lens, the ?nse peaking in 20–30 minutes and subsiding by 45–60 ?tes. Blebs are asymptomatic and of little clinical ?icance. Blebs appear to be due to an acidic pH change ? endothelium causing oedema of the nuclear area of ?intracellular fluid vacuoles and fluid spaces between ?Thus endothelial blebs are probably the result of a ?oedema phenomenon whereby the posterior surface of ?lebbed' endothelial cell bulges backwards towards the ?us and alters the reflected image. (From Holden, ?ams and Zantos (1985), *Invest. Ophthal. Vis. Sci.*, **26**, ?, with kind permission)

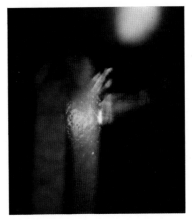

Plate 65 Corneal endothelial guttata. (Courtesy of J. Bergmanson)

Plate 66 Endothelial guttata seen at higher magnification than in *Plate 65* represent areas of missing endothelium that have occurred naturally, e.g. as a congenital deformity or dystrophic condition. They can be differentiated from blebs by their outline, and persistence even with no lens in place. (Courtesy of B. Holden and H. Swarbrick)

Plate 67 Striae begin to occur when approximately 5–6% corneal oedema occurs. They are fine, usually vertically orientated greyish-white, wispy lines that appear in the posterior stroma. They need to be differentiated from nerve fibres, the latter being more regular in appearance and with obvious bifurcations. Striae are thought to represent a refractile effect due to fluid separation of fine, vertically orientated collagen fibrils in the posterior stroma. This one appears as a vertical curved line in the posterior stroma (*see also Plate 89* showing striae in keratoconus). (From Zantos and Holden (1978), *Aust. J. Optom.*, **61**, 418, with kind permission)

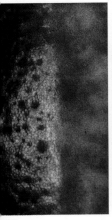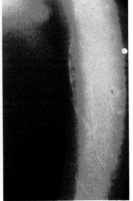

? 66   **Plate 67**

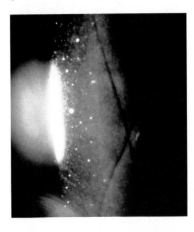

? **68** Stromal folds in a conspicuous 'black cross' pattern ?in the posterior stroma and Descement's membrane ? corneal oedema reaches more than 10–12%. They are ?ght to represent a physical buckling of the posterior ?eal layers as in this case of a patient with 19.6% central ?al oedema induced by a tightly fitting soft lens. They ?est observed using specular reflection and are a danger ?indicating gross physiological insult. Contact lens-?ced corneal oedema, whether from daily or extended ?, should never exceed 10–12%. (From Zantos and ?en (1978), *Aust. J. Optom.*, **61**, 418, with kind ?ission)

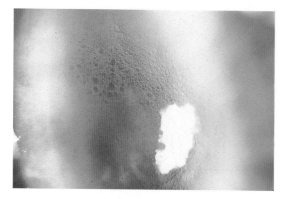

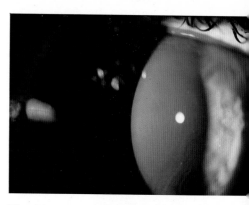

Plate 69 Intense oedema and bullae (superiorly) in the epithelium resulting in this case from a ruptured Descemet's membrane causing hydrops in keratoconus. (Courtesy of C. McMonnies)

Plate 70 Epithelial wrinkling is an infrequent condition sometimes encountered with the wearing of hydrogel and other lenses. It is also sometimes seen in the superior cornea area of keratoconics corrected by RGP lenses, perhaps caused by slight cone pressure from the lens. True corneal staining does not result, the fluorescein simply collecting in the epithelial furrows. This is quickly lost by the sluicing action of the tears (*see also Plates 22, 34* and *94*). (Courtesy A. J. Phillips)

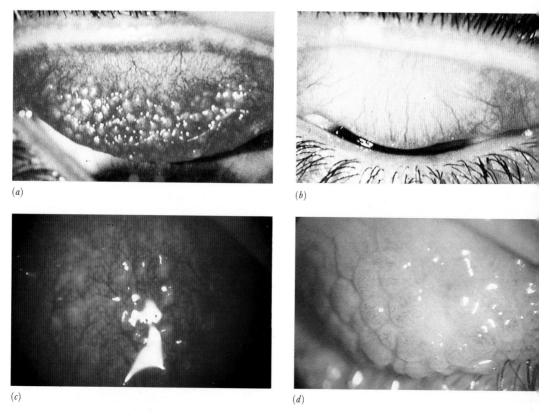

(a)

(b)

(c)

(d)

Plate 71 Giant (GPC) or contact lens-induced papillary conjunctivitis (CLPC) of the upper palpebral conjunctiva due to contact lens wear shown in (a) and compared to the normal conjunctiva in (b). Shown in (c) is the early 'tapioca' granule appearance of early GPC compared to the more advanced papillary formations shown in (d). ((a, b) Courtesy of M. R. Allansmith and (c, d) courtesy of D. J. Coster)

Chapter 13

The verification of hydrogel contact lenses

D. F. C. Loran

Hydrogel contact lenses are flexible and if exposed to the atmosphere they dehydrate and alter their contour; thus, conventional methods of measuring hard lens parameters are not applicable to this type of contact lens. As a consequence, practitioners may feel unable to check the specification of these lenses conveniently and this may, in turn, result in frustration and disappointment if a lens received from the laboratory does not provide the expected performance *in situ*. Such a situation is obviously most unsatisfactory and practitioners are urged to verify the parameters of soft contact lenses within the limitations of present instrumentation.

Undoubtedly, it is most convenient to check soft lens parameters directly in air using conventional instruments, although such methods may present inaccuracies due to surface deformation, shrinkage of the hydrogel on dehydration and also accumulation of surface moisture. In order to overcome these artefacts liquid cells as shown in *Figures 13.1* and *13.2* have been utilized to measure the parameters of soft lenses.

The British Standards *Specifications for Contact Lenses* (1978), now withdrawn, recommends that, following equilibrium, soft contact lenses should be measured in physiological (normal) saline at a temperature of $20.0 \pm 0.5°C$. However, as the lens equilibrates it will continuously change shape which is a potentially error-prone part of the measuring process.

If hydrogel lenses are mounted in a transparent cell containing a compatible medium such as sterile physiological saline solution (without a preservative) then the lens should assume its natural, undistorted form. Masnick and Holden (1972) ascertained that changes in pH and tonicity of the lens environment produced clinically significant alterations in the water content with associated parametric variations. Measurements of the total diameter and also

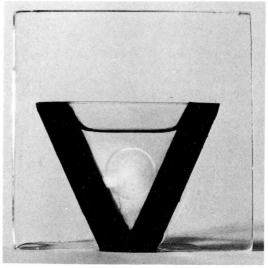

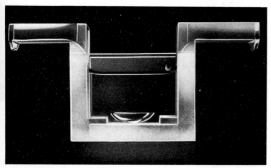

Figure 13.1 Hydrogel lens immersed in physiological saline solution in a liquid cell. (Photograph by courtesy of Söhnges Optik)

Figure 13.2 Liquid cell, showing an immersed lens, used to determine power of lens in saline solution, to measure diameters with a band magnifier, or for surface inspection

primary sagitta of soft lenses by Poster and Skolnik (1974) indicated that these changes varied with tonicity, but not pH, while Masnick and Holden (1972) observed a decrease in total diameter in acidic and an increase in total diameter in alkaline solutions. Port (1982b) noted that, as the pH of the ambient saline is increased, the back optic zone radii flatten significantly and consequently physiological, buffered saline is recommended as the test medium (Kemp, 1979). Phillips (A. J., 1987, personal communication) suggests this flattening is caused by an increase in water content which is more likely to occur in polymers containing methacrylic acid and which are more pH sensitive.

Furthermore the refractive index increases and the water content reduces with increased temperature (Fatt and Chaston, 1980). As water is lost the lens becomes thinner and less positive powered but this is more than offset by the increase in positive power of plus lenses as the refractive index increases. Thus, the accumulative effect is towards more positive power. In general these parametric changes are greater for high water content lenses and these findings emphasize that environmental factors need to be specified, standardized and carefully controlled when measuring soft lens parameters.

In a comprehensive survey Harris, Hall and Oye (1973) checked soft lenses in air and concluded that, with the notable exception of radii, these parameters could be checked in air with a reasonable degree of accuracy. Mandell (1974a) recommends the following procedure for air measurement of soft lens power:

(1) The lens should be removed from its liquid environment using a sterile spatula or soft plastics-protected forceps.
(2) The lens is then placed on a lint-free tissue and the tissue folded over the uppermost convex surface of the lens.
(3) The lens is transferred onto a dry area of tissue and step (2) repeated to make sure that both surfaces are blotted dry.
(4) The lens is dried in air with forceps.
(5) The lens surfaces are examined macroscopically and, if smudges are present, the process is repeated.
(6) Although it is probably preferable to check the lens within an overall period of one minute of air exposure (Titmus Eurocon,

1974), the lens essentially maintains its contour within clinical limits for up to four minutes during which time the measurements should be completed.

Before considering the verification of soft contact lenses, however, it is expedient to consider the lens specification which, in turn, is predetermined by the method of manufacture which may be spin-casting, lathe-cutting or moulding.

Manufacture of hydrogel contact lenses

Spin-casting

The Bausch & Lomb Soflens (Polymacon) is produced by a computer-controlled method of axial spin-casting originally introduced by Wichterle and Lim (1960) for the Czechoslovakian Geltakt lens.

Liquid monomers of 2-hydroxyethyl methacrylate and ethylene diglycol methacrylate are stored at a temperature of $-5°C$ and injected through a polythene tube into a rotating female mould where polymerization occurs in a carbon dioxide atmosphere at a temperature of $65°C$ (Hartstein, 1973).

By controlling three variables — mould diameter, spin-speed and the volume of monomer injected — it is possible to produce a variety of shapes and curves. As illustrated in *Figure 13.3*, the lens is formed front surface downwards through the action of centripetal force and gravity (Bausch & Lomb Ltd, 1975, personal communication from R. Myers). The front curve is therefore determined by the shape of the female mould and at the time of writing the front optic zone radii range from 8.60 to 10.08 mm with a centre thickness which varies from 0.035 to 0.300 mm. These lenses are available in three total diameters, 12.50 mm, 13.50 mm and 14.50 mm with primary sagitta values from 2.84 to 4.10 mm. The lenses may be described by a series code which at present is as follows: F, B3, B4, U, U3, U4, O3, O4, −HO3, −HO4, SOFSPIN, +M3, +M4, +H3, +H4, Plano U, Plano U3, Plano B4, Plano O4, and Plano T. (The suffixes '3' and '4' denote the 13.50 mm and 14.50 mm total diameters respectively.)

In addition the toric and the P.A.1. aspheric bifocals produced by Bausch & Lomb and the Hydron S.C. lenses are also spun-cast, while the

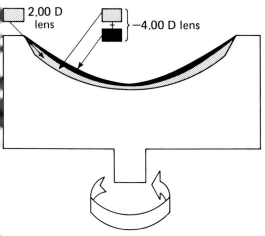

Figure 13.3 Axial spin-casting method of producing the Geltakt and the Bausch & Lomb Soflens by injecting liquid monomers into a rotating mould where polymerization occurs. The lens is indicated by the grey shaded area within the concave mould. The darker area above indicates the lens shape and the additional minus power produced either by a higher speed of mould rotation or a greater injection pressure

Bausch & Lomb Optima has a spun-cast front surface with a lathed back surface. Chapter 11 includes greater details of these lenses (*see* for example, *Table 11.20* and *Figures 11.27–11.30*).

As the injection pressure or the speed of rotation is increased, more material is projected towards the periphery thereby increasing the edge thickness. Consequently, as negative power is increased for a given series the back surface steepens and the lens fits more tightly, the reverse occurring as negative power is reduced or positive power is increased.

The spin-casting process is fully automatic and produces smooth, reproducible surfaces free from tool marks, peripheral grooves and other imperfections which may occur in the polishing and finishing of lathe-cut lenses.

Lathe-cut lenses

Traditionally hydrogel contact lenses are lathed in a similar manner to hard lenses except that the lathing process is slower, and non-toxic, aluminium oxide-based polishes* are used. This technique offers a broad spectrum of parameters

*Examples of soft lenses polishes are: XPAL, or Alox 721 manufactured by Cerium Chemical Co., CCPI manufactured by City Crown, and SP1 or SP2 manufactured by C.L.M. Group Ltd.

as dictated by a patient's fitting and refractive considerations. However, with the advent of thinner and/or higher water content soft lenses, often based on a uni-fit philosophy, there is now a trend towards alternative methods of manufacture. Spin-casting, spin-casting one surface and lathing the other, cast-moulding or stabilized soft moulding may all yield more reproducible lenses and are methods which may be more readily adapted to computer-controlled mass production techniques. However, lens lathing technology has also been considerably improved and updated. In the lathing method of production the front and back optic radii are cut and polished from stress-free, dehydrated buttons, allowance being made for a predetermined linear swell on hydration. Consequently the radii are steeper and the thickness less by a known amount in the dry state, than in the hydrated state.

The linear swell may be defined (H. Gee, 1980, personal communication) as:

$$\text{Linear swell } (\%) = \frac{L_g}{L_p} \times 100 = \frac{V_g}{V_p} \times 100$$

where L_g = linear dimension of the hydrated polymer

L_p = linear dimension of the dehydrated polymer

V_g = volume of hydrated polymer

V_p = volume of the dehydrated polymer

It has been shown that, provided ambient variables such as temperature and humidity are carefully controlled during manufacture, then the hydrated parameters such as centre thickness can be predicted with reasonable accuracy from the linear swell value (Loran, French and Auerbach, 1982).

Moulding

A moulded contact lens is produced by pressing, usually between dies, and is defined as one manufactured basically by a shaping process without the removal of material (British Standard, 1979). Moulded scleral lenses have been produced for many years by heating a Perspex laminate to softening point and it is then pressed onto a hard cast. Kelvin Lenses Ltd and Zeiss (Wöhlk) Contact Lenses Ltd mould hard corneal lenses both in polymethyl methacrylate and cellulose acetate butyrate.

Provided that plastic memory can be controlled then moulding is generally considered to be a satisfactory manufacturing process and may result in relatively thin, smooth and reproducible surfaces. Indeed, most polymers if they are not cross-linked are basically suitable for moulding (H. Gee, 1980, personal communication) and consequently this process has also been used to produce soft contact lenses. Silicone lenses such as Tesicon produced by CIBA Vision (Titmus Eurocon) and the Silflex lens produced by Zeiss (Wöhlk) Contact Lenses Ltd are both moulded and a hydrogel lens manufactured by the International Lens Corporation (ILC) is moulded between dyes from liquid monomers.

Current fitting philosophy appears to be directed towards thin, permeable lenses worn for extended periods and possibly discarded when removed from the eye. If this concept is desired then it is conceivable that moulding could be considered as a suitable manufacturing process to produce relatively inexpensive lenses to fulfil these criteria.

Lens specification

Although manufacturers and practitioners may specify lenses in an abbreviated form, the British Standard 3521 1979 (now withdrawn) recommended a more detailed specification, examples of which are as follows:

(a) Single curve soft hydrophilic corneal lens

L Cl Hyd/8.40:13.00/−3.50/t_c 0.15/FOD 12.00/HEMA 38%
  (i)   (ii)   (iii)   (iv)   (v)   (vi)

which denotes the following:
(i)   Left single curve soft hydrophilic contact lens.
(ii) Back optic zone radius and total diameter.
(iii) Back vertex power.
(iv) Centre thickness.
(v)   Front optic (zone) diameter.
(vi) PHEMA (polyhydroxyethyl methacrylate) with 38% water content.

(b) Bi-curve soft hydrophilic scleral lens

R S2 Hyd/8.50:11.00/9.70:14.50/+4.00/t_e 0.17/HEMA 60%
  (i)   (ii)   (iii)   (iv)   (v)   (vi)

which implies:

(i)   Right scleral bi-curve soft hydrophilic contact lens.

(ii) Back optic zone radius and back optic zone diameter.
(iii) Back peripheral radius and total diameter.
(iv) Back vertex power.
(v)   Edge thickness.
(vi) PHEMA with 60% water content.

Definitions

Before considering the verification of soft contact lens parameters, it would perhaps be helpful to define some of the terms used. In practice, however, this is not entirely straightforward as confusion exists in the terminology used, not only between the layman and the scientist, but also perhaps more significantly between one science and another (e.g. physics and psychology). It is hoped that standardization and agreement will occur with the fullness of time.

Error

Error (e) is the difference between a measured and a 'true' value and may either be greater than the true value in which case it is positive, or negative if less.

$$e = x - x'$$

whereby x = true value; x' = measured value.

Random error

A random error (Re) has an equal probability of being positive or negative and may be reduced by learning, operator skill or taking a series of measurements. Examples of random error include the judging of alignment or just contact between two surfaces.

Systematic error

A systematic error (Se) is one due to bias and which tends to be constant or in one direction only. It will persist over a series of measurements and is equally likely to be either positive or negative and may be minimized by good experimental design such as correct calibration. An operator reading a scale from an oblique angle or prejudiced observations are examples of systematic errors.

Accuracy

Accuracy refers to the degree of agreement between a measured and a true value (C. N. French, 1986, personal communication) or how close a measured value is to the true value (M. Sheridan, 1986, personal communication); in psychological science this term is usually referred to as validity. Guillon, Crosbie-Walsh and Byrnes (1986), however, using meteorological terminology define accuracy (A) as the sum of the quadrature precision (R) and the systematic uncertainties (S) so that:

$$A = \sqrt{R^2 + S^2}$$

For a fuller discussion of errors in physical and psychological sciences, reference should be made to appropriate texts, for example Anastasi (1961) or Bevington (1969).

Validity

Validity refers to the extent by which a supplied value deviates from the ordered value and measuring instruments should be calibrated against a range of known standards and a compensation factor applied where necessary.

Reliability

Reliability, repeatability or precision refers to the stability or consistency of a reading when it is repeated and may be expressed in terms of the standard deviation of these repeated readings, more properly referred to as the standard error of measurement.

Standard deviation

Standard deviation (σ)

$$= \sqrt{\Sigma(\bar{x} - x)^2/(N - 1)}$$

in which x = any measurement, $\bar{x}$ = the mean of the measurements, N = the number of measurements.

The standard error of the mean

The standard error of measurement should not be confused with the standard error of the mean which is the standard deviation divided by the square root of N.

Calibration

Calibration is a process of supplementing a measuring instrument with a complementary statement regarding likely errors inherent in the system (British Standard, 1986).

Gauge mechanisms

These should eliminate backlash so that this source of error need not be considered if readings are taken in one direction only.

Tolerance

Tolerance is the maximum permissible difference by which a parameter is allowed to deviate from the stated or ordered value. The tolerance should be twice the accuracy of the measuring instrument and the test method should be stated (British Standard, 1986).

Tolerance limit

Tolerance limit refers to the upper and lower bounds of permissible deviation from a prescribed value (British Standard, 1986).

In psychological terminology, accuracy is usually referred to as validity, but in physical science accuracy is a function of both validity and reliability. Reliability, repeatability or precision are all the same thing, although precision and accuracy are often confused and incorrectly used synonymously. In attempting to verify soft contact lens parameters, this licence is perhaps understandable as validation is at present difficult if not impossible to establish. The accuracy of a measuring instrument may be determined against a test object such as a thickness gauge or a master sphere which has previously been measured with a high precision instrument and certified by a recognized, authoritative body such as the National Physical Laboratory. A series of measurements on test objects may then be made to calibrate the measuring instrument over a range of anticipated parameters and a compensation factor then applied as appropriate.

American standards for soft contact lens tolerances are now available (American National Standard Z80.8, 1986) and are illustrated in *Table 13.1*. These were based on a survey involving manufacturers and practitioners and conclude that, as the lens becomes thinner or as

Table 13.1 Soft contact lens tolerances (American National Standard Z80.8 — 1986)

Parameter	Water content		
	11–49%	*50–69%*	*70% and above*
Base curve (CPC) (mm)	±0.15	±0.20	±0.25
Diameter, total (chord or curved) (mm)	±0.20	±0.25	±0.25
Central thickness (mm)			
up to 0.15	±0.02	±0.02	±0.03
from 0.16 to 0.25	±0.03	±0.03	±0.04
0.26 and above	±0.04	±0.04	±0.05
Vertex power in air (D)*†			
0–10.0	±0.25	±0.25	±0.25
10.25–20.0	±0.50	±0.50	±0.50
above 20.0	±0.75	±0.75	±0.75
Prismatic power (Δ)			
0–10.0	±0.25	±0.25	±0.25
above 10.0	±0.50	±0.50	±0.50
Cylinder power (D)‡			
0–5.0	±0.25	±0.25	±0.25
above 5.0	±0.50	±0.50	±0.50
Cylinder axis (°)*			
Reference point is cylinder axis (°)			
0.50–1.50 D	±8	±8	±8
above 1.50 D	±5	±5	±5
Truncation (°)¶			
Reference point is prism axis (°)	±5	±5	±5

*Tolerances are greater than those accepted for spectacle ophthalmic lenses but represent the current state of the art of measuring soft lenses in the hydrated state.
†Conventionally, most soft lenses are specified with back vertex power, although the difference between respective vertex powers may be negligible. In those cases in which the difference may be meaningful, the manufacturer shall provide proper notification to the practitioner.
‡For measurement purposes, spherocylinder powers will be transformed to meridional powers and that tolerance applied to each individual power.
¶For truncations that appear to be arcs rather than chords, the truncation line will be assumed to be the chord connecting the ends of the arc.

the water content increases, a more generous tolerance of back optic zone radius is permissible. This is not an unreasonable suggestion, because as a soft lens becomes thinner or as the water content increases, it becomes more flexible (Layland, Sweeney and Holden, 1980).

Having considered the manufacture and specification of soft hydrophilic lenses it is now in order to consider the quality control of these parameters, namely radii, diameters and linear parameters, thickness, back vertex power and surfaces.

Verification procedures

Radii

The use of reflected light to determine soft contact lens radii

The optic zone radii are probably the most clinically significant variables in fitting standard thickness soft contact lenses, but paradoxically they are the most difficult to check. An undistorted lens is a necessity for the measurement of soft contact lens radii and because of the inherent flexibility of the material it is preferable, if not essential, to support the lens in a liquid-filled, parallel, flat-surfaced cell in order to determine radii, which may be measured by reflected light, microspherometry or optical gauging.

Keratometers

A keratometer is essential in the armamentarium of the contact lens practitioner, and its use has therefore been considered in determining the radii of hydrogel lenses (Chaston, 1973) and an accuracy of ±0.10 mm is claimed (Forst, 1974). It is essential that the lens is mounted in a liquid cell and the mire images are then

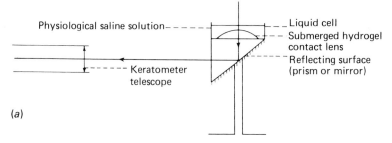

(a)

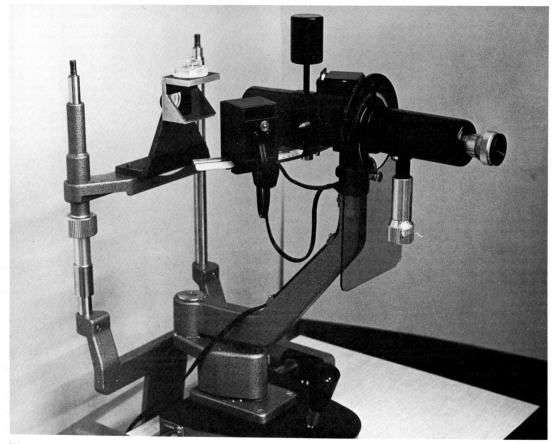

(b)

Figure 13.4 (*a*) Measurement of the back optic zone radius of a soft contact lens by keratometry. (*b*) Soft contact lens immersed in saline solution and mounted on a Javal–Schiötz keratometer. (Photograph by courtesy of Smith & Nephew Research Ltd)

reflected into the telescope either by a prism as illustrated in *Figure 13.4a* or, alternatively, by an inclined mirror, as shown in *Figure 13.4b*.

The lens is completely immersed in physiological saline solution of refractive index 1.336 but separated from the telescope by air. The contact lens/liquid lens air system thus acts as an equivalent mirror (Chaston, 1973) so that the vertex of the mirror and the centre of curvature of the equivalent mirror are displaced towards each other as illustrated in *Figure 13.5*. Consequently, the measured radius of curvature is shorter than the true radius of curvature by an amount dependent on the refractive index of the saline solution. Furthermore, a keratometer calibrated for convex surfaces will slightly underestimate the radii of concave surfaces by approximately 0.03 mm (Emsley, 1963; Bennett, 1966).

Therefore: $r = nr' + Y$

where r is the radius of curvature in air
    r' is the radius of curvature in liquid
    n is the refractive index of saline solution = $1.336 \simeq \frac{4}{3}$
and Y is the concave compensation factor so that

$$r = \frac{4r'}{3} + (\simeq) \, 0.03$$

Thus:

	Corrected values (Bausch &
$\frac{4}{3} \times r'$	Lomb) for concave surfaces
7.00 mm	7.02 mm
7.50 mm	7.525 mm
8.00 mm	8.030 mm
8.50 mm	8.535 mm

The radius of curvature of the lens in air, however, may be more easily determined from a graph as shown in *Figure 13.6*.

It is suggested that an instrument for checking soft lens radii should have a range from 7.40 to 9.50 mm which by liquid immersion is transferred to the range 5.40 to 7.10 mm. *Table 13.2* illustrates the range of radii of keratometers chosen at random and from this it is noted that the radii are too flat to measure soft lenses in 50% of the instruments. However, as pointed out by Hartstein (1973), it is possible by placing a +1.25 D spherical auxiliary lens over the telescope objective, to extend the range of

steeper radii measured by approximately 1.30 mm. This topic is also covered in Chapters 6 and 12.

Further complications, as listed below, arise in the use of keratometers with liquid immersion.

(1) In a liquid environment less light is reflected from each lens surface than when the lens is in air. Fresnel's law for light of normal incidence is:

$$R = \left[\frac{n' - n}{n' + n} \right]^2 \times 100\%$$

where R is the percentage of reflected light, n is the refractive index of the surrounding medium (= 1.336 for saline solution and 1.00 for air), n' is the refractive index of the second medium ($\simeq$ 1.430 for hydrogel material). In air, therefore, $R = 3.13\%$, and in saline solution $R = 0.115\%$.

The luminosity of the mires has therefore to be significantly increased to compensate for the reduction in intensity of the reflected light when a lens is measured in a saline solution cell.

(2) In order to increase the luminosity it is feasible that excessive heat could be generated, and Loran (1974) has shown that the manifestation of an increased ambient temperature of the liquid is to steepen the radii. Ideally, soft lens parameters should be checked at the environmental temperature of the conjunctival sac. The temperature of the cornea exceeds that of the atmosphere, but is slightly below body temperature (Mandell, 1974b) although

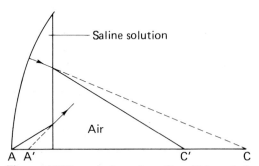

Figure 13.5 The equivalent mirror effect which results in a reduced back optic zone radius when a liquid-immersed lens is measured by keratometry. (From Chaston, 1973)

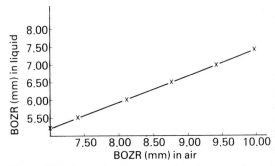

Figure 13.6 Conversion from the back optic zone radius measured in saline solution by the keratometer to the back optic zone radius in air

Table 13.2 Steepest soft lens radii capable of checking by keratometry due to the limitations set by the steep end of the scale of various instruments

Instrument	Steepest scale reading in air = soft lens radius measured in saline solution (mm)	Corresponding soft lens radius in air = radius in saline solution × 1.336 (mm)
Guilbert Routit (topographical)	4.60	6.15
Zeiss (Jena) (East German)	5.00	6.70
Carl Zeiss (West German) (Oberkochen)	5.50	7.35
Gambs	5.50	7.35
Sbisa (Javal–Schiötz)	5.60	7.50
American Optical	5.60	7.50
Guilbert Routit (Javal–Schiötz)	6.00	8.05
Bausch & Lomb	6.40	8.55

Note: keratometer scales can be extended (*see* p. 470).

when a soft lens is inserted into the eye a temperature gradient is manifested which may vary from 37°C on the back surface to 20–25°C on the front (Ruben, 1973, 1974). Furthermore, the temperature of the conjunctival sac may vary with factors such as lid closure, blepharospasm and palpebral aperture size (Hill and Leighton, 1964).

(3) If an attempt is made to utilize reflected light to measure the radii of a submerged lens then a double image is formed by reflections at the front and back surfaces of the lens, respectively, so that the operator must first identify, and secondly ignore the unwanted image. The image formed by the surface proximal to the mires will be brighter, and if the back vertex power of the lens is negative the back surface will produce the smaller image; the reverse occurring with positive lenses (Forst, 1974).

Although the above-mentioned limitations are not confined to keratometry it is obvious that this technique is not entirely straightforward and practice is necessary to achieve the claimed reliability.

Many modern keratometers are illuminated with brightness controlled halogen bulbs and provide scale intervals of 0.01 mm which read to radii of 5.0 mm or less. Some instruments such as the Carl Zeiss (Jena) Ophthalmometer CZ110 provide a wet cell as a standard accessory whilst the Rodenstock C.E.S. keratometer incorporates an additional objective lens mounted on a turret on the telescope to measure directly the radii of soft lenses in saline.

Radiuscopes

In employing a radiuscope to determine the back optic zone radii of a hard lens the front of the lens is immersed in a liquid-filled concave holder which avoids distortion of the lens and also eliminates unwanted reflections from the front surface. A similar technique for hydrogel soft lenses has been suggested by Stone (J., 1975, personal communication) who recommends blotting the back surface dry and carefully floating the convex surface in a concave holder filled with saline solution. Capillary attraction, however, between the lens and the holder tends to tilt and distort the lens and accumulation of surface moisture often precludes a clear image. Tajiri (1974) has designed a conical corral-type holder which permits a clear radiuscope reading. Its lattice structure is apparently not unlike the basket holder of many hard lens soaking cases, and maintains the lens contour parallel to the saline surface and also acts as a pump to suspend the lens at the liquid–air surface. If a clear image of the radiuscope lamp filament is obtainable the examiner is able to obtain a clear image of the radiuscope target and the radius is determined in the normal way.

A specially designed soft lens radiuscope has been produced by Chamarro Tormo (1974) which claims to overcome the previously mentioned difficulties. The Ultra Radiuscope is illustrated in *Figure 13.7* which shows the lens centred in a liquid cell into which the waterproof objective lens of a travelling microscope is immersed. Although a high luminosity is

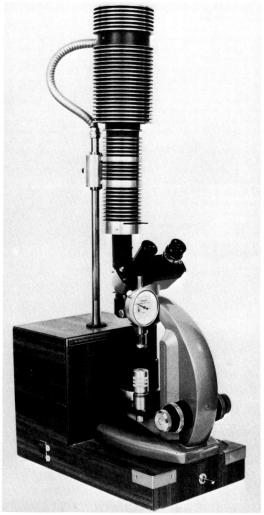

Figure 13.7 The Ultra Radiuscope produced by Conoptica Laboratory, Madrid. The lens is mounted in a liquid cell and the objective is immersed into the saline solution. The back optic zone radius is read directly from the instrument. (Photograph by courtesy of G. Nissel & Co.)

required in this instrument the reflected light only travels through a single refracting medium and a direct reading through saline solution is taken in a similar manner to a conventional radiuscope, resulting in a reliability of ±0.02 mm (G. Nissel, 1975, personal communication). In order to attain the required brightness it is necessary to incorporate a 200-watt halogen bulb into the instrument which normally only has a working life of 25 hours, although this can be doubled by using sub-maximum

voltage supplied to the instrument in gradual stages (G. Nissel, 1975, personal communication).

Garner (1981) describes a modification of the radiuscope to measure the sag of a soft lens in air mounted convex side upward on a lens support. The total sag is defined as the distance between the microscope focused on the edge of the lens support and the front vertex of the lens while the sag to be measured is the total sag less the centre thickness which is measured in the conventional way with the microscope. Although this method is time consuming and requires operator skill, it nevertheless shows a repeatability similar to that obtained with instruments such as the Neitz (Softometer) SM 100 designed specifically to measure soft lens radii.

Autostigmatic Microscope

The Autostigmatic Microscope (Steele and Freund, 1985) is illustrated in *Figure 13.8*. This is another example of a conventional Drysdale microscope modified to measure soft lens parameters. The beam splitter is relocated in front of the objective and is dipped into the saline of the wet cell into which the lens is mounted concave surface upwards. To enhance light intensity, one of the prisms is anti-reflection coated and the wet cell which is made of clear plastic incorporates a black plastic light trap below. Location of the target graticule is assisted by surrounding it with a clear wire ring which can be closed down by an iris diaphragm when the image has been found thus further reducing stray light. The radii are measured as with a conventional radiuscope giving a population standard deviation of ±0.07 mm on repeated measurements of the back optic zone radius (Carney, Ungerer and Brennan, 1985).

Microspherometry

Contact lens radii are steep and the curvatures represent a small part of a complete sphere. In such circumstances the radii may be determined indirectly by microspherometry.

In *Figure 13.9*, *AB* represents a small portion of a spherical curve where C is the centre of curvature, r is the radius of curvature, and h is the primary sagitta (or sag) given chord $2y$ so that:

$$r^2 = y^2 + (r - h)^2 \text{ and } r = y^2/2h + h/2$$

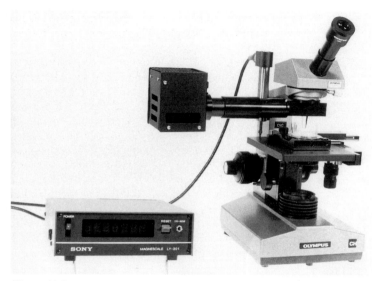

Figure 13.8 The Autostigmatic Microscope based on the Drysdale principle incorporating a clear Perspex wet cell with a light trap. The height of the microscope stage is shown on the digital probe. (From Steele and Freund (1985) with kind permission)

Thus, if the chord diameter and the primary sag can be measured for a given segment it is possible to deduce the radius of curvature. Alternatively, a lens surface of known diameter may be specified in terms of its sag (e.g. Bausch & Lomb Optima lenses – *see* Chapter 11). The lens is usually placed on an anvil, the diameter of which is critical to the measurement of the sagitta. When a lens is mounted this way it may flatten due to gravitational sag, a phenomenon referred to as 'the slumping problem' (Loran and Hough, 1987). Small changes in the measured sagittal height will cause larger (implied) changes in the parameter of interest which is the back optic radius. For example, consider a soft contact lens which, when placed on an anvil of 6.25 mm diameter, slumps downwards by 0.02 mm; although the actual back optic zone radius may be 8.60 mm, the implied radius will be 8.90 mm, but this obviously depends on the anvil diameter $2y$.

If $h = r - \sqrt{r^2 - y^2}$

Then $\dfrac{\mathrm{d}h}{\mathrm{d}r} = 1 - \dfrac{r}{\sqrt{r^2 - y^2}}$

This suggests that for an anvil diameter of 10 mm, an error in sag height yields four times the error in the back optic zone radius (Loran and Hough, 1987, citing Campbell, 1987). A tolerance of $\pm$ 0.05 mm on sagittal height measurement is suggested.

The principle of microsphometry is used in the Abbé spherometer and is also utilized in the following instruments.

The Wet Cell Radius Gauge (C.L.M. Group Ltd)

This instrument, illustrated in *Figure 13.10*, is a magnified vertex depth gauge which permits approximate determination of the back optic zone radius of a spherical hydrogel contact lens in the hydrated state.

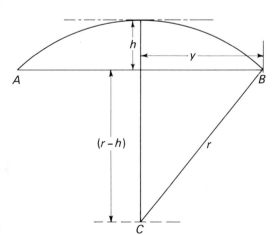

Figure 13.9 Principle of microsphometry

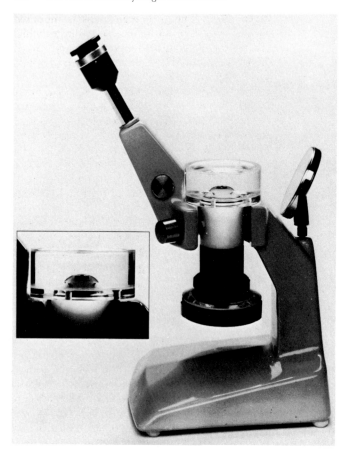

Figure 13.10 The Wet Cell Gauge produced by C.L.M. Group Ltd, which utilizes microspherometry to determine the approximate radius of curvature of a liquid-immersed contact lens. Inset: soft lens in place in saline cell. The supporting ring, oblique centring posts and central probe can be seen. (Photograph by courtesy of C.L.M. Group Ltd)

The lens rests on a support ring which determines the chord diameter and is centred in physiological saline solution by four obliquely directed posts covered with soft plastic sleeves. A sagittal section of the lens is then viewed through an inclined, externally illuminated monocular microscope. A micrometer probe is now viewed, and adjusted vertically upwards through the support ring until contact is made with the back surface of the lens. The upward probe movement is continued until one or both sides of the lens are just perceptibly raised from the support ring. The probe movement necessary to lift the lens represents the sag for a known chord diameter, and the back optic zone radius is directly read off the micrometer adjustment screw. Although this instrument is now obsolete, it was one of the earliest instruments designed to measure the back optic zone radius of soft lenses. It shows a remarkable reliability for such a simple and inexpensive instrument (± 0.10 mm: Contact Lenses (Manufacturing) Ltd, 1975; ± 0.096 mm: Loran and French, 1978) and also shows a high operator agreement of 90% (Jenkins, 1981).

The Wöhlk microspherometer

This instrument is illustrated in *Figure 13.11*. Like the Wet Cell Radius Gauge it also determines the primary sag, but unlike other microspherometers it measures the back optic zone radius of soft lenses in air.

The lens is removed from its storage solution and excess fluid is eliminated first by shaking and secondly by wiping the back surface with the finger. The lens is then placed, convex side up, onto the holding ring which locates a chord diameter of 10 mm. The upward motion of the central probe is observed through a magnifier from above. The back optic zone radius is read in millimetres from a clock dial when the probe

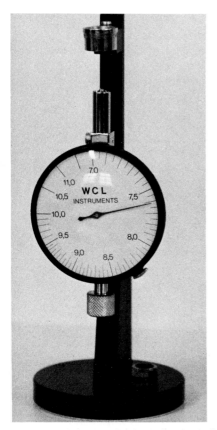

Figure 13.11 The Wöhlk Microspherometer determines the primary sag for a predetermined chord diameter of a soft contact lens in air. The back optic zone radius which corresponds to a specific sag height is directly read off a clock dial. (Photograph by courtesy of Wöhlk Contact Lenses Ltd, – now Zeiss)

just contacts the back surface of the lens. The manufacturers (Wöhlk-Contact-Linsen, Kiel) stress that this initial point of contact is critical and the operator must therefore cease upward movement of the probe immediately contact occurs. Furthermore, in common with all measurements of soft lens parameters made in air, the measurement should be made reasonably quickly. The instrument is calibrated against a concave quartz master sphere and with practice an accuracy of ±0.05 mm is claimed (D. Burns, 1975, personal communication).

The Basescope

This instrument is produced in Japan by the Union Optical Company and is illustrated in

Figure 13.12. The submerged lens is mounted, convex side up, on a 6 mm column, which locates the chord diameter with an accuracy of 0.50 μm (micrometres) and is circumferentially supported by a Y-shaped transparent funnel, thus facilitating rapid and precise centration as illustrated in *Figure 13.13*. A sagittal section of the lens is seen reflected through a 45° inclined mirror and viewed at ×30 magnification through a binocular microscope. The sag from the chord diameter to the lens vertex is now displayed in micrometres on a digital counter (*Figure 13.12*), compensation having been made for lens thickness.

The back optic zone radius is now read off either from tables or from a graph, and an accuracy of ±0.015 to ±0.025 mm is claimed for this precision instrument (Nakijima *et al.*, 1974; A. Hirando, 1975, personal communication).

Electronic microspherometers

Electric circuit microspherometry utilizes the hydrogel property of conducting electricity in order to facilitate the critical point of contact between the palpating pin and the back surface of the lens (Forst, 1979; Chaston and Fatt, 1980).

The upward movement of the probe is monitored and displayed continuously on a digital read-out and, at the point of contact, an electrical pathway is established between the support ring and the probe where a difference in potential is maintained. A signal is then relayed back to the measuring device which it blocks and the corresponding sag value appears on the read-out display. Electronic microspherometers currently on the market include the B.C. Tronic (Médicornéa), the B.C.O.R. Electrogauge (Kelvin Lenses Ltd), the Rehder Gauge (The Rehder Development Co.) and the S.M. 100 Softometer (Neitz Optical Co.) (Chaston and Fatt, 1980).

The Kelvin Soft Lens Gauge

This instrument which is illustrated in *Figure 13.14* measures the sag of a lens in saline employing a process known as proximity gauging. As the glass probe approaches the back vertex of the lens, the electric circuit is completed and a light-emitting diode is illuminated. At this point, the operator then ceases

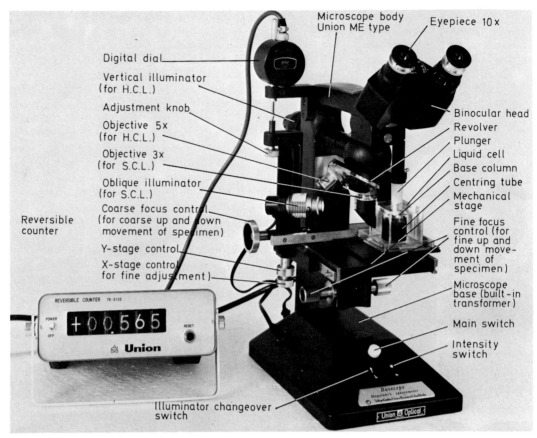

Figure 13.12 The Basescope, produced by Union Optical Co., is a precision instrument utilizing microspherometry to measure the back optic zone radius. The primary sag is read off a digital counter and the radius determined from tables or from a graph. (Photograph by courtesy of Union Optical Co.)

movement of the motorized probe just prior to actual contact occurring. Due to the fact that the probe stops at a predetermined distance from the vertex of the lens, this has to be allowed for in calculating the true sag and subsequently the

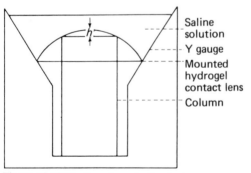

Figure 13.13 The Cuvette centration device used to centre and mount the hydrogel lens in saline solution in the Basescope

back optic zone radius which is displayed on a digital read-out. Because there is no actual physical contact with the lens, there is virtually no surface distortion and, therefore, the reported measurement consistency of ±0.02 mm is excellent (Port, 1983). However the water content of the lens affects the electrical field generated by the approaching probe and consequently the instrument cannot be calibrated against a rigid master sphere. Consequently, radii may only be compared (not strictly speaking measured) and the instrument has therefore to be readjusted for different materials.

Ultrasonography

The sagittal height of a lens may be measured in saline employing ultrasound. The lens is mounted on a support and ultrasonic pulses

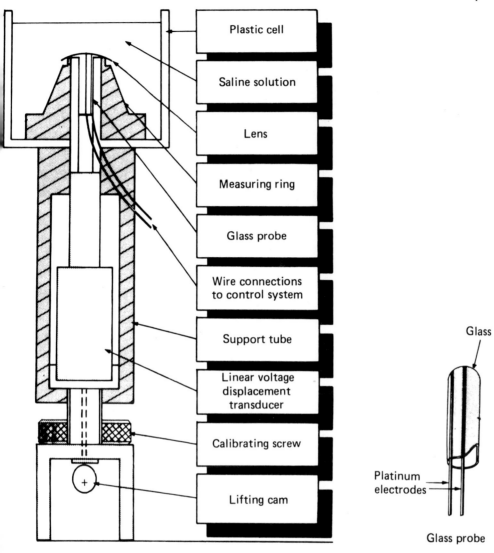

Figure 13.14 Cross-section of the Kelvin Soft Lens Measuring Gauge showing the essential components. (From Port (1983) with kind permission)

emitted from a transducer to the back surface of the lens are reflected back and electronically analysed. The time for the signal to travel from the back vertex of the lens to a reference plane is a function of the speed of sound in saline and the distance travelled, the latter being the sag for that specific chord. The following soft lens radius meters utilize ultrasound: The Panometrics Ultrasound System (Patella *et al.*, 1982) showing an average standard deviation of ±0.02 mm; the A.M.S. Optison (±0.03 mm at an ambient temperature of 24.0°C (Port, 1982a)

and the Neitz (Softometer) S.M.100 giving a reliability of ±0.10 mm (Port, 1981b).

Interferometry

Interferometry has been suggested as an accurate and reproducible method to measure the radii of both hard and soft contact lenses (El-Nasher and Larke, 1980). A lens is suspended in physiological saline and the interference patterns formed by incident monochromatic light are measured with a

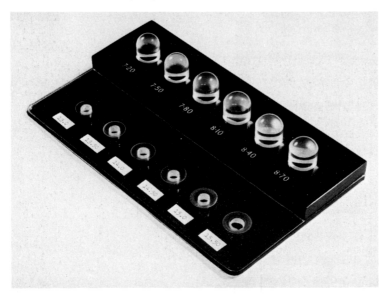

Figure 13.15 The Lensmaster, formerly produced by Contactalens Ltd, which uses optical gauging to determine the approximate back optic zone radius in air, using the hemispheres at the back and total diameter using the circles engraved at the front, known as a comparator

microdensitometer and converted mathematically into radii. This system produced a maximum coefficient of variability between 0.6% for back optic zone radii and 2.0% for the front optic zone radii compared to the manufacturers' published results.

Optical gauging

Master spheres

One of the simplest methods of obtaining an approximate value for the radius of a soft contact lens is to utilize master spheres and apply a system known as optical gauging. The lens, in the hydrated state, is placed with its convex face upwards onto one of a series of accurately made acrylic spheres of known radii. If the two surfaces are not aligned, a bubble forms and its location determines the relative curvature of the hydrogel lens with respect to the master sphere. If the back optic zone radius is steeper than the master sphere a bubble forms centrally, whereas a peripheral bubble indicates that the back surface of the lens is flatter than the test plate. The Lensmaster is an example of this type of system and is shown in *Figure 13.15*. This system is relatively inexpensive, is rapid and simple and has the advantage of allowing

the checking to be done in air, but according to Harris, Hall and Oye (1973) only produces a reliability of ±0.30 mm. Hampson (1973) attributed inaccuracies to capillary attraction and also to stretching between the master spheres and the hydrogel material. For these reasons, assessment of the relative curvature should be made within a few seconds of placing the lens on the master sphere. Ultrathin and hyperthin lenses cannot be checked in this way.

The Söhnges control and projection system

Söhnges Optik (1974) projects the profile of a fluid-immersed lens onto a screen by means of a projector incorporating a high luminosity 24 volt/250 watt halogen bulb and a cooling system. The screen is engraved with horizontal and vertical linear millimetre scales and a series of annuli graded from 7.20 to 9.50 mm in 0.10-mm steps which may be adjusted vertically. The projection distance is approximately 1 m and is determined by calibrating the instrument against a known test plate. The profile of the lens is projected onto the graticules which are adjusted vertically until alignment is achieved (*Figure 13.16*).

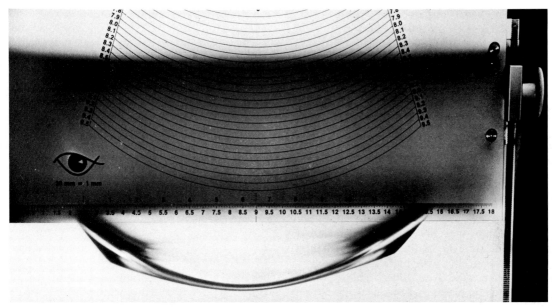

Figure 13.16 The image of the sagittal section of an immersed lens projected in the Söhnges System onto a screen containing annuli which may be adjusted vertically until alignment is achieved. (Photograph by courtesy of Söhnges Optik and reproduced by kind permission of the National Eye Research Foundation)

Inaccuracies may occur with the Söhnges system due to an increase in the ambient temperature of the saline solution and also from eccentricity of projection. Loran (1974) and Loran and French (1978) claimed an error of measurement of −0.107 mm in measuring production lenses and a reliability of ±0.10 mm for this instrument.

The Optimec Soft Lens Analyser

This is a projection system which is essentially available in two forms, both providing temperature control of the wet cell and also saline filtration (Port, 1981a) as available extras. The original model, the J.C.B., employs back projection while the J.C.F. model illustrated in *Figure 13.17* is a front projection system. In either model, the lens is mounted convex surface upwards in saline on a 8.50 mm diameter cylinder and centred. The lens profile is then viewed on a built-in screen at × 15 magnification and a probe manually advanced until contact is confirmed by the observer detecting a just perceptible edge lift. The probe is then lowered by the same amount and the back optic zone radius read directly in millimetres. Port

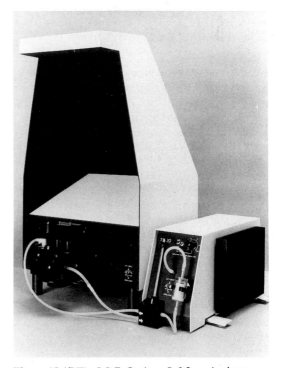

Figure 13.17 The J.C.F. Optimec Soft Lens Analyser, Front Projection Model with temperature control and saline filtration. (Photograph courtesy of Optimec Ltd)

(1981a) states that the centration system is both easy to use and efficient and believes that the Optimec is the most efficient and useful system currently available. For lenses of 40% water content, the reported precision for the J.C.B. model without temperature control is ±0.03 mm and ±0.05 mm for the J.C.F. with temperature control (Port, 1982b). Although one would expect a smaller standard deviation when temperature is controlled, these findings do not confirm this assumption. According to Port (M. J. A., 1987, personal communication), there was only a small variation of temperature in either experiment, back projection is more reliable than front projection and day-to-day variation in repeatability may have occurred. Certainly, careful control of the ambient variables is very important especially with higher water content lenses. Grant (1987) calibrated an Optimec, J.C.B. with temperature control against three PMMA buttons previously verified with a radiuscope and then measured three Weicon 38E (Ciba Vision) lenses 10 times each at a temperature of 21°C. The reported precision of the instrument was ±0.07 mm and the accuracy of the readings ±0.02 mm

Measurement of parameters in air

Lathe-cut hydrogel lenses are made in the hard state and are then smaller and steeper than in their final form. In the xerogel state, parameters may be checked in air, using conventional instruments, to achieve a similar tolerance to hard lenses, as shown in *Table 13.3*. After xerogel verification, the lenses are rigorously sterilized, the assumption being made that a known and predetermined expansion factor may be applied to determine the hydrated parameters. Unfortunately, however, the hydrogel material does not possess plastic memory and, if allowed to dry spontaneously in air, does not normally

Table 13.3 Manufacturer's tolerances of xerogel parameters

Parameter	Reliability
Back optic zone radius (mm)	±0.04
Back vertex power (D)	±0.12
Centre thickness (mm)	±0.02
Diameter (mm)	±0.05

Hydron (U.K.), 1975.

contract in a regular manner because of differential hydration across the lens surface due to differences in lens thickness. If, however, the ambient humidity is monitored and slowly reduced in a controlled environment, then the lens may dehydrate without significant distortion and, indeed, limited modifications may be possible (Bier and Lowther, 1977).

Consequently, although xerogel lenses may be verified with a high degree of accuracy, there is normally no way this tolerance may be checked once the lens is received by the practitioner in the hydrated state. It might therefore be argued that the accuracy claimed by the manufacturers is to some extent academic.

Diameters

Diameters are important considerations in specifying, fitting and duplicating contact lenses and a tolerance of ±0.05 mm to ±0.10 mm is suggested for hard lenses and ±0.20 mm to ±0.25 mm for hydrated soft lenses. Soft contact lenses are often mono-curve on one surface and bi-curve on the opposite surface, and while verifying diameters it is important to examine the transition between adjacent radii which, in the author's experience, are sometimes sharp. If sharp transitions are present in soft semi-scleral contact lenses, they may present a potential source of limbal indentation, corneal anoxia and abrasion.

The back optic zone diameter is a significant parameter in determining the primary sag and hence the physical and physiological fit of the lens. A complete lens specification should perhaps include total and intermediate diameters. In practice, however, it is more convenient to specify the total diameter, which for a given edge form and thickness varies directly with the back optic zone diameter.

Ruben (1974) and Bailey (1975) suggest that diameters should be measured in a liquid, while Stone (J., 1975, personal communication) and Mandell (1974c) believe checking in air to be clinically adequate and certainly more convenient. It should be pointed out, however, that diameters measured in air may differ from those measured in liquid and account for apparent discrepancies between the laboratory and the practitioner if different measuring techniques are used. If diameters are measured in air it is normal to dry the lens which, in turn, is mounted on a plane surface such as a microscope slide. Initially, the lens size increases due to surface tension and adhesion between the lens and the glass mount (Bailey, 1975) followed by contraction on dehydration.

Band magnifier

It is without doubt more convenient to check diameters and, indeed, all soft lens parameters in air using conventional instrumentation, and for measuring the total diameter and intermediate diameters the band magnifier is recommended (Bailey, 1975; J. Stone, 1975, personal communication).

The air-dried lens is mounted horizontally and, orientating the axis of the instrument vertically, the lens is measured against an external light source; with this technique one may expect a reliability of approximately ±0.10 mm which is similar to that achieved for the diameters of hard lenses.

Bailey (1975) measures the transverse section of a liquid-immersed soft lens with a band

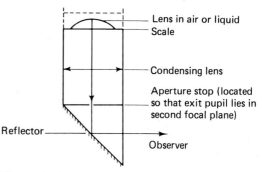

Figure 13.18 Modification of a band magnifier to determine the diameters of a hydrogel lens in a liquid or in air

magnifier placed in contact with the liquid cell wall which should be as thin as possible to reduce parallax errors. A microscope slide offers reasonable optical quality and is recommended for this purpose.

If a band magnifier is modified as illustrated in *Figure 13.18*, it is possible to examine the transverse lens section either in air or liquid with the examiner's head in a normal, comfortable position. The scale and the lens plane

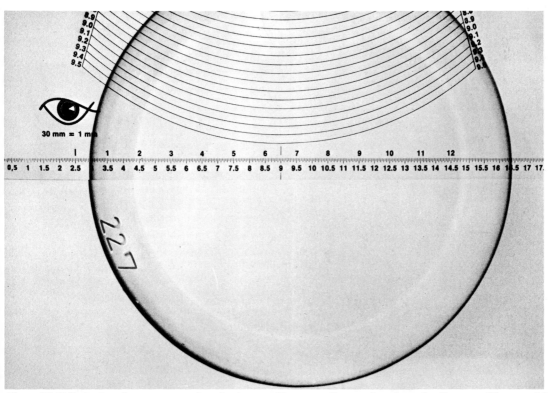

Figure 13.19 Projection of a transverse section of an immersed lens onto a linear scale to determine diameters. (Photograph by courtesy of Söhnges Optik and reproduced by kind permission of the National Eye Research Foundation)

almost coincide, and the telecentric principle may be incorporated by placing an aperture stop in the second focal plane of the lens thereby overcoming most of the objections previously mentioned.

Projection

Both the Söhnges and Optimec provide an efficient and reasonably accurate method of determining the back and front surface optic zone diameters and also the total diameter of a liquid-submerged lens. Either a sagittal or transverse section may be projected as illustrated in *Figures 13.16* and *13.19*, respectively and the pertinent diameters read off a millimetre scale previously calibrated against a test plate to

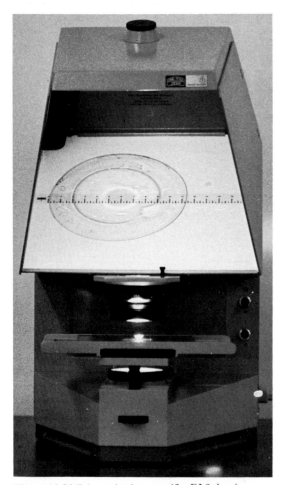

Figure 13.20 Zeiss projection magnifier DL2 showing projection of a soft lens. (Photograph reproduced by kind permission of Wöhlk Contact Lenses Ltd)

determine the correct projection distance. Microfilm projectors may also be used, preferably suitably adapted to take a parallel optically flat-surfaced cell containing the lens in saline solution. A millimetre scale, engraved on one surface of the cell against which the edges of the lens rest, is magnified along with the lens and thus the appropriate diameters may be read off on the receiving screen. This is an excellent system used by some of the lens manufacturers. An example of such a projection magnifier is shown in *Figure 13.20*, but here the scale is printed on the screen.

Travelling microscope

Ruben (1974) recommends the use of a travelling microscope to measure the total diameter of a liquid-immersed soft lens, and, although the reliability of this method is not stated, one must assume it to be accurate.

V gauge

The V gauge illustrated in *Figure 13.2* has been designed to hold the lens while the back vertex power in a liquid is determined, but could presumably be modified by incorporating a millimetre scale adjacent to the channel, from which the total diameter could be quickly and conveniently read off.

Comparators

An example of a comparator is illustrated in *Figure 13.15* and comprises a series of translucent annuli inscribed in a translucent Perspex base. The air-dried lens is simply superimposed onto the test circle to which the total diameter is compared. This method is quick and simple but it is not logical to expect an accuracy better than ±0.25 mm as the graduations are in 0.50 mm steps.

Thickness

Centre thickness

The thickness of a hydrogel contact lens is a significant parameter which contributes to the oxygen transmissibility, optical stability and durability of a lens, and Barradell (1975) suggests that soft lenses should be as thin as

Table 13.4 Some ultrathin hydrogel contact lenses

Lens	Manufacturer	Approximate centre thickness at $-3.00\,D$ (mm)
Hydroflex S.D.	Wöhlk Contact Lenses Ltd (Zeiss)	0.08
Eurothin	Kelvin Lenses (CooperVision)	0.07
Superthin	Averlan	0.07
U Series Soflens	Bausch & Lomb	0.07
Cooperthin	CooperVision	0.07
C.S.I.D.W.	Pilkington/Syntex Ophthalmics	0.07
Gelflex U.T.	Gelflex Laboratories	0.06
Gelflex Membrane	Gelflex Laboratories	0.06
Zero 6	Hydron	0.06
T40	Hoya	0.06
Extra thin	Focus	0.05
Hydrocurve 11/S.T.	Hydrocurve Soft Contact Lenses	0.04
Zero 4	Hydron	0.04
C.S.I.E.W.	Pilkington/Syntex Ophthalmics	0.035
O Series Soflens	Bausch & Lomb	0.035

Other manufacturers produce lenses of similar centre thickness.

durability will permit. As thickness is reduced, a hydrogel lens becomes fragile and more difficult to handle. Conversely, thinner lenses offer the advantages of greater oxygen transmissibility, improved comfort and better centration. At the time of writing ultrathin hydrogel lenses are widely fitted and those currently available are listed in *Table 13.4*.

The practitioner should be capable of examining the lenticulation and also measuring the thickness within reasonable limits, from the centre to the periphery. Due to the fragility and distensible nature of the hydrogel matrix, however, normal thickness measuring devices such as micrometers, verniers or thickness gauges cannot be utilized, but instead indirect measurements which may employ reflected light, optical doubling or projection are relied on.

Radiuscope

The conventional radiuscope, which employs Drysdale's method to determine the radii of reflecting surfaces, may be used to measure lens thickness by focusing the vertically travelling microscope first on the centre of one surface of the lens, and then on the centre of the other surface. Hartstein (1973) recommends the following procedure:

(1) Mount the lens, back surface down, on a master sphere with a steeper curvature than the lens being measured so that centre contact occurs.

(2) The target is first focused on the sphere and the dial gauge zeroed. This may be done with or without the lens in place.

(3) The radiuscope is now refocused on the front surface of the lens and the travel noted on the dial.

(4) Although not mentioned by Hartstein, if step (2) is carried out with the lens in place, the apparent thickness should now be multiplied by the refractive index of the hydrogel material to obtain the real thickness. If step (2) is carried out without the lens in place, step (3) will give the real thickness directly.

The accuracy of this technqiue depends on the location and precise focusing of the two images of the radiuscope target and this process has been improved by employing a special holder known as a bisurfaced hydrogel lens platform (BHLP). This is essentially an aluminium cylinder, one half of which is highly polished and the other half dull. The lens is dried and mounted in air concave side upwards on the platform which fits over the lens holder part of the microscope. The radiuscope is first focused on the polished half of the cylinder and then on the back surface of the lens by observing the target against the dull side of the holder (Paramore and Wechsler, 1978; Wechsler and Paramore, 1978).

The radiuscope has the dual advantage of air checking and also utilizing conventional instrumentation and according to Paramore and Wechsler (1978) and Wechsler and Paramore (1978) the use of BHLP produced a repeatability range of ±0.01 mm. The last published tolerance of centre thickness in the UK was ±0.05 mm, but this has now been temporarily withdrawn (British Standard, 1978). The 1986 American National Standards (Z80.8–1986) for soft contact lens tolerances are illustrated in *Table 13.1* and suggest a range of acceptable tolerances for centre thickness. If the water content is below 70% and the stated centre thickness is below 0.15 mm, a tolerance of ±0.02 mm is recommended compared to ±0.05 mm for lenses with a water content above 70% and a centre thickness of 0.26 mm or greater. A survey by Loran and Hough (1987) covering 30 laboratories, practitioners and academics suggested that a tolerance range of ±0.012 mm for lenses of under 50% water content and less than 0.05 mm centre thickness to ±0.028 mm for those of above 70% water content with a centre thickness of 0.20 mm and above was both realistic and within the accuracy of available instrumentation (*Table 13.5*).

Table 13.5 Soft contact lens tolerances: survey of 30 practitioners, laboratories and academics to recommend acceptable realistic soft contact lens tolerances

Back optic zone radius

Centre thickness (mm)	Tolerances (mm) for lenses of water content		
	<50%	50–69%	>70%
<0.05	±0.18	±0.23	±0.27
0.06–0.10	±0.16	±0.21	±0.25
0.11–0.15	±0.14	±0.17	±0.21
0.16–0.20	±0.12	±0.18	±0.21
>0.20	±0.10	±0.16	±0.19
	Mean ±0.14	Mean ±0.19	Mean ±0.23

Centre thickness

Ordered (mm)	Tolerances (mm) for lenses of water content		
	<50%	50–69%	>70%
<0.05	±0.012	±0.012	±0.012
0.06–0.109	±0.012	±0.017	±0.02
0.11–0.15	±0.014	±0.020	±0.028
>0.20	±0.018	±0.022	±0.028

Back vertex power

BVP in air (D)	Tolerances (D) for lenses of water content		
	<50%	50–69%	>70%
>10.00	±0.21	±0.23	±0.32
10.25–20.00	±0.337	±0.40	±0.52
<20.00	±0.57	±0.57	±0.70

From Loran and Hough, 1987.

Pachometry

This is the method recommended by Ruben (1974) to give an approximate thickness of a hydrogel lens mounted on a scleral contact lens in saline solution. The apparent thickness of the lens is measured with the pachometry attachment of a Haag–Streit slit lamp, and while this technique is subject to errors, a reliability of ±0.02 mm is claimed. Although the thickness of a soft contact lens in both air and liquid is of theoretical interest, it could be argued that it is the lens dimensions *in situ* which are significant, and these may alter with environmental variables such as osmolarity, pH, tear evaporation and temperature. Presumably the thickness of the lens could also be measured *in situ* using pachometry.

Projection

In addition to the annuli, and the horizontal millimetre scale, the screen of the Söhnges' system also incorporates a vertical millimetre scale which is adjusted to determine the edge and the centre thickness of the lens profile.

Electric circuit micrometry

Water-bearing hydrogels conduct electricity and this property has been utilized in a modified micrometer which it is claimed will measure the thickness of a hydrogel contact lens to an accuracy of ±0.003 mm (Fatt, 1977).

The probes which are made of plastics incorporate an electric wire cast into the centre line so that when the probes just make contact an electric circuit is completed. An ohm-meter is incorporated into the circuit so that when the probes either just contact each other, or the front and back surfaces of a hydrogel lens, a deflection is recorded on the needle. The probes are first brought into contact, the deflection noted and the instrument zeroed. The probes are next separated and a hydrogel lens is mounted convex side up on the lower support; the upper probe is now lowered until the ohm-meter needle is again deflected and the thickness read from the micrometer.

Average thickness

The specification of central thickness is convenient and reasonably representative in low-powered lenses but, when the back vertex power exceeds $\pm 1.50\,\mathrm{D}$, it does not reflect the true thickness across the lens diameter. The concept of specifying both centre and edge thicknesses certainly provides a better overall view, but as one approaches the periphery, thickness measurement, while still possible, is more difficult. Specifying the average thickness (t_a) however is clearly more meaningful and may be approximated by (Fatt, 1979):

$$t_a = \tfrac{1}{3}\text{ Centre thickness} + \tfrac{2}{3}\text{ Edge thickness}$$

(across a specific chord)

The edge thickness may be specified either axially or radially whereby axial edge thickness is measured parallel to the axis of symmetry and radial edge thickness normal to the front lens surface, both parameters specified at a point near to the edge (Pearson, 1986). The radial edge concept is generally considered to be the more meaningful measurement as heat, water and gases flow normally to the lens surface.

The arithmetical mean thickness (t_{am}) is given by Fatt (1979) as:

$$t_{am} = \frac{1}{A \int L \mathrm{d}A}$$

in which A is the area under consideration and L is the minimum lens thickness within that area.

An alternative concept of harmonic mean thickness (t_{hm}) has been suggested by Sammons (1981) in which the lens is considered as a series of annuli and:

$$t_{hm} = \frac{N}{\dfrac{1}{t_1} + \dfrac{1}{t_2} + \dfrac{1}{t_3} \ldots \ldots + \dfrac{1}{t_N}}$$

Further and more complex calculations have also been published (Fatt, 1979; Sammons, 1981; Brennan, 1984a) which consider a number of continuous variables over the area at which the average thickness is to be calculated. It would clearly be more convenient if this information could be simplified, but graphs unfortunately do not traditionally lend themselves to presenting more than two variables. Brennan (1984b) overcame this dilemma by structuring the necessary information in the form of nomograms in which these continuous variables, including back vertex power, centre and average thickness, the optic zone diameter, water content and minimum centre thickness for a specific water content, are included. Using the nomogram illustrated in *Figure 13.21* for negative lenses and a similar but separate one for positive lenses, the average thickness can be estimated to less than 5% for negative lenses, and generally less than 5% for positive lenses compared to the calculated value (Efron and Brennan, 1985).

Laboratory measurement

The average thickness of a soft contact lens may be determined *in vitro* by measuring the total diameter and accurately weighing the lens which has been suitably blotted dry. If the specific gravity is either known or measured (Refojo and Leong, 1984) and if we equate the hydrogel spherical cap to a disc then the average thickness (W. N. Charman, 1987, personal communication):

$$t_a = \frac{m}{(\phi/2)^2 \pi \rho}$$

where ϕ is the total diameter of the lens; ρ is the specific gravity, and m is the mass of the lens.

Water content

The water content of a hydrogel contact lens is an important parameter which affects lens flexibility, comfort, dehydration characteristics and permeability and, consequently, it would be most helpful if the water content could be verified. The water in a lens is expressed as a percentage of the total mass of the lens in its hydrated state under equilibrium conditions with physiological saline solution containing

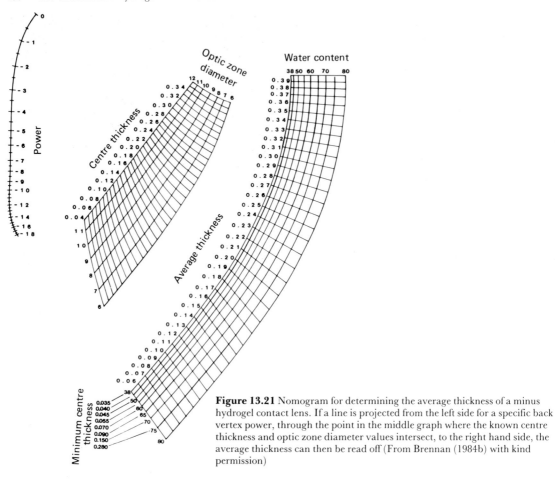

Figure 13.21 Nomogram for determining the average thickness of a minus hydrogel contact lens. If a line is projected from the left side for a specific back vertex power, through the point in the middle graph where the known centre thickness and optic zone diameter values intersect, to the right hand side, the average thickness can then be read off (From Brennan (1984b) with kind permission)

9 g/l sodium chloride at a temperature of $20 \pm 0.5°C$ with a stated pH value (British Standard, 1978):

Percentage water content =

$$\frac{\text{Mass of water}}{\begin{array}{c}\text{Mass of the hydrated lens}\\ \text{(including solids)}\end{array}} \times 100$$

and

$$= \frac{\begin{array}{c}\text{(Mass of the hydrated)} -\\ \text{(Mass of dehydrated lens)}\end{array}}{\begin{array}{c}\text{Mass of the hydrated lens}\\ \text{(including solids)}\end{array}} \times 100$$

The water content may be measured *in vitro* using a sensitive microbalance to determine the mass of the hydrated lens which has been blotted dry and the dehydrated lens fully dried

in a vacuum or in a microwave oven. Limitations of this technique (which is clearly unsuitable for the practice, office or smaller manufacturing laboratories), include the use of expensive equipment, the fact that it is time consuming and lens destructive, and that there is difficulty in accurate and reproducible surface blotting of the hydrogel lens surface.

An alternative and simpler technique has been suggested to estimate the water content indirectly by measuring the refractive index (Brennan, 1983; Efron and Brennan, 1985). As the water content of a hydrogel increases, the refractive index reduces and there is a close correlation between these variables especially in the range between 30 and 70% water content (Fatt and Chaston, 1980; Teuerle, 1984). It is postulated, therefore, that the measurement of refractive index could then provide a rapid and non-destructive method of estimating the water content. The refractive index under specific environmental conditions and for a given wavelength is the sine of the angle of incidence divided by the sine of the angle of reflection and the angle at which internal reflection occurs can be easily measured using a hand-held Abbé Refractometer (Brennan, 1983; Efron and Brennan, 1985). The hydrated lens is blotted dry and, using a glass daylight plate, is applanated onto the fixed prism of the refractometer as illustrated in *Figure 13.22*. The instrument is then directed towards an external light source and the border between the dark and light fields is viewed in the eyepiece; the water content is then read directly from the scale as shown in *Figure 13.23* (Efron and Brennan, 1985). This system assumes that the hydrogel acts as a simple solvent and, providing the instrument is periodically calibrated against a medium of known refractive index (e.g. saturated sodium chloride) and the ambient temperature is controlled and specified, then the estimated refractive index correlates well with both measured and manufactured stated values (Brennan, 1983). The reported reliability of this instrument is ±1.0% (Efron, 1987).

Oxygen transmissibility

Although there is considerable debate on the oxygen requirements of the human cornea, which shows significant individual variation, it is nevertheless agreed that the critical oxygen performance ranges from 8% to avoid loss of corneal sensitivity (Millodot and O'Leary, 1980), 10% equivalent oxygen performance to avoid oedema (Holden, Sweeney and Sanderson, 1984), 13% to maintain epithelial mitosis

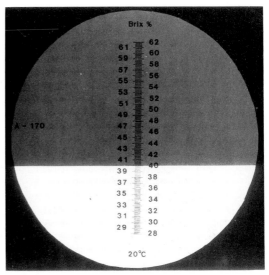

Figure 13.23 Scale of the Atago CL-1 Soft Contact Lens Refractometer as seen by the operator in which the upper field appears dark and the lower field clear. The boundary between the upper and lower portions of the field indicates the water content of the lens which is read directly from the scale. (From N. Efron (1987) with kind permission)

and avoid lactate accumulating in the anterior chambers (Hamano *et al.*, 1983), to 15% to avoid the formation of microcysts and polymegathism in extended lens wear (Holden, 1986). The passage of oxygen to the cornea through the water phase of hydrogels is therefore of critical significance and may be quantified in terms of transmissibility in which:

$$\text{Transmissibility} = \frac{Dk}{t} \left(\text{or } \frac{Dk}{L} \right)$$

where t (or L) refers to the lens thickness and Dk the rate of flow of a gas, usually oxygen, at a

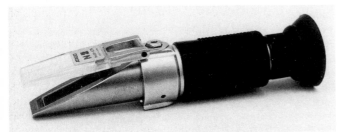

Figure 13.22 The Atago CL-1 Soft Lens Refractometer showing the clear Perspex daylight plate which applanates the hydrogel lens onto the opposing prism face. The rim adjacent to the rubber eye cup may be adjusted to focus the eyepiece. (From Efron and Brennan (1985) with kind permission)

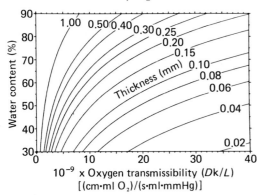

Figure 13.24 Graph illustrating the relationship between percentage water content and oxygen transmissibility (*Dk*/*L* or *Dk*/*t*) for a lens of specific average or centre thickness. (From Efron and Brennan (1985) with kind permission)

specified temperature through a unit area of unit thickness of the lens and subject to a specified unit pressure difference. So

$$Dk = \frac{\text{Amount of gas (ml } O_2) \times \text{Thickness (cm)}}{\text{Area (cm}^2) \times \text{Time (s)} \times \text{Pressure difference (mmHg)}}$$

It is clearly advantageous for the practitioner to know and, if possible, measure or estimate the transmissibility of a lens of known material. This important information facilitates the design, identification and verification of the chosen lens and affects the dehydration, monitoring and after-care of the patient. By measuring the centre thickness or preferably determining the average thickness with the Brennan nomogram (*see Figure 13.21*) and knowing the water content, the centre or average transmissibility may be conveniently read off the graph in *Figure 13.24*. Although *Dk*/*t* (also referred to as *Dk*/*L*) is the generally accepted parameter for oxygen transmissibility, Flynn, Quinn and Hill (1983) have suggested the hydration/thickness (*H*/*t*) index as an alternative which gives a correlation coefficient of +0.90 with oxygen performance and is easily calculated. The *H*/*t* index is defined as the quotient of water content and centre thickness. However, thick and thin lenses should not be inter-compared by the *H*/*t* index. Also the *H*/*t* index does not indicate the effect of flexibility or oxygen transmission in the midperiphery or the periphery of the lens (A. J. Phillips, 1987, personal communication). If the centre thickness were to be replaced by average thickness then both the average transmissibility (*Dk*/t_{av})

and the average hydration index (*H*/t_{av}) would be more meaningful values, albeit more difficult to measure and calculate.

Power

A possible limitation of hydrogel contact lenses is that the visual acuity with the contact lens may be less than the equivalent acuity obtained with spectacles or hard contact lenses. It is therefore important that the refraction is accurate, the lens is fully settled on the eye (to allow for ambient environmental factors), before an over-refraction is attempted and, finally, that the back vertex power of the lens has been accurately worked and verified.

Focimetry

Liquid cells

In measuring the back vertex power of a soft contact lens, it is preferable that a projection focimeter is utilized to enhance the accuracy of the reading, and Nakijima *et al.* (1974) recommend mounting the lens in a liquid cell or cuvette and reading off the power of the resultant thick polymer-liquid lens on a projection focimeter.

In order to determine the back vertex power in air of a lens measured in liquid a compensation factor, K, must be applied (Poster, 1971).

If *n* is the refractive index of air = 1.00
n' is the refractive index of the saline solution = 1.336
n'' is the refractive index of the hydrogel material ≃ 1.430
F_1 is the back vertex power in air
F_2 is the back vertex power in the liquid
Then $F_1 = F_2 K$
Where, approximately,

$$K = \frac{(n'' - n)}{(n'' - n')} = \frac{1.43 - 1.00}{1.43 - 1.336} = 4.57$$

The Poster conversion factor which converts the lens power in saline to the power in air only applies to thin lenses (Pearson, 1980, citing Wray, personal communication). Although complex equations may be applied to thick lenses (Wichterle, 1965) these pre-assume an accurate knowledge of the front optic zone radius, back optic zone radius and centre thickness.

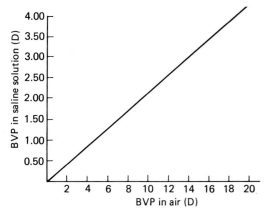

Figure 13.25 Conversion from back vertex power in liquid to back vertex power in air

Thus, the back vertex power measured through the liquid cell must be multiplied by the compensation factor. This may be more conveniently read off from tables or from a graph as illustrated in *Figure 13.25*. This means that the accuracy of focimetry must be improved by 457% and the required sensitivity necessitates readings of 0.05 D. Thus, an error of 0.12 D in the focimeter reading would lead to an error of over 0.50 D in the actual lens power in air. Hampson (1973) also points out that surface distortions of the hydrogel lens may be masked by the ambient saline solution; furthermore pseudocylinders, prisms and other distortions may be introduced by the cell walls. In view of

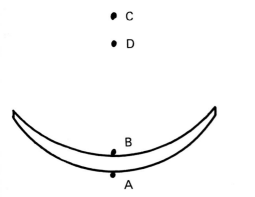

Figure 13.26 Measurement of back vertex power of a soft contact lens in saline using the Autostigmatic Microscope (*see Figure 13.8*). The target is focused in turn on A and B which represent the front (lower) and back (upper) surfaces of the lens; C is the centre of curvature of the upper surface while D is the image of the centre of curvature of the lower as viewed through the upper surface. (From Steele and Freund (1985) with kind permission)

these limitations it is doubtful if liquid immersion offers substantial advantages for checking the power of soft contact lenses.

By using the Autostigmatic Microscope (*see Figure 13.8*), the BVP of the saline-immersed lens mounted with the back surface upwards may be calculated. A focused target image is seen on the front lens surface A, at its apparent centre of curvature D, also at the back lens surface B and at its centre of curvature C (Steele and Freund, 1985, and personal communication, 1989).

From *Figure 13.26* the back vertex power may be calculated thus:

$$BVP = (n - 1) \left(\frac{1}{b} - \frac{1}{r} - \frac{S}{(nb^2 + bS)} \right)$$

in which
$S = AB$
$r = BC$
$t = BD$
n = the refractive index of the lens
n' = the refractive index of saline
b = distance from D to actual centre of curvature of front surface

and $\dfrac{1}{b} = \dfrac{n'}{nt} + \dfrac{(n - n')}{nr}$

The average standard deviation of the BVP of lenses ranging from 38% to 70% water content, from +4.25 D to −4.00 D and any thickness is ±0.37 D.

Air checking

This has been recommended by Isen (1972), Gasset (1972), Hampson (1973), Ruben (1974), Mandell (1974a) and Stone (J., 1975, personal communication) for which a projection focimeter is recommended. There is a critical period of the first minute after removing the lens from the saline solution during which the reading should be taken. For 30 seconds this image is hazy (Isen, 1972), although shrinkage on dehydration does not substantially affect the readings for a period of 4 minutes (Mandell, 1974a). The focimeter scale is initially set to the expected reading (J. Stone, 1975, personal communication), the lens carefully dried and placed convex side upward either on a reduced aperture focimeter or a conical contact lens holder, and the reading taken in air. With practice a reasonably clear image can usually be obtained with this method for which a reliability of ±0.25 D is claimed (Harris, Hall and Oye, 1973). Pearson (1980) found a standard error of measurement of BVP of ±0.09 D in air and ±0.05 D in saline and while recommending wet cell checking acknowledged the problems of converting wet to air power.

Surface inspection

Hydrogel contact lenses are inherently fragile, especially in the higher water content polymers recommended for extended wear (de Carle, 1972), and are also liable to exogenous and endogenous contamination, examples of which are given in *Figures 13.27, 13.28* and *13.29* and in *Tables 13.6, 13.7* and *13.8*. It is generally accepted that continuous irrigation is an efficient method of removing debris and microorganisms, and this important function is performed in the conjunctival sac by the tears. If the irrigation interface (and this includes the cornea or the contact lens) presents an irregular surface resulting, for example, from scratches, crevices and other lesions (*see Plate 30*), the surface may harbour microorganisms which collect and multiply away from the natural protective mechanisms (Tripathi and Ruben, 1972/73). It

therefore follows that the importance of inspection of the surfaces and edges of hydrogel contact lenses both on and off the eye cannot be over-emphasized. *Plates 29–46* should be studied with this in mind.

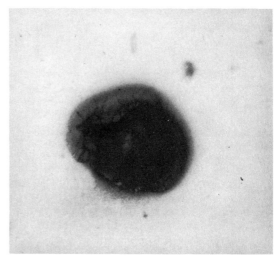

Figure 13.28 Contaminant embedded on the front surface of a semi-dehydrated hydrogel contact lens in contact with a saline solution droplet. × 40

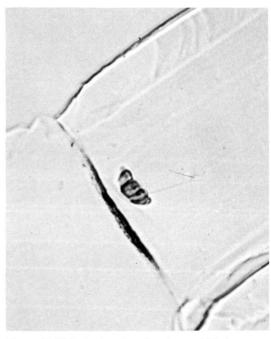

Figure 13.29 Sagittal section of a red spot which shows a deeply embedded ferrous particle of unknown aetiology. The location of the contaminant, however, suggests an endogenous aetiology possibly introduced during spin-casting

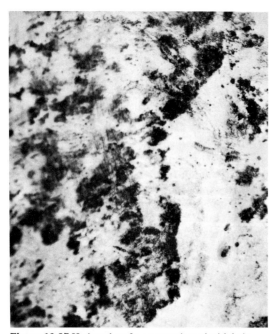

Figure 13.27 Hydrogel surface contaminated with hair rinse

Table 13.6 Potential lesions of hydrogel surfaces

Lesion	Possible cause	Possible effect	Possible remedy
Tears, cracks and splits*	Mishandling or manufacturing defect	Accumulation of debris. Discomfort, abrasions and infection	Replacement lens
Linear indentations*	Polishing marks in manufacture	Accumulation of debris. Discomfort, abrasions and infection	Replacement lens
Lens engraving	Inscribed in xerogel state	Accumulation of debris. Discomfort, abrasions and infection	Replacement lens although debris may be removed by surfactant cleaning followed by boiling, enzyme or oxidative cleaning
Foreign bodies	Airborne debris	Discomfort, lacrimation, abrasions and infection	Massage and irrigation with 0.9% saline solution
Aerosol sprays	Make-up incorrectly applied	Discomfort and reduced wetting	Surfactant cleaning followed by boiling or oxidative cleaning. Replacement lens often necessary
Fungi (Filippi, Pfister and Hill, 1973)	Poor hygiene	Enzymatic degradation of material	Asepticization. Replacement lens often necessary
Microbes (Phillips, 1980)	Exogenous or endogenous aetiology	Infection	Surfactant cleaning followed by heat or chemical disinfection
Chemical binding	Incorrect or incompatible solution (for example, hard lens solution, eyedrops and medications)	Eye irritation, chemosis, infection	Discontinue soft lens wear and seek medical treatment. If binding is due to protein deposits on lenses, clean lenses to remove deposits
Surface crazing and cracks (Bier and Lowther, 1977)	Hydrogel dehydration followed by stress. Incomplete polymerization or degradation of the material	Accumulation of debris and microbes. Discomfort, abrasion and infection	Replacement lens

*Most lenses carry a manufacturer's warranty against mechanical defects.
See also Chapters 3 and 4.

Table 13.7 Potential surface films on hydrogel lenses

Lesion	Possible cause	Possible effect	Possible remedy
Tenacious milky film which may appear green on phase contrast microscopy (*see Figure 13.35*)	Proteins deposited on the lens surface which may become denatured, especially if heat disinfected. May contain albumin, γ-globulin, α_1-lipoprotein, mucopolysaccharides, lipids and phospholipids. Predisposition to the build-up of other inorganic materials (for example, chlorhexidine binding) and inactivation of anti-microbial additives	Impaired wettability, reduced contact lens acuity. Red eye reaction, tarsal papillae (protein or giant cell conjunctivitis), mucus discharge, itching and increased lens movement	Non-denatured protein build-up may be prevented by surfactant cleaning or treatment by electrical pull copolymers. Denatured proteins may be treated by broad-spectrum proteolytic enzyme cleaners, bleaching (for example, chlorine), or hydrogen peroxide. Lipoprotein treated by lipase cleaners and phospholipids by phospholipase cleaners
Greasing	Meibomian secretions, sebaceous secretions or tear cholesterol	Intermittent blurring, reduced acuity and adhesion of pathogens	Surfactant cleaning. Lipase and phospholipase cleaners

See also Chapters 3 and 4.

Table 13.8 Potential discolouration of hydrogel lens material

Lesion	Possible cause	Possible effect	Possible remedy
White spots (Ruben, 1976)	Tear calcium. Crystalline deposits from solutions prepared from non-purified water	Lens intolerance	Possible treatment with calcareous chelating agent such as EDTA or oxidization cleaners
Red spots (Loran, 1973)	Ferrous particles endogenously or exogenously induced. The ambient saline solution and also heat sterilization make them highly susceptible to corrosion	No known adverse effects to date, although the possibility of ocular siderosis must be considered	Probably replacement lens though possibly inhibited by ferrous chelating agents such as desferrioxamine (CIBA), EDTA or oxidization cleaners
Green film (Bier and Lowther, 1977)	Accidental contamination with fluorescein	Discolouration of lens, and possibly exogenous infection by pathogenic microbes such as *Pseudomonas aeruginosa*	Heat or boil in physiological saline solution. If heavily stained then soak in Milton* for 15–30 minutes. Place in a vial containing sterile, physiological saline solution and boil for 30 minutes. Transfer to a clean vial and fresh saline solution and repeat the boiling process (up to four times) until the pH returns to normal. Finally, rehydrate in appropriate solution
Red film (F. A. B. Hodd, 1975, personal communication)	Accidental contamination with rose bengal	Discolouration of lens. Possible exogenous infection	Nor normally removed by boiling
Yellow/brown discolouration (Stewart, 1978; Phillips, 1980)	Tobacco smoke. Aromatic compounds in tears. Chlorhexidine reaction especially with chlorinated cleaners	Reduced acuity, discomfort and possible infection	Boiling in saline solution followed by the use of strong oxidization cleaners

*Milton (Richardson-Merrell).
See also Chapters 3 and 4.

494

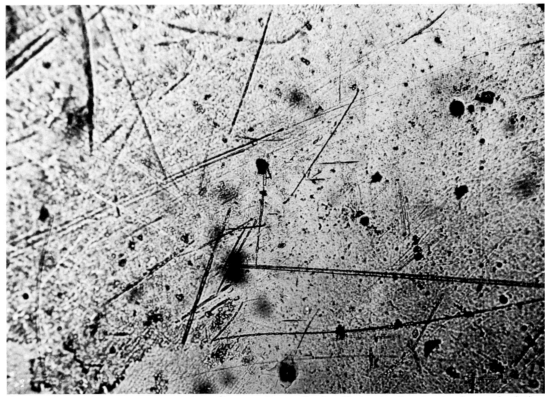

Figure 13.30 Polishing marks seen on a lathe-cut lens at × 40 magnification. (Reduced to three-quarters in reproduction)

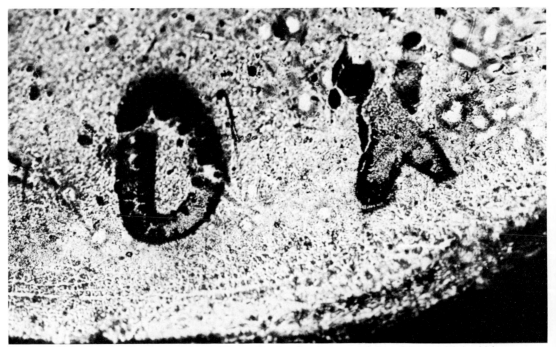

Figure 13.31 Appearance of lens engraving at × 40 magnification showing accumulation of dirt and debris which may harbour pathogenic microbes. (Reduced to three-quarters in reproduction)

Light microscopy

The surface area of a soft contact lens varies from approximately 140 to 200 mm^2 and clinically it is necessary to scan the hydrogel surface not only with reasonable speed but also to employ high magnification to critically evaluate suspect areas such as those illustrated in *Figures 13.30* and *13.31* which show how easily debris can accumulate in scratches and engravings. In practice a range from × 5 to × 40 is adequate and the slit lamp biomicroscope performs the function admirably, although, if preferred, a separate stereomicroscope can be used.

When the lenses are inspected in air they should be shaken or blotted dry and examined under magnification, preferably on glass, against a white background. For this purpose, the lens may be mounted on a microscope slide with a white adhesive background (*Figure 13.32* and *Plate 35*) or, alternatively, the test plate of the slit lamp may be modified as shown in *Figure 13.33*. It should be pointed out, however, that if the test plate is mounted on the body of the slit lamp in the normal manner, then the lens plane is displaced forward slightly from the focal plane of the microscope and the lens surface is permanently out of focus unless the microscope has an independent focusing control. It may therefore be necessary to hold the lens mount by hand which may be tilted and moved as necessary. By employing conventional variations in slit lamp illumination the lens surface may be examined and evaluated. Brandreth (1975) recommends that the examiner use moderate magnification with direct focal illumination, 'sclerotic scatter', to evaluate the edges, and parallelepiped illumination with moderate magnification for inspection of the lens surfaces.

Dark-field illumination is also useful, where

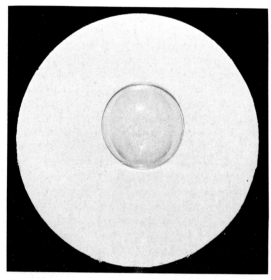

Figure 13.33 Lens mounted on a slit lamp test plate (with white background) for air surface inspection

the lens is illuminated by the slit beam against a dark background. Imperfections and deposits on the lens then show up light against the dark background much as corneal irregularities may show up against the dark background of the pupil. Some deposits or irregularities not seen against a light background may show up in this way (*see Plate 36* and *Figure 4.12d*).

If the practitioner wishes to employ even higher magnification, Brandreth also suggests modifying the slit lamp in the following manner. The lens is mounted on a glass slide or held by hand in the region of the head-rest directly in the beam of light. The illuminating system is aligned with the axis of the microscope set opposite to each other at a zero reading, so that the contact lens is located between the light

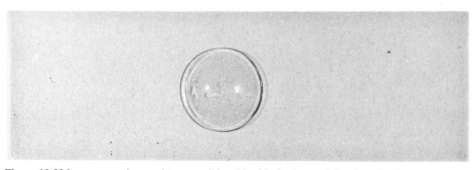

Figure 13.32 Lens mounted on a microscope slide, with white background, for air surface inspection

source and one of the microscope objectives. By moving the eyepiece, if necessary, a greatly magnified image may now be projected onto a convenient wall and examined for imperfections.

Degradation of the lens surfaces can and does occur in wear as *Figures 13.34* and *13.35* illustrate, and such lesions may not only interfere with vision or cause discomfort but may be extremely hazardous. It is therefore necessary for the practitioner to critically examine the lens surfaces each and every time the patient is seen for soft lens after-care. The practitioner would normally employ the slit lamp while the lenses are *in situ* to evaluate centration, lag and conjunctival disturbances. It is suggested that at the same time the lens surfaces should be examined (*see Plates 31* and *32*). The lens should also be examined out of the eye as previously explained either using the slit lamp or a stereomicroscope.

Electron optics

Light microscopy is limited by the wavelength of light to a magnification of approximately × 1000 and a resolution from 100 to 200 nm which is considerably greater than is required clinically. In research, however, greater magnification may be necessary to make ultrastructural studies of the hydrogel polymer (Matas, Spencer and Hayes, 1972; Tripathi and Ruben, 1972/73; Filppi, Pfister and Hill, 1973; Loran, 1973; Holden, Pain and Zantos, 1974).

If it is necessary to employ higher magnification, electron optics must be used, which is that branch of physics concerned with the projection of the electron beam. Electron microscopy permits 1000 times greater resolution than light microscopy so that magnification of up to × 100 000 may be achieved. The beam is focused directly onto a suitably sectioned specimen through electron lenses in transmission electron microscopy, or arranged to scan the specimen in scanning electron microscopy, the latter technique being recommended by Holden, Pain and Zantos (1974) for hydrogel contact lenses. The reflected electrons are then picked up by a suitable detector and finally the signal is amplified and is displayed on a cathode ray tube where the electron image may be photographed as a micrograph as shown in *Figures 13.36* and *13.37*.

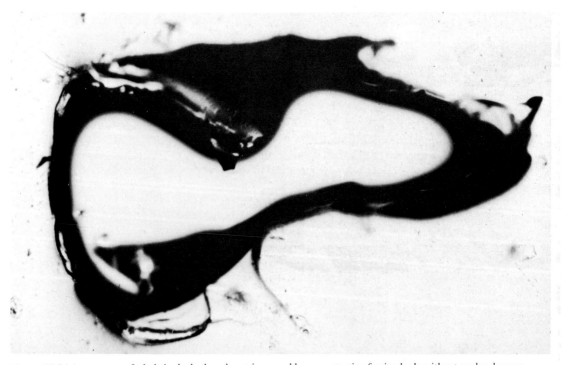

Figure 13.34 Appearance of a hole in the hydrogel matrix caused by a penetrating foreign body without ocular damage

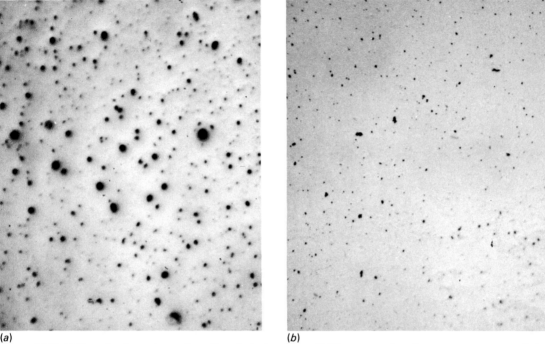

(a) (b)

Figure 13.35 (*a*) Coagulated proteins on the surface of a hydrogel lens. (*b*) The same surface after treatment by a proteolytic enzyme cleaner

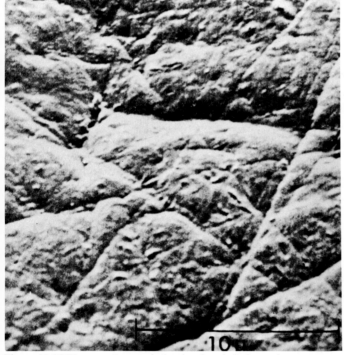

Figure 13.36 Electron micrograph showing the relatively rough appearance of a lathe-cut lens at × 3000 magnification. (From Matas, Spencer and Hayes (1972) and reproduced by kind permission of the American Medical Association; reduced to three-quarters in reproduction)

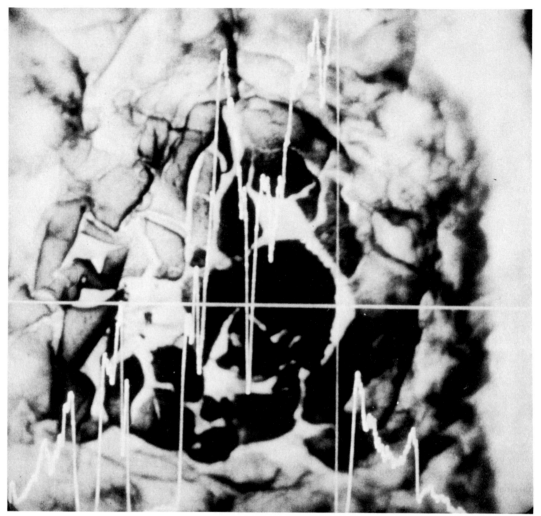

Figure 13.37 Electron microprobe analysis of the contaminant illustrated in *Figure 13.28* which was coated with a thin layer of carbon to enhance conductivity of the electrons. The subsequent X-ray scan was superimposed on a × 300 electron image and shows strong iron radiation in the alpha (mean) component of the K band of the spectrum. A less intense oxygen radiation was also present. (From Loran (1973); reduced to three-quarters in reproduction)

It is also possible to identify some hydrogel contaminants by a technique known as electron microprobe analysis in which the electron probe scans a prepared specimen, which, subsequent to excitation, emits characteristic X-rays. The latter may then be analysed and identified by crystal spectrometry. An example of an X-ray scan superimposed on an electron image of ferrous contamination of a hydrogel lens is illustrated in *Figure 13.37*.

Conclusion

Contact lenses may only be manufactured and prescribed as accurately as they may be checked, and in attempting to establish an acceptable system of tolerances for contact lens parameters, it is necessary first to establish fitting criteria which should then be correlated with the cost of manufacture and also the reliability and validity of available quality

Table 13.9 Summary of the reliability of verifying the back optic zone radius of soft contact lenses

Method	Instrument	Reliability	Source
Master spheres	Lensmaster	±0.30	Harris, Hall and Oye (1973)
Sagometry in saline	C.L.M. Wet Cell Gauge	±0.10	Contact Lenses (Manufacturing) Ltd (1975)
Sagometry in saline	C.L.M. Wet Cell Gauge	±0.09	Loran and French (1978)
Sagometry in saline	Cell Gauge Basescope	±0.02	Nakijima et al. (1974)
Sagometry in air	Wöhlk Microspherometer	±0.02	Campbell Burns (D., 1975, personal communication)
Sagometry in air	Wöhlk Microspherometer	±0.17	Loran and French (1978)
Radiuscope in saline	Ultra Radiuscope	±0.02	Nissel (G., 1970, personal communication)
Radiuscope in saline	Ultra Radiuscope	±0.023	Loran and French (1978)
Radiuscope in saline	Autostigmatic Microscope	±0.07	Carney, Ungerer and Brennan (1985)
Radiuscope in saline	Radiuscope	±0.10	Garner (1981)
Keratometry in saline	Zeiss Ophthalmometer	±0.05	Holden et al. (1977) Loran and French (1978)
Sagometry in saline	Hydrovue Soft Lens Analyser	±0.10	Harris, Hatashita and Matsumoto (1981) Davies and Anderson (1979)
Sagometry in saline	Optimec J.C.B. with no temperature control (lenses under 40% water content)	±0.03	Port (1981a)
Sagometry in saline	Optimec J.C.F. with temperature control (lenses under 40% water content)	±0.05	Port (1982b)
Sagometry in saline	Optimec J.C.B. with temperature control	±0.07	Grant (1987)
Electric circuit microscopy	B.C. Tronic	±0.10	Koetting (1981)
Ultrasonic sagometry	Neitz (Softometer)	±0.13	Harris, Hatashita and Matsumoto (1981)
	SM 100	±0.10	Port (1981b)
Ultrasonic sagometry	Panametric system	±0.034	Patella et al. (1982)
Ultrasonic sagometry	A.M.S. Optison (No temperature control)	±0.03	Port (1982a)
Ultrasonic sagometry	A.M.S. Optison (Temperature control)	±0.04	Port (1982b)
Projection in liquid	Sohnges Projection system	±0.10	Loran (1974) Loran and French (1978)
		Mean ±0.08	Range ±0.02–±0.30

control instrumentation. Fitting criteria and cost considerations must take into account the opinions of those personnel engaged in the manufacture and prescribing of contact lenses. A cross-section of the views of manufacturers, practitioners and academics to recommend acceptable and realistic tolerances is illustrated in *Table 13.5* (Loran and Hough, 1987). A summary of the probable reliability of existing soft lens verification methods is also shown in

Table 13.10 Summary of the reliability of checking the centre thickness of hydrogel contact lenses

Method	Instrument	Reliability (mm)	Source
Travelling microscope in air	Radiuscope	±0.03	Titmus Eurocon (now CIBA Vision) (1974)
Travelling microscope in air	Radiuscope	±0.01	Harris, Hall and Oye (1973)
Electronic circuit microscope in air	Micrometer	±0.03	Fatt (1977)
Pachometry in liquid	Pachometer	±0.02	Ruben (1974)
Travelling microscope in air	Bisurfaced hydrogel lens platform	±0.02	Paramore and Wechsler (1978) Wechsler and Paramore (1978)
Sagometry in liquid	Autostigmatic Microscope	±0.008 <0.10 mm centre thickness ±0.012 >0.10 mm centre thickness ±0.010 for 38% water ±0.015 for 70% water	Carney, Ungerer and Brennan (1985)
		Mean ±0.017 mm	Range 0.01–0.03

Tables 13.9–13.12. These results essentially endorse the views of the American National Standard (Z80.8 – 1986) for soft contact lens prescription requirements (*see Table 13.1*) that:

(1) A more generous tolerance for back optic zone radii is permissible on more flexible materials which are inherently more gas transmissible by virtue of being thinner, or having a higher water content, or both.

(2) As lenses are made thinner, the proportional effect on transmissibility and oxygen supply is greater and hence stricter tolerances on thickness are necessary.

It is interesting to note that in the Loran and Hough findings (1987), the tolerances suggested as acceptable by laboratories were either similar to or even stricter than those agreed by academics and practitioners.

The checking of soft lenses in air is more convenient and adequate for verification of most parameters and, where possible, the practitioner obviously prefers to utilize conventional instruments. Holden (1977), however, suggests that the only satisfactory way to check soft lens parameters is in the hydrated state. In 1984, the existing British Standards for soft contact lenses (British Standard, 1978; 1979) were considered outdated and were withdrawn until validity

considerations could become established. However, 2 years later, American soft lens tolerances (American National Standards Z80.8 – 1986) based on an agreed consensus of experts was published. These recommendations, illustrated in *Table 13.1*, attempt to relate the characteristics of soft contact lenses to a patient's needs and are based on the current art of measuring soft contact lenses. However, at the time of writing there is no authoritative experimental evidence available to substantiate basic validity considerations such as how accurately do soft contact lenses need to be prescribed and how accurately can their parameters actually be measured. Until such questions can be answered, recommended tolerances based on consensus can only be considered as an 'educated guess'.

The current recommendations of the American National Standards (Z80.8 – 1986) together with the views of other National Standards Institutes are currently being debated by the International Organisation for Standardisation who intend to prepare and publish an agreed standard in due course. For the present, however, it is suggested that the *Soft Lens Tolerances*, published by the American National Standards Institute (Z80.8 – 1986) (*see Table 13.1*, p. 468) should act as a working guide for laboratories, teachers and practitioners.

Table 13.11 Summary of the reliability of verifying diameters of soft contact lenses

Method	Instrument	Reliability (mm)	Source
Measurement in air	Band Magnifier	±0.10	Titmus Eurocon (now (Ciba Vision) (1974)
Projection in saline	Projector	±0.10	Farlow (1980)
Projection	J.C.B. Optimec analyser (not temperature controlled)	±0.05	Port (1981a)
		Mean ±0.08	Range ±0.05–±0.10 mm

Table 13.12 Summary of the reliability of verifying the back vertex power of soft contact lenses

Method	Instrument	Reliability (D)	Source
Air checking	Focimeter	±0.50	Ruben (1974)
Air checking	Focimeter	±0.25	Harris, Hall and Oye (1973)
Air checking	Focimeter	±0.12	Titmus Eurocon (now Ciba Vision) (1974)
In saline	Focimeter	±0.223	Pearson (1986)
Sagometry in saline	Autostigmatic Microscope	±0.350 for 38% water ±0.41 for 45% water ±0.32 for 52% water ±0.20 for 70% water	Carney, Ungerer and Brennan (1985)
		Mean +0.29	Range +0.125 to +0.50

Acknowledgements

At the time of writing there are no international glossaries of terms, tolerances or methods of specification applicable to soft hydrophilic contact lenses. Furthermore, many instruments are still in the development stage and often not available for personal evaluation by the author.

Consequently, I am most grateful to those authors and laboratories who supplied photographs of their instruments and to the publishers who kindly granted permission for the reproduction of these illustrations in the text. I should also like to acknowledge the assistance of those colleagues cited under personal communications, to Dr Chris French for his helpful suggestions in the definitions section and also to Michael Sheridan on his guidance on the deliberation of the British Standards Institute and the International Standards Organisation. Finally I should like to thank Mrs Freda Taylor and Mrs Janice Patrick for the typing of the manuscript.

References

AMERICAN NATIONAL STANDARD (1986). Prescription requirements for first quality soft contact lenses. American National Standard Requirements for Soft Contact Lenses Z80.8 — 1986. National Standards Institute for Ophthalmics

ANASTASI, A. (1961). *Psychological Testing*, 2nd edn. London: Collier-Macmillan

BAILEY, N. J. (1975). Inspection of hydrogel lenses. *Int. Contact Lens Clin.* **2**(1), 42–48

BARRADELL, M. J. (1975). Re-appraisal of attitudes in prescribing soft lenses. *Optician* **170**(4393), 20–26

BAUSCH & LOMB SOFLENS DIVISION (1977). *Soflens International Fitting Guide*. New York: Bausch & Lomb

BENNETT, A. G. (1966). The calibration of keratometers. *Optician* **151**, 317–321

BEVINGTON, D. R. (1969). *Data Reductions and Error Analysis for the Physical Sciences*. New York: McGraw-Hill

BIER, N. and LOWTHER, G. E. (1977). *Contact Lens Correction*, p. 422. London: Butterworths

BRANDRETH, R. H. (1975). Biomicroscopic techniques for hydrogel lenses. *Int. Contact Lens Clin.* **2**(1), 33–41

BRENNAN, N. A. (1983). A simple instrument for measuring the water content of hydrogel lenses. *Int. Contact Lens Clin.* **10**, 357–361

BRENNAN, N. A. (1984a). Average thickness of a hydrogel lens for gas transmissibility calculations. *Am. J. Optom. physiol. Optics* **61**, 627–635

BRENNAN, N. A. (1984b). Application of hydrogel lens average thickness. *Am. J. Optom. physiol. Optics* **61**, 636–642

BRITISH STANDARD 5562 (1978). *Specification for Contact Lenses.** London: British Standards Institution

BRITISH STANDARD 5321. PART III (1979). *Glossary of Terms Relating to Contact Lenses.* London: British Standards Institution

BRITISH STANDARD (1986). Draft British Standards specification for rigid contact lenses (OES/78/1). London: British Standards Institution

DE CARLE, J. (1972). Developing hydrophilic contact lenses for continuous wear. *Contacto* **16**(1), 39–42

CARNEY, L. G., UNGERER, J. L. and BRENNAN, N. A. (1985). Validation of a new instrument for measurement of flexible contact lenses. *Aust. J. Optom.* **68**, 100–103

CHAMARRO TORMO, C. J. (1974). Las lentes de contacto flexibles, merced a un sencillo sistema optico, pueden ser medidas y controladas. *J. Gaceta. Optica* **36**, 31–35

CHASTON, J. (1973). A method of measuring the radius of curvature of a soft contact lens. *Optician* **165**(4271), 8–12

CHASTON, J. (1977). In-office measurements of soft contact lenses. *Am. J. Optom. physiol. Optics* **54**, 286–291

CHASTON, J. and FATT, I. (1980). Survey of commercially available instruments for measuring the back radius of soft contact lenses. *Optician* **18**(179), 19–44

CONTACT LENSES (MANUFACTURING) LTD (1975). The wet cell instruction sheet

DAVIES, H. E. and ANDERSON, D. J. (1979). An investigation of the reliability of hydrogel lens parameters. *Int. Contact Lens Clin.* **6**, 136–142

DEDONATO, L. M. (1981). Determination of the average thickness of a contact lens. *Am. J. Optom. physiol. Optics* **58**, 846–847

DRIEFUS, M. (1968). A new hydrogel lens made from polyglycolmonomethacrylate. *Augen. Optik* **85**, 35–39

EFRON, N. (1987). A closer look at hydrogel dehydration. Paper delivered to the European Symposium on Contact Lenses. Barcelona, Spain

EFRON, N. and BRENNAN, N. A. (1985). Simple measurement of oxygen transmissibility. *Aust. J. Optom.* **68**, 27–35

EL-NASHER, N. and LARKE, J. K. (1980). Interference measurements of soft lenses. *J. Br. Contact Lens Ass.* **3**, 64–70

EMSLEY, H. H. (1963). The keratometer: measurement of concave surfaces. *Optician* **146**, 161–168

FARLOW, D. W. (1980). Soft lens measurement. *J. Br. Contact Lens Ass.* **3**, 98–100

FATT, I. (1977). A simple electric device for measuring thickness and sagittal height of gel contact lenses. *Optician* **173**(4474), 23–24

FATT, I. (1979). The definition of thickness for a lens. *Am. J. Optom. physiol. Optics* **56**, 324–337

FATT, I. and CHASTON, J. (1980). The effect of temperature on refractive index, water content and central thickness of hydrogel contact lenses. *Int. Contact Lens Clin.* **7**, 250–255

FILPPI, J. A., PFISTER, R. M. and HILL, R. M. (1973). Penetration of hydrophilic lenses by *Aspergillus fumagatus*. *Am. J. Optom.* **50**, 553–557

FLYNN, W. J., QUINN, T. G. and HILL, R. M. (1983). Oxygen comparison made easy. *Contact Lens Forum* **8**, 57–59

FORST, G. (1974). New methods of measurement for controlling soft lens quality. *Contacto* **18**(6), 6–9

FORST, G. (1979). Prufung der MeBgenauigkeit eines elektronischen Spharometers. Sonderdruck aus der Fachzeitschrift. *Die Contactlinse,* Heft 5/1979. 13 Jahrgang

GARNER, L. F. (1981). A comparison of two methods for measurement of the sagittal height of soft contact lenses. *Int. Contact Lens Clin.* **8**(5), 19–23

GASSET, A. R. (1972). The Griffin Naturalens: basic concepts and fitting techniques. In *Soft Contact Lens,* edited by A. R. Gasset and H. E. Kaufman, Chap. 12. St Louis: C. V. Mosby

GRANT, R. (1987). Measurement of elliptical soft contact lenses. Unpublished workshop paper delivered to the British Contact Lens Association Annual Clinical Conference

GUILLON, M., CROSBIE-WALSH, J. and BYRNES, D. (1986). Application of pachometry to the measurement of hard contact lens edge profile. *Transactions of the British Contact Lens Association Clinical Conference,* pp. 56–59

HAMANO, M., HORI, M., HAMANO, T., KAWABE, H., MIKAM, M., MITSUNGA, S. and HAMANO, T. (1983). Effects of contact lens wear on mitosis of corneal epithelium and lactate content in aqueous humour of rabbit. *Jap. J. Ophthal.* (58), 434

HAMPSON, R. (1973). Considerations in the checking and predictability of hydrophilic lenses. *Optician* **165**(4283), 4–16

HARRIS, M. G., HATASHITA, M. B. and MATSUMOTO, D. M. (1981). Base curve measurements of soft contact lenses. *Am. J. Optom. physiol. Optics* **58**, 951–959

HARRIS, M. G., HALL, K. and OYE, R. (1973). The measurement and stability of hydrophilic lens dimensions. *Am. J. Optom.* **50**, 546–552

HARTSTEIN, J. (1973). *Questions and Answers on Contact Lens Practice,* 2nd edn, pp. 155–157. St Louis: C. V. Mosby

HILL, R. M. and LEIGHTON, A. J. (1964). Physiological time courses associated with contact lenses — temperature. *Am. J. Optom.* **41**, 3–9

HOLDEN, B. A. (1977). Checking soft contact lens parameters. *Aust. J. Optom.* **60**, 175–182

HOLDEN, B. A. (1986). Effects of contact lens induced hypoxia on the cornea. Paper delivered to the European Symposium on Contact Lenses, Nice, France

* This Standard is now withdrawn but is due to be published in revised form in 1989. A draft Standard (1986) (see above) is available.

HOLDEN, B. A., PAIN, P. and ZANTOS, S. (1974). Observations on scanning electron microscopy of hydrophilic contact lenses. *Aust. J. Optom.* **57**, 100–106

HOLDEN, B. A., SWEENEY, D. F. and SANDERSON, G. (1984). The minimum precorneal oxygen tension to avoid corneal oedema. *Invest. Ophthal. Vis. Sci.* **25**, 476–480

HOLDEN, B. A., COOPER, G. N., VAEGAN, K. and ALEXANDER, J. A. (1977). The accuracy and validity of measurements of the B.C.O.R. of hydrated soft contact lenses using a Zeiss keratometer and Holden wet cell. *Aust. J. Optom.* **60**, 46–51

HOLLY, F. J. and REFOJO, M. F. (1972). Oxygen permeability of hydrogel contact lenses. *Am. J. optom. Ass.* **43**, 1173–1180

HYDRON SOFT LENS (1975). *Technical Report*, Vol. 2

ISEN, A. A. (1972). The Bionite Naturalens. In *Symposium on the Flexible Lens*, Part III, The Griffin Laboratories Flexible Lens, edited by J. L. Bitonte and R. H. Keates, Chap. 5, pp. 35–51. St Louis: C. V. Mosby

JENKINS, G. (1981). A clinical and scientific comparison of contact lens analysis. *J. Br. Contact Lens Ass.* **4**, 28–32

KEMP, B. (1979). Soaking solutions and base curve variations. *Contact Lens Forum* **4**(6), 55–65

KOETTING, R. A. (1981). Clinical use of the Medicornea B.C. Tronic for measuring soft lenses. *Am. J. Optom. physiol. Optics* **58**, 631–632

LAYLAND, B., SWEENEY, D. and HOLDEN, B. A. (1980). Factors that affect or correlate with hydrogel lens flexibility. *Undergraduate Project*, School of Optometry, University of New South Wales

LORAN, D. F. C. (1973). Surface corrosion of hydrogel contact lenses. *Contact Lens* **4**(4), 3–10

LORAN, D. F. C. (1974). The determination of hydrogel contact lens radii by projection. *Ophthal. Optician* **14**, 980–985

LORAN, D. F. C. and FRENCH, C. N. (1978). The efficacy of verifying the base curve of hydrogel contact lenses. *Int. Contact Lens Clin.* **5**, 276–281

LORAN, D. F. C. and HOUGH, D. A. (1987). How realistic are soft contact lens tolerances. *Transactions of British Contact Lens Association*, vol. 4, p. 70

LORAN, D. F. C., FRENCH, C. N. and AUERBACH, D. (1982). The validity of determining thickness from the swell factor. *Ophthal. physiol. Optics* **2**, 231–235

MANDELL, R. B. (1974a). Can gel lens power be measured accurately? *Int. Contact Lens Clin.* **1**(1), 36–37

MANDELL, R. B. (1974b). *Contact Lens Practice: Hard and Flexible Lenses*, 2nd edn. Springfield, IL: C. C. Thomas

MANDELL, R. B. (1974c). Lathe-cut hydrogel lenses. *Int. Contact Lens Clin.* **1**(1), 53–62

MASNICK, K. B. and HOLDEN, B. A. (1972). Studies of water content and parametric variations of hydrophilic contact lenses. *Aust. J. Optom.* **55**, 481–487

MATAS, B. R., SPENCER, W. H. and HAYES, T. L. (1972). Scanning electron microscopy of hydrophilic contact lenses. *Archs Ophthal.* **88**, 287–295

MILLODOT, M. and O'LEARY, D. J. (1980). Effect of corneal deprivation on corneal sensitivity. *Acta ophthal.* **58**, 434–439

NAKIJIMA, A., SHIBATA, H., MAGATANI, H., HIRANO, A. and TERAO, T. (1974). A method of soft contact lens measurement. *J. Jap. Contact Lens Soc.* **16**, 123–131

PARAMORE, J. E. and WECHSLER, S. (1978). Reliability and repeatability study of a technique for measuring the centre thickness of a hydrogel lens. *J. Am. optom. Ass.* **49**, 272–274

PATELLA, V. M., HARRIS, M. G., WONG, V. A. and YUEN, D. C. (1982). Ultrasonic measurement of soft contact lens base curves. *Int. Contact Lens Clin.* **9**, 41–53

PEARSON, R. M. (1980). Wet cell measurement of soft lens powers. *J. Br. Contact Lens Ass.* **3**(1), 15–16

PEARSON, R. M. (1986). How thick is a contact lens? *Transactions of the British Contact Lens Association Conference*, pp. 82–85

PHILLIPS, A. J. (1980). The cleaning of hydrogel contact lenses. *Ophthal. Optician* **20**(11), 375–388

PORT, M. J. A. (1975). The radius measurements of hydrophilic contact lenses using ultrasonics. *MSc Thesis*, University of Aston in Birmingham

PORT, M. J. A. (1976). New methods of measuring hydrophilic lenses. *Ophthal. Optician* **16**, 1079–1082

PORT, M. J. A. (1981a). The Optimec Contact Lens Analyser. *Optician* **181**(4683), 11–14

PORT, M. J. A. (1981b). The radius measurement of soft contact lenses in air. *J. Br. Contact Lens Ass.* **5**, 168–176

PORT, M. J. A. (1982a). Assessing a new soft lens radiuscope: The AMS Optison. *Optician* **183**(4726), 11–14

PORT, M. J. A. (1982b). A comparison of two soft lens radiuscopes. *J. Br. Contact Lens Ass.* **5**, 107, 110–116

PORT, M. J. A. (1983). The measurement of soft lens radii by proximity gauging. *Ophthal. physiol. Optics* **3**, 167–174

POSTER, M. G. (1971). Hydrated method of determining dioptric power of all hydrophilic lenses. *J. Am. optom. Ass.* **43**, 287–299

POSTER, M. G. and SKOLNIK, A. J. (1974). Effect of pH and tonicity change on some parameters of a soft lens (T.M.). *J. Am. optom. Ass.* **45**, 311–314

REFOJO, M. F. (1972). A critical review of properties and application of soft hydrogel contact lenses. *Surv. Ophthal.* **16**, 233–246

REFOJO, M. F. and LEONG, F. L. (1984). Identification of hard contact lenses by their specific gravity. *Int. Contact Lens Clin.* **11**(2), 79–82

RUBEN, M. (1973). Soft lenses 1. *Optician* **166**(4296), 9–12, 15–16, 19–20

RUBEN, M. (1974). Soft lenses: the physico-chemical characteristics. *Contacto* **18**(5), 11–23

RUBEN, M. (1976). Biochemical aspects of soft contact lenses. *Optician* **172**(4462), 34–35

SAMMONS, W. A. (1981). Thin lens design anad average thickness. *J. Br. Contact Lens Ass.* **4**(3), 90–97

SÖHNGES OPTIK (1974). Information Deutsche Kontactlinsen Gamb. No. 9, Deutsche Kontactlinsen GMBH, 8 München 2, Postfach 202207, W. Germany

STEELE, W. H. and FREUND, C. H. (1985). A microscope for measuring soft contact lenses. *Aust. J. Optom.* **68**(3), 96–99

STEWART, B. V. (1978). Soft contact lens discoloration and the use of tobacco. *Int. Contact Lens Clin.* **15**(6), 269–275

TAJIRI, A. (1974). Measurement of the hydrogel lens with a

radiuscope. *Symposium on Contact Lenses*, pp. 118–120. Japan: Toyo Contact Lens Company

TEUERLE, W. (1984). Refractive index calculation of hydrogel contact lenses. *Int. Contact Lens Clin.* **11**, 625–628

TITMUS EUROCON (1974). Information sheet of Titmus Eurocon Kontactlinsen K. G., D-8750 Aschaffenburg, P.O. Box 74, Goldbacher Strasse 57, W. Germany

TRIPATHI, R. and RUBEN, M. (1972/73). Degenerative changes in a soft hydrophilic contact lens. *Ophthal. Res.* **4**, 185–192

WECHSLER, S. and PARAMORE, J. (1978). Accuracy of manufacturers' stated centre thickness of hydrogel contact lenses. *Am. J. Optom.* **55**, 677–680

WICHTERLE, O. (1965). Les Lentille de Contact Souples. Geltakt: Problems, Techniques et Chimiques. *Les Cahiers des Verres de Contact* **4**(6), 7–12

WICHTERLE, O. and LIM, D. (1960). Hydrophilic gels for biological uses. *Nature* **185**, 117–119

Chapter 14

Toric contact lens fitting

D. Westerhout

Toric forms of contact lenses have been in use for many years, and now that laboratories are prepared to devote more time and resources to the manufacture of such lens forms, they are being used much more widely.

It appears that many practitioners attempting to fit a patient for whom a toric lens might be of value are reluctant to actually use one, partly due to their lack of experience of such lenses as well as the acknowledged difficulty in having them manufactured accurately, and the high cost involved.

There is no doubt that the accurate manufacture of a contact lens incorporating a toroidal optical surface is extremely difficult, although the 1980s have seen an improvement in production methods and machinery. This difficulty is more than doubled if two toroidal optical surfaces are used, and the problems become still greater if other toroidal surfaces are involved as in, for example, the case of a bi-toric corneal lens with a multi-curved back surface toroidal peripheral zone.

Manufacturing costs of such a lens are related to the difficulty of production, and are therefore linked to the number of toroidal surfaces used in the final construction of the lens

Fitting toric hard corneal lenses

Indications for the use of toric contact lenses

The main uses of toric lenses are as follows:

(1) To improve the vision in cases where a lens employing spherical front and back optic zone radii is unable to provide adequate refractive correction.
(2) To improve the physical fit in cases where a lens with a spherical back optic zone radius (BOZR) and spherical back peripheral zone radii fails to provide an adequate physical fit. The terms 'spherical BOZR' and 'spherical back peripheral zone radii' include, in this context, any lens of any construction whether it be aspheric, conoidal or using any non-spherical curves, provided that the BOZR specifications are the same in any two meridians at right-angles to one another and the peripheral construction has the same specification in all meridians.

These two main uses of toroidal surfaces on contact lenses are usually distinct, and a lens is normally employed for either a physical or an optical reason. There are occasions on which the two types of use overlap — notably, when the front surface of a contact lens has to be made toroidal to correct the astigmatism induced when a lens with a toroidal back optic zone is worn on a cornea in order to produce a good physical fit. This is known as a compensated bi-toric contact lens.

Forms of toric lens

There are seven main varieties of toric corneal lens available to the practitioner, as follows:

(1) With toroidal back optic zone and peripheral zone.
(2) With toroidal back optic zone and spherical peripheral zone.

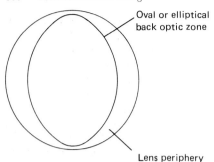

Oval or elliptical
back optic zone

Lens periphery

Figure 14.1 The radii of the toroidal peripheral zone incorrectly worked at right-angles to the corresponding BOZR, i.e. C2 Toric/$\dfrac{8.00}{7.50}$:6.50/$\dfrac{\mathbf{8.00}}{\mathbf{8.50}}$:9.50 instead of C2 Toric/$\dfrac{8.00}{7.50}$:6.50/$\dfrac{\mathbf{8.50}}{\mathbf{8.00}}$:9.50

(3) With spherical back optic zone and toroidal peripheral zone.

(4)–(7) Each of the first three varieties can be produced with or without a toroidal front optic surface, as can a lens with a spherical back optic zone and spherical peripheral zone.

This classification may be subdivided as follows.

A lens which has a toroidal back optic zone and a toroidal front surface has a bi-toric construction. If the principal meridians of the toroidal front and back surfaces are not parallel then the lens is of oblique bi-toric construction.

With respect to toric contact lenses, British Standard 3521 (1979) stated that a toroidal surface should be specified by the radii of curvature in its two principal meridians, the radius in the flatter meridian being written above a line and the radius in the steeper meridian below it (as in *Figure 14.1*), and where it is necessary to specify the orientation, the direction of the flatter meridian in standard axis notation should be written after the longer radius, prefixed by the letter 'm' to denote meridian. The abbreviation Tor may be used with BS to denote back surface, FS to denote front surface, OZ for optic zone and PZ for peripheral zone so as to indicate which surface is toroidal.

As, at present, International Standard ISO 8320-1986 does not include recommended methods of specification, the system outlined in BS 3521 (1979) will be adhered to in this chapter.

Lenses with toroidal back optic and peripheral zones

This type of lens is generally used in attempting to obtain a good physical fit on a cornea which is too astigmatic to allow a good fit with a lens having a spherical BOZR and spherical peripheral radii.

Although corneal lenses in general may be successfully fitted with either apical clearance or apical contact, it is generally more satisfactory to fit lenses with toroidal back optic zones in or near alignment. Fitting in alignment is difficult to define, and many practitioners differ in their interpretation of this term. It is often held to mean fitting with a BOZR of the same radius as the corneal radius in its flattest meridian as found by keratometer (or K) reading. This may be a reasonably accurate interpretation when the cornea to be fitted is almost spherical, but 'fitting on flattest K' is unlikely to represent alignment in medium or high degrees of corneal astigmatism. Alignment, to some practitioners, may mean a situation in which the lens fitted shows no apical clearance with fluorescein, but if the BOZR is decreased or the BOZD is increased by clinically significant amounts, then the fluorescein picture would change to one of apical clearance (Westerhout, 1969).

Since the lens form under discussion is made with a toroidal back optic zone to fit the contour of an astigmatic cornea, it may be seen that there is sound reasoning in trying to match the BOZR* to the corneal radii. This generally means fitting on or near the keratometer reading in each meridian. Such a lens usually gives a good physical fit in close alignment, especially if the peripheral toroidal curves are fitted with similar consideration to the difference in peripheral radii of the corneal principal meridians.

Such a lens frequently gives a physical fit, as denoted by the fluorescein pattern, similar to that seen with a well-fitted spherical lens in alignment to a cornea devoid of clinically significant astigmatism. However, a lens in such close alignment is sometimes likely to create physiological problems. A lens with both spherical BOZR and peripheral radii fitted to an eye with a clinically significant degree of corneal astigmatism does have an inbuilt advantage in that the slight looseness in the meridian of

*BOZR indicates back optic zone radius for a spherical surface and back optic zone radii for a toroidal surface.

steepest corneal curvature helps the lens to rock slightly on the flattest corneal curve, thus aiding the interchange of tears across the cornea behind the lens. Indeed, this rocking motion tends to act as a pump, and it is interesting to watch the flow of tears behind such a lens with a slit lamp biomicroscope — especially as the lens moves with and between blinks.

Conversely, it may happen that a spherical lens closely fitted to a spherical cornea, or an astigmatic cornea fitted with a lens utilizing toroidal back optic and peripheral curves, may give a poor liquid interchange, and it may be necessary to aid the maintenance of normal corneal metabolism by using a slightly modified lens form.

In the case of the closely aligning toric lens, the following possibilities exist:

(1) The use of a toroidal back optic zone fitted slightly flatter (longer radii) than the corneal radii. Either or both radii may be made flatter, and it is common for the steeper radius of the pair to be fitted a little flatter than the appropriate corneal radius to assist the interchange of tears.

(2) The use of spherical peripheral radii with a toroidal back optic zone. These peripheral radii may be chosen to give a conventional clearance and fit along the meridian of the flattest corneal curve (*see* Chapter 10). This tends to produce a looser peripheral fit in the meridian at right-angles which may aid the flow of tears behind the lens, especially if the cornea has astigmatism 'with-the-rule'. In such cases, the peripheral clearance is greater in the vertical meridian — which is probably the most helpful position if the lacrimal flow behind the lens is to be improved. This method also simplifies the lens production and reduces its cost. In the production of lenses with both toroidal back optic and peripheral curves, it is not uncommon for a laboratory to cut and polish the peripheral radii so that they do not lie along the same meridians as the corresponding BOZR, i.e. the flatter peripheral radius does not lie along the same meridian as the flatter BOZR. This results in a lens which appears to have a markedly elliptical or oval back optic zone (*Figure 14.1*). A properly made lens with a toroidal back optic zone and toroidal peripheral

curves which differ by the same amount from the corresponding BOZR has a similar appearance to a lens with a spherical BOZR and spherical peripheral radii. In both cases, the transition between the back optic zone and the peripheral zone is circular, or almost so.

(3) The toroidal peripheral zone may be made substantially flatter in relation to the BOZR than might normally be used for a spherical lens.

(4) The back optic zone diameter and/or the total diameter may be kept as small as is consistent with adequate visual acuity and comfort.

(5) The lens may be fenestrated. With a toroidal back optic zone, a central 0.2–0.4 mm hole is often found to be most effective.

(6) A more oxygen-permeable or better wetting material may be used.

Lenses with both toroidal back optic and peripheral curves are much easier to fit if keratometer readings are available, and still easier if the practitioner has a fitting set of such lenses. Such fitting sets are rarely used by practitioners, possibly because of their high cost and number of potential parameters. Many practitioners have, however, accumulated a series of prescription lenses which have had to be rejected when new replacement lenses have been prescribed. Such lenses are very useful, both for fitting and refraction purposes.

An example of the type of physical fitting which might be derived from keratometer readings is shown below, related to two different types of peripheral fit used for reasonably spherical corneas.

Example 1

Spherical cornea, keratometer reading 8.00 mm

Practitioner A might prescribe:
C2/8.00:6.50/9.00:9.50

Practitioner B might prescribe:
C4/8.00:6.50/8.50:7.50/9.00:8.50/9.50:9.50

Toric cornea, keratometer readings
8.00 mm along 180
7.50 mm along 90

Using the same approach to the physical fitting as for spherical corneas:

Practitioner A might prescribe:
C2 Toric/8.00:6.50/9.00:9.50
$$\underline{7.50} \quad \underline{8.50}$$

Practitioner B might prescribe:
C4 Toric/8.00:6.50/8.50:7.50/9.00:8.50/9.50:9.50
$$\underline{7.50} \quad \underline{8.00} \quad \underline{8.50} \quad \underline{9.00}$$

The refraction of such an eye wearing a lens with either an 8.00 mm BOZR or 8.00 mm × 7.50 mm BOZR is very different with the two types of correction. This is dealt with on p. 513.

In the event of keratometer readings not being available in the case of a toroidal cornea, such as that considered in Example 1, the lens could be fitted by observing conventional lenses having spherical back surface curves.

An experienced or skilful practitioner observing only the flatter meridian would probably find that an 8.00 mm BOZR combined with his favoured peripheral fit would fit very well along that particular meridian. By observing the degree of flatness in the vertical meridian and/or by consideration of the spectacle astigmatism and degree of residual astigmatism, it is possible to estimate the required fit in the vertical meridian with a fair degree of accuracy. Fitting in this way usually produces a sufficiently good physical fit, but may make it difficult to quantitatively predict the refractive effect of the lens. A more precise method of prescribing by consideration of the spectacle refraction and the use of spherical trial lenses is shown on p. 518, Example 5.

Since corneal lenses with both spherical BOZR and peripheral radii are often used successfully on corneas with a medium to high degree of astigmatism, it is important to decide what degree of astigmatism should indicate the use of toroidal back optic zones. In general, these should only be used when a lens with a spherical BOZR cannot be made to fit successfully. It is rare to find that toroidal back optic zones are necessary unless the difference in the corneal radii, as measured with a keratometer, exceeds 0.5 mm.

A great deal depends on factors other than corneal astigmatism. Lid positions and tension are important. In a case of high corneal astigmatism, with-the-rule, and a low, loose lower lid, a toroidal back optic zone may be needed to obtain a good physical fit and centration. But a similar eye with a firm, high lower lid may well be successfully fitted using a lens with spherical back surface curves.

Consideration should also be given to the likely moulding effect of a spherical lens on a toroidal cornea. The undesirable difficulties which may occur with spectacle blur and variations in visual acuity and refractive error (*see* Chapters 19 and 20) if the wearing of the contact lens has to be ceased for any reason, must be carefully weighed against the advantages of fitting a spherical lens. When such a lens is fitted, the post-wear refractive error should be carefully monitored at all after-care visits, and modification to the fit carried out if gross changes occur.

The majority of cases of corneal astigmatism are found with the steeper corneal curve in the vertical (with-the-rule). If an attempt is made to fit such an eye with a spherical BOZR, the lens often drops low on the cornea, causing physical discomfort and/or poor vision. Such an example is illustrated in *Figure 14.2*. If the same eye is fitted using a lens with toroidal back optic and peripheral curves, then the physical fit and centration are usually much improved (*Figure 14.3*).

Sometimes, with such astigmatism, it is found that a lens with a spherical BOZR is lifted high on the cornea by the top lid. This may give a reasonable standard of steady vision but can cause physiological problems through its immobility and tendency to cause a stagnant pool of tears just below the upper limbus.

A fitting set of lenses with both toroidal back optic and peripheral curves is extremely valuable, as already mentioned. Even a limited set

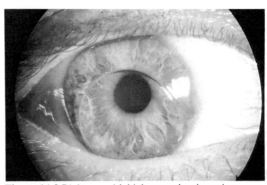

Figure 14.2 Right eye with high corneal astigmatism. Keratometer reading 7.86 mm along 2.5, 7.26 mm along 92.5. Optimum fit with spherical BOZR showing lens centring very badly

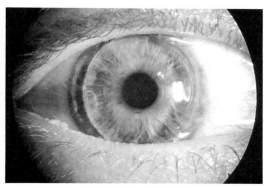

Figure 14.3 Same right eye as in *Figure 14.2* wearing an alignment fitted corneal lens using a toroidal back optic zone of BOZR 7.85 × 7.25 mm. Note: this PMMA lens now centres well, but requires fenestration (or use of RGP material) for adequate tear exchange and physiological fit

can be of great value. A suggestion for a minimum set is one covering the range 7.5 × 7.00 mm to 8.5 × 8.0 mm BOZR in 0.1 mm increments in both meridians.

The peripheral radii may be chosen to reflect the type of peripheral fit usually preferred by the practitioner concerned. Each meridian is considered separately, and the peripheral fittings in the two principal meridians are selected to provide the same difference between back optic and peripheral radii most commonly used by the practitioner in fitting spherical corneas.

Since the cutting and polishing of each pair of peripheral radii on a toroidal surface is such a complicated and costly process it is best to choose the simplest possible form of peripheral fit preferred. If a tri-curve periphery, i.e. a tetra-curve lens is normally used when fitting only spherical back surface zones, a less sophisticated lens with just one pair of toroidal peripheral curves, i.e. a bi-curve lens in each principal meridian, may be advantageous.

Since such a fitting set is extremely useful for refraction purposes as well as for observation of the fluorescein pattern, the back optic zone diameters should be between 6.5 and 7.0 mm when using PMMA lenses and 7.2–7.8 mm when using rigid gas permeable (RGP) lenses. (Total diameters of 9.0–9.5 mm are appropriate in any hard material.)

Lenses with toroidal back optic zones and spherical peripheral zones

As already mentioned, it can be useful to use spherical peripheral radii with the intention of improving the circulation of tears beneath these lenses. However, when this is done, it is possible that the lens may become less stable with regard to resisting rotation. A fully toroidal peripheral zone may assist in preventing excessive lens rotation, and this can be helpful if it is necessary to hold the lens in a non-rotating position to correct residual astigmatism or to correctly position a bifocal segment.

One difficulty that may arise with the use of a toroidal back optic zone and a spherical front surface, is that there is a variation of edge thickness, which may give rise to discomfort. The use of spherical peripheral radii makes it easier for the laboratory to produce a more uniform edge thickness, and this may be of some slight physical advantage in certain cases.

It is often said that toric lenses cannot be adjusted, but this is not correct. If, for example, a lens with toroidal back optic and peripheral curves provides too little tear flow behind the lens, it is possible to re-cut or polish the peripheral radii to spherical form using a radius or radii identical to those used for the original flatter meridian. The radii can also be made flatter than the original flatter radius or radii. The steeper peripheral radii may also be made only a little flatter, but not as much as the flatter meridian.

In theory, if a lens with an all toroidal back surface rotates, then the steeper peripheral radii may come to rest along the flatter corneal meridian. In this position, they are far too tight and may cause corneal abrasions or disturbance. This is seldom seen as a problem in practice, but if encountered, it may provide an indication for the use of spherical peripheral radii.

The back surface specification of a useful fitting set having the first back peripheral curve toroidal, as well as the back optic zone, but with the two most peripheral curves being spherical, is given in *Table 14.1*. Some practitioners may prefer the latter two curves to be even flatter to encourage tear interchange.

Lenses with spherical back optic zones and toroidal peripheral zones

These lenses are frequently used as a means of attempting to improve the physical fit of a lens on an astigmatic cornea without the optical complications inherent in the use of lenses with toroidal back optic zones.

Table 14.1 Fitting set of toroidal back surface corneal lenses, but with two final spherical peripheral curves

Toroidal BOZR (mm)	: BOZD (mm)	Toroidal BPR_1 (mm)	: BPD_1 (mm)	Spherical BPR_2 (mm)	: BPD_2 (mm)	Spherical BPR_3 (mm)	: TD (mm)
7.00×7.60	: 7.00/	7.55×8.30	: 7.80/	8.70	: 8.60/	9.30	: 9.00
7.10×7.70		7.70×8.45		8.90		9.60	
7.20×7.80		7.80×8.55		9.00		9.90	
7.30×7.90		7.95×8.70		9.20		10.10	
7.40×8.00		8.10×8.80		9.40		10.30	
7.50×8.10		8.20×8.95		9.60		10.50	
7.60×8.20		8.30×9.05		9.80		10.70	
7.70×8.30		8.45×9.25		10.00		11.00	
7.80×8.40		8.55×9.30		10.20		11.30	
7.90×8.50		8.70×9.50		10.30		11.50	
8.00×8.60		8.80×9.60		10.50		11.80	
7.00×8.00		7.55×8.80		9.10		9.90	
7.10×8.10		7.70×8.95		9.30		10.10	
7.20×8.20		7.80×9.05		9.50		10.30	
7.30×8.30		7.95×9.25		9.60		10.50	
7.40×8.40		8.10×9.30		9.80		10.80	
7.50×8.50		8.20×9.50		10.00		11.00	
7.60×8.60		8.30×9.60		10.30		11.30	
7.70×8.70		8.45×9.80		10.50		11.60	

BVP of all lenses: -3.00 D on flattest meridian

Since the BOZR of such a lens has to align as well as possible with a toroidal cornea, these lenses are usually fitted fairly small and centrally rather steeper than the flatter corneal meridian. Many practitioners favour fitting steeper than the flatter keratometer reading by about one-third of the difference between the keratometer readings. Back optic zone diameters are usually around 6.5 mm, with a commonly encountered range of between 6.0 and 7.0 mm. Total diameters tend to be between 8.5 and 9.5 mm, with larger values being used for RGP lenses.

The toroidal peripheral zones are chosen in much the same way as when fitting lenses with all toroidal back surface curves. The practitioner, however, is using a spherical BOZR and is able to observe his fitting set lenses on the cornea with fluorescein. Observing the peripheral fit along the flatter corneal meridian, assists the choice of an appropriate radius or radii for the steeper peripheral meridian by consideration of the keratometer reading and/or the fluorescein pattern.

A typical case might be as follows:

K readings: 8.00 mm along 180
                7.40 mm along 90
BOZR chosen: 7.80 mm

Consider the philosophies of peripheral fitting by practitioners A and B in Example 1 (p. 507).

Both *A* and *B* might find that a fitting lens with a BOZR of 7.90 mm gives good alignment and peripheral fit in the 180 meridian.

If the optimum BOZD and TD were chosen to be 6.5 mm and 9.5 mm respectively, the final specifications might be as follows:

Practitioner A
C2/7.80:6.50/8.90:9.50
              8.30

Practitioner B:
C4/7.80:6.50/8.40:7.50/8.90:8.50/9.40:9.50
              7.80   8.30   8.80

These lenses have a vertical oval back optic zone such as that illustrated in *Figure 14.1*.

This type of lens can be very useful in certain cases where a fully spherical lens is not adequate, but the toroidal peripheral zones are, at best, only an attempt at a compromise. Such lenses frequently rotate sufficiently to cause difficulty in stabilizing a correction for residual astigmatism or for keeping a bifocal addition in the correct position. They often rotate more than lenses with all toroidal back surface curves, and the steeper peripheral radii occasionally end up in close proximity to the flatter corneal meridian, thus causing slight corneal abuse. This occurs more often than in a lens utilizing a fully toroidal back surface.

It is comparatively easy to see if the lens is rotating much by observing the peripheral fit with fluorescein, but the inexperienced practitioner may find it helpful to have the steeper peripheral meridian marked with two dots, one at each edge of the lens. Two dots are much more useful than one for this purpose. Temporary dots may be put on with waterproof fibre pen.

Optical considerations of toroidal back optic zones

It is important that the fundamentals of the optics of contact lenses are understood if some of the complications of toroidal optic surfaces on corneal lenses are to be appreciated. With the advent of personal computers and programmable calculators the tedious calculations involved in determining the necessary radii and powers of these lenses are now no longer a problem (see Chapter 5). However, a basic understanding is still essential.

To help understand and perform some of the calculations needed in toric lens work the reader is referred to Chapter 5, particularly pp. 219–221, and also to *Optics of Contact Lenses*, 5th edition by A. G. Bennett (1985), and to *Contact Lens Optics* by W. A. Douthwaite (1987). This topic is, therefore, covered here in somewhat abbreviated form and consists mainly of the different approaches to the problems concerned.

The most useful basis for the consideration of toric corneas and lenses is Gullstrand's Schematic Eye (No. 1, Exact). The refractive indices used in this eye are:

Cornea   1.376
Tears   1.336
Aqueous   1.336

The tear lens does not, therefore, fully neutralize the refractive effect of the *front surface* of the cornea, as some imagine, but only 0.336/0.376 (approximately nine-tenths) of its power.

Considered in relation to contact lenses, this does not adversely affect the prescribing of a lens with a spherical back optic zone radius as any necessary correction may be worked on the front optic surface of the lens, but it does mean that only nine-tenths of the *front surface* corneal astigmatism is corrected by the tear lens, the remaining tenth probably in most cases being corrected by the back surface of the cornea, as shown below.

The back surface of the cornea is seldom considered as relevant to contact lens work, but it should be considered if all the optical complications of contact lens prescribing are to be appreciated.

It is difficult to know whether or not the back surface of the cornea follows the same trends in contour and shape as its front surface, but on the evidence available it seems reasonable to assume that there is at least a similarity.

If the back corneal surface does follow the same curve as the front surface, then the astigmatism created by the back surface is opposite in effect to that of the front surface. This can be seen in an example using Gullstrand's Schematic Eye (No. 1, Exact) and assuming a certain degree of corneal astigmatism (Westerhout, 1969; Bennett, 1985).

Assuming corneal astigmatism, with-the-rule, of 5% on the front surface and a similar contour on the back surface:

Front corneal surface

Vertical radius of curvature = 7.70 mm
Horizontal radius of curvature = 7.70 mm + 5%
= 8.085 mm

This is equivalent to

$$\frac{1000(1.376 - 1)}{7.70} - \frac{1000(1.376 - 1)}{8.085} \, \text{D}$$

astigmatism with-the-rule = 2.35 D   (1)

Corneal astigmatism measured with a keratometer calibrated for a nominal refractive index of 1.3375 is:

$$\frac{1000(1.3375 - 1)}{7.70} - \frac{1000(1.3375 - 1)}{8.085} \, \text{D}$$

astigmatism with-the-rule = 2.08 D
= approximately nine-tenths of (1) .... (3)

Back corneal surface

Vertical radius of curvature = 6.80 mm
Horizontal radius of curvature = 6.80 mm + 5%
= 7.14 mm

This is equivalent to

$$\frac{1000(1.336 - 1.376)}{6.80} - \frac{1000(1.336 - 1.376)}{7.14} \, \text{D}$$

astigmatism against-the-rule = 0.28 D   (2)

Note that (1) + (2) = 2.07 D
= (approximately) keratometer reading, 2.08 D   (3)

The tears then neutralize all but one-tenth of the front surface corneal astigmatism, and this is likely to be corrected by the back surface corneal astigmatism, which may be about equal to approximately one-tenth of the front surface astigmatism and opposite in effect.

The index of calibration of most keratometers (1.3375) is chosen to take this effect of the corneal back surface into account, in order to give the user a guide to the total refractive effect of the cornea.

In contact lens practice, this refractive index is very helpful because it is so close to that of the tears (1.336). Thus, the corneal astigmatism measured with the keratometer should be completely corrected by the liquid lens between the cornea and contact lens, provided the back of the contact lens is spherical (see Chapter 5, p. 205).

Expected residual astigmatism

If the practitioner measures a degree of corneal astigmatism which is very different from the cylinder element in the most accurate spectacle prescription, then a certain amount of residual astigmatism may be expected. The degree of this residual astigmatism should, in theory, be equal to the difference between the corneal astigmatism and spectacle astigmatism (provided that the vertex distance is allowed for). It is difficult, however, to think of an aspect of visual optics in which theory and practice are so far divorced. It is common to find an estimated residual astigmatism of over 1.00 D by calculation, only to discover that the actual residual astigmatism measured by refraction over a corneal lens is no more than 0.25–0.50 D.

Many examples of the lack of correlation between calculated and measured residual astigmatism can be quoted, and it has been estimated that in no more than 38% of eyes do the two closely approximate (Fairmaid, 1967).

This is due, in part, to the fact that the estimated residual error is based on measurement of corneal astigmatism over a small area of the corneal surface, whereas the refractive effect of the cornea is also influenced by other areas of the surface than those used by the keratometer.

The amount of residual astigmatism is also based on two measurements of astigmatism — one taken from spectacle refraction of the eye and the other taken from a refraction over a contact lens. These measurements are almost invariably fully or partly subjective, and are thus hardly scientifically measured quantities. It may well be that closer correlation between estimated and actual residual astigmatism would be found if the calculations were based on objective measurements of refraction with and without the lens in place. Retinoscope or eye refractometer measurements could be used, or perhaps a combination of both types. However, in practice, it is the subjective amount which is important.

Unfortunately, the term 'residual astigmatism' is often used loosely and is frequently confused with induced astigmatism or corneal astigmatism. Residual astigmatism has been variously defined (Goldberg, 1964) but may be said to be the astigmatic component of a lens required to fully correct an eye wearing a spherical powered hard contact lens with a spherical back optic zone radius. However, it is not quite as simple as this since the degree and axis of residual astigmatism varies with different lenses. If the parameters of the lens *in situ* for refraction are changed, then the measured residual astigmatism is also likely to alter. In particular, changing the back optic zone diameter, total diameter, amount of prism, back optic zone radius, thickness, and position on the cornea are likely to have a noticeable effect on the measured residual astigmatism.

When stating the degree of residual error, therefore, it is as well to state the specification of the lens through which the astigmatism has been measured.

Residual astigmatism is probably most commonly anatomical, the site of which may be in the cornea, crystalline lens or retina. The effect may be due to irregularities in the refractive index of the transparent media of the cornea and/or crystalline lens, or due to obliquity of one or more of the surfaces to the direction of the incident light.

Residual astigmatism measured over a lens having a spherical BOZR may also be induced by the following:

(1) An irregular tear film caused by a tilted or poorly centred lens.
(2) The obliquity of a tilted lens to the incident light.
(3) Irregular refractive index of the liquid lens caused by stagnation or partial evaporation of the tear liquid.

(4) Warping of a lens due to bad handling, or even under the influence of heavy lid pressure. The effects of the latter are discussed on p. 530 and in Chapter 5.

There are other factors which individually or collectively may have an influence on residual astigmatism (Goldberg, 1964), but the most important aspect of this subject is its clinical significance and correction, which is dealt with on p. 515.

Refraction with toroidal back optic zones

The main purpose of fitting such a lens is to obtain a good physical fit in cases of high or medium astigmatism. Unfortunately, its use is complicated by the introduction of induced astigmatism.

Induced astigmatism, in this context, may be taken as the astigmatic effect created in the contact lens/tear liquid system by the toroidal back optic zone bounding two surfaces of different refractive index — 1.49 and 1.336 (Westerhout, 1969), assuming a lens of PMMA material is used.

With rigid gas permeable materials, many of which have a lower refractive index than PMMA, varying from 1.445 to 1.49 (*see* Chapter 3, p. 117, *Table 3.5*), the amount of induced astigmatism is significantly less.

Induced astigmatism is introduced into the system every time toroidal back optic zone surfaces are used and, despite all the methods of attempting to reduce its effect, it remains one of the biggest problems to be overcome with this form of lens. It is due only to the lens/tear boundary, as the following example shows, and it occurs even though the liquid lens itself is of negligible power.

As with spherical lenses, the power of the contact lens in air, plus the power of the liquid lens in air, should add up to the ocular refraction, but with toric lenses the two separate meridians must be considered.

Example 2

Spectacle *Rx*: −2.00/−3.00 × 180
Keratometry: 8.20 mm along 180
7.70 mm along 90

An afocal corneal lens of BOZR 8.20 mm might be inserted and a refraction of −2.00 DS found with this lens *in situ*. (The back surface of the tears neutralizes the front and back surface corneal astigmatism as shown in Example 1.)

If, however, the lens is changed to one having a toroidal back optic zone to align with the cornea, the power of the surface combining the lens BOZR and tear liquid is as follows.

In the vertical meridian

Lens back surface power in air:

$$\frac{1000(1 - 1.49)}{+7.70} = -63.64\,\text{D}$$

Tear front surface power in air:

$$\frac{1000(1.336 - 1)}{+7.70} = +43.64\,\text{D}$$

Total power in vertical meridian = −20.00 D

In the horizontal meridian

Lens back surface power in air:

$$\frac{1000(1 - 1.49)}{+8.20} = -59.76\,\text{D}$$

Tear front surface power in air:

$$\frac{1000(1.336 - 1)}{+8.20} = +40.98\,\text{D}$$

Total power in horizontal meridian = −18.78 D

Total effect of lens/tear surface =
−18.78 DS with −1.22 DC × 180

The back surface of the tears remains unchanged in its effect.

Thus, if the front surface of the contact lens remains spherical, a spectacle lens of +1.22 DC × 180 is needed in front of the contact lens to fully correct the eye. (With an RGP material of refractive index 1.45, a reduced cylinder of +0.90 DC × 180 would be needed.)

It is possible for this cylinder to be added to the front surface of the contact lens; but this addition, although easy to calculate and prescribe, is often very difficult to fabricate in the laboratory and its effect in practice is not always as anticipated.

It is worth noting at this point that Example 2 deals with the most commonly encountered type of case — namely, corneal and spectacle astigmatism with-the-rule. The induced astigmatism is, however, against-the-rule (positive cylinder axis horizontal), which is of the same form that the majority of residual astigmatism takes.

It is often thought that the induced astigmatism created by using a toroidal back optic zone surface on an eye with corneal astigmatism and residual astigmatism will fortuitously cancel out the residual astigmatism. In practice, however, this is most unlikely to occur in more than a few cases. Indeed, the induced astigmatism usually exaggerates the effect of the residual astigmatism.

Very occasionally, however, an example of induced and residual astigmatism cancelling out one another is encountered, as in the following case met in practice.

Keratometry:
RE   8.03 mm along 147, 7.65 mm along 57
LE   8.07 mm along 27, 7.57 mm along 117

Residual astigmatism over spherical lenses:
RE -1.00 DC $\times$ 130
LE -1.25 DC $\times$ 45

Calculated induced astigmatism with aligned toroidal back optic zone:
RE -0.95 DC $\times$ 147
LE -1.26 DC $\times$ 27
i.e. this virtually cancels out the residual error.

Actual total residual error measured over lenses with toroidal back optic zones:
RE -0.25 DC $\times$ 75
LE   plano

In the calculation of induced astigmatism, it is not necessary to go to the trouble of calculating the surface powers in air for plastics and tears separately. It is quicker to use the appropriate radii considered with the change in refractive effect travelling from plastics to tears, i.e. power of PMMA lens/tear boundary:

$$= \frac{1000(1.336 - 1.49)}{r}$$

$$= \frac{-1000(0.154)}{r}$$

$$= \frac{-154}{r}$$

where r = radius in mm.

By subtracting the values found of $-154/r$ for one principal meridian from the other, the value for the induced astigmatism may be obtained directly. With RGP materials of refractive index less than 1.49, the figure of $-1.54/r$ no longer applies; for example a refractive index of 1.45 would yield a figure of $114/r$ for determining the surface power at the lens/tear boundary.

Reference to Appendix B, *Table B.I*, which gives surface powers for various radii and refractive index differences, enables the induced astigmatism to be determined from the surface

powers in the two principal meridians. If PMMA is being used the astigmatic difference can be obtained directly from Appendix B, *Table B.VIII*, making the calculations in Example 2 unnecessary.

In Example 2 it is useful to consider the power of the final bi-toric lens in steps:

Power meridians shown relative to back optic zone meridians:

Spherical front surface — giving -2.00 D on 8.20 mm BOZR

Back surface lens astigmatism

$$= \frac{1000(1 - 1.49)}{8.20} - \frac{1000(1 - 1.49)}{7.70}$$

$$= -3.88 \text{ DC} \times 180$$

Thus total power $= -5.88$ D on 7.70 mm BOZR

This is shown diagrammatically in *Figure 14.4a*.

Lens after adding $+1.22$ DC $\times$ 180 *to front surface* (*Figure 14.4b*):

Powers   are -2.00 D on 8.20 mm BOZR
         and -4.66 D on 7.70 mm BOZR

(In practice, $+1.25$ DC would be added.)

In this example, the lens described should give a reasonable visual acuity with very little residual error.

It is frequently thought that a bi-toric lens should not rotate at all, or certainly not more than a few degrees (Capelli, 1964). It is also felt by many practitioners that such a lens, when it does rotate, creates a visually disturbing, constantly changing cylindrical correction before the eye. In fact, however, in the type of case given in this example, the correction for induced astigmatism is only necessary because the toroidal back optic zone creates the induced astigmatism along its principal meridians. With such a lens, made with a spherical front surface, the axis of the induced astigmatism depends only on the position of the principal meridians of the back optic zone before the eye. With the lens under discussion, if it rotates until the 8.20 mm BOZR lies along the 45 meridian, then the axis of the $+1.22$ DC is also required along this meridian. If, therefore, the front surface cylinder power is ground on to the lens in the correct meridian relative to the principal meridians of the back optic zone, then it does not matter if the lens does rotate as the lens carries its correction for induced astigmatism with it when it moves away from its intended position. This is worth

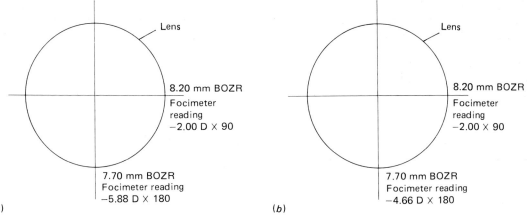

Figure 14.4 (*a*) Focimeter readings of a toric lens with BOZR 8.20 × 7.70 mm and BVP −2.00 D along the flatter meridian. (*b*) Focimeter readings of the same lens shown in (*a*) with +1.22 DC × 180 added to the front surface. (Note: focimeter targets are invariably in focus along a *power axis, not* a *power meridian*)

remembering when correcting an eye with a bi-toric lens containing a front surface cylinder for the correction of induced astigmatism only, i.e. a 'compensated bi-toric' contact lens.

It may well be that many practitioners believe that bi-toric lenses must not rotate, due to their experiences when refracting over lenses with toroidal back optic zone surfaces and spherical front zone surfaces. When refracting over such a lens, the cylinder addition is frequently found to fluctuate in axis with the lens rotation. This gives the impression that the lens must not be permitted to rotate, but this does not matter once the correction for induced astigmatism is ground on the front of the lens in the appropriate meridian as the correcting cylinder then rotates with the surface inducing the astigmatism.

Most eyes, however, do have some residual astigmatism. Therefore, while going to the trouble of having a front surface cylinder ground on to the lens to make it bi-toric, it is good practice in certain cases to incorporate a correction for residual astigmatism (*see* calculations on p. 520). When this is done, however, the lens must not rotate more than a few degrees as the axis of correction for the residual astigmatism remains fixed in relation to the eye. This limitation on rotation is important, for when residual astigmatism is of a low degree, from the clinical standpoint, then it is not worth while incorporating its correction with that for the induced astigmatism.

For residual astigmatism of 0.50 D or more, if the patient can obtain good visual acuity without its correction, it is probably not worth while adding a front surface cylinder to correct more than the calculated induced astigmatic error. If, however, the residual astigmatism is clinically significant, then it is worth incorporating provided that lens rotation can be kept to a minimum (*Figures 14.5* and *14.6*).

Probably the easiest method of estimating the significance of the induced and residual astigmatic errors is not by calculation but by the use

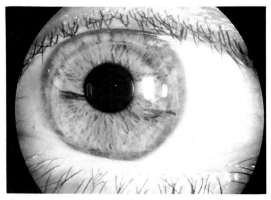

Figure 14.5 A left lens with a toroidal back optic zone fitted in alignment. Keratometer reading: 8.16 mm along 175, 7.60 mm along 85. Lens BOZR 8.15 × 7.60 mm. The 8.15 meridian is marked with grease pencil and can be seen aligning well with the 175 meridian. There is no significant rotation, thus permitting accurate correction of residual astigmatism, as well as induced astigmatism, with a front surface cylinder

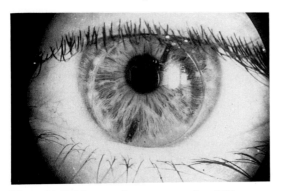

Figure 14.6 Right eye — keratometer reading: 8.27 mm along 175, 7.70 mm along 85. BOZR 8.25 × 7.70 mm with 8.25 meridian marked with grease pencil. This should be located along the 175 meridian, but, as shown, this lens rotates badly, thus permitting only the accurate correction of induced astigmatism with a front surface cylinder

of a fitting set of lenses with toroidal back optic zones, as mentioned previously. Frequently, a discrepancy is found between the estimated and actual effects. If the refraction over such a lens reveals an astigmatic component not more than 0.50 D different from the calculated induced astigmatism, then it is almost certainly not worth while adding more than a correction for the latter to the front surface of the lens. A great deal also depends on the amount of rotation of the toroidal back surface of the trial lens used. If such trial lenses are not available, it is reasonable to expect lenses with a small difference between the principal back optic zone radii to rotate more than lenses with a large difference.

The value of trial fitting lenses with toroidal back optic zone surfaces cannot be over-estimated and, almost invariably, it is found that the best visual results are obtained where they have been used. They certainly help to obviate the need for resolving obliquely crossed cylinders, which frequently needs to be done in calculating the powers required.

For example, in the case just considered, a refraction is performed over the BOZR 8.20 mm × 7.70 mm (with a spherical front surface giving −2.00 D along the 8.20 mm meridian):

Refraction +2.00 DC × 30

The lens does not rotate more than a few degrees and, thus, the full cylinder effect is desired on the front surface.

It may be best to order the lens by sketching the requirements as shown in *Figure 14.7a,b*.

It may also be useful to calculate the resolved effect and give the laboratory the final focimeter reading and axis expected. Laboratories often seem to have difficulty in working this out and it must not be forgotten that some contact lens technicians are not familiar with standard notation and the transposition of sphero-cylinders and are confused by the fact that focimeter targets are in focus along the power axis and not the power meridian.. An unambiguous order is therefore very helpful.

It is important to have clear marks on the lenses to denote the position of one of the principal meridians of the back surface. These marks should be permanent as they provide a check on the amount of rotation with the lens *in situ* and also provide an axis of orientation about

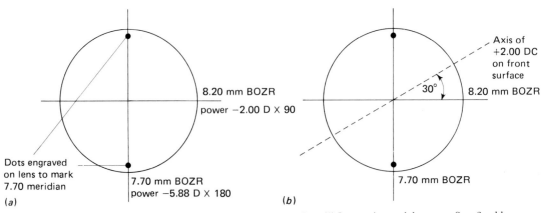

Figure 14.7 (*a*) Instructions to laboratory. Step 1: spherical front surface. (*b*) Instructions to laboratory. Step 2: add +2.00 DC × 30

which the accuracy of the powers and axes of the surfaces produced by the laboratory can be checked.

Some laboratories mark the axis with fluorescent dots which show up under ultraviolet illumination. These are not as good as permanent marks as they are removed when a front surface cylinder is added. The best marking is a pair of engraved dots along the steepest (shortest) back surface meridian. This is the thicker meridian near the periphery and usually has ample substance for such engraving. The small pits fill with fluorescein, and during examination with ultraviolet illumination they thus provide an easily visible reference meridian.

Calculation of the salient points in bi-toric hard corneal lens work follows in the form of examples.

Example 3: Calculating the back vertex power of a bi-toric lens

Spectacle refraction (vertex distance ignored):
−2.00/−3.00 × 180

Keratometer reading: 8.10 mm, 41.62 D along 180
7.60 mm, 44.37 D along 90

A contour, multi-curve or similar trial lens is placed on the cornea and the fit is examined along the flattest corneal curve (horizontal). The peripheral fit is examined in this meridian only to select the appropriate peripheral radii.

Having chosen an appropriate spherical lens to fit this meridian (say, for example, C2/8.10:6.50/ 8.70:9.00/−2.00 D) then a refraction with this lens *in situ* is carried out.

Spectacle refraction and visual acuity with contact lens: plano, 6/6 (no residual astigmatism)

Rx along 180 meridian: C2/8.10:6.50/8.70:9.00/ −2.00 D

This lens is approximately in alignment with the horizontal meridian, and from the keratometer reading the BOZR 7.60 mm might be chosen to fit the vertical meridian.

The front surface of the tear lens has radii of: 8.10 mm in the horizontal, 7.60 mm in the vertical.

Knowing this, the power of the front surface of the tear lens is calculated from its refractive index (1.336). Thus (*see* Appendix B, *Table B.V*):

$$F = \frac{(1.336 - 1)1000}{r}$$

Tears: dioptric value of 7.60 mm radius = +44.21 D
Tears: dioptric value of 8.10 mm radius = +41.48 D
Therefore, tear lens front surface astigmatism =
+2.73 D = C × 180

The steeper meridian is more positive in power by this amount. Therefore, total lens power required in the vertical meridian is:

−2.00 D + (−2.73 D) = −4.73 D

Final *Rx* of lens:

BOZR 8.10 m 180, −2.00 D
BOZR 7.60 m 90, −4.75 D

Since the principal meridians of the front and back toroidal surfaces have the same orientation the full specification of the lens is as follows.

C2 Parallel bi-toric/8.10 m 180:6.50/8.70:9.00
          7.60   8.20
−2.00/−2.75 × 180

This represents the same power as the spectacle refraction had vertex distance been taken into account. This is what is expected when the BOZRs correspond to the corneal radii, for the liquid lens power is then negligible.

Example 4

If refraction with the 8.10 mm − 2.00 D lens used in Example 3 had been plano/−1.00 × 90 then power along flattest meridian (180) = −3.00 D. Required meridional powers with 8.10 mm BOZR are as shown in *Figure 14.8*.

Consider the steepest meridian (as in Example 3) with BOZR 7.60 m 90:

Converting radii to dioptres (*n* = 1.336)
7.60 mm   = +44.21 D
8.10 mm   = +41.48 D
Difference = +2.73 D

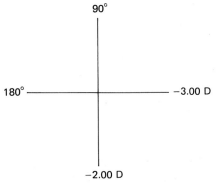

Figure 14.8 Meridional powers required in Example 4

Refraction along 90 with 8.10 mm BOZR = -2.00 D
(*see above*)
Along this meridian, the liquid lens is more positive
by $+2.73$ D
Therefore, additional BVP required along 90 =
-2.73 D

Therefore, required power along 90 = -4.73 D

Full *Rx* = 8.10 m 180, -3.00 D
    7.60 m 90, -4.73 D

In Examples 3 and 4, the powers specified are
the back vertex powers of the bi-toric lens in the
appropriate meridians. These are the powers
read by the laboratory when checking the lens
on a focimeter if the image quality is good
enough.

Example 5

Keratometer readings not known. Bi-toric specification is based on spectacle *Rx* and trial corneal lenses
with spherical BOZR.

Spectacle *Rx* = $-2.00/-3.00 \times 45$
(vertex distance ignored)

As in previous examples, the flattest meridian is
fitted in a conventional manner with a spherical
BOZR and a refraction is performed with such a lens
in situ. This enables the corneal radii to be
determined.

Flattest meridian (*45*)
BOZR of trial contact lens used = 7.70 mm (power
-2.00 DS)

Spectacle addition over this trial lens = -1.00 DS
with no residual astigmatism

Total required power with 7.70 mm BOZR =
-3.00 DS

Therefore, liquid lens power = $+1.00$ D

But liquid lens front surface power of the 7.70 mm
meridian ($n = 1.336$) = $+43.64$ D

Therefore, liquid lens back surface power ($+1.00$ D
-43.64 D) = -42.64 D

Therefore, radius of back surface of liquid lens ($n =$
1.336) = 7.88 mm

This must be the same as the corneal radius.
Therefore, BOZR chosen to align with flattest corneal
radius for a bi-toric lens might thus be 7.90 mm. *Rx* in
this 45 meridian: 7.90 mm, -2.00 D.

Steepest meridian (135)
Flattest meridian of 7.88 mm radius has a power of
42.64 D for $n = 1.336$. Spectacle *Rx* indicates corneal
astigmatism (no residual astigmatism detected)

corrected by -3.00 DC $\times$ 45, which has all been
corrected by the liquid lens.

Thus, the 135 meridian must be steeper than the 45
meridian by approximately this amount, and the back
surface of the liquid lens has a power along 135 =
-42.64 D -3.00 D = -45.64 D. Therefore, liquid
lens radius along 135 = 7.36 mm ($n = 1.336$) and
corneal radius = 7.36 mm.

The BOZR chosen for alignment along 135
meridian might thus be 7.35 mm. Power required for
correction of refractive error in this meridian is power
required along 45 meridian plus power of liquid lens
cylinder

$$= -2.00 \text{ D} + (-3.00 \text{ D}) = -5.00 \text{ D}$$

Therefore, *Rx* for steepest meridian (7.35 mm) =
-5.00 D.
Complete lens *Rx* with BOZR and back vertex
powers in the meridians appropriate to the radii is:

7.90 m 45, -2.00 D
7.35 m 135, -5.00 D

This is the same as the spectacle *Rx*.
If residual astigmatism had been found when
refracting with the original 7.70 mm BOZR -2.00 DS
lens *in situ*, an allowance would merely have to be
made for this when calculating the corneal astigmatism.
If the refraction over this lens had been $-1.00/$
-1.00×45, then clearly -1.00 D of the -3.00 DC $\times$
45 spectacle *Rx* would not have been due to corneal
astigmatism, and thus the correction for corneal
astigmatism would have been estimated at -2.00 DC
$\times$ 45.
Thus, the 135 meridian would be steeper than the
45 meridian by 2.00 D and its power would be

$$+42.64 \text{ D} + 2.00 \text{ D} = +44.64 \text{ D}$$

Therefore, radius of 135 meridian = 7.53 mm.

If residual astigmatism is measured in negative
cylinder form and has its axis parallel to the
negative cylinder axis in the spectacle *Rx*, then
the estimated corneal astigmatism is reduced by
the amount of the residual astigmatism. If the
residual negative cylinder axis is perpendicular
to the negative cylinder axis in the spectacle *Rx*,
then the estimated corneal astigmatism is
increased by the amount of the residual
astigmatism. Unfortunately, the calculations
involved are not always quite as simple as those
shown above. It is rare, for example, for the axis
of the residual astigmatism to correspond
exactly with one of the principal meridians of
curvature of the cornea. This means that

resolution of obliquely crossed cylinders is frequently necessary before completing the calculations. It is also rare for the estimated corneal astigmatism, as in the last example, to agree with the corneal astigmatism found with the keratometer. In clinical practice, it is unusual for residual astigmatism, measured by refraction through a spherical corneal lens, to equal exactly that expected from consideration of the spectacle correction and keratometer readings.

The calculations so far have not considered the effect of vertex distance, which must be taken into account if this distance is great or if the refractive power in either meridian exceeds 3.00 D.

It is frequently useful, in considering bi-toric lenses, to draw a representation of meridional powers to ensure that simple errors in confusing axes and meridians are not made. A slightly more complicated example is now shown, in which the BOZRs of the toric lens do not exactly agree with the principal corneal radii, and the axes of the spectacle refraction do not correspond with the principal meridians of corneal curvature.

Example 6

Spectacle $Rx = -4.50/-3.50 \times 180$
Vertex distance = 14 mm
Ocular refraction = $-4.23\,DC \times 90$, $-7.19\,DC \times 180$
Ocular astigmatism = $-2.96\,DC \times 180$
Meridional powers (ocular refraction) are shown in *Figure 14.9*.

Keratometer reading: 8.50 mm along 20
8.05 mm along 110

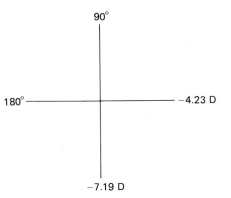

Figure 14.9 Meridional powers required in Example 5

BOZR chosen for the toroidal back surface of the lens:

8.45 mm on 20
8.10 mm on 110

Surface powers of tear lens in air given by

$$F = \frac{(1.336 - 1)1000}{r}$$

Power of back surface of tear lens (taken from keratometer radii)

= -39.53 D along 20,
-41.74 D along 110

Front surface power of tear lens (taken from lens BOZR)

= $+39.76$ D along 20,
$+41.48$ D along 110

Tear lens total power

= $+0.23$ D along 20,
-0.26 D along 110
= $+0.23/-0.49 \times 20$

Back vertex power required on bi-toric lens to correct ametropia = ocular refraction − power of tear lens

Back vertex power with:

BOZR 8.45 mm on 20
8.10 mm on 110
= $-7.19/+2.96 \times 90$
$-(+0.23/-0.49 \times 20)$
= $-7.42/+2.96 \times 90$ with
$+0.49 \times 20$

These oblique cylinders must be resolved (*see* Stokes' construction: Stokes, 1883) (*Figure 14.10*).

Sphere/cylinder effect of resolved cylinders = $+0.41/+2.62 \times 86.5$

Total back vertex power of bi-toric lens = $-7.01/+2.62 \times 86.5$

This type of lens specification is very interesting but difficult for the laboratory to interpret and convert to lens fabrication specifications.

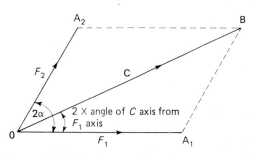

Figure 14.10 Stokes' construction

This prescription for a lens involves the principal meridians of the back optic zone oblique to the principal meridians of the back vertex power (an oblique bi-toric contact lens). The greatest use of such a specification is to allow the laboratory to mount the final bi-toric lens on a focimeter with the toroidal back optic zone surface orientated along the appropriate axes in order to check the focimeter readings against the back vertex power ordered.

In the case of Example 6, there are three different pairs of principal meridians relative to the horizontal meridian. The toroidal back optic zone has principal meridians at 20 and 110, the back vertex power at 86.5 and 176.5 and those of the toroidal front surface are different again — all this on a thin piece of plastic with an optic zone diameter of between 6.00 mm and 7.50 mm. It should not be difficult to understand the problems involved in both making and checking such lenses.

Stokes' construction

This is an excellent method of resolving two cylinders F_1 and F_2, with an angle between their axes of α, into an equivalent sphere/cylinder power (*Figure 14.10*).

A parallelogram is constructed with the two sides OA_1 and OA_2 proportional to F_1 and F_2, with the angle between them 2α

The parallelogram is completed and the resultant OB drawn. This is proportional to the resultant cylinder C. The angle between OB and OA_1 being twice the angle between the axis of C and that of F_1, where

S = equivalent sphere
C = equivalent cylinder
S = ½ $(F_1 + F_2 - C)$

Another approach to the calculation of the final power of bi-toric lenses is shown in Example 7.

Example 7

In this example, all measurements and quantities are rounded off to clinically significant amounts, and it is assumed to be a PMMA lens.

Keratometer reading:
7.65 mm, 44.12 D along 90
8.16 mm, 41.37 D along 180

Spherical trial lens (BOZR 8.15 mm) placed on cornea, BVP = −2.25 DS

Refraction through lens = −1.50/−1.00 × 180

Thus, total power through 8.15 mm lens = −3.75/−1.00 × 180

BOZR 8.15 mm × 7.65 mm used for final lens

These radii give induced astigmatism = −1.25 × 180

Therefore, cylinder power to be placed on front surface of lens = +0.25 × 180   (a)

Sphere power required = −3.75 D   (b)

Cylindrical effect of back surface of lens (measured in air) = −4.00 × 180 (c)

Thus, final total power of lens = a + b + c = −3.75/−3.75 × 180

It is also possible to calculate the power of a bi-toric lens by considering a theoretical emmetropic cornea (Capelli, 1964) as shown in Example 8.

Example 8

Keratometer reading:
7.42 mm, 45.50 D along 90
7.94 mm, 42.50 D along 180
Corneal power = +42.50/+3.00 × 180
Ocular refraction = −3.00/−1.50 × 180

Thus, theoretical corneal power to produce emmetropia = +39.50/+1.50 × 180

Back surface power of lens (BOZR 7.95 mm × 7.40 mm) plastic/tear boundary (relative n = 0.154) = −19.37/−1.44 × 180

Therefore, required front surface power of lens = +58.87/+2.94 × 180

Back surface power of lens in air (BOZR 7.95 mm × 7.40 mm) = −61.64/−4.58 × 180

And final total lens power = −2.75/−1.62 × 180

Toroidal front surfaces combined with spherical back optic zones

Residual astigmatism frequently needs to be corrected in cases where the patient is fitted well, physically, with a lens utilizing a spherical back optic zone. Such a lens therefore requires a toroidal front surface but must not be allowed to rotate sufficiently to cause the changing cylinder effect to give rise to visual discomfort.

Rotation is normally prevented by the use of prism ballast or by the use of truncation to align with the lower or upper lids, or both.

Prism ballast is most commonly used and the lens is prescribed in the normal manner with the addition of between 1 and 3 Δ. When ordering the lens, some practitioners assume that the weight or prism ballast orientates the lens in a certain fixed position on the cornea and order the cylinder axis with respect to this position.

Alternatively, the lens can be made without the front cylinder but with the position of the prism base marked with a small permanent dot. The spherical power is calculated to give the necessary cylinder in positive form. A refraction is performed over the lens *in situ* and the average position of the dot in normal, common directions of gaze is estimated. The laboratory is then asked to add the residual refractive error — expressed in positive cylinder form — to the front of the lens, using the dot position as a point of reference for the cylinder axis.

To avoid recording the prism base position as 'down along 90' or 'down along 100', its actual location is recorded as being at 270 or 280 respectively.

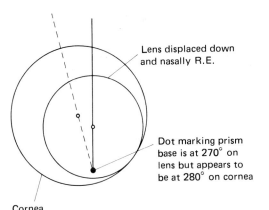

Figure 14.11 The importance of the position of the prism base–apex line is indicated relative to the lens when the latter is off-centre. The position of the prism base relative to the cornea is irrelevant

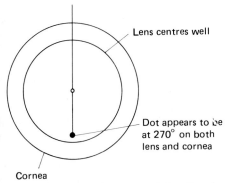

Figure 14.12 If the lens centres well then the prism base–apex line is at the same angle with respect to either the lens or cornea

It is important to realize that it is the angular position of the dot on the lens that is significant and not the position of the dot on the cornea. This is illustrated in *Figures 14.11* and *14.12*.

It is difficult to assess accurately the position of the dot on the lens. One of the best methods is to photograph the lens on the cornea in the desired direction of gaze and enlarge the photographs, or project slides on to a screen where they can be superimposed on a protractor and the angle measured easily and accurately. These photographs are easily taken through slit lamp biomicroscopes with photographic attachments.

The illustrations in this chapter were taken from transparencies obtained in this manner.

This type of photograph can be useful for assessing the angle of eyelid contact with the lens and for measuring the eye if an appropriate scale is photographed. A lens of known total diameter *in situ* acts as a useful unit on which to base measurements.

The most commonly used method of assessing the axis taken up by the prism base–apex line is to place a trial frame before the eye and hold a transparent ruler through the dot and through the middle of the lens. Alternatively, a transparent plastic disc or afocal trial case lens, with a diagonal line finely drawn upon it, can be placed in the frame and rotated until the line passes through the dot and contact lens centre. The angles are read from the trial frame protractor.

It must not be forgotten that it is impossible to add a negative front surface cylinder to the lens without transposing to positive cylinder form and altering the sphere power. Only positive cylinders, therefore, should be prescribed.

If it is intended to use a prism ballasted lens with a toroidal front surface, it is important when refracting to use a trial lens with almost identical specifications to the lens to be prescribed. BOZR, BOZD and TD should be the same, if possible. The trial lens should also contain the appropriate amount of prism, if such a lens is available. It is common to measure different degrees of residual astigmatism with lenses of different specifications, as the following case record shows.

Mrs R. C. (left eye)

Keratometer reading: 8.03 mm along 180
7.86 mm along 90

Spectacle refraction: −5.00/−0.50 × 95

Rx over trial lens,
C4/8.00:6.50/8.50:7.50/9.00:8.50/9.50:9.50/−2.00 D
= −2.50/−1.50 × 95, VA = 6/6

Prescription lens made up to the following:
C4/8.00:6.50/8.50:7.50/9.00:8.50/9.50:9.50/−6.00 D
with 1 Δ base-down

Refraction with this lens = +1.00/−0.50 × 75, VA
= 6/6

Refraction with
C4/8.00:7.00/8.50:7.80/9.00:8.60/9.50:9.50/−5.00 D
= +0.25/−1.50 × 100, VA = 6/6 (no prism ballast
used)

Ideally, the contact lens with which to measure residual astigmatism should be worn for a few hours for several consecutive days and refraction carried out on each occasion. The measured degree and axis of astigmatism is often found to change significantly during this period.

A fitting set of prism ballasted lenses is very useful in order to assess likely prism position. If the position of the prism appears stable and predictable, then a lens can often be made up

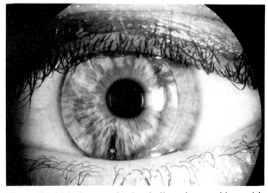

Figure 14.13 Right eye and prism ballasted corneal lens with base–apex along an average angle of 100°

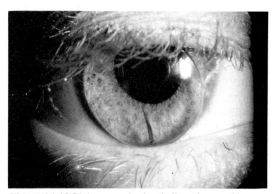

Figure 14.14 Left eye and prism ballasted corneal lens with base–apex along an average angle of 80°

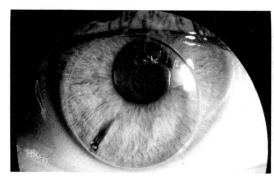

Figure 14.15 Right eye and prism ballasted lens with base–apex along 35° (prism base at 215°). This is some 45° off the expected position

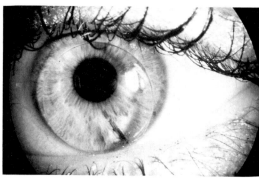

Figure 14.16 Left eye and prism ballasted lens with base–apex along an angle of 120°. This is some 40° off the expected position

straight away with both prism and front toroidal surface, missing out the intermediate stage.

It is difficult to predict the final position of the prism base and the effect of the nasal rise of the lower lid. This latter has been estimated at 10–15° (Fairmaid, 1967), while the former has been quoted as being 20° displacement nasally (Goldberg, 1964) and 10° nasally (Westerhout, 1971a). The differences in these figures may be accounted for by the fact that the authorities quoted used different lens designs, sizes, thicknesses and amounts of prism ballast.

One of the disadvantages of fitting a prism ballasted lens with a spherical front surface and subsequently adding a front cylinder is that the altered lighter lens may well take up an entirely different position on the cornea — especially if a positive cylinder is added with its axis horizontal, thus thinning the upper and lower edges. The influence of the lids may well be altered.

The average positions of the prism base and wide variations from the normal are shown in *Figures 14.13–14.16*.

It will be seen from the variations shown in *Figures 14.15* and *14.16* that it is unwise to place too much reliance on the expected positions of the prism base unless a trial prism ballasted lens has been observed after several hours of use.

If the patient has an occupation involving unusual positions of gaze, the prism base position should also be observed with the eyes held in an appropriate direction. If the direction of gaze influences the dot position greatly, consideration must be given to this fact in prescribing the cylinder axis on the lens.

When asking the laboratory to add a front cylinder at a certain axis, it is worth drawing a sketch showing the corrected position of the axis with the dot at 6 o'clock (or at 270). If, for example, the dot marking the ballast position is found to settle at 280 and the required cylinder axis is 120, the axis is ordered as 110 with the dot at 6 o'clock (at 270).

It should be mentioned that a lens which is physically comfortable before the cylinder is added to the front surface frequently becomes uncomfortable after the addition of the toroidal surface. This is usually because the addition of a cylinder has materially altered the edge finish and this may not have been reworked and repolished sufficiently. Since the upper edge of a prism ballasted lens is very thin, it may well be worth while ordering the original lens about 0.2 mm larger in total diameter to allow for re-edging after the cylinder is added. This same suggestion remains valid even if the lens is not prism ballasted.

A common laboratory error is to mark the dot some way off the position of the prism base. This does not matter greatly provided that the cylinder axis is prescribed relative to the dot, which should remain visible so that the added cylinder axis can be checked.

Checking hard toric lenses

Although covered in Chapter 12, a brief resumé of verification techniques for hard toric lenses is appropriate here, with elaboration of certain points. Many of the parameters of toric lenses are checked as for spherical lenses. Total diameter and thickness are measured in the conventional way, not forgetting that truncated lenses need to have their total diameter dimensions measured along the major and minor axes,

and the edge finish in the truncated area should be checked to ensure that it is satisfactory. Similarly, lenses with spherical back optic zones and toroidal peripheral zones, or vice versa, should have both diameters of the back optic zone measured. Lenses with toroidal back optic zones and toroidal peripheral zones may also appear to have slightly oval back optic zones, if the difference between the two BOZRs is very large, or the difference between BOZR and peripheral radius in one meridian is different from that in the other meridian.

Toroidal back optic zone surfaces are usually measured on a radiuscope, and as in focimetry, it is useful to remember that on most instruments the line in focus is at right-angles to the meridian whose radius is being measured when the target image is formed at the centre of curvature. (In order to locate the meridians accurately, the lens must be rotated until one of the target lines is sharply in focus.) This is probably the reason why the dots marking the required meridian are so often found at right-angles to their correct position. The dots are also often found 5–15° off the true meridian, even if the meridian approximates to the required one. This may well be due to the fact that it is difficult to mount a lens on a radiuscope lens holder in such a way as to facilitate the exact marking of the meridians. It is better for the laboratory to mark the lens directly, with respect to the axis of the holding device, while the lens is mounted for cutting and polishing the BOZR. Unfortunately, not all laboratories have efficient methods of cutting and polishing toroidal surfaces and some still resort to a flexed lens (i.e. one in which the lens is physically distorted, or bent, to give the required astigmatic surface: it is then cut to a spherical curvature and, when the pressure on the lens is released, it slowly returns to its original state and assumes an equal but opposite astigmatic surface to that produced by the bending).

It is difficult for the checking to be done with the meridian-identification dots at an exactly set position on the radiuscope lens holder. If the lens has a toroidal back optic zone, the best procedure is to measure the radii on a radiuscope and check the meridians of the radii relative to the dots by mounting the lens on a keratometer. There are many methods of mounting the lens. A simple one, shown in *Figure 14.17*, is to place the lens on a 45°

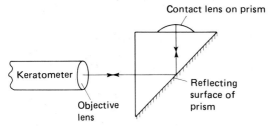

Figure 14.17 The use of a 45° reflecting prism to position a contact lens in order to measure its BOZR and principal meridians with a keratometer

reflecting prism. The lens is then adjusted until the dots appear horizontal. This can be done by marking permanent lines on the prism, which remain horizontal with the prism in position. The keratometer is racked forward to focus the lens and dots while the lens is being adjusted. The instrument is then moved back to focus on the mire images, and the radii and their axes are read off on the keratometer protractor scale. With the magnification provided by the keratometer and the use of its accurate protractor scale, far greater accuracy can be achieved than with the radiuscope alone. Even a rotation test using a crossed line chart does not provide a high degree of accuracy.

One difficulty which is hard to overcome is that on a small lens the dots themselves subtend quite a large angle.

The keratometer and prism mount are also useful for checking the actual cylinder power added to the front surface of a lens. The lens point of reference (dot or dots) is mounted in a set position, which is checked by focusing on the lens surface. The front surface radii and axes of their meridians are then measured with the lens mounted on water to prevent reflections from the back surface. The radii are then converted to dioptric power using a refractive index of 1.49 if PMMA is used — *see* Appendix B, *Table B.II.* (The dioptric scale on the keratometer cannot be used.) This is an excellent way of measuring the added cylinder. The focimeter is very useful for checking toric corneal lenses, but it does have several disadvantages. The main disadvantage is that the focimeter images are rarely perfectly clear and are usually considerably off-centre due to the prisms often used. If the lens is bi-toric, the relatively small front surface cylinder is completely dwarfed by the invariably much larger back surface cylinder, which does

not need to be checked since it is automatically created by the toroidal back optic zone surface. It is also difficult to mount the reference points in a precise position on the focimeter.

It is common to find discrepancies between front cylinder measurements taken with the keratometer and focimeter. If there is a discrepancy, it is often found that the keratometer reading is more compatible with the result obtained from refraction with the lens *in situ*.

Some examples found in clinical practice serve to illustrate this point. To simplify the examples, the peripheral radii are not specified.

Miss M. (left eye)
All lenses of TD 9.50 mm and BOZD 7.00 mm
Spectacle refraction: −1.00/−2.00 × 80
Trial lens: 8.00 mm BOZR, −2.00 D, Add = −1.25 × 85
Lens ordered: 8.00 mm BOZR, −2.00 D 1 Δ (base dotted)
Rx with this lens: +0.50/−2.00 × 85, dot at 265
This power added as −1.50/+2.00 × 175 to the front surface

(*Note:* it would have been more satisfactory to order −3.25 DS in the first place.)

After addition
Rx with lens: plano/−0.50 × 85
Focimeter reading: (dot at 6 o'clock)
  −1.50/−2.00 × 85
Front surface cylinder checked on keratometer (dot at 6 o'clock): +1.40 × 180

Frequently, the most baffling results are obtained where no measurements seem compatible. In such cases, the focimeter images are frequently found to be of poor quality.

Mrs L.
All lenses of TD 8.50 mm and BOZD 6.50 mm

Spectacle refraction: RE −3.50/−0.50 × 25
             LE −4.00/−0.50 × 170

Keratometer reading: RE 7.02 mm along 170
             6.81 mm along 80
             LE 7.02 mm along 180
             6.78 mm along 90

Trial lens
R 7.00 mm BOZR, −3.00 D 1 Δ (base dotted)
Add = +0.75/−1.25 × 75, dot at 300
L 7.00 mm BOZR, −3.00 D 1 Δ (base dotted)
Add = plano/−1.50 × 100, dot at 280

Lenses ordered
R 7.00 mm BOZR, −2.25/−1.25 × 45, 1 Δ base at 6 o'clock (at 270)
L 7.00 mm BOZR, −3.00/−1.50 × 90, 1 Δ base at 6 o'clock (at 270)

Lenses checked on focimeter with prism base dots at 6 o'clock
R −2.25/−1.50 × 45
L −3.50/−1.50 × 90
Refraction with lenses *in situ*
R +0.25/−1.00 × 105, dot at 280
L +0.75/−1.50 × 115, dot at 280
Front surface cylinders checked on keratometer with dots at 6 o'clock (at 270)
R −1.62 × 45
L −1.12 × 90

It is relatively rare to find an oblique bi-toric lens with clear focimeter images and so the keratometer cylinder measurements can be very helpful.

It may be said that, in checking toric lenses, the focimeter readings are a useful guide but should not be relied upon too fully. They are useful to relate to the refractive effect upon the eye. Apparently identical lenses, as measured with the focimeter, may give entirely different effects on the eye; but in such cases, the keratometer or radiuscope readings usually reveal differences in front surface cylinder and optical quality.

Frequently, the cylinder added to the front surface of a lens is inaccurate and, if the lens has enough substance, one feels inclined to ask the laboratory, rather than reworking the cylinder to repolish the surface to a spherical power so that the refraction can be checked with the lens *in situ* once again. This process is often unsuccessful for, frequently, the polishing appears to follow the contour of the cylinder, and the intermediate stage is an irregular and undetermined toricity. Since many lenses with front surface cylinders also have prism ballast, it is very difficult to remount the lens on the polishing tools without producing irregularity.

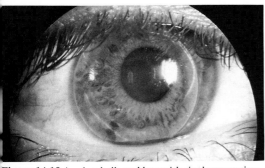

Figure 14.18 A prism ballasted lens with single truncation. This often proves very successful in preventing unwanted rotation

Truncation and double truncation

Truncation of corneal lenses has long been used as a method of attempting to secure freedom from rotation in stabilizing bifocal and toroidal front surface lenses. It is generally found associated with prism ballast, and the combination of both methods is frequently very effective.

The usual method with truncated prism ballasted lenses is to prescribe the lens in the normal way with the addition of the front surface cylinder at the correct angle relative to the estimated or observed position of the prism base. The relationship of the lower lid to the edge of the lens is observed and a truncation is then to cut to align with the lower lid (*Figures 14.18–14.20*).

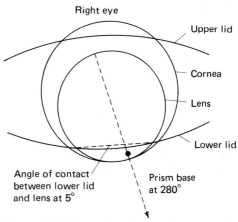

Figure 14.19 The position of contact between a prism ballasted corneal lens and the lower lid margin

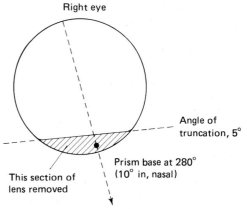

Figure 14.20 The lens shown in *Figure 14.19* has been truncated to enable the lower edge of the lens to align with the lower lid margin

In *Figures 14.19* and *14.20*, the lower lid chord makes an angle of 5° to the horizontal at its contact with the lens, and the truncation might well be cut at that angle. The lower edge is thick at the truncation, and thus the lens is unlikely to slip below the lower lid and tends to be influenced by it. If the nasal rise of the lower lid during blinking is excessive, then in the case illustrated, the angled truncation may cause the lens to rise too much nasally. A truncation at 10° may be more effective in these circumstances.

Much depends on the position of the lower lid. Clearly, if the lower lid is situated well below the lower limbus, or even below the average position of the lens, it cannot be depended on to give a great deal of stable support for the lens. This type of truncation works mainly by the support given by the lower lid between blinks. Knowledge of the patient's occupation is also important in these cases as it obviously influences the lid/lens relationship. A clerical worker, with his visual axes depressed throughout much of the day, needs to be examined with the eyes in this position and the lid angles and their influence assessed. Some degree of support from the lower lid can almost certainly be counted on with the patient looking down; but unfortunately, the resultant position of the lens may be entirely different from that taken up in distance vision. This is probably one of the reasons why some patients wearing a high correction for residual astigmatism which is stabilized by prism and/or truncation complain that either distance or near vision is poor in comparison with the other. It is not always, as one supposes, a mere over- or under-correction of the basic refractive error. In addition there are other problems encountered during close work by wearers of toric or non-toric lenses (Stone, 1967).

Prism ballasted lenses, with or without truncation, are not always as physically comfortable as non-prism lenses. Fortunately, therefore, it is possible to use truncation or double truncation to stabilize a lens without the use of a prism. Such truncations often work extremely well even if the lower lid position is very low and well below the limbus. This type of lens relies on the effect of blinking on the truncations and is not required to rest almost constantly on the lower lid.

Very little interest appears to exist in double truncation but, if fully exploited, it can give better comfort and visual acuity than the more common forms of stabilization.

Large lenses, and prism ballasted lenses in particular, are heavy and therefore tend to locate low on the cornea. Lenses also tend to be made thicker by the laboratories if they contain a cylinder correction.

It is a natural inclination to attempt to prescribe double truncated lenses as large as possible due to the loss of so much of the vertical dimension. This is a mistake. The lenses are usually found to work best if prescribed in alignment or with slight apical clearance and with the horizontal total diameter about 0.5 mm larger than would normally be used for a conventional lens. The most common horizontal total diameters are between 8.80 and 9.70 mm and the vertical ones between 7.50 and 8.50 mm, depending on the palpebral aperture size and pupil diameter. The vertical total diameter should be as small as possible consistent with good visual acuity, and considering possible use for night driving. The greater the discrepancy between horizontal and vertical total diameters the better, since this gives a greater truncated chord length on which the lids can act.

The BOZD of this lens design is usually between 6.50 and 7.20 mm, and edge thickness needs to be carefully controlled. Edge thickness depends on the size and power of the lens, and so the final edge finish may have to be carefully modified by a good technician. The general principle is that the edge finish must permit the lid to slide over it comfortably while still influencing the truncated edge and aligning it.

It would appear that an edge thickness of about 0.15–0.20 mm for the non-truncated edge is helpful, with the truncated area in the region of 0.17–0.25 mm thick. Much depends on the degree and axis of the front surface cylinder. The vertical edges tend to be thinner with the addition of a positive cylinder axis horizontal. The peak of the edge is best arranged to fall nearer the front surface of the lens on the truncated area, and the edge does not need to be as blunt as in bifocal truncation.

The longer axis of the double truncated lens almost invariably aligns with the flattest corneal meridian, which is usually nearly horizontal. If this is nasally slightly down (i.e. at 170 in the right eye), then the effect is counteracted by the tendency for the lower lid to rise nasally. Fairmaid (1967) states that he has never observed a lens with truncation stabilized downward nasally and that most lenses, when settled, stabilize so that it is within a degree or two of the horizontal.

The upper lid influences the lens when blinking and assists in aligning it. The lens rises with the upper lid after the downward movement of the blink and may rotate nasally up during that movement. It may have been noticed that most corneal lenses tend to resist sliding far over the upper limbus on to the conjunctiva. The upper junction of cornea and conjunctiva and the irregular thickness of tissue at the limbus tend to act as stabilizing factors if the lens rises this far on blinking. Even if it does not rise on blinking the lens tends to rise on the cornea on depression of the visual axis, as during clerical work, and this may assist with stabilization. There may be a case for cutting the upper truncation on a line using a radius equal to that of half the corneal diameter. This may well be appropriate if the lens locates high and is almost constantly under the top lid, so that the truncation lines up with the limbus as shown in *Figure 14.21*.

Truncations are, however, usually most effective if cut straight, parallel and horizontal with only the corners rounded off. This rounding off should only be a smoothing and should not result in an oval lens. In many cases, it seems unnecessary to cut the truncations to correspond with the lid angles, and unless the nasal rise of the lower lid is excessive, it is best to cut the truncations horizontal — especially if the

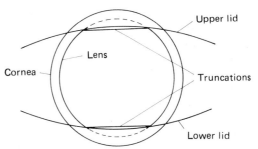

Figure 14.22 The correct positions for double truncations to permit upper and lower edges of the lenses to align with the lid margins

practitioner has little experience in judging the effect of lids upon truncations. It is foolish, however, to ignore wide departures from normal lid orientation, and especially so if the front surface cylinder is high.

A lens which is overlapped by one or both of the eyelids in normal use can be converted to an interpalpebral design by double truncation (*Figure 14.22*).

A small interpalpebral lens in its round state can also be double truncated to produce an

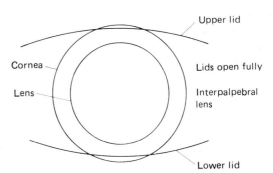

Figure 14.23 An interpalpebral lens shown on a right eye with the lids in a relaxed, fully open position prior to blinking

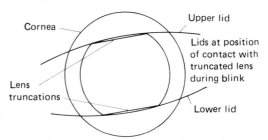

Figure 14.24 The same right eye as in *Figure 14.23* during the act of blinking. Note that during a blink the angle of the lid margin contact with the lens is different from that expected from the relaxed position. The truncation is cut accordingly

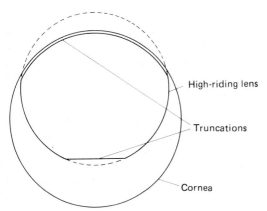

Figure 14.21 The upper truncation of a high riding lens cut to run parallel with the upper limbus. This type of truncation also assists a bifocal corneal lens to rise adequately for near vision

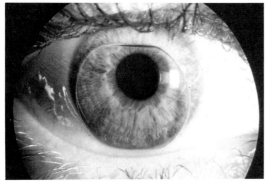

Figure 14.25 A double truncated lens without prism. This lens contains a front surface cylinder correction of 1.50 D which remains stable and gives a visual acuity of 6/4.5 and complete comfort. The patient had previously had seven other pairs of unsuccessful lenses from various sources

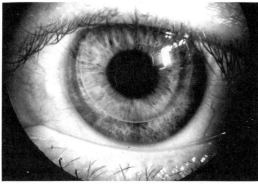

Figure 14.26 High corneal astigmatism does not always require correction with a toroidal back optic zone. This cornea has keratometer readings of 8.23 mm along 180, 7.43 mm along 90. The corneal lens has a BOZR of 8.10 mm and a power of +3.00 D. It centres extremely well and gives a visual acuity of 6/4.5

effective control of rotation; but when calculating the angles at which the truncations must be cut, it is worth considering the angles of the lids at the moment when they just contact the lens during a blink. The lid angle, relative to the horizontal, may be found to change considerably in comparison with the non-blinking state (*Figures 14.23–14.26*).

Physiological problems

The use of toric forms of lens often produces severe physiological problems. The use of a toroidal back optic zone to align the cornea closely, or of a prism ballasted lens can often produce excessive oedema during the adaptive stage.

Westerhout (1971b) found that in a group of cases fitted with toroidal back optic zones the incidence of oedema after 2 weeks of adaptation rose from an expected 38% with spherical back surfaces to 83% with the toroidal forms. Westerhout also found that if prism ballasted lenses were to be exchanged for non-prism ballasted lenses after 2 weeks' adaptation, the incidence of oedema was as high as 92% after a further 2 weeks of adaptation, compared with an expected incidence of approximately 20% with spherical non-ballasted lenses at that stage. All these results were obtained with PMMA lenses and would be less of a problem with gas permeable lenses, provided they were thin enough.

The same survey indicated that if a patient suffering from oedema with prism ballasted lenses were to be refitted with double truncated lenses without prisms then 80% of these eyes would lose their oedema after 4 more days of wearing.

Clearly, the use of toric forms of corneal lens can be made difficult for other than optical considerations.

The author has found that although central fenestrations of 0.2–0.4 mm can be helpful physiologically (*see* p. 357, Chapter 10), it is usually better to employ one or more fenestrations of 0.2–0.3 mm in the midperiphery of the lens. Central fenestrations tend to cause visual disturbances, possibly from tear fluid passing through the holes and cascading down the front of the lens in front of the pupil.

Midperipheral fenestrations are usually better visually, and if a lens stabilizes well, such as that in *Figure 14.3*, then it is possible to place the fenestrations beside the pupil area without much risk of their covering the pupil region.

As is well known, fenestrations can produce additional adhesion to the cornea in alignment fitted lenses (because of the additional tear meniscus created between lens and cornea) and tend to work best in central clearance fittings.

Rigid gas permeable materials

The relief of oedema, in cases such as those referred to in the preceding paragraphs, is often made considerably easier by using rigid gas permeable materials. The same design and optical principles apply whatever material is used, but calculations must, of course, take account of the different refractive indices of the many and varied gas permeable materials now available.

Many of the gas permeable materials are capable of giving equivalent oxygen performance of well over 7% when made with a central thickness of 0.12 (Hill, 1975). This figure is comparable to the findings of Fatt, Freeman and Lin (1974) who estimated that during sleep the cornea receives between 7% and 8% oxygen.

Unfortunately, however, the use of gas permeable lenses is not an instant panacea to all the physiological problems of fitting various forms of toric rigid lenses. In the case of prism ballasted lenses the average thickness is considerable and the transmission of oxygen through such a thick lens is not always sufficient to remove all oedema problems. Gas permeable lenses are also much more prone to flex when thin and very few of the gas permeable lenses can be made thin enough to be able to exploit their potential for permeability.

Many toric lens manufacturers produce their lenses by crimping lens blanks during manufacture and it is by no means certain that this is satisfactory with some of the gas permeable, but highly unstable, materials. Due to the difficulty of manufacturing toric lenses it is rare to be able to make them thin even in PMMA material. This thicker form of lens in gas permeable material greatly limits the oxygen transmission capabilities.

One of the advantages of gas permeable materials is that many of them have lower refractive indices than the 1.49 of PMMA. Thus the induced astigmatism created by a gas permeable toroidal back surface is usually less than that for PMMA material. The author has, for years, advocated trying to make lenses from a material with a refractive index of 1.336, or as near as possible to that figure (e.g. vinyl trifluoroacetate (Westerhout, 1976b) which has a refractive index of 1.3106). If this were to be done then a perfectly fitting toroidal back surface and spherical front surface could be used to correct large degrees of corneal astigmatism with no induced astigmatism.

The physiological requirements of the corneal surface are not all met by using a permeable lens which provides an adequate oxygen supply. Regrettably the preoccupation with corneal oxygen requirements and lens permeability has led manufacturers and practitioners to largely ignore the tear film circulation between lens and cornea. Many of today's gas permeable lens designs have inadequate tear circulation and this is often seen at its worst when closely aligning toroidal back surfaces are used. Sufficient peripheral clearance must always be used with all forms of rigid lenses, especially when a fully toroidal back surface is used. The trend towards poor design is largely due to the fact that, in many countries, practitioners no longer design a lens, complete with suitable edge clearance, to fit an eye, but prefer to use a standard laboratory designed lens in the hope that it will fit acceptably, rather than optimally.

Flexing of rigid corneal lenses

Many practitioners will have noticed that visual acuity with very thin lenses is often variable and poor. Refraction over these lenses can be very unreliable and often irregular retinoscopic reflexes are seen through such lenses.

There is no doubt that very thin lenses flex with lid movement and pressure, and the warping effect induces an astigmatic component in the system. Harris and Chu (1972) investigated 10 cases and found that PMMA corneal lenses with a central thickness of less than 0.13 mm flexed toroidally on a toroidal cornea and changed the residual astigmatism in a predictable fashion. They reasoned, therefore, that residual astigmatism could be altered by changing the central thickness of the corneal lens (*see* Chapter 5). They produced ingenious graphs showing how much change in residual astigmatism could be produced, for a given change in central thickness, for a known toricity.

For example, on a cornea having 4 D of astigmatism with-the-rule, changing the central thickness from 0.15 to 0.08 mm induces a 1.25 D cylinder, with-the-rule, which would cancel out 1.25 D of residual astigmatism against-the-rule (if the latter were present with the thicker lens).

This is very useful and certainly a thin lens can be used to reduce residual astigmatism when the residual astigmatism with a thick lens and corneal astigmatism are in opposite directions, which is the usual case. Unfortunately, many cases of residual astigmatism occur with fairly spherical corneas.

Westerhout (1976a) investigated 24 cases of 'thin' corneal lens wearers and found that there was very little relationship between lens flexure and corneal astigmatism and that there was no evidence of the highest changes in flexure occurring with the highest corneal astigmatism.

It is, however, worth trying much thinner lenses if the conditions are right (*see* Chapter 5).

Flexing and distortion of rigid gas permeable materials

Since the advent of gas permeable corneal lenses the problem of flexing has become more serious. It is well known that gas permeable materials flex much more than PMMA and that, in general, the higher the *Dk* value the higher the flexibility. CAB (cellulose acetate butyrate), however, is very flexible despite a low *Dk* value.

Although PMMA lenses of centre thickness of 0.13 mm and above do not flex significantly on a toroidal cornea the lower-to-medium *Dk* materials will have to be made from 0.16 mm to 0.20 mm thick to avoid flexure. Higher *Dk* materials may have to be made as thick as 0.25 mm to avoid flexure problems. Corneal lenses are not as comfortable in these thicknesses. Most laboratories and manufacturers, for obvious reasons, publish *Dk* and *Dk/t* figures which look excellent. High *Dk* materials with an impressive *Dk/t* figure for a centre thickness of 0.1 or 0.15 mm are presented which would be impracticable in clinical practice due to the flexing of the lens.

At present there is no standard published factor for rigid gas permeable materials, to enable prediction of the expected flexing with different thicknesses. This problem needs to be addressed urgently.

The problem of flexing is greatly oversimplified by many workers in this field who seem to assume that the flexing effect on the cornea is a constant factor once the lens has settled. Nothing could be further from the truth. The effects of lid tension, palpebral aperture, lens total diameter, and flatness or steepness of fitting all need to be considered.

Westerhout (1976b), while investigating flexure of thin rigid PMMA lenses on toroidal corneas, found that 16 results out of 40 had to be rejected due to the unstable and variable results which could not be incorporated into the study. In this study all lenses were fitted in alignment. It was found that the palpebral aperture relative to lens total diameter had a large influence on flexure, especially for astigmatism with-the-rule.

Studies in which the lid aperture effects, or the fitting philosophy used, are not considered have little validity.

A recent study by Harris *et al.* (1987) investigated flexure with two brands of gas permeable lenses on 12 toroidal corneas. Central thicknesses were varied between 0.1 mm and 0.2 mm. The results indicated that thinner lenses flexed more. The critical thickness to avoid flexure seemed to be 0.15 mm. All the subjects in the study had with-the-rule astigmatism of between 1.75 D and 3.25 D, but were all fitted with the same BOZR of 7.74 mm and a total diameter of 9.0 mm irrespective of corneal curvature. Harris *et al.* found no relationship between the corneal toricity and flexure with the two gas permeable materials used. They found the results contradicted flexure results with PMMA (Harris and Chu, 1972) which showed a relationship between corneal toricity and lens flexure. They attributed this to the limited range of toricities in the study of gas permeable materials. This study, however, was conducted on 12 subject eyes, whereas the earlier PMMA study was conducted on 10 subject eyes. Westerhout (1976b) obtained results which appeared to contradict the findings of Harris and Chu (1972) in that toricity did not appear to be related to flexure with thin lenses. Indeed, in 22 cases of corneal astigmatism with-the-rule, 5 of these cases showed flexure against-the-rule. These results are more compatible with Harris *et al.*'s (1987) gas permeable results.

When keratometry measurements are taken on the front surface of a thin, rigid contact lens, the author has noticed considerable variations in keratometer readings, during the act of blinking. Patients often complain that visual acuity changes with blinks while wearing rigid lenses and, although this is usually attributed to wetting or re-wetting during the act of blinking, the author is of the opinion that some of these variable vision experiences are as a result of flexure changes during blinking.

Certainly Herman (1983, 1986) and Stone and Collins (1984) have suggested that the upper eyelid is a major factor in lens flexure, but Kimball and Mandell (1974) using small, ultrathin PMMA lenses (t_c 0.08 mm and TD 8.0–8.3 mm) found large degrees of lens flexure despite the intrapalpebral nature of the fitting. Harris and Applequist (1974) showed that varying the range of total diameters of corneal lenses from 8.0 mm to 10.0 mm had no effect on the degree of flexure for a given eye. Lydon and Tait (1988) in a detailed review of the effects of lid pressure concluded as follows: 'It now remains to be seen whether the forces required to produce rigid lens flexure are within the capabilities of the average eyelid.'

Clinicians are, of course, inclined to believe what they see and for those many practitioners who have taken keratometer readings over a well-wetted, thin rigid lens and watched the mire reflections changing rapidly on blinking, it will be difficult to convince them that the lids do not affect flexure.

Practitioners should not be fearful of flexure effects, but should rather learn how to exploit them. In the case of a patient with significant corneal astigmatism and no residual astigmatism, a thin gas permeable lens may flex and the over-refraction may show residual astigmatism. The practitioner may be tempted to make a front surface cylinder to correct this and stabilize it with a prism ballast. The use of prism ballast substantially increases thickness (by 0.05–0.1 mm depending on the power of the prism and the size of the lens). This increase in thickness prevents the lens from flexing and then there is no residual astigmatism created by flexure. The use of the prism would also reduce the amount of oxygen able to reach the cornea.

If the patient has significant corneal astigmatism (especially with-the-rule) and a spherical refraction, then the use of a soft lens would normally be indicated as it should wrap around the cornea and produce a toroidal front surface which neutralizes the residual (lenticular) astigmatism. The use of a rigid PMMA lens (t_c 0.14 mm) or RGP lens (t_c 0.18 mm) would prevent the lens from flexing and then residual astigmatism would be experienced by the patient. If a rigid gas permeable lens was required for some other reason, then it would be best to attempt the use of a very flexible material made rather thin. This would hopefully flex on the cornea thus negating the residual (lenticular) astigmatism.

Fitting toric soft lenses

Soft contact lenses have made a very big impact on contact lens practice since their introduction by Wichterle and Lim (1960). The unique form of the soft lens material has enabled a large number of difficult cases to be fitted, many of whom had failed to wear well-made hard corneal lenses. Nevertheless throughout the many years of their use it has always been held, until fairly recently, that a contra-indication for soft lenses is the presence of significant astigmatism.

It is clear that a soft flexible material tends to follow the curvature of the underlying cornea and thus any corneal astigmatism tends to be transferred through the lens material. In the early years of the development of soft lenses, various ideas for overcoming the problems of astigmatism were postulated and detailed results were described involving the use of thick lenses to reduce the amount of corneal astigmatism transferred to the front surface of the soft lens. It is obvious, however, that attempts to use a thick soft lens may well result in poor physiological performance as thickness is un-doubtedly a most significant factor in successful long-term use of soft contact lenses (Hill and Jeppe, 1975). Numerous manufacturers of soft contact lenses have made extremely optimistic, perhaps irresponsible, claims of their lenses being able to correct, satisfactorily, astigmatism of between 1 and 2 D. Only rarely is this achieved, and in reality, most experienced practitioners are now well aware that the most helpful indication of the likely residual astigmatism found while wearing a spherical soft contact lens is the ocular astigmatism determined from an accurate subjective spectacle refraction.

The optimistic and misleading claims of the ability of a spherical soft lens to correct astigmatism has resulted in a very large number of soft contact lens wearers who are only partially successful and who basically wear their lenses for social use without really adequate visual acuity. In the initial euphoria of early soft lens wearing, when their great comfort is so much enjoyed by the wearer, the limitations of visual acuity are often not noticed, but after a relatively short period these patients become aware of the fact that their visual acuity is poorer than with their spectacles, particularly for near vision.

It is ironic that one of the reasons why this limitation is noticed is due to the absence of spectacle blur following the removal of the majority of soft lenses. Most hard contact lens wearers suffer from some degree of spectacle blur and often report that their spectacle visual acuity is worse than with their contact lenses (*see* Chapter 20). They are unaware of the spectacle blur effect and compare their spectacle visual acuity, on contact lens removal, with their contact lens visual acuity before removal.

Now that there is such a large number of soft contact lens wearers, it is clear that more and more patients need a correction for the residual astigmatic errors present when the soft lens is being worn.

As soft contact lenses became more viable, several workers began experimenting with toric forms of soft lens in the early 1970s. Strachan (1975) described early development work on toric lenses in 1972 as did Hirst (G., 1975, personal communication). Much of the earlier development of toric soft lenses took place in Australia and New Zealand. Useful forms of toric soft lens became available in the UK in 1975 but from that time onwards, there has been development in many countries.

Indications

Due to the complexity and expense of manufacturing toric forms of soft lens, most practitioners are inclined to prescribe them only when it is absolutely necessary. Obviously, orthodox hard corneal lenses are able to cope with a large variety of astigmatic problems but in many instances the patient may be unable to wear such a lens with sufficient comfort.

However, if a soft lens is preferred by a practitioner, or patient, for physical reasons and the resultant residual astigmatism is significant, then a toric soft lens should at least be considered, even if subsequently rejected on the grounds of cost or the difficulty of manufacturing the complex lens design required.

There are other obvious indications for a spherical soft lens such as the classic case in which the patient manifests a spherical spectacle refraction, but has appreciable corneal astigmatism. In this instance it is clear that the use of a spherical hard corneal lens would result in a correction for residual astigmatism being necessary, whereas a spherical soft lens immediately provides an adequate correction.

The incidence of astigmatism in a sample of ametropes is of interest, as it gives some indication of the likely requirement for toric soft lenses. The author reviewed a group of 500 consecutive eyes examined in practice, excluding only postoperative conditions, and found the percentage incidence of spectacle astigmatism to be as follows:

Astigmatism (in D)				
0–0.50	0.75–1.00	1.25–2.00	2.25–3.00	>3.00
Percentage incidence				
36	40	13	9	2

Holden and Garner (1976), in discussing the criteria for the prescribing of toric lenses, gave a statistical analysis showing that 45% of the population required a cylindrical correction of up to 0.75 D and 25% of the population required a correction of 1.00 D or more.

Forms of toric soft lens

Some of the most common types of toric soft lens fitting have already been discussed briefly in Chapter 11. A more comprehensive discussion of this form of lens now follows.

Westerhout (1976b) has described 12 different forms of toric soft lens, the principal categories being as follows:

(1) Toroidal back surface with a spherical front surface
(2) Toroidal back surface with toroidal front surface (bi-toric).
(3) Spherical back surface with toroidal front surface.

It should be noted that the toroidal back surface can be prescribed without any other form of stabilization save that of the back surface toricity, but that all three varieties of lens described above can be stabilized with either prism ballast or truncation, or a combination of both prism ballast and truncation.

(4) Another variety of lens utilizes what is termed dynamic stabilization (Fanti, 1975) in which the upper and lower portions of the

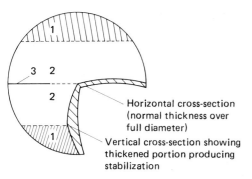

1
3 2
2
Horizontal cross-section (normal thickness over full diameter)
1
Vertical cross-section showing thickened portion producing stabilization

Figure 14.27 Weicon-T lens showing the form and position of the dynamic stabilization zones. This diagram shows a plano lens with a cylinder of −3.00 D × 180, worked on as +3.00 D × 90. (1) Dynamic stabilization zones; (2) optic zone; (3) engraved line marking axis of stabilization

front surface of the lens are chamfered (*Figure 14.27*) to allow the action of the lids, moving over the thickened and chamfered portions during blinking, to orientate the lens.

(5) A combination of a hard lens on top of a soft lens could be construed as a method of correcting astigmatism with a soft contact lens (Westerhout, 1973).

Principles of fitting

If an accurate spectacle refraction indicates a degree of astigmatism similar to that found with keratometry, then it is clear that the astigmatic error is mostly corneal. If, therefore, it is possible to prescribe accurately a lens with a toroidal back surface, to align with the corneal curvatures in each meridian, then the back surface of the lens may wrap itself sufficiently precisely onto the cornea to enable the front spherical surface of the lens to remain spherical. In this instance it is assumed that the spherical front surface of the contact lens corrects the ametropia and the toroidal back surface of the lens corrects the astigmatism. This is the principle now used by many practitioners. The optical considerations are little different from those encountered when using hard corneal lenses, because the total optical effect of the tear film in contact with the front surface of the cornea remains as it would be in using a toroidal back surface hard lens. However, the toroidal back surface of the soft lens in contact with the tear film is somewhat different because its refractive index is lower than that of a hard lens. The refractive indices of soft lens materials vary considerably and although they are closer than PMMA to that of the tears, there is still sufficient difference in most cases to leave an induced astigmatic effect at this soft lens/tears –cornea interface.

The same principle applies as has already been dealt with in the section dealing with corneal lenses on p. 513. Even if the toroidal back surface soft lens aligns exactly with the toroidal cornea there is still some induced astigmatism despite the front surface of the lens remaining spherical. Hence, many of the principles employed by some clinicians appear to be based on a false premise. However, by making the back surface of a soft lens less toroidal than the cornea, when it flexes to match the cornea, the front surface of the lens also becomes slightly toroidal. Thus, with care and careful calculation, the undercorrection of the astigmatism by the front surface of the soft lens can be made to neutralize (or largely so) the overcorrection by the back surface.

Other faulty considerations apply to the assumption that if a soft lens wraps itself onto the cornea in close alignment, any change in the back surface radius gives rise to an almost equal change in the front surface radius. Most of these assumptions (Strachan, 1973; Baron, 1975) do not appear to have been supported by theoretically correct arguments.

Bennett (1976) has, however, produced a mathematical method of calculating the power changes expected when a soft lens flexes (*see* Chapter 5, p. 214). Bennett's results indicate that the power changes are likely to be much greater in magnitude and even different in sign to those predicted by the use of the 'wrap factor' (Strachan, 1973).

If it is assumed that the principal meridians of the toroidal back surface of the contact lens align with the principal meridians of the cornea, then it can readily be seen that this method of correction is only applicable in the absence of any significant lenticular or residual astigmatism. It must also be assumed that the lens will orientate accurately in the correct meridian, as it is rarely found that toroidal back surfaces align accurately without additional methods of stabilization such as prisms or truncation.

If there is a significant difference between the spectacle refraction cylinder and the keratometric cylinder, then clearly residual astigmatism will result and a straightforward toroidal back surface and spherical front surface is inadequate. In this case a bi-toric soft lens can be prescribed in which the toroidal back surface corrects the corneal astigmatism and the toroidal front surface corrects the lenticular or residual astigmatism together with any induced astigmatism. Such a lens is extremely difficult to manufacture accurately, especially if the residual astigmatism is at an axis different from the principal meridians of the cornea. If the axis of the residual astigmatism corresponds to one of the corneal principal meridians then the lens may not be too complex, but as this is not often encountered the lens becomes extremely complicated, especially if it is inclined to rotate despite methods used to stabilize it.

In some cases, where the residual astigmatism and the corneal astigmatism have parallel axes, it is possible to order the toroidal back surface radii so that they are not the same as the corneal radii. As described for the correction of corneal astigmatism above, this results in the lens wrapping itself around the cornea in such a way that the increased or decreased astigmatic effect from the back surface of the lens is transferred through the flexible material to induce front surface astigmatism on the contact lens. By careful selection this may be made to correct any residual error. This is clearly impossible to achieve if the residual astigmatism is at a different axis from that of the cornea.

Spherical back surfaces

A spherical back surface is normally employed with a toroidal front surface to correct a variety of types of residual astigmatism found by refraction while a spherical soft contact lens is being worn. If such a lens can be made to stabilize precisely with an accurately made toroidal front surface, it may be utilized to correct any form of regular astigmatism. It does not matter whether the astigmatism is totally corneal, residual (lenticular) or induced, provided the front surface of the lens corrects the astigmatism found by refraction over a spherical lens. This is clearly a great advantage over the other more complex forms of lens all of which have a limited application.

Stabilization

All forms of astigmatic soft lens need to be stabilized to prevent unnecessary rotation. It has already been stated that even a fairly toroidal back surface, without other forms of stabilization, is unlikely to prove satisfactory. With many years of experience of stabilizing hard corneal lenses it is only natural for practitioners and laboratories to turn to the existing methods which are well known and tried.

The use of prism ballast

The use of prism ballast is well known in stabilizing toric forms of lens but it does have certain disadvantages when applied to soft lens designs. Since many forms of soft lens are relatively thick in comparison to hard lenses, and are made larger than the corneal diameter, the additional thickness brought about by the use of a prism can be a problem with regard to oxygen permeability. The additional thickness can also cause physical discomfort in patients with sensitive lids, but a great deal depends on the position of the lids relative to the edge of the contact lens. Fortunately, the thicker edge in the region of the prism base can be thinned during the manufacturing stage without negating the effect of the prism ballast. The thickest portion of the lens is also usually situated underneath the lower lid.

One of the difficulties which arises with the use of prism ballast is that if it is going to be prescribed monocularly it may well cause vertical prismatic effects which may make the patient uncomfortable. This then requires the use of a similar prism for the other eye. Although this is not a serious difficulty if that eye is also to wear a contact lens, it can be an inconvenience if the other eye is emmetropic. Fortunately, however, prism ballast does not often give rise to binocular problems (Gasson, 1977).

The principle of the use of prism ballast is to balance the forces acting on the lens in order to stabilize it. The effect of the centre of gravity being displaced away from the geometric centre helps to rotate the lens around the geometric centre and it is very important, therefore, that the lens be fairly free-moving. A tight lens will not move freely and be influenced by the prism ballast, and such lenses are to be avoided. A reasonably loose, free-moving lens is important if the prism ballast is to work satisfactorily.

The effects of prisms

For many years it was thought that prism ballast effectively stabilized lenses through the gravity effects of the heavier base of the lens. Although it is now known that this is not always the case, weight effects cannot be entirely discounted. In the earlier days of toric hard corneal lenses, many manufacturers ballasted their lenses with small metal weights and the author has found several patients who experience a rotation of the prism ballasted lens when they tilt their head towards their shoulder. The effects of such head tilting makes the base–apex line of the prism ballasted lens remain almost vertical and at an angle to the lower lid position which is now tilted away from the horizontal.

Many workers have observed that patients who are turned upside down still have the prism base at the lower lid position, despite the fact that the heavier part of the lens is now higher than the lighter, prism apex.

On occasion, a prism ballasted lens will turn upside-down and perhaps stay there all day. This upside-down effect is also noticed with truncated lenses with and without prism ballast.

The simple clinical fact is that any area on a lens which offers an obstruction to smooth lid movement, helps to orientate the lens relative to the lid position. This applies to both lids and is also dependent on the lid position, lid angle, palpebral aperture and lid tension. The orientating obstruction can be in the form of a thick prism base, a 'slab-off' zone, a 'thin zone' or 'thick zone' taper, a 'comfort chamfer', an off-centre lenticulation or a truncation. It can also be a combination of any of these factors.

Truncation

Truncation has already been described in the section dealing with corneal lenses and is a very well-tried and successful method of stabilizing lenses. Many practitioners (Strachan, 1975; Holden and Garner, 1976) advocate the use of double truncation although Fanti (1975) has described the difficulties that apply when truncation is utilized. Whereas double truncation is preferred by some practitioners for most

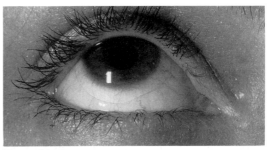

Figure 14.28 A repaired soft lens showing truncation effect. This is atypical in that it is not aligning near the horizontal

of their cases, other practitioners (Davy, 1976; Hodd, 1976) appear to prefer single truncation. It is certainly true that a proportion of patients are less comfortable with a single or double truncated soft lens than they are with a non-truncated lens. The author's first experience of truncation occurred inadvertently when, in the earlier days of 1970, numerous damaged or torn soft lenses were partly truncated in an attempt to repair them and make them useful for wear. These truncated regions usually stabilized when situated at an angle parallel with that of one of the lid margins but rotation nasally, as with hard lenses, also occurred as shown in *Figure 14.28*.

These earlier, accidentally truncated soft lenses were not prism ballasted and yet appeared to stabilize well and there is no doubt that many lenses do stabilize satisfactorily in this way. A great deal depends on the lid tension, position and angle and, in truncating a lens, consideration to these details must be given.

One of the greatest difficulties with truncations is the instability which can occur when truncation is used with oblique cylinders. The uneven thickness produced by oblique cylinders can then make the lens very difficult to stabilize successfully.

Dynamic stabilization

This ingenious method of stabilization developed by Fanti (1975) utilizes a similar principle to truncation in that lid action is made use of to stabilize the lenses. In this instance, however, Fanti has been able to retain the comfortable, round shape of the lens and, in effect, has moved his truncated action areas within the periphery of the lens to form what he terms dynamic stabilization areas. *Figure 14.27* shows the construction of such a lens. In this particular method, movement of the eyes or lids results in pressure being applied superiorly and inferiorly to help stabilize the lens. This has a very wide application and as it avoids the complications of truncation and prism ballast it appears to be a practical method in many instances. Although originally considered difficult to make, recent improvements in lathing technology and lens design are making this form of toric soft lens the one of first choice. The excessive lower thickness of prism ballast lenses can be avoided and by producing toroidal back surfaces the average lens thickness can be made only slightly more than that of spherical designs. Improvements, in the last few years, in reproducibility and stability of orientation have been impressive.

Principles of correction

It is clear that to produce a stable ocular correction for the astigmatic eye, the lens must align closely over the central cornea in front of the pupil. It is important that the lens does not flex more than the anticipated amount in this vital central, optical area because it is well known that flexing of a contact lens produces a power change. Although this is no great problem if the power of the final lens is similar to the trial, spherical lens, it can be a problem with a final toric lens, as the meridional powers are different. For lenses incorporating cylinders of up to 2.50 D it is possible to have cylindrical errors of 0.50–0.75 D induced by the flexure of the lens.

The lens must provide the correct power while it is *in situ*.

The lens must stabilize effectively to prevent the rotation of the meridional powers away from their correct meridians.

Alignment

To achieve what has been referred to in the previous section, certain factors must be taken into account.

Table 14.2 Residual refractive error induced by mislocation of toric lenses of various cylindrical powers

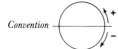

Convention   (1) Axes in standard axis notation
(2) Anti-clockwise is +ve, clockwise −ve

Example: (a) −2.00 × 180 required refractive correction
(b) −2.00 × 170 obtained, i.e. −10° mislocation
(c) Residual cylinder axis is +40°
(d) Residual spherocylinder power is +0.35/−0.69
(e) Expected residual error +0.35/−0.69 × 40

Mislocation (degrees)	−1.00 D	−2.00 D (×2)
5	+0.08/−0.16 × 42.5	+0.17/−0.34 × 42.5
10	+0.17/−0.34 × 40	+0.35/−0.69 × 40
15	+0.26/−0.52 × 37.5	+0.52/−1.04 × 37.5
20	+0.34/−0.69 × 35	+0.68/−1.37 × 35
25	+0.43/−0.85 × 32.5	+0.85/−1.69 × 32.5
30	+0.50/−1.00 × 30	+1.00/−2.00 × 30
35	+0.57/−1.14 × 27.5	+1.14/−2.29 × 27.5
40	+0.64/−1.28 × 25	+1.29/−2.57 × 25
45	+0.71/−1.42 × 22.5	+1.41/−2.83 × 22.5
50	+0.76/−1.53 × 20	+1.53/−3.06 × 20
55	+0.82/−1.64 × 17.5	+1.64/−3.28 × 17.5
60	+0.87/−1.73 × 15	+1.73/−3.46 × 15
65	+0.90/−1.82 × 12.5	+1.81/−3.63 × 12.5
70	+0.94/−1.88 × 10	+1.88/−3.76 × 10
75	+0.96/−1.93 × 7.5	+1.93/−3.85 × 7.5
80	+0.98/−1.97 × 5	+1.97/−3.94 × 5
85	+0.99/−1.99 × 2.5	+1.99/−3.98 × 2.5
90	+1.00/−2.00 × 180	+2.00/−4.00 × 180

Reproduced by kind permission of Holden and Frauenfelder (1973).

The material of which the lens is made is of vital importance. Some materials are very much softer and more flexible than others, thus allowing closer moulding to the corneal shape. Other materials are more elastic and springy in action and this can make a lens somewhat erratic in its alignment, especially if the lens is a little steep in relation to corneal curvature.

The total diameter of the lens is clearly relevant because this parameter determines to some degree how stable the lens will be in centration and thus also in alignment. The relationship of the BOZR of the soft lens to the corneal shape is very important in achieving alignment. In general, flat fitting lenses tend to give better alignment than steep fitting lenses. If the lens is inclined to give apical corneal clearance, there tends to be a springing back-wards and forwards of the soft lens on and off the corneal apex during the act of blinking.

The central thickness and variations in thickness of the lens greatly influence alignment. Variations in thickness such as occur with the use of prisms or lenticular forms are therefore clearly important.

Effect of lens rotation

It is surprising how much induced cylindrical error is produced when a lens does not stabilize satisfactorily and rotates. Holden and Frauen-felder (1973) have produced a table indicating the degree of error induced when a lens rotates (*Table 14.2*). If the correction requires $-2.00\,DC \times 180$, the table reveals that a mislocation of the axis by $10°$ results in a cylindrical error of $-0.69\,D \times 40$. A $20°$ movement gives a cylindrical error of $-1.37\,D \times 35$ and a $25°$ rotation gives a cylindrical error of $-1.65\,D \times 32.5$. These errors are considerable, but use can be made of this table in assessing the amount of rotation of the lens (provided that the lens is well made) by carrying out an accurate refraction with the lens *in situ*. The cylindrical error thus determined can then be related to the induced error in the table to show the degree of lens rotation.

Prescribing and fitting of toric soft lenses

This has been covered briefly in Chapter 11 but is dealt with here in greater detail.

Spherical back surface combined with toroidal front surface using prism ballast stabilization and/or truncation

In this category may be included lenses having a non-toroidal back surface which is not truly spherical. This would include lenses having aspherical back surfaces, as were commonly used in Australia and New Zealand (Hirst, 1975). Such lenses may be fitted with or without truncation. For this reason it may well be worth while ordering the lens with prism ballast, but without truncation, as the truncation can easily be added later either in single or double form.

Since there are different options available in the use of this lens, and the lens can be adjusted after manufacture, it is more constructive and avoids repetition to consider the two approaches involved separately; these follow below.

The use of a spherical back surface and toroidal front surface combined with truncation but without prism ballast

Hirst (1975) has stated that it has been shown clinically that if the position of the truncation can be judged accurately while the trial lens is on the eye, prism ballasting may not be necessary or, if necessary, a small amount of prism (no more than $1\,\Delta$) may be used to give the correct location.

In the fitting of this lens it is suggested that a single truncated, non-toric, non-ballasted trial lens should be used, and fitted using the same principles as those the practitioner would normally use with an orthodox spherical, soft lens (Hirst, 1975). It is not suggested that the practitioner change his normal principles of soft lens fitting because the lens fitted is in a truncated form. It is, as always, helpful if the prescription of the spherical trial lens is as near as possible to that of the final prescription lens.

In the selection of the total diameter of the truncated soft lens it is generally found that the major axis is up to 0.5 mm larger than a conventional, round, soft lens fitting in the same eye. The minor axis perpendicular to the truncation is between 1.0 and 1.5 mm shorter than the longer axis. It is seldom necessary to make these lenses with more than a 1.5 mm truncation and the average total diameter is 14 mm × 12.5 mm.

A careful refraction is carried out over the

single truncated or circular, soft trial lens after the lens has settled for a period in excess of half an hour. In general terms, the longer the lens has settled on the eye before refraction, the more accurate the results are likely to be.

Axis rotation

When the truncated lens is carefully observed on the eye, it may be seen that the truncation has swung nasally 5° or more from the horizontal axis. If a rotational movement is noted its extent should be measured and the prescribing of the cylinder axis in the final lens will have to be modified to compensate for this rotation. There is, of course, no need to describe the rotational swing to the laboratory provided this rotation is provided for in the final prescription.

Example

The refraction over a plano prescription trial lens is found to be −3.00/−1.50 × 180. During the fitting, the right truncation located at approximately 10° instead of the expected 180° position. Thus, the prescription ordered from the laboratory should read: −3.00/−1.50 × 170. This means that with the lens *in situ*, the truncation will rotate to a position along approximately 10°, thus rotating the cylinder axis to approximately its correct position at 180°.

If the final lens is made up accurately to the practitioner's satisfaction and yet is found to rotate in an unpredictable fashion, evident by direct observation and over-refraction, it may be possible to modify the truncation on the lens to attempt to bring it to its correct orientation, rather than ordering another lens.

The angle of the truncation relative to the cylinder axis can be modified by cutting the lens with scissors in its wet state, dehydrating the lens and repolishing the newly truncated area with a soft lens polishing paste while in its dry state and then rehydrating the lens. The author has found this a very satisfactory way in which to deal with the problem.

If the single truncation, despite modification, proves to be unsatisfactory, then the lens can be double truncated by removing between 1.0 and 1.5 mm in the superior region. Before this is done, however, a careful observation of the lid angle of the middle third of the upper and lower lids should be made as this information may well be utilized in cutting the truncations. *Figures 14.29* and *14.30* illustrate this point.

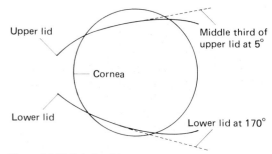

Figure 14.29 Relationship of upper and lower lid angles to the cornea

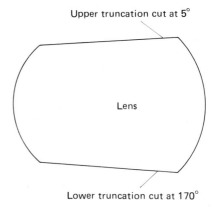

Figure 14.30 Truncations cut on a soft lens to fit the eye illustrated in *Figure 14.29*

Unlike the use of truncation for bifocal fitting, where it is normally necessary that the truncation be cut square so as to rest on the lower lid, this is not the case with toric soft lenses. Indeed, as the lower lid margin is generally found to lie near to or above the position of the lower limbus, and if the lens were forced to ride above this position by being constantly in contact with the margin of the lower lid, the patient could well suffer from irritation caused by the truncation.

The author finds that in the majority of cases it is better if the truncated area rests on the conjunctiva below the lower limbus even if this is well below the position of the lower lid margin.

With these points in mind it must be said that the use of truncation in soft lens fitting is totally different from that used in hard corneal lens fitting. Indeed it can be observed that only in pronounced vertical movements of the eyes do the lid margins actually have any direct contact with the truncated edge or edges. This point is illustrated in *Figure 14.31*.

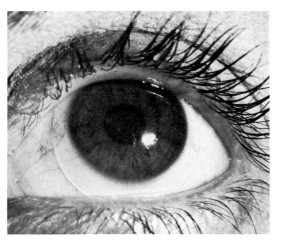

Figure 14.31 This is a prism ballast, single truncated, soft lens with a spherical back surface and toroidal front surface. The lower truncation has been cut at the angle of the middle third of the lower lid, but it can be seen how far below the lower limbus it is situated. In this photograph the patient had to look up in order to bring the truncation near the lower lid. The lid margin may thus only have a limited effect on the truncation

For this reason observation of the angle of the middle third of the lower lid may be better noted with the eyes looking up and noting the lid angle at the point of expected contact with the truncation. The upper lid angle is then noted while looking down using the same principle.

The exact method by which the lids act on the soft lens truncations is not fully understood. Possibly the action of the palpebral orbicularis muscle fibres which run parallel to the lid margins have a similar effect on truncated soft lenses as do the lid margins on truncated hard lenses.

If, as stated by Hirst (1975), the lens is still found to be unsatisfactory due to rotational movement, the lens may be re-ordered with the addition of prism of between 1 and 1.5 Δ.

Since rotation of toric lenses is the main problem encountered in this form of prescribing it would seem that many practitioners are currently using a combination of both prism ballast and truncation for the initial prescription lens.

Truncation positions in successful fittings

The majority of lower lid margins are situated just at or above the lower limbus. It follows, therefore, that the majority of soft lens trunca-

tions situated at, or just below, the lower limbus (depending on the total diameter of the lens and the amount of truncation) are located at or beneath the level of the lower lid margin.

Many practitioners appear to believe that in order to have an effect on the truncation, the lower lid must be just below it and impinge on it during movement. The fact that this is not necessary is concluded from the fact that superior truncations are always overlapped by the upper lid and yet are frequently effective. Other clinicians appear to feel that it is uncomfortable to have the lower truncations situated on or above the limbus, as drying of the lower cornea may occur when the lower lid does not cover this area.

Many hundreds of very successful toric soft lens cases have been seen where the truncation

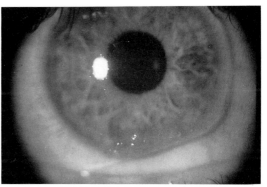

Figure 14.32 A successful toric soft lens with the lower truncation orientated at an entirely different angle from the lower lid. Despite this, however, the lens does not rotate. Note the deposits just above the truncation, a common site for such deposits

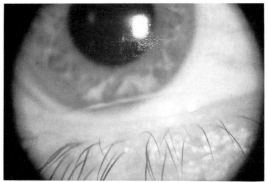

Figure 14.33 A successful toric soft lens with the lower truncation positioned above the limbus. Despite this position the lens is entirely comfortable

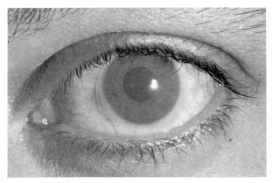

Figure 14.34 A patient with a very low lower lid wearing a very successful toric soft lens. This left lens has been stained with fluorescein to better illustrate the position closely aligning the lower lid. Very little rotation was observed

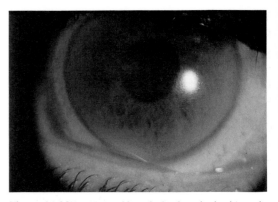

Figure 14.36 A truncated lens drying later in the day and standing off from the globe. Such a condition can be irritating for the lower lid

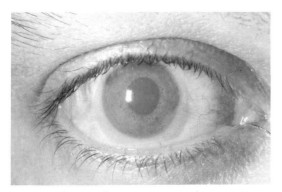

Figure 14.35 Right eye of the same patient as in *Figure 14.34* showing very different orientation of truncation. Very little rotation was observed

is situated in an unusual position, in which it might be expected to cause discomfort or unstable orientation. Two such cases are illustrated in *Figures 14.32* and *14.33*. The two eyes of the same patient often behave rather differently as may be seen in *Figures 14.34* and *14.35*.

A common problem with lower truncations is that, although the lens may be well fitted and perform well in the earlier part of the day, later in the day the lens begins to dry out and the truncation often stands away from the globe forming a small bubble and often irritating the lower lid (*Figure 14.36*).

Spherical back surface with toroidal front surface combined with prism ballast and truncation

It should be noted that as it is frequently desirable, with such complex and expensive lenses, to order lenses capable of modification, it

may be better for the novice practitioner to order the lenses with prism ballast but without truncation. If the truncation is then required subsequently, it can be added in the manner already described. Similarly it is helpful if the spherical lens used for fitting is prism ballasted but not truncated.

The initial fitting of the trial lens should be done as if fitting an orthodox soft spherical lens with no provision made for the fact that the lens may be made truncated or with a toroidal front surface. It is highly desirable that marks are made on the contact lens to indicate the position of the prism base, and when the lens is settled for at least half an hour the position of the prism base is noted. If the lens is to be prescribed in truncated form then the angle of the middle third of the lower eyelid should be noted relative to the position of the prism base. The truncation is then ordered to be cut at this angle.

A careful refraction is then carried out and the final prescription written, making allowance for the position of the prism base. It should be unnecessary to state the position of the prism base provided that this is done.

Example

If the prescription is RE −1.00/−2.00 × 10 and the prism base is found to locate at 280°, the lens is then ordered with the cylinder axis at 180° with the prism base at 270°. When the lens is in position on the eye the prism base will rotate 10° up nasally, from 270° to 280°, thus allowing the cylinder axis to return to its correct position at 10°. It is generally found more satisfactory and less confusing to order the prism base at the 6 o'clock (270°) position.

Toroidal back surface lenses, stabilized by one or two truncations

Such a lens may be made with or without a toroidal front surface to correct lenticular or induced astigmatism. The somewhat complex calculations involved in prescribing these lenses are generally left to the laboratory, especially as different materials are used in the manufacture and the refractive index of these materials varies considerably. The principle of fitting is as follows.

The practitioner fits the patient with the flattest spherical trial lens that will remain stable on the eye. The stability and centration should be at least as good as that found with an orthodox spherical soft lens to be fitted to the same eye. The patient is then carefully refracted after the lens has settled for at least half an hour, followed by keratometric readings taken from the front surface of the contact lens *in situ*. The angle of the middle third of the lower and upper lids is estimated, relative to the horizontal, as these will be used for the cutting of the truncations.

When the final lens arrives from the laboratory and has been checked for accuracy, it is inserted and allowed to settle. If it is found to rotate, judged by over-refraction and observation, then the truncation can be added, if this has not already been done. If no truncation has been used, any additional nasal swing of the prism base can be compensated for by cutting a truncation along the angle of the middle third of the lower lid. This should be done with the

prism base at the correct position to obtain orientation of the cylinder at the required axis. In the above example the truncation would be cut with the prism base at 280°.

Once the truncation is cut, however, it is often found that the influence of the lids is not as expected and the truncation may not orientate parallel to the lower lid. Any such additional rotation may sometimes be compensated for by cutting a second truncation at a different angle to attempt to reorientate the lens. This principle is illustrated in *Figures 14.37–14.39*.

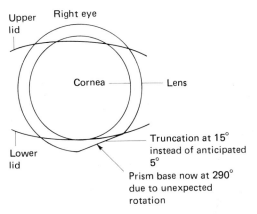

Figure 14.38 The prism base of the lens illustrated in *Figure 14.37* unexpectedly rotates a further 10° nasally. The cylinder is now 10° off-axis. This may sometimes be corrected as shown in *Figure 14.39*

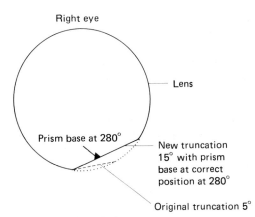

Figure 14.39 The faulty lens positioning (*see Figure 14.38*) may be corrected in some cases by cutting a new truncation. Here the new truncation is cut at an angle of 15°, with the prism base at 280°. If the truncation has more influence than the prism, the truncation may orientate in the same position as in *Figure 14.38*, thus allowing the prism base to settle in its correct position at 280° with the truncation at 15°

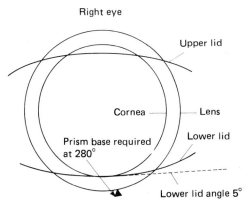

Figure 14.37 With the lower lid angle at 5°, the lower truncation would be cut initially at 5° to allow the prism base to position at 280° thus allowing the cylinder to take up the correct axis

The techniques described above for the spherical back surface and toroidal front surface appear to be satisfactory methods of correcting astigmatic errors, especially as the relationship of lenticular to corneal astigmatism is irrelevant with such lenses. The lens is simply stabilized and the front surface cylinder added to correct the overall cylindrical refractive effect.

If, however, the lenses are uncomfortable and the patient proves to be intolerant to the use of prisms, with or without truncation, then other methods of correction may have to be found.

Another type of toric lens incorporating a front toroidal surface with a spherical back surface is that utilizing dynamic stabilization, but this is dealt with separately on pp. 535 and 546. A description of those techniques which make use of a toroidal back surface now follows.

From the above results the laboratory then calculates the back surface toricity to correct the astigmatism. Holden and Garner (1976) recommend the double truncation of such lenses for stabilization, but it may be worth while, in view of the complexity of the lens to order initially a lens with a single lower truncation, with the upper truncation to be added later if the lens is not sufficiently stable. If the lens is double truncated the average size is between 11.5 mm × 13 mm and 12 mm × 14 mm. As can be seen, each truncation is normally in the region of 1 mm.

Unfortunately, due to their complex design, these lenses are frequently found to be very unstable and need to be made rather large in order to work satisfactorily. As toroidal surfaces are always difficult to work on a very thin lens, the combination of a thick lens in a large size may prove to be physiologically unsatisfactory. Very often such lenses prove to be unstable optically, but if the lens is held in a stable position on the cornea with the fingers, good visual acuity may be obtained. As soon as the support of the fingers is removed, however, the lens may rotate and provide poor and unstable acuity. The visual acuity is most likely to be satisfactory if the lens has only to correct corneal astigmatism, and least likely to be satisfactory if the lens has to correct more than this. If the lens is made in bi-toric form then, clearly, its complexity is a major problem if it cannot be stabilized to prevent rotation.

Back surface toroidal lenses without prism or truncation

Once again this form of lens can be made with or without a toroidal front surface to correct residual or induced astigmatism and, due to the wide variety of materials used and the variations in refractive index, most laboratories prefer the practitioner to supply basic information for the calculation of the toroidal back surfaces. These are suitably cut in the dehydrated state to allow for the increase in radii and lowering of refractive index with hydration.

Mathematical formulae for these calculations have been presented (Holden and Garner, 1976) but despite this, most laboratories prefer to work with basic information, rather than be told by the practitioner what radii to use on the lens. For the fitting of this type of lens the laboratories require to be given accurate keratometric readings and an accurate refraction. The corneal diameter is also carefully measured. The lens is made up by the laboratory with a toroidal back surface to correct corneal astigmatism, without the use of truncation or prism. If the ocular astigmatism is different from the corneal astigmatism then the laboratory will make a bi-toric lens to correct the residual astigmatism. As, however, in this instance the residual astigmatism has only been calculated rather than determined *in situ*, errors may arise, as mentioned in the section dealing with hard corneal toric lenses. The great difficulty with this type of lens, as with the previous variety, is that with toroidal back surfaces it is almost impossible to check the lenses accurately. Optimistic attempts have been made to do this, and claims have been made that lenses can be checked very accurately by keratometric methods involving the suspension of the lens in a saline solution bath. Some authorities, however, are somewhat unhappy with the accuracy of this method, even with a spherical surface, and the task of measuring a toric soft lens becomes even more difficult.

This type of lens, without additional stabilization, usually produces poor results. The lens frequently rotates between 10° and 30° (usually excyclorotation) with resultant poor and variable acuity. Generally speaking lenses which give poor but stable acuity are more acceptable than those which give moments of clear vision followed by moments of poor vision as the lens rotates.

When the lens rotates it also flexes differently in the different meridians, and this also produces fluctuations in the effective power on the eye. If the lens rotates in an unpredictable fashion then it can be truncated by the practitioner in the manner already described. Either one or two truncations can be added, and this is frequently sufficient to stabilize the lens enough to give satisfactory vision.

Back surface toroidal lenses with prism ballast

Lenses of this type have been made to prescription by several laboratories and are also manufactured under the trade name Hydroflex/m-T. The latter lens was originally designed by the German laboratory of Wöhlk, now part of the Zeiss (West German) organization, and consists of a toroidal back surface which is stabilized on the eye by means of prism ballast of approximately 1.5 Δ. The lens is designed for use in cases of corneal astigmatism only, although it is possible to modify the back surface toricity to cope with residual astigmatism, provided the axis of the residual astigmatism is similar to that of the corneal astigmatism. Such lenses can be made in a full range of powers from −20.00 to +20.00 D with cylinders from 0.75 to 6.00 D. With this form of lens, as with most of those having toroidal back surfaces, special fitting lenses are not necessary. When ordering the final lens the laboratory may either be given the necessary information to design it to correct the manifest astigmatism, or the practitioner can work out the back surface radii required from a table of radii and surface powers for a refractive index of 1.4448 (*see* Appendix B, *Table B.I*). This method is preferred by the laboratory. In the former case the laboratory requires accurate corneal radii and meridians, the exact refraction of the eye, with the cylinder expressed in negative cylinder form and the specification of the orthodox Hydroflex/m lens giving the best physical fit in as large a total diameter as possible. Wöhlk used to claim that in approximately 70% of cases the desired result could be achieved with the very first pair of lenses, although Hodd (1976) reported a success rate somewhat lower than this. As is common with all forms of toroidal back surface soft lens, considerable skill and experience is required in fitting these lenses.

Laboratories can, or should, be able to make their lenses with any marks requested by the practitioner, and the Hydroflex/m-T is provided with two small marks at the edge. These are only visible using magnification. The base of the prism lies at an angle of 90° to an imaginary line drawn between these two marks, the latter normally being expected to lie along the 180° meridian. If this is not the case in the final prescription lens the amount of divergence from the 180° meridian should be determined and the laboratory should be notified of this divergence. The lens is then remade, taking this variation into account, so that, although the markings of the second lens do not lie along 180°, its cylinder axis should locate correctly. One of the difficulties of lenses of this type is that they are almost invariably rather thick, which often leads to poor physiological results. Within the total diameter range available for Hydroflex/m lenses the Hydroflex/m-T lens is fitted as large and flat as possible (average total diameter of 13.0 mm). By so doing it is inclined to give a somewhat better physiological result than larger more steeply fitted lenses; also because the lenses are reasonably thin. A Hydroflex/m-T lens of −3.00 D with a 1.5 Δ prism and a total diameter of 12.5 mm would have a central thickness of 0.2 mm. Unfortunately, some of the smaller soft lenses of this thickness can give considerable discomfort in the conjunctival region adjacent to the limbus and also on the lid margins, which may offset their other physiological advantages.

Despite these problems, however, which are common to most types of toric soft lens, the lenses are well made and provide a logical way of dealing with manifest corneal astigmatism. It is, again, important that the refraction over the spherical trial lens be performed with a lens as near to the final prescription as possible.

These lenses can be fitted as large as 13.5 mm total diameter although the majority are in the region of 12.5 mm. As the toroidal back surface is the primary form of stabilization, the greater the corneal astigmatism the more likely the lens is to stabilize. Unfortunately, however, the higher the corneal astigmatism, the smaller the degree of rotation the patient will tolerate optically. It is obviously necessary for the spectacle refraction cylinder and keratometer cylinder to be almost identical for accurate results. Skilful changing of the prescription of the toroidal back surface can also give an induced front surface cylinder to correct residual astigmatism. Hodd (1976) found that with the use of the Hydroflex/m-T lens for the correction of corneal astigmatism, fair to good visual acuity was obtained in 19 out of 40 lenses made for 24 eyes. With the same type of lens used for the correction of lenticular astigmatism he reported only obtaining fair to good visual acuity in 3 cases out of 15 lenses made for 10 eyes. Hodd also reported that in a group of 14 cases, for which this lens was indicated, only one was able to achieve constant wearing time with visual acuity equivalent to that of spectacles.

The lens appears to work somewhat better in the hyperopic eye than in the myopic eye and this may well be due to the increased thickness and thus more stable lens form. Possibly for this very reason Wöhlk (now Zeiss) also make a larger, prism ballasted and truncated toroidal back surface lens which is slightly thicker and more stable. It is known as the Hydroflex-TS lens. It is often necessary to use a vertical prism in both eyes if lenses are to be equally comfortable and in order to prevent an induced vertical heterophoria. Gasson (1977), however, finds that it is often possible to omit the prism when the contralateral eye is fitted with a non-toric lens.

A clinical rationale for the use of a toroidal back surface soft lens with spherical front surfaces

As an example consider the case of a patient with a corneal cylinder of:

−2.50 D with-the-rule
The corneal radii differ by approximately 0.5 mm
No residual (lenticular) astigmatism present

Then visualize a medium thickness soft lens, suitable to fit such a cornea, being placed on a finger tip and being sufficiently rigid to hold its shape.

Placing such a lens on the cornea and allowing it to settle will force the lens to flex much more in the vertical than in the horizontal. Given the springy nature of such material, the vertical meridian will tend to spring back to its flatter initial shape, although, in the main, it will remain wrapped around the cornea.

Its tendency to spring back off the steeper meridian will depend on:

(1) The elasticity of the material.
(2) The thickness.
(3) Variation in thickness (e.g. use of prism).
(4) Use or absence of truncation.
(5) Lid tension.
(6) Lid aperture.
(7) Blinking.

If, however, a lens is used which has been cut from a blank to produce a toroidal back surface with a 0.5 mm difference in radii, then it will 'wrap' onto the toroidal cornea, without the need to flex. The vertical meridian will not have to flex more than the horizontal meridian and thus there is no tendency to 'spring back' to a spherical shape. This normally makes such lenses more predictable in their performance and much less prone to cause variations in acuity due to instability and flexure.

If the lens back surface aligns with the cornea it is less likely to be affected by lids, blinking, degree of astigmatism and thickness.

In the case under consideration with a PMMA lens having a toroidal back surface, with a 0.5 mm difference in radii and a spherical front surface, then the induced astigmatism would measure approximately:

−1.25 DC × 90

This is created by the difference in the refractive indices, of the tears (1.336) and lens (1.49) at the toroidal surface with a 0.5 mm difference in radii.

Fortunately soft lens materials have lower refractive indices than PMMA and range mainly between 1.44 and 1.37, depending on water content.

The use of a 60% water content material with a refractive index of 1.39 is recommended to give a good compromise between stability and low refractive index.

Reconsidering the case above, fitted with a toroidal back surface soft lens instead of a PMMA lens, the induced astigmatism would be greatly reduced:

(1) Using a HEMA lens of refractive index 1.44, the induced astigmatism would reduce to approximately 0.75 D.
(2) With a 60% water content material of refractive index 1.39, the induced astigmatism reduces to less than 0.50 D.

In most cases of significant corneal astigmatism, it is clinically best to try to use a toroidal back surface and spherical front surface with a low refractive index material. In such an instance there is only a very low induced cylinder to contend with, which can often be ignored.

Clinical experience indicates that, as the back surface matches the corneal shape better, the lens flexes less, fits the cornea better and rotates less. In such cases small lens rotations of 5–10° appear to give very little change in the front surface keratometry reading with the lens *in situ*. The clinical evidence of good visual acuity and stable front surface K readings seem to indicate that toroidal back surface lenses can rotate more than toroidal front surface lenses without adversely affecting the visual results.

If the visual acuity is poor and the front surface K reading reveals a small cylinder in the original axis direction, then the lens is prescribed with a greater difference in the radii of the back surface of the lens in an attempt to achieve a spherical front surface K reading.

Example

Original corneal cylinder $-2.50\,D \times 180$
Lens back surface radii: 0.5 mm difference
Front surface K: $-1.00\,DC \times 180$
Since 0.05 mm difference in radius is approximately equivalent to 0.5 D, a new lens is supplied with back surface radii difference of 0.6 mm

It is recommended that more reliance is placed on the front surface K reading *in situ* than on over-refraction as visual acuity is usually best when the front surface of the lens shows spherical K readings. It is, of course, possible to manipulate the chosen back surface radii to compensate for residual or induced astigmatism. For example, if the corneal cylindrical correction is $-5.00\,D \times 180$, then the difference in corneal radii is about 0.9 mm. If a lens is fitted with a full 0.9 mm difference in back surface radii, the induced cylinder needs to be corrected by approximately -0.75 to $-1.00\,D \times 90$ with a lens of refractive index 1.39.

With a back surface difference in radii of 0.8 mm then the slightly flatter vertical back surface radius would have to flex slightly to fit the steeper vertical meridian of the cornea and this would produce a lens with front surface astigmatism with-the-rule, which would tend to compensate the induced against-the-rule astigmatism.

Great success can be achieved with this system and visual acuities of 6/6 (20/20) have been obtained in cases of prescriptions as high as $+1.00/-8.50 \times 30$ and $+17.00/-6.00 \times 90$.

With the multiplicity of available lens designs and materials the practitioner can manipulate the fittings relative to the refractive index of the material to obtain the best possible results.

Several queries have been raised as to whether or not toroidal back surface lenses stabilize better than those with toroidal front surfaces. Tomlinson, Chang and Hitchcock (1986) compared a series of cases fitted with toroidal back surface lenses and toroidal front surface lenses. Little difference was found in the stability and ability to resist rotation between the two lens types but it was found that the toroidal front surface design was less comfortable.

However, excellent results with toroidal back surfaces are only possible when using very high quality lenses from laboratories who will make any combination of radii required by the practitioner. It is also necessary to have more than one total diameter available.

It can be readily understood that more sophisticated and complex fittings, such as torics and bifocals, need to be fitted with even greater care and subtlety than ordinary spherical fittings. This implies a need for a wider range of parameters being available for the complex cases, and unfortunately the reverse is normally true.

Tomlinson, Chang and Hitchcock (1986), for example, used the Hydrocurve II and Durasoft 2 lenses in their investigations. According to Tyler's guide (Tyler, 1987) the Hydrocurve II lens (toroidal back surface) is available with a BOZR of 8.6 mm in a total diameter of 13.5 mm, and a BOZR of 8.9 mm in a total diameter of 14.5 mm. The Durasoft 2, however, is available with BOZRs of 8.3 and 8.6 mm in a TD of 14.5 mm and BOZRs of 8.2 and 8.5 mm in a TD of 13.5 mm. A custom-made BOZR of 9.0 mm in a TD of 14.5 mm is also available. It would, therefore, have been very hard for the investigators to obtain great subtlety of fitting and it would appear that the Durasoft 2 lens should be capable of being fitted more accurately in view of its wider range of parameters.

Such limited parameters which force practitioners to constantly compromise preclude the possibility of a high success rate. Unfortunately the larger American laboratories and manufacturers produce a very limited range of parameters for their toric lenses, whereas European practitioners have had the benefit of virtually unlimited parameters since the mid-1970s.

Dynamic stabilization

This technique (Fanti, 1975) has been used to considerable advantage as the lens design is not stabilized by gravity or adhesion but, as explained on p. 535 and in Chapter 11, by the kinetic forces associated with blinking. Such lenses were made by Titmus Eurocon (now part of the CIBA Vision group) under the name Weicon-T. Several similar designs, referred to as 'double slab-off' or 'thin zone' stabilized or reverse prism stabilized, are now manufactured by other laboratories

There are two segments, one each at the top and bottom of the lens, as illustrated in *Figure 14.27*. The remaining central portion of the front surface is toroidal. The dynamic stabilization axis (known as the DS axis) is symmetrical to these two zones and passes through both the optical and geometric centres of the lens. The method in which the lens is inserted is not important since the action of the lids during blinking stabilizes the lens very quickly. *Figures 14.27* and *14.40* indicate that the action of the lids on the superior and inferior lens chamfers are inclined to stabilize the lens with the DS axis approximately horizontal.

In designs produced by other laboratories a longer, i.e. larger, thinned zone is provided superiorly to utilize the fact that most of the

blink action is performed by the upper eyelid. With these designs it is more important that the lens is inserted the correct way up. To facilitate this lenses are commonly laser marked at the lower edge with one or more lines, e.g. three lines showing the vertical and 10° or 15° either side. These also aid practitioner determination of lens rotation.

Even if such a lens is put into the eye with the DS axis vertical, the lens will normally rotate within 30 seconds to bring it to its stable axis position. Advantages of this type of lens are that the lens is very smooth and round in shape which gives the patient a very good reaction initially, comparable to that of orthodox soft spherical lenses.

Due to the unique nature of the lens it is necessary that the lens be fitted with a fitting set of lenses with the dynamic stabilization periphery. The fitting lenses are spherical and are marked with the DS axis (*Figure 14.40*). Due to the large size of the lens it is fitted approximately 1.2 mm flatter than the mean of the principal K readings and it is recommended that such a lens be fitted a little tighter than the simple spherical form. In general, the fit can be considered optimum if the lens centres satisfactorily and shows minimal movement with blinking. The author usually fits these lenses as tight as possible consistent with finding no indentation of the conjunctiva underneath the extreme periphery of the lens when the lens is gently moved with digital pressure.

A diagnostic fitting set normally has BOZR in steps of 0.2 or 0.3 mm ranging from 8.2 to 9.4 mm. Most diagnostic lenses are made in −3.00 D power with total diameter of 14.0 or 14.5 mm.

This lens design is very satisfactory for the correction of astigmatic errors in myopes of over 3.00 D and if careful selection of the right patient is made, the success rate should be very high. The visual acuity is almost always extremely good with very little rotation. Lenses which orientate with the DS axis more than 20° from the horizontal should be considered with suspicion as the lens may not be stable in its final form. Frequently, if fitting lenses are found to rotate in an unsatisfactory manner, the difficulty can be overcome by fitting a slightly tighter lens. If so, consideration must be given to the possible adverse physiological effects. (Poor physiological results occurred with some high positive

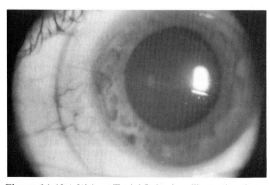

Figure 14.40 A Weicon-T trial fitting lens illustrating the engraved line (DS axis) with reference to which the cylinder axis is prescribed. The conjunctival injection is normal in this particular patient even in the absence of a contact lens

experimental lenses made for the author with cylinders of up to −7.00 D. The focimeter images with these lenses were comparable with those of orthodox spectacle lenses, so the optical quality was very good.)

The prescribing of the final cylinder axis is relative to the DS axis which is assumed to be horizontal for the purposes of prescribing. Thus, if the cylindrical error, during over-refraction, is found to be at an axis of 45° and the DS axis is at an angle of 10°, then the final prescription lens must be ordered with the cylindrical axis at 35°. When the lens rotates to its correct DS axis of 10° on the eye, the cylindrical component will rotate to its true position of 45°.

Indications for this lens include both corneal and residual astigmatism, or combinations of the above. The real advantages of this form of lens are its ability to stabilize reliably and the ability to prescribe both for corneal and residual astigmatism.

Contra-indications to this type of lens are unstable positioning on the eye with whatever fitting is attempted and any unusual lid action or closure. It is also contra-indicated in irregular astigmatism.

The use of the Weicon-T lens is made considerably easier if the practitioner has a reliable and accurate method of measuring the axis of the dynamic stabilization region. The fitting lenses are engraved with a broken line along this axis, but it is often extremely difficult to view this line in the eye (*Figure 14.40*). If it is visible its orientation can be measured by placing before the eye a plano glass trial lens with an engraved line across the middle of the lens. This is aligned with the engraved line on the Weicon-T lens and the angle is read on a trial frame. However, if the engraved lines cannot be seen clearly through the plano trial lens, the patient is then best observed with a slit lamp biomicroscope using low magnification. Although there is limited depth of focus the microscope can be racked back and forth slightly to focus first the contact lens axis then the engraved glass trial lens, the axis of which can be read off on the trial frame.

An even better method involves the use of a special biomicroscope eyepiece containing a graticule ruled as a protractor, on which the DS axis of the Weicon-T lens can be read off directly. Another method described by Fanti (1975) is to use a slit lamp microscope with a

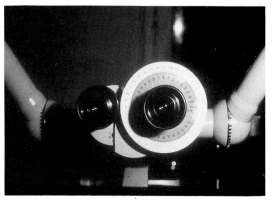

Figure 14.41 A protractor mounted on a slit lamp eyepiece for measuring rotation and orientation position

measuring graticule which is connected to a protractor fixed on the outside of the eyepiece of the instrument. The measuring graticule is then turned to correspond with the angle of the DS axis seen through the microscope and the axis can then be read on the protractor (*Figure 14.41*).

A further excellent method of measuring the angle of the DS axis accurately is to use an ophthalmometer employing the Javal principle with the doubling device in only one meridian. If such an instrument is focused onto the engraved DS reference line, with the eye well illuminated via an external light source, the observer will generally detect the doubled image of the lens and the DS axis line. If the instrument is rotated, as for normal axis determination, until the two images coincide and can be superimposed, then only one line will be visible. The axis of the DS line can now be read off on the ophthalmometer scale.

It is extremely useful to observe what happens to the soft trial lens when the patient blinks in different directions of gaze. Frequently, the lens remains stable, but if the patient looks down and blinks the lens may rotate 10° or more. If this recurs when the test is repeated it may be taken as a contra-indication, especially if the astigmatism is high and if the patient's work involves a lot of looking down such as carrying out clerical tasks.

Any lens which is found to rotate more than 10° will almost certainly be unsatisfactory in its final form. Obviously, a great deal depends on the power of the cylinder to be incorporated on the front surface. Wearers of high cylinders are not able to tolerate much rotation.

The reliability of stabilization of the Weicon-T lens is also dependent on the degree of myopia present in the correction. From *Figure 14.27*, illustrating the form and principle of the lens, it will be seen that the more myopic the patient the thicker is the peripheral region, thus giving greater stabilization by permitting better chamfering at the top and bottom of the lens. Tests by the author indicate that a lens of approximately −3.00 D stabilizes on the eye in approximately 5–10 minutes, but may still then rotate by some 5–7°. A lens of −10.00 D will stabilize almost immediately and often remain almost immobile in terms of rotation.

However, the DS axis of the final lens may differ from that of the spherical trial lens due to the effect on edge thickness of the front surface cylinder and its axis (*see* pp. 535–536 and 551).

Stock lenses *vs* custom-made lenses

It is regrettable that whilst most practitioners pride themselves on the accuracy of their refraction, they are prepared to accept toric lenses available in only one or two cylindrical powers set at perhaps six or eight axes. This has arisen because the thousands of permutations of possible cylindrical powers and axes do not lend themselves to the mass production techniques and inventory supply of the large international laboratories. Further, since many of these laboratories manufacture in one country and then export lenses to several other countries where subinventories are held, it would be impossible to produce lenses and have them available everywhere in all possible permutations, and equally impossible to provide a custom-made service. The larger laboratories therefore typically produce lenses of two cylindrical powers such as −1.25 D and −1.75 D, set at eight axes, usually 20°, 10°, 180°, 170°, 160°, 80°, 90° and 100°. As most patients accept cylindrical corrections that are within ±0.25 D of the correct power, and since cylinders of under −1.00 D need correcting only infrequently (provided that it is assumed that up to 0.75 D of astigmatism may be corrected with a spherical lens), this effectively covers astigmatic errors up to 2.00 D in most of the common axes.

As all practitioners fitting appreciable numbers of contact lenses are bound to come across patients rquiring cylindrical corrections not covered by the above range, it is essential to have access to a laboratory which can produce lenses to any required parameter. The small independent laboratories are generally the only ones offering this facility, and the personalized service they provide has been mutually beneficial, often ensuring their continued existence.

Many practitioners prefer to use custom-made toric lenses for all astigmatic patients. This enables them to alter parameters in any possible direction if the lens rotates or prescription changes. Nevertheless the cheaper mass-produced toric lenses, although of limited parameters, enable rapid supply, easy exchange facility and high reproducibility. It is also possible for practitioners to hold a selection of lenses in their own inventory permitting a more accurate assessment of the effects of lens rotation by using a lens of almost correct power and axis on the eye. A large number of practitioners therefore fit both mass-produced and custom-made toric lenses.

The practitioner with only limited experience of toric soft lens fitting is also well advised to use a laboratory offering exchange facilities. Remba (1986) found an average of 1.8 lenses per eye in successful cases, and 2.6 lenses per eye if both successful and unsuccessful cases were considered.

Irregular astigmatism

None of the previously mentioned forms of soft lens is capable of being used to correct irregular astigmatism. Conventionally, astigmatic errors of this nature are corrected with hard lenses but in some severe types of irregular astigmatism, such as that encountered in moderate or advanced keratoconus, some patients are physically unable to wear such lenses satisfactorily. One solution to this problem is the use of a lens with a rigid centre which corrects the irregular astigmatism, and a soft periphery which is flexible and fits the irregular cornea and limbus with comfort while holding the rigid central portion in place. Gumpelmayer (1986, personal communication) made such experimental lenses in the 1970s, but found them too fragile. More recently, the Saturn lens (manufactured by Pilkington Barnes–Hind in the USA) has been produced in this form, and the Russians discussed such a lens with the author in Moscow in 1980.

Usually, however, the 'combination' or 'piggy-back' system is preferable due to its great flexibility and unlimited range of parameters. When the Saturn lens is available in a wider range of parameters it should prove very useful for it seems probable that such lenses with hard centres and soft peripheries will become a major form of correction for astigmatism in the future. Both the Saturn lens and the combination system are discussed in Chapter 21 in the section on the fitting of keratoconus.

The 'combination' system (Westerhout, 1973) is a means of overcoming irregular astigmatism by fitting the eye conventionally with a soft lens so as to provide an artificial cornea over which an orthodox hard lens can then be fitted, as shown in *Plates 121* and *122*. Naturally enough, in severe keratoconus, the fitting of the soft lens can produce certain difficulties but most lathe-cut lenses can be made sufficiently steep to deal with this problem.

Once a suitable soft lens has been fitted and is found capable of being worn comfortably for daily use, the front surface of the soft lens is then measured with a keratometer, and forms an artificial cornea to which the hard lens is then fitted. Gas permeable hard corneal lenses are preferable to PMMA lenses for this purpose.

Westerhout (1973) has recommended that the soft lens used should be of fairly high negative power in order that its front surface radii are lengthened so as to approach more closely the average, normal fitting range of hard lenses. The 'combination lens' has been used very successfully in a large number of cases of irregular astigmatism and keratoconus and will continue to be a viable proposition.

Checking soft toric lenses

Methods of checking soft lenses are covered in Chapter 13 but a few points are worthy of emphasis here. The special features of lenses with toroidal surfaces apply as much to soft lenses as hard lenses and the approach to verification is similar (*see* p. 523). Because of the relative fragility of the soft lens material it is important to look for areas of damage to the lens where axis markings or other engravings have been made. These areas are also more likely to become contaminated during use.

Many practitioners feel very apprehensive about dispensing a new toric soft lens to a patient. As a result of numerous bad experiences and disappointments, practitioners have almost come to expect mediocre visual results, especially if they are unable to check the lenses accurately.

With a little care and ingenuity, however, it is possible to check lenses accurately. Projection focimeters, with small aperture stops, are best for this purpose, although the problem of orientating the identification marks is difficult to solve without a satisfactory way of holding or supporting the lens.

Many toric soft lenses may be made accurately in power and axis direction relative to prism or stabilizing zones, but may be wrongly marked. If a wet cell is not used, the basic difficulty in checking the power of a soft lens is to attempt to dry the lens in such a way as to leave it lint or dust free.

Wet cells

Wet cells have been used with effect for many years for soft lens checking and inspection and in the early 1970s were marketed by several European soft lens manufacturers. Their advantages and disadvantages are discussed in Chapter 13. They are probably best reserved for inspecting and measuring surface quality, diameter and radius on special instruments.

Checking a surface-dried lens

Lint-free filter paper is the most effective if a soft lens is to be dried before inspection. Unfortunately, however, the dried lens rapidly dehydrates causing its power to change. It is essential, therefore, to carry out the mounting of the lens on the instrument and the subsequent power measurement as quickly as possible. This is difficult with a toric soft lens. When a lens is placed on the small stop of a focimeter it tends to droop over the stop causing distortion. Especially if they are thin, lenses tend to wrinkle and fold up, and even if they can be placed on the stop without distortion, they cannot be placed with the orientation marks in a specific, accurate direction.

In consequence of these problems the most common form of toric soft lens check is to place the lens on the eye and check the visual acuity.

The Tori-Check

This device is a simple but effective tool to facilitate the support of a soft contact lens on a focimeter and permit the practitioner to position the orientation marks accurately, before the power and axis are read. The lens is first blotted dry (*Figure 14.42*), and mounted on the rotatable disc which is turned so that the lens marks are in an appropriate position — usually vertical or horizontal (*Figure 14.43*).

The Tori-Check handle is then placed on the spectacle frame platform to orientate it horizontally (as shown in *Figure 14.44*) and the measurements are then taken on the instrument.

If it is found that a lens is mismarked, with respect to stabilization zones, prisms or axes (*Figure 14.45*), the handle is placed on a compatible protractor and the marking error

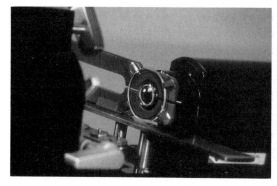

Figure 14.44 Use of Tori-Check for checking toric soft lens power. The handle on the instrument is placed on the spectacle frame platform, or held parallel to the platform, with the rotatable disc centred on the lens stop

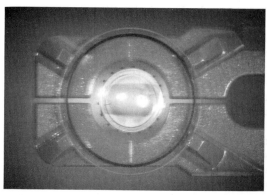

Figure 14.45 Incorrectly marked 'thin-zone' soft toric lens on a Tori-Check instrument. The 'thin-zone' lens has been rotated so that the shadows indicating the thin zones are parallel to the instrument axis. The orientation marks are incorrectly engraved and can be seen at approximately 10° off-axis

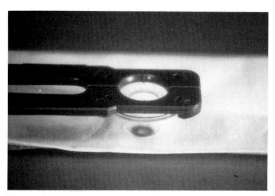

Figure 14.42 Use of the Tori-Check instrument. The instrument is inverted and brought into contact with the blotted lens. The lens adheres to the clear rotatable disc seen under the grey handle

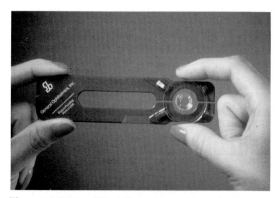

Figure 14.43 Use of Tori-Check for checking toric soft lenses. The rotatable disc is turned so that the orientation marks or truncations are in the desired position (usually in the horizontal or vertical)

can then be measured, and reported to the laboratory or used as a basis for re-ordering.

This simple device is very helpful, especially if toric soft lenses are to be checked by auxiliary staff with limited experience.

As with any type of lens, particularly those of medium to high power, it is essential to know whether or not the manufacturer uses front or back vertex powers, the latter being recommended. Ideally the practitioner should know the methods used for checking, as well as the instruments employed by the laboratory. As discussed in Chapter 12, unless the back vertex of the lens can be placed in the correct plane, a steeply curved and high powered lens supported on a wide focimeter stop suffers a larger power error due to the sagitta of the lens compared to the same lens on a narrower stop. Such differences may lead to disagreement between practitioner and laboratory.

Markings on lenses

The original Weicon toric lens developed in the early 1970s by Fanti (1975) was engraved with straight lines across the horizontal meridian. These lines were quite visible with the lens on the eye and the practitioner was able to observe the orientation of the lens easily and accurately.

It is of greater importance that the lines should be observable without the patient taking up an unnatural posture or the lids being retracted. As the orientation of toric lenses depends largely on lid action, it is clearly unsatisfactory to have to retract the lids and thereby lose the effect of lid and lens interaction, in order to observe the marks. It is also important to be able to see the markings or points of reference without the patient making unnatural head movements which may influence the lid position and lens orientation. Many recent designs of toric lens have marks which are so difficult to find that they can only be seen with a slit lamp biomicroscope, and often only when the lower lids are withdrawn, which risks the patient being in a slightly abnormal posture.

Westerhout (1976a) has drawn attention to the changes in measured cylinder effects varying in different directions of gaze, so that if the patient is going to be engaged in prolonged close work with the visual axes directed down, then it is usually worth while checking the required cylinder power and axis, and lens orientation, with the eyes directed down in this working position, i.e. with chin raised if being observed with the biomicroscope.

The use of the keratometer or ophthalmometer for observation of lens markings has been dealt with on p. 547. The American Optical Company has marketed a combined keratometer and observation instrument permitting keratometer readings to be taken in one mode, then at the turn of a lever, a magnified view of the eye is obtained. Although the latter mode of use of the instrument is of limited value for observation of subtle corneal changes it is most useful for observing the orientation marks on a toric contact lens. Having lined up the instrument with the contact lens orientation marks,

the lever is turned and the axis read off on the protractor scale.

Slit lamps can also be modified to measure angles of rotation (*see* p. 547 and *Figure 14.41*).

Variations in astigmatism

Unfortunately the prescribing of toric soft lenses is made more complex by the fact that the astigmatism may vary with different directions of gaze. These changes are mainly due to the varying effects of the lids in different positions of gaze.

Westerhout (1976a) has reported variations in the degree and axis of astigmatism in transferring the gaze from distance to near. He reported one patient who manifested a residual cylinder of $-2.50\,D \times 165$ for distance and $-4.00\,D \times 150$ for near. Analysis of 40 eyes revealed that the change in astigmatism on looking down varied from a shift towards with-the-rule astigmatism of a maximum of $1.25\,D$ (mean $0.72\,D$) to a shift towards against-the-rule astigmatism of a maximum of $0.50\,D$ (mean $0.29\,D$).

Clearly these problems are additional complications in the use of toric forms of soft lens. It should also be noted that even if accurate trial lenses are used for the fitting of soft toric lenses, the stabilization may well be different when the edge and centre thickness vary in the final lens form. A notable example of this is in the use of the Weicon-T lens where, if the trial lens is found to stabilize accurately and the prescription lens is made up with a high cylinder correction for astigmatism against-the-rule, the reduction of the thickness in the stabilization areas, in the vertical meridian, may considerably affect the lens stabilization because adequate chamfering of the lens may be difficult to achieve. Results may be still worse if the axis of the cylinder is oblique. In this case the edges may vary enormously in thickness and may have a profound effect on the rotation of the lens. Similar variations with oblique cylinders on lenses with toroidal back surfaces can also produce unreliable and unpredictable rotational effects.

All toric soft lenses are difficult to manufacture and the material used in manufacture is, therefore, very important. Laboratory technicians find that some soft lens blanks in their hard form can be cut and polished with far more accuracy than others and these better materials are therefore clearly worth using when manufacturing such complicated lenses. Oxygen permeability is, however, a factor to consider as such lenses are thicker than normal. The ideal material for toric soft lens manufacture is, therefore, a material of high oxygen permeability, great flexibility and ease of accurate cutting and polishing.

Trends in toric soft lens design

The conventional means of stabilizing toric soft lenses have already been discussed elsewhere in this chapter. Analysis of the lens designs currently available reveals very little radical change during the last 10 years. Most lenses are still orientated with prism ballast although fewer seem to be truncated. Increasingly lenses are being used with dynamic stabilization or zonal thinning.

Most of the lenses designed in the 1970s suffered from problems of irregular and unpredictable edge thickness. Many of the modern lenses avoid this difficulty which aids stability and freedom from unwanted rotation.

Most of the low water content prism ballasted lenses produce undesirable physiological results, on occasion, due to their thickness. This problem has been addressed in a variety of ways which improve performance.

Several designs have been made where the prism does not exist in the optic zone containing the toric prescription. Perhaps the first of these was the toric optic cap (TOC) lens made by Hirst of New Zealand. This lens contained a lenticular toric optic zone with no prism and a peripheral carrier zone with a prism, but no prescription. This provided a thin and constant edge profile, regardless of power, and more predictable fitting characteristics than previous lenses. It also removed the possibility of the prism giving rise to vertical heterophoria.

A more recent version of this type of lens is the Hydron Z6T which also has a central prism-free optic zone and is stabilized by a peripheral prism zone, including a 'comfort chamfer' which appears to be a modification of the thin-zone principle.

This lens is available in four BOZRs and has the advantage of being only 0.06 mm in central thickness in minus powers. This reduction in thickness, over previous designs, substantially reduces the physiological problems previously discussed (*see* p. 534).

Custom-made lenses produced in higher water content materials such as the Duragel 60% material of the late 1970s have also helped to solve the physiological problems, so common with the thick, low water content toric lenses of the past. In 1977 the author had several toric lenses made up from this material in powers up to $+8.00$ D and they performed very well. There is now a multiplicity of other materials available which can be used to produce more oxygen-permeable toric soft lenses. Indeed, in the USA, there are now several extended wear, toric soft lenses. This implies that their oxygen delivery to the cornea must be adequate, despite the fact that their water content is only in the 55–60% range.

Making lenses in lower water content materials is still the easiest method of manufacture and such lenses work well from the physiological standpoint provided that they are thin, as in the case of the Hydron Z6T lens.

Other laboratories are also in the process of developing sophisticated toric lenses in more permeable designs or materials. Zeiss (formerly Wöhlk of West Germany), known for many years for the accuracy and wide parameter range of their 38.6% water content toric soft lenses, is also developing more permeable toric soft lenses. Titmus Eurocon (CIBA Vision), the manufacturers of the original Weicon T lens, are now providing a smaller, thinner version although the range of parameters is limited.

Summary

It has been requested that a brief and simplified summary of the appropriate types of toric lens fittings be included at the end of this chapter.

Over-simplification is never desirable in a clinical subject, but the brief notes below may be of assistance to some.

Toric hard corneal lens fittings

The required initial information is as follows:

(1) An accurate subjective spectacle refraction.
(2) An accurate keratometric reading with radii, powers and axes.

In the following discussion the term 'compatible' means that a comparison of the cylinder elements in the refraction and keratometric readings reveals a discrepancy of 0.75 D or less. It is clearly up to the clinician to decide whether or not a residual cylinder of 1.00 D or greater, is going to be acceptable to his patient. 'Compatible axes' means axes which are similar, and it is clear that patients may well be able to tolerate the visual limitations of axes varying by larger angular discrepancies with low cylinders than they would with high cylinders. In general, compatible, in this context, means approximately plus or minus 10°.

Principal clinical indications

(1) The refraction cylinder is compatible with the keratometric cylinder. Here a spherical corneal lens can be used if the amount of toricity is small enough to permit its fitting.
(2) The refraction and keratometric cylinders are compatible but highly toroidal. Here a toroidal back surface may be required physically, in a lens of compensated bi-toric form.
(3) The refraction cylinder is not compatible with the keratometric cylinder which may be very small. This gives rise to residual astigmatism with a spherical lens and may thus require a stabilized lens with toroidal front surface.
(4) The keratometric cylinder is high with the refraction cylinder not compatible, but axes are similar. Here a parallel bi-toric lens may be found useful.
(5) The keratometric cylinder is high, but the refraction cylinder axes are not compatible. Here an oblique bi-toric lens may be required.
(6) The keratometric cylinder is high, but the refraction cylinder is higher, such that the residual astigmatism with a spherical lens is cancelled out by the cylinder induced by a toroidal back surface. This occurs when the ocular astigmatism is about 50% greater than the corneal astigmatism and the axes are similar. Here a toroidal back surface with a spherical front surface may suffice.

Toric soft lens fittings

(1) Low refraction cylinder. A spherical soft lens is indicated whether or not the keratometric cylinder is high or low.
(2) A high refraction cylinder, but the keratometric cylinder is low. In this case a toroidal front surface is indicated or, if axes are compatible, the more complex toroidal back surface to induce a toroidal front surface. Either form must be stabilized by prism ballast and/or truncation.
(3) A high refraction cylinder compatible with keratometric cylinder in power and axes. Here a toroidal front surface, or a toroidal back surface to correct corneal astigmatism, may prove successful. Stabilization in some form is likely to be necessary.
(4) A high refraction cylinder with keratometric cylinder at different axes. A toroidal front surface lens is the only lens likely to succeed, although an oblique bi-toric lens could be attempted, as, in theory, it is the better proposition, but is extremely difficult to make. Either type would need to be stabilized.
(5) A high refraction cylinder and high keratometric cylinder, although not compatible. If the axes are compatible then a parallel bi-toric lens may suffice, although a toroidal front surface is simpler and easier to prescribe and manufacture. If the axes are not compatible, fit as in (4) above.
(6) A high refraction cylinder, but a high keratometric cylinder not compatible and with different axes. Here an oblique bi-toric soft lens may prove successful, although a toroidal front surface lens is preferable. Again stabilization is likely to be necessary.

Acknowledgements

I am indebted to my father, Mr N. E. Westerhout, for all the line drawings of *Figures 14.1–14.24* and also to Mrs V. Campbell for the line drawings of *Figures 14.27–14.39*. I am also grateful to the many laboratory technicians who have so skilfully made complex forms of toric contact lens for me.

References

BARON, H. (1975). Some remarks on the correction of astigmatic eyes by means of soft contact lenses. *Contacto* **19**(6), 4–8

BENNETT, A. G. (1976). Power changes in soft contact lenses due to bending. *Ophthal. Optician* **16**, 939–945

BENNETT, A. G. (1985). *Optics of Contact Lenses*, 5th edn. London: Association of Dispensing Opticians

BRITISH STANDARD 5562 (1978). *Specification for Contact Lenses — BS 5562:1978*. London: British Standards Institution

BRITISH STANDARD 3521 (1979). *Glossary of Terms Relating to Ophthalmic Lenses and Spectacle Frames — BS 3521:1979. Part 3. Glossary of Terms Relating to Contact Lenses*. London: British Standards Institution

CAPPELLI, Q. A. (1964). Determining final power of bitoric lenses. *Br. J. physiol. Optics* **21**, 256–263

DAVY, M. W. (1976). Success for toric soft lenses. Letter in *Optician* **172**(4451), 33

DOUTHWAITE, W. A. (1987). *Contact Lens Optics*. London: Butterworths

FAIRMAID, J. A. (1967). The correction of residual astigmatism with double truncated front surface toric corneal lenses. *Ophthal. Optician* **7**, 1046–1050

FANTI, P. (1975). The fitting of a soft toroidal contact lens. *Optician* **169**(4376), 8–9, 13, 15–16

FATT, I., FREEMAN, R. D. and LIN, D. (1974). Oxygen tension distributions in the cornea: A re-examination. *Expl Eye Res.* **18**, 357–365

GASSON, A. P. (1977). Back surface toric soft lenses. *Optician* **174**(4491), 6–7, 9, 11

GOLDBERG, J. B. (1964). The correction of residual astigmatism with corneal contact lenses. *Br. J. physiol. Optics* **21**, 169–174

GULLSTRAND, A. (1924). Appendices II and IV in *Helmholtz's Treatise on Physiological Optics, Vol. I*, edited by J. P. C. Southall. New York: Optical Society of America (reprinted by Dover Publications, New York, 1962)

HARRIS, M. G. and CHU, C. S. (1972). The effects of contact lens thickness and corneal toricity on lens flexure and residual astigmatism. *Am. J. Optom.* **49**, 304–307

HARRIS, M. G. and APPLEQUIST, T. D. (1974). The effect of contact lens diameter and power on flexure and residual astigmatism. *Am. J. Optom. physiol. Optics* **51**, 266–270

HARRIS, M. G., GALE, B., GANSEL, K. and SLETTE, C. (1987). Flexure and residual astigmatism with Paraperm O₂ and Boston II lenses on toric corneas. *Am. J. Optom. physiol. Optics* **64**, 269–273

HERMAN, J. P. (1983). Flexure of rigid contact lenses on toric corneas as a function of base curve fitting relationship. *J. Am. optom. Ass.* **54**, 209–213

HERMAN, J. P. (1986). Flexure. In *Rigid Gas-Permeable Contact Lenses*, edited by E. S. Bennett and R. M. Grohe. New York: Professional Press

HILL, R. M. (1975). Can you teach an old ('rigid') lens new tricks? *Aust. J. Optom.* **58**, 322–325

HILL, R. M. and JEPPE, W. H. (1975). Hydrogels: is a pump still necessary? *Int. Contact Lens Clin.* **2**(4), 27–29

HODD, N. F. B. (1976). Clinical appraisal of toric soft lenses. *Optician* **172**(4445), 8, 11, 13

HOLDEN, B. A. and FRAUENFELDER, G. (1973). The principles and practice of correcting astigmatism with soft contact lenses. *Aust. J. Optom.* **58**, 279–299

KIMBALL, D. and MANDELL, R. B. (1974). Clinical performance of ultrathin lenses. *Int. Contact Lens Clin.* **1**, 99–107

LYDON, D. and TAIT, A. (1988). Lid pressure: its measurement and probable effects on the shape and form of the cornea — rigid contact lens system. *J. Br. Contact Lens Ass.* **11**(1), 11–22

REMBA, M. (1986). Clinical evaluation of contemporary soft toric lenses. *Optician* **192**(5066), 17–19, 24

STOKES, G. G. (1883). *Mathematical and Physical Papers, Vol. 2*, pp. 172–175. Cambridge: Cambridge University Press

STONE, J. (1967). Near vision difficulties in non-presbyopic corneal lens wearers. *Contact Lens* **1**(2), 14–16, 24–25

STONE, J. and COLLINS, C. (1984). Flexure of gas permeable lenses on toroidal corneas. *Optician* **188**(4951), 8–10

STRACHAN, J. P. F. (1973). Some principles of the optics of hydrophilic lenses and geometrical optics applied to flexible lenses. *Aust. J. Optom.* **56**, 25–33

STRACHAN, J. P. F. (1975). Correction of astigmatism with hydrophilic lenses. *Optician* **170**(4402), 8–11

TOMLINSON, A., CHANG, F. and HITCHCOCK, J. (1986). A comparison of the stability of front and back surface toric soft lenses. *Int. Eyecare* **2**(4) April, 218–222

TYLER, T. (Ed.) (1987). *Tyler's Quarterly Soft Contact Lens Parameter Guide*. Vol. 4, No. 2

WESTERHOUT, D. I. (1969). Clinical observations in fitting bi-toric and toric forms of corneal lenses. *Contact Lens* **2**(3), 5–6, 8–9

WESTERHOUT, D. I. (1971a). The first toric back optic multifocal corneal lens. *Br. J. physiol. Optics* **26**, 143–149

WESTERHOUT, D. I. (1971b). A clinical survey of oedema, its signs, symptoms and incidence. *Contact Lens* **3**(2), 3–14, 18–22, 24–25

WESTERHOUT, D. I. (1973). 'The combination lens' and therapeutic uses of soft lenses. *Contact Lens* **4**(5), 3–10, 12, 16–18, 20, 22

WESTERHOUT, D. I. (1976a). Contact lenses: corneal, residual and induced astigmatism. *Int. Contact Lens Clin.* **3**(3), 52–61

WESTERHOUT, D. I. (1976b). Lecture to Maryland Optometric Association, June 1976, University of Maryland

WESTERHOUT, D. I. (1986). Paper delivered to American Academy of Optometry, Dec. 1986, Toronto

WICHTERLE, O. and LIM, D. (1960). Hydrophilic gels for biological use. *Nature* **185**, 117–118

Chapter 15

Extended wear lenses

Brien A. Holden and Helen A. Swarbrick

Extended wear of contact lenses can be defined as the wearing of lenses without removal during eye closure, for periods ranging from occasional overnight wear up to 30 days or more of continuous wear. Extended wear has long held considerable attraction for prospective contact lens wearers because of the possibility of being totally free of spectacles. Continuous contact lens wear holds the promise of normal vision without glasses, or as some patients put it: 'a chance for new eyes'. Certainly, wherever extended wear is publicized, patient demand is extremely high because of the attraction of this alternative modality of contact lens wear.

Over the years, there have been anecdotal reports of patients sleeping in lenses, including polymethyl methacrylate (PMMA) lenses. In spite of the extremely disadvantageous physiological conditions imposed by this activity, a few patients appear to be able to tolerate this stress, at least in the short term. However, contact lenses were first intentionally used on an extended wear basis as bandage lenses (Gasset and Kaufman, 1970) to minimize patient discomfort and promote wound healing of the cornea in cases of trauma or corneal perforation due to disease and following surgical procedures. The advantage of minimal handling with this mode of lens wear led to the use of extended wear lenses for elderly aphakes who had difficulty in inserting and removing lenses on a daily basis. In recent years, extended wear lenses have become increasingly popular for cosmetic use by patients with a wide range of refractive errors.

Up until relatively recently, hydrogel or silicone elastomer lenses were the lenses of choice for extended wear. Compared to daily wear lenses, extended wear lenses must transmit considerably more oxygen in order to minimize disruption to corneal physiology during closed-eye wear. This has led to the formulation of a wide range of hydrogel lens materials with high water content, and correspondingly greater oxygen permeability, and the development of techniques to manufacture very thin lenses in low water content materials. Silicone elastomer lenses, which have very high oxygen transmissibility, have also been in use since the mid-1970s for aphakic and cosmetic extended wear, particularly in Europe and Japan.

The aggressive marketing of '30-day lenses', particularly in the USA, led to considerable consumer pressure for extended wear lenses. Press reports of devastating corneal infections associated with extended wear lenses, however, have led to a re-evaluation of the safety of this wearing modality. In addition, increasing practitioner awareness of factors predisposing the patient to acute complications, and dissemination of information on the subtle long-term effects of hydrogel extended wear lenses on corneal structure and function, have emphasized the need for a more conservative attitude to extended wear (Holden, 1986). In particular, this has meant a re-orientation in attitude to the '30-day lens' concept, and it is now widely accepted that more frequent lens removal, at least once a week and preferably more often, is imperative in order to minimize the risks of both short- and long-term complications of hydrogel extended lens wear.

The development of rigid gas permeable (RGP) materials with high oxygen permeability has encouraged investigation of the feasibility of RGP lenses for extended wear. These lenses have been shown to have a number of advantages over hydrogel lenses for extended wear, and it is likely that they will gain more widespread acceptance for this type of use at least until hydrogel materials with higher oxygen permeability become available for use in this modality in the near future.

The ocular environment

Oxygen needs and supply

When the eye is open, oxygen is supplied to the cornea directly from the atmosphere (Smelser and Ozanics, 1952; Hill and Fatt, 1964). The concentration of oxygen in the atmosphere is approximately 21%, corresponding to a partial pressure (Po_2) of 155 mmHg (21 kPa) at sea level. During eye closure, oxygen is provided to the cornea almost exclusively from the capillary plexus of the palpebral conjunctiva, but at much reduced levels (Po_2 = 60 mmHg or 8 kPa; Efron and Carney, 1979; Holden and Sweeney, 1985).

An adequate supply of oxygen is essential to maintain normal epithelial aerobic metabolism. When the level of oxygen at the anterior corneal surface is reduced, there is a decrease in the rate of aerobic metabolism, and a consequent increase in the rate of anaerobic metabolic activity in the epithelium. One major metabolic waste product of anaerobic glycolysis is lactate, which is usually oxidized in the presence of oxygen, but which accumulates in the epithelium and stroma under hypoxic conditions, as it gradually moves towards the aqueous where it is eliminated from the tissue. According to the theory of Klyce (1981), the increased concentration of lactate in the corneal tissue during hypoxia osmotically induces an influx of fluid into the stroma, leading to corneal swelling or oedema.

Controversy exists as to the minimum level of oxygen required at the anterior corneal surface to maintain normal epithelial metabolism and thus to prevent oedema. Polse and Mandell (1970) found that an atmospheric level of only 1.5–2.5% oxygen (11–19 mmHg or 1.5–2.5 kPa) was required to avoid corneal oedema. However, more recent studies have suggested that, in fact, much higher levels of oxygen are necessary. Holden, Sweeney and Sanderson (1984) found that in the majority of patients at least 10% oxygen must be provided to the cornea to prevent oedema (*Figure 15.1*). Their results are supported by findings from other laboratories. For example, Hamano *et al.* (1983) found that the rate of epithelial mitosis was reduced, and lactate began to accumulate in the aqueous if less than 13% oxygen was supplied to the anterior corneal surface. Millodot and O'Leary (1980) report that corneal sensitivity is decreased when the eyelid is closed and oxygen

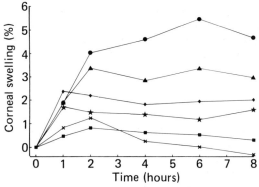

Figure 15.1 Average corneal swelling versus time for a range of precorneal oxygen concentrations. Gas-goggles were used to expose the cornea to gases of various oxygen tensions over an 8-hour period. Eight human subjects were used. (×) 21.4% O_2; (■) 10.1% O_2; (★) 7.5% O_2; (♦) 4.9% O_2; (▲) 2.5% O_2; (●) 1.0% O_2. (From Holden, Sweeney and Sanderson (1984) with kind permission)

availability falls to 8% oxygen. In addition, Williams (1986) reports that an endothelial bleb response is generally induced if oxygen levels fall below 15% oxygen. There are considerable individual variations in the minimum oxygen requirement; Holden, Sweeney and Sanderson (1984) report that a range of between 7.5 and 21% oxygen was required to avoid oedema in their eight subjects.

During contact lens wear, the passage of oxygen to the anterior corneal surface is impeded by the lens. This is particularly significant during overnight wear of lenses, as less oxygen is available from the palpebral conjunctival vessels. Thus, most contact lenses induce a state of relative hypoxia, particularly during overnight wear.

Oxygen can reach the cornea during contact lens wear via two mechanisms: by circulation of oxygen-rich tears behind the lens, driven by a lid-activated tear pump, or by diffusion of oxygen through the lens material.

The tear pump is active only during open-eye lens wear. Although it has been suggested that tear circulation due to eye movements during rapid eye movement (REM) sleep may provide some corneal oxygenation, Benjamin and Rasmussen (1985) have shown that such a mechanism is unlikely to supplement oxygen availability to any significant extent.

During closed-eye wear, therefore, oxygen is supplied to the anterior corneal surface predominantly by diffusion through the lens material. The rate of diffusion of oxygen (j) is dependent upon the diffusivity (D) and solubility (k) of oxygen in the lens material, and the lens thickness (t), and can be expressed by the equation:

$$j = \frac{Dk}{t} \ (P_1 - P_2)$$

where P_1 and P_2 are the oxygen tensions at the anterior and posterior lens surfaces (Fatt and St Helen, 1971). The term Dk represents the oxygen permeability of the lens material, and Dk/t represents the oxygen transmissibility of the lens itself. Lenses with higher Dk/t values provide more oxygen to the cornea, and thus induce less corneal oedema. Corneal oedema can therefore be minimized by using a lens material with a high Dk value, or by reducing lens thickness to increase the Dk/t value of the lens itself.

Efron and Carney (1979) have demonstrated that oxygen diffusion through current-generation hydrogel lenses under closed-eye conditions is insufficient to maintain normal epithelial functioning, and that some corneal oedema during sleep is therefore inevitable. This has been confirmed by the work of Holden, Mertz and McNally (1983). The same is true of many RGP lenses currently available for extended wear (LaHood, Sweeney and Holden, 1986), although advances in the field of polymer chemistry hold the promise of new materials with Dk properties similar to those of silicone elastomer lenses which apparently avoid overnight corneal oedema (Sweeney and Holden, 1987).

The major difference between hydrogel and RGP lenses in the mechanism of oxygen provision to the anterior corneal surface becomes apparent when the eyes are opened after overnight wear. Both lens types provide oxygen to the cornea during closed-eye wear by diffusion through the lens material. Thus hydrogel and RGP lenses of comparable 'effective' Dk/t will induce similar levels of overnight oedema. However, the lid-activated tear pump mechanism with rigid lenses is considerably more efficient than with hydrogel lenses. An estimated 10–20% tear exchange occurs under a rigid lens with each blink (Cuklanz and Hill, 1969; Fatt and Hill, 1970). However, Polse (1979) estimates a tear exchange per blink of only 1% under hydrogel lenses, due to their greater flexibility. Thus, when the eye is opened after overnight wear, oxygen is provided to the anterior cornea much more efficiently with RGP lenses compared to hydrogels, facilitating rapid corneal recovery from overnight hypoxic stress. Andrasko (1986) has demonstrated that the cornea deswells more rapidly after overnight wear of RGP lenses than with hydrogel lenses, as a result of the greater tear pumping efficiency of rigid lenses. He also suggests that the smaller area of the cornea covered by RGP lenses, and possible differences in the anterior–posterior distribution of oedema through the cornea with RGP lenses may also contribute to the more rapid deswelling.

The cornea appears to be able to eliminate approximately 8% corneal oedema during the open-eye phase following overnight wear of hydrogel lenses (Holden, Mertz and McNally, 1983). Thus hydrogel lenses which induce more than 8% overnight oedema will induce a state of chronic low-level daytime oedema. The cornea then undergoes an 'oedema cycle' of high overnight swelling, followed by partial recovery during the open-eye phase (*Figure 15.2*).

The amount of oedema that the cornea is able to eliminate following RGP overnight wear has yet to be established, as it varies with the relative efficiency of the tear pump, which in turn is a function of the fit of the lenses and the blink frequency (Fatt, 1969). However, data from a study reported by Holden *et al.* (1988) suggest that approximately 10% oedema can be eliminated within 5 hours of eye opening following overnight RGP lens wear. It is reasonable that a greater amount of oedema can be eliminated with these lenses because of the supplementation of corneal oxygenation by the tear pump. However, an oedema cycle similar to that accompanying hydrogel extended wear can also occur with RGP extended wear.

It has been suggested (Kenyon *et al.*, 1986) that an 'average edema index' (AEI), which gives an estimate of the average level of oedema experienced over a 24-hour cycle, may provide a more meaningful measure of the overall hypoxic stress experienced during extended wear than the overnight swelling response.

Elimination of waste products

As well as impeding the supply of oxygen to the anterior corneal surface, contact lenses may also

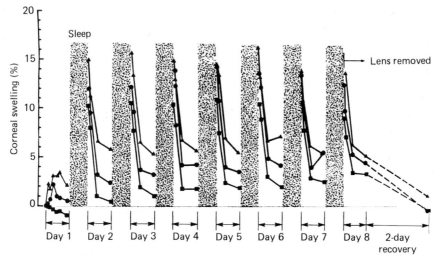

Figure 15.2 Average corneal swelling versus time for 10 unadapted subjects wearing Bausch & Lomb Soflens O4 series contact lenses continuously for a period of one week. All subjects wore −1.25 D lenses on one eye, half wore −6.00 D lenses and half wore −9.00 D lenses on the other eye. (■) −1.25 D; (●) −6.00 D; (▲) −9.00 D. (From Holden, Mertz and McNally (1983) with kind permission)

provide a barrier to the elimination of waste products from the anterior cornea, in particular carbon dioxide and cellular debris.

Carbon dioxide

For many years, it was widely accepted that hydrogel contact lenses do not restrict carbon dioxide efflux from the cornea, as it has been stated that the carbon dioxide permeability of hydrogel materials is in the order of 20 times that of oxygen (Fatt, Bieber and Pye, 1969). However, a recent study by Holden, Ross and Jenkins (1987) suggests that even very thin

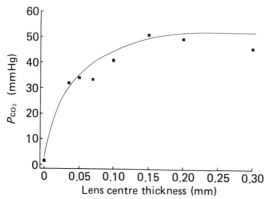

Figure 15.3 Carbon dioxide partial pressure at the anterior corneal surface immediately following 10 minutes wear of hydrogel (HEMA) lenses of various centre thicknesses. (From Holden, Ross and Jenkins (1987) with kind permission)

(0.035 mm) hydrogel lenses provide a significant barrier to carbon dioxide efflux (*Figure 15.3*). This suggests that during extended contact lens wear, the cornea may experience chronically raised levels of carbon dioxide, with little opportunity for recovery to normal open-eye levels.

The effects of chronically raised carbon dioxide levels on corneal physiology are not known. Increased carbon dioxide concentration is likely to lead to a reduction in stromal pH, due to an increase in the concentration of carbonic acid in the tissue. Holden, Williams and Zantos (1985) have suggested that such a pH change may be responsible for the endothelial bleb response (*Plate 64*). It is also possible that chronic reductions in stromal pH may contribute to changes in stromal thickness and endothelial cell morphology accompanying long-term hydrogel extended wear (Holden *et al.*, 1985b).

Cellular debris

The corneal epithelium is continually replenishing cells by mitosis. These cells are produced at the basal layer and move towards the corneal surface until they are eventually sloughed off and washed away in the tears.

During rigid lens wear, this cellular debris is readily flushed out from behind the lens. However, debris is more likely to become trapped behind a hydrogel lens because of the lower rate of tear exchange (*Plate 46b*). Enzymes released during breakdown of this cellular material have the potential to provoke a toxic reaction from the epithelium. This mechanism has been implicated in the acute red eye reaction (*Plate 47*) seen in some hydrogel extended lens wearers (Zantos and Holden, 1978; Mertz and Holden, 1981). RGP extended wear lenses have less potential to provoke such a response as debris trapped behind the lens during overnight wear is more rapidly removed after eye opening due to the greater tear exchange with these lenses. However, RGP lenses may occasionally provoke an acute red eye reaction if the lens remains 'bound' or adherent to the cornea following eye opening (Schnider, Zabkiewicz and Holden, 1988) (*see Plates 19* and *46a*).

Environmental changes under the closed lid

Overnight corneal oedema (no lens)

Following 8 hours of overnight eye closure without contact lenses, the cornea normally exhibits 3–4% corneal oedema. Because the capillary plexus of the palpebral conjunctiva supplies oxygen to the cornea at a lower level (8%) than that required to avoid corneal oedema (10%; Holden, Sweeney and Sanderson, 1984), it is reasonable to assume that this relative hypoxia during eye closure contributes to the normal, no-lens overnight corneal oedema response. However, Holden, Sweeney and Sanderson (1984) found that a gas mixture containing 7.5% oxygen, approximately the level of oxygen available during eye closure, induced an average of less than 2% corneal oedema over 8 hours of exposure to the gas. This suggests that other factors, such as changes in temperature, tear pH and tonicity under the closed lid may also contribute to the overnight swelling response (Hill, 1977).

Temperature

The temperature of the anterior corneal surface of the open eye lies in the range 33–36°C (Fatt and Chaston, 1980). When the eye is closed, however, and the cornea exposed to the palpebral conjunctiva at a temperature of 36.2°C (Holden and Sweeney, 1985), the corneal surface temperature increases by approximately 3°C to lie in the range 35.6–36.5°C (Fatt and Chaston, 1980). This increase in corneal temperature influences the rate of metabolic activity in the epithelium (Freeman and Fatt, 1973), and therefore the epithelial oxygen consumption rises. Thus during closed-eye wear of contact lenses, the effects of reduced oxygen availability at the anterior cornea may be exacerbated by an increased epithelial demand for oxygen. In this way, temperature effects may contribute to overnight corneal swelling accompanying extended lens wear.

Holden *et al.* (1981) have also reported that the level of corneal oedema induced by gaseous anoxia is increased if the temperature of the circulating anoxic gas is increased.

Tear pH

Carney and Hill (1976) have established that tear pH usually exhibits a pattern of diurnal variation about a mean of 7.45 ± 0.16 in the open eye, with a general increase in alkalinity during the day. When the eye is closed, the tear pH shows an acid shift; immediately on eye opening after sleep, tear pH is reduced on average to approximately 7.25, and recovers to average open-eye levels within 3–4 hours of eye opening.

Tear pH may also be reduced in neophyte contact lens wearers (Hamano, 1978), although attempts to determine long-term changes in tear pH with contact lens wear have been less conclusive. It is probable that reductions in tear pH with eye closure and contact lens wear are due in part to the restriction of carbon dioxide efflux from the cornea under these conditions.

Changes in ambient pH have been shown to alter the ion transport properties of the epithelium (Fischer *et al.*, 1978), and may therefore affect corneal hydration. Thus the normal acid shift in tear pH during eye closure, possibly compounded by reduced pH accompanying contact lens wear, could contribute to the overnight swelling of the cornea. It has been suggested, however, that an acidic environment may decrease corneal oxygen consumption (Carney and Efron, 1980). Furthermore, both Carney (1974) and Holden, Williams and Zantos (1985) found that exposure of the cornea to carbon dioxide gas, which would be expected to lower corneal pH, did not induce corneal oedema.

Tear osmolarity

Terry and Hill (1978) found a shift in tear tonicity from 0.97 ± 0.02% NaCl in the open eye to 0.89 ± 0.01% NaCl following sleep periods of 6–8 hours. This overnight hypotonic shift may be explained by reduced tear evaporation during the closed-eye phase. O'Neal and Polse (1985) have demonstrated that corneal thickness recovery from induced oedema in a 100% humidity environment is significantly impeded when compared to recovery in a normal (60% humidity) environment; this confirms the role of tear film evaporation in the control of normal corneal thickness.

Rigid contact lens wear also induces a hypotonic shift in tear tonicity, particularly during adaptation due to reflex tearing (Harris and Mandell, 1969), although hydrogel lenses induce only transient changes in tear osmolarity (Martin and Holden, 1983), probably because of their greater 'on-eye' comfort. As changes in the tonicity of the precorneal environment can osmotically induce changes in corneal thickness, osmotic swelling during overnight contact lens wear due to a hypotonic tear shift probably contributes to the overall closed-eye swelling response.

In summary, environmental changes under the closed lid may have a subtle influence on corneal physiology, and contribute to the slight swelling of the cornea during sleep. Hypoxia due to reduced oxygen availability, and tonicity changes due to the elimination of tear evaporation during eye closure, are probably the most significant contributors to this normal overnight corneal swelling.

Overnight contact lens wear, which further reduces oxygen availability, may also exert an influence on other aspects of the precorneal environment and thus exacerbate the overnight swelling response. However, the extent to which corneal function is compromised by these subtle alterations in corneal environment during overnight contact lens wear is generally masked by the more prominent effects of restricted oxygen availability.

Hydrogel extended wear

Historical review

The development of a hydrophilic material suitable for contact lens applications was first reported by Wichterle and Lim in 1960. Hydrophilic lenses achieved widespread use as daily wear lenses, and were also found to be useful as bandage lenses for the treatment of ocular diseases such as bullous keratopathy, recurrent corneal erosions, corneal ulcers and perforation, and dry eye syndromes. As it became apparent that these bandage lenses could be worn for 24 hours a day, and with their increasing use for aphakic patients with postsurgical complications, it was recognized that aphakic extended wear was a viable alternative to aphakic spectacle correction, intraocular lens implantation and daily contact lens wear. Although in use in some countries since the mid-1970s, extended wear lenses for aphakic correction first received FDA (Food and Drugs Administration) approval in the USA in 1979, and in 1981 hydrogel lenses were approved for cosmetic extended wear.

The development of high water content hydrophilic lenses for extended wear was pioneered by John de Carle in England in the early 1970s. The early promising performance of the Permalens, a 71% water content lens, stimulated further developments in this area, including the Sauflon lens (promoted by Philip Cordrey), and the Duragel material (developed by Highgate and Frankland), investigated by Klas Nilsson and marketed in Sweden under the trade name Scanlens. As oxygen permeates through the water contained in the polymer, the high water content of these early lenses increased the amount of oxygen reaching the anterior corneal surface compared with daily wear low water content materials. With the development of more sophisticated manufacturing techniques, it became possible to produce very thin lenses in low water content materials which rivalled the high water content lenses in their ability to transmit oxygen to the cornea. Both lens types are currently used for extended wear; their relative advantages and disadvantages will be discussed later.

In the last decade, cosmetic extended wear lenses have grown enormously in popularity, due in part to aggressive consumer marketing of these lenses particularly in the USA. By 1983, it was estimated that more than 500 000 people in the USA were wearing extended wear lenses, with 40 000 new fittings every month, resulting in approximately 4 million extended lens wearers by 1985. The rapid growth in the use of these lenses, however, has not been without problems due in part to poor follow-up and patient advice by some practitioners. Early reports from England (Ruben, 1976) and Australia (Cooper and Constable, 1977; Zantos and Holden, 1978) suggested that these lenses could induce severe corneal complications. These warnings went largely unheeded at first in the USA, until the issue was raised by Barry Weissman in 1983. Clinical reports of corneal infections associated with extended wear then began to appear with increasing frequency in the US scientific literature. Recent US media reports of gross corneal infections and subsequent litigation have since led to a re-evaluation of the safety of this modality, and a down-turn in patient pressure for extended wear.

Early research on hydrogel extended wear placed much emphasis on the oxygen-transmitting properties of these lenses, particularly during overnight wear. The relative simplicity of fitting hydrogel lenses, and the ready patient acceptance due to improved comfort and minimal handling, suggested that all that was required to guarantee success was the provision of adequate oxygen to the anterior corneal surface to maintain normal epithelial functioning. While this aspect of lens performance is of major importance, it soon became apparent that the fit of hydrogel lenses plays a subtle but very important role in maintaining corneal health. Hydrogel lens material properties and design are significant factors in the clearing of debris that collects behind the lens, in minimizing deposit formation, and in the provision of tear-carried metabolites essential for the maintenance of epithelial growth and repair during extended wear.

With increasing knowledge of the subtle long-term effects of hydrogel extended wear, and of the factors which may predispose the cornea to acute complications, it has become clear that careful patient selection and instruction, rigorous follow-up, strict care and maintenance procedures, frequent overnight rest periods and regular replacement of lenses are vital factors in maintaining corneal health and maximizing extended wear success.

Advantages and disadvantages

The principal advantage of extended wear over daily wear of contact lenses is that of convenience. As the lenses do not have to be inserted and removed each day, extended wear is of considerable benefit for patients who would have difficulty in handling the lenses, such as elderly patients and children. In these two groups, extended wear lenses are particularly useful for aphakic correction. Ellis (1983) and others have also reported considerable extended wear success with highly myopic and anisometropic children.

Many ametropic patients are also attracted to the convenience of the extended wear modality, and the commercial advertising of the '30-day lens', particularly in the USA, has fostered a considerable consumer demand for extended wear. The attractive prospect of being able to see well immediately on awakening, while not considered important by many emmetropes, is often mentioned by prospective extended wearers, and is a particular advantage in many occupations, such as in the military service (Nilsson and Rengstorff, 1979), where time-consuming lens insertion may be more than an inconvenience.

It is important, however, that extended wear patients are made aware that extended wear does not mean continuous wear and that, although lens handling is minimal, the lenses must be removed periodically for routine cleaning and to rest the cornea. Thus it is imperative that patients are able to handle the lenses, and at the very least are competent themselves or have someone available to remove the lenses if problems such as unusual discomfort, redness or persistent blurred vision occur.

Extended wear hydrogel lenses are not without their disadvantages. As well as acute complications, which will be discussed in detail later, other less serious but troublesome problems may occur in some patients, including persistent deposit formation on lenses, poor vision due to lens flexure and undercorrected astigmatism, and lens damage during handling. As the incidence of these problems is frequently related to the water content of the hydrogel lens material, the advantages and disadvantages of various hydrogel lens types will be discussed below. Silicone elastomer lenses, although not hydrogels as they contain virtually no water, will also be discussed in this section.

High water content lenses

The first hydrogel lenses used for extended wear were made from materials containing a high proportion of water (Permalens, 75%, Sauflon, 85%). As oxygen is transmitted through the water contained in the polymer, it was thought at the time that these lenses could be made fairly thick (0.14–0.30 mm) and still transmit enough oxygen to be considered for extended wear.

The relative thickness of high water content extended wear lenses means that they retain their shape and are therefore easier to handle and to locate if accidentally dropped or dislodged from the eye. However, the fragility of some high water content polymers can lead to more frequent tearing and other damage than with low water content daily wear lenses.

Contamination and deposit formation on high water content lenses is also a significant problem. This is probably due to the large pore size in these polymers (Fatt, 1978), which allows small contaminating molecules to penetrate the polymer matrix (Refojo and Leong, 1979), and provides a more substantial 'toehold' for larger molecules to adsorb on to the lens surface. 'Jellybump' deposits, also known as 'mulberry' deposits, lens calculi or calcium deposits, are a particular problem with high water content lenses. These round nodular deposits, which are composed of calcium and lipid (Caroline *et al.*, 1985), can cause ocular irritation and poor visual acuity and, because they are difficult to remove without damaging the lens surface, lens replacement is usually necessary (*see Plates 38 and 39*).

Low water content lenses

Thin, low water content lenses became available in 1980 as an alternative to high water content lenses for extended wear. The thinness of these lenses allows sufficient oxygen to diffuse through the lens for them to be considered for extended wear. The first lenses of this type, the Bausch & Lomb 'O series' lenses, were made from HEMA (hydroxyethyl methacrylate) material (38.6% water content) with a centre thickness of 0.035 mm. More recently lenses in other materials with similar water content and centre thickness (for example, CSI-T and Permathin) have been developed for extended wear applications.

The advantages of low water content lenses include increased durability of the polymer and less deposit accumulation within the lens due to the denser polymer matrix. However the ex-

treme thinness of these lenses for extended wear can make them difficult to handle, particularly in low powers, and also more vulnerable to damage such as tearing (Klein, 1983). In addition, the tendency of these lenses to 'drape' onto the cornea results in less lens movement than with thicker high water content lenses, which in some patients may hinder the flushing of debris from behind the lens. However, Holden and Sweeney (1987) have suggested that as little as 0.2 mm movement may be adequate with these lenses provided it is maintained during lens wear.

Hydrogel alternatives

In an attempt to minimize the problems associated with high and low water content lenses, many extended wear lenses available today are made from medium water content materials (45–60%) with moderate centre thickness in the range 0.05–0.12 mm. As would be expected, the properties of these lenses provide a compromise between those of thin, low water and thick, high water content extended wear lenses.

Thin, high water content lenses have also been investigated for extended wear use. In theory, the high water content (70–75%) combined with a reduced centre thickness (0.03–0.08 mm) should greatly enhance the oxygen transmission characteristics of the lenses. In practice, however, the lenses are extremely fragile and difficult to handle, and may induce epithelial erosions (*Plate 58*) due to on-eye dehydration which causes epithelial dessication (Holden, Sweeney and Seger, 1986).

Silicone lenses

Silicone has been used for many years as a biomaterial for medical applications and, because of its inherent high oxygen permeability, there has been considerable interest in its use as a contact lens material. Silicone elastomer lenses have been available for aphakic and cosmetic extended wear use in Japan and Europe since the mid-1970s, but have gained FDA approval in the USA for aphakic use only at the time of writing.

The high oxygen permeability of the silicone elastomer material, although in lens form probably not as high as the manufacturers' claim of $300\text{--}400 \times 10^{-11}$ Dk units where a Dk unit is measured in $(\text{cm}\,\text{ml}\,O_2)/(\text{cm}^2\,\text{s}\,\text{mmHg})$ for (amount of oxygen × thickness)/(area × time × pressure difference) (Glasser and Weissman, 1983), is a major advantage for maintaining corneal function during extended wear. The lenses are also very durable and easy to handle, being approximately five times more rigid than an equivalent 50% water content hydrogel lens (Ruben and Guillon, 1979).

Silicone is by nature hydrophobic; thus current-generation silicone elastomer lenses are surface treated to render them hydrophilic. In spite of this, deterioration of surface wettability (*Plate 44*) has been reported (Ruben and Guillon, 1979; Fanti, 1980; Josephson and Caffery, 1980) and, in general, silicone lenses have a life expectancy of about 12 months before requiring replacement. Lens deposits are also a problem (Ruben and Guillon, 1979; Fanti, 1980; Blackhurst, 1985), possibly due to the hydrophilicity of the treated surface, although stronger cleaning solutions (*Plate 45*) can be used with these lenses than with hydrogels (Josephson and Caffery, 1980).

Patient awareness of silicone elastomer lenses is generally greater than with hydrogels, particularly during the adaptation period (Hill *et al.*, 1983; Mannarino, Belin and Weiner, 1985). Silicone lenses also require a more discriminating fitting procedure than hydrogel lenses. Fluorescein can be used to assess lens fit without discolouring the lenses (*Plates 41–43*). If adequate lens movement is not maintained, however, these lenses have a tendency to adhere or 'suck on' to the cornea (Fanti, 1980; Josephson and Caffery, 1980). Fatt (1979) has suggested that this phenomenon is due to the high modulus of elasticity of the material, which can store energy in the deformed state. When the lens is pressed by the lid against the cornea, a large positive pressure at the lens edge and a negative pressure or suction under the lens results, leading to lens adherence. Other authors (Fanti, 1980; Josephson and Caffery, 1980) have suggested that 'contact adhesion' between a hydrophobic lens surface and the bare cells of the epithelium, which are also hydrophobic, may contribute to this phenomenon. Refojo and Leong (1981) have also suggested pervaporation through the lens as a possible mechanism for silicone lens adherence.

Acute complications of hydrogel extended wear

Stromal oedema

Corneal stromal swelling or oedema during contact lens wear indicates that insufficient oxygen is being supplied to the anterior corneal surface to maintain normal epithelial aerobic metabolism. Thus stromal oedema is an important physiological indicator of epithelial hypoxic stress. Corneal oedema has been suggested as an aetiological factor in corneal neovascularization (Cogan, 1949), limbal injection (Tomlinson and Haas, 1980) and changes in corneal curvature (Mandell, 1975). In addition, chronic hypoxia, of which stromal oedema is an important index, can have a significant effect on corneal structure and function in the long term (Holden *et al.*, 1985b). Thus it is intuitively desirable to attempt to eliminate or reduce contact lens-induced stromal oedema.

Stromal oedema accompanying hydrogel lens wear is evenly distributed across most of the cornea, although there is significantly less swelling in the extreme periphery than in the central cornea (Bonanno and Polse, 1985; Holden *et al.*, 1985a), as shown in *Figure 15.4*. The lower swelling response of the peripheral cornea is thought to reflect a reduced swelling capability due to physical restraint in the limbal region.

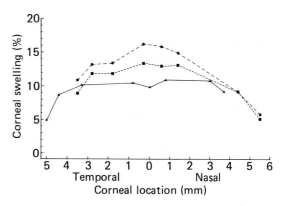

Figure 15.4 Average overnight corneal swelling *vs* horizontal corneal location for 10 unadapted subjects wearing Bausch & Lomb Soflens O4 series contact lenses continuously for a period of one week. All subjects wore $-1.25\,\text{D}$ lenses on one eye; half wore $-6.00\,\text{D}$ lenses and half wore $-9.00\,\text{D}$ lenses on the other eye. (●--●) $-9.00\,\text{D}$; (■--■) $-6.00\,\text{D}$; (▲—▲) $-1.25\,\text{D}$. (From Holden *et al.* (1985a) with kind permission)

The diffuse nature of hydrogel lens-induced stromal oedema makes it difficult to see with the slit lamp, as there is minimal light scatter in the stroma unless the oedema is severe. Moderate levels of stromal oedema are also unlikely to give rise to significant patient symptoms or reductions in visual acuity. However, when the cornea swells more than 4–6%, fine striae appear at the level of the posterior stroma and Descemet's membrane (Sarver, 1971; Polse and Mandell, 1976); the striae are usually vertical, but may be horizontal or oblique (*Plate 67*). The presence of these fine stress lines may therefore be used to infer the existence of stromal oedema. If the stromal oedema is severe (over 15%), dark lines resembling folds in Descemet's membrane may also be observed (Holden, 1977; *Plate 68*). Folds in Descemet's membrane represent a more severe buckling at the posterior stroma than striae, and usually suggest that stromal oedema has reached clinically unacceptable levels.

The most direct way of quantifying stromal oedema is by measuring changes in corneal thickness using a pachometer (*see* Chapter 6). Although not widely used in clinical practice, pachometry provides a valuable means to detect and monitor subtle levels of stromal oedema which may not be detectable by visual acuity measurement or slit lamp examination.

Efron and Carney (1979) found that current-generation hydrogel lenses do not provide enough oxygen during overnight wear to maintain normal epithelial functioning. Thus some corneal oedema is invariably present on eye opening during hydrogel extended wear. Holden, Mertz and McNally (1983) found average overnight oedema levels of 9.7–15.1% with a range of extended wear hydrogel lenses. They also found that the level of oedema reduced quite rapidly following eye opening to reach levels of 1.6–5.8% after 12 hours of open-eye wear. This 'oedema cycle', shown in *Figure 15.2*, of high overnight swelling, followed by partial recovery during the open-eye phase, is repeated with each overnight wear.

Zantos and Holden (1978) and Schoessler and Barr (1980) report that corneal swelling accompanying extended wear reaches a peak during the first week of wear and declines thereafter, suggesting some adaptation to the reduced oxygen supply. However, Holden *et al.* (1985b) refute this suggestion as stromal thinning due to chronic hypoxia masks stromal

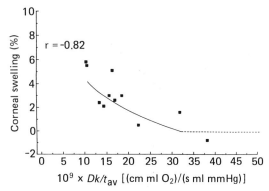

Figure 15.5 Residual corneal swelling (12 hours after eye opening following overnight lens wear or day 2) *vs* average lens oxygen transmissibility (Dk/t_{av}) for 11 lens types. Dk/t_{av} values were calculated using published polymer oxygen permeability (Dk) data or manufacturers' specifications, and measured lens thickness. Critical Dk/t_{av} and equivalent oxygen performance (EOP) values necessary to reduce residual overnight swelling to zero are 34.3×10^{-9} and 12.1%, respectively. (From Holden and Mertz (1984) with kind permission)

oedema to some extent after long-term extended wear, and a period without lens wear is needed in order to determine the true level of contact lens-induced oedema.

Holden and Mertz (1984) have derived the critical hydrogel lens oxygen transmissibility needed to limit overnight corneal oedema to 4%, the level experienced without a contact lens on the eye. This ideal level of oxygen transmissibility (Dk/t), based on published nominal Dk values for hydrogel lenses, was found to be 87×10^{-9} (cm ml O_2)/(s ml mmHg). This cannot be provided by current hydrogel lens materials, as average lens thickness would have to be reduced well below the limits of manufacturing feasibility. These authors therefore proposed an interim alternative criterion for acceptability of hydrogel lenses for extended wear. This compromise criterion of zero residual swelling, allowing 8% overnight oedema with subsequent recovery of normal corneal thickness during daytime wear, yielded a minimum desirable oxygen transmissibility of 34×10^{-9} (cm ml O_2)/(s ml mmHg) (*Figure 15.5*). The lens thickness necessary to achieve this Dk/t appears to be feasible from a manufacturing point of view, at least for high water content lenses where a maximum average lens thickness of 0.117 mm is indicated.

The acute red eye reaction

The contact lens-induced acute red eye reaction, also occasionally called the 'tight lens' syndrome or non-ulcerative keratitis, is an alarming acute complication of extended hydrogel lens wear for both patient and practitioner. The patient symptoms are characteristic — sudden onset, with the patient usually waking in the night with unilateral pain, ocular redness, tearing and photophobia. Clinical signs include marked conjunctival hyperaemia and small patches of subepithelial infiltrates (*Plates 53, 54* and *57*) invading the cornea from the limbus. The typical clinical appearance of an acute red eye reaction is shown in *Figure 15.6* and *Plate 47*). If the patient has not removed the lens, in most cases the lens is relatively tight and immobile, and often large flakes of debris can be observed apparently trapped behind the lens (Mertz and Holden, 1981). On lens removal, epithelial staining may be present, often corresponding to the pattern of tear debris. In severe cases a uveal response may be triggered, with aqueous flare and keratic precipitates.

Zantos and Holden (1978) have suggested that this condition represents an inflammatory reaction to toxic substances released by the breakdown of debris which has accumulated behind the lens. The presence of large numbers of inflammatory cells (neutrophils) together with mucus and squamous epithelial cells in post-lens debris recovered from a 'red eye' patient, as reported by Mertz and Holden (1981), lends support to this hypothesis. The concurrent appearance of infiltrates, which indicates that leucocytes have been mobilized to invade the cornea from the limbal vessels (Josephson and Caffery, 1979), further underlines the inflammatory nature of this response. It is also possible that substances absorbed into or adsorbed on to the lens material (*Plate 56*) may precipitate this acute inflammatory response (Kotow, Grant and Holden, 1987), although Phillips *et al.* (1986) were unable to simulate a red eye reaction in rabbits using endotoxin-coated lenses.

Extended wear patients should be advised to remove their lenses immediately if a red eye reaction occurs, and to consult their practitioner promptly in the morning. Lens removal generally gives some relief from symptoms, although patching may be necessary to relieve ocular discomfort. Patients should be seen again later

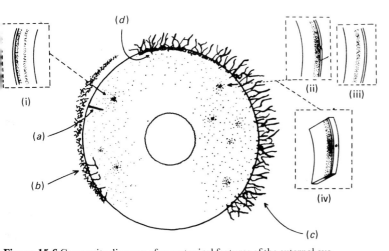

Figure 15.6 Composite diagram of some typical features of the external eye appearance in patients with an acute red eye reaction during extended lens wear. (*a*) Midstromal blood vessel invasion; (*b*) perilimbal ring of vessel injection; (*c*) marked engorgement of bulbar conjunctival and ciliary blood vessels; (*d*) engorgement of limbal capillary plexus. Insets: (i) optic section near epithelial lesion, showing two distinct depths of stromal infiltrates separated by a layer of clear stroma; (ii) epithelial lesion with associated anterior stromal infiltrates; (iii) deeper stromal infiltrates adjacent to epithelial lesion in (ii); (iv) parallelepiped of section (ii) showing sharp demarcation between infiltrated and clear stroma. (From Zantos and Holden (1977a) with kind permission)

Table 15.1 Adverse response rates (per annum) with extended lens wear — from CCLRU clinical studies, using a variety of care and maintenance regimens

Response	High water content lenses		Low water content lenses		RGP lenses	
	No. of eyes	%	No. of eyes	%	No. of eyes	%
Total seen	145		135		200	
Acute red eye	32	22.1	16	11.9	2	1.0
CLPC	11	7.6	21	15.6	1	0.5
Corneal ulcer	2	1.4	1	0.7	1	0.5

in the day following the episode and, if the epithelium has not healed or if there are signs of a sustained uveal reaction, referral to an ophthalmologist is advisable. The patient may notice some ocular irritation, photophobia and tearing over the following 2 days, and infiltrates may take weeks to resolve. Lens wear should be discontinued during this period, and a new lens should be issued when lens wear recommences once the cornea is clear.

A summary of the incidence per annum of acute red eye reactions found during hydrogel extended wear studies conducted at the Cornea and Contact Lens Research Unit (CCLRU), Sydney, is shown in *Table 15.1*. Using the most careful lens fitting and care and maintenance procedures, the incidence of acute red eye reactions can be reduced to as low as 2% per annum (Kotow, Grant and Holden, 1987).

There are several ways in which the incidence of acute red eye reactions can be minimized. It is essential to ensure that the lens moves freely over the cornea to facilitate the flushing of tear debris from behind the lens. It must be kept in mind that environmental changes under the closed lid will often tighten a lens fit (Weissman, 1982) leading to inadequate lens movement on awakening. Rigorous care and maintenance procedures, including frequent overnight lens removal, careful lens cleaning and disinfection, use of an enzymatic cleaner and regular replacement of lenses, also reduce the incidence of red eye reactions (Kotow, Grant and Holden, 1987). These authors report a disturbingly high incidence of red eye reactions (56% after 12 months of extended wear) in patients using heat disinfection with high water content lenses, suggesting that heat is not an appropriate method of disinfecting these lenses. The incidence of red eye reactions generally appears to be greater with high water content lenses. This

may be due to their propensity to absorb contaminants more easily than low water content lenses, and their more rapid ageing and spoiling.

Giant papillary conjunctivitis

Giant papillary conjunctivitis (GPC) is characterized by pronounced papillary hypertrophy and hyperaemia of the upper tarsal conjunctiva (*Plate 71*), with excess mucous discharge and ocular itching and discomfort. This condition has been likened to vernal conjunctivitis (Allansmith *et al.*, 1977; Collin, 1980, 1981), and is precipitated by both hard and soft contact lens wear (Allansmith *et al.*, 1977), ocular prostheses (Srinivasan *et al.*, 1979), and protruding suture ends following anterior ocular surgery (Reynolds, 1978). In association with contact lens wear, GPC generally causes reduced lens tolerance and may result in temporary or permanent discontinuation of lens wear. Although the condition may be unilateral, both eyes are usually affected.

GPC was first described by Spring (1974) who reported 78 cases in a population of 170 long-term daily wear soft contact lens wearers. Allansmith *et al.* (1977) described the condition in more detail and reported its occurrence with both hard and soft contact lens wear. More recently, there have been a number of reports of GPC in association with extended soft lens wear (Mackie and Wright, 1978; Coon, Miller and Meier, 1979; Kotow, Grant and Holden, 1987). The incidence per annum of papillary changes occurring during hydrogel extended wear studies conducted at the CCLRU is shown in *Table 15.1*.

In its early stages, GPC is characterized more by mild patient symptoms than by obvious clinical signs. Often direct questioning of the patient is necessary to elicit early symptoms which include mild mucous discharge evident in the nasal corner of the eye on awakening, and itching of the eyes on lens removal. As the condition progresses, however, the patient will complain of increasing stringy mucous discharge and watering during the day, blurring of vision due to lens deposits or excess mucus, excessive lens movement and occasional lens displacement, and intense itching and lens awareness after a period of lens wear, which may become severe enough to limit wearing times and eventually lead to complete lens intolerance.

The clinical signs of GPC also follow a progressive course, although the severity of symptoms is not always related to the clinical picture. Eversion of the upper eyelid is necessary to detect GPC in what may otherwise appear as a normal quiet eye. The instillation of fluorescein is often useful in revealing early papillary changes during slit lamp examination, because the fluorescein collects in the channels between the papillae.

Allansmith et al. (1977) have categorized tarsal conjunctival appearance into four categories corresponding to stages in the development of the condition. In the early stages, the palpebral conjunctiva may retain its normal satin-smooth appearance free of papillary changes in the presence of mild symptoms of GPC. The next stage, which is accompanied by moderate symptoms of mucous discharge and itching, is characterized by the appearance of uniform small elevated papillae (4–8 per mm), and mild hyperaemia of the palpebral conjunctiva. As the condition progresses, larger non-uniform papillae develop, and increased lens awareness, mucous discharge and excessive lens movement or displacement are often reported. In association with soft lens wear, the papillae are typically localized over the tarsus above the tarsal fold. The appearance of 'giant' papillae, 1 mm or more in diameter, often covering all zones of the tarsal conjunctiva, marks the terminal stage in the development of GPC, and is associated with excessive stringy mucous discharge, ocular discomfort and often complete intolerance to lens wear.

Because patient symptoms and changes in the appearance of the palpebral conjunctiva may be noted well before the condition reaches its terminal stage with the appearance of 'giant' papillae, it has been suggested (Barishak et al., 1984; Kotow, Grant and Holden, 1987) that it is more appropriate to describe the condition, in association with contact lens wear, as 'contact lens-induced papillary conjunctivitis' or CLPC.

The aetiology of CLPC is not fully understood. Allansmith et al. (1977) suggest that the condition is immunological in origin and noted, on the basis of their histological findings, that it shows the characteristics of a cutaneous basophilic hypersensitivity reaction. They hypothesized that the antigen initiating the tissue response is a product of deposits on the lens surface rather than the lens material itself. Fowler, Greiner and Allansmith (1979) noted that surface deposits on soft lenses worn by patients with CLPC were indistinguishable from those on lenses worn by asymptomatic patients, suggesting that individual patient susceptibility may be an important factor. Because the condition may be stimulated by trauma from exposed suture ends, for example, a mechanical component has also been suggested (Mackie and Wright, 1978; Reynolds, 1978). It is possible, therefore, that irritation of the palpebral conjunctiva by the contact lens edge or deposits or irregularities on the lens surface allows access of the antigen to the mucous membrane, initiating the hypersensitivity reaction in susceptible individuals (Molinari, 1983).

A number of approaches to the management of CLPC have been proposed. Early recognition of the condition and prompt initiation of appropriate therapeutic measures are important factors in arresting its progression. Cessation of lens wear generally leads to relief of symptoms within 2–5 days (Allansmith et al., 1977). However, clinical signs may persist for weeks or months, and resumption of lens wear will frequently precipitate the return of symptoms. Unfortunately, a significant number of patients who develop CLPC are unable to resume lens wear at all in spite of intensive therapeutic measures.

Dispensing a fresh lens of the same material and design may allow resumption of lens wear in some patients in the early stages of the condition (Spring, 1974; Allansmith et al., 1977). A change in the lens polymer or design may also interrupt progression of the condition (Mackie and Wright, 1978; Molinari, 1981), as may changes in the solutions used to disinfect the lens (Molinari, 1981), and regular use of an enzymatic papain-based cleaner (Allansmith *et al.*, 1977; Mackie and Wright, 1978). Resolution of symptoms has also been reported with the use of systemic tetracycline (Mackie and Wright, 1978), or sodium cromoglycate ophthalmic solution (Meisler, Krachmer and Goeken, 1981; Molinari, 1983), particularly in atopic patients. Regular replacement of lenses may also reduce the incidence of CLPC (Holden, Kotow and Swarbrick, 1986). However, until the aetiology of the condition is more fully understood, management of CLPC in the clinical situation requires a trial and error approach to identify the most appropriate measures to relieve patient symptoms and encourage resumption of lens wear in each individual case (*see also* Chapter 19).

Corneal infection

The acute complication of contact lens wear which causes the most concern is corneal infection. When corneal ulceration occurs involving the stroma, corneal scarring remains after resolution of the infection; if the scar is located in the central cornea, vision will be affected and keratoplasty may be required to restore useful vision.

Corneal infection may be initiated by a variety of pathogens of viral, fungal and bacterial origin. The pathogen most feared, however, is *Pseudomonas aeruginosa*, because of the rapid course of the infective process and its devastating effects, which in the worst case may lead to corneal perforation and loss of the eye (Raber *et al.*, 1981). Gram-negative bacterial organisms such as *Pseudomonas* sp. are the most common pathogens causing corneal infections in contact lens wearers (Adams *et al.*, 1983; Galentine *et al.*, 1984; Weissman *et al.*, 1984).

The cornea is normally protected from infection by antibacterial agents in the tears, in particular lysozyme, and by the barrier properties of the epithelium. Under certain conditions, however, contact lens wear can compromise the epithelial barrier function, allowing pathogens to invade the corneal tissue. Thus any occurrence of corneal abrasion, erosion or trauma may predispose the cornea to infection. In addition, more subtle compromise of epithelial function, due to the effects of chronic hypoxia for example, may impair the normal epithelial defence against invading

organisms (Holden *et al.*, 1985b). Furthermore, Madigan, Holden and Kwok (1987) have recently reported that soft contact lens-induced hypoxia can significantly reduce epithelial adhesion. This may provide an explanation for the recently described SLACH syndrome (soft lens-associated corneal hypoxia syndrome; Wallace, 1986), whereby there is spontaneous loss of up to 40% of the epithelial surface during lens wear (*Plate 60*).

Fortunately, the incidence of corneal infections with contact lens wear is low. Although corneal infections have been reported in hard contact lens wearers (Golden, Fingerman and Allen, 1971), this mode of lens wear appears to carry the least risk. Chalupa *et al.* (1987), in a 2-year survey, reported no corneal infections associated with daily hard lens wear in an estimated wearing population of 5000. The incidence of corneal infections in the soft lens daily wearing population of approximately 15 000 was 34 (or 0.2%); one infection was severe enough to eventually necessitate keratoplasty to retain useful vision. However, these workers found that extended wear considerably increases the risk of serious corneal infection. Although the overall incidence of corneal infection of 21 in a population of 15 000 (or 0.1%) was lower than with daily soft lens wear, five of these infections were particularly severe, and visual acuity was significantly reduced after resolution of the infective process. The large number of reports of corneal infections in association with extended lens wear over recent years in scientific journals (Cooper and Constable, 1977; Adams *et al.*, 1983; Salz and Schlanger, 1983; Spoor *et al.*, 1984; Weissman *et al.*, 1984, to cite a few) and in the popular press (*Time*, Jan. 27, 1986, p. 57) confirms the impression that extended wear carries a considerably greater risk of severe corneal infection than do other modes of lens wear.

Soft contact lenses are easily contaminated due to their water-containing nature and the ease with which contaminants can invade the polymer matrix. Inadequate disinfection procedures and contaminated lens storage solutions, therefore, are frequently identified as the source of the invading pathogen in cases of corneal infection (Cooper and Constable, 1977; Weissman *et al.*, 1984). During daily wear, handling of the lenses with unwashed fingers may also introduce pathogens to the eye

(Cooper and Constable, 1977; Galentine *et al.*, 1984). In addition, the low tear exchange behind hydrogel lenses ensures that any introduced pathogens remain in proximity to the cornea (Galentine *et al.*, 1984).

Because of reduced lens handling during extended wear, it would be expected that there is less opportunity for pathogens to contaminate the lens than during daily wear. It is significant that many corneal infections with extended wear are associated with recent manipulation of the lens (Adams *et al.*, 1983; Galentine *et al.*, 1984). However, other factors may exacerbate the severity of extended wear infections. Perhaps the most significant factor is the reduced epithelial metabolic activity induced by chronic hypoxia (Holden *et al.*, 1985b), which may compromise the epithelial barrier and reduce the ability of the cornea to resist invading organisms. Delay in removing lenses and in seeking treatment have also been identified as particularly significant predisposing factors (Cooper and Constable, 1977; Salz and Schlanger, 1983; Lemp *et al.*, 1984). Unfortunately, in some cases this delay is attributable to inadequate patient instruction and poor patient follow-up by practitioners. Furthermore, many extended wear patients are elderly aphakes, with reduced corneal sensitivity and tear secretion (Salz and Schlanger, 1983; Galentine *et al.*, 1984), and concomitant diseases such as arthritis, keratoconjunctivitis sicca and blepharitis (Lemp *et al.*, 1984). Many of these patients have difficulty in handling lenses; indeed this is often the initial reason for prescribing extended wear lenses, but consequently the lenses may not be removed immediately if problems such as discomfort, redness or blurred vision occur. Other factors which appear to increase the risk of a severe progression of corneal infection include diabetes (Eichenbaum, Feldstein and Podos, 1982; Spoor *et al.*, 1984), lens wear in warm climates (Leisegang and Forster, 1980; Sjostrand *et al.*, 1981), and the initiation of inappropriate antibiotic (Galentine *et al.*, 1984) or corticosteroid therapy (Eichenbaum, Feldstein and Podos, 1982; Adams *et al.*, 1983; Chalupa *et al.*, 1987).

The clinical detection of corneal infection is often initiated by patient symptoms, which may range from mild ocular discomfort and foreign body sensation through to severe ocular pain, redness and heavy discharge. Any corneal erosion accompanied by corneal infiltrates should be treated as a potential corneal infection. In severe cases, corneal erosion with dense stromal infiltration, severe conjunctival hyperaemia and mucopurulent discharge may be noted. Hypopyon and aqueous flare may also be present. Immediate lens removal and prompt referral for ophthalmological treatment are imperative because of the frequent presence of highly virulent organisms. Treatment usually involves intensive and aggressive topical and subconjunctival antibiotic therapy, prescribed on the basis of culture of corneal scrapings which will frequently determine the drug sensitivity of the infective organism. Hospitalization in severe cases is often necessary. The use of intravenous medication may be indicated if the integrity of the globe is threatened. Sequelae in the form of peripheral or central corneal opacities are to be expected if the stroma is involved, and further surgical intervention, such as keratoplasty, may be necessary after resolution of the infection in order to restore useful vision.

The risk of corneal infection can be reduced by careful patient management. It is important to emphasize to extended wear patients that lenses must be removed and the practitioner contacted immediately if any unusual redness, discomfort or blurred vision occurs, particularly in one eye only. In particular, the practitioner should ensure, in the case of elderly aphakic patients, that a competent companion or family member is available to remove the lenses under these circumstances. Rigorous patient instruction on lens disinfection and handling procedures is also necessary to reduce the risk of introducing pathogens into the eye. Although it has been suggested that the risk of corneal infection may be reduced by limiting the frequency of lens removal and handling during extended wear (Adams *et al.*, 1983; Galentine *et al.*, 1984), the authors believe that, in fact, regular overnight lens removal, at least once a week, for lens disinfection and to rest the cornea, is a more appropriate way of ensuring lens hygiene and maintaining corneal health. In fact, Grant, Kotow and Holden (1987) report that serious complications are significantly reduced if hydrogel extended wear is limited to 1–2 nights per week. Finally, minimizing the chronic hypoxic stress experienced by the cornea during extended wear will help to maintain epithelial integrity. This can be achieved with hydrogel lenses by fitting lenses with high Dk/t values, ensuring adequate lens movement, and instituting a care regimen of frequent overnight lens removal and regular lens replacement. Alternatively, RGP lenses with high Dk/t values may be fitted to increase corneal oxygenation during lens wear (Schnider *et al.*, 1986a).

Other acute responses

Corneal neovascularization

The growth of new blood vessels into the normally avascular cornea is a sign that the cornea is under stress and may, in itself, threaten the integrity of the tissue. Corneal neovascularization has been reported in association with therapeutic (Schecter, Emery and Soper, 1975) and aphakic extended wear (Stein and Slatt, 1977), but less frequently in association with cosmetic extended wear, possibly because the cornea is not compromised by an underlying abnormal condition or surgical intervention.

The aetiology of corneal neovascularization is not clear, and appears to be complex and multifactorial. A variety of predisposing or triggering mechanisms have been proposed, including peripheral corneal oedema, which reduces stromal tissue compactness (Cogan, 1949), and vasostimulatory factors released by inflammatory cells (Fromer and Klintworth, 1976), damaged epithelial cells (Eliason, 1978), or the by-products of altered corneal metabolism under hypoxic conditions (Imre, 1972). These stimuli may all be present during hydrogel contact lens wear.

Extended lens wear appears to carry a greater risk of corneal neovascularization than daily wear. This may be because of the continual presence of the lens on the eye. The chronic increased limbal vessel injection and proliferation found in extended lens wearers (Holden *et al.*, 1986b) may also increase the risk of new vessel growth in response to a precipitating stimulus, because of the presence of an established active vascular plexus close to the corneal tissue.

Increased limbal vessel proliferation and hyperaemia are normal, if undesirable, findings in association with extended hydrogel lens wear (Holden *et al.*, 1986b). Limbal vessels may be distinguished from corneal vessels by locating the translucent limbal transition zone (*Plates 53*

and *54*) using marginal retroillumination with the slit lamp (McMonnies, Chapman-Davies and Holden, 1982). Vessels extending beyond this zone, particularly if unlooped, should be viewed with concern, and cessation of lens wear is advised. McMonnies (1983) suggests that, although established corneal vessels may empty to become ghost vessels, they rarely regress and may refill rapidly once the vasoproliferative stimulus reoccurs. Resumption of lens wear once the invading vessels have emptied, therefore, should be undertaken with caution, after elimination of all possible causes for the initial vessel proliferation, such as hypoxia, toxic effects from lens or solutions, or traumatic causes such as damaged or heavily deposited lenses.

Corneal infiltrates

Although infiltrative keratitis is a known clinical entity in the general population, its occurrence in association with hydrogel lens wear is of concern because of the exacerbating influence of the lens. The incidence of corneal infiltrates in the hydrogel lens-wearing population has been estimated as 4–5% (Josephson and Caffery, 1979; Gordon and Kracher, 1985). Infiltrative keratitis represents an inflammatory response of the cornea, stimulating the release from the limbal vasculature of leucocytes which invade the cornea from the limbus; the tear film has also been suggested as a source of the invading leucocytes (Josephson and Caffery, 1979). The chemotactic stimulus to leucocytic invasion may be traumatic, viral, allergic or toxic, and may be associated with solution preservatives, poor lens fit or condition, or toxic environmental stimuli. Infiltrates are a typical finding in association with an acute red eye reaction, but may also occur in the absence of any identifiable stimulus.

Corneal infiltrates are usually subepithelial or stromal, although they may also occur in the epithelium (Zantos and Holden, 1977a, 1978; Zantos, 1981). They may be focal or diffuse, but in extended wear are typically focal and appear as round, well-demarcated, greyish-white areas, 0.5–2.0 mm in diameter, and are usually separated from the limbus by a clear zone (*Plate 57*). Infiltrates associated with extended lens wear often occur in the superior region of the cornea covered by the upper eyelid (Gordon and Kracher, 1985), although in association with an acute red eye reaction, they are generally more widespread (Zantos and Holden, 1977a). While infiltrates do not usually stain with fluorescein, staining suggests that the overlying epithelium is compromised, and this is cause for concern because of the risk of opportunistic infection.

The presence of corneal infiltrates requires cessation of lens wear until the cornea is clear. Recovery time is related to the severity of the infiltration; severe stromal infiltrates may take up to 3 months to clear (Josephson and Caffery, 1979), while mild infiltrates may resolve within 1–2 weeks (Zantos and Holden, 1977a). Before recommencing lens wear, it is advisable to attempt to identify and eliminate any predisposing factors such as a tight lens fit, excessive lens deposition or solution preservatives; dispensing a fresh lens is a recommended procedure.

Epithelial microcysts

Epithelial microcysts are a common clinical finding in hydrogel extended lens wearers and are best detected with the slit lamp using high magnification and marginal retroillumination (Zantos and Holden, 1978; Zantos, 1983). They appear as tiny translucent irregular dots, approximately 10–90 µm in diameter (*Figure 15.7* and *Plates 61* and *62*), and are usually distributed in an annulus in the corneal midperiphery (Zantos and Holden, 1978; Zantos, 1983) (*Figure 15.8*). It is thought that microcysts contain disorganized cellular material and are formed in the deeper layers of the epithelium, moving gradually towards the epithelial surface, where they may stain with fluorescein as they break through.

Microcysts normally develop within 3 months of commencing extended lens wear, and are thought to reflect compromise of epithelial function due to chronic hypoxic stress. The number of microcysts may fluctuate during lens wear, in some cases reaching as many as several hundred. Following cessation of lens wear, the number of microcysts increases temporarily, due to the resurgence of normal epithelial metabolic activity and the increased rate of elimination of metabolic waste products (Holden *et al.*, 1985b). As normal metabolism is re-established, the number of microcysts decreases, and complete recovery usually occurs within 3 months (Zantos and Holden, 1978; Humphreys, Larke and Parrish, 1980; Holden *et al.*, 1985c).

Although microcysts indicate that the epithelium is compromised, it has been suggested that they can be considered to be a normal consequence of hydrogel extended lens wear, and should not cause concern unless marked epithelial disruption or more than 50 microcysts are present (Zantos, 1983). In these circum-

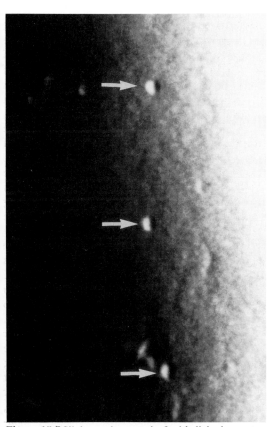

Figure 15.7 Slit lamp photograph of epithelial microcysts (arrows) in the corneal epithelium of a lens-wearing eye. Note that the microcysts display reversed illumination, i.e. the distribution of light within the microcysts is opposite to that of the background. This suggests that microcysts represent pockets of cellular debris. Magnification × 200 (reduced by 30% on reproduction). (From Holden *et al.* (1985b) with kind permission)

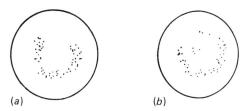

(a)   (b)

Figure 15.8 Schematic representation of the distribution of epithelial microcysts, in an annulus in the corneal midperiphery, in one patient after 23 weeks of extended hydrogel contact lens wear. (a) Right eye; (b) left eye. (From Zantos and Holden (1978) with kind permission)

stances it may be advisable to return the patient to daily wear until the epithelium regains a more normal clinical appearance. Recurrent excessive microcystic development should be managed by refitting the patient with a lens of higher Dk/t value, reducing the number of nights of lens wear (Grant, Kotow and Holden, 1987) or by returning the patient to a daily wearing schedule.

The endothelial bleb response

The transient endothelial bleb response was first reported in 1977 by Zantos and Holden (1977b), who observed the appearance of small dark spots distributed over the endothelium of an unadapted subject soon after the insertion of a thick soft contact lens. This observation has since been substantiated by a number of authors (Barr and Schoessler, 1980; Kamiya, 1980; Vannas et al., 1981; Schoessler, Woloschak and Mauger, 1982). Both hard and soft lenses can induce this transient response, as can lid closure (Khodadoust and Hirst, 1984), and exposure to atmospheric anoxia (Holden and Zantos, 1981) and carbon dioxide (Holden, Williams and Zantos, 1985).

Endothelial blebs appear as small, dark, non-reflective areas scattered over the endothe-lial mosaic (*Plate 64*), and increase in size and number with continued exposure to the stimulus, reaching a peak after approximately 30 minutes. The bleb response then decreases to a steady level and disappears rapidly following removal of the stimulus. During extended lens wear, the bleb response shows a biphasic diurnal cycle, with a reduction in the number of blebs after eye opening, and a second phase of increased response in the late afternoon and evening (Williams and Holden, 1986; *Figure 15.9*). The bleb response also shows adaptation with continued lens wear (Barr and Schoessler, 1980; Kamiya, 1980; Williams and Holden, 1986).

The nature and aetiology of the bleb response are not fully understood. However, histological studies (Vannas, Holden and Makitie, 1984) indicate that the change in appearance of the endothelial mosaic is due to cellular oedema which causes bulging of the posterior endothe-lial cell membrane, altering its specular reflect-ing properties. Holden, Williams and Zantos (1985) have established that reduction in stromal pH due to carbon dioxide and/or lactate accumulation is the most likely cause for this response.

The clinical significance of the endothelial bleb response is not clear. It has been suggested

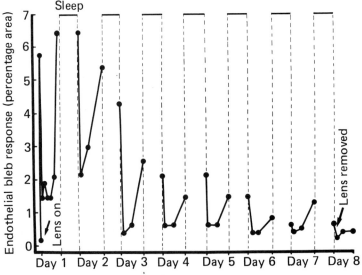

Figure 15.9 Typical pattern of endothelial bleb response in one subject who wore a hydrogel lens continuously for a period of one week. Note the biphasic diurnal variation, and the adaptation of the bleb response with continued wear. (From Williams and Holden (1986) with kind permission)

that patients who exhibit a persistent bleb response to contact lenses may show poor adaptation to extended wear (Holden, 1983). However, the endothelial bleb response does not appear to affect the endothelial pump or barrier functions, at least in the short term, as blebs can be induced in the absence of corneal swelling, and no correlation between the amount of corneal oedema and the magnitude of the bleb response has been established (Holden, Williams and Zantos, 1985).

Long-term effects of hydrogel extended wear

In a recent study, the CCLRU–Goteborg study, Holden *et al.* (1985b) demonstrated that long-term hydrogel extended wear causes subtle changes in corneal structure and function. Holden and his co-workers examined the corneas of 27 patients who had been wearing a high water content hydrogel lens in one eye only (because of amblyopia or anisometropia) on an extended wear basis for an average of 5 years. Compared to the non-lens-wearing fellow eye, the lens-wearing eye showed significant reductions in epithelial thickness and oxygen uptake rate, more epithelial microcysts, stromal thinning, and increased endothelial polymegathism (variation in endothelial cell area). No interocular differences in endothelial cell density were found.

In order to investigate the time course of recovery from these corneal changes, patients in the study were asked to discontinue lens wear

for one month. During this time epithelial thickness and oxygen uptake rate returned to levels found in the non-lens-wearing eye. The number of epithelial microcysts increased in the lens-wearing eye in the week following lens removal and subsequently decreased in number. This recovery of normal epithelial function is shown in *Figure 15.10*. The stromal and endothelial changes, however, were more long lasting. Continued follow-up of several of the study patients over 6 months without lens wear showed little recovery in stromal thickness or endothelial cell regularity (Holden *et al.*, 1985c). MacRae *et al.* (1986) also found little evidence of a reduction in lens-induced endothelial polymegathism 4 years after discontinuation of PMMA contact lens wear.

The clinical significance of these subtle alterations in corneal structure and function has yet to be clarified. Holden *et al.* (1985b) believe that the lens-induced reduction in epithelial metabolic rate, as evidenced by epithelial thinning and decreased epithelial oxygen demand, may compromise the ability of the epithelium to withstand invading organisms, thus predisposing the cornea to infection. Furthermore, epithelial adhesion to the basement membrane may be reduced by extended hydrogel lens wear (Madigan, Holden and Kwok, 1987), suggesting that the epithelium

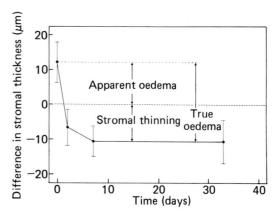

Figure 15.11 Changes in stromal thickness of the lens-wearing eye, relative to the control (non-lens-wearing) eye (dotted line), after cessation of long-term extended wear of high water content hydrogel contact lenses. Data on day 0 were obtained immediately following lens removal. Error bars represent the standard error. The apparent oedema on lens removal, stromal thinning, and true oedema are indicated. (Adapted from Holden *et al.* (1985b) with kind permission)

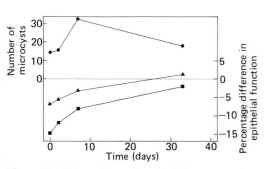

Figure 15.10 Mean changes in epithelial oxygen uptake (■), epithelial thickness (▲) and epithelial microcysts (●) after cessation of long-term extended wear of high water content hydrogel contact lenses. Data on day 0 were obtained within 2 hours of lens removal. The dotted line represents the control (non-lens-wearing) eye data. (From Holden *et al.* (1985b) with kind permission)

may be more susceptible to trauma. The changes in epithelial characteristics after cessation of lens wear are thought to reflect the resurgence in epithelial metabolic activity which has been depressed as a result of chronic lens-induced hypoxia.

In the CCLRU–Goteborg study the amount of stromal thinning found after 5 years of extended wear was approximately 11 μm, which represents a thinning rate of only 2 μm per year. No structural abnormalities of the stroma were observed on biomicroscopic examination in patients exhibiting stromal thinning, nor was visual acuity affected. Thus the long-term significance of stromal thinning is unclear. However, the authors suggest that stromal thinning may partially explain the apparent reduction in corneal oedema accompanying extended wear, as reported by Schoessler and Barr (1980) and Lebow and Plishka (1980). Indeed, Holden and co-workers found that immediately upon lens removal, the stroma of the lens-wearing eye was 2.5% thicker than in the fellow non-lens-wearing eye; after 7 days without lens wear, the lens-induced oedema had subsided to reveal stromal thinning in the eye that had been wearing the lens (*Figure 15.11*).

Increased endothelial polymegathism in association with extended contact lens wear (*Figure 15.12*) has been reported previously by Schoessler (1983). Other studies have reported similar changes in endothelial morphology with long-term PMMA (Schoessler and Woloschak, 1981; Hirst *et al.*, 1984; Stocker and Schoessler, 1985; MacRae *et al.*, 1986) and daily soft lens wear (MacRae *et al.*, 1986). Interestingly, Schoessler, Barr and Freson (1984) reported no change in endothelial polymegathism in patients wearing silicone elastomer contact lenses, which have extremely high Dk/t values. Although this suggests that chronic lens-induced hypoxia plays a role in the aetiology of endothelial polymegathous changes, the mechanism may in fact be more complex. A recent study by Holden, Williams and Zantos (1985) has shown that the transient endothelial bleb response is caused by a reduction in stromal pH due to either lactate accumulation under hypoxic conditions, or restriction of carbon dioxide efflux during lens wear (Holden, Ross and Jenkins, 1987). Indeed, such a reduction in stromal pH during eye closure and contact lens wear has been demonstrated by Bonanno and Polse (1987a,b). It is possible, therefore, that chronic reductions in

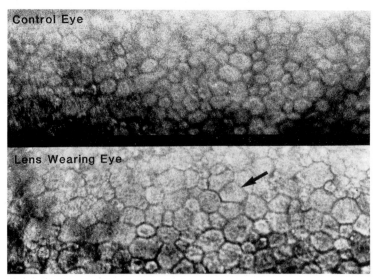

Figure 15.12 Endothelial photograph of the non-lens-wearing eye (top) and lens-wearing eye (bottom) of a patient who had worn a hydrogel lens on an extended wear basis in one eye only for 79 months. A greater variation in endothelial cell size (polymegathism) is evident in the lens-wearing eye. Also evident in that eye are a number of rosette formations (arrow); these are thought to occur following injury of a single endothelial cell, whereby neighbouring cells radiate towards the centre of the damaged cell (compare *Figures 6.11, 6.12* and *7.9*). (Adapted from Holden *et al.* (1985b) with kind permission)

stromal pH during lens wear contribute to long-term changes in endothelial morphology, such as endothelial polymegathism.

Rao *et al.* (1984) have established that patients with higher degrees of preoperative endothelial polymegathism have significantly greater postsurgical complications following intraocular lens implantation. This suggests that the functional reserve of the endothelium may be compromised with higher degrees of polymegathism, although it is unclear whether the functional integrity of the endothelium is threatened in the absence of the added stress of surgery. The full significance of contact lens-induced polymegathism may not be clarified until the present generation of contact lens wearers age, and their response to procedures such as intraocular surgery is assessed.

Clinical management of hydrogel extended wear

Patient selection

Patients who may be considered for extended wear fall into the three broad categories shown below.

Patients who require therapeutic or 'bandage' lenses due to corneal conditions

Extended contact lens wear may be recommended to patients in this category where it is anticipated that the contact lens will promote corneal healing or alleviate ocular discomfort. Conditions which may benefit from application of a bandage lens include bullous keratopathy, indolent corneal ulcers, neuroparalytic conditions, exposure keratitis, penetrating corneal wounds and recent keratoplasty. Extended wear rather than daily wear is often indicated if regular manipulation of the lens may re-traumatize the healing cornea. As the use of contact lenses in ocular pathology is covered in detail in Chapter 21, this application of hydrogel extended wear will not be discussed further.

Patients who would benefit from contact lens correction, but have difficulty in handling lenses on a daily basis

Extended contact lens wear is a particular advantage for this reason for elderly aphakic patients or young children with aphakia (*see* Chapter 21), anisometropia or high refractive errors.

Opinion has been expressed widely in the literature that patients in this category can be left with the lens *in situ* for several months between practitioner visits for lens removal and cleaning. Considering the susceptibility of elderly patients to corneal insult due to concomitant external eye conditions such as decreased tear flow and chronic blepharoconjunctivitis, and reduced corneal sensitivity following cataract surgery, the authors feel that this approach to patient after-care is a recipe for disaster. Corneal surgery has been shown to decrease epithelial metabolic activity (Holden *et al.*, 1982; Vannas *et al.*, 1985), which may render the cornea more susceptible to infection. In addition, an elderly patient may not, for a number of reasons, appreciate the early warning signs of an acute corneal complication, and may be unable or unwilling to remove the lens even if symptoms are recognized. There is, therefore, a risk of progression of the corneal insult before practitioner contact is initiated. As stated previously, patient delay in seeking treatment is a major factor in the development of vision-threatening corneal infections.

Patient selection for aphakic extended wear should therefore involve careful evaluation of the risk:benefit ratio in each individual case. The patient's mental alertness, manual dexterity, personal hygiene and social environment should be considered. If the patient has reduced mental competence, or is unable to manipulate the lenses if necessary, it is advisable that a relative or attendant be instructed to examine the patient's eyes periodically for unusual redness or discharge, and be trained to remove the lenses for regular cleaning or if signs or symptoms of corneal complications occur.

Following cataract extraction, many aphakic patients exhibit a certain amount of corneal astigmatism, which is not easily corrected by a hydrogel contact lens unless a toric fitting is attempted. However, in spite of the reduced visual acuity due to uncorrected astigmatism, contact lens correction provides many visual benefits over aphakic spectacle correction, including wider visual fields, and decreased distortion and prismatic effects. Provision of an appropriate spectacle over-correction to correct the cylindrical element, and/or to provide reading correction will often prove acceptable to the aphakic extended wear patient.

Contact lenses often prove beneficial for visual correction of high refractive errors, aphakia and anisometropia in very young children. However, care must be taken, when prescribing extended wear lenses in this age group, to ensure that the parents or guardians are thoroughly trained in handling the contact lenses and in detecting early warning signs of acute complications. Parents should also be advised that the need for lens replacement, due to lens damage or loss, and also due to rapid changes in corneal curvature and diameter (Ellis, 1983), is more frequent in this age group, and the financial commitment will therefore be greater (see also Chapter 21).

Patients with moderate refractive errors who desire extended wear for cosmetic reasons

Most extended lens wearers fall into this category. A wide variety of refractive errors can be corrected with extended wear hydrogel lenses, although undoubtedly the majority of these patients are myopic.

The convenience of extended wear is a major advantage in some occupational groups, such as military personnel, ambulance drivers and physicians on call, where time-consuming lens insertion under certain circumstances would be disadvantageous. Extended lens wear may also prove an advantage in certain leisure pursuits such as camping or ocean sailing where adequate provision for daily lens removal is awkward or inconvenient. Due to the aggressive consumer advertising of extended wear lenses, however, most patients seeking cosmetic extended wear, at least in the USA, are attracted primarily by the prospect of not having to handle the lenses on a routine basis, and often anticipate trouble-free, comfortable, clear visual correction with these lenses for extended periods of wear of 30 days or more.

The primary responsibility of the contact lens practitioner, therefore, is to educate the prospective cosmetic extended wear patient in the risks, benefits and realities of extended wear. Potential acute complications and long-term effects should be clearly explained, and emphasis should be placed on the need for regular overnight lens removal, meticulous lens hygiene and disinfection procedures, and the importance of immediate lens removal and professional advice should unusual redness, discomfort or blurred vision occur. It is advisable to reinforce this preliminary discussion with a written summary detailing the patient's responsibilities and the risks involved. In particular, it is important that the patient realizes that extended wear does not mean continuous wear, and that by proceeding with extended wear, the patient is committed to a substantial continuing investment in terms of time and money.

Undoubtedly, some practitioners will be more willing to fit cosmetic extended wear than others. This, of course, is primarily a matter for the individual practitioner to decide, based on his or her perception of professional responsibility and personal competence and interest. The authors believe that, if a patient can be talked into daily contact lens wear or occasional overnight lens wear with frequent overnight lens removal, then this course should be followed in preference to extended wear. If the patient wishes to proceed with extended wear, the practitioner should carefully evaluate factors such as the patient's mental alertness, manual dexterity and personal hygiene before proceeding with lens fitting. A careful slit lamp examination of the external eye and a detailed history including previous ocular complications, allergic conditions and general health are essential to exclude patients with contra-indications for extended wear, such as reduced tear flow, ocular allergy, structural abnormalities of the lids, diabetes or the use of ocular medications. Care should be taken when recommending extended wear to patients with moderate or high degrees of hyperopia, as the greater thickness of plus lenses will reduce oxygen transmission through these lenses.

Attempts to predict which individual patients are more likely to suffer acute complications or long-term effects have generally been inconclusive. An analysis of data collected during the CCLRU–Goteborg study (Holden et al., 1985b) indicated that long-term lens-induced changes in corneal structure and function were less apparent in patients with thinner corneas and structurally regular endothelium prior to commencing extended lens wear. Sarver, Polse and Baggett (1983) and Efron (1986) have suggested that hypoxic stress testing of prospective extended lens wearers, either by 3 hours' wear of thick hydrogel lenses, or short-term exposure to gaseous anoxia, may identify those individuals more susceptible to excessive corneal oedema during contact lens wear. However, in the short term, the most direct way of evaluating an individual patient's response to extended wear is to monitor the corneal response closely during the first weeks of extended lens wear.

Lens fitting

The fitting of soft contact lenses is discussed in detail in Chapter 11. There are no major differences in the approach to fitting hydrogel extended wear lenses compared with daily wear lenses, except in two areas.

First, consideration must be given to maximizing the oxygen transmission characteristics of the lenses. Thus selection of either a high water content lens, or a very thin, low water content lens is indicated. The refractive error of the patient may influence this choice. Because of their greater average thickness, plus lenses or high-minus lenses will transmit less oxygen than the more commonly prescribed low-minus lenses. Holden *et al.* (1985a) found that high-minus lenses in a low water content material induced greater midperipheral corneal swelling than in a high water content material, presumably because of the greater Dk/t differential with low water content lenses between centre and periphery. Thus high water content lenses are preferable for patients with higher degrees of refractive error.

Secondly, the provision of adequate lens movement is considered to be an important factor in avoiding complications such as acute red eye reactions. More specifically, the lens should not fit tightly or become tight with wear, and should move across the cornea with ease when pushed by the eyelid. With high water content lenses, lens movement on a blink should be in the region of 0.4 mm. Thin low water content lenses move less on the eye because they tend to 'drape' on to the cornea; however, lens movement of approximately 0.2 mm on a blink is desirable. It must be kept in mind that lenses often tighten up during wear. This tends to be a greater problem with high water content lenses due to their more rapid ageing. It is therefore recommended that the practitioner should attempt to fit the flattest possible lens consistent with acceptable patient comfort and stable vision.

Care and maintenance

Rigorous care and maintenance procedures are a key factor in maximizing extended wear success. As well as maintaining good patient comfort and vision, the removal of lens deposits and regular lens disinfection ensure that bacteria and other pathogens are less likely to adhere to the lens surface or persist within the polymer matrix, thus reducing the risk of corneal infection. In susceptible individuals, deposits on the front surface of the lens may also precipitate papillary changes in the upper palpebral conjunctiva; maintenance of a clean front lens surface, therefore, may avoid or halt the progression of this tissue response.

Regular overnight removal of extended wear lenses is desirable, in order to carry out lens cleaning and disinfection procedures, and to rest the cornea from chronic hypoxic stress. The authors recommend that extended wear lenses should be removed for a minimum of 16 hours, including a period when the eye is open, at least once a week. In fact, from a physiological point of view it is preferable to limit overnight wear with current hydrogel lenses to 1–2 nights per week if possible (Grant, Kotow and Holden, 1987). Establishment of a routine timetable for overnight lens removal will reinforce the maintenance of regular lens cleaning and disinfection habits.

The care and maintenance regimens recommended for high and low water content lenses are summarized in *Table 15.2*. A surfactant cleaner should be used initially to remove loose surface deposits and debris, followed by enzymatic cleaning on a weekly basis to remove persistent deposits. The lenses should then be

Table 15.2 Recommended care and maintenance regimens for hydrogel extended wear lenses

High water content	Low water content
Weekly removal	Weekly removal
Surfactant cleaner	Surfactant cleaner
Unpreserved saline rinse[a]	Unpreserved saline rinse
Enzymatic cleaner	Enzymatic cleaner
Repeat surfactant cleaner	Repeat surfactant cleaner
Peroxide disinfection	Heat or peroxide disinfection
16-hour rest period	16-hour rest period
Replacement every 1–3 months	Quarterly replacement

[a] Aerosol or single dose saline.

disinfected using either heat or peroxide, to destroy contaminating bacteria and other pathogens. Recent studies suggest that the use of peroxide results in a lower adverse response rate than heat disinfection, particularly for high water content lenses (Kotow, Grant and Holden, 1987). Because of the possibility of allergic and toxic reactions to preservatives, the authors recommend that non-preserved saline (unit dose or aerosol) be used to rinse the lenses during the cleaning process. Scrupulous attention should be paid to cleanliness of the hands to avoid recontaminating the lenses during handling. It is advisable to review cleaning procedures routinely with the patient during after-care visits to ensure patient compliance.

There is evidence to suggest that regular replacement of extended wear lenses may reduce the risk of both acute complications (Holden, Kotow and Swarbrick, 1986; Kotow, Holden and Grant, 1987) and long-term effects (Holden et al., 1985b). Replacement of the lenses helps to avoid problems related to the build-up of stubborn deposits, and lens ageing and spoiling. The concept of regular replacement was originated by Klas Nilsson (1983) in Sweden, with high water content lenses, and by Ake Gustafsson with low water content lenses. Nilsson's care system, developed over 10 years' experience with hydrogel extended wear, includes 6-monthly replacement of lenses, avoidance of preserved solutions, and the use of oxidizing disinfection systems. The complication rates found using this system are encouraging. Holden et al. (1985b) report an incidence of acute red eye reactions of 7% per year. In recognition of the benefits of regular lens replacement, some US contact lens companies have adopted Nilsson's system, with the establishment of regular replacement services, whereby fresh lenses are automatically issued to every extended wear patient on a regular basis. The use of disposable contact lenses has also begun in some countries, although a trial programme utilizing this concept in Denmark foundered, due mainly to problems with parameter reproducibility and variable packaging standards (Benjamin, Bergmanson and Estrada, 1985). Although frequent lens replacement may increase the patient's financial commitment, the authors recommend that fresh extended wear lenses should be issued routinely at least every 6 months, and as often as every 1–3 months,

depending on the material used, for those patients who show persistent stubborn lens deposits or rapid lens spoiling.

Patient advice and management

Before the lenses are dispensed, it is important to ensure that the patient is competent in lens handling or at the very least, where handling difficulties are apparent, that a family member or companion is trained to insert and remove the lenses. In most cases, a daily wear adaptation period is not essential, as adaptation is generally rapid.

It is important to see patients early in the morning following the first overnight wear of the lenses, in order to assess the patient's response to overnight hypoxic stress. A careful slit lamp examination should be performed to evaluate the corneal oedema response; the presence of striae or folds more than 2 hours after eye opening should be taken as a warning sign of high levels of overnight corneal swelling. The fitting characteristics of the lenses should also be assessed to ensure that adequate lens movement has been maintained.

Follow-up visits after 3 days, 1 week and 2 weeks of extended wear are then advised. Discussion and reinforcement of lens handling and care and maintenance procedures at these visits are suggested in order to emphasize the importance of these to the patient. If no problems are apparent, monthly after-care visits should follow.

Yamane and Kuwabara (1987) suggest that extended wear patients should be encouraged to check their eyes daily to ensure that they 'feel good, look good, and see good'; if these criteria are not met, the patients should remove their lenses and consult their practitioner.

From clinical studies at the CCLRU, the following measures have been found to lead to safer extended wear (Holden, 1986).

Patient advice

(1) Remove the lenses if there is any unusual redness, irritation or blurred vision, especially in one eye only.
(2) Instil sterile saline in the morning and evening.
(3) Remove lenses during a cold, influenza or hospitalization.

(4) When swimming in fresh water wear swimming goggles and in salt water remove the lenses.

Patient management by the clinician

(1) If corneal erosions occur, remove the lenses and refer for ophthalmological attention.
(2) A corneal erosion with infiltrates may well indicate a corneal infection and referral to an ophthalmologist with experience in contact lens-related problems is imperative.
(3) If significant corneal staining is noted, remove the lenses for at least 48 hours and review.
(4) If asymptomatic infiltrates are present, remove the lenses for 3 days and review. No lens wear is advised until the infiltrates disappear. A fresh lens should be issued.
(5) If corneal striae/folds are present 2–3 hours after waking, return the patient to daily wear or try a lens with higher oxygen transmissibility.
(6) A drop in visual acuity of one line or more requires an over-refraction and a check of lens condition. Replace the lenses if necessary.
(7) Acute red eye warrants immediate lens removal (if the eye is painful, patching may help). Infiltrates must be resolved before recommencing lens wear. New lenses should be issued when resuming lens wear.
(8) The development of CLPC requires lens removal and review every 3–4 weeks. Re-fitting with RGP lenses for extended wear may be more successful in avoiding CLPC than re-fitting with a new soft contact lens, or a different hydrogel material.

RGP extended wear

Historical review

Rigid gas permeable (RGP) lenses have been available for daily wear since the mid-1970s. The first rigid oxygen-permeable material, cellulose acetate butyrate (CAB; marketed initially as RX-56, Meso and Cabcurve), provided little additional oxygen by diffusion through the lens material, and was soon replaced by a new generation of RGP materials made of co-polymers of silicone and methyl methacrylate. The first of these was the Polycon

material, developed by Leonard Seidner, and approved for daily wear in the USA in January 1979. New silicone – acrylate materials were soon to follow, including the Boston material (Polymer Technology Corp.), and the Calgary and Alberta materials (Corneal Contact Lens Co., Canada). Today over 30 RGP materials of various compositions are available for daily wear.

Although there are anecdotal reports of patients achieving continuous wear with oxygen-impermeable PMMA lenses (reviewed by Young, 1985), it is now well known that the cornea requires oxygen during closed-eye wear in order to maintain its integrity in both the short and long term. The use of RGP lenses for aphakic extended wear was first reported by Garcia in 1976, but the development of hydrogel extended wear lenses effectively stifled interest in this modality for several years. However, with increasing reports of adverse acute and chronic effects with hydrogel extended wear, and with the development of new RGP materials with oxygen transmission characteristics rivalling those of hydrogel extended wear materials, interest in RGP extended wear was revived.

In 1983, Levy reported the successful use of RGP lenses for cosmetic extended wear in an elderly myope, and commented that 'preliminary results indicate that rigid gas permeable materials are a viable alternative to the high water content hydrophilic materials currently in use for extended wear'. The following year, Fonn (at the Eighth European Research Symposium, Interlaken, Switzerland) reported a pilot study in which 10 subjects were fitted for extended wear with a hydrogel lens in one eye, and an RGP lens in the other. He found that the acute adverse response rate and physiological effects were less in the RGP lens-wearing eye; these findings were confirmed in a follow-up study with a further 30 subjects (Fonn and Holden, 1988). Since these reports, the interest in RGP extended wear has grown enormously, and has stimulated the development of many new RGP materials which combine increased oxygen transmission properties with improved wettability, stability and deposit resistance. RGP extended wear lenses are now in clinical use in many parts of the world, and have received FDA approval in the USA.

Materials used for RGP extended wear lenses can be broadly classified as silicone–acrylate polymers, fluoropolymers or fluorosilicone–acrylate polymers (*see* Chapter 3). Silicone–acrylate materials contain siloxane units to enhance oxygen permeability, methacrylic acid or HEMA for wettability, and methyl methacrylate to give good mechanical and optical properties (Caroline and Ellis, 1986). Cross-linking agents are added to the polymer to give the material additional strength and dimensional stability. In general, differences between silicone–acrylate materials arise from variations in the proportions of these monomers in the polymer matrix. The more recently developed fluoropolymers (Keates, Ihlenfeld and Isaacson, 1984) incorporate fluorine in the backbone of the polymer chain to enhance oxygen permeability, surface wettability and deposit resistance. Other co-monomers are also incorporated such as *N*-vinyl pyrrolidone to enhance wetting and methyl methacrylate for added strength. The ratio of these co-monomers can be manipulated to alter the physical and physiological properties of the material. A third family of RGP materials which comprise copolymers of silicone, fluorocarbon and methyl methacrylate (e.g. Equalens, Quantum 1, Alberta N) have also become available (*see* Chapters 3 and 10).

Advantages and disadvantages

The interest in RGP extended wear has been spurred primarily by the potential of RGP lenses to transmit more oxygen to the cornea than is possible with current-generation hydrogel materials. Early studies of RGP extended wear utilized lenses with oxygen transmissibilities equivalent to those provided by hydrogel extended wear lenses (Sweeney and Holden, 1983; Benjamin and Simons, 1984; Kenyon, Polse and O'Neal, 1985; Koetting, Castellano and Nelson, 1985; Levy, 1985; Port, 1985; Zantos and Zantos, 1985; Zabkiewicz, Swarbrick and Holden, 1986). Not surprisingly, similar levels of overnight corneal oedema were obtained as with hydrogel lenses, and Sweeney and Holden (1983) cautioned that RGP lenses should have a *Dk/t* value of at least 25 in order to be considered for extended wear. It was found, however, that the cornea could eliminate overnight oedema at a faster rate with RGP lenses than with hydrogel lenses, due principally to the oxygenation provided by the tear pump

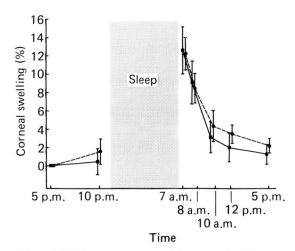

Figure 15.13 Average corneal swelling *vs* time for 10 unadapted subjects wearing an RGP (Boston IV) lens (■) on one eye and a soft (Permalens) lens (●) on the other eye over a 24-hour wake/sleep cycle. (From Holden *et al.* (1988) with kind permission)

on eye opening (Andrasko, 1986; Holden *et al.*, 1988) (*Figure 15.13*). Thus, during extended wear, the cornea is likely to experience less chronic hypoxic stress with RGP compared to hydrogel lenses of comparable *Dk/t* value.

Developments in the field of polymer chemistry have resulted in RGP materials with higher *Dk* values than hydrogel extended wear materials. Early clinical trials with these second-generation moderate *Dk* materials, termed 'super-permeables', suggest that hypoxia-induced corneal changes, such as striae and epithelial microcysts, are less frequent than with lower *Dk* RGP and hydrogel materials. Overnight corneal oedema also appeared to be considerably reduced; levels in the range of 5–7% were reported initially (Mandell and Liberman, 1985), comparing favourably with the normal overnight swelling response of 3–4% without lens wear. These encouraging initial reports, however, were based on the results from patched-eye studies, which significantly underestimate the true level of overnight oedema present on eye opening. Holden, LaHood and Sweeney (1985) found that overnight oedema levels with these materials were in fact closer to 10% when measured immediately on eye opening; more recent work by Seger and Mutti (1986) and LaHood, Sweeney and Holden (1988) has confirmed this higher oedema response. However, technological developments are now providing RGP lenses with far higher *Dk/t* values, thus further reducing the hypoxic stress on the cornea during extended wear (Terry *et al.*, 1986).

As clinical trials of RGP extended wear have progressed, other advantages of this modality have become apparent. Compared with hydrogel extended wear, there appears to be a much lower incidence of acute complications such as acute red eye reactions, CLPC and corneal infection (Fonn and Holden, 1988). In RGP extended wear clinical studies conducted at the CCLRU, involving a patient population of over 150 (200 eyes), the authors have observed two (1%) acute red eye reactions, both associated with an adherent lens and occurring in previous soft lens problem patients, and four cases of CLPC, three of which also occurred in previous soft lens wearers with this complication prior to commencing RGP extended wear, giving an incidence of RGP-induced CLPC of 0.5% (Schnider, Zabkiewicz and Holden, 1988). These results compare favourably with the adverse response rates of approximately 17% acute red eye reactions, and 11% CLPC in association with hydrogel extended wear (Grant, Kotow and Holden, 1987; *see Table 15.1*). In addition, there have been only two reports to date of corneal ulceration during RGP extended wear (Levy, 1985; Schnider, Zabkiewicz and Holden, 1988).

The reasons for the low incidence of acute complications with RGP extended wear are two-fold. First, because of the efficient tear pump with rigid lenses, tear debris and contaminants are readily flushed from behind the lens. This may explain the low rate of acute red eye reactions, which are thought to be triggered by breakdown products of retained back surface debris. Secondly, RGP lenses attract less deposits and are more easily cleaned, and therefore build up fewer stubborn deposits on the lens surface than hydrogel lenses. Thus inflammatory reactions to lens deposits, such as CLPC, are minimized, and bacteria and other pathogens are less likely to be retained on the lens surface, thus reducing the risks of corneal infection. In addition, the lower hypoxic stress experienced by the cornea during RGP as compared to hydrogel extended wear probably reduces compromise of epithelial metabolism, and the epithelium is therefore more able to withstand invading organisms.

Because of their rigidity, RGP lenses generally provide better vision than hydrogel lenses, as they do not flex as much on the cornea; corneal astigmatism of up to 3 D can be corrected with these lenses, depending on the flexibility of the lens material. The greater ease of cleaning and maintenance, combined with enhanced deposit resistance compared to hydrogel lenses, particularly with the fluoropolymer materials, is also of considerable benefit for many patients in terms of improved vision, comfort and convenience. In general, RGP lenses are more durable than hydrogels, more stable under varying environmental conditions, and are able to be modified or polished.

RGP extended wear is not without its drawbacks, however. It is important to bear in mind that many years of clinical experience with hydrogel extended wear were necessary before the adverse effects and problems associated with it became apparent. Therefore, caution is advised with RGP extended wear until its long-term safety and efficacy are established. Potential problems with RGP extended wear include corneal distortion or moulding, lens binding and corneal staining; these complications will be discussed in detail in the following sections. As with hydrogel extended wear, acute red eye reactions, CLPC and corneal infections may also occur in association with RGP extended wear. Other minor complications have also been identified. Lens discomfort and intolerance have been noted in some patients, although once adaptation is achieved, comfort is usually very good, and may be superior to that with hydrogel lenses (Fonn and Holden, 1988). The edge profile of the lens appears to be a significant factor determining RGP lens comfort, with a rounded front edge being the most important factor in providing good subjective comfort (LaHood, 1988). Abrasions due to foreign bodies, lens mishandling or dislodgement also occur with greater frequency than with hydrogel lenses. Careful patient instruction may circumvent these problems to some extent. Fonn and Holden (1986) have also reported the development of transient eyelid ptosis in association with RGP extended wear. They postulate that the ptosis is caused by lid oedema or inflammation due to chronic irritation of the eyelid by the lens edge or deposits on the lens surface.

Acute complications of RGP extended wear

Stromal oedema

As with hydrogel extended wear, overnight wear of low or moderate Dk/t RGP lenses may give rise to significant levels of overnight corneal oedema. Because the oedema accompanying RGP lens wear is usually localized in the central 6 mm of the cornea (Fonn *et al.*, 1984), it may be detected with the slit lamp using the technique of sclerotic scatter (*see* Chapter 6 and *Plate* 23). However, oedema associated with RGP overnight lens wear resolves rapidly following eye opening due to the circulation of oxygenated tears behind the lens; unless the patient is seen within one hour of eye opening, therefore, there may be little evidence of residual oedema. As with hydrogel lens-induced oedema, the presence of striae or folds in the posterior stroma which persist for more than 2 hours following eye opening can be used to infer the occurrence of clinically unacceptable levels of overnight corneal swelling.

The selection of an RGP lens material which will provide adequate corneal oxygenation during sleep is usually based on the clinician's knowledge of the Dk value of the material. At the CCLRU, RGP lens materials that have been assessed to date can be classified as either low Dk [$<40 \times 10^{-11}$ $(cm^2\ ml\ O_2)/(s\ ml\ mmHg)$], moderate Dk (40–70) or high Dk (>70) (*Table 15.3*). The authors believe that, while consideration must be given to other lens properties, it is advisable to prescribe only high Dk RGP lens materials for extended wear, in order to maximize oxygen availability to the cornea during sleep, and thus reduce the chronic hypoxic stress experienced by the cornea in the long term.

Information on the nominal Dk value of RGP materials is generally supplied by the marketing company and, until recently, has been based on Dk measurements performed using the technique described by Fatt (1984). However, recent controversy (Guillon, 1985; Hamano, Kawabe and Mitsunaga, 1985; Holden, LaHood and Sweeney, 1985; Brennan, Efron and Holden, 1986a, b; Fatt, 1986a,b; Holden, Kotow and Swarbrick, 1986) has stimulated a re-examination of both the measurement of Dk/t and the derivation of Dk from these measurements. At this time, the role of barrier and surface effects (Hwang, Tang and Kammermeyer, 1971), edge effects (Melpolder, personal communication; Brennan, Efron and Holden, 1986b) and other factors affecting both Dk/t measurement *in vitro* and prediction of Dk/t *in vivo* have not been clarified. For example, Holden, LaHood and Sweeney (1985) observed that Paraperm EW, a silicone–acrylate material with a nominal Dk value of 56×10^{-11} units, in a thickness of 0.17 mm (i.e. nominal Dk/t of 33×10^{-9} units) induced 10% overnight oedema, equivalent to the level induced by a hydrogel lens with a Dk/t of 22×10^{-9} units. This implies that the on-eye or 'effective' Dk value of Paraperm EW is closer to 37×10^{-11} units. It is now apparent, therefore, that early estimates of the Dk/t of RGP lenses (Fatt, 1984) overestimated the true Dk/t values of these lenses on the eye. This emphasizes the importance of monitoring individual patient responses to RGP extended wear in order to identify those patients who may be susceptible to excessive overnight corneal swelling.

Table 15.3 Rigid gas permeable contact lens materials for extended wear

Dk *range*	*Material*	*Polymer type*	Dk[a, c]	Dk[b, c]
Low (<40)[c]	Boston IV	Silicone acrylate	18	24
	Paraperm EW	Silicone acrylate	33	49
Moderate (40–70)[c]	Equalens	Fluorosilicone acrylate	59	55
	Quantum 1	Fluorosilicone acrylate	59	55
	Optacryl Z	Fluorosilicone acrylate	70	67
High (>70)[c]	Oxylens 2	Fluorosilicone acrylate	>100	133
	Flurofocon A	Fluoropolymer	>100	95

[a]Measured using the technique described by Brennan, Efron and Holden (1986a).
[b]Measured using Fatt's technique (Fatt, 1984).
[c]Units are $(cm^2\ ml\ O_2)/(s\ ml\ mmHg) \times 10^{-11}$

Corneal moulding and distortion

Because of the rigidity of RGP compared to hydrogel lenses, it has been suspected that corneal distortion or moulding of corneal curvature may result from overnight wear of these lenses, due to the sustained pressure exerted by the eyelid on the lens and the cornea beneath it. Distortion of the cornea under these circumstances may possibly be facilitated in a 'softened' or swollen cornea during closed-eye wear.

Clinical investigators have indeed reported slight corneal moulding with RGP extended wear. The trend appears to be towards a slight change in corneal curvature in the direction of the back surface curvature of the lens, which occurs to a greater extent with more astigmatic corneas. In general, the steeper corneal meridian appears to be more affected, resulting in a trend towards reduced corneal toricity (Benjamin and Simons, 1984; Kenyon, Polse and O'Neal, 1985; Mandell and Liberman, 1985; Schnider *et al.*, 1987).

The long-term significance of these subtle changes in corneal curvature is presently unclear, and further work is needed. However, slight corneal moulding does not appear to cause detectable structural changes in the cornea and, in general, corrected visual acuity is unaffected.

Temporary localized corneal distortion and spectacle blur have been reported in association with lens binding, and other physiological disturbances such as corneal oedema and vacuoles (Zabkiewicz, Swarbrick and Holden, 1986). Appropriate clinical management of the underlying condition is likely to eliminate the distortion in these cases.

Lens binding

A number of investigators have reported the phenomenon of lens binding or adherence in association with RGP extended wear, whereby the lens is tightly adherent to the cornea on eye opening (Zantos and Zantos, 1985; Seger and Mutti, 1986; Zabkiewicz, Swarbrick and Holden, 1986; Polse *et al.*, 1987; Schnider, 1987; Swarbrick and Holden, 1987; Swarbrick, 1988). The lens is typically decentred, usually in the nasal position and often overlapping the limbus, and causes little discomfort or subjective symp-

toms. Spontaneous lens movement generally occurs within the first hour of open-eye wear, due to increased tear secretion and lid action, although in some cases the lens may remain bound to the cornea for 5 hours or more (Swarbrick and Holden, 1987). On lens removal, the epithelium may display some central punctate staining, and a complete or partial indentation or compression ring (*Plate 19*) corresponding to the lens edge is usually observed. The compression ring rarely stains with fluorescein; more typically fluorescein pools in the indentation, or appears to thin in this area if the indentation is shallow. Lens binding has been estimated to occur in between 10 and 50% of RGP extended lens wearers (Rosenthal, 1986; Seger and Mutti, 1986; Swarbrick and Holden, 1987), although the incidence may increase with time (Zabkiewicz *et al.*, 1987).

Lens binding is a significant complication of RGP extended wear for two main reasons. First, epithelial compression by the lens edge causes significant localized corneal distortion (*Figure 15.14*), which may persist for some hours. Lens binding also exacerbates 3 and 9 o'clock staining, which may show rapid progression to dellen and peripheral corneal ulceration. Levy

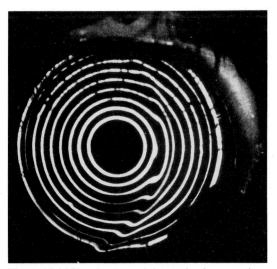

Figure 15.14 Photokeratoscopic image showing corneal distortion associated with corneal indentation induced by the edge of a bound RGP lens. The photograph was taken immediately following lens removal. (From Swarbrick and Holden (1987) with kind permission, © The American Academy of Optometry, 1987)

(1985) first reported the development of bilateral peripheral corneal ulceration in one of his subjects in association with lens binding; fortunately the ulcers healed without affecting vision. A disturbing aspect of this incident was that the patient did not experience any subjective symptoms. Schnider, Zabkiewicz and Holden (1988) also reported a case of peripheral corneal ulceration precipitated by severe 3 and 9 o'clock staining which developed in association with a bound lens.

The other cause for concern with lens binding is that, while the lens is adherent, there is no circulation of tears behind the lens. Consequently corneal deswelling after overnight hypoxic stress may be impeded, although this may not cause significant problems with high Dk/t lenses. More importantly, however, tear debris and mucus remain trapped behind the lens, typically collecting in a ring behind the midperiphery of the lens (*Plate 46a*; Zantos and Zantos, 1985). This trapped debris has the potential to provoke an acute red eye reaction; such a course of events has been noted in two RGP extended lens wearers participating in CCLRU clinical trials (Schnider, Zabkiewicz and Holden, 1988).

In a retrospective analysis of factors influencing lens binding, Swarbrick and Holden (1987) reported an incidence of lens binding of 22%. Lens binding was more frequent with large diameter, flat base curve lenses with little edge lift. Lenses fitted on-K or slightly flatter than central K, or which showed insufficient lens movement before eye closure, were also more likely to bind. These authors also noted that some patients had a greater propensity to exhibit repeated lens binding, suggesting that factors such as peripheral corneal topography, tear film characteristics or eyelid pressure may influence this phenomenon.

The aetiology of lens binding is unclear, although several theories have been advanced, based on mechanisms proposed to explain silicone elastomer lens adhesion. The negative pressure or 'suction cup' effect proposed by Fatt (1979) has been discussed in relation to RGP lens binding. However, steeply fitted RGP lenses in fact show a reduced incidence of lens binding (Swarbrick and Holden, 1987), and lens fenestration, which would be expected to reduce the suction effect, appears to have little influence on lens binding (Swarbrick, 1988). Contact adhesion between the back surface of the lens and the corneal epithelium, as discussed by Josephson and Caffery (1980) in relation to silicone elastomer lens adhesion, has also been proposed as a mechanism. One would anticipate that such intimate contact would induce epithelial staining; however, although central punctate staining may accompany lens binding, it is not a necessary finding even after prolonged periods of adherence (Swarbrick, 1988), and is rarely observed in the area of indentation, where contact between lens and cornea is usually heaviest.

Recent evidence (Swarbrick, 1988) suggests that lens binding may be precipitated by expulsion of the aqueous phase of the tear layer from between lens and cornea during eye closure. The resultant very thin, highly viscous layer of mucus-rich tears then acts as an adhesive which sticks the lens to the cornea. On eye opening, the force required to initiate lens movement may exceed that exerted by the eyelid during blinking, and the lens will remain bound until the mucous layer is thickened and diluted by gradual penetration of aqueous tears behind the lens.

Because of the potential for serious consequences with repeated episodes of lens binding, clinicians should examine RGP extended wear patients as early as possible in the morning. Although an adherent lens will rarely be observed, as spontaneous lens movement is generally rapid, the presence of a corneal indentation ring should be considered as a positive diagnostic sign. Reliable strategies for controlling lens binding have yet to be determined, and attempts to manage the consistent lens binder can prove frustrating. Various clinical approaches have been advocated, including manipulation of the edge and peripheral design to provide a wider peripheral and edge clearance, increasing lens thickness (although this will reduce the Dk/t value of the lens; Polse *et al.*, 1987), decreasing back optic zone diameter, adding a moderate to heavy midperipheral blend, and the use of in-eye wetting drops (Bennett and Egan, 1986; Henry, Bennett and Forrest, 1987). Alerting the patient to the phenomenon, so that lens movement can be initiated on eye opening by irrigation with saline solution and gentle lens manipulation, may reduce the risk of complications. However, in many cases, the most practical clinical option is to change the patient to a daily wearing schedule.

Corneal staining

Significant corneal staining with fluorescein, in particular 3 and 9 o'clock desiccation staining (*Plate 20*), may occur in association with RGP extended wear (Zantos and Zantos, 1985; Seger and Mutti, 1986; Zabkiewicz, Swarbrick and Holden, 1986; Schnider, 1987; Schnider, Zabkiewicz and Holden, 1988). In general, 3 and 9 o'clock staining can be attributed to peripheral corneal desiccation resulting from inappropriate lens design and fitting, rather than to the lens material itself. During daily wear, it is most commonly due to excessive edge lift of the lens, which creates a pool of tears under the lens edge which draws tears from adjacent areas, and also causes a bridging effect whereby the eyelid cannot properly resurface the cornea adjacent to the lens edge with mucin or rewet the peripheral cornea, leading to localized drying and desiccation (Zabkiewicz, Swarbrick and Holden, 1986; Schnider, Zabkiewciz and Holden, 1988). This situation may be exacerbated by a high-riding lens, or by inadequate blinking and low tear secretion and break-up time; these factors may also induce inferior corneal exposure keratitis and associated desiccation staining (Zabkiewicz, Swarbrick and Holden, 1986). In extended wear, however, insufficient mid-peripheral or peripheral clearance may result in a sudden increase in peripheral staining, due to lens adherence and the associated peripheral corneal distortion.

If 3 and 9 o'clock staining is persistent and severe, the localized drying of the cornea may lead to dellen formation and corneal thinning (Seger and Mutti, 1986) and, in extreme cases, epithelial erosion, neovascularization or corneal infection may ensue. Although mild 3 and 9 o'clock staining is not unusual with RGP extended wear, severe cases must be managed promptly by reducing wearing time until the staining resolves, and by increasing and widening the peripheral clearance to minimize lens adherence; however, for daily wear, incorporation of a thinner, steeper tapered edge profile may be more successful (Bennett, 1985; *see also* Chapter 19).

Another type of corneal staining, termed the Fischer–Schweitzer polygonal mosaic, is also frequently noted immediately upon lens removal following RGP extended lens wear (Benjamin and Simons, 1984; Levy, 1985; Zantos and Zantos, 1985; Zabkiewicz, Swarbrick and Holden, 1986). This phenomenon does not generally involve true staining of the epithelium, but rather manifests itself as a polygonal meshwork of fluorescein pooling in the central or superior regions of the cornea. The aetiology of the phenomenon has been described by Bron and Tripathi (1969), who consider that external pressure exerted on the cornea, or a reduction in the intraocular pressure, causes ridges to form in Bowman's layer as the cornea flattens. Following removal of the stimulus, Bowman's layer regains its normal curvature, leaving grooves where epithelial cells have been compressed above the ridges during flattening. The corneal mosaic normally disappears within 10 minutes following removal of the stimulus. Although not of concern in itself, the appearance of this corneal mosaic pattern in RGP extended lens wearers suggests that the contact lens may be exerting undue pressure on the cornea during wear, possibly indicating an excessively flat fit.

Corneal staining due to foreign bodies, lens mishandling or dislodgement, lens binding or damaged lenses may also be noted during RGP extended wear. In severe cases (*see Plate 59*), it is wise to discontinue lens wear until the epithelial defect has resolved. Appropriate clinical management and patient education may reduce the incidence of these complications.

Long-term effects of RGP extended wear

Because RGP extended wear is relatively new, little is known of its long-term effects on corneal physiology. It is thought that the long-term changes accompanying hydrogel extended wear are induced directly or indirectly by chronic hypoxic stress on the corneal tissue (Holden *et al.*, 1985b). Therefore, it could be anticipated that similar changes would occur with long-term extended wear of RGP contact lenses of comparable Dk/t values.

As RGP lenses of higher Dk/t value become used increasingly for extended wear, however, it might be expected that changes such as epithelial thinning and microcystic development, reduced epithelial oxygen uptake, stromal thinning and endothelial polymegathism, would be less apparent with these lenses. Indeed, early results from CCLRU RGP extended wear studies indicate that epithelial changes with high Dk/t RGP lenses are considerably less severe than with hydrogel lenses (Holden *et al.*, 1986a, 1970; Schnider *et al.*, 1986a, b; Schnider, 1987). Epithelial microcysts, which are invariably seen in hydrogel extended lens wearers after 3 months of wear, are infrequent in high *Dk/t* RGP lens wearers (Terry *et al.*, 1986; Holden *et al.*, 1987; Schnider *et al.*, 1987), and increases in endothelial polymegathism, which may be noted after only 2 weeks of hydrogel extended wear (Holden *et al.*, 1985c), are expected to be minimal with high *Dk* RGP extended wear. The significance of other potential chronic effects, such as reduced corneal and lid margin sensitivity, and eyelid ptosis (Fonn and Holden, 1986) has yet to be determined. Longer-term studies are needed to detail the extent of these and other chronic changes which may be induced by RGP extended wear, and to ensure that the extended wear of high *Dk* RGP materials continues to be a safe and efficacious means of vision correction.

Clinical management of RGP extended wear

Patient selection

Because RGP lenses do not cover the cornea completely, and may induce mechanical trauma to a compromised cornea, the use of these lenses for bandage purposes is unlikely to be beneficial, and is therefore not recommended. However, RGP lenses have been used successfully for both aphakic (Benjamin and Simons, 1984; Elie, 1986) and cosmetic extended wear (Levy, 1985; Mandell and Liberman, 1985; Port, 1985; Zabkiewicz, Swarbrick and Holden, 1986; Holden and Sweeney, 1987; Schnider *et al.*, 1987).

The criteria for patient selection for hydrogel extended wear have been outlined in a previous section; these criteria also apply to the selection of potential patients for RGP extended wear. As with hydrogel extended wear, the risk:benefit ratio for each individual patient should be considered carefully before proceeding with RGP extended wear, and thorough patient education and instruction are essential in order to emphasize the realities of extended wear, including the need for regular lens cleaning and maintenance, frequent overnight lens removal to rest the cornea and prompt contact with the practitioner should unusual redness, discomfort or blurred vision occur.

More latitude is available for correcting corneal astigmatism with RGP lenses compared to hydrogel lenses, although the centre thickness of the lenses may have to be increased to minimize on-eye flexure which may cause fluctuating vision on blinking (*see* Chapter 10). It must be remembered, however, that increasing lens thickness will reduce the *Dk/t* value of the lenses. In general, the use of ocular medications in conjunction with RGP extended wear does not present a problem because of the non-porous nature of the polymer. However, solutions containing benzalkonium chloride should be avoided as it has been suggested that this chemical may bind to the lens surface (Rosenthal *et al.*, 1986), although this has been questioned, at least for low *Dk* materials, by Wong, Dziabo and Kiral (1986) (*see also* Chapter 4).

Patients with dry eye problems or poor blinking habits may have poor success with RGP extended wear, particularly if the lens fit is less than optimal. It has been suggested that hydrogel extended lens wearers who are forced to discontinue lens wear due to the development of CLPC may be successfully re-fitted with RGP lenses for extended wear. However, it has been the experience at the CCLRU that although patient symptoms may be reduced initially, there is frequently a recurrence of CLPC after a period of RGP lens wear (Schnider, Zabkiewicz and Holden, 1988).

Lens fitting

Techniques for fitting RGP lenses are discussed in Chapter 10, and therefore will not be considered in detail in this section. In general, RGP lens fitting for extended wear requires more care and expertise than hydrogel lens fitting, and follows slightly different principles from those originally employed for PMMA daily wear lenses.

Large diameter lenses can be used as less reliance needs to be placed on tear exchange for provision of oxygen to the anterior corneal surface. Lens total diameters in the range of 9.4–10.2 mm are now most frequently employed. These large diameter lenses allow for greater back optic zone diameters, in the range 8.0–8.2 mm, giving the advantages of less flare in younger patients with large pupils, particularly under conditions of low illumination, and increased comfort.

It is advisable to aim for an alignment fitting which minimizes the bearing pressure on any particular corneal location, in particular the midperiphery, in order to encourage an even tear flow beneath the lens and to minimize lens-induced corneal distortion. Tri-curve or multi-curve back surface designs with well-blended transition zones, or aspheric lens designs, can be used to achieve this type of fitting, which is best verified using fluorescein fitting techniques. A tapered edge design incorporating two to three peripheral curves is suggested. On fluorescein evaluation the peripheral clearance should be approximately 0.4–0.5 mm wide and edge clearance 70–80 μm deep (*see* Chapter 10). Excessive edge clearance or edge thickness may exacerbate 3 and 9 o'clock desiccation staining, while a narrow tight edge may encourage lens adherence.

Lens movement or lag following a blink should be smooth, without apical rotation or excessive lens–lid interaction. Although there is less dependence on the tear pump for corneal oxygenation, lens movement following a blink should be in the order of 0.75–1.50 mm in order to permit efficient flushing of debris and waste products from behind the lens. Good centration of the lens between blinks is also desirable; it may be necessary to steepen the BOZR very slightly in some cases to achieve this.

The choice of RGP lens material will influence the long-term physiological performance of the lens for extended wear. In the short term, moderate *Dk* materials, such as Equalens and Quantum 1, appear to perform reasonably well for extended wear for most patients, but are not likely to stand the test of time in physiological terms. We believe that the oxygen requirements of the cornea during extended wear can be fully met only with RGP materials with a *Dk* approaching 100×10^{-11} units (using the method described by Brennan, Efron and Holden, 1986a), and that these materials should be used in preference to low or moderate *Dk* materials which are more likely to induce long-term changes in corneal physiology. However, other aspects of on-eye lens performance are also critical for long-term extended wear success, including lens wettability and deposit formation. These characteristics appear to vary between individual patients, and should be evaluated carefully before a final decision on lens material is made.

Lens centre thickness will also influence the physiological performance of the lens. However, a balance must be achieved between enhancing the oxygen transmission characteristics of the lens and minimizing on-eye lens flexure, particularly on astigmatic corneas. An increase in lens thickness of 0.02 mm for every dioptre of uncorrected corneal cylinder has been suggested as a rule of thumb (Bennett, 1985; *see also* Chapter 10).

Care and maintenance

Because of the non-porous nature of RGP lens materials, contaminants are unable to penetrate the polymer matrix. Thus the care and maintenance procedures for RGP extended wear lenses are considerably less complicated and time consuming than those required with hydrogel lenses.

Contaminants and deposits which adsorb onto the lens surface are usually easily removed using a surfactant cleaner. Cleaning solutions incorporating a fine particulate suspension may prove advantageous for the removal of stubborn surface deposits through friction, as may the textured cleaning pads which have been developed (for example, 3M, Minnesota). Because of the propensity of RGP materials to bind tear proteins (*see Plates 24–26*), some practitioners also recommend the use of enzymatic cleaners to enhance lens cleanliness in those patients with significant deposit problems. Other alternatives, such as the use of peroxide disinfection, are currently under investigation.

Overnight lens storage solutions should be used when the lens is off the eye to maintain lens hydration and enhance surface wettability. An antibacterial agent is generally incorporated in the storage solution to inhibit bacterial contamination. Although it has been suggested that the preservative benzalkonium chloride may bind to the surface of silicone–acrylate materials (Rosenthal *et al.*, 1986), it probably does not reach concentrations which are toxic to the eye, at least for low *Dk* materials (Wong, Dziabo and Kiral, 1986). Wetting solutions can be used to maximize lens wetting and patient comfort on lens insertion. The current trend appears to be towards combination storage/wetting solutions, which considerably simplify lens care for the patient. In-eye 'comfort' drops for re-wetting and cleaning the lenses on the eye may also be used to maintain patient comfort during lens wear (see Chapter 4).

Because we believe that a conservative approach to RGP extended wear is advisable, we recommend that patients be advised to remove their lenses overnight at least once a week to rest the cornea from hypoxic stress. Within this framework patients should be encouraged to remove their lenses as often as they desire. As with hydrogel extended wear, occasional overnight wear is preferable to continuous wear for long periods without lens removal, although with very high Dk materials such as the Flurofocon A (3M, Minnesota) and Oxylens 2 (Contex, California) materials, true continuous wear remains a possibility (Terry et al., 1986).

Regular lens replacement is probably not as beneficial as with hydrogel extended wear, because RGP lenses do not absorb contaminants or age as rapidly as do hydrogel lenses. However, there is some clinical evidence that certain RGP lenses may spontaneously develop surface 'crazing' or 'cracking' (Plate 27) after a period of time (Klein, 1986; Schnider, 1987), although further work is needed to clarify this phenomenon (see Chapter 10). Obviously, replacement of damaged or scratched lenses is essential to avoid corneal or lid trauma.

Patient advice and management

As with hydrogel extended wear, it is essential that patients are able to handle their RGP lenses competently before these are dispensed. A period of daily wear of 1–2 weeks is often useful to reinforce the patient's lens handling techniques, and is advisable if there are any doubts about the lens fit, which must be optimal before an extended wear regimen is initiated. During the daily wear adaptation period, problems with lens wettability and deposit formation may also be identified and changes in lens material or care and maintenance procedures instituted before extended wear begins. Adaptation to RGP lenses is generally rapid, and full-time daily wear is often possible from the first day. However, there will be greater lens awareness during the first few days than with hydrogel lenses and previous hydrogel lens wearers should be warned of this.

Patients should be seen early in the day following the first overnight wear of their RGP lenses. At this visit, the practitioner should examine the cornea carefully for signs of residual corneal oedema (striae and folds) and lens binding (compression ring). Follow-up visits after 3 days, 1 week and 2 weeks of extended wear are then advised, and if no problems are apparent, monthly after-care visits should follow.

Patient advice and management procedures are similar to those suggested for hydrogel extended lens wearers. It is essential to emphasize to the patient that if unusual redness, discomfort or blurred vision develops, particularly in one eye only, the patient should remove the lenses and consult the practitioner immediately.

The future of extended wear

Extended or continuous wear is the desired mode of contact lens wear for the majority of prospective contact lens patients. In a recent survey of contact lens patients, Holden and Sweeney (unpublished data) found that 41% desired continuous wear (without lens removal), 35% were happy with 6 nights of wear per week, 21% preferred occasional extended wear, and only 3% wanted daily wear.

Whether safe, comfortable continuous wear lenses will ever be developed depends upon a number of factors. In a recent paper, Holden and Sweeney (1987) outlined the prerequisites for safe extended wear. These include provision of adequate oxygen to the cornea during sleep, maintenance of fluid movement behind the lens during waking hours, and physical and mechanical compatibility of the lens with the ocular tissue. The highest Dk RGP lenses used in CCLRU extended wear studies provide an equivalent oxygen performance of approximately 15% oxygen under static conditions (according to the measurements of Hill, Brezinski and Flynn, 1985), 17% oxygen during open-eye wear, and 3–4% oxygen when the eyes are closed. This level of oxygen and the amount of lens movement with these lenses is adequate to avoid a clinically significant microcystic response even after 2 years of extended wear (Holden et al., 1987; Schnider et al., 1987). This indicates that these are the first lenses (apart from silicone elastomer lenses) to meet corneal oxygen needs in the majority of patients. In addition, according to Schnider (1987), the tear exchange is sufficient and the deposit levels limited enough to result in an extremely low adverse response rate. Although these physiological results are promising, comfort, 3 and 9 o'clock staining, lens binding, changes in corneal shape and curvature, and lens wettability remain as problems which need careful monitoring and long-term follow-up.

As yet, clinically viable high *Dk* flexible lenses have not become available for clinical testing, and extended wear of currently available hydrogel lenses needs to be restricted to as little as 1–2 nights of wear per week in order to avoid chronic corneal effects (Holden *et al.*, 1987). However, research and development in the area of extended wear is still very active, and if the progress made in the last 5 years in understanding this very complex field is maintained, the future will certainly be very exciting.

References

ADAMS, C. P., COHEN, E. J., LAIBSON, P. R., GALENTINE, P. and ARENTSEN, J. J. (1983). Corneal ulcers in patients with cosmetic extended-wear contact lenses. *Am. J. Ophthal.* **96**, 705–709

ALLANSMITH, M. R., KORB, D. R., GREINER, J. V., HENRIQUEZ, A. S., SIMON, M. A. and FINNEMORE, V. M. (1977). Giant papillary conjunctivitis in contact lens wearers. *Am. J. Ophthal.* **83**, 697–708

ANDRASKO, G. J. (1986). Corneal deswelling response to hard and hydrogel extended wear lenses. *Invest. Ophthal. Vis. Sci.* **27**, 20–23

BARISHAK, Y., ZAVARO, A., SAMRA, Z. and SOMPOLINSKY, D. (1984). An immunologic study of papillary conjunctivitis due to contact lenses. *Current Eye Res.* **3**, 1161–1168

BARR, J. T. and SCHOESSLER, J. P. (1980). Corneal endothelial response to rigid contact lenses. *Am. J. Optom.* **57**, 267–274

BENJAMIN, W. J. and RASMUSSEN, M. A. (1985). The closed-lid tear pump: oxygenation? *Int. Eyecare* **1**, 251–256

BENJAMIN, W. J. and SIMONS, M. H. (1984). Extended wear of oxygen-permeable rigid lenses in aphakia. *Int. Contact Lens Clin.* **11**, 547–560

BENJAMIN, W. J., BERGMANSON, J. P. G. and ESTRADA, P. J. (1985). Disposable 'eight-packs'. *Int. Eyecare* **1**, 494–497

BENNETT, E. S. (1985). Silicone/acrylate lens design. *Int. Contact Lens Clin.* **12**, 45–53

BENNETT, E. S. and EGAN, D. J. (1986). Rigid gas-permeable lens problem solving. *J. Am. optom. Ass.* **57**, 504–511

BLACKHURST, R. T. (1985). Personal experience with hydrogel and silicone extended wear lenses. *Contact Lens Ass. Ophthal. J.* **11**, 136–137

BONANNO, J. A. and POLSE, K. A. (1985). Central and peripheral corneal swelling accompanying soft lens extended wear. *Am. J. Optom.* **62**, 74–81

BONANNO, J. A. and POLSE, K. A. (1987a). Measurement of in vivo human corneal stromal pH: open and closed eye. *Invest. Ophthal. Vis. Sci.* **28**, 522–530

BONANNO, J. A. and POLSE, K. A. (1987b). Corneal acidosis during contact lens wear: effects of hypoxia and CO_2. *Invest. Ophthal. Vis. Sci.* **28**, 1514–1520

BRENNAN, N. A., EFRON, N. and HOLDEN, B. A. (1986a). Oxygen permeability of hard gas permeable contact lens materials. *Clin. expl Optom.* **69**, 82–89

BRENNAN, N. A., EFRON, N. and HOLDEN, B. A. (1986b). Oxygen transmissibility of hard gas permeable and hydrophilic contact lenses (abstract). *Am. J. Optom.* **63**(10), 4P

BRON, A. J. and TRIPATHI, R. C. (1969). Anterior corneal mosaic — further observations. *Br. J. Ophthal.* **53**, 760–764

CARNEY, L. G. (1974). Studies on the basis of ocular changes during contact lens wear. *PhD Thesis*, University of Melbourne, Melbourne, Australia

CARNEY, L. G. and EFRON, N. (1980). pH ambient et flux d'oxygene corneen. *J. fr. Ophthal.* **3**, 125–126

CARNEY, L. G. and HILL, R. M. (1976). Human tear pH. *Archs Ophthal.* **94**, 821–924

CAROLINE, P. J. and ELLIS, E. J. (1986). Review of the mechanisms of oxygen transport through rigid gas permeable lenses. *Int. Eyecare* **2**, 210–213

CAROLINE, P. J., ROBIN, J. B., GINDI, J. J., PICKFORD, M. S., OLSON, A. P. and SCHANZLIN, D. J. (1985). Microscopic and elemental analysis of deposits on extended wear soft contact lenses. *Contact Lens Ass. Ophthal J.* **11**, 311–316

CHALUPA, E., SWARBRICK, H. A., HOLDEN, B. A. and SJOSTRAND, J. (1987). Severe corneal infections associated with contact lens wear. *Ophthalmology* **94**, 17–22

COTAN, D. G. (1949). Vascularization of the cornea. *Archs Ophthal.* **41**, 406–416

COLLIN, H. B. (1980). Vernal and giant papillary conjunctivitis. Part 1. *Aust. J. Optom.* **63**, 251–257

COLLIN, H. B. (1981). Vernal and giant papillary conjunctivitis. Parts 2 and 3. *Aust. J. Optom.* **64**, 4–8; 71–76

COON, L. J., MILLER, J. P. and MEIER, R. F. (1979). Overview of extended wear contact lenses. *J. Am. optom. Ass.* **50**, 745–749

COOPER, R. L. and CONSTABLE, I. J. (1977). Infective keratitis in soft contact lens wearers. *Br. J. Ophthal.* **61**, 250–254

CUKLANZ, H. D. and HILL, R. M. (1969). Oxygen requirements of corneal contact lens systems. *Am. J. Optom.* **46**, 228–230

EFRON, N. (1986). Intersubject variability in corneal swelling response to anoxia. *Acta ophthal.* **64**, 302–305

EFRON, N. and CARNEY, L. G. (1979). Oxygen levels beneath the closed eyelid. *Invest. Ophthal. Vis. Sci.* **18**, 93–95

EICHENBAUM, J. W., FELDSTEIN, M. and PODOS, S. M. (1982). Extended-wear aphakic soft contact lenses and corneal ulcers. *Br. J. Ophthal.* **66**, 663–666

ELIASON, J. A. (1978). Leukocytes and experimental corneal vascularization. *Invest. Ophthal. Vis. Sci.* **17**, 1087–1095

ELIE, G. (1986). Gas permeable extended wear lenses: an excellent solution for aphakic patients. *Contact Lens Ass. Ophthal. J.* **12**, 51–53

ELLIS, P. (1983). Extended wear contact lenses in paediatric ophthalmology. *Contact Lens Ass. Ophthal. J.* **9**, 317–321

FANTI, P. (1980). Gas permeable lenses in Germany. *Contact Lens Forum* **5**(11), 29–41

FATT, I. (1969). Oxygen tension under a contact lens during blinking. *Am. J. Optom.* **46**, 654–661

FATT, I. (1978). Water flow conductivity and pore diameter in extended-wear gel lens materials. *Am. J. Optom.* **55**, 43–47

FATT, I. (1979). Negative pressure under silicone rubber contact lenses. *Contacto* **23**, 6–9

FATT, I. (1984). Oxygen transmissibility and permeability of gas permeable hard contact lenses and materials. *Int. Contact Lens Clin.* **11**, 175–183

FATT, I. (1986a). Some comments on methods used for measuring oxygen permeability (Dk) of contact lens materials. *Contact Lens Ass. Ophthal. J.* **12**, 36–38

FATT, I. (1986b). Now do we need 'effective permeability'? *Contax* July, 6–23

FATT, I. and CHASTON, J. (1980). Temperature of a contact lens on the eye. *Int. Contact Lens Clin.* **7**, 195–198

FATT, I. and HILL, R. M. (1970). Oxygen tension under a contact lens during blinking — a comparison of theory and experimental observations. *Am. J. Optom.* **47**, 50–55

FATT, I. and ST HELEN, R. (1971). Oxygen tension under an oxygen-permeable contact lens. *Am. J. Optom.* **48**, 545–555

FATT, I., BIEBER, M. T. and PYE, S. D. (1969). Steady state distribution of oxygen and carbon dioxide in the in vivo cornea of an eye covered by a gas-permeable contact lens. *Am. J. Optom.* **46**, 3–14

FISCHER, F. H., SCHMITZ, L., HOFF, W., SCHARTL, S., LIEGL, O. and WIEDERHOLT, M. (1978). Sodium and chloride transport in the isolated human cornea. *Pflüger's Arch.* **373**, 179–188

FONN, D. and HOLDEN, B. A. (1986). Extended wear of hard gas permeable contact lenses can induce ptosis. *Contact Lens Ass. Ophthal. J.* **12**, 93–94

FONN, D. and HOLDEN, B. A. (1988). Rigid gas permeable vs hydrogel contact lenses for extended wear. *Am. J. Optom. physiol. Optics* **65**, 536–544

FONN, D., HOLDEN, B. A., ROTH, P., GOOLEY, G. and KENEFICK, J. (1984). Comparative physiologic performance of polymethyl methacrylate and gas-permeable contact lenses. *Archs Ophthal.* **102**, 760–764

FOWLER, S. A., GREINER, J. V. and ALLANSMITH, M. R. (1979). Soft contact lenses from patients with giant papillary conjunctivitis. *Am. J. Ophthal.* **88**, 1056–1061

FREEMAN, R. D. and FATT, I. (1973). Environmental influences on ocular temperature. *Invest. Ophthal.* **12**, 596–602

FROMER, C. H. and KLINTWORTH, G. K. (1976). An evaluation of the role of leukocytes in the pathogenesis of experimentally induced corneal vascularization. III. Studies related to the vasoproliferative capability of polymorphonuclear leukocytes and lymphocytes. *Am. J. Pathol.* **82**, 157–167

GALENTINE, P. G., COHEN, E. J., LAIBSON, P. R., ADAMS, C. P., MICHAUD, R. and ARENTSEN, J. J. (1984). Corneal ulcers associated with contact lens wear. *Archs Ophthal.* **102**, 891–894

GARCIA, G. E. (1976). Continuous wear of gas-permeable lenses in aphakia. *Contact Intraoc. Lens med. J.* **2**, 29–34

GASSET, A. R. and KAUFMAN, H. E. (1970). Therapeutic uses of hydrophilic contact lenses. *Am. J. Ophthal.* **69**, 252–259

GOLDEN, B., FINGERMAN, L. H. and ALLEN, H. F. (1971). Pseudomonas corneal ulcers in contact lens wearers. *Archs Ophthal.* **85**, 543–547

GORDON, A. and KRACHER, G. P. (1985). Corneal infiltrates and extended wear contact lenses. *J. Am. optom. Ass.* **56**, 198–201

GRANT, T., KOTOW, M. and HOLDEN, B. A. (1986). The comparative clinical performance and adverse response rates with high and low water content lenses for extended wear (abstract). *Am. J. Optom.* **63**(10), 57P

GRANT, T., KOTOW, M. and HOLDEN, B. A. (1987). Hydrogel extended wear: current performance and future options. *Contax* May, 5–8

GUILLON, M. (1985). The HGP Dk controversy. *Int. Eyecare* **1**, 505

HAMANO, H. (1978). Fundamental researches on the effect of contact lenses on the eye. In *Soft Contact Lenses — Clinical and Applied Technology*, edited by M. Ruben, pp. 121–141. London: Ballière Tindall

HAMANO, H., KAWABE, H. and MITSUNAGA, S. (1985). Reproducible measurement of oxygen permeability (Dk) of contact lens materials. *Contact Lens Ass. Ophthal. J.* **11**, 221–226

HAMANO, H., HORI, M., HAMANO, T., KAWABE, H., MIKAMI, M., MITSUNAGA, S. et al. (1983). Effects of contact lens wear on mitosis of corneal epithelium and lactate content of aqueous humor of rabbit. *Jap. J. Ophthal.* **27**, 451–458

HARRIS, M. G. and MANDELL, R. B. (1969). Contact lens adaptation: osmotic theory. *Am. J. Optom.* **46**, 196–202

HENRY, V. A., BENNETT, E. S. and FORREST, J. F. (1987). Clinical investigation of the Paraperm EW rigid gas-permeable contact lens. *Am. J. Optom.* **64**, 313–320

HILL, J. F., ANDERSON, F. L., JOHNSON, T. K., RIGEL, L. E. and SEELYE, R. R. (1983). Eighteen-month clinical experience with extended wear silicone contact lenses on 400 patients. *Am. J. Optom.* **60**, 578–581

HILL, R. M. (1977). Behind the closed lid. *Int. Contact Lens Clin.* **4**(1), 68–70

HILL, R. M. and FATT, I. (1964). How dependent is the cornea on the atmosphere? *J. Am. optom. Ass.* **35**, 873–875

HILL, R. M., BREZINSKI, S. and FLYNN, W. J. (1985). The rigid 'super-permeables'. *Contact Lens Forum* **10**(1), 35–39

HIRST, L. W., AUER, C., COHN, J., TSENG, S. C. G. and KHODADOUST, A. A. (1984). Specular microscopy of hard contact lens wearers. *Ophthalmology* **91**, 1147–1153

HOLDEN, B. A. (1977). High magnification examination and photography with the slit lamp. In *Clinical Slit Lamp Biomicroscopy*, edited by R. H. Brandreth, p. 335. San Leandro, California: Blaco

HOLDEN, B. A. (1983). Ocular changes associated with the extended wear of contact lenses. *Ophthal. Optician* **23**, 140–142

HOLDEN, B. A. (1986). Weaning patients from long-term extended wear. *Contact Lens Spect.* **1**(6), 38–39

HOLDEN, B. A. and MERTZ, G. W. (1984). Critical oxygen

levels to avoid corneal edema for daily and extended wear contact lenses. *Invest. Ophthal. Vis. Sci.* **25**, 1161–1167

HOLDEN, B. A. and SWEENEY, D. F. (1985). The oxygen tension and temperature of the superior palpebral conjunctiva. *Acta ophthal.* **63**, 100–103

HOLDEN, B. A. and SWEENEY, D. F. (1987). The ocular requirements for extended wear. *Contax* May, 13–18

HOLDEN, B. A. and ZANTOS, S. G. (1981). Corneal endothelium: transient changes with atmospheric anoxia. In *The Cornea in Health and Disease* (Sixth Congress of the European Society of Ophthalmology), Royal Society of Medicine International Congress and Symposium Series No. 40, pp. 79–83. London: Academic Press and Royal Society of Medicine

HOLDEN, B. A., KOTOW, M. and SWARBRICK, H. A. (1986). The current status of extended wear. *Contax* Mar./Apr., 21–24

HOLDEN, B. A., LaHOOD, D. and SWEENEY, D. (1985). Does *Dk/L* measurement accurately predict overnight edema response? (abstract) *Am. J. Optom.* **62**(10), 95P

HOLDEN, B. A., MERTZ, G. W. and McNALLY, J. J. (1983). Corneal swelling response to contact lenses worn under extended wear conditions. *Invest. Ophthal. Vis. Sci.* **24**, 218–226

HOLDEN, B. A., ROSS, R. and JENKINS, J. (1987). Hydrogel contact lenses impede carbon dioxide efflux from the human cornea. *Current Eye Res.* **6**, 1283–1290

HOLDEN, B. A., SWEENEY, D. F. and SANDERSON, G. (1984). The minimum precorneal oxygen tension to avoid corneal edema. *Invest. Ophthal. Vis. Sci.* **25**, 476–480

HOLDEN, B. A., SWEENEY, D. F. and SEGER, R. G. (1986). Epithelial erosions caused by thin high water content lenses. *Clin. expl Optom.* **69**, 103–107

HOLDEN, B. A., WILLIAMS, L. and ZANTOS, S. G. (1985). The etiology of transient endothelial changes in the human cornea. *Invest. Ophthal. Vis. Sci.* **26**, 1354–1359

HOLDEN, B. A., SWEENEY, D., JENKINS, J., ROSS, R., MARTIN, D. K. and SMITH, K. (1981). Factors contributing to contact lens induced edema. *Am. J. Optom.* **58**, 1010

HOLDEN, B. A., POLSE, K. A., FONN, D. and MERTZ, G. W. (1982). Effects of cataract surgery on corneal function. *Invest. Ophthal. Vis. Sci.* **22**, 343–350

HOLDEN, B. A., McNALLY, J. J., MERTZ, G. W. and SWARBRICK, H. A. (1985a). Topographical corneal oedema. *Acta ophthal.* **63**, 684–691

HOLDEN, B. A., SWEENEY, D. F., VANNAS, A., NILSSON, K. T. and EFRON, N. (1985b). Effects of long-term extended contact lens wear on the human cornea. *Invest. Ophthal. Vis. Sci.* **26**, 1489–1501

HOLDEN, B. A., VANNAS, A., NILSSON, K., EFRON, N., SWEENEY, D., KOTOW, M. *et al.* (1985c). Epithelial and endothelial effects from the extended wear of contact lenses. *Current Eye Res.* **4**, 739–742

HOLDEN, B. A., LaHOOD, D., SWEENEY, D., SCHNIDER, C. and KENYON, E. (1986a). The critical oxygen levels required with rigid gas permeable lenses to avoid adverse physiological effects on extended wear (abstract). *Am. J. Optom.* **63**(10), 5P

HOLDEN, B. A., SWEENEY, D. F., SWARBRICK, H. A., VANNAS, A., NILSSON, K. T. and EFRON, N. (1986b). The vascular

response to long-term extended contact lens wear. *Clin. expl Optom.* **69**, 112–119

HOLDEN, B. A., GRANT, T., KOTOW, M., SCHNIDER, C. and SWEENEY, D. (1987). Epithelial microcysts with daily and extended wear of hydrogel and rigid gas permeable contact lenses. *Invest. Ophthal. Vis. Sci.* **28** (Suppl.), 372

HOLDEN, B. A., SWEENEY, D. F., LaHOOD, D. and KENYON, E. (1988). Corneal deswelling following overnight wear of rigid and hydrogel contact lenses. *Current Eye Res.* **7**, 49–53

HUMPHREYS, J. A., LARKE, J. R. and PARRISH, S. T. (1980). Microepithelial cysts observed in extended contact-lens wearing subjects. *Br. J. Ophthal.* **64**, 888–889

HWANG, S-T., TANG, T. E. S. and KAMMERMEYER, K. (1971). Transport of dissolved oxygen through silicone rubber membrane. *J. macromol. Sci. Phys.* **B5**(1), 1–10

IMRE, G. (1972). Neovascularization of the eye. In *Contemporary Ophthalmology*, edited by J. G. Bellows, pp. 88–91. Baltimore: Williams and Wilkins Co.

JOSEPHSON, J. E. and CAFFERY, B. E. (1979). Infiltrative keratitis in hydrogel lens wearers. *Int. Contact Lens Clin.* **6**, 223–242

JOSEPHSON, J. E. and CAFFERY, B. E. (1980). Clinical experiences with the Tesicon™ silicone lens. *Int. Contact Lens Clin.* **7**, 235–245

KAMIYA, C. (1980). Temporary changes in corneal endothelial mosaic observed soon after wearing contact lenses. *J. Jap. Contact Lens Soc.* **22**, 269–277

KEATES, R. H., IHLENFELD, J. V. and ISAACSON, W. B. (1984). An introduction to fluoropolymer contact lenses; a new class of materials. *Contact Lens Ass. Ophthal. J.* **10**, 332–334

KENYON, E., POLSE, K. A. and O'NEAL, M. R. (1985). Ocular response to extended wear of hard gas-permeable lenses. *Contact Lens Ass. Ophthal. J.* **11**, 119–123

KENYON, E., SWEENEY, D. F., HOLDEN, B. A. and LaHOOD, D. (1986). An average edema index for hard and soft extended wear lenses. *Invest. Ophthal. Vis. Sci.* **27** (suppl.), 140

KHODADOUST, A. A. and HIRST, L. W. (1984). Diurnal variation in corneal endothelial morphology. *Ophthalmology* **91**, 1125–1128

KLEIN, P. (1983). Use of hyper-thin, low water content hydrophilic lenses for extended wear. *Am. J. Optom.* **60**, 783–787

KLEIN, P. (1986). Surface adsorption phenomena. Readers' views. *Contact Lens Spect.* **1**(12), 62

KLYCE, S. D. (1981). Stromal lactate accumulation can account for corneal oedema osmotically following epithelial hypoxia in the rabbit. *J. Physiol.* **321**, 49–64

KOETTING, R. A., CASTELLANO, C. F. and NELSON, D. W. (1985). A hard lens with extended wear possibilities. *J. Am. optom. Ass.* **56**, 208–211

KOTOW, M., GRANT, T. and HOLDEN, B. A. (1987). Avoiding ocular complications during hydrogel extended wear. *Int. Contact Lens Clin.* **14**, 95–99

KOTOW, M., HOLDEN, B. A. and GRANT, T. (1987). The value of regular replacement of low water content contact lenses for extended wear. *J. Am. optom. Ass.* **58**, 461–464

LaHOOD, D. (1988). Edge shape and comfort of rigid lenses. *Am. J. Optom. physiol. Optics* **65**, 613–618

LaHOOD, D., SWEENEY, D. F. and HOLDEN, B. A. (1988). Overnight corneal edema with hydrogel, rigid gas permeable and silicone elastomer contact lenses. *Int. Contact Lens Clin.* **15**, 149–154

LEBOW, K. A. and PLISHKA, K. (1980). Ocular changes associated with extended-wear contact lenses. *Int. Contact Lens Clin.* **7**, 49–55

LEISEGANG, T. J. and FORSTER, R. K. (1980). Spectrum of microbial keratitis in South Florida. *Am. J. Ophthal.* **90**, 38–47

LEMP, M. A., BLACKMAN, H. J., WILSON, L. A. and LEVEILLE, A. S. (1984). Gram-negative corneal ulcers in elderly aphakic eyes with extended-wear lenses. *Ophthalmology* **91**, 60–63

LEVY, B. (1983). The use of a gas permeable hard lens for extended wear. *Am. J. Optom.* **60**, 408–409

LEVY, B. (1985). Rigid gas-permeable lenses for extended wear — a 1-year clinical evaluation. *Am. J. Optom.* **62**, 889–894

MACKIE, I. A. and WRIGHT, P. (1978). Giant papillary conjunctivitis (secondary vernal) in association with contact lens wear. *Trans. Ophthal. Soc. UK* **98**, 3–9

McMONNIES, C. W. (1983). Contact lens-induced corneal vascularization. *Int. Contact Lens Clin.* **10**, 12–21

McMONNIES, C. W., CHAPMAN-DAVIES, A. and HOLDEN, B. A. (1982). The vascular response to contact lens wear. *Am. J. Optom.* **59**, 795–799

MacRAE, S. M., MATSUDA, M., SHELLANS, S. and RICH, L. F. (1986). The effects of hard and soft contact lenses on the corneal endothelium. *Am. J. Ophthal.* **102**, 50–57

MADIGAN, M. C., HOLDEN, B. A. and KWOK, L. S. (1987). Extended wear of contact lenses can compromise corneal epithelial adhesion. *Current Eye Res.* **6**, 1257–1260

MANDELL, R. B. (1975). Corneal edema and curvature changes from gel lenses. *Int. Contact Lens Clin.* **2**, 88–98

MANDELL, R. B. and LIBERMAN, G. (1985). Paraperm E.W. — a superpermeable for extended wear. *Contact Lens J.* **13**(10), 3–6

MANNARINO, A. P., BELIN, M. W. and WEINER, B. M. (1985). Clinical fitting characteristics of extended wear silicone (Silsight) lenses. *Contact Lens Ass. Ophthal. J.* **11**, 339–342

MARTIN, D. K. and HOLDEN, B. A. (1983). Variations in tear osmolality, chord diameter and movement during wear of high water content hydrogel contact lenses. *Int. Contact Lens Clin.* **10**, 323–342

MEISLER, D. M., KRACHMER, J. H. and GOEKEN, J. A. (1981). Giant papillary conjunctivitis. *Am. J. Ophthal.* **92**, 368–371

MERTZ, G. W. and HOLDEN, B. A. (1981). Clinical implications of extended wear research. *Can. J. Optom.* **43**, 203–205

MILLODOT, M. and O'LEARY, D. J. (1980). Effect of oxygen deprivation on corneal sensitivity. *Acta ophthal.* **58**, 434–439

MOLINARI, J. F. (1981). The clinical management of giant papillary conjunctivitis. *Am. J. Optom.* **58**, 886–891

MOLINARI, J. F. (1983). Review: giant papillary conjunctivitis. *Aust. J. Optom.* **66**, 59–67

NILSSON, K. T. (1983). Preventing extended wear problems, the Swedish way. *Contact Lens Forum* **8**(3), 21–29

NILSSON, K. and RENGSTORFF, R. H. (1979). Continuous wearing of Duragel contact lenses by Swedish Air Force pilots. *Am. J. Optom.* **56**, 356–358

O'NEAL, M. R. and POLSE, K. A. (1985). In vivo assessment of mechanisms controlling corneal hydration. *Invest. Ophthal. Vis. Sci.* **26**, 849–856

PHILLIPS, A. J., BADENOCH, P. R., GRUTZMACHER, R. and ROUSSEL, T. J. (1986). Microbial contamination of extended-wear contact lenses: an investigation of endotoxin as a cause of the acute ocular inflammation reaction. *Int. Eyecare* **2**, 469–475

POLSE, K. A. (1979). Tear flow under hydrogel contact lenses. *Invest. Ophthal. Vis. Sci.* **18**, 409–413

POLSE, K. A. and MANDELL, R. M. (1970). Critical oxygen tension at the corneal surface. *Archs Ophthal.* **84**, 505–508

POLSE, K. A. and MANDELL, R. B. (1976). Etiology of corneal striae accompanying hydrogel lens wear. *Invest. Ophthal.* **15**, 553–556

POLSE, K. A., SARVER, M. D., KENYON, E. and BONANNO, J. (1987). Gas permeable hard contact lens extended wear: ocular and visual responses to a 6-month period of wear. *Contact Lens Ass. Ophthal. J.* **13**, 31–38

PORT, M. J. A. (1985). Rigid lenses in extended wear. *Transactions of the British Contact Lens Association Conference*, pp. 18–20

RABER, I. M., LAIBSON, P. R., KURZ, G. H. and BERNARDINO, V. B. (1981). Pseudomonas corneoscleral ulcers. *Am. J. Ophthal.* **92**, 353–362

RAO, G. N., AQUAVELLA, J. V., GOLDBERG, S. H. and BERK, M. L. (1984). Pseudophakic bullous keratopathy — relationship to preoperative corneal endothelial status. *Ophthalmology* **91**, 1135–1140

REFOJO, M. F. and LEONG, F-L. (1979). Microscopic determination of the penetration of proteins and polysaccharides into poly(hydroxyethyl methacrylate) and similar hydrogels. *J. polymer Sci.* **66**, 227–237

REFOJO, M. F. and LEONG, F-L. (1981). Water pervaporation through silicone rubber contact lenses: a possible cause of complications. *Contact Lens* **7**, 226–233

REYNOLDS, R. M. P. (1978). Giant papillary conjunctivitis — a mechanical aetiology. *Aust. J. Optom.* **61**, 320–323

ROSENTHAL, P. (1986). Clinical performance and fitting principles of 'rigid' superpermeable contact lenses. *Transactions of the British Contact Lens Association Conference*, pp. 88–90

ROSENTHAL, P., CHOU, M. H., SALAMONE, J. C. and ISRAEL, S. C. (1986). Quantitative analysis of chlorhexidine gluconate and benzalkonium chloride adsorption on silicone/acrylate polymers. *Contact Lens Ass. Ophthal. J.* **12**, 43–50

RUBEN, M. (1976). Acute eye disease secondary to contact lens wear. *Lancet* **i**, 138–140

RUBEN, M. and GUILLON, M. (1979). Silicone rubber lenses in aphakia. *Br. J. Ophthal.* **63**, 471–474

SALZ, J. J. and SCHLANGER, J. L. (1983). Complications of aphakic extended wear lenses encountered during a seven-year period in 100 eyes. *Contact Lens Ass. Ophthal. J.* **9**, 241–244

SARVER, M. D. (1971). Striate corneal lines among patients wearing hydrophilic contact lenses. *Am. J. Optom.* **48**, 762–763

SARVER, M. D., POLSE, K. A. and BAGGETT, D. A. (1983).

Intersubject difference in corneal edema response to hypoxia. *Am. J. Optom.* **60**, 128–131

SCHECTER, D. R., EMERY, J. M. and SOPER, J. W. (1975). Corneal vascularization in therapeutic soft lens wear. *Contact Intraoc. Lens med. J.* **1**, 141–145

SCHNIDER, C. M. (1987). An overview of RGP extended wear. *Contax*, May 10–12

SCHNIDER, C. M., ZABKIEWICZ, K. and HOLDEN, B. A. (1988). Unusual complications associated with RGP extended wear. *Int. Contact Lens Clin.* **15**, 124–128

SCHNIDER, C., HOLDEN, B. A., LaHOOD, D., TERRY, R., ZABKIEWICZ, K. and SWARBRICK, H. (1986a). Critical factors in avoiding adverse responses with hard gas permeable (HGP) extended wear. *Invest. Ophthal. Vis. Sci.* **27** (suppl.), 139

SCHNIDER, C., ZABKIEWICZ, K., TERRY, R., LaHOOD, D. and HOLDEN, B. A. (1986b). Unusual complications of RGP extended wear (abstract). *Am. J. Optom.* **63**(10), 35P

SCHNIDER, C., HOLDEN, B. A., TERRY, R., ZABKIEWICZ, K. and LaHOOD, D. (1987). One and two year results from large scale clinical studies of RGP EW lenses. *Invest. Ophthal. Vis Sci.* **28** (suppl.), 372

SCHOESSLER, J. P. (1983). Corneal endothelial polymegathism associated with extended wear. *Int. Contact Lens Clin.* **10**, 148–155

SCHOESSLER, J. P. and BARR, J. T. (1980). Corneal thickness changes with extended contact lens wear. *Am. J. Optom.* **57**, 729–733

SCHOESSLER, J. P. and WOLOSCHAK, M. J. (1981). Corneal endothelium in veteran PMMA contact lens wearers. *Int. Contact Lens Clin.* **8**(6), 19–25

SCHOESSLER, J. P., BARR, J. T. and FRESON, D. R. (1984). Corneal endothelial observations of silicone elastomer contact lens wearers. *Int. Contact Lens Clin.* **11**, 337–340

SCHOESSLER, J. P., WOLOSCHAK, M. J. and MAUGER, T. F. (1982). Transient endothelial changes produced by hydrophilic contact lenses. *Am. J. Optom.* **59**, 764–765

SEGER, R. G. and MUTTI, D. O. (1986). Corneal swelling and epithelial compromise with hard gas permeable contact lenses. *Transactions of the British Contact Lens Association Conference*, pp. 92–94

SJOSTRAND, J., LINNER, E., NYGREN, B., KAIJSER, B. and BRORSON, J-E. (1981). Severe corneal infection in a contact lens wearer. *Lancet* **i**, 149–150

SMELSER, G. K. and OZANICS, V. (1952). Importance of atmospheric oxygen for maintenance of the optical properties of the human cornea. *Science* **115**, 140

SPOOR, T. C., HARTEL, W. C., WYNN, P. and SPOOR, D. K. (1984). Complications of continuous-wear soft contact lenses in a nonreferral population. *Archs Ophthal.* **102**, 1312–1313

SPRING, T. F. (1974). Reactions to hydrophilic lenses. *Med. J. Aust.* **1**, 449–450

SRINIVASAN, B. D., TAKOBIEC, F. A., IWAMOTO, T. and DeVOE, G. (1979). Giant papillary conjunctivitis with ocular prostheses. *Archs Ophthal.* **97**, 892–895

STEIN, H. A. and SLATT, B. J. (1977). Extended wear soft contact lenses in perspective. *Int. Contact Lens Clin.* **4**, 35–40

STOCKER, E. G. and SCHOESSLER, J. P. (1985). Corneal endothelial polymegathism induced by PMMA contact lens wear. *Invest. Ophthal. Vis. Sci.* **26**, 857–863

SWARBRICK, H. A. (1988). A possible etiology for RGP lens binding (adherence). *Int. Contact Lens Clin.* **15**(1), 13–19

SWARBRICK, H. A. and HOLDEN, B. A. (1987). Rigid gas permeable lens binding: significance and contributing factors. *Am. J. Optom. physiol Optics* **64**, 815–823

SWEENEY, D. F. and HOLDEN, B. A. (1983). The closed-eye swelling response of the cornea to Polycon and Menicon O_2 gas-permeable hard lenses. *Aust. J. Optom.* **66**, 186–189

SWEENEY, D. F. and HOLDEN, B. A. (1987). Silicone elastomer lens wear induces less overnight corneal edema than sleep without lens wear. *Current Eye Res.* **6**, 1391–1394

TERRY, J. E. and HILL, R. M. (1978). Human tear osmotic pressure: diurnal variation and the closed lid. *Archs Ophthal.* **96**, 120–122

TERRY, R., LaHOOD, D., SCHNIDER, C. and HOLDEN, B. A. (1986). Continuous wear of a high Dk gas permeable lens (abstract). *Am. J. Optom.* **63**(10), 6P

TOMLINSON, A. and HAAS, D. D. (1980). Changes in corneal thickness and circumcorneal vascularization with contact lens wear. *Int. Contact Lens Clin.* **7**, 26–37

VANNAS, A., HOLDEN, B. A. and MAKITIE, J. (1984). The ultrastructure of contact lens induced changes. *Acta ophthal.* **62**, 320–333

VANNAS, A., MAKITIE, J., SULONEN, J., AHONEN, R. and JARVINEN, E. (1981). Contact lens induced transient changes in corneal endothelium. *Acta ophthal.* **59**, 552–559

VANNAS, A., HOLDEN, B. A., SWEENEY, D. F. and POLSE, K. A. (1985). Surgical incision alters the swelling response of the human cornea. *Invest. Ophthal. Vis. Sci.* **26**, 864–868

WALLACE, W. (1986). The SLACH syndrome. *Int. Eyecare* **1**, 220

WEISSMAN, B. A. (1982). An introduction to extended-wear contact lenses. *J. Am. optom. Ass.* **53**, 183–186

WEISSMAN, B. A. (1983). Danger: EXW. *Optom. Monthly* **74**, 21–22

WEISSMAN, B. A., MONDINO, W. C., PETTIT, T. H. and HOFBAUER, J. D. (1984). Corneal ulcers associated with extended-wear soft contact lenses. *Am. J. Ophthal.* **97**, 476–481

WICHTERLE, O. and LIM, D. (1960). Hydrophilic gels for biological use. *Nature* **185**, 117–118

WILLIAMS, L. J. (1986). Transient endothelial changes in the in vivo human cornea. *PhD Thesis*, University of New South Wales, Sydney, Australia

WILLIAMS, L. and HOLDEN, B. A. (1986). The bleb response of the endothelium decreases with extended wear of contact lenses. *Clin. expl. Optom.* **69**, 90–92

WONG, M. P., DZIABO, A. J. and KIRAL, R. M. (1986). Dynamics of BAK adsorption by silicone acrylate lenses. *Contact Lens Spect.* **1**(11), 49–53

YAMANE, S. J. and KUWABARA, D. M. (1987). Ensuring compliance in patients wearing contact lenses on an extended-wear basis. *Int. Contact Lens Clin.* **14**, 108–112

YOUNG, G. (1985). Overview on rigid lens extended wear before 1974. *J. Br. Contact Lens Ass.* **8**, 71–77

ZABKIEWICZ, K., SWARBRICK, H. and HOLDEN, B. A. (1986).

Clinical experiences with low to moderate Dk hard gas-permeable lenses for extended wear. *Transactions of the British Contact Lens Association Conference*, pp. 101–102

ZABKIEWICZ, K., TERRY, R., HOLDEN, B. A. and SCHNIDER, C. (1987). The frequency of rigid lens binding in extended wear increases with time (abstract). *Am. J. Optom.* **64**(10), 110P

ZANTOS, S. G. (1981). The ocular response to continuous wear of contact lenses. *PhD Thesis*, University of New South Wales, Sydney, Australia

ZANTOS, S. G. (1983). Cystic formations in the corneal epithelium during extended wear of contact lenses. *Int. Contact Lens Clin.* **10**, 128–146

ZANTOS, S. G. and HOLDEN, B. A. (1977a). Research techniques and materials for continuous wear of contact lenses. *Aust. J. Optom.* **60**, 86–95

ZANTOS, S. G. and HOLDEN, B. A. (1977b). Transient endothelial changes soon after wearing soft contact lenses. *Am. J. Optom.* **54**, 856–858

ZANTOS, S. G. and HOLDEN, B. A. (1978). Ocular changes associated with continuous wear of contact lenses. *Aust. J. Optom.* **61**, 418–426

ZANTOS, S. G. and ZANTOS, P. O. (1985). Extended wear feasibility of gas-permeable hard lenses for myopes. *Int. Eyecare* **1**, 66–75

Chapter 16

Bifocal and multifocal contact lenses

J. T. de Carle

Introduction and history

The presbyopic patient presents a problem to all contact lens practitioners and it is important to discuss this problem with the patient at the initial visit. Such patients may be fitted with single vision contact lenses, corrected for distance, and wear a pair of additional glasses for near vision (this correction could be made up in the form of plano distance bifocal spectacles), or they may be fitted with bifocal or multifocal contact lenses. Possibly the biggest problem occurs with early presbyopes who are just becoming aware of the fact that they are experiencing difficulty with near vision and have only been wearing single vision spectacles or contact lenses. It is sometimes difficult to convince such patients that it is necessary to change from single vision spectacle lenses to single vision contact lenses plus spectacles, or to bifocal contact lenses. In these cases, it may be preferable to fit them with contact lenses with +0.50 D added to aid near vision, at the same time explaining that presbyopia happens to everybody and that these changes occur whether or not they have contact lenses; also it should be explained that reading spectacles in addition to the contact lenses will be needed after a short time, or bifocal contact lenses.

A number of practitioners have given a single vision distance contact lens to the dominant eye and a single vision near contact lens to the non-dominant eye. Although this technique, known as 'monovision', has been popular over the years, patients should be selected with care and the slight loss of stereopsis taken into account.

Generally, patients who would be considered suitable for single vision lenses should be suitable for bifocals. But care must be taken with neurotic patients who might just pass suitability tests for single vision lenses but would prove unsuitable for the more complicated bifocal lenses.

The first reference to bifocal contact lenses is credited to Feinbloom of New York, who showed diagrams of bifocal and trifocal segments in the optic zone of scleral contact lenses in a patent specification in 1938 (*Figure 16.1*). F. A. Williamson-Noble (1951), a British ophthalmologist, mentioned his own work on bifocal contact lenses when he gave the presidential address to the Contact Lens Society in 1950. He had become interested in the possibility of these lenses after seeing a patient aged 71 years who could read small print easily, both with and without a +2.25 D near addition. Slight lens opacities had made the crystalline lens, in effect, bifocal and it occurred to him that something similar might be possible with a contact lens. A lens was made with a central portion 2.00 D more convex than the remainder

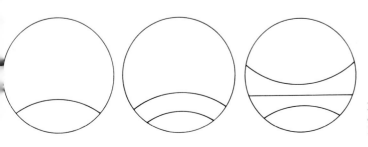

Figure 16.1 Bifocal and trifocal constructions in the optic portion of scleral lenses as suggested by Feinbloom (1938)

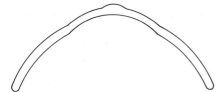

Figure 16.2 Bifocal scleral lenses suggested by Williamson-Noble (1950) with a small convex central near portion on the front surface

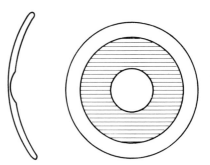

Figure 16.4 De Carle concentric back surface bifocal (1957) with a 2.0–4.0 mm central distance portion surrounded by the near portion used as a bearing surface

of the front surface (*Figure 16.2*). This lens was tried on his own eye but at first did not work in the way he had hoped. However, he found that if he kept his eye open for some time the print gradually became clearer. This was felt to be due to the front surface of the lens becoming dry and then allowing the near addition to have its proper effect; also that an accumulation of tear liquid around the small near addition prevented the lens from working properly. It was therefore suggested that a fused bifocal would probably be the answer.

Pinhole lenses have been suggested as a means of giving a presbyopic patient clear vision from distance to a normal near working position (Freeman, 1952). This can be easily achieved with contact lenses, half the normal near addition being added to the distance prescription (*Figure 16.3*). The diameter of the aperture is between 1.00 and 2.00 mm, according to the near addition: the higher the near addition the smaller the aperture needs to be to achieve an acceptable degree of vision by reducing the size of the blur circles. Unfortunately, this cannot be done without a number of disadvantages as follows:

(1) Considerable loss of light. A 1.00 mm aperture is the equivalent of a very dark-tinted spectacle lens.

(2) Reducing field of view; this could be as little as 15°, depending on the depth of the anterior chamber, i.e. the distance of the lens from the eye's entrance pupil.
(3) Poor cosmetic appearance.
(4) A lens with a minimum of movement is essential. This is often difficult to achieve without sacrificing comfort and upsetting corneal metabolism.

De Carle (1959) considered all these experiments in 1957 and, because of the difficulties involved in making a fused bifocal, decided that a similar effect could be achieved by putting the bifocal surface on the back of the lens so that the partial neutralization effect of the tears would be constant. De Carle also reversed the positions of the near and distance portions so that there was now a small distance portion in the centre (*Figure 16.4*). Provided that the distance portion was small (2.00–4.00 mm was usual), the fact that the back central curve was much steeper than the cornea did not create problems. (Large distance portions, particularly with the higher near additions, were found not to be practical as a bubble or bubbles would form between the lens and the eye.) In this type of concentric bifocal lens, the patient looked through both the distance and near portions at the same time.

The de Carle bifocal may best be visualized as a near vision contact lens with a small portion in the centre of the back surface, ground and polished to a much steeper radius for distance vision use. This creates a positive tear lens between the central portion of the lens and the cornea. The power difference in air between the distance portion and the near portion is just over three times the near addition actually required

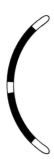

Figure 16.3 Cross-section of a pinhole contact lens with opaque areas of the lens shown in black

(*see* Chapter 5), for example:

Distance *Rx* +2.00 D
Near addition +2.50 D
Distance BCOZR 6.92 mm
Near BPOZR 7.80 mm
Distance BVP of lens in air −3.50 D
Near BVP of lens in air +4.50 D

To some extent most multi-curve corneal lenses act as back surface bifocals, for the BVP through the periphery of the lens is more positive, or less negative, than through the optic zone, due to the back surface peripheral flattening.

In 1957–1958, Wesley and Jessen of Chicago (Jessen, 1960) were also working on a concentric bifocal lens with a central distance portion. One difference between their bifocal and the de Carle bifocal was that the bifocal surface was worked on to the front surface. A second difference was that the distance portion was larger (*Figure 16.5*). The Wesley–Jessen bifocal had the same power difference in air between the distance and near portions as the near addition actually required. As the difference in radii on a de Carle bifocal is three times greater than that on a Wesley–Jessen bifocal, the manufacturing problems are slightly less as there is less tendency for the two curves to blend together when being polished. Also, any errors of this nature are two-thirds eliminated by the tear liquid on the de Carle bifocal.

The main effect of the difference in sizes of the distance portions of these two lenses conveniently illustrates the two ways in which bifocal contact lenses work. The average distance portion diameter of the de Carle bifocal is 3.00 mm and the lens is fitted so that this completely covers the pupil with only a small amount of movement. The distance portion

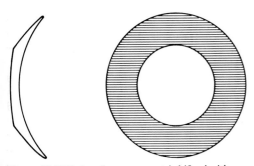

Figure 16.5 Wesley–Jessen concentric bifocal with a relatively flat distance portion on the front surface surrounded by a more convex near portion

diameter is determined by the pupil size so that approximately the same amount of light enters the eye through the distance portion as the near portion. This is the 'bivision' principle. When viewing distant objects, there is a sharp image from the distance portion and, superimposed over it, a very blurred image from the near portion, and vice versa when the patient reads or does close work. This has the advantage that the patient does not have to hold his reading matter in any particular position to read. The main disadvantage is that the vision is not as sharp because of the side-effects from the superimposed images, although this is not as bad as might be expected and has proved to be quite acceptable to many patients. The Wesley–Jessen bifocal originally had a 6.00 mm distance portion, but this was later reduced slightly to 5.00 mm to increase the near portion. The near portion on this lens can only cover the pupil by movement of the lens — the 'alternating vision' principle. This normally occurs by the patient looking down to read and the lens being pushed upwards by the lower lid. The advantage is sharper image formation with less visual side-effects — the disadvantage being that some lower lids are very loose, so that the lens tends to slide between the lid and the eye and is therefore not pushed upwards sufficiently. These lenses are often fitted slightly lower than average to allow them to move up easily. This can have the disadvantage that the near portion may partly cover the pupil immediately after a blink — probably for a second or less, but enough to be very disturbing to the patient.

Wesley (1962, personal communication) developed a very unusual and ingenious lens, utilizing the chromatic aberration of the eye: red light being brought to a focus beyond blue. The near portion of his lens was of a blue or violet plastics material and the distance portion was tinted red. Simply by using different colours, the dioptric difference on the eye, between the distance and the near portions, can be varied. The greater the difference between the two main wavelengths of light transmitted the greater the dioptric difference.

When non-tinted plastic material is used for the distance portion, of the wavelengths this transmits, the eye is most sensitive to 550 nm. With blue plastics used for the near portion, the wavelength of maximum transmission is 486 nm. This gives an effective near vision addition of 0.45 D. By using red plastics of approximately 656 nm maximum transmission for distance instead of clear plastics, this can be increased to 0.85 D.

Even greater dioptric differences can be obtained by using violet at 400 nm and red at 700 nm, but these lenses are darker and rather impractical for use indoors. This idea of varying the colour used for the two portions, instead of the curvature, works in the same way as the red and green duochrome test used by many refractionists.

The lenses can be made to any design, such as concentric or prism ballasted. It is obvious that their use would be mainly for early presbyopes. If it were possible to surface tint one portion of an existing bifocal successfully, it should be possible to increase the effective near addition by about 0.50 D. This could be very useful if an early presbyope who had had bifocals a year or so needed a slight increase in the near addition.

The dioptric difference obtained with these lenses is only apparent on the eye. If a single vision lens is tinted in this way, it will not alter the focimeter reading.

In 1967, Wesley announced another ingenious lens to achieve a bifocal effect (Plastics Contact Lens Company, 1970). Essentially, it has a small central distance portion with a plurality of light-transmitting apertures in the opaque remainder (*Figure 16.6*). This corrected one of the major objections to pinhole lenses, namely, the restricted field of view. Many different patterns of apertures have been tried,

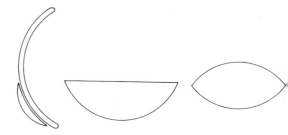

Figure 16.7 McKay Taylor additive bifocal. A small supplementary additional lens is placed on top of the carrier lens *in situ*. Two suggested shapes for additive lenses are shown on the right of a cross-section through carrier and additive lens (left)

the average width of the slits being 0.8 mm. The central transparent portion has been made as large as 3.00 mm. The distance correction is the same as would be prescribed for a single vision distance lens, the near vision focus being achieved by the reduced blur circles from the peripheral apertures.

A further type of bifocal lens was suggested by McKay Taylor (1962) and consisted of a small lens placed on top of a contact lens *in situ* (*Figure 16.7*). The lens was held in place by the surface tension of the tears and was made with a single back surface curve slightly flatter than the front radius of the carrier lens to allow a certain amount of movement of the additive lens. When the parent lens was a corneal contact lens, it was necessary to flatten the peripheral curve of the front surface slightly to prevent the additive lens from sliding off entirely. The combined weight caused the corneal lens to rotate in the same way as a prism ballasted lens. When the patient wished to see only in the distance, he removed the small additive lens with a suction holder.

From about 1960, bifocal contact lenses resembling spectacle bifocals became increasingly popular. The segment shapes were mostly very similar to their spectacle lens counterparts. Nearly all the lenses were prevented from rotating and kept in their correct position by the use of a prism which settled base-down. *Figure 16.8* shows two of the first of these lenses, both worked on the front surface. *Figure 16.9* shows a decentred de Carle bifocal incorporating prism with the distance portion decentred upwards relative to the base of the prism. *Figure 16.10* shows some solid bifocal lenses designed by Hodd (1967) that are theoretically excellent visually but extremely difficult to make in

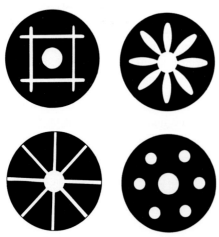

Figure 16.6 Multiple aperture lenses for distance and near vision use suggested by Wesley in 1967

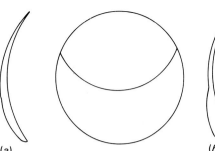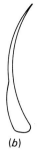

(a)   (b)

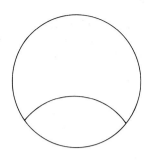

Figure 16.8 Two early suggested front surface solid prism ballasted bifocals

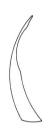

Figure 16.9 De Carle back surface concentric bifocal incorporating prism ballast and with the distance portion decentred upwards relative to the base of the prism

practice. In fact, all these lenses and variations of them appear to suffer from some disadvantages. Because the two front surface curves are so similar, front surface bifocals are very difficult to make to ensure a sharp focimeter image right up to the transition, with no blending of the two curves at all. Nevertheless, some excellent lenses of this type have been made. The main difficulty is that vision is not always as definite as with single vision lenses. This is probably for the reason given by Williamson-Noble in 1950, i.e. the accumulation of tear liquid prevents the bifocal from working properly. Back surface bifocals do not have this disadvantage, but the type shown in *Figures 16.4* and *16.9* must either have a small distance portion to avoid bubbles becoming trapped or be fitted so that the radius on the back surface for the near portion is flatter than the cornea. This results in the transition touching the cornea, which could cause corneal abrasion. Corneal abrasion from the edge of the recessed portion of the lens shown in *Figure 16.10a* could be a problem, the segment needing to be recessed as the radius of curvature of the near portion has to be flatter than the distance

portion. Blending is undesirable as it creates an area of blurred vision.

Mandell (1966) was commissioned by a laboratory (Kontur Kontact) to design a prism ballast bifocal to try and eliminate the problems encountered with earlier front surface bifocals.

The result is the Mandell 'No-Jump' bifocal, and it is probably the most successful of the front surface bifocals.

The making of this lens is an example of contact lens manufacturing technique at its finest. The near portion is cut into the front surface so that there is a slight 'ledge' between the distance portion and the near portion (similar to a semi-visible centre controlled spectacle bifocal, but on the front surface). The amount of this ledge increases towards the edge

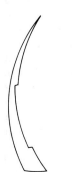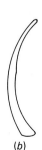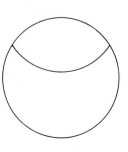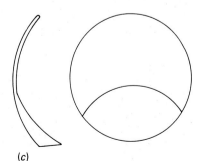

(a)

(b)

(c)

Figure 16.10 Some solid bifocal contact lenses suggested by Hodd (1967). (a) With recessed near portion on the back surface; (b) an upcurve prism ballasted back surface bifocal; (c) a downcurve prism ballasted back surface bifocal

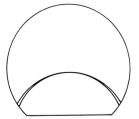

Figure 16.11 Mandell 'No-Jump' front surface bifocal lens

of the lens and is absent in the centre (*Figure 16.11*). This ledge does not appear to cause irritation of the upper lid.

Monocentric fused bifocals should give an equal performance and have the advantage that the front surface can, within reason, be repolished or have a small power change carried out. Due to the very precise nature of the front surface of the Mandell bifocal, repolishing is not advised.

A bifocal with an inserted segment of a higher refractive index, or a fused bifocal as shown in *Figure 16.12* would overcome the objections to the back and front surface solid bifocals. The French company of Ysoptic have made an inserted segment type of lens (Guilbert,

1969a,b). This lens has a unique back surface. The distance and near portions have the same radius but are set at a slight angle to each other so that the lens can rock on the cornea. This is intended to anchor the lens more firmly for distance or near use (*Figure 16.12b*). Ysoptic also make a bifocal measuring lens for determining segment heights (*Figure 16.13*). Fused bifocals, on the other hand, are nearly always made so that the segment is worked from the back surface and can be made slightly thinner than lenses with an inserted segment as depicted in *Figure 16.12a,b*. Their construction and manufacture has been described by Bryant (1973).

A variety of segment shapes can be made as shown in *Figure 16.14*. The first segment (*a*) has the disadvantage that near vision becomes blurred if the lens slips slightly to one side. The second segment (*b*) largely overcomes this problem, but the optical centre of the near portion is a greater distance from the optical centre of the distance portion so that a 'jump' is

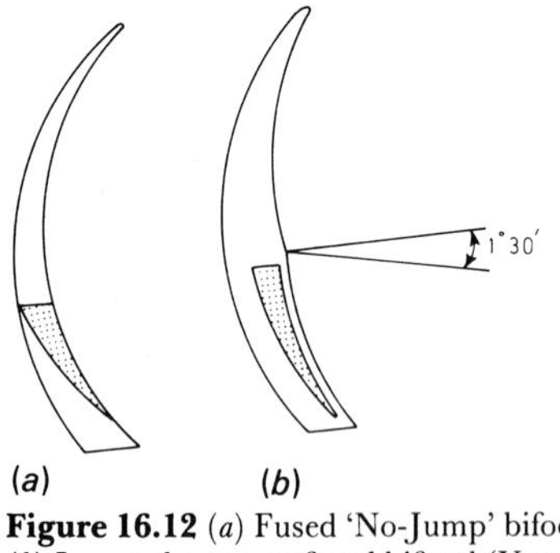

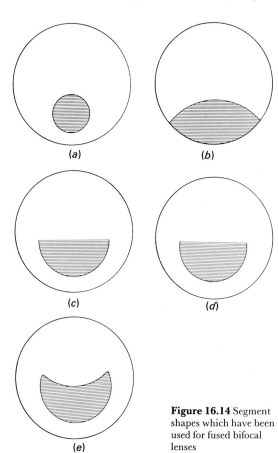

Figure 16.14 Segment shapes which have been used for fused bifocal lenses

Figure 16.12 (*a*) Fused 'No-Jump' bifocal (cross-section). (*b*) Inserted segment fused bifocal (Ysoptic Laboratories) with a double back optic surface to help locate the lens with the desired optic portion in front of the pupil

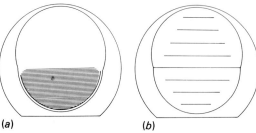

Figure 16.13 (*a*) Front view of the Ysoptic inserted fused bifocal; (*b*) Ysoptic measuring lens for determining segment height

created as the visual axis passes from one portion to the other. The third segment (*c*) is theoretically monocentric so that there should be no 'jump', and the width of the segment is therefore exactly twice the height. This sometimes limits the height of the segment as an increase in size would increase the thickness, which might be undesirable in negative lenses. The fourth segment (*d*) is a good compromise, not theoretically monocentric but the 'jump' is so slight that it is no problem in practice. The fifth segment (*e*) is also monocentric, the aim of the up-curved top of the segment being to ensure that the centre of the segment top is always in the same position in relation to the pupil if the lens swings slightly in a pendulum manner on the eye (Goldberg, 1969). Theoretically, the radius of curvature of the top of the segment should be the same as half the overall lens size. The disadvantage of this type of segment is the possibility of slight peripheral blur at the sides when using distance vision.

Theoretical basis of bifocal contact lenses

Bifocal contact lenses can be divided into five different categories but some designs incorporate features from two categories.

(1) Simultaneous vision or bivision bifocals.
(2) Translating or alternating vision bifocals.
(3) Monovision.
(4) Multizone bifocals.
(5) Non-refractive bifocals:
    (a) pinhole lenses;
    (b) spherical aberration correcting lenses;
    (c) diffractive lenses.

Simultaneous vision or bivision bifocals

Light enters the eye from both the distance and near portions at the same time. When viewing distance objects, there is a sharp image from the distance portion and, superimposed over it, a very blurred image from the near portion, and vice versa, when the patient reads or does close work. This has the advantage that the patient does not have to hold his reading matter in any particular position to read. The main disadvantages are that the vision is not as sharp as with a single vision lens because of the side-effects from the superimposed images, although this is not as bad as might be expected. Also the ratio of light entering the eye from the two portions varies with different pupil sizes and thus different lighting conditions. (Multizone bifocals are being developed to try and overcome these problems, especially the problem of varying pupil sizes. The Diffrax lens, made by Pilkington, has a 5 mm diameter central diffractive zone on the back surface, which provides both distance and near powers all over this area — *see* p. 615. This effectively overcomes any problem with varying pupil sizes.)

Lenses with separate portions can be made with the central portion for either distance or near. A disadvantage of the near central portion is during bright lighting conditions, for example, when the sun comes from behind a cloud while driving, when good distance vision is essential. In this situation the pupil constricts thereby limiting vision to the near portion and making distance vision blurred. This can be improved by wearing sunglasses.

Breger (1980) has suggested that if the central portion is small, between 1 mm and 2 mm in diameter, the blur circle from the out-of-focus image will be reduced. The writer believes that the ideal diameter of the central portion is determined by the pupil diameter and the distance from the anterior surface of the cornea to the pupil. Light entering the eye should be divided as nearly as possible so that there is 50% from the distance portion and 50% from the near portion. In normal lighting conditions this results in an average size of 3.00 mm for the central portion. Erickson and Robboy (1985) found that the best diameters for simultaneous vision with a central distance portion were from 2.25 mm to 3.00 mm.

A variation of these designs is possible using a lens with an aspherical back surface with the distance power located in the lens centre.

Translating or alternating vision bifocals

Theoretically, these bifocals provide alternating vision, the patient looking through the distance portion for distance vision, the lens moving upwards for close work through the near portion. A prism ballast of approximately 1.5 Δ base-down is often incorporated to orientate the lens correctly and in addition the lens is sometimes truncated. In practice, achieving the correct amount of movement is difficult. The lens must move up easily when the eye looks down for close work but the lens must not be so loose that the lens rides up when looking straight ahead causing the near portion to cover the pupil.

Monovision

Although strictly speaking not a bifocal technique, monovision is the generally accepted name for the method of correcting presbyopia by using a distance contact lens for one eye and a near contact lens for the other eye. It has proved popular over the years due to the simplicity of the system, the minimal additional cost involved and its reasonable success rate. In addition, the success rate with earlier bifocal designs has been mediocre or poor. The monovision principle does not work well with spectacles due to the difference in prismatic effects between the two eyes on version movements and the small difference in magnification between the two eyes. These problems are minimal with contact lenses and for this reason it works well in many cases.

Objections to monovision are that binocular vision is degraded and that the patient must learn to suppress the central vision of each eye alternately. In practice the distance lens is usually fitted to the dominant eye in order to minimize the distance blur effect of the 'reading' lens. This is important for such activities as driving. For patients doing a large amount of close work the dominant eye may be fitted with the 'reading' lens.

An investigation by Loshin, Loshin and Cromer (1982), using contrast sensitivity, revealed that as the power of the near addition is increased, the binocular contrast sensitivity is reduced until it is almost a monocular function. In practice, it is found that most patients have little difficulty in accepting an addition of +1.00 D in the non-dominant eye. As the addition is increased further, the blur becomes more noticeable and they often feel giddy and unbalanced. It is the author's opinion that monovision should only be used for early presbyopes, and that as better and cheaper bifocal contact lenses become available the idea of monovision will cease to be used. An interesting legal situation might arise for a car driver who had a road accident while driving wearing monovision contact lenses, although

many uncorrected ametropes are effectively in a similar binocular refractive situation.

Before trying a near lens in the non-dominant eye it is necessary to determine which is the dominant eye. It is usually the right eye if the patient is right handed and vice versa but it must not be assumed that this is the case. Testing for dominancy is quick and simple: ask the patient to clasp both hands together interlocking the fingers but leaving a hole between the thumbs and first fingers, then, without closing one eye, ask the patient to raise the arms with hands as far away as possible and to sight an object such as the large letter at the top of the distance chart in the centre of the hole. Occluding one eye soon shows which eye is dominant. If this test is done with one hand only there is sometimes a tendency to turn and sight the target on the same side.

The strength of the near addition should be as low as possible commensurate with visual needs. Too weak a near addition, however, may cause problems as the patient will then read at arms' length and may become visually confused as to which eye should be used. The 'reading' addition can often be found by refraction in the normal way, adding plus power slowly to the non-dominant eye with a pair of single vision contact lenses in place. The effect on both distance and near vision binocularly can be assessed. It is essential to explain exactly how monovision works and what is being done. Despite doing this comments such as 'when I shut my right eye my distance vision is all blurred' are quite common, both at the time of explanation and later!

If the patient is still interested a 'reading' lens of the indicated power should be tried. It is a good idea to ask patients to walk outside as a lens which is acceptable in the consulting room may prove unacceptable in a busy street. Phillips (A. J., 1987, personal communication) has stated that approximately 50% of monovision wearers required supplementary single vision or bifocal spectacles to balance vision for concentrated distance, near, or both visual situations.

Multizone bifocals

The one factor that causes the most difficulties with the fitting and success of bifocal contact lenses is the pupil size. In recent years there have been several attempts to design and make a lens where the optical effects would not be affected by (1) the difference in pupil size from one presbyope to another, or (2) variations in the pupil size due to different lighting conditions.

One theoretical way of overcoming this problem is a bifocal lens with a large number of distance and reading portions, the advantage being that as the pupil size varied, more or less portions would be used and the 50:50 ratio maintained. Little or no lens movement would be ideal. Good centration would be preferable but, in theory, the 50:50 ratio could be maintained even if the lens was badly decentred.

In 1977, Cohen, in the USA applied for a patent for a zonal bifocal contact lens. This consisted of concentric rings, alternately powered for distance and near, the adjacent zones interfaced continuously so that there were no steps. The bifocal surface was on the lens front surface and he suggested that the partial neutralization of this surface by tears could be corrected by changing the relationship of one zone with the next, so that an overlying tear

layer would form a surface matching the distance and near curvatures as closely as possible. The patent does not state if this would be achieved by blending the junctions.

In 1983, de Carle, in the UK applied for a patent for a multizone bifocal contact lens. He was unaware of the work of Cohen, and as well as applying for a similar design (*Figure 16.15a*) he also applied for two other designs as shown in *Figure 16.15b,c*. Appreciating the problems that can be created by tears on the anterior surface and not being convinced that changing the design of the front surface would be sufficient to eliminate them, as the quantity of tears can vary from second to second, he suggested that the designs could also be made in fused form or on the posterior surface.

All multizone designs are very hard to make and only economical if moulded. The advantages are that they are easy to fit. The practitioner is then only concerned with obtaining the correct near addition, good centration and minimum movement. Also there should be no side-effects from a fluctuating pupil size. With experimental lenses, rings around lights have been noticed corresponding to the number of distance and near portions on the lens. Experiments are continuing. These lenses are not yet available commercially.

Non-refractive bifocals

A non-refractive 'bifocal' is a lens that acts as a distance and near correction but with either no corrective power at all in the lens, or else a single vision prescription only; alternatively it may achieve the bifocal effect by some other means.

Pinhole lenses

The simplest non-refractive 'bifocal' is the pinhole lens, as described earlier (*see Figure 16.3*). In theory there should be no need for a refractive element; a thin lens made from black plastic with a small central hole should provide good visual acuity for both distance and near vision, but in practice a power midway between the distance and near powers is best. However, the drawbacks are that the light has to be very bright for adequate vision to be achieved, and there is only a small central visual field. Also pinholes, if too small, give rise to diffraction haloes which degrade the retinal image.

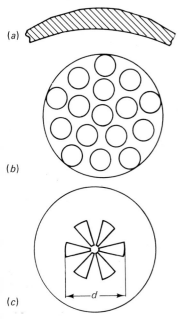

Figure 16.15 De Carle multizone bifocal lens design. (*a*) Multizone front surface bifocal; (*b*) multizone design to maintain an approximately equal ratio of distance to near power in front of the pupil during lens movement. (*c*) As (*b*) with diameter *d* intended to be larger than the pupil diameter to allow for lens movement

An improvement on the pinhole lens would be a plurality of apertures (*see Figure 16.6*), but there would still be a reduction in the light reaching the retina, and possible diffraction haloes. There is also a risk of multiple images if the pupil is large, because of the variation in power of the eye (spherical aberration) across the pupil.

All such pinhole lenses are really therefore of only academic interest but could, on the rare occasion, be useful.

Spherical aberration correcting lenses

A good camera lens is corrected for spherical aberration. The human eye is not. A cheap camera lens that has not been corrected for spherical aberration produces an image which is not perfectly sharp. Rays refracted through the periphery of such an 'uncorrected' lens focus in front of the rays from the centre of the lens. It follows that if a contact lens can be produced which will correct the spherical aberration of the eye (and also in higher powers the spherical aberration of the contact lens itself), then the retinal image should be sharper. This should have the effect of increasing the depth of focus and therefore of effectively increasing amplitude of accommodation, but if the pupil size is too large or the eye suffers from irregular aberrations the effect may be negated.

Kaplan (1967) used models to show that a front aspherical surface would help to correct presbyopia and astigmatism. At least two lenses have been developed using this principle. One is the CALS lens, the result of work by Carl and Thomas Evans (Evans and Evans, 1981; Evans, 1983; Evans, Mayers and Szabocsik, 1988) of Canada. The other is the PS45 lens, developed in England in 1987 by Nissels from original work done in the USA.

Whereas the positive power of aspheric bifocal lenses (e.g. Hydrocurve II) increases towards the periphery, with the CALS and PS45 lenses it decreases towards the periphery. It should be emphasized that these lenses are not an attempt to make a bifocal lens by a method which is the reverse of the aspheric bifocal. In fact these lenses are not bifocals at all, but by reducing spherical aberration the visual acuity of presbyopic and astigmatic patients, as well as some patients with visual problems, should be improved. The central power of the lens, which can only be accurately checked with a very small aperture (e.g. 1.5 mm) on the focimeter, should be that required for a point dioptrically half way between the distance and near powers.

Evans (1983) refers to the blur circle tolerance range (BCTR). It has been suggested that the BCTR of the eye is 2.00 D, and if that is so the lens prescription would be $+1.00$ D added to the distance power. The best focus should then be at 1 metre from the eye, where the blur circle should be so small as to be almost non-existent. At infinity and 50 cm from the eye the blur circle would be at its largest within the range considered to be 'in focus'. As the pupil size affects the depth of focus, it is doubtful whether a presbyope with a large pupil would agree that objects at infinity and 50 cm were both in focus. The author found that both the PS45 lens and CALS lens gave him effectively only 0.75 D of additional accommodation.

These lenses should be useful for early presbyopes needing a near addition of up to $+1.50$ D. Their usefulness in patients needing a higher near addition probably depends on their pupil size and occupational vision requirements.

All bifocal contact lenses have some side-effects. Many of these could probably be reduced if they employed this principle of having an aspherical front surface to reduce spherical aberration. Such combination lenses may produce better bifocals than any available today.

Diffractive bifocals

A diffractive lens is one which breaks up each ray of light into dark and light bands or into colours of the spectrum. A ray of light normally travels in a straight line but can be bent by diffraction; the longer the wavelength the more it is bent. Red light which has the longest wavelength of the visible spectrum is therefore deviated more than blue. This is the opposite way round to the chromatism produced by a prism or lens or, for that matter, the eye itself.

In 1981, Freeman in the UK, applied for a patent for a contact lens with a transmission hologram providing diffractive power on a wavelength and/or amplitude selective basis, whereby light from both distance and near objects could be focused on the retina of a presbyopic wearer. This permits an equal amount of light to be used for distance vision and near vision whatever the pupil size.

He suggested several ways in which this could be achieved. The hologram could be on either surface or on a layer inside the lens. The hologram could be generated by using two lasers, the effective near addition being created by the distance of the light sources. For example, if one beam was at infinity and the other at 33 cm they would have a divergence of 3 D. The laser beams would interfere within photosensitive material in or on the lens, creating interference fringes.

A Fresnel zone plate uses a similar principle, the zones being alternately clear and opaque, and a lens could be made in this form. Such a lens would suffer the same disadvantages as a multiple pinhole. However, the opaque zones can be changed into transparent ones if the thickness of the optical path has been increased by a half wavelength. Freeman has taken this a step further by changing this extra thickness smoothly across the width of each zone from nil to one wavelength (or some fraction of a wavelength depending on the colour). The power of the superimposed zones provides the diffractive near addition. The near addition varies for different colours. For example, if the addition is $+2.00$ D with a wavelength of 400 nm (blue), it will be approximately $+3.50$ D with a wavelength of 700 nm (red). Fortunately, the majority of this effect is neutralized by the chromatic aberration of the eye but is apparent on a focimeter with the lens in air (*see* Chapter 12). Pilkington have now marketed such a lens — the Diffrax lens — which is fitted much as a conventional single vision gas permeable lens (*see* p. 615).

Choice of bifocal type

The patient's occupation is a very important consideration which should help to determine whether or not to supply him with bifocal contact lenses and also the type of lens. This is an area where the practitioner's skill and experience is invaluable. It is important that the practitioner realizes that there is no one design of bifocal or trifocal lens that is ideal for every single patient. This point has been elaborated by Hodd (1974) who has published some case histories illustrating the use of different types of bifocal lens, which he also describes. By the correct choice of the type of lens, a very high percentage of patients should be successfully

fitted. It is important to question the patient carefully regarding his near and intermediate distance visual requirements and, if necessary, give a demonstration of these requirements. These should fall into one of the following categories.

Good distance vision essential (for flying, driving etc.)

Good peripheral vision will also be essential, so the concentric type of bifocal should not be fitted to these patients. A prism ballasted bifocal should give the best results, and to ensure that the near portion does not ride up or rotate on the eye when the patient is using distance vision, slightly more prism ballast should be given and the near portion should possibly be fitted slightly lower than average. This latter situation is not possible if the patient insists on very good near vision.

Diffractive bifocals or multizone bifocals may well prove to become the lens of first choice, as they too satisfy the demand for good distance vision.

Very good near vision required for long periods of time

A concentric bifocal with a small distance portion should be tried and compared against a prism ballasted bifocal with the largest possible near portion. The latter should be fitted so that the near portion is as high as possible without interfering with the distance vision.

An alternative is to specify the lens for the non-dominant eye biased towards the near vision so that the distance vision is reduced by approximately one line. This is usually preferable to the much greater effect upon distance vision that monovision would have.

Good intermediate vision at, or slightly below, eye level

Musicians are examples of this type of patient. One approach is to make the near portion suitably powered for the intermediate distance. However, there are very few patients who are satisfied with poor near vision.

A concentric aspheric bifocal should be considered. Alternatively, a lens with the addition for the intermediate focus in the dominant eye and for the near focus in the non-dominant eye may be successful.

Good intermediate vision required above eye level

An example of this type of patient is a chemist with bottles on high shelves to be seen continuously throughout the day. In this case, a concentric lens with the addition for the intermediate focus in the dominent eye may be successful.

Good near vision required above eye level

Usually, a concentric bifocal with a peripheral near portion fitted to give alternating vision is the most satisfactory lens, particularly if it tends to settle below the central position on the cornea.

Lenses required mainly for social reasons

In such cases, long-sustained critical near vision is not usually carried out with the bifocal contact lenses. Possibly, nothing more critical than reading a menu or theatre programme is required. This can usually be achieved with a concentric bifocal. However, if the patient is a keen bridge player, two different powered additions (intermediate and near) may be the answer, one for each eye.

Two anatomical features are of importance with bifocal contact lenses that are of lesser importance with single vision lenses. These are the pupil diameter and the position and tightness of the lower lid, the latter being of even greater importance in hard lens fitting than in soft. The pupil diameter may be a very important factor if it fluctuates very considerably between bright and dark conditions. This particularly applies when considering concentric bifocals. It has sometimes been stated that patients with small pupils are unsuitable for bifocal contact lenses; but back surface concentric bifocals with distance segments as small as 1.50 mm have been successfully fitted. The larger the pupil diameter the greater the difficulty in fitting prism ballasted bifocals because the possibility of achieving good alternating vision becomes harder and some degree of bivision has to be accepted.

The lower lid should be carefully examined, particularly if prism ballasted bifocals are being considered. The lower lid is essential to raise the lens when the patient lowers his eyes for near vision. A very loose lower lid or a lower lid below the limbus may be unable to do this sufficiently to obtain enough vertical movement of the lens. In such cases, a concentric bifocal fitted on the bivision principle will probably be the lens of choice.

Fitting procedures

Hard and gas permeable lenses

Back surface concentric bifocals with central distance portion

Utilizing the simultaneous vision method of fitting these lenses (*see Figure 16.4* and p. 601) must be fitted so that they centre well with the minimum amount of movement that is acceptable to the patient and practitioner. This can be done by fitting the lenses larger, steeper or thinner than usual. All three methods could result in an uncomfortable lens, so considerable care is required by the practitioner. Such lenses often need to be fenestrated, if made of PMMA or gas permeable materials with very low oxygen transmission. A lens that rides up very slightly is preferable to one that settles slightly below centre. A low fitting lens makes near vision difficult, although patients may be able to read quite well if they hold the reading matter above eye level (*Figure 16.16*).

The BPOZR is the main fitting radius and with the front surface radius determines the near portion power. The BCOZR is calculated to determine the correct distance portion power (*see*

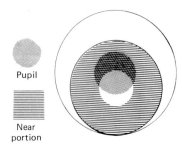

Figure 16.16 A low fitting concentric bifocal interferes with good distance vision and makes near vision difficult unless looking above eye level

Table 16.1 Recommended diameter of the distance portion in concentric bifocals related to the pupil diameter

Pupil diameter (mm)	Distance portion diameter (mm)	Pupil diameter (mm)	Distance portion diameter (mm)
4.5	3.20	3.2	2.25
4.4	3.10	3.1	2.20
4.3	3.05	3.0	2.10
4.2	2.95	2.9	2.05
4.1	2.90	2.8	2.00
4.0	2.80	2.7	1.90
3.9	2.75	2.6	1.85
3.8	2.70	2.5	1.75
3.7	2.60	2.4	1.70
3.6	2.55	2.3	1.65
3.5	2.45	2.2	1.55
3.4	2.40	2.1	1.50
3.3	2.30	2.0	1.45

Chapter 5) and has a negligible effect on the fit. The BPOZD needs to be 7.50–8.00 mm, and the back peripheral radii and total diameter are selected to achieve good centration with adequate tear exchange, as when fitting a large single vision gas permeable lens (*see* Chapter 10).

The diameter of the distance portion (BCOZD) is mainly dependent upon the pupil diameter and should cover approximately half the area of the pupil. One method is to measure the pupil in low illumination and order the distance portion according to *Table 16.1*. The pupil is difficult to measure with a scale, however, in low illumination (although ultraviolet illumination is useful as the crystalline lens fluoresces). The most accurate method is by photography. A scale — preferably divided into 0.1-mm graduations — is held in approximately the same plane as the iris and photographed, using a flash gun. The pupil does not contract until immediately after the flash has taken place. Another method is to measure the pupil diameter when a bright light is shone into the patient's eye and order the distance portion of the same diameter. Where both methods are used, some practitioners order a distance portion diameter half way between the two diameters indicated. A laboratory can usually slightly reduce the diameter of the distance portion on the finished lens, if necessary, but cannot increase the diameter satisfactorily. *Figure 16.17* shows how a well-fitted lens can move approximately 1.00 mm and still have all the distance portion over the pupil and the same percentage of the pupil area covered by the near portion.

Trial lenses with different sized distance portions are preferable as an added check on these calculations. However, with the advent of other types of bifocal, back surface bifocals are now seldom fitted, so the outlay on a fitting set may not be considered justified. Nevertheless, these lenses can be very useful when the prism ballasted type has been found unsatisfactory because of a very loose lower lid.

The distance portion diameter can also be varied according to the patient's visual requirements. For example, a person who needs bifocals only to see to read a menu or a theatre programme can be given a larger distance portion than a person who needs to read small print for long periods of time.

Although, in theory, this type of lens could be fitted flatter and used as an alternating vision concentric bifocal, the larger distance portion than required would, in practice, lead to an increased risk of central bubble formation or a stagnant central pool of tears likely to cause central corneal oedema.

The alternating vision type of concentric bifocal is better fitted where the near addition is worked on the front surface. A description of this now follows.

Front surface concentric bifocals

Figure 16.5 shows one of these lenses and the fitting principles are discussed on pp. 601 and 602. The BOZR is determined by the flattest keratometer reading. If the BOZR is flatter than

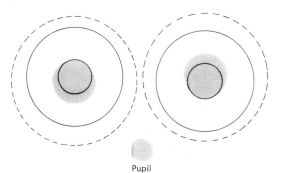

Pupil

Figure 16.17 A well-fitting concentric bifocal can move up to 1.0 mm and still have all the distance portion in front of the pupil (shaded)

this, the lens may have a tendency to ride slightly high on the cornea so that the distance portion is displaced upwards. Conversely, if the BOZR is made steeper the lens may tend to remain in a central position, and for near vision the patient will have difficulty in getting the lens to move in order to use the near portion.

The BOZD should be as large as possible, but at the same time, the intermediate and peripheral curves must be sufficiently flat to allow a moderate amount of lens movement. The total diameter is usually increased to 0.30 mm larger than a single vision lens, and the thickness is approximately 0.05 mm thicker than the equivalent single vision lens except with higher powered negative lenses. Most positive lenses should be made in a lenticular form to prevent very thin edges as the lower lid must move the lens slightly upwards when the patient is looking at a near object. Bronstein (1959) recommended putting an empirical 1.00 D of additional positive power on the near addition. This was presumably to compensate for a slight negative tear lens on the front surface (*see* p. 222, Chapter 5).

The diameter of the distance portion (FCOZD) must be carefully measured. If the distance portion is too large, the lens will not be able to move sufficiently to allow the patient to look through the near portion. If the distance portion diameter is too small, the patient will have a noticeable blur surrounding distant objects and this becomes aggravating when the lens moves during blinking. The FCOZD should not be smaller than the pupil size in a normal artificially lit room. If the pupil is larger than 5 mm, it is preferable to fit these lenses steeper by the bivision method; but with smaller pupils, they are normally always fitted using the alternating vision principle, although a certain amount of simultaneous vision invariably occurs.

An alternative method of arriving at the distance portion diameter is to measure the distance from the bottom edge of the lens (or lower lid margin) to the bottom edge of the pupil, then double this value and subtract it from the total diameter (TD) of the lens. For example, if the bottom edge of the lens is 2.50 mm from the lower edge of the pupil, the number doubled equals 5.00 mm and subtracted from a trial lens of 9.50 mm TD it gives a distance portion diameter of 4.50 mm.

Prism ballasted bifocals

Figures 16.8–16.14 illustrate these types of bifocal. The fitting requirements are the same whether the lens is a front surface, back surface or fused bifocal. In addition to all the information required when ordering a single vision lens the practitioner needs to calculate the following:

(1) Near addition.
(2) Size and shape of segment.
(3) Height of segment above the lower edge of the lens.
(4) Amount of prism ballast and thickness of the lower edge.
(5) Vertical total diameter.

These are examined in detail below.

Near addition

This varies according to the type of lens being ordered. When Wesley and Jessen (Jessen, 1960) introduced their front surface concentric bifocal, they also suggested that the near addition should be made 1.00 D stronger than that actually required. Some practitioners have continued this practice with solid front surface prism ballast bifocals but the majority claim it is unnecessary. With solid back surface bifocals of every design, it is necessary to allow for the fact that the tears neutralize just over two-thirds of the difference in power between the two areas (*see* Chapter 5). For example, to achieve a near addition of 2.50 D, the dioptric difference in air between the distance and the near portion needs to be approximately 8.00 D. For fused bifocals, the near addition should definitely be no stronger than that which would be ordered for spectacle bifocals.

Size and shape of segment

The segment should normally be the largest possible without increasing the thickness. However, there is no point in having a segment that is so large that it extends beyond the back optic zone diameter or is cut into by the lower edge of the lens. This particularly applies to fused bifocals, where the vertical dimension of the segment should not be made greater than the height of the top of the segment above the bottom of the lens. Occasionally, it is necessary to increase the thickness of a lens slightly to

Table 16.2 Minimum central thicknesses recommended for fused bifocals according to segment width (or diameter) and near addition

Near (reading) addition (D)	Minimum central thickness (mm)					
	Segment widths (mm)					
	5.00	5.50	6.00	6.50	7.00	7.50
+1.50	0.12	0.14	0.17	0.20	0.23	0.28
+1.75	0.14	0.16	0.19	0.23	0.27	0.32
+2.00	0.16	0.18	0.22	0.26	0.31	0.37
+2.25	0.17	0.20	0.25	0.29	0.35	0.42
+2.50	0.19	0.23	0.27	0.33	0.40	0.47
+2.75	0.21	0.25	0.30	0.36	0.44	0.52
+3.00	0.22	0.27	0.33	0.40	0.48	0.57

Table 16.3 Minimum central thicknesses for prism ballasted lenses of 9.00 mm total diameter according to back vertex power (and prism ballast in negative powered lenses)

Positive lenses, 9.00 mm total diameter all 1.5 Δ prism ballast		Negative lenses, 9.00 mm total diameter		
BVP (D)	Central thickness (mm)	BVP (D)	Central thickness (mm)	Prism (Δ)
0.00	0.32			
+0.50	0.34	−0.50	0.31	1.5
+1.00	0.35	−1.00	0.30	1.5
+1.25	0.35	−1.00	0.30	1.5
+1.50	0.36	−1.50	0.29	1.5
+2.00	0.37	−2.00	0.27	1.5
+2.50	0.39	−2.50	0.26	1.5
+3.00	0.40	−3.00	0.25	1.5
+3.50	0.41	−3.50	0.24	1.5
+4.00	0.42	−4.00	0.25	2
+4.50	0.44	−4.50	0.25	2
+5.00	0.45	−5.00	0.24	2
+5.50	0.46	−5.50	0.23	2
+6.00	0.47	−6.00	0.22	2
+6.50	0.49	−6.50	0.25	2.5
+7.00	0.50	−7.00	0.24	2.5
+7.50	0.51	−7.50	0.23	2.5
+8.00	0.52	−8.00	0.22	2.5
+8.50	0.54	−8.50	0.25	3
+9.00	0.55	−9.00	0.24	3
+9.50	0.56	−9.50	0.23	3
+10.00	0.57	−10.00	0.22	3
+10.50	0.59	−10.50	0.25	3.5
+11.00	0.60	−11.00	0.24	3.5
+11.50	0.61	−11.50	0.23	3.5
+12.00	0.62	−12.00	0.22	3.5
+12.50	0.64	−12.50	0.25	4
+13.00	0.65	−13.00	0.24	4
+13.50	0.66	−13.50	0.23	4
+14.00	0.67	−14.00	0.22	4

obtain a sufficiently large segment. This particularly applies to fused bifocals and could occur, for example, with the combination of a large pupil, a high near addition, and myopia (i.e. with a flat top segment and the thickest part of the segment coinciding with the thinnest part of a negative lens). *Table 16.2* gives the minimum thicknesses advised by one manufacturer of fused bifocals for certain segment widths and near additions. If this table is used in conjunction with *Table 16.3*, it may easily be determined if a particular reading addition and segment width are possible without increasing the central thickness.

The segment shape is usually determined by the type of lens which the practitioner has decided is likely to give the best performance. As the lens moves with the eye, many of the criteria that are used to determine the size and shape of spectacle bifocal segments do not apply to contact lens bifocals. For instance, whether a book-keeper can see books on both sides of the desk will depend as much on whether the lenses are stable and remain over the pupil area as on the segment width. It is interesting to note that patients complain far less about seeing the segment when they walk, go up stairs etc., than those with bifocal spectacles. The author's preference is for slightly upcurved fused segments, the particular dimensions being calculated for each case.

Height of segment above the lower edge of the lens

The height of the segment can be stated in two ways:

(1) In relation to the centre of the lens (with a truncated lens this is taken as that of the round lens prior to truncation).
(2) As the height above the lower edge of the finished lens.

The author strongly recommends the second method.

The higher the segment without having any noticeable effect on the distance vision the better. In this way, the amount by which the lens has to rise to allow good near vision is reduced. It has been found, in practice, that the top of the segment can be one-quarter of the pupil diameter above the lower edge of the pupil without causing visual annoyance. In other words, if the pupil diameter is 4.00 mm, the top of the segment can be 1.00 mm above the bottom of the pupil when the patient is looking straight ahead (*Plate 87a*).

It is therefore necessary to measure the distance from the lower lid to the bottom of the pupil and then add one-quarter of the pupil diameter. When the lower lid is below the limbus, a prism ballasted lens — not necessarily a bifocal but one of approximately the correct thickness — should be placed on the eye so that the practitioner may observe the lowest point that the lower edge reaches. The position of the lower edge in relation to the edge of the iris should be noted to aid this measurement. Due to the added weight of a prism ballasted lens, and the fact that a tight lens is unlikely to move sufficiently for a satisfactory visual result, prism ballasted lenses normally rest on the lower lid if this is on or above the limbus. (Occasionally, they will actually depress a flaccid lower lid and an allowance for this may have to be made.) However, it is not very easy to measure this with a scale as the eye does not keep still. An accuracy of 0.50 mm is as much as can normally be attained. The height of the segment is one of the most important factors in the successful fitting of prism ballasted bifocals and an accuracy of 0.10 mm is desirable. Photography is the most accurate method. An ordinary camera with an auxiliary lens may be used at 25–35 cm from the eye, with a scale divided into 0.10-mm divisions placed close to the eye. It is important that this is held at the same distance from the camera as the pupil and iris. The photograph is taken in ordinary room illumination with a flashlight. Fortunately pupil contrac-

tion occurs after the photograph has been taken, so that the normal pupil diameter is recorded. The main disadvantage is waiting for the film to be developed. Ideally, to obtain the measurements most accurately, it should then be projected on to a screen. The author has had a Polaroid camera specially made so that it takes a photograph of the eye five times the normal size (*Figure 16.18*). Special devices have had to be made to ensure that the eye is exactly the correct distance from the camera lens when the photograph is taken; even an error of 1.00 mm would make an appreciable difference in the measurements.

Bifocal trial lenses are also an excellent method of assessing the segment height, as well as other factors. However, unless an extremely large trial set is available, estimation is needed in deciding the segment height. The use of trial lenses also enables a subjective visual check on the segment height to be carried out. It is not possible with trial lenses to adhere exactly to the rule of the segment top being one-quarter of the pupil diameter above the bottom of the pupil, but the segment height may be varied by pushing the lens upwards with the lower lid. If the vision with the trial lens is reasonably good, the patient should be able to make valuable comments on the effect of the near portion on his distance vision. An assistant may be able to hold a trial spectacle lens in front of the eye to see if this improves the distance visual acuity. In most cases, the segment may be lowered by pulling down the lower lid. It is essential for the practitioner to be able to see the top of the segment, and this may be done by marking the top line with instant drying waterproof ink or a

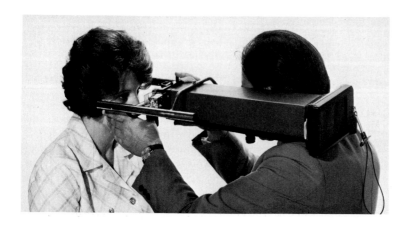

Figure 16.18 Camera designed by the writer for photography of the external eye (photographed by kind permission of Contactasol Ltd)

grease pencil. The entire segment area may also be coloured in with waterproof ink, which has the advantage of permitting the patient to notice a colour change, as soon as the visual axis enters the segment area, thus checking the segment position. This is particularly useful if the trial lens segment is of insufficient power (or even when a single vision trial lens — without a segment — is used). A fluorescent mark may also be used. One advantage of fused bifocals is that the whole segment may be made slightly fluorescent (Bier, 1965), although an ultraviolet lamp is needed to show it up (*Plate 86*). The top of flat-top fused bifocal segments can also be seen quite easily with an ophthalmoscope or slit lamp. It has been suggested that a scale placed in the focal plane of the eyepiece of a slit lamp biomicroscope would be a useful way of determining the segment height. Such graticule eyepieces are available as accessories to most slit lamp biomicroscopes.

If in doubt, it is best to err on the high side when ordering the segment height — but not excessively so, if the patient is not to notice any deleterious effect on his distance vision. The segment may usually be lowered by removing material from the bottom of the lens (i.e. by truncating the lens) but material cannot be added to raise the segment. The segment height may be as small as 2.50 mm above the lower edge, if the lower lid is tight and high above the lower limbus, or as big as 5.00 mm on a large eye with a loose or low lower lid. Giving an average in every case will result in many failures.

Amount of prism ballast and thickness of the lower edge

This can usually be left to the laboratory. *Table 16.3* gives details of average centre thicknesses and prisms. These may need to be modified, for example, if ordering negative lenses for a patient where there is a considerable prescription difference between the two eyes. The prism must normally be the same for the two lenses.

Advocates of small, thin single vision lenses must modify their techniques when fitting bifocals. The extra thickness often helps to keep the lens from riding up every time the patient blinks, which can be so annoying visually; but unnecessary thickness beyond this point usually reduces the comfort, and may give rise to corneal oedema.

The portion of the edge just below the segment is of extreme importance. It is this part of the lens that is pushed upwards by the lower lid when the patient looks down to read. Positive lenses obviously create the biggest problem of how to increase the lower edge thickness without increasing the overall thickness and weight more than is absolutely essential. Unless the patient has a very tight lower lid most positive lenses are better made in a decentred convex carrier lenticular form (*Figure 16.19*). This keeps the weight down but increases the lower edge thickness.

The greater the prism the poorer the focimeter image. However, in many cases, this would appear to be preferable to the alternatives of either a very thick lens or a lens which does not ride up when the patient is reading because the lens slips under the lower lid. For the same reason, no lower edge thinning should be attempted except on very high negative lenses. This gives an edge similar to the one shown in *Figure 16.20*, which would seem to be a highly undesirable edge to those who have studied edge forms for single vision lenses (Shanks, 1966). In practice, it is found that — provided that this unusual edge does not continue right around the lens and there is a normal corneal lens edge at the top — the lens is perfectly comfortable to wear and, when inserted, quickly rotates to the correct position.

Vertical total diameter

The factors determining the vertical total diameter are quite different from those that determine the total diameter of a single vision lens. The main factor is that the lens must be

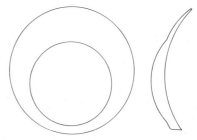

Figure 16.19 Positive lens with a prism ballasted convex carrier peripheral portion and decentred downwards with respect to the base of the prism. Such a lens has a sufficiently thick lower edge to rest on the lower lid without being excessively heavy and may therefore be made in bifocal form

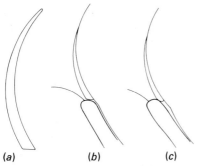

(a)   (b)   (c)

Figure 16.20 (*a*) Diagrammatic representation of the ideal inferior edge shape in a prism ballasted lens to be made in bifocal form. (*b*) The 'square' edge shown in (*a*) rests on the lower lid (shown in cross-section) and moves upwards and downwards on the cornea as the eye is depressed or elevated. (*c*) Excessive rounding of the inferior edge enables the lens to pass behind the lower lid and the near portion may not then move in front of the pupil on depression of the gaze

able to move vertically by not less than half the pupil diameter. This is to enable the lens to rise upwards from the position where the segment covers one-quarter of the pupil diameter to covering three-quarters of the pupil diameter as shown in *Plate 87*. If the lens has more movement than this, it may be considered excessive. If there is less movement than this, the patient will have near vision difficulty. Trial lenses can also be a help in assessing the vertical total diameter.

The practitioner new to prism ballasted bifocals usually visualizes them moving as illustrated in *Figure 16.21*. On closer examination, it can be seen that this is not normally possible. A lens of 8.00 mm total diameter on an

11.50 mm diameter cornea can move approximately 4.00 mm, allowing for the fact that it is on a curved surface. However, if the pupil diameter is 4.00 mm, an average size for a presbyopic patient, it will be seen that the pupil can only be covered entirely by the distance or near portions if the lens has moved from the extreme lower area of the cornea to the extreme upper area; also there is no room on this lens for peripheral and intermediate curves so that a situation of completely alternating vision is only possible when the pupil is very small. For most patients, we must accept the fact that there will be a combination of 'alternating vision' and 'bivision'.

Figure 16.22 shows a larger lens where the upper edge of the near portion coincides with the lower edge of the pupil. However, the lens is only able to move vertically by 2.00 mm, and on a 4.00 mm pupil this means that only half the pupil area is covered by the near portion when the patient looks down for near vision.

In *Figure 16.23*, the top of the near portion covers 1.00 mm of the 4.00 mm pupil when the lens is in the low position. When the lens rises by 2.00 mm, the near portion covers 3.00 mm of the 4.00 mm pupil. It can be shown mathematically that when this lens is in the position for maximum distance vision, 80% of the pupil area is covered by the distance portion of the lens. Similarly, when the lens is in the near position, 80% of the pupil area is covered by the near portion. This is the method of fitting preferred by the author.

Prism ballasted bifocals can be truncated, but

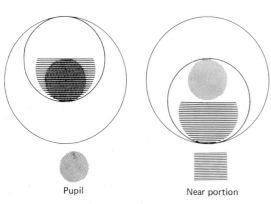

Pupil   Near portion

Figure 16.21 The theoretical ideal for a bifocal contact lens where the entire distance portion is centred before the pupil for distance (right) and the entire near portion centred for close work (left)

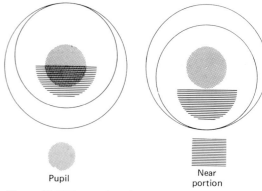

Pupil   Near portion

Figure 16.22 In practice, a lens made with the top of the near portion level with the bottom of the pupil (right) usually only covers half of the pupil when the gaze is depressed (left)

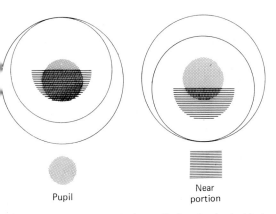

Pupil

Near portion

Figure 16.23 A compromise is usually found to be the ideal so that 80% of the pupil area is covered by the distance portion of the lens during distance vision (right) and a similar proportion is covered by the segment during near vision (left). (*See also Plates 86 and 87*)

this does not necessarily keep them in their correct position. In fact, some lenses of this type have occasionally rotated through 180° showing no tendency to return to the normal position. One advantage of a truncation is to increase the area of edge to be raised by the lower lid, but edge thickness and shape are probably of greater importance. The truncation should preferably not be straight but slightly curved to match the radius of curvature of the lower lid (*Figure 16.24*). Examination of photographs of the eye has shown this radius to be between 15.0 and 21.0 mm. A radius of 18.0 mm is a good average.

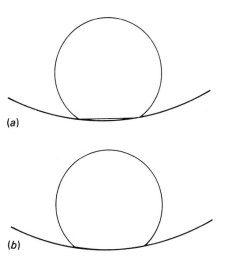

(a)

(b)

Figure 16.24 The lower edge of a truncated prism ballasted lens should not be straight as shown in (*a*) but curved to match the line of the lower lid as shown in (*b*)

Lenses may be stabilized by other means (Gates, Ewell and Remba, 1961), the principal methods are as follows:

(1) An oval lens or a double truncation. The BOZR should be approximately the same as the keratometer reading at 180° if it is intended to keep the long axis horizontal. It must be remembered that there is a strong tendency for the long axis of the lens to settle along the meridian of the cornea with a similar curvature and for this reason the method is unsuitable in cases of oblique or 'against-the-rule' astigmatism.

(2) A spherical BOZR combined with toroidal peripheral curves on the back surface (only appropriate for toroidal corneas).

(3) A small metal weight embedded in the plastics near the edge, which should rotate to the 6 o'clock position, but this is rarely, if ever, used and is not hygienic.

Methods (1), (2) and (3) all lose the advantage of the prism ballasted lens for bifocals, namely, increased thickness at the lower edge to enable the lower lid to raise the lens. Methods (1) and (2) also have the disadvantage that the lenses can fit in two positions at 180° to each other, so that a bifocal near portion would be correct in one position but upside down in the other.

Adjusting prism ballasted bifocal lenses

A number of adjustments are possible to these lenses; despite the most accurate measurements, it is often necessary to adjust them to obtain the best possible results. The following are the most common problems and the adjustments that will usually correct them.

Good distance vision with poor near vision

Assuming that the reason is not an incorrect prescription, it is usually due to the near portion not covering the pupil sufficiently when the patient looks downwards. This may be caused by one of the following:

(1) If the lens is unable to move up sufficiently when the patient's gaze is directed downwards. The adjustment in this case would be to remove material from the top of the lens in order to reduce the vertical total

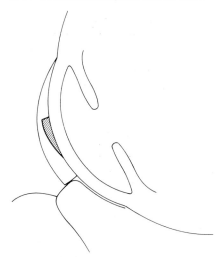

Figure 16.25 A fused bifocal which rises too high on the depression of gaze causes the patient to look through the distance portion below the segment as well as partly through the segment

diameter to allow the lens to ride up higher or, if the lens is not moving up to the upper limbus, to flatten the back surface intermediate and peripheral curves at the upper part of the lens. It is not essential — and, in fact, is often inadvisable — to flatten these curves all the way round the lens. By carefully masking the lower portion of the lens on the back surface with thin tape and then holding the lens on to the appropriate tool of the adjustment kit, it is possible to flatten the curves only at the top of the back surface of the lens. Sometimes, a reduction in both total diameter and flattening of the curves is needed.

(2) If the near portion rises too high when the patient looks down, the patient will look partly through the near portion and partly through the area below the segment (*Figure 16.25*). This tends to happen particularly if the patient's lower lid is well above the lower limbus. In this condition, it is important to have as little non-optical area below the near portion as possible. The method of rectification is to remove material from the bottom of the lens, but not so much that the lower edge actually cuts into the near portion. This is usually done by a slightly curved truncation, and it is recommended that no more than 0.50 mm is removed before trying out the lens again. If necessary, more can be removed; but if too

much material is removed, a new lens will have to be ordered, so it is better to do a little at a time. The vertical extent of the near portion is often no greater than the pupil diameter, and sometimes smaller. It is very important that this is positioned as closely as possible over the pupil area when the patient looks down in his normal position for near work. A difference of 0.50 mm up or down can often make a great deal of difference. As the horizontal width is often considerably larger than the pupil diameter, a little movement laterally is usually of small consequence visually. It is also surprising that it is often possible for the lens to twist considerably on the cornea and for the patient still to obtain good vision. The critical factor seems to be how much of the pupil area is covered by the near portion when it is required to see at near.

Good near vision with poor distance vision

This is almost certainly caused by the near portion being too high and covering too large an area of the pupil. First, it is important to determine whether this is due to the near portion height being too great or to the lens settling above the lower lid when the gaze is directed straight ahead. If it is the former, the only adjustment possible is to remove material from the lower edge so that if the lens continues to rest on the lower lid the segment height will be lowered by the same amount that is removed from the lower edge of the lens. If it is the latter, there is no one answer. High-riding single vision lenses often settle higher still if the intermediate and peripheral curves on the back surface are flattened, and a steeper lens is required to achieve better centration. This may apply to bifocals; but generally, the increased weight due to the prism helps the lens to settle low so that flattening the intermediate and peripheral curves may have the desired effect.

If not, re-ordering a lens with an increased prism is indicated.

Poor vision due to excessive lens movement

Thinning the edge on the front surface, being careful not to reduce the lower edge thickness, may help. However, it is nearly always necessay to order a larger lens by at least 0.50 mm. (The total diameter can always be reduced later, if necessary.)

General discomfort

It would be wrong to assume that a prism ballasted bifocal is far more uncomfortable than a normal single vision lens. The edge should be checked with a microscope (*see* Chapter 12) to make sure that there are no sharp areas. Although a truncated edge is flat its intersection with front and back surfaces should be well polished and the lateral limits of the truncation should be well rounded. The intermediate and peripheral back surface curves should be adjusted in the usual way, if necessary; but care must be taken to ensure that the BOZD is not reduced. It is always advisable to make several small adjustments — trying the lens on the eye in between — rather than one large adjustment.

Diffractive bifocals

Recently introduced as the Diffrax lens by Pilkington, these were first described by Freeman and Stone in 1987 followed by clinical papers on their use and fitting by Walker and Churms (1987), Churms *et al.* (1987), and by Stone (1988). Of those patients accepted as suitable at initial assessment, a success rate of 75% is reported by Walker and Churms.

Available lens parameters are given in *Table 16.4*, and standard fitting sets consist of 16 lenses, all with +2.00 D near addition, 8 each of distance BVP +3.00 D and −3.00 D. With both positive and negative lenses the range of effective BOZRs in the fitting set is from 7.4 to

Table 16.4 Parameters of the Diffrax lens

Material type	Polycon II (*Dk* = 12 Fatt units)
BOZD (mm)	7.00
TD (mm)	9.50
BOZR (equivalent) (mm)	7.00–8.40 in 0.10-mm steps
Hologram diameter (mm)	5.00
Back peripheral zone	5 curves giving AEL 0.11 ± 0.01 mm, REL 0.09 mm
Near additions (D)	+1.00 to +3.00 in 0.50-D steps
Distance BVP (D)	−10.00 to +8.00 in 0.25-D steps
Centre thickness (mm)	Varying from 0.12 at −10.00 D
Edge thickness (mm)	0.12 (radial)

8.1 mm in 0.1-mm steps, but the available range is from 7.0 mm to 8.4 mm.

The BOZR over the diffractive zone or hologram is referred to as the 'effective' or 'equivalent' BOZR because it is a non-existent curve (*Figure 16.26*). Freeman (1987, personal communication) has drawn the analogy between that and a tiled roof: the tiles are set at one angle and yet the roof angle which they create is different. The 'effective' BOZR is comparable to the 'roof angle' and the diffractive zones are analogous to the 'tiles'. The number of diffractive zones, which appear as rings (*Figure 16.27*), varies with the near addition power, being 6, 8, 11, 14 and 17 for near addition values of +1.00 D, +1.50 D, +2.00 D, +2.50 D and +3.00 D, respectively.

The lens is fitted like a single vision lens with apical and peripheral clearance. The diffractive zone is designed to give the correct near addition power effect in tears, so apical clearance is essential. Pilkington recommend that the first lens selected for fitting should have an effective BOZR 0.1 mm steeper than the flattest keratometer reading for corneal astigmatism of up to 2 D, and 0.2 mm steeper for corneal astigmatism

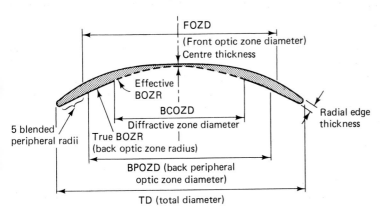

FOZD (Front optic zone diameter)
Centre thickness
Effective BOZR
BCOZD
Diffractive zone diameter
True BOZR (back optic zone radius)
5 blended peripheral radii
Radial edge thickness
BPOZD (back peripheral optic zone diameter)
TD (total diameter)

Figure 16.26 Cross-section of a negative powered Diffrax lens

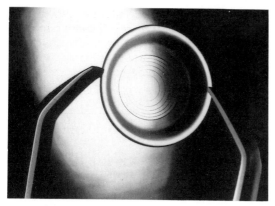

Figure 16.27 A Diffrax lens with a near addition of +1.00 D, having six rings or diffractive zones. (Reproduced by kind permission of Pilkington)

of 2–3 D. It is essential to get good centration to within 1 mm, and movement with blinking should be within 1.5 mm. The fitting recommendations may have to be varied to achieve this.

Because of the apical clearance method of fitting, and the fact that RGP materials flex more on toroidal corneas when fitted steeper than flattest K reading (*see* Chapter 10), highly toroidal corneas cannot be fitted satisfactorily with this lens. However the material is more rigid than some RGP materials, and this, coupled with the broad midperipheral bearing area leads to less flexure than expected.

From the wearer's point of view the lens acts as a simultaneous vision bifocal with the advantage that variations in pupil size do not affect the 1:1 ratio between distance and near images which occur with concentric simultaneous vision bifocals. The slight background blur due to the non-focused image gives rise to a small loss of contrast, as with all lenses of this type, and this precludes the fitting of people with existing degraded vision due to media opacities or macular changes. Most patients adapt to this slight reduction in contrast within 3–4 weeks. If the lens does decentre the out-of-focus image can form a blurred 'ghost' image above or below the observed image, according to whether the lens is displaced up or down respectively, during near vision. In distance vision a reverse movement of the 'ghost' image occurs, but it is rarely noticed at distance, and at near it is usually only conspicuous with black print on a white background. It is more definite with the lower

near additions because of the small dioptric difference between the two foci. The absence or presence of this ghost image, and its location with respect to the clear image, forms a useful subjective clinical guide to the position of the lens during near vision. Because this effect is rarely noticed in distance vision, good centration of the lens is more important during near vision than during distance vision. As most lenses tend to move up as the gaze is depressed for near vision, a lens which positions a little low with the eye in the primary position is preferable to a high riding lens. Thus lenses with the centre of gravity well forward such as positive lenses and those with flatter BOZRs (*see* Chapter 10) are likely to perform slightly better for near vision than negative lenses and those with steep BOZRs (Stone, 1988).

Patients with continuous excessively critical visual tasks to perform may find that near vision with the lenses is just not quite good enough, although the majority of wearers can achieve N5.

Careful binocular balancing of distance and near powers is emphasized, particularly if the near addition is a low one, to prevent the accommodative mechanism 'hunting' between one image and the other — which can cause confusion. This applies to any simultaneous vision bifocal lens. The greater the presbyopia and the higher the near addition, the less this is likely to occur.

Occasionally slight lateral lens decentration can lead to a three-dimensional effect when reading, making the print stand clear of the page. This is a binocular effect and is usually due to temporal displacement of one or both lenses as the person looks down and in to read. The background ghost image is then displaced nasally on each retina, which is interpreted binocularly as coming from a more remote point than the object of regard (Stone, 1988). Again this is a feature common to all simultaneous vision bifocal contact lenses.

As with all RGP lenses they should only be fitted to those who are physiologically suitable — adequate tears being essential. The diffractive zone has a fine ripple effect of a few micrometres depth (less than that of many scratches) which may encourage deposition of debris if careful cleaning is not carried out. The lens should be inserted carefully so that no central air bubbles are entrapped which would render the diffractive zone optically incorrect, as well as breaking up into froth and giving rise to dimpling of the central corneal epithelium.

Existing wearers of PMMA and RGP lenses adapt more quickly to the optical effect of the lens than do previous non-wearers, whose initial foreign body reaction of increased tear output can cause excessive movement of the lens leading to ghost images, but this applies to all rigid simultaneous vision bifocals. Physical adaptation to a single vision lens first may be necessary for some patients.

The main problem the author has found has been to obtain good near vision with some patients, and this is probably when the patient has relatively large pupils so that light enters the eye from beyond the 5.00 mm central holographic zone. This area has the distance prescription only and the 1:1 ratio between distance and near images cannot then be maintained.

The methods of verifying the lens parameters are covered in Chapter 12, but because of its unique optical design some comments on methods of checking the BVP and near addition are appropriate here.

Checking distance BVP and near addition

The lens is designed to give the correct power effect in tears, so that in air the reversed chromatic aberration due to the diffractive element shows up giving rise to several coloured images. This results in several prescriptions being read on the focimeter, the middle one being exactly equidistant between the two extremes. None of them is the distance or near back vertex power, but if so interpreted could make the near addition appear to be considerably more than ordered. To obtain the true near addition a hard single vision contact lens which has a front surface of approximately the same radius as the back surface of the Diffrax lens should be selected. A drop of water is then placed in the back diffractive surface of the bifocal and the hard lens dropped into it. The lenses should stick together without a bubble. It will then be found that the true near addition is easily assessed, being the difference between the two power readings now obtained on the focimeter, the intermediate power having disappeared. The Diffrax lens is then dried and placed on the focimeter in air. Having estab-

lished the correct near addition power (also determined by counting the diffractive zones — see Chapter 12) the distance BVP is found by subtracting twice the near addition power from the maximum positive (green) focimeter reading in air.

Scleral bifocal lenses

These are now almost of historic interest only. However, it is remotely possible that the advent of rigid gas permeable materials will lead to their reintroduction.

All the forms of corneal lens bifocals are theoretically possible with scleral lenses. The type recommended by the author is an upcurved near portion worked on the back surface. This design has been suggested by Hodd (1967) for corneal lenses but has the disadvantage that the back surface may be unacceptable in contact with the cornea. However, as the back optic surface of a scleral lens clears the cornea, this does not apply; and there is a major advantage in that the lens can be made in distance form first. The BOZR should be up to 0.25 mm steeper than would normally be ordered but with the usual apical clearance, so some slight limbal touch can be expected. The lens can be adjusted, if necessary, and a line then marked on the front optic surface one-quarter of the pupil diameter above the lower pupil margin. The lens is returned to the laboratory for a second back optic radius (BOR) to be cut and polished, decentred inferiorly (*Figure 16.28*). For example:

BOZR	8.00 mm
Near add	+2.25 D
Second BOR	9.05 mm

This will ease the limbal touch considerably. The lens should be fitted and allowed to settle before any further adjustments are considered.

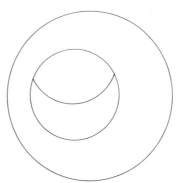

Figure 16.28 Upcurve back surface solid bifocal scleral lens

Adjustments to aid the comfort of the lens at this stage may affect the visual performance.

If the lens is not being raised sufficiently for the patient to obtain good near vision when the direction of gaze is lowered, the vertical total diameter should be reduced by removing material from the upper edge. Not more than 1.00 mm should be removed at a time. Increasing the inferior limbal clearance may also help slightly.

If the near portion is too high and affecting the distance vision, removal of material from the lower edge should help to lower the lens slightly. Care must be taken, because if too much material is removed it is possible for the lower edge to rise above the lower lid on an upward gaze and to hold the lower lid down when looking normally again. Removing material from the lower back scleral surface or increasing the superior limbal clearance should also help to lower the lens slightly.

Multifocal contact lenses

The first multifocal contact lens, to the author's knowledge, was made by accident. In 1958, Jessen, of America (personal communication), suggested that it should be possible to make and fit a concentric back surface bifocal by fitting a single vision corneal lens corrected to the patient's near vision and then setting this up on a lathe and cutting a small steep central curve on the back surface. This necessitated removing approximately 0.01–0.02 mm of material, which was extremely difficult. Polishing this area was even more difficult. When the final lenses were checked, it was found that the focimeter target remained in focus over a range of 8 D, although fainter than normal. By blending the two curves together, a multifocal lens had inadvertently been produced with a range of focus from infinity to about 25 cm. Unfortunately, the side-effects experienced with this lens were so great that it was not a practical proposition.

In 1972, Wesley, of America, suggested a new lens that was almost identical in concept to the one described above, that had been made accidentally 16 years before. The idea had been forgotten and by strange coincidence, was re-invented by Dr Jessen's partner Newton K. Wesley. The new lenses should succeed where others failed because of new methods of manufacture. This lens is the result of research

into fitting using the PEK method (*see* Chapters 6, 7 and 10).

In 1959, Jessen (personal communication) produced a lens which was a combination of a back surface concentric bifocal and a front surface concentric bifocal. By making the diameter of the distance portion on the back surface smaller than the distance portion on the front surface, a trifocal effect was achieved.

Söhnges (1962, 1963) developed a blended multifocal lens on the front surface consisting of a small central distance portion and concentric rings 0.50 mm wide, each ring 0.50 D more positive in power than the one before it, so that the positive addition increased gradually towards the edge of the lens.

The problem with any type of blended multifocal lens, or varifocal lens, must be that the majority of the light entering the pupil has passed through an optical area that is not correctly focused for the distance in use. There is a sharp image with a blurred image superimposed over it. This also happens with the de Carle concentric back surface bifocal and the Diffrax lens, but to a lesser extent, and the patient usually learns to accept the side-effects and ignore them. The greater the varifocal effect the greater the side-effects. The brain can ignore the side-effects to some extent (the fact that we are not normally aware of our blind spot in monocular vision is proof of that) but patients are unable to adapt if the side-effects are too obvious.

These comments also apply to another back surface bifocal, the Presbycon lens, developed by Compucon Contact Lens Laboratory in the USA. It is a corneal lens having an entirely aspherical back surface with three possible variations of that asphericity. The peripheral flattening of the back surface provides a continuously variable near addition. Due to the rapid degree of flattening the posterior apical radius of the lens is fitted some 0.20–0.25 mm steeper than the flattest corneal keratometer reading (El Hage, 1976). To provide maximum near addition the greatest degree of peripheral flattening, or asphericity must be used, and this can result in too mobile a lens even though fitted centrally steeper than the cornea. In general, results with the lens are reported to be good, and it has even been used to relieve symptoms of near esophoria and esotropia in young patients (El Hage and Cook, 1976).

From the author's experience, it is preferable, for good vision, for the area in front of the pupil to be at least 60% of one power so that using a combination of alternating vision and bivision, a trifocal lens should be possible in many cases, particularly if the pupil diameter is not greater than 4.00 mm.

Hydrophilic bifocal contact lenses

With the increased usage of hydrophilic contact lenses it was inevitable that attention would turn to manufacturing bifocal and multifocal lenses in this interesting material. A fused hydrophilic bifocal lens has not been made but all the solid designs that have been made in hard materials have been made in hydrophilic form. One advantage is that the larger total diameter enables the practitioner to achieve better control of centration and lens movement.

Simultaneous vision bifocals

These are concentric bifocals and rely for their success, on good centration and patients with larger than average pupil sizes. The CIBA Bi-Soft lens was the first lens of this type to be approved in the USA by the Food and Drugs Administration (FDA) and has a distance portion of approximately 3.20 mm diameter. Unfortunately, one diameter is not suitable for everyone. The author has used small specialist laboratories to make concentric bifocals with distance portions varying from 2.20 mm to 4.00 mm. Lenses with unusual dimensions can also be ordered to try and improve the visual result. For example, if a lens settles inferiorly, the patient may find reading in the normal position difficult but excellent above eye level. A larger or steeper lens can often help achieve better centration.

The majority of the simultaneous vision lenses fitted are of this type but there is one interesting alternative. The Alges bifocal has a central near portion similar to the lens first tried in 1951 by Williamson-Noble and uses the principle of pupil constriction with close work. The diameters originally available for the near portions were small, 2.12 mm and 2.35 mm, probably to avoid the dangers from poor distance vision. Unfortunately, some patients found that their vision for close work was not helped because their pupils were too large. The author found that his vision for close work was actually worse with a lens having a 2.35 mm portion than with a simple distance lens of the same prescription. To overcome this problem three larger near portions are now available: 2.55 mm, 3.00 mm and 3.50 mm.

Obviously, the smaller the near portion the better. When driving, for example, patients should be advised to wear sunglasses, where appropriate, to avoid the situation of sudden pupil constriction and blurred distance vision should the sun shine on the drivers' eyes.

The Alges bifocal is available with BOZR values of 8.60 and 8.90 mm with a total diameter of 14.00 mm.

Some practitioners have tried one lens of each design on the same patient, fitting a concentric lens with a central distance portion on the dominent eye and a central near portion on the non-dominant eye. This interesting idea overcomes some of the criticisms of monovision, and of bifocals with central near portions.

Translating or alternating vision bifocals

The Bausch & Lomb Cresent bifocals and the Wesley–Jessen bifocals with an upswept crescent near portion which are prevented from rotating by a base-down prism and truncation, are typical of many lenses of this type now available. Some lenses, such as the Bausch & Lomb Crescent bifocals have additional features such as a negative angle truncation but the basic principles are the same (*Figure 16.29*). *Table 16.5* shows the parameters available for the Bausch & Lomb upcurve crescent bifocal. Small specialist laboratories are often prepared to make similar lenses beyond the range of parameters available from the large laboratories.

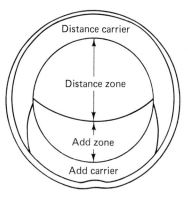

Figure 16.29 Bausch & Lomb crescent bifocal

Table 16.5 Available parameters of the Bausch & Lomb crescent bifocal

Material	Hefilcon B
Water content (%)	45
Manufacture	Lathe cut
BOZR (mm)	8.6 and 8.9
Centre thickness (mm)	0.30–0.39 (plano to +6.00 D)
	0.29–0.16 (−0.25 D to −6.00 D)
Total diameters (mm)	14.00: −0.25 D to −6.00 D
	13.5: plano to +6.00 D
Distance powers (D)	−5.00 to +5.00 in 0.25 steps
	±5.50 and ±6.00
Near add (D)	+1.50, +2.00, +2.50

Madden & Layman Ltd manufacture a similar lens — the R segment soft bifocal lens (*see Plate 88a* and *b*) in which the segment top may be specified at any position. It is normally fitted 0.50 mm flatter than the flattest K reading and can be supplied with the segment top unmarked, or marked in blue or brown, the latter fading away after a minute.

Fitting requirements

(1) The lens must move upwards easily when the patient looks down.
(2) The lens must resume the normal position immediately upon looking straight ahead.
(3) The vertical lens movement when looking straight ahead must be minimal.
(4) The lens must settle quickly in the correct position and not rotate.

Practitioners are strongly advised to try all types of bifocal contact lenses on their own eyes. It is not necessary to be presbyopic to notice the side-effects. This particularly applies to translating bifocals. They can be excellent but fitting the lens so that the near portion does not cover the pupil immediately after a blink when looking straight ahead, is sometimes difficult.

The vertical translation of the lens for close work is mainly controlled by the lower lid. As the position of the lower lid varies from over 1.00 mm below the corneal limbus to over 1.00 mm above, the effectiveness is bound to vary considerably. Consequently, as many lenses are only available in a very small range of total diameters, with variables such as the height of the near portion often fixed at one position only, one particular type of lens will be unsuitable for a large number of patients. This

can be partly overcome by using lenses from several manufacturers.

With hard and gas permeable lenses many adjustments are possible and can often make the difference between a successful and an unsuccessful fitting. With hydrophilic lenses no adjustments are possible. Fitting becomes a matter of trial and error and the more different trial lenses which are available the greater the chance of success.

The height of the near portion in relation to the geometric centre is important. With a combination of a high lower lid and lid tightness, the lens is likely to settle 1.00–2.00 mm above a normal position and the near portion is likely to interfere with the distance vision. A lens with an equal amount of extra truncation may prevent this, provided that the smaller vertical diameter does not allow the lens to move excessively. Alternatively, a lens with the same specification but the near portion further below the geometric centre may achieve the same result without unwanted movement.

The reverse situation can occur, with a very loose lower lid, or a lower lid 1.00 mm or more below the corneal limbus, or a combination of both factors. The lens may then settle below the normal position when looking straight ahead and not translate sufficiently when the patient looks down. A larger lens or a lens with a steeper back surface could make it centre properly but the vertical movement might then be reduced so that it did not translate sufficiently when looking down for close work. A lens with the near portion closer to the geometric centre or even above it should then be tried.

The fitting of translating bifocals is not easy and many practitioners try a few standard lenses and then change to simultaneous vision bifocals or monovision if they do not appear to be successful almost immediately.

Concentric 'multifocal' lenses

These rely on the simultaneous vision principle and therefore require good centration and a fairly large pupil size.

By using an aspherical back surface it is possible to produce a lens with the distance power in the centre and the near power progressively stronger outwards from the centre (the reverse of the CALS and PS45 lenses — *see* p. 604). Two soft lenses of this type are the

Hydrocurve II bifocal contact lens and the Bausch & Lomb PA1 lens which has a nominal +1.25 D addition.

Lenses of this type should be tried when the patient requires the lenses primarily for social reasons. The intermediate power is useful, for example, for playing cards and the piano. However, patients requiring lenses for sustained reading will probably prefer bifocal lenses to these 'multifocals'. It is possible, however, to fit this type of lens on the monovision principle, by making the lens for the non-dominant eye +0.50 D to ±1.00 D too strong centrally, which slightly blurs distance vision but allows good intermediate and near vision, the dominant eye achieving good distance and intermediate vision.

Fitting sets

The large successful contact lens practice will have no difficulty in purchasing a variety of sets so that many different types of bifocal lenses can be offered (*Tables 16.4–16.9*). For the practitioner with a small contact lens practice the financial outlay would not be justified. How then can bifocal contact lens fitting be started?

One way is to order one or a pair of bifocals basing the specification on the best fitting single vision lens of a similar material and total diameter. For example, if a hard bifocal contact lens is required the choice might be between a fused bifocal and a Diffrax bifocal. The lenses are so different that it would not be practical to wear one type on one eye and the other type on the other eye. However, one of each could be ordered for the same eye and the second lens ordered after a short trial in the consulting room comparing the lenses. One advantage over a

fitting set is that the prescription should be correct, which should give the patient a much better idea of the visual performance than a fitting lens with an additional spectacle lens held in front.

Lenses not used will form the basis of a useful fitting set. The practitioner is advised to quote a total fee at least 60% more than the fee for single vision lenses.

Hard and rigid gas permeable bifocal fitting sets

A fitting set of fused bifocals (*Table 16.6*), although not essential, is most useful as the top of the segment shows very clearly, which helps considerably in judging both the correct segment height and the correct amount of lens movement. If necessary the lens may then be ordered in another form, for example, the two lenses shown in *Figure 16.14d,e*. It is suggested that the basic fitting set should consist of round lenses only, but truncated lenses are sometimes required for patients with high lower lids, and a second set of truncated lenses would certainly be very useful, as shown in *Table 16.7*.

Details of the fitting set used for fitting Diffrax lenses has already been given on p. 615. These are essential when prescribing that type of bifocal contact lens.

Hydrophilic bifocal fitting sets

If only one set of lenses could be afforded it would be preferable to make up a set with a few lenses of several types rather than a full range of one type. For suggestions of such hydrophilic bifocal lenses *see Table 16.8. Table 16.9* gives details of a few comprehensive fitting sets available from some of the larger laboratories.

Table 16.6 Basic fused bifocal fitting set

BOZR (mm)	*BOZD* (mm)	*BPR$_1$* (mm)	*TD* (mm)	
7.20	7.00	7.80	8.80	BPR$_2$ 12.25 mm
7.35	7.00	7.95	8.90	All lenses round
7.50	7.00	8.10	9.00	Segment on datum
7.65	7.25	8.35	9.10	Suggested *Rx*: Distance plano
7.80	7.25	8.50	9.20	Near addition +2.50 D
7.95	7.25	8.65	9.30	Prism: 2 Δ base-down
8.10	7.50	8.90	9.40	Upper edge as thin as possible
8.25	7.50	9.05	9.50	Lower edge as shown in *Figure 16.20a*
8.40	7.50	9.20	9.60	

Table 16.7 Additional truncated fused bifocal fitting set

BOZR (mm)	BOZD (mm)	BPR₁ (mm)	Horizontal TD (mm)	Truncation	
7.20	7.00	7.80	9.00	0.70	BPR₂: 12.25 mm
7.35	7.00	7.95	9.10	0.75	Radius of truncation 18.00 mm as
7.50	7.00	8.10	9.20	0.80	shown in *Figure 16.24b*
7.65	7.25	8.35	9.30	0.85	Segment on datum before truncation
7.80	7.25	8.50	9.40	0.90	Suggested *Rx*: Distance plano
7.95	7.25	8.65	9.50	0.95	Near addition +2.50 D
8.10	7.50	8.90	9.60	1.00	Prism: 2Δ base-down
8.25	7.50	9.05	9.70	1.05	Upper edge as thin as possible
8.40	7.50	9.20	9.80	1.10	Lower edge as shown in *Figure 16.20a*

Table 16.8 A minimum selection of various types of hydrophilic bifocal fitting lenses

Barnes-Hind Hydrocurve II

BOZR (mm)	TD (mm)	Distance Rx (D)	Near add (D)
9.00	14.80	−3.00	Fixed
9.00	14.80	+3.00	Fixed

Bausch & Lomb PA1

BOZR (mm)	TD (mm)	Distance Rx (D)	Near add (D)
Varies	13.50	−3.00	Fixed at a nominal value
with *Rx*	13.50	+3.00	of +1.25 D

CIBA Bi-Soft

BOZR (mm)	TD (mm)	Distance Rx (D)	Near add (D)
8.30	13.80	−3.00	+2.50
8.60	13.80	−3.00	+2.50
8.60	13.80	+3.00	+2.50
8.90	13.80	+3.00	+2.50

Alges

BOZR (mm)	TD (mm)	Distance Rx (D)	Near add (D)	Diameter (mm)
8.60	14.00	−3.00	+2.50	2.35
8.60	14.00	−3.00	+2.50	3.00
8.90	14.00	+3.00	+2.50	2.35
8.90	14.00	+3.00	+2.50	3.00

Bausch & Lomb Crescent

BOZR (mm)	TD (mm)	Distance Rx (D)	Near add (D)
8.60	14.00	−3.00	+2.50
8.90	14.00	−3.00	+2.50
8.60	14.00	+3.00	+2.50
8.90	14.00	+3.00	+2.50

Table 16.9 Some comprehensive fitting sets of bifocal hydrophilic lenses as available from some of the larger laboratories

---

Barnes-Hind Hydrocurve II

---

30 and 50 lens fitting sets are available in a range of powers
For parameters *see Table 16.8*

Bausch & Lomb PA1
Available in distance powers of up to ±6.00 D   4 lenses
As in *Table 16.8* but two lenses of each distance power
12 and 24 lens fitting sets are also available

CIBA Bi-Soft
Available in distance powers of up to ±7.00 D   12 lenses
with near additions of +1.50 D to +3.00 D in 0.25 D steps
TD of 13.00 and 13.80 mm
FCOZD of 3.2 and 3.8 mm

BOZR (mm)	TD (mm)	Distance Rx (D)	Near add (D)
8.30	13.80	−3.00	+2.00
8.30	13.80	−3.00	+2.50
8.30	13.80	−3.00	+3.00
8.60	13.80	−3.00	+2.00
8.60	13.80	−3.00	+2.50
8.60	13.80	−3.00	+3.00
8.60	13.80	+3.00	+2.00
8.60	13.80	+3.00	+2.50
8.60	13.80	+3.00	+3.00
8.90	13.80	+3.00	+2.00
8.90	13.80	+3.00	+2.50
8.90	13.80	+3.00	+3.00

Alges
Available in distance powers of up to ±6.00 D   20 lenses
with near additions of +2.00 D to +3.50 D in 0.50 D steps

BOZR (mm)	TD (mm)	Distance Rx (D)	Near add (D)	Diameter (mm)
8.60	14.00	±3.00	+2.50	2.12
8.60	14.00	±3.00	+2.50	2.35
8.60	14.00	±3.00	+2.50	2.55
8.60	14.00	±3.00	+2.50	3.00
8.60	14.00	±3.00	+2.50	3.50
8.90	14.00	±3.00	+2.50	2.12
8.90	14.00	±3.00	+2.50	2.35
8.90	14.00	±3.00	+2.50	2.55
8.90	14.00	±3.00	+2.50	3.00
8.90	14.00	±3.00	+2.50	3.50

Bausch & Lomb Crescent
Available in powers of up to ±6.00 D   4 lenses
with near additions of +1.50 D, +2.00 D and +2.50 D
As in *Table 16.8*
24 lens fitting set also available

Nissel PS45
Available in powers from +1.50 D to +2.50 D in 0.25 D steps, then 0.50 D steps to +5.50 D
Effective near addition of +2.00 D covering distance powers from −0.50 D to +3.50 D
BOZR 8.70 mm, TD 14.00 mm
Twelve lens fitting set available with two of each power from +1.50 D to +3.00 D in 0.50 D steps and +4.00 D and +5.00 D

References

BIER, N. (1965). Prescribing for presbyopia with contact lenses. *Ophthal. Optician* **5**, 439–454

BREGER, J. L. (1980). Improved bivision contact lens for the treatment of presbyopia. British Patent Application 2086605

BRONSTEIN, L. (1959). Bicon lenses. *CLAO Papers* **1**, 13–20

BRYANT, P. G. (1973). Construction and manufacture of a fused bifocal lens. *Ophthal. Optician* **13**, 1052–1056

CHURMS, P. W., FREEMAN, M. H., MELLING, J., STONE, J. and WALKER, P. J. C. (1987). The development and clinical performance of a new diffractive bifocal contact lens. *Optometry Today* **27**(22), 721–724

COHEN, A. L. (1977). Zonal bifocal contact lens. United States Patent 4162122. Application 1977, granted 14 September 1979

DE CARLE, J. T. (1957). A bifocal contact lens. British Patent 831546. Application 1957, granted 9 April 1958

DE CARLE, J. T. (1959). The de Carle bifocal contact lens. *Contacto* **3**, 5–9

DE CARLE, J. T. (1983). Bifocal contact lenses. British Patent 2129155. Application 1983, granted 20 May 1987

EL HAGE, S. G. (1976). Clinical evaluation of the Presbycon aspheric contact lens. *Int. Contact Lens Clin.* **3**(2), 65–74

EL HAGE, S. G. and COOK, J. L. (1976). The effect of the aspheric Presbycon contact lenses on esophoric patients. *Int. Contact Lens Clin.* **3**(4), 42–47

ERICKSON, P. and ROBBOY, M. (1985). Performance characteristics of a hydrophilic concentric bifocal contact lens. *Am. J. Optom.* **62**, 702–708

EVANS, T. C. (1983). The CALS lens: optical and perceptual considerations in aspheric topography. *Can. J. Optom.* **45**(1), 21–23, 26–27

EVANS, C. H. and EVANS, T. C. (1981). The CALS soft lens: an introductory clinical study. *Can. J. Optom.* **43**(4), 166–169, 190

EVANS, T. C., MAYERS, H. B. and SZABOCSIK, J. M. (1988). The CALS lens/Unilens — a front aspheric hydrogel contact lens for the correction of presbyopia and astigmia. *Optom. Today* **28**, 622–628

FEINBLOOM, W. (1938). United States Patent 2,129,305. Application 21 August, patented 6 September, 1938

FREEMAN, E. (1952). Pinhole contact lenses. *Am. J. Optom.* **29**, 347–352

FREEMAN, M. H. (1981). UK Patent GB2101764B assigned to Pilkington PE Limited

FREEMAN, M. H. and STONE, J. (1987). A new diffractive bifocal contact lens. *Transactions of the British Contact Lens Association Conference*, pp. 15–22

GATES, H., EWELL, D. G. and REMBA, M. J. (1961). Bifocal contact lenses. *Ophthal. Optician* **1**, 1045–1053

GOLDBERG, J. B. (1969). A comprehensive method for fitting monocentric crescent bifocal contact lenses. *Optom. Wkly* **60**, 24–26

GUILBERT, J. (1969a). *Biaptal Bifocal Lenses*. News Bulletin, Laboratories Ysoptic, Paris

GUILBERT, J. (1969b). La lentille bifocale. Paper read at The Contact Lens Society's World Congress, Eastbourne

HODD, F. A .B. (1967). Bifocal and multifocal contact lenses. Presidential address to The Contact Lens Society in *Transactions of The Contact Lens Society 1967–70*, pp. 1–20. Also published (1969). A design study of bifocal corneal contact lenses. *Ophthal. Optician* **9**, 450–454, 467–469, 588–592, 597–560, 644–648, 651–653, 700–702; and published as a monograph with the same title by The British Optical Association

HODD, F. A. B. (1974). Bifocal contact lens practice. *Ophthal. Optician* **14**, 315–320, 325–326, 378–380, 385–388; and published as a monograph with the same title by The British Optical Association

JESSEN, G. N. (1960). Bifocal contact lenses. *Br. J. physiol. Optics* **17**, 217–221

KAPLAN, M. M. (1967). The aplanatic contact lens. *Optom. Weekly* **58**(6), 25–29, 42–45

LOSHIN, D. S., LOSHIN, M. S. and COMER, G. (1982). Binocular summation with monovision contact lens correction for presbyopia. *Int. Contact Lens Clin.* **9**, 161–165

MANDELL, R. B. (1966). *No-Jump Bifocal*. Technical memorandum, Kontur Kontact Lens Co. Inc., U.S.A.

McKAY TAYLOR, C. (1962). The McKay Taylor additive bifocal. *Optician* **143**, 585–587

Plastics Contact Lens Company (1970). British Patent 1,178,211. Application 20 April, 1967, patented 21 January, 1970

SHANKS, K. R. (1966). Subjective comparison of corneal lens edges. *Br. J. physiol. Optics* **23**, 55–58

SÖHNGES, W. P. (1962). Multifocal micro-pupil lens. *Contacto* **6**, 156–159

SÖHNGES, W. P. (1963). British Patent 939,016. Patented 9 October, 1963

SOKEL, E. (1961). Improvements in or relating to corneal lenses. British Patent 910455. Application 1961, granted 14 November 1962

STONE, J. (1988). Experience with the Diffrax lens. *Optician* **195**(5138), 21–23, 25, 28, 33–34, 36

WALKER, P. and CHURMS, P. (1987). The diffractive bifocal contact lens. *Optician* **194**(5117), 21–24

WESLEY, N. K. (1972). Multi focal contact lens. US Patent 3794414. Application 1972, granted 26 February 1974

WILLIAMSON-NOBLE, F. A. (1951). Contact lenses — what of the future? *Br. J. physiol. Optics* **8**, 244–246

Chapter 17

Preformed scleral lens fitting techniques

E. G. Woodward

During the two decades since the first edition of this book appeared, the number of scleral lenses fitted has declined precipitously. In general optometric practice they are rarely fitted, only occasionally in specialist contact lens practice and only in some hospital contact lens clinics. Notwithstanding this, they are part of the contact lens practitioner's armamentarium and a knowledge of their basic principles is essential for the practitioner. There are a significant number of patients still wearing this type of lens and, without an understanding of fitting criteria, proper after-care is not possible. Furthermore, an appreciation of the subtleties of preformed scleral lens fitting gives an understanding of corneal and anterior scleral topography which is not acquired fitting other types of lenses. Finally, development of new materials may lead to a resurrection of this lens type much as happened to corneal lenses when PMMA became available.

The preformed method of fitting scleral contact lenses is one which is difficult to justify in theoretical terms particularly in a country where the use of local anaesthetics by those who are not medical practitioners is legal. Additionally, the great majority of eyes fitted with scleral lenses are of an irregular shape and the basic assumptions on which most of the preformed sets were designed no longer appear to be valid. These factors would suggest that the impression technique is the only successful method of fitting scleral lenses but this has not proved to be the case. The rather surprising survival of the preformed method may be explained in two ways:

(1) Assumptions which have since been proved to be incorrect have nearly all related to the contour of the sclera and hence to the shape of the scleral zone of the lens. Paradoxically in a scleral lens the fit of the portion which rests on the sclera is relatively unimportant. Large departures from a 'glove fit' in the scleral zone cause no problems whatsoever providing the optic zone is well balanced in relation to the cornea geometrically and hydraulically. Tolerance to this departure is explained by distortion and compression of the bulbar conjunctiva concealing large variations in the scleral fit.

(2) Impression techniques have been perfected for many years and now, with modern materials, it is comparatively easy to obtain an accurate reproduction of the anterior surface of the globe. But to produce a wearable lens from the cast demands, not only considerable experience, but a degree of manual dexterity which many practitioners simply do not possess.

Having now established the essentially pragmatic nature of preformed scleral lens fitting, the detailed advantages and limitations of this technique can be considered. However, some mention should first be made regarding new standard terminology. Since previous editions of this book were written, the major change in terminology affecting this chapter is the use of the term 'scleral zone' to replace 'haptic portion'.*

Advantages

(1) Before ordering any lenses specifically for the patient, the practitioner can put on the patient's eye a lens which, even at its worst, is an approximate fit for the eye. Thus, the patient is given the 'feel' of a scleral lens — a most useful experience at the preliminary

*See Glossary of terms at the beginning of the book.

investigation. This is vital for tolerance trials.

(2) Whatever method of fitting is used, a scleral lens is needed to carry out a contact lens refraction. This lens is preformed in so far as the characteristics of the optic zone are known. Use of a corneal lens, or resort to inexact calculations using ocular refraction and keratometer readings, is a poor alternative.

(3) Specifications having been decided upon, the lens can be ordered by telephone or mail. There is no need to send or preserve casts at this stage.

(4) A preformed scleral lens allows the most accurate interpretation of the practitioner's instructions. Even more important, in most cases, the way in which instructions have been obeyed by the manufacturer can be checked.

(5) The specification of a preformed lens is a set of figures. If optic grind-outs or other adjustments have to be made, appropriate alterations can be made to the original specification. Thus, theoretically, it should be possible to reproduce a lens exactly when a replacement lens is necessary. But in actual practice, few if any manufacturers can produce two lenses which have identical specifications and have the same corneal clearance on the eye. Even so, replacement lenses are a comparatively simple proposition.

(6) Some preformed scleral lenses can be turned from solid material, which can give a thinner lens than one moulded over a cast.

(7) In certain cases, such as patients with one blind eye, fitting by the impression technique may become very difficult due to visual fixation problems. The preformed method avoids this. Cases of nystagmus may give better results with preformed lenses, and the taking of impressions on high myopes carries a small but definite risk of retinal detachment.

Limitations

The limitations of the preformed method are mainly financial and organizational. If unlimited funds were available, preformed lenses of every possible combination of parameters could be made in the form of a huge trial case.

This would allow selection of the one correct trial lens, among many thousands, for each eye fitted. In practice, enough trial lenses must be available to make the method feasible without having a prohibitively large number of lenses. With a basic fitting set of eight scleral zone fitting lenses and 28 fenestrated lenses for optic measurement (FLOM), practically any eye worth fitting with preformed lenses can be fitted. If preformed scleral lens fitting is the only method in use, a much larger fitting set is required. Irregular eyes cannot be fitted with preformed lenses unless the latter are subsequently modified so much that they cease to be preformed.

Types of preformed lens

A preformed scleral lens is a contact lens, not an impression lens, whose back surface is of some predetermined form. The latter is a mathematical form, thus excluding from consideration the Dallos 'type shells', which are shells based on impressions of different sizes and shapes of eye (Dallos, 1937). The appropriate 'type' lens is selected on the basis of the type of eye being fitted (*see* Chapter 1).

'True' preformed scleral lenses fall broadly into two main groups, as follows.

(1) Those in which the scleral fitting and optic fitting are done with the same lenses.
(2) Those in which the scleral zone is fitted with one set of lenses and the optic zone fitted with an entirely different type of optic measuring lens.

Group I

Conical lenses

These were developed by William Feinbloom (1936) from 1936 onwards. Each consists of a spherical optic zone, a scleral zone of which the major part is conical, and a crescent on the temporal side which has a spherical curve (*Figure 17.1*).

In the original 'Tangent Cone' series of lenses there were three variables:

(1) The angle of the cone.
(2) The radius of the temporal crescent.
(3) The back scleral size.

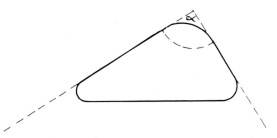

Figure 17.1 Feinbloom conical lens (cone angle $\alpha/2$)

The choice of cone angles was restricted to 43°, 46° and 49°, and the radius of the temporal portion varied from 20 to 38 mm. Later, the range was extended to give a choice of primary optic diameters, and 'double cones' were included to fit toroidal eyes.

These lenses are not usually very comfortable as the lens only rests on the sclera where this is tangential to the conical section — and, except on a very flat scleral curve, this is not a very large area.

Some of these lenses are still being fitted, but they are no longer widely used.

Wide angle lenses

These lenses were introduced by G. Nissel in 1947 and an introductory paper was written by Cowan in 1948 (Jenkin and Tyler-Jones, 1964). The design is a composite one based on the ground spherical lens and the Feinbloom cone lens, the aim being to combine the 'firm scleral fit' of a spherical lens with the good limbal clearance of Feinbloom's cone lens (*Figure 17.2*).

As can be seen in *Figure 17.2*, the optic and scleral zones are spherical but the transition is conical. The 'corneal chord' (BOZD) is standardized at 11.5 mm and the 'limbal chord' at 16 mm. The terms 'corneal' and 'limbal' chord are used rather than the normal nomenclature

because, as the lens is usually pressed out over a master tool, the more usual measurement of the primary optic diameter cannot readily be made. If the lens is produced by cutting from solid, the terms 'back optic zone diameter' and 'peripheral diameter of cone' may be substituted for 'corneal chord' and 'limbal chord' respectively.

The variables in this lens are the back optic zone radius, the back scleral zone radius and the cone angle of the transition. The cone angles vary from 45° to 54° in 1.5° steps for each 0.25 mm change in back optic zone radius from 7.50 to 9.00 mm. Based on the assumption that the best transitional form is one in which the transition is tangential to the back optic curve, an attempt has been made to pair each angle with a particular back optic zone radius. For example, a 7.50 mm back optic zone radius is joined by a transition of cone angle 45°, and a 7.75 mm radius with 46.5° and so on. The selection of these relationships is empirical. The lenses are pressed from master tools with a predetermined scleral form and interchangeable optic zones whose primary sags can be varied. Unless the lens is specially made, there is no choice of the transition cone angle. Another disadvantage with this method of manufacture — the usual one for wide angle lenses — is that after the lens is pressed it is then mounted and the optic zone first ground with a diamond impregnated tool and then polished with a wax polisher. The amount of material removed in this process is an unknown quantity and could vary considerably with the skill of the operator. Thus, lenses with apparently identical specifications could have varying primary sags.

Wide angle hapticon lenses

This lens, developed by S. M. Braff (1965), may be considered as a more sophisticated version of the original wide angle lens. In its production, the die is made up of three parts instead of only two as in the wide angle lens. The extra part is the transitional portion, which in the original version is allowed to free form by suspension over a void. This extra part gives better control over the form of the transition. In the later version of this lens, the transition is no longer a flat angled section but is a spherically arched section. The optic and limbal chords are still kept the same as in the original wide angle series.

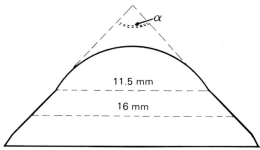

Figure 17.2 Wide angle lens (cone angle $\alpha/2$)

In the manufacture of this lens, after the die and plastics blank have been pre-heated, the blank is moulded to the die under air pressure. This is claimed to give much greater accuracy than the type of hand-operated press and infrared heater lamps commonly used in England to manufacture wide angle lenses.

Group II

Spherical preformed lenses

This type of lens is a direct descendant of the original Zeiss ground lens, developed in 1912–13 (von Rohr and Boegehold, 1934). The lens, in its present form, is based on Bier's transcurve lens (Bier and Cole, 1948), and both back optic and scleral curves are spherical and are joined by a spherical transition whose radius of curvature is the mean of the back optic and scleral radii and of 2 mm width. The great advantage of this type of lens construction is that it lends itself to the method of cutting from solid material. These lenses can probably be made more accurately than any others. Once made, they can also be checked with greater certainty than those which have been pressed out over a die. When fitted, however, they do seem to need more adjustment in the transitional region than some of the other types of lens.

The fit of the optic zone is measured with FLOM lenses as described on p. 635.

Offset lenses

These very interesting lenses, developed by the late A. J. Forknall between 1947 and 1951, were first described in a paper given to the Contact Lens Society in December, 1951 (Forknall, 1953). The basis of their design was the so-called 'spherical rule' connecting the back scleral size with scleral curvature. This rule states that, to maintain the same fit, any increase in back scleral size must be accompanied by a corresponding increase in back scleral zone radius and the converse. Approximately 1.5 mm increase in back scleral size requires 0.25 mm extra on the back scleral zone radius. Forknall drew, on a larger scale, a series of curves following this rule and joined them together with a single curve (*Figure 17.3*).

He found that the resultant curve needed a larger radius than the component radii, and also

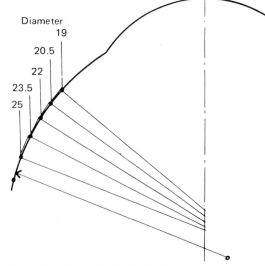

Figure 17.3 Forknall 'offset lens' design

that its centre of curvature had to be 'offset' to the distal side of the axis of symmetry. This was the nature of the curve used in the design of these lenses. There have been two sets of offset lenses: the original ones were used for several years and then Forknall decided that they tended to give slightly too much stand off on the temporal edge and, using slightly different data, he designed the '*x* offsets', which he claimed were more satisfactory in this respect.

Like spherical preformed scleral lenses, the offset lenses are used in conjunction with a FLOM fitting set, but with more possibility of a discrepancy in the process of manufacture. As in the wide angle lenses, the shells were originally pressed out over a die with interchangeable (protruding) steel balls to form the optic zone. A back optic zone diameter is specified, but the primary sag may vary somewhat according to the allowance made by the operator in adjusting the height of the steel ball to allow for subsequent 'take-up' of the polishing tool.

BSD lenses (bi-sphériques décentrés)

Developed by Henry Biri (1968), these lenses may be regarded as a further sophistication of the Forknall Offset lens. The elaboration is that the scleral zone consists of two spherical curves of which only the second has its centre of curvature decentred nasally with respect to the axis of symmetry of the lens (*Figure 17.4*).

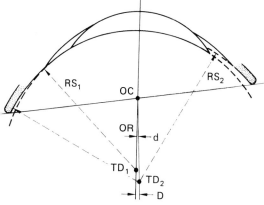

Figure 17.4 BSD lens. (Reproduced from Les Cahiers des Verres de Contact, by kind permission of H. Biri, les Fréres Lissac, Paris)

The variables in these lenses are the first scleral radius (RS_1), the second scleral radius (RS_2), the displacement of the centre of curvature of the second scleral radius from the lens axis (D). The second scleral radius is flatter than the first by 0.50–1.00 mm, the greater difference being on the flatter lenses. For example, the trial lens equivalents to spherical lenses of 12.50 mm, 13.75 mm and 14.25 mm back scleral zone radii would be 12.25/12.75 mm, 13.50/14.25 mm and 14.00/15.00 mm respectively.

The displacement of the centre of curvature of the second scleral radius from the lens axis varies between 0.20 and 0.40 mm. The transition is spherical and of radius equal to the mean of the first scleral radius and back optic zone radius, plus 0.75 mm. The centre of curvature of the transition is displaced by approximately half the displacement of the second scleral radius from the lens axis. The lenses are usually made horizontally oval with 1 mm difference in back scleral size between the major and minor axes. All trial lenses have back scleral sizes of 23.50 × 22.50 mm or 24.50 × 23.50 mm.

Variation of the displacement of the centre of curvature of the second scleral radius from the lens axis is used when, although the scleral fit appears good, there is excessive clearance at the temporal limbus with nasal limbal tightness on the slightest convergence. This very familiar picture with spherical preformed lenses can be radically altered by this extra variable available with BSD lenses.

Although FLOM lenses are used in conjunction with this lens, the back optic zone radius and primary optic diameter so obtained are not used directly in the final lens characteristics. The designer of this lens has prepared a table (*Table 17.5*) which gives the optic zone characteristics for the final lens for a given FLOM fitting, and the final lens has a steeper back optic zone radius than that of the FLOM lens, usually by about 0.25 mm. *Table 17.5* is at the end of the section on FLOM fitting (p. 639).

Fitting sets

The absolute prerequisite for fitting preformed scleral contact lenses is a fitting set. In the UK, at the time of writing, most preformed lenses are wide angle, spherical or offset. There follows a discussion of the fitting sets for these three types of lens.

Wide angle fitting sets

The optic zone is fitted simultaneously with the scleral zone, and a fairly large fitting set is obviously necessary. The minimum desirable set is shown in *Table 17.1*.

It is known that making a lens round or oval does not make such a great difference to the fit as was once thought. Most pracitioners eventually fit oval lenses because they find them more stable in wear, and it is probably best to order horizontally oval lenses. If a 2 mm difference is used between principal meridians, the horizontal back scleral size can be 23 mm in the steeper part of the range and up to 24.5 mm in the flatter lenses.

Table 17.1 Minimum wide angle fitting set

Back scleral zone radius (mm)	Back optic zone radius (mm)				
12.50	8.00	8.25	8.50		
12.75	8.00	8.25	8.50		
13.00	8.00	8.25	8.50	8.75	
13.25	8.00	8.25	8.50	8.75	9.00
13.50	8.00	8.25	8.50	8.75	9.00
13.75		8.25	8.50	8.75	9.00
14.00			8.50	8.75	9.00
14.25			8.50	8.75	9.00

(30 lenses)

Spherical preformed fitting sets

The lenses used for obtaining the scleral fit in this set have a very steep back optic zone radius (8.00 or 8.25 mm) to avoid resting on the cornea, which would create a pseudo-scleral fit. Virtually all cases that can be fitted with preformed scleral lenses are within the range of estimation of eight fitting lenses (*Table 17.2*).

Table 17.2 Minimum spherical fitting set

Back scleral size (mm)	Back scleral radius (mm)				
22.50	12.50	13.00	13.50	14.00	
24.00		13.00	13.50	14.00	14.50

Steps of 0.25 mm are not essential because it is a fairly easy matter to estimate when an intermediate lens is needed from the flatter and steeper lenses. Round or oval lenses can be used with spherical preformed lenses as with wide angle lenses. Most stock fitting sets sold by manufacturers contain too many lenses in the steeper range and not enough in the flatter range. For the type of patient usually fitted with scleral lenses, a back scleral radius of 14.25 and 14.50 mm is quite a common requirement, yet not many fitting sets contain such lenses.

Offset fitting sets

The basic offset fitting set originally consisted of 13 lenses marked with two letters. The first letter gave the 'equivalent' conventional spherical back scleral zone radius. It must be emphasized that it was an equivalent because the curve of the scleral portion, although spherical, is a much flatter one with an 'offset' centre of curvature. The second letter designated the back scleral size (*Table 17.3*).

These lenses have a steep optic zone and are used with separate FLOM lenses.

FLOM lenses

These lenses were first described by Bier (1948), using the term 'corneal ventilated trial lenses'. They consist of an optic zone with a narrow scleral rim of approximately 2 mm width. This scleral zone portion is usually of approximately 13 mm radius, which is almost invariably flatter than the scleral in the limbal region, so that

Table 17.3 Offset trial set markings

First code letter and equivalent back scleral zone radius (mm)		(mm)	Second code letter, back scleral size and displacement of optic zone (mm)
A	11.00	H 12.75	
B	11.25	J 13.00	
C	11.50	K 13.25	E = 22 D 1.5
D	11.75	L 13.50	L = 23.5 × 22.5 D 2
E	12.00	M 13.75	T = 24.5 × 23.5 D 1.5
F	12.25	N 14.00	
G	12.50		

there should be no possibility of the scleral rim influencing the corneal fit. This avoids a false impression of corneal clearance being given. The lens is designed to rest on the eye at the transition between the back optic zone surface and the scleral rim. This transition is deliberately left sharp, although this makes these lenses somewhat uncomfortable (*Figure 17.5*).

The FLOM is identified by the back optic zone radius and the primary optic diameter. If all or some lenses of each back optic zone radius are optically worked, these lenses can be used for refraction purposes. This avoids having to find for refraction a scleral lens which fills properly with tears to provide a liquid lens. It

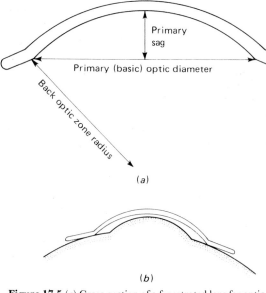

Figure 17.5 (a) Cross-section of a fenestrated lens for optic measurement (FLOM). (b) Diagrammatic representation showing how a FLOM transition rests on the sclera and avoids creating pseudo-fit

Table 17.4 FLOM fitting set

Back optic zone radius (mm)	Primary optic diameter (mm)							
8.00	13.00							
8.25	13.00	13.25	13.50	13.75	14.00			
8.50		13.25	13.50	13.75	14.00	14.25		
8.75			13.50	13.75	14.00	14.25	14.50	
9.00			13.50	13.75	14.00	14.25	14.50	14.75
9.25				13.75	14.00	14.25	14.50	14.75
9.50								14.75

also eliminates the calculations involved when such a lens does not have the same back optic zone radius as the one to be ordered. Twenty-eight FLOM lenses, as shown in *Table 17.4*, are usually adequate.

A large (1.5 mm) fenestration hole is provided in each lens, and the front transition should be smooth to permit handling with a suction holder.

General considerations in scleral fitting

The scleral zone of the lens is only there to hold the optic zone in the correct position. Provided that the scleral zone keeps the optic zone reasonably centred during ocular excursions of up to 30°, with an apical corneal clearance of approximately 0.07 mm, and is neither uncomfortable nor cosmetically ugly, the means and reasons whereby this is achieved are relatively unimportant. Much has been written on the fitting and adjustment of the scleral zone, but less attention has been paid to the optic zone and transitional fits which, somewhat paradoxically, are the most important aspects of scleral lens fitting.

The easily compressed bulbar conjunctiva absorbs minor imperfections in the scleral fit and, provided that the optic zone centres well, the basic principles are as follows:

(1) The lens should be comfortable, with the weight, as far as possible, evenly distributed. To achieve this, the maximum possible surface area should rest on the bulbar conjunctiva, as long as the lower scleral zone is not so large as to cause the lens edge to be supported by the inferior fornix.
(2) The lens should not move on the globe any more than necessary. Extreme lateral move-ments can cause the bubble under the optic zone to move excessively and disturb vision. Undue rotation of the lens can cause the fenestration to be covered by one of the lids for far too long, thereby upsetting corneal metabolism.
(3) The lens should be as large as possible without bumping on either the caruncle or the lateral check ligaments on version movements. This is cosmetically desirable and distributes the weight of the lens over as large an area as possible

The technique of fitting the scleral zone

It is important to emphasize that the fitting of this zone of the lens is very simple. If the third or fourth trial lens inserted is not the correct one, the practitioner should be in a position to say that the patient is not suitable for preformed scleral lenses. An impression should then be taken. The so-called 'spherical rule' has tended to complicate the fitting of this portion. It suggests that the sclera is hyperbolic in shape, not spherical, and thus, to maintain the same fit, the back scleral zone radius must be varied as the back scleral size is altered. The relationship is that for an increase of 1.5 mm in back scleral size the radius must be lengthened by 0.25 mm (although some practitioners make a 0.25 mm increase in back scleral zone radius for each 1 mm increase in back scleral size, which appears to be more realistic).

Marriott (1966) indicates that the temporal anterior sclera is, in fact, roughly spherical but with a much larger radius than previously thought and with a centre of curvature not necessarily on the axis of symmetry of the cornea. When the back scleral size is increased by 0.75 mm, the increase in back scleral zone radius, for example, from 13.50 to 13.62 mm is less than 1%, suggesting an insignificant amount which in fact appears to make no difference. In recent years, some practitioners have ignored this rule completely. Its only application might be when ordering a lens considerably larger than the largest trial lens available or when fitting an oval spherical lens to a toroidal eye, as explained below. It also applies only to spherical lenses and not to any of the offset types.

As Marriott (1966) states, the sclera is much flatter than the back scleral zone radii fitted to it. There may therefore be some justification for using the rule. Any increase in back scleral size must introduce extra clearance of the lens from the eye unless the back scleral radius is flattened at the same time. The theory is similar to that of FLOM fitting. *Figure 17.12* illustrates the increase in clearance given by an increase in size, and *Figure 17.11* illustrates the reduction in clearance obtained by using a flatter radius. Thus, one alteration can be used to counteract the other, or each may be used separately to improve the fit of the scleral zone.

Theoretically, in fitting a spherical lens to a toroidal eye, a steeper back scleral zone radius than that which aligns the flatter meridian of the sclera may be used providing the back scleral size is reduced along this flatter meridian. The reduction in size along the flatter meridian allows the lens to rest close to the eye and the steeper back scleral radius allows a compromise fit between the two meridians.

In practice, horizontal, oval, preformed, spherical lenses do give a slightly better fit on eyes with 'against-the-rule' toricity, but vertical, oval, preformed, spherical lenses do not usually locate correctly on eyes having 'with-the-rule' toricity. As the latter is the more common state of affairs, the possibility of fitting toroidal eyes with spherical lenses by varying their shape is so remote as to be rarely worth considering.

The sequence of events in fitting the scleral zone follows.

The object is to determine the back scleral zone radius, back scleral size and the optic displacement. Provided there is no corneal touch (giving a pseudo-scleral fit), the optic zone is of little interest at this stage. A lens with a steep back optic zone radius should therefore be chosen in order to give corneal clearance.

Patient preparation

The patient should be told what is about to happen, and that his cornea is very sensitive and his sclera relatively insensitive. If he follows instructions and looks in the direction indicated, corneal touch can be avoided. It often helps at this stage to touch the bulbar conjunctiva lightly with the edge of a scleral lens, after assuring the patient that the lens is not going to be inserted. The fact that he can hardly feel this usually boosts the patient's morale. Local anaesthetics are contra-indicated at this stage of the fitting. They are not needed, and the patient's subjective reactions are a useful guide.

Choice of first lens

The eye to be fitted should be examined and an estimate made of its relative flatness or steepness; a lens is chosen accordingly. A surprisingly good estimate of radius can be made with very little practice. Eyes having steep corneas also tend to have steep scleras etc., so that keratometry may give a guide to the relative steepness or flatness of the eye.

Insertion of lens first chosen

At this stage, only two dimensions — back scleral size and back scleral zone radius — need be considered. If the back scleral size is too small, it has little effect on the radius. If it is too big, the lens may be lifted by the caruncle and/or the lateral check ligament, giving an erroneous picture. It is important to watch for any such fitting. Too large a lens tends to remain stationary as the eye moves behind. The lens should be large enough for the edges to remain invisible in the palpebral aperture during normal eye movements.

If the eye can be fitted with spherical preformed scleral lenses, the radius may be too steep, too flat or correct (*Figure 17.6*). Following the instillation of fluorescein, the fit may be observed with white light and ultraviolet illumination, having made sure that there is no corneal touch which would invalidate the fit of the scleral zone.

(1) If the back scleral zone radius is too steep, the lens is tight at the edges and may cause blanching of the conjunctival blood vessels, and fluorescein or air extends from the optic

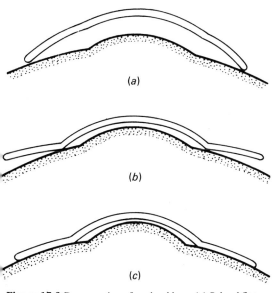

Figure 17.6 Cross-section of a scleral lens. (*a*) Scleral fit too steep; (*b*) scleral fit too flat; (*c*) correct

too far towards the periphery of the lens, i.e. well past the transition.

(2) If the back scleral zone radius is too flat, the edges stand off the eye, there is mid-scleral blanching of the bulbar conjunctival vessels, and fluorescein is restricted to within the limbal region. The lens is first examined with white light and the following noted.

(3) Total diameter and back scleral size of lens: the lens should be as large as possible. If it is ordered too large, the back scleral size can be reduced — but the converse does not apply.

(4) Blanching: where local pressure is exerted by the lens upon the conjunctiva and the episclera, the blood columns in smaller vessels are squeezed, producing blanching or whiteness in excess of normal (*Figure 17.7* and *Plate 77*). Peripheral blanching indicates too steep a lens. Midscleral blanching usually accompanies an edge which 'stands off', indicating too flat a lens.

(5) Frothing: a collection of fine bubbles usually indicates a channel.

(6) Edge 'stand-off': looseness or stand-off at the edge of the scleral zone may admit a bubble locally, or trap a pocket or annulus of tear liquid.

Fluorescein picture

The lens is then examined, using fluorescein and an ultraviolet source. The insertion of fluorescein demonstrates that a preformed scleral lens fit is never a 'textbook' picture, which should not be expected. If the lens fits well over three-quarters of the scleral zone, this is usually adequate. Pooling in the lower nasal quadrant occurs frequently and can initially be ignored if the scleral zone fits elsewhere.

Fluorescein pictures indicate steepness or flatness of the lens, as shown in *Figure 17.8*.

If the the lens is too steep, there is a large central pool (*Figure 17.8a*).

If the lens is too flat, there is a small central pool, and perhaps pooling round the edges (depending on how the lens tilts on its supporting annulus of sclera) associated with mid-scleral blanching (*Figure 17.8b*).

In an ideal fit, the pool extends evenly just beyond the optic zone (*Figure 17.8c* and *Plate 79*).

It cannot be emphasized too strongly that during the determination of the scleral zone fit (with the optic zone clearing the cornea) the depth of the central fluorescein pool is of no interest; only its size is of importance.

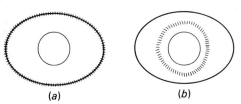

Figure 17.7 Blanching (indicated by lines) in (*a*) steep and (*b*) flat scleral fits (compare *Figure 17.6*)

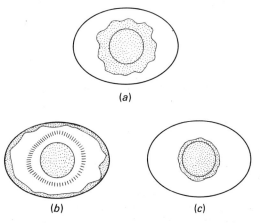

Figure 17.8 Fluorescein pictures with (*a*) steep, (*b*) flat and (*c*) correct scleral zone fittings, respectively. Blanching is indicated by the line shading and fluorescein by dot shading

Displacement of optic

The required optic displacement is estimated by putting a suitable lens of known displacement on the eye. Normal displacements fall within the range 0.5–2.5 mm. The lens is inserted, bearing in mind possible alterations of optic displacement and their effects on the disposition of the scleral zone on either side of the cornea. The trial of alternative lenses with different displacements serves well. For example, too large a nasal scleral zone may cause nasal corneal touch which disappears when a lens of the same back scleral size but bigger displacement of optic is used (*see Plate 72*).

If the ideal fit described above is not obtainable, the eye is rather irregular or toroidal. An irregular eye requires an impression lens. Toroidal fitting sets are available for preformed spherical, conical, wide angle and offset scleral lenses. The impression method is also suitable for these cases and, consequently, there appears to be no advantage in using toric preformed lenses. For satisfactory results, a large and expensive fitting is needed — hardly justifiable on economic grounds.

It is possible to estimate and order a toric lens by estimation from the spherical lens which aligns with the flattest meridian.

Forknall (1959) claimed that nearly all toroidal eyes could be fitted with either 0.50 mm or 0.75 mm difference in back scleral zone radius between the principal meridians. It is often possible, therefore, to align the flattest meridian and order a lens such that the meridian in which the edge stands off most is 0.50 mm steeper and obtain a satisfactory final lens. Low degrees of

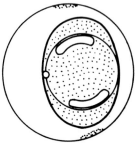

Figure 17.9 Static bubbles in the upper and lower limbal region when an eye having fairly marked corneal astigmatism (with-the-rule) is fitted with a spherical lens. The fluorescein picture is a typical vertical oval with slight vertical edge stand-off (shown by dot shading). In more marked astigmatism, the fluorescein pool would break through to the edge

toricity can be dealt with by lens adjustment. For example, a spherical lens on an eye having with-the-rule scleral and corneal toricity may give the best fit when the lens aligns the horizontal meridian of the eye but allows a large vertical oval-shaped fluorescein pool extending well beyond the upper and lower cornea accompanied by slight stand-off of the upper and lower edges. This additional limbal space may encourage air bubbles to collect and remain at the 6 and 12 o'clock positions of the limbal region. As such immobile bubbles may cause corneal dessication, such a lens (*Figure 17.9*) would then need a localized back scleral zone grind-out on either side of the fluorescein pool horizontally followed possibly by slight grinding out of the back scleral zone near the upper and lower 'mid-rim' portions of the lens. As these back scleral zone grind-outs permit the lens to settle back on to the eye, localized transitional grind-outs at 3 and 9 o'clock may also then be needed to relieve limbal touch, followed by a possible back optic grind-out to relieve subsequent central corneal touch.

This demonstrates why large amounts of toricity are best fitted with toric lenses or impressions taken.

Scleral zone fitting determines the dimensions of the back scleral zone radius, back scleral size and optic displacement. The next step is the determination of the optic zone specifications. As explained earlier, some types of preformed trial lens are arranged in sets in which both the optic and scleral zone specifications vary, so that the same lenses are used for fitting both scleral and optic zones. In which case a lens with the correct back scleral zone radius but with a flatter back optic zone radius than used during scleral zone fitting, is selected, until the correct optic and scleral zone fit is achieved — *see Figures 17.8c and 17.15*. This is the procedure adopted in fitting wide angle lenses. Otherwise, the optic fitting is continued with FLOM lenses.

The technique of obtaining optic zone specifications with FLOMs

Fenestrated lenses for optic measurement are not fitted in the sense that they represent a lens to be worn. They simulate the optic zone of a complete scleral lens. The FLOM is simply a measuring device and it may be legitimate to instil a local anaesthetic with a sensitive patient, for the following reasons.

First, these lenses are not comfortable to wear and the patient's subjective response is of no particular value. Secondly, the FLOM giving the desired corneal clearance is not necessarily any more comfortable than any other FLOM. Thirdly, a lens permits a more accurate refraction, with less chance of ciliary spasm, if it is not too uncomfortable. Finally, corneal abrasions caused while inserting and removing the trial lenses are less likely if the patient is relaxed and not apprehensive.

The purpose of FLOM fitting is as follows. It is required to arrive at a curve (or series of curves) which clear the centre of the cornea by an amount between 0.04 and 0.08 mm, with adequate clearance in the limbal region (Marriott and Woodward, 1964).

A suitable back optic zone radius must be considerably flatter than the mean corneal radius (*Figure 17.10*). The difference in radius between the back optic zone of the lens and the keratometer reading is usually in the region of 0.50–0.70 mm, which dictates the back optic zone radius of the first trial lens to be inserted. Corneal clearance is achieved in two ways. A lens with a single back optic zone radius has two variables — the radius of curvature and the primary optic diameter — both of which affect the clearance of the lens from the cornea.

Decreasing the back optic zone radius without altering the primary optic diameter increases the corneal clearance and vice versa (*Figure 17.11*).

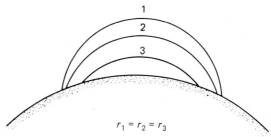

Figure 17.12 The effect on clearance of increasing and decreasing diameter, keeping radius constant

Decreasing the primary optic diameter without altering the back optic zone radius reduces the corneal clearance and vice versa (*Figure 17.12*).

Alteration of both variables at once produces either an additive or a subtractive result, or preserves the status quo. In practice, often, a given apical corneal clearance must be maintained while the variables are altered for other reasons — for example, to increase or decrease limbal clearance. Usually, there is a simple relationship (*Figure 17.13*) which allows variation of radius and diameter to give the required apical and limbal clearance. A FLOM lens (a in *Figure 17.13*) lying on a flat surface has a certain primary sagitta. If the radius of curvature is increased (b in *Figure 17.13*) to maintain the same primary sagitta, its diameter must be increased. The sagitta formula dictates that, for the typical values encountered in FLOM fitting, if the back optic zone radius is increased by 0.50 mm the primary optic zone diameter must be increased by the same amount to give approximately the same primary sagitta. This relationship, although not exact, works well in general.

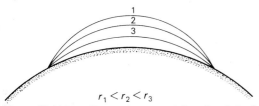

Figure 17.10 Cross-section of the desired corneal clearance

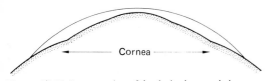

Figure 17.11 The effect on clearance of alterations in back optic (or scleral) zone radius when primary optic zone diameter (or back scleral size) is kept constant

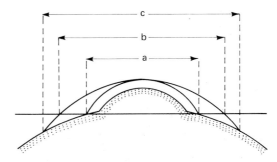

Figure 17.13 The relationship between radius and diameter for a given clearance

However, a lens fitted to an eye is not resting on a flat surface but on a curved surface, flatter than the lens itself. *Figure 17.13* shows that if the back optic zone radius is flattened, an even greater diameter (c) is needed than on a flat surface (b) to preserve the same corneal clearance. Clinically, it is found that if the back optic zone radius is increased by a certain amount, then the primary optic diameter must be increased by *twice* that amount to preserve the same corneal clearance. For example, FLOM 8.00/13.00, 8.25/13.50 and 8.75/14.50 all give the same apical corneal clearance on a certain eye. Because of this, such lenses are known as *clinical equivalents* (although they give different limbal clearances).

The best method of inserting the FLOM is for the patient to look straight ahead while the practitioner gently parts the lids and places the lens symmetrically on the cornea and limbus as if inserting a large corneal lens. If a local anaesthetic has been used, this is perfectly straightforward; otherwise, it is sometimes necessary to place the lens in the upper fornix and then slide it down, with a much greater risk of corneal abrasion. The use of a suction holder allows easier manipulation of the lens during its placement on the eye.

First trial lens

To choose the back optic zone radius of this first lens, 0.50–0.70 mm is added to the mean keratometer reading and a lens of the nearest radius is used. If, for example, the mean keratometer reading is 8.00 mm, an 8.50 mm or 8.75 mm radius is indicated. In a FLOM fitting set there are usually five lenses of each radius, with diameters, in this example, from 13.25 to 14.50 mm. A lens in the middle of this diameter range (probably an 8.75/14.00) is the first FLOM to insert. It has been suggested that the visible iris diameter is a guide to primary optic diameter, but as this is not a measurement which can be determined accurately and the primary optic diameter range of FLOMs of a given radius only extends over 1 mm there is little or no help from this measurement.

The first FLOM, after cleaning, is inserted without solution and left for up to 5 minutes to see whether it fills with tear liquid, at what rate it fills, and with what shaped bubble. If the radius is too steep, the bubble tends to cross the

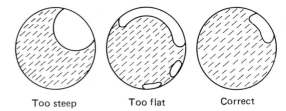

Figure 17.14 Bubble shapes in FLOM fitting

pupil; if the radius is too flat, a ring bubble extends a considerable way round the limbus region; if the fit is correct, a small kidney-shaped bubble forms with its concave surface inwards. The bubble shape is an indication of the relationship between the back optic zone radius and the corneal radius — a round bubble indicating too steep a lens and an annular bubble too flat a lens. The size of the bubble is an indication of the amount of clearance (*Figure 17.14*). *Plate 73* shows a FLOM with excessive apical clearance and insufficient limbal clearance.

If the bubble shape indicates that the radius is too steep, the primary optic diameter is maintained but the radius is flattened by one step (0.25 mm). A bubble shape indicating that the radius is too flat must be confirmed with fluorescein. If the lens does not fill at all, the primary optic diameter is reduced until the lens does fill or, if this does not have the desired effect, the radius is flattened. At this stage, one variable at a time should be altered — otherwise, it may not be clear which is having the greater effect. In theory, a flattening of 0.25 mm in radius has twice the effect of a 0.25 mm reduction in diameter in reducing the apical corneal clearance (*see Figure 17.13*).

White light inspection takes the fitting to the stage where a lens has been selected which fills with tear liquid within 2 or 3 minutes and has a satisfactory bubble. Fluorescein is then instilled and the fit is observed under ultraviolet light, enabling two factors to be checked which are not easily observed with any other method: the presence or absence of corneal touch; and the clearance at the limbus.

These two factors must be considered in relation to each other. There are now four possible situations in the typical case, as follows.

(1) Central corneal touch with limbal tightness (*Figure 17.15a*). The same radius is main-

tained and the primary optic diameter is increased to give more clearance until both the touch and tightness are eased.

(2) Central corneal touch with adequate limbal clearance, requiring a shorter radius with the same primary optic diameter (*Figure 17.15b*).

(3) Limbal tightness with correct central corneal clearance (*Figure 17.15c*). This requires an increase in primary optic diameter with a compensatory increase in the radius of curvature to preserve the same central corneal clearance. Thus, if the lens which gives limbal tightness with correct apical corneal clearance is 8.50/13.50, the diameter may be increased to 14.00 mm while altering the radius to 8.75 mm to preserve the same apical corneal clearance.

(4) The correct lens shows neither signs of limbal tightness nor apical corneal touch (*Figure 17.15d*). The bubble circulates freely around the limbus on eye movements, bubble position being opposite to the direction of gaze.

Gentle pressure, for example, with a glass rod, on the apex of the correctly fitting FLOM should demonstrate minimal apical corneal touch while limbal clearance is still maintained.

Figure 17.16 shows diagrammatically the possible sequence of events and the action to take.

The desired optic fit is now represented by two measurements towards the final specification. The only value these figures have in isolation is possibly when FLOM lenses are used to determine the required radius of curvature for the back optic surface of an impression lens.

Multiple curve optics

Occasionally, there occurs an eye on which it is impossible to achieve the required fit and reach the desired final specification with ordinary FLOM lenses. There is perhaps the correct shaped bubble and good limbal clearance, but it is impossible to avoid central touch no matter how the radius and primary optic diameter are varied. These are the cases in which multiple back surface radii are needed (*Figure 17.17*).

Multiple curve fitting sets are available, but they are difficult to check and are needed fairly infrequently. A method of fitting which avoids recourse to these fitting sets and is adequate for the average practice is as follows.

The eye is fitted with single curve FLOMs, in the normal way, to find the lens which gives adequate limbal clearance with correct bubble size and shape but which still touches centrally. The diameter of the touch area is then measured and 2 mm is added to determine the diameter of the new central back optic zone, whose radius is 0.50 mm steeper.

If, for example, the first lens is 9.00/14.50, giving a touch area of 6 mm in diameter, an optic with 8.50 mm radius and a central back optic zone diameter of 8.00 mm is ordered with a 9.00 mm back peripheral radius and primary optic diameter of 14.50 mm. (For refraction purposes, an 8.50 mm radius lens must be used or the appropriate power allowance made.)

This method works well in practice and avoids using a double curve fitting set of doubtful veracity.

Interpretation of results

A lens may then be ordered. There are normally no allowances to be made in the specification of the scleral zone. The back scleral zone radius is the one that was chosen as the best fit — or, if the exact trial lens required was not available, the one deduced by interpolation.

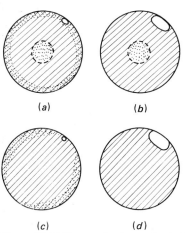

(a)   (b)

(c)   (d)

Figure 17.15 Fluorescein pictures in FLOM fitting (*see* text). Line shading indicates fluorescence, and dot shading corneal touch

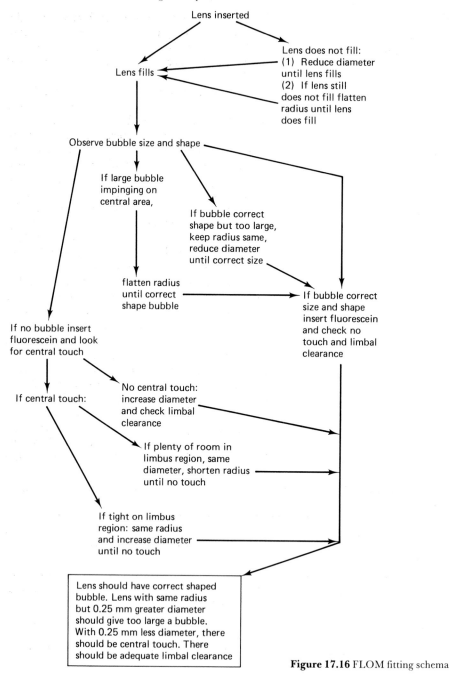

Figure 17.16 FLOM fitting schema

If composite fitting lenses were used, it may be necessary to order the final lens with a primary optic sag varied by ±0.05–0.10 mm because the range of lenses giving the correct scleral fit may not give the correct central corneal clearance. Estimation based on the apical touch and other factors such as bubble size may be required.

Possibly because of the relatively imperfect fit on the sclera, preformed scleral lenses settle closer to the eye after a period of time. More corneal clearance is required initially than may

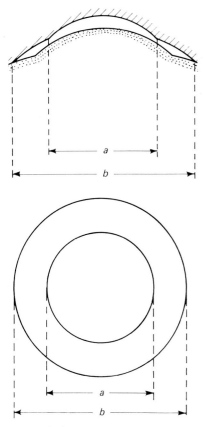

be acceptable in the finally fitted lenses in order to allow for settling to take place. The amount of settling varies considerably from patient to patient, being most on big, soft eyes often found in high myopes.

Settling is compensated for by ordering a primary optic diameter larger than that of the correctly fitting FLOM lens. Elaborate guides have been given (for example, Bier, 1957) for the allowances to be made in a particular case, but an addition of 0.25 mm suffices in most cases. For example, if the final FLOM is 8.75/13.75, then the optic specification 8.75/14.00 should be ordered. If a greater allowance is made, the patient is likely to be bothered by excessively large bubbles in the first few weeks of wear. It is no great comfort for the patient to be told that these bubbles should diminish in a few weeks if they are at that moment interfering with his daily life. Most patients have to earn a living, and they find it difficult to wear such lenses enough for them to settle sufficiently. The extra 0.25 mm may not give sufficient extra clearance — in which case, the lens may give apical corneal touch after some weeks of wear. It is then a relatively simple matter to grind 0.05 or 0.10 mm from the back optic zone with modern modification tools (*see* Chapters 22 and 23).

An ideally fitting fully settled scleral lens has a central corneal clearance between 0.04 and 0.08 mm with no bubble when the eye is in the

Figure 17.17 Cross-section and plan view of a multiple curve optic. *a* is the central back optic zone diameter and *b* the back peripheral diameter (primary optic diameter)

Table 17.5 Suggested back optic zone radii and primary optic diameters (POD) to be ordered in relation to the ideal fitting set lens parameters when fitting BSD lenses

FLOM fitting set BOZR (mm)	*FLOM fitting set POD* (mm)						
	12.75	13.00	13.25	13.50	13.75	14.00	14.25
8.00	7.75/13.00	7.75/13.50 −0.02	7.80/13.50	7.80/13.75 −0.02	7.87/14.00 +0.02	7.87/14.25 +0.02	7.87/14.50
8.25	8.00/13.00 +0.02	8.00/13.25	8.00/13.50	8.00/13.75 −0.02	8.05/14.00	8.05/14.25 −0.02	8.12/14.50
8.50	8.25/13.00 +0.02	8.20/13.25	8.25/13.50 +0.02	8.25/13.75	8.25/14.00	8.50/14.25 −0.02	8.50/14.50
8.75	8.37/13.00	8.37/13.25 −0.02	8.45/13.50 +0.02	8.50/13.75 +0.02	8.50/14.00	8.50/14.25	8.50/14.50
9.00	8.62/13.00 +0.02	8.62/13.50	8.62/13.50 −0.02	8.70/13.75	8.75/14.00 −0.02	8.75/14.25	8.75/14.50

It will be seen from the table that the final lens invariably has a steeper BOZR than the FLOM lens fitting indicated, and the degree of steepening is greater on the smaller primary optic diameters.

When figures such as +0.02 or −0.02 are seen, these are instructions to the manufacturer to give this much more or less primary sag, the amount being measured in millimetres.

primary position. Bubbles appear on version movements but should rotate freely around the limbus and then disappear when the eye has returned to the primary position for a few seconds. This is shown in *Plates 72* and *79a,b*.

As mentioned previously, when fitting BSD lenses the optic characteristics are obtained from a table prepared by the designer, and not as in the method just described (*Table 17.5*).

Refraction

Refraction is best carried out using a FLOM which has a known back vertex power. The lens used should fulfil the following four requirements:

(1) It should have the same back optic zone radius as the prescription lens. Alternatively, the nearest radius available is used and the necessary calculations are made (*see* Chapter 5, pp. 206–207).
(2) The lens must fill adequately.
(3) There must be adequate and, as near as possible, correct corneal clearance. Excessive corneal touch may flatten and distort the cornea, giving a false refraction. Too much clearance introduces too large a bubble or at least provides another source of error, the thicker tear layer having an optical effect different from that which is required.
(4) The front surface of the lens must stay wet, wetting solutions being used if necessary.

Ideally the lens should also be as near as possible to the final back vertex power required (*see* Chapter 5).

Any favoured refractive technique may be used, and if two suitable powered lenses are available the refraction should be binocular.

Residual astigmatism should be measured but, at this stage, only the best sphere ordered. Residual astigmatism may vary or even disappear when the lenses have been worn for a while. If it does not disappear, it is still necessary for the lenses to assume their final resting position before the axis may be marked with the lens *in situ*, as even horizontal oval, preformed scleral lenses rarely lay with the major axis exactly along the horizontal meridian.

The vertex distance of the supplementary trial lens from the eye must be measured and its effective power at the cornea calculated (*see* Appendix A). With a knowledge of the keratometric findings, the approximate power of the liquid lens can be calculated and, thus, the contact lens power compared with the spectacle prescription. Any large discrepancies found must be investigated. On the higher positive powers, the thickness of the trial contact lens used must also be taken into account. This part of the procedure of fitting preformed scleral lenses is the part where there is the least excuse for error.

Fenestration and local adjustments

At this stage, the lenses have arrived from the laboratory and been checked, and the patient has returned for final fitting.

Insertion of the lenses is preceded by an explanation that, until the lenses are fenestrated, vision is likely to be unclear. If necessary, the lenses can be inserted filled with liquid to avoid this.

The fit of the lenses is then checked with white light and with fluorescein to detect gross errors of fitting. Minor areas of tightness and leaks may safely be left until after fenestration because they may then alter or disappear. Fenestration helps to equalize the pressure in front of and behind the lens, allowing it to settle back on the eye. The back scleral size must be corrected before fenestration, particularly if it is too large. Also, if the back scleral size is too great in any one meridian this must be remedied before fenestration, otherwise the fenestration may come to rest in the wrong place with respect to the lids. If the lens is too small, there is no remedy and the lens should be re-ordered.

The back scleral size can be reduced on a grindstone or grinding ball, or with a file — the latter method being slower but safer. The edge is then reshaped with a narrow file, or fine carborundum ball, and smoothed with fine sandpaper. Final polishing is carried out on a soft buff (*see* Chapter 23).

Assuming that the size is now correct, the lens is re-inserted, after a grease pencil or waterproof line has been drawn along the proposed horizontal meridian. A lens with grease pencil on the outer surface may feel gritty, and the patient should be warned of this. (Waterproof fibre pens are more satisfactory, but paraffin or methylated spirits have to be used to remove the marking.) The patient is then instructed to look in every direction in turn and execute some rapid eye movements. It does not matter if the lens rotates a little, provided that it always returns promptly to the same position. If it does not do this, the back scleral size is probably still too big. Alternatively, corneal touch may be present, causing the lens to spin on the cornea, or there may be an area of heavy scleral touch acting as a pivot for the lens. This must be remedied. When the lens is stable, it is ready for fenestration.

The fenestration should be positioned on the optic zone on the temporal side in the shadow of the upper lid when the eye is in the primary position. If it is placed too far towards the centre of the cornea, it may subsequently cause a localized area of dimpling. If it overlies the sclera, it becomes too readily visible. With a small hole of 0.50–0.70 mm correctly positioned just in front of the iris pattern, the fenestration should be visible only to the trained observer. This size appears optimum as a larger diameter gives a poor cosmetic effect and a smaller diameter tends to clog with mucus fairly easily.

Marking the fenestration position may be done while the patient looks straight ahead — a cross being made with a grease pencil or waterproof fibre pen to indicate the correct position. An alternative method is to draw a squared grid in the appropriate limbal area before the lens is inserted. When the lens is inserted, it is simply a matter of making a mental note in which square of the grid the hole should be drilled. In *Figure 17.18*, the hole would be correctly positioned in the centre square of the centre row.

The hole is best made by hand, using a 0.50 mm or 0.70 mm drill mounted in a pin-vice.

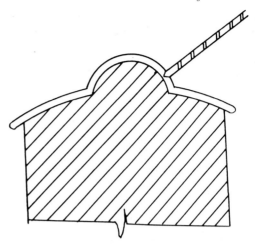

Figure 17.19 Drilling a fenestration with the lens mounted on a cast

It is better to make a slight mark on the front surface first with a sharply pointed tool to stop the drill slipping sideways. With thinner lenses and smaller holes, the angle of the hole is of little significance and it is drilled at right-angles to the front surface. If the lens is hand held, the hole can be drilled from the back, but by mounting the lens on a plaster mount, good contact is obtained by boring from the front (*Figure 17.19*).

The hole is countersunk at both ends with a small dental ball tool and then polished, as described in greater detail in Chapter 23.

The lens and fenestration hole are thoroughly cleaned and the lens is placed without solution on the patient's eye. Minor tight and loose areas should not be modified at this stage because they may alter after a few hours' wear. Initially the patient may notice a clicking noise as air is expressed or enters via the fenestration hole during eye movements and blinking. This usually goes as the lens settles. The lens should only be adjusted under the circumstances listed below.

(1) The lens does not fill. It must be settled by evenly grinding out the back scleral zone until it fills well enough to give reasonable visual acuity.
(2) There is corneal touch. As this is likely increase after a few hours' wear, a back optic grind-out must be performed immediately.

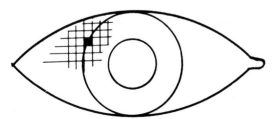

Figure 17.18 Cross-hatching drawn on a scleral lens to mark the fenestration position (upper lid slightly retracted)

(3) There is limbal tightness. This must be relieved before the patient wears the lens.

(4) The back scleral size is still too large. The size must be reduced, particularly if it causes heavy nasal bumping on the limbus region on convergence.

(5) The power is more than ±0.75 DS incorrect. A correction is then necessary before the lens is worn.

All other adjustments should be carried out at subsequent visits — probably on the first visit at which the patient arrives having worn the lenses for a few hours. It is important that all transitions are smooth and well blended, the fenestration hole well polished, and that the final corneal and limbal clearance are correct, otherwise frothing of the bubble may occur with resultant dimpling of the corneal epithelium, and dimple 'veil' occur after lens removal (*see* Chapter 16 and *Plate 22*).

Insertion and removal

The only acceptable method of insertion is by the use of the fingers. Suction holders are generally unnecessary and unaesthetic. The only acceptable method of removal is by using the upper lid. Methods involving hooking the lens out with the fingernails are dangerous.

Insertion and removal is best taught by the practitioner, who first demonstrates with his own lenses. It is made clear to the patient that, in both insertion and removal, he should keep his sensitive cornea out of harm's way. With regard to positioning of the lens, the patient is told that the fenestration hole goes on the side towards the ear (*see* Chapter 9).

Lens ordering

The result of a preformed scleral lens fitting being simply a set of figures, and not a cast as in impression fitting, it is very important that these figures are conveyed to the prescription laboratory (or anyone else) in a form which is unambiguous and universally accepted.

At the time of writing the British Standards relating to preformed scleral lenses are BS 5562:1978, and BS 3521:1988:Part 3; the latter is based on the International Standard ISO 8320–1986.

The essentials of their recommendations regarding back surface specification are as follows.

Spherical preformed lenses

Dimensions (in millimetres) and orientations are invariably to be given in the following order:

(*i*) Eye and preformed scleral lens (S denotes scleral).

(*ii*) Back optic zone radius.

(*iii*) Back optic zone diameter (primary optic diameter if no peripheral zone present).

(*iv*) Back peripheral radius of optic, if present.

(*v*) External diameter of back peripheral zone (if applicable), i.e. primary optic diameter.

(*vi*) Back scleral zone radius.

(*vii*) Back scleral size (BSS) or total diameter (TD) and long and short axes. (*Note:* Where BSS is specified it should be preceded by a letter B, otherwise the dimension is assumed to be the TD.)

(*viii*) Orientation of long axis in standard axis notation.

(*ix*) Displacement of optic and direction.

(*x*) Details of transitions.

Example:

LS/8.50: 11.50/11.00: 13.50/13.50:
(*i*) (*ii*) (*iii*) (*iv*) (*v*) (*vi*)

B24.00 *X* 22.00/L 10/D 1.00 in/sharp transitions
(*vii*)   (*viii*) (*ix*)   (*x*)

An earlier British Standard recommendation was written in 1962 and then the back surface specification was written in the sequence required by a technician cutting the lens from solid material, namely:

(*i*) Radius of back scleral surface.

(*ii*) Radius of back optic zone.

(*iii*) Primary optic diameter.

(*iv*) (Subsidiary optic dimensions.)

(*v*) Back scleral size or total diameter.

(*vi*) Orientation of long axis.

(*vii*) Displacement of optic.

Example:

14.00/8.50/13.50/B24 D1 in:
(*i*)   (*ii*)   (*iii*)   (*v*)   (*vii*)

Most fitting sets still (in 1988) have lenses labelled in this old sequence. Great care is therefore necessary to avoid confusion, particularly where parameters of similar dimensions such as back scleral zone radius and primary optic diameter could be inadvertently interchanged. Now the above dimensions would be written in this order:

(1) Radius of back optic zone.
(2) Primary optic diameter.
(3) Radius of back scleral surface.
(4) Back scleral size.
(5) Displacement of optic.

The example previously written would then become:

8.50/13.50/14.00/B 24 D1 in:
  (1)   (2)   (3)   (4)   (5)

Wide angle lenses

The corneal and limbal chords being standardized on these lenses, the specifications to be given are as follows.

(1) Back optic zone radius.
(2) Back scleral zone radius.
(3) Back scleral size.
(4) Displacement of optic.

In the old system back scleral zone radius was written first followed by back optic zone radius and most fitting sets available are labelled using the old system.

As this is a 'composite' type of lens, where the scleral and optic specifications are obtained with the same lens, the final lens required is often not in the fitting set. The nearest lens is usually ordered, together with the instructions 'raise (or lower) optic by x-tenths of a mm' according to whether greater or less corneal clearance is required.

Offset lenses

These lenses are ordered in the following way.

(1) Back optic zone radius.
(2) Primary optic diameter.
(3) The first letter on the fitting set lens (i.e. the 'equivalent' back scleral zone radius).
(4) The 'size' letter (*see Table 17.3*).

Example:

8 / 13 / K / T
(1)   (2)   (3)   (4)

whereas the old system was to give 'K/8/13/T' which is still used on these fitting sets.

BSD lenses

These lenses are ordered in a similar way to spherical preformed lenses but, in addition, the displacement of the centre of curvature of the second scleral zone radius from the axis of symmetry must be specified.

With all types of preformed lens the power of the lens is to be given in the back vertex form. Lens thickness is easily controlled with preformed lenses and this can be ordered as desired; 0.50–0.60 mm is a good thickness to aim for after doing any necessary modifications.

Materials

The scleral lens has the longest history of any contact lens design, but until comparatively recently has only been manufactured from polymethyl methacrylate, or originally, glass. In view of its propensity to cause neovascularization if worn regularly for long periods, despite various expedients to improve tear flow beneath the lens, it is not surprising that the advent of rigid gas permeable materials aroused interest among scleral lens practitioners. The main problem has been the lack of availability of sheets of RGP material because these are normally made in rods from which small buttons are cut.

In 1983, Ezekiel reported on scleral lenses manufactured from Boston II material, a siloxanyl/acrylate polymer with a *Dk* value of 16.4 and a receding wetting angle of 21.5°. As the material is heat sensitive the lenses were lathe-turned following conventional preformed fitting using FLOM lenses as described earlier. The lenses were fenestrated and fitted in the conventional manner with minimum corneal clearance and a small circulating bubble. Patients found these lenses much more acceptable than similar lenses manufactured from polymethyl methacrylate, whether this was due to the oxygen permeability or the low wetting angle of the material was not clear.

Ruben and Benjamin (1985) used the same material to investigate oxygenation of the cornea underneath a gas permeable scleral lens. They found, by measuring the corneal oxygen uptake rate immediately after lens removal, an equivalent oxygen percentage of 2.3% with a Boston II lens of centre thickness 0.64 mm as compared with 0.3% with a polymethyl methacrylate of centre thickness of 0.81 mm. A lens was then lathe cut from Boston EW material ($Dk = 27$) with a centre thickness of 0.11 mm and a transitional thickness of 0.10 mm. This lens gave an equivalent oxygen percentage of 3.6%, this being theoretically sufficient to prevent corneal oedema and anaerobic metabolism. Furthermore, none of these lenses was fenestrated which would have provided additional sources of corneal oxygenation.

Geyer (1987) reported the use of both preformed and impression scleral lenses manufactured from gas permeable material in the fitting of keratoconic patients. The material used was a polymer blend of cellulose acetate butyrate and ethyl vinyl acetate with a Dk value of 4.3. The mean thickness of the lenses was 0.40 mm; some were fenestrated, others not. Tolerance was reported to be good and a trial set has been manufactured from this material. In view of the relatively low Dk value of the material such success is rather surprising. This may be due to the rather unusual tear flow characteristics found between scleral lenses and keratoconic corneas. Chapter 19 gives additional information on moulded gas permeable scleral lenses.

The advent of more highly oxygen permeable polymers which may be lathe cut into thin scleral lenses offer interesting possibilities to future scleral lens practitioners. With materials currently available the fragility of such thin lenses can pose a problem but more flexibility might overcome this.

Summary

The most significant factor limiting the wider dissemination of scleral lenses has been the manual dexterity and time demanded in their fitting. In the majority of cases both impression and preformed scleral lenses demand hand work to fully refine the fit. This situation may change.

As Ruben and Benjamin (1985) wrote:

Modern precision semiautomated lathes are able to produce lenses thin enough to transmit oxygen and provide excellent flexibility in the haptic zone of the lenses.

Fitting of preformed scleral lenses is an exercise in applying simple rules and accepting the limitations of each lens type. If thin preformed scleral lenses can readily be produced by lathing or moulding highly oxygen permeable polymers, their flexibility and oxygen transmission may render many of the adjustments necessary with polymethyl methacrylate redundant. The benefits of scleral lenses may then begin to outweigh their more complex and time-consuming fitting techniques.. This could considerably increase their use, especially where medical, optical, vocational or recreational indications would make them the lens of choice.

The renaissance of scleral lenses may yet be on the horizon.

References

BIER, N. (1948). The practice of ventilated contact lenses. *Optician* **116**, 497–501

BIER, N. (1957). *Contact Lens Routine and Practice*, 2nd edn. London: Butterworths

BIER, N. and COLE, P. J. (1948). The transcurve contact lens fitting shell. *Optician* **115**, 605–606, 610

BIRI, H. (1968). Le B.S.D. nouveau verre scléral de form géométrique. *Cah. Verres Contact* **16**, 8–16

BRAFF, S. (1965). The design and development of a scleral lens. *J. Am. optom. Ass.* **36**, 217–223

British Standard 3521 (1988). *Glossary of Terms Relating to Ophthalmic Lenses and Spectacle Frames. BS 3521: 1988. Part 3. Glossary of terms relating to contact lenses.* London: British Standards Institution

COWAN, J. M. (1948). The wide angle contact lens. *Optician* **115**, 359

DALLOS, J. (1937). The individual fitting of contact glasses. *Trans. Ophthal. Soc. UK* **57**, 509–520

EZEKIEL, D. (1983). Gas permeable haptic lenses. *J. Br. Contact Lens Ass.* **6**(4), 158–161

FEINBLOOM, W. (1936). A plastic contact lens. *Trans. 15th Congress Am. Acad. Optom.* **10**, 44

FORKNALL, A. J. (1953). Pre-formed lenses, corneal fit, with a note on the slit lamp. *Br. J. physiol. Optics* **10**, 15–22, 49

FORKNALL, A. J. (1959). Some notes on haptic lenses. *Br. J. physiol. Optics* **16**, 96–115

GEYER, O. CHR. (1987). La correction du keratocone par des lentilles de contact sclero-corneennes rigides. *Contactologia* **4**(9), 191–194

JENKIN, L. and TYLER-JONES, R. (1964). *Theory and Practice of Contact Lens Fitting*, pp. 15–16. London: Hatton Press

MARRIOTT, P. J. (1966). An analysis of global contours and haptic lens fitting. *Br. J. physiol. Optics* **23**, 3–40

MARRIOTT, P. J. and WOODWARD, E. G. (1964). A method of measuring the corneal clearance of a haptic lens. *Br. J. physiol. Optics* **21**, 61–83

VON ROHR, M. and BOEGEHOLD, H. (1934). *Das Brillenglas als Optisches Instrument*, p. 17. Berlin: Springer

RUBEN, M. and BENJAMIN, W. J. (1985). Scleral contact lenses: preliminary report on oxygen-permeable materials. *Contact Lens J.* **13**(2), 5–9

Eye impressions, production and fitting of scleral lenses and patient management

Kenneth W. Pullum

This chapter is an amalgamation and update of two chapters in the second edition written by Peter Marriott.

Introduction

Scleral contact lenses are highly occlusive as they prevent atmospheric oxygen being dissolved by the precorneal tear film. As most of the anterior eye is covered by a non-permeable shell, no other lens form can claim this undesirable drawback so completely. However, it can be overcome.

Early workers in contact lens practice showed that the vision became misty after up to 4 hours wear of a sealed scleral lens. This is the result of corneal hypoxia, but the mechanism was not understood at the time. Onset might have been expected immediately after insertion, but the delay demonstrates that the oxygen dissolved in the tear pool is sufficient to maintain a nearly normal metabolism for a limited period. The natural tear film is disrupted and replaced by a partially adequate corneal environment, but replenishment of the dissolved oxygen is necessary for longer periods of wear.

A recovery period as long as or longer than the duration of lens wear may be needed to re-establish normality. To prevent or retard the onset of hypoxia, it is necessary to create an even coverage and a continuous flow of tears behind the lens. If the scleral zone is in close apposition to the globe, with the weight of the lens evenly distributed over the sclera, the optic zone will be supported more accurately and securely in position. Taking an impression of the anterior

eye provides for both the optimum fit of the scleral zone and the basis for production of the physiologically most acceptable back optic zone curvature.

Indications for scleral lens fitting

Corneal or hydrogel lenses are preferable in the vast majority of cases, but there remain some instances when a scleral lens provides a functional result after all other options have proved to be unsatisfactory. As this is so in spite of the sophistication of contact lens technology, it seems probable that an alternative always will be necessary on occasions.

There are some vocational and recreational reasons for fitting scleral lenses. Active sportsmen, especially those involved in any kind of water sport, or people whose occupations demand that lenses do not fall out, may benefit. Otherwise, scleral lenses would normally only be fitted when there is a clinical indication for contact lenses. They can provide an alternative to some surgical procedures in ophthalmology including corneal grafting, secondary implantation of an intraocular lens (IOL) and refractive surgery. On occasion, it is valuable that the conservative and reversible option is seen to have been offered, even if surgery is ultimately necessary.

Advantages of scleral lenses

Scleral lenses have a number of advantages which can make them lenses of choice:

(1) They are held in place by the eyelids and by capillary attraction between the sclera and

the lens, so they do not move or fall out. They do not rely upon capillary attraction to the cornea for centration, making irregular corneal topography less of a problem. It is rarely, if ever, necessary to use a toroidal back optic zone. They are not affected by traction which may draw high negative corneal lenses under the upper lid, or by the alteration in the position of the centre of gravity which tends to make high positive corneal lenses ride low.

(2) The optic zones are nearly always larger and flatter than those of corneal lenses, making scleral lenses better able to bridge both topographical and optical irregularities of the cornea. Therefore, correction of visual disorders which are corneal in origin is maximized by their use. Chapter 5 fully describes neutralization of the cornea by the liquid lens with a contact lens *in situ*.

(3) They may be more comfortable than corneal lenses over short durations of wear because of reduced lid sensation. Foreign bodies are less easily trapped behind scleral lenses than behind corneals. This may be advantageous for contact lens wearers who have to work in dusty conditions.

(4) Maintenance is very straightforward. Cleaning with dilute liquid detergent, rinsing with potable tap water and dry storage is a perfectly acceptable regimen. Wetting solutions may assist initial cushioning, but this is not always necessary and is sometimes unhelpful because of the increase in viscosity. If so, soft lens rinsing solutions may be substituted or may be used to wash away some of the wetting solution. There is no risk of infection arising from contamination of soaking solutions as none is used and there need be no problem of reaction to preservative if aerosol or unit dose sterile saline is used for rinsing. There is none of the problems of splitting and spoilation associated with hydrogel lens wear and they are not subject to alterations in hydration. Because of their more substantial nature, polishing carries less risk of distortion compared to corneal lenses.

(5) They are usually easier for patients who are clumsy handlers of corneal or hydrogel lenses and are less easily lost or broken.

(6) They cover most of the anterior eye within the palpebral aperture. This is an advantage for some therapeutic uses of scleral lenses.

(7) Small amounts of prism, perhaps up to 5 or 6 Δ, can be incorporated into a scleral lens, and can be orientated as desired.

Limitations of preformed lenses

Preformed scleral lenses have been fitted extensively in the past, but impression techniques are far more practical for unusual or abnormal eyes which now account for the majority of scleral lens fittings. The asymmetrical contour of the sclera also does not lend itself readily to any preformed fitting set. Preformed sets are cumbersome, and the procedures may be quite time consuming if many different lenses have to be inspected on the eye. In addition, many modifications may be required as the precision of the impression method is lacking. Fenestrated lenses for optic measurements (FLOMs; *see* Chapter 17) are often used to determine the specifications of the back optic zone, but their behaviour *in situ* is not always sufficiently comparable to that of the final lens because of the dissimilarity of the bearing surfaces.

Type casts and shells   Josef Dallos was an advocate of a fitting technique which could be described as a combination of both philosophies, a system of type casts and shells. Having accumulated hundreds of casts over many years of scleral lens practice, he would select a cast with a shape similar to the patient's eye and use it to produce a shell (*see* Chapter 1). In this way he moved towards the idea of preformed fitting, but retained some of the benefits of impressions. This has some advantages, but it is not really practical today as scleral lenses are much less frequently used. In any event, it is debatable that selecting a cast in the manner described is a significant saving in time compared to taking a new impression.

Anterior ocular anatomy relevant to scleral lens fitting

The technique of constructing and fitting a scleral lens by means of making an impression of the eye requires a knowledge of the conjunctival, corneal and scleral topography, the positions of the extraocular muscle insertions, and the configuration of the orbit.

The conjunctiva

The nasal bulbar conjunctiva terminates at the caruncle. Therefore, when the eye turns nasally, the conjunctiva bunches more than when the eye turns in any other direction.

The sclera

From observation of casts of normal eyes (Marriott, 1966), it can be seen that the contour is not spherical or symmetrical about the visual axis of the eye, especially in the horizontal meridian. The nasal sclera is flatter, and the centre of curvature of the steeper temporal sclera is also contralaterally offset, making the nasal limbal sulcus more pronounced while the temporal sclera is nearer to being tangential to the cornea, as in *Figure 18.1* (Chapter 17, p. 628, gives a further explanation of the effect of offset centres of curvature). *Figure 18.2* is a photograph of the cast of the author's eye which has a nearly spherical corneal radius of 8.25 mm. The

Figure 18.2 Photograph of outline of cast of the author's eye showing the more pronounced nasal limbus (on the left hand side). Keratometry: 8.25 mm spherical

Figure 18.3 Outline of a cast of the same eye as in *Figure 18.2*, but in the vertical meridian. There is little difference between the upper and lower curvatures of the sclera, and the limbus is almost symmetrical. Note that the limbus (arrowed) is not sharply defined in either *Figures 18.2* or *18.3*

vertical meridian is more symmetrical, with a radius about midway between that of the temporal and nasal sclera. *Figure 18.3* is a photograph of the vertical meridian of the author's eye.

The horizontal recti muscles

The positions of insertion of the medial and lateral recti muscles are important because the periphery of the final lens may lie over them. The insertions of the superior and inferior recti and the obliques do not have a significant effect. A diagrammatic representation of the recti muscle insertions is shown in *Figure 18.4*.

The position of the origins of the medial and lateral recti are at the apex of the orbit which is nasally placed relative to the globe, as *Figure 18.5* shows. Because of this, the lateral rectus wraps itself around the globe towards the equator, while the medial rectus tends to come away from the globe just posterior to its point of insertion. The lateral rectus remains in contact with the globe during all eye movements whereas the medial rectus separates from the globe with nasal gaze, as shown in *Figure 18.6*. This and the conjunctival bunching result in a flattening of the nasal contours.

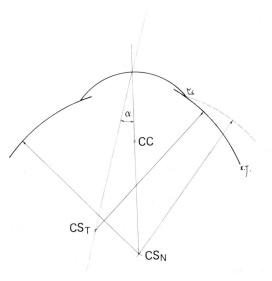

Figure 18.1 Diagrammatic representation of the difference between the nasal and temporal scleral contours. The less pronounced limbus on the temporal side is because the centre of curvature of the temporal sclera is contralaterally offset. In this diagram, the nasal and temporal radii have been made equal to show solely the effect of this offset. Sometimes the nasal scleral radius is actually flatter, which accentuates this effect. CC = centre of corneal curvature; CS_T = centre of curvature of temporal sclera; CS_N = centre of curvature of nasal sclera; α = angle of offset; $\triangledown$ = temporal limbus. The dotted line indicates the continuation of the nasal sclera on the temporal side

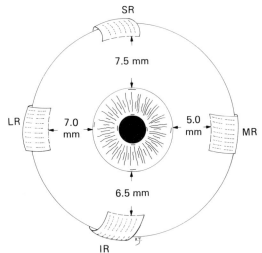

Figure 18.4 Diagrammatic representation of the extraocular muscle insertions showing their positions in relation to the limbus. LR = lateral rectus; MR = medial rectus; IR = inferior rectus; SR = superior rectus. The oblique muscle insertions are not included as they do not have a significant effect

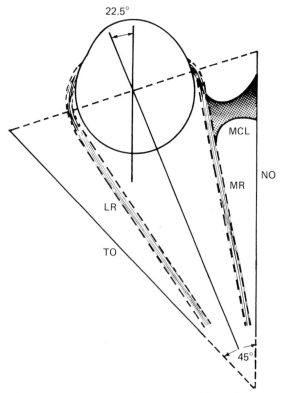

Figure 18.5 Configuration of the lateral and the medial rectus muscles in the orbit (left eye seen from above). LR = lateral rectus; MR = medial rectus; NO = nasal orbital wall; TO = temporal orbital wall; MCL = medial check ligament

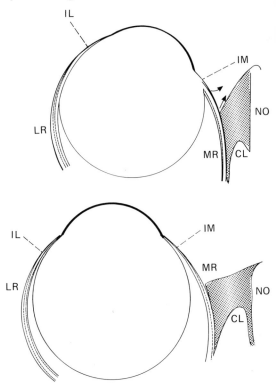

Figure 18.6 Effect on the scleral contours during gaze movements to the nasal side, when the medial rectus departs from the globe. The upper diagram shows the eye turned nasally and the lower diagram the eye in the primary position. IM = medial rectus insertion; IL = lateral rectus insertion; MR = medial rectus; LR = lateral rectus; NO = nasal orbital wall; CL = medial check ligament

The impression procedure and production of the cast

The prerequisite for fabrication of a scleral lens from an impression of the eye is that an accurate reproduction of the anterior contours of the eye can be made.

Production of the impression

The method of production of the impression is a similar procedure to that of taking a mould in dental work. It requires that a substance with gelling properties is held in contact with the anterior eye so that its contours are reproduced as exactly as possible. The gelling time of the material must be short enough to ensure that small eye movements do not blur the detail. The equipment and drugs necessary are listed below.

Equipment

Flexible sided rubber or plastic bowls (it is difficult to mix alginates and stone powder in porcelain bowls)
A curved stainless steel spatula
A selection of impression trays
One 10 ml syringe per eye to be moulded
Measuring cylinders or spoons
Tissues
A waterproof fibre pen
A stand for holding the trays after the impression has been taken

Drugs

Topical anaesthetic
Fluorescein
A prophylactic for instillation after the impression if necessary
A disinfecting agent
Unit dose saline for irrigating the eye after the impression
(*See also* Chapter 4)

Materials

Fresh Kromopan (Wright Dental Co. Ltd, Dundee, UK) or alternative impression material
Fresh distilled water or unit dose saline to mix with the alginate
Dental stone powder and plaster of Paris
Water to mix dental stone and plaster of Paris

Impression materials

Kromopan

Some dental alginates can be used to take impressions of eyes. They are soft enough to minimize abrasion of the cornea and separate easily from moist surfaces. Alginate powder mixes with water to form a thick creamy fluid which gels in a few seconds to the consistency of the white of a boiled egg. There are many available, but Kromopan is the one most frequently used today for contact lens work because of its very smooth texture and rapid gelling time.

Panasil

Some silicone-based products have been produced in recent years for dentistry. Storey and

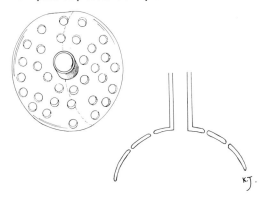

Figure 18.7 Back view and cross-section of an impression tray

Vale (1970) described an early attempt to use them in contact lens practice. Panasil (Kettenbach Dental Co., Eschenburg, Germany) is one proprietary brand which has gained popularity for eye impressions. Presentation is in paste form in a soft tube. A separate smaller tube of hardener is supplied which must be mixed with the paste to initiate the gelling process.

Support of the impression on the eye

Impression trays are used to hold the impression material in contact with the eye. About 20 countersunk holes, 1–1.5 mm in diameter are drilled in the tray. A tube, about 25 mm long and 5 mm in diameter, is attached to the front. *Figure 18.7* diagrammatically illustrates a tray.

The optimum thickness is about 0.6–0.8 mm. If thinner than this, there is a risk that it may distort or break. A greater thickness protrudes more, causing more lid pressure and making the impression more difficult to remove. The tray should be such a shape that it rests on the eye only at its extremities, and is otherwise just clear of the eye, as in *Figure 18.8*, resulting in an impression which is thicker over the cornea and limbus. The largest tray that can be inserted and removed should be used as this gives the largest supported impression. It should be remembered that the bulk of the impression material may make removal of the tray more difficult.

Sets of trays

A range of different diameters is needed to accommodate the variety of sizes of palpebral

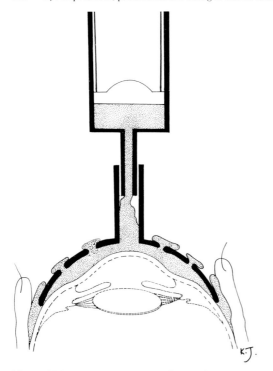

Figure 18.8 Impression tray *in situ*. Contact is only at the extreme periphery. The thickness of the impression is greatest over the cornea and limbus. The impression material extrudes through the holes in the tray to lock the gelled impression and the tray together

apertures. The temporal and superior portions of the tray should both be about 2 mm larger than the nasal and inferior. A set of trays, three or four for each eye, with diameters between 21 and 27 mm, should be adequate to be able to mould most eyes. The radius of the inside surface should be 12.5–13 mm to ensure that the tray is not too flat when resting on the globe. Special large, small, steep or flat trays can be made if required.

Preparation for taking the impression

A full eye examination should have been carried out already. This reveals any abnormalities that may be relevant to the taking of an impression. Any superficial irregularities are noted, and later should be evident on the cast. Having an impression taken may be a daunting prospect for patients, so a full explanation of what is about to happen helps to put them at their ease. A state of relaxation is conducive to achieving a good end result. The patient should be seated,

with back straight and the head comfortably supported in an upright position. There is less than a minute available from the start of the process to the end, so it is vital to ensure that all the necessary items are ready to hand.

Selection of tray

A tray is selected and cleaned. Its size is determined partly by the palpebral aperture, but not by this alone. Sometimes a much larger tray than expected can be inserted into the space to the temporal side of the outer canthus, if the lids can be stretched apart easily. Topical anaesthetic is then instilled. More than one drop is usually needed, and a good guide for adequate anaesthesia is that no further stinging is felt with subsequent drops. A trial insertion of the tray ensures that it is the correct size. It is then removed and the top marked 'R' or 'L' as appropriate with a waterproof fibre pen.

Establishing correct visual fixation

The method of fixation must ensure that the position of the eye is not affected by head movements or heterophorias and heterotropias. The eye to be moulded will be occluded during impression taking so the fellow eye is used for fixation.

(1) The eye to be moulded is covered so that the fellow eye takes up fixation, but in such a way that the practitioner can still see the covered eye.
(2) The patient is asked to fixate on his own finger, which the practitioner moves into position so that the eye to be moulded is in the desired position.
(3) The eyelid immediately below the pupil of the fixing eye, i.e. the eye not having the impression taken, is marked with a waterproof fibre pen.
(4) When the impression is taken, the patient is asked to look at his or her own finger, which is repositioned until the pupil is lined up with the mark made on the eyelid.

If there is no fellow eye, or if the fellow eye does not have good enough fixating ability, the correct positioning is arranged by asking the patients to look at their own index finger. During impression taking, patients are asked to maintain fixation at the point where they think their finger is located. This uses the function of innate hand–eye proprioception. It is usually possible to achieve a satisfactory result.

If the impression is taken with the eye turned towards the nasal side, the cast records a bunched up conjunctiva and any flattening of the nasal sclera due to contraction of the medial rectus, so the final shell will be loose on the nasal side when the eye is in the primary position. If the primary position is chosen for fixation, the lens may lift off to some extent when the eye is turned in. The most important consideration in practical terms is to ensure that the impression of the cornea is reasonably well centred.

Mixing impression materials

Kromopan

The optimum consistency is obtained by mixing 2 g powder to 7 ml water. Mixing briskly in a soft-sided rubber or plastic bowl makes a homogeneous cream. The spatula is best made of stainless steel and curved to enable stropping against the side of the bowl. The colour of the mix changes during spatulation, from purple, which indicates when the syringe should be charged, through pink, when it should be injected into the tray and finally to white. However, experienced users usually find it is more satisfactory to assess the viscosity changes by sense of touch. The main advantage of the colour change is that unmixed particles show up in the syringe because they do not change colour as quickly. If the syringe is held upright and the plunger is pressed slowly, the particles will remain static and the free-flowing homogeneous paste will pass them in the body of the syringe, preventing them blocking the nozzle or passing onto the eye, as shown in *Figure 18.9*. The cream does not remain free flowing for more than about a minute, in which time spatulation and injection must be finished. It takes some practice to mix alginates fully in that time. The material gels 20–30 seconds after turning white and can be removed after another 30 seconds. All alginates, being hygroscopic, change over a period of time, and Kromopan is no exception. The gelling time may lengthen and the quality of the final impression may suffer if the powder is not reasonably fresh. Ambient temperature and humidity also have an effect. Gelling is much quicker in warm, humid conditions and it

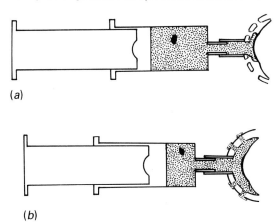

(a)

(b)

Figure 18.9 Diagrammatic representation of the relatively slow movement of a particle of unmixed alginate in the syringe. (*a*) At the start of injection into the impression tray on the eye; (*b*) almost at the conclusion of injection with the anterior eye completely covered by impression material

may be necessary to use refrigerated water. In addition, the gelling property may vary from batch to batch. Sometimes it is necessary to add more water if it is too viscous during the spatulation. If in doubt it is useful to do a trial mix to assess gelling time.

Panasil

Everything necessary for correct mixing is provided with the package. This includes paper on which the Panasil is mixed with the hardener. The correct length of the Panasil is mapped out in a grid drawn on the paper. A length of Panasil is squeezed from the tube onto the grid as in *Figure 18.10*, and an equal length of hardener, or with Panasil C a drop of hardener for each grid square, is added. The two substances are mixed on the paper surface with a spatula. It is easier to obtain a uniform consistency than with Kromopan. The texture of Panasil is rather more sticky than Kromopan in the transitional phase of gelling, which makes

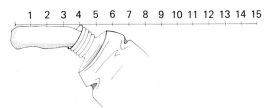

Figure 18.10 Panasil mixing sheet

it less popular with some practitioners. However, it is less subject to deterioration when stored after the tube has been opened, so may be preferred if scleral lens fitting is carried out only occasionally. The effect of humidity changes is also less than with Kromopan. Storey (1987) has reviewed the use of Panasil in greater detail.

Taking the impression

Injecting

When the impression material is ready for mixing, the tray is replaced under the lids. Some practitioners prefer to delay re-inserting the tray until the impression material is finally mixed. This reduces the time the tray is in place, which may be more comfortable for the patient, but leaves less time available for spatulation. A syringe is charged with the homogeneous impression material. This is injected through the tubular handle into the space between the tray and the eye. Fixation is maintained throughout, and it is verified that it is still correct when sufficient material has been injected. The tray should be held away from the globe slightly while injecting, and it helps to fully cover the whole of the anterior eye by injecting from all directions. This is done by moving the tray up, down, left and right in a continuous action as the plunger is pressed.

Insertion method

As an alternative to injecting, the tray can be inserted filled with mixed impression material. The largest tray that can be put in place under the lids easily and quickly is selected. The patient's head has to be bent forwards until facing the floor. If this is not done, the impression material drops away from the upper part of the tray. Panasil is sometimes the preferred moulding material because of its stickier texture. The impression should be of more even thickness than if the injection method is used, so the back radius of the tray should nearly match the eye. A range of trays with different radii as well as total diameters is desirable. Some practitioners are of the opinion that the less bulky impression gives improved definition.

Injection is usually the simpler choice with patients whose eyes are more difficult to mould.

The tray is already on the eye, so there is no risk of gelling before the tray can be inserted, e.g. because of an unexpected blepharospasm. Also, larger trays can be used which help to maximize the coverage of the globe. Inserting the tray is not made easier when it is also necessary to avoid spilling the impression material.

Removal of impression

Excess material is removed from the lids and long lashes are pulled from the impression by partially everting the lid. Muscle hooks are not necessary for this. If the tray has rotated, the new top position should be marked. The patient is asked to look up as far as possible. The lower lid is pulled down below the impression, and pressed gently into the sclera, relieving the suction. A slight twist also helps removal. The tray is allowed to slide down over the lower lid. If the tray is pulled sharply away from the globe, there is the risk of separation of the impression from the tray.

Inspection of impression

The impression is inspected. The corneal area should be clearly defined and its position central or displaced slightly to the nasal side. Small flaws are not necessarily a reason for rejection as these can often be removed from the dental stone cast. The impression tray is placed in a suitable holder until it is cast with dental stone. Filling a Kromopan impression with water helps to slow down shrinkage and dehydration.

Precautions

Corneal distortion

It has been suggested that the cornea is compressed by the bulk of impression material as it covers the anterior globe. This is not easy to prove or disprove, and it is debatable that it happens to a clinically significant extent. However, it is worth bearing this in mind when dealing with eyes which may have reduced corneal rigidity. It could happen if the impression material had almost fully gelled before injecting, but when free flowing, there is very little pressure on the cornea. *Figure 18.11* is an outline of two casts of the same keratoconic eye, the first clearly demonstrating that some distortion had taken place. It was thought that the

(a)

(b)

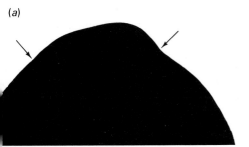
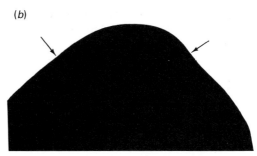

Figure 18.11 (*a*) Photograph of the outline of a cast showing corneal distortion after injection of alginate that had gelled too quickly, depressing the central area of a keratoconic cornea with below average rigidity. (*b*) This shows a more accurate impression of the same eye. ↓ indicates the limbus

(a)

(b)

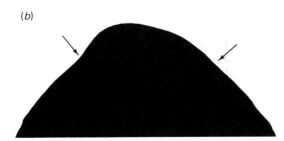

Figure 18.12 (*a*) Photograph of the outline of a cast made from an impression taken immediately following scleral lens wear. The cornea has been made more spherical to some degree by the scleral lens that had been worn. (*b*) A photograph of the outline of a cast of the same eye made from an impression taken after the lens was left out for 15 hours. ↓ indicates the limbus

Note: *Figures 18.11* and *18.12* are the left and right eyes, respectively, of the same keratoconic patient. The impressions were taken during a normal clinical session, and not specially contrived to demonstrate these points. This illustrates that mishaps can happen, and the practitioner should be alert to their occurrences

alginate had partially gelled as it was being injected.

Another possible cause of distortion of the impression exists when an eye already wearing a scleral lens has another impression taken. If the original lens is bearing on the cornea, as is frequently the case with keratoconus (*see* p. 682 and *Plate 76*) some distortion of the new impression may occur if the cornea is not allowed to resume its usual shape first. This is illustrated in *Figure 18.12*, which shows outlines of two casts of an eye, one from an impression taken immediately after removal of the patient's own scleral lens, and the other taken when the lens had not been worn for 15 hours. The more regular shape is the cast of the impression taken when the lens had just been removed. The other is a more accurate reproduction of the true contours of the eye. *Figures 18.11* and *18.12* were the left and right eyes respectively of the same patient. This

was not done intentionally for demonstration purposes, but does illustrate that mishaps occur sometimes when taking impressions.

Collapse of impression under the weight of the dental stone

If the impression is not well enough supported, there is a chance that it will collapse when filled with dental stone. *Figure 18.13* shows an unsupported section of the impression collapsing under the weight of the liquid dental stone as it is poured in. The central section of the unsupported impression tends to collapse outwards, while both sides collapse inwards. The result is something of an egg-shaped cast. An area of loose scleral fitting bordered on both sides by a tight area could well be attributable to such poor support. *Figure 18.14a,b* illustrates the casts of a patient's right and left eyes which were

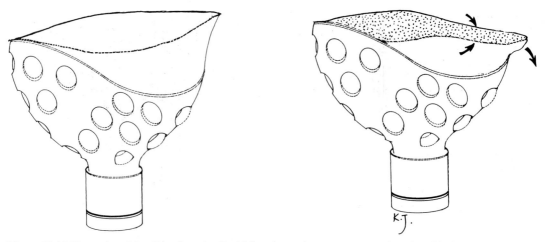

Figure 18.13 Illustration of the effect of pouring liquid dental stone into an unsupported section of the impression. Note the collapse outwards, in the right hand diagram, of the weakest part of the impression, with inward collapse of the adjacent areas, as arrowed. ↓ indicates collapse of impression

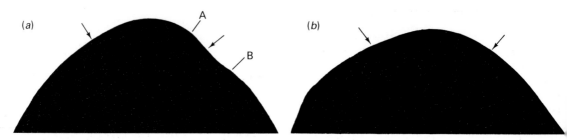

Figure 18.14 (*a*) Photograph of the outline of a cast made from a left eye impression that had collapsed at the limbus between points A and B. Final fitting of the lens was impossible. (*b*) A photograph of the outline of a cast made from an impression of the fellow eye which was nearly symmetrical and of almost exactly the same contours. The left eye was reasonably well fitted by turning the cast of the right eye upside down to make a shell. The indication for scleral lens fitting was bilateral aphakia following congenital rubella cataract. Note that the limbus is barely perceptible in the cast made for the right eye, which was an accurate representation of the contours. ↓ indicates limbus

almost totally symmetrical, both photographed from the temporal side at the same angle. The pronounced depression superior to the limbal margin is an artefact.

Omission of impression of parts of the globe

Care must be taken to avoid failing to cover a section of the globe with impression material. For example, there may be a marked Bell's reaction on taking an eye impression, when the whole superior sclera may be missed.

The liquid dental stone adheres to any particles of unmixed alginate on the surface of the impression and, on setting, leaves an irregular cavity in the cast which has to be filled

in. A gap or an air bubble in the impression will be filled by the dental stone, giving rise to an unwanted proud area which has to be scraped away. Both entail some guesswork as to what the shape would have been, so only small defects can be rectified in this way.

Post-impression examination

The eye should be examined for any residual impression material in the conjunctival sac. If any remains, it usually forms a sliver which is easily seen and removed. Irrigation of the eye helps to flush out any particles. Inspection of the cornea using the slit lamp and fluorescein will reveal any abrasions. If these are serious, instillation of prophylactics may be indicated. A single drop will not keep the conjunctival sac sterile for the whole of the time it takes for the cornea to heal. If there is a likelihood of an abrasion becoming infected, repeated instillations of eye drops are necessary. Ointment remains in contact with the eye for much longer so may be better.

Preparation of the cast from the impression

There is only time for a single cast to be made from a Kromopan impression, so this must be done correctly and without delay. This does not apply to casts made from Panasil which does not dehydrate and shrink as its water content is zero.

Casting with liquid dental stone

Cold water is added to dental stone powder and stirred in a rubber bowl until the mixture is creamy and even in texture. The proportion by volume is about one part water to five parts powder, but this varies with different types of stone. Most air bubbles can be brought to the surface by tapping the bowl against a table top, or with an agitating machine. A drop of the liquid stone is lowered gently into the middle of the impression. More is added to it to make it creep up the side to prevent introduction of bubbles. If a section of the impression is not supported, stone can only be laid against it if it can be seen that the weight of the stone is not bending the impression. If air has been introduced, there is still time at this stage to wash out the liquid dental stone and start again.

A plaster of Paris base added afterwards provides a solid foundation. Leaving a spur in the middle of the dental stone cast, as in *Figure 18.15*, helps to lock the dental stone to the plaster. A more viscous mix may be needed for the spur to retain its shape.

Marking and trimming the cast

When the cast sets, which for most types of stone is at least 45 minutes, the back is marked 'R' or 'L' at the top corresponding to the position of the mark on the tray, and with the patient's reference. It is then separated from the impression. If the stone has fully set, there is never any

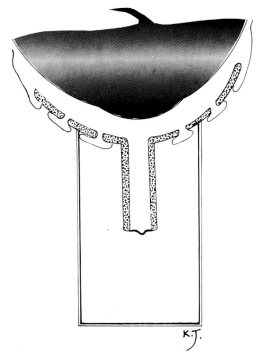

Figure 18.15 Spur left on the base of the dental stone cast as it is poured into the inverted impression

adhesion, except when there is some unmixed alginate on the surface of the impression. With some dental stone powders, a granular texture of the surface of the cast results if it is removed from the impression too soon.

The front is marked at the top with 'R' or 'L'. The limbus can be delineated and the nasal and temporal sides indicated if desired. If the dental stone spilled over the perimeter of the impression, this surplus material should be removed. This is a simple task if done quickly, but if left for too long the stone becomes very hard and it is much more difficult to remove unwanted ridges or to trim the edge without biting chunks out of the cast with the plaster knife. Conjunctival folds and vessels are faithfully recorded on the cast. These are not helpful and should also be removed promptly by scraping lightly with the blade of the plaster knife.

Mounting the cast

The back of the stone cast is placed in freshly mixed plaster of Paris on a sheet of Perspex to give a final flat base. Plaster of Paris sets in a few minutes and, just before it finally hardens, can

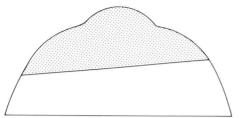

Figure 18.16 The cornea is usually not in the centre of the impression but nearer to the nasal side. The temporal sclera is generally wider than the nasal, so when mounted on a plaster of Paris base, the bottom of the dental stone cast (shown shaded) is not parallel to the plaster of Paris base if the cornea is sited centrally and uppermost

be easily shaped to conform to the outer edges of the cast. The corneal section of the cast must be situated uppermost and, as it may be displaced to the nasal side, the bottom of the cast is not necessarily parallel to the bottom of the plaster base, as in *Figure 18.16*.

When the plaster of Paris is set, the flat base is marked with the relevant details. Shells and lenses can now be produced in any style.

Production and fitting of shells and lenses

For best results, as much handwork on the shell as possible should be carried out by the practitioners or under their immediate supervision, especially with the more complex pathological cases which now account for the majority of scleral lens fittings. Sending the shell to a laboratory for this to be done means that many more fitting sessions are necessary and is not conducive to making the best final lens. If it is very inconvenient to have a small adjustment carried out, it may be tempting to leave it in the original state. This never needs to be so if full manufacturing equipment is to hand.

Equipment necessary

(1) Variable speed suspension motor — up to 12 000 rev./min.
(2) Flexible drive attachment.
(3) A selection of dental tools mounted on mandrels or on fixed mounts designed to fit the flexible drive:
  rose burrs of various sizes from 0.3 mm to 2 mm in diameter;
  fissure burrs or special cutters;
  flat discs about 25 mm in diameter and 5 mm wide;
  conical shapes about 12 mm long and 8 mm wide tapering to a blunted point;
  hard packed felt wheels for polishing;
  loose rag wheels for buffing
  (*Figure 23.6* illustrates some of these tools).
(4) Block of PMMA polish.
(5) Powerful bench motor of at least one-third horse power, or a dental lathe. A two-speed model is preferable, approximately 1200 rev./min and 2500 rev./min.
(6) Rag wheels both tightly and loosely packed, fitted to the bench motor.
(7) Eye protectors, which should be worn at all times when using high velocity wheels on both types of motor.
(8) Clinical quality PMMA sheets, of thickness between 1 mm and 3 mm in 0.5 mm increments.
(9) A device for heating and pressing PMMA sheets over the cast — *see Figures 18.17, 18.18* and *18.19*.
(10) Contact lens thickness gauge — *Figure 18.20* shows the thickness of a scleral lens being measured.
(11) Selection of diamond-coated lapping stones, as shown in *Figures 18.21* and *18.22*. Radii of 6.00 mm to 9.50 mm in 0.25 mm increments is the minimum workable range. It is better to have 0.1 mm increments, and also useful to have both coarse and fine grit stones available. The cheaper alternative to diamond-coated stones is to apply carborundum powder to smooth stones, but this is very time consuming.
(12) Vertical bench spindle — *see Figure 18.21*.
(13) Polishing tools: a range of brass or hard plastic tools made to match the diamond tools, also shown in *Figure 18.21*. These are covered with an adhesive cloth, e.g. zinc oxide plaster tape, to absorb the polish. The correct tool is slightly steeper than the diamond tool to allow for the thickness of the cloth, as in *Figure 18.23*. Individually made wax polishing tools can be cut to the desired radius by using a female gauge (*Figure 18.24*) selected from a range matching the diamond stones. However, even experienced technicians find it difficult to

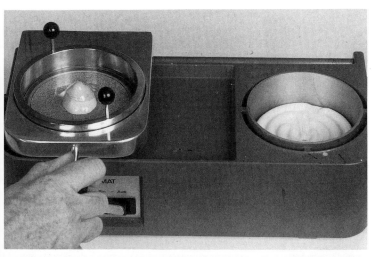

Figure 18.17 Integrated heating and vacuum press in operation

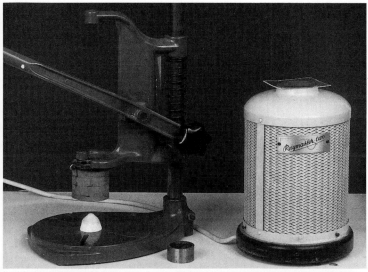

Figure 18.18 Infrared heating unit and mechanical press (power drill support). Alternatively, a simple rigid metal cylinder can be used to press out a shell

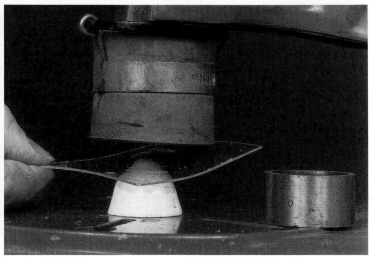

Figure 18.19 Heated PMMA sheet about to be pressed over a cast using a cylinder mounted on a press

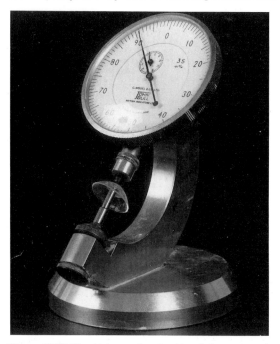

Figure 18.20 The thickness of a scleral lens being measured on a standard thickness gauge

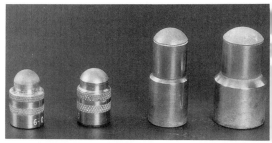

Figure 18.22 Four lapping tools to show difference between the curvatures

cut a consistently true curve by this method. Lathe cutting is much more satisfactory — *see* Chapter 22 and *Figure 22.6*.

(14) Polish: silver polish is quite workable, but special Perspex polish, which is thicker, may be preferable.

(15) Riders for holding the shell: corneal lens buttons can be used. One surface should be flat, the other concave, of radius between 6.5 mm and 8.5 mm. The button with a radius approximating to the front surface of the shell is selected. A small central hollow is made in the flat surface, to take a pencil point.

(16) Double-sided adhesive tape.

Success or failure may hinge upon fine adjustments which are not easily described. Even experienced observers need to inspect the shell *in situ* before a final judgement can be made on whether or not a modification has had the desired effect.

Four stages of production and fitting procedures now follow: production of the flush fitting basic shell; cutting the primary optic zone; shell fitting; manufacture and modification of the finished lens.

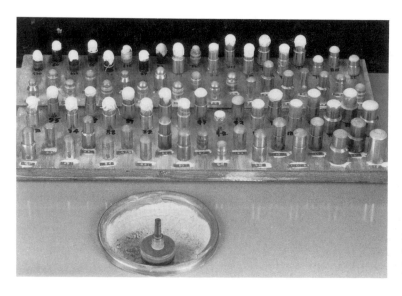

Figure 18.21 Range of diamond lapping tools and cloth-covered polishing tools with vertical bench spindle

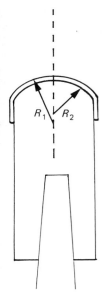

Figure 18.23 Cloth-covered spherical brass polishing tool. An allowance must be made for the thickness of the cloth which makes the radius slightly greater when in use. Erring on the flat side polishes more towards the periphery of the back optic zone, on the steep side towards the centre. R_2 = radius of brass tool plus thickness of cloth; R_1 = radius of brass tool

Production of the flush fitting basic shell

A clinical quality PMMA sheet is selected. The usual thickness is approximately 1.5 mm. A thicker sheet may be necessary to produce a lens of high power, especially if a large optic zone diameter is required for a high positive lens. The maximum thickness necessary is about 2.00 mm unless the lens is also intended to serve as a ptosis prop (pp. 693–695). It may be possible to use sheets only 1.00 mm thick if it is anticipated that the final power will be plano to about -5.00 D, or if making a copy lens which needs very little substance removed from the back surface.

The sheet is softened by heating to about 140°C and pressed over the cast. Purpose-designed vacuum presses with integrated heating elements are excellent, but expensive. *Figure 18.17* illustrates such a device in use. An infrared lamp is adequate for heating. Care must be taken to avoid overheating, which causes bubbles in the PMMA sheet. A simple way to press out a shell is to use a rigid cylinder, the diameter of which must be greater than the cast but less than the width of the sheet. The cylinder can be mounted on a drill stand if desired. *Figures 18.18* and *18.19* show this equipment in use.

The perimeter of the shell is marked using a waterproof pen according to the line previously drawn marking the edge of the cast, as in *Figure 18.25*. This basic shape is then cut using a fissure burr or cutter mounted in the flexible drive as in *Figures 18.26, 18.27* and *18.28*.

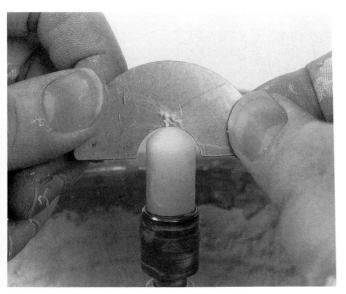

Figure 18.24 Cutting a wax polishing tool with a female gauge

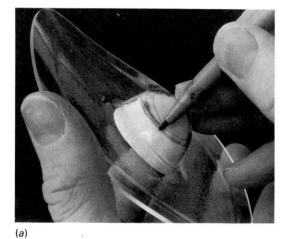

(a)

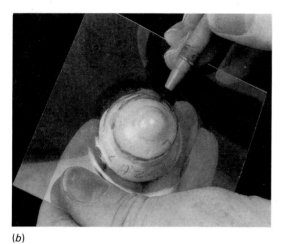

(b)

Figure 18.25 Marking the periphery of the shell according to marks made on the cast. (a) Side view; (b) top view

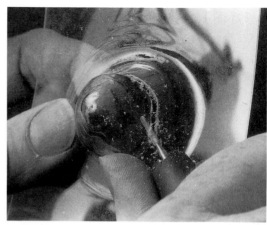

Figure 18.27 Photograph to show cutting the shell from the moulded PMMA sheet

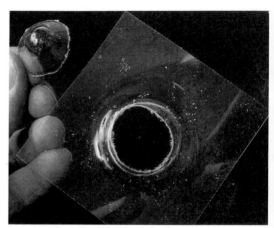

Figure 18.28 The rough-edged shell taken from the moulded PMMA sheet

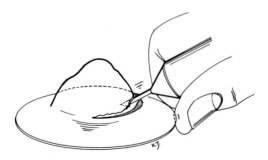

Figure 18.26 Use of cutting tool or fissure burr mounted into the flexible drive of a suspension motor to cut the shell from the moulded sheet of PMMA. This leaves a rough edge

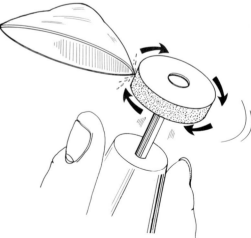

Figure 18.29 Use of a disc-shaped abrasive tool to give the desired size of the shell

A disc-shaped tool is used to trim the shell more precisely to the desired size (*Figures 18.29* and *18.30*). The same tool can be used to commence the edge thinning and shaping process (*Figure 18.31*) and a conical-shaped tool to continue shaping the edge on the inside (*Figures 18.32* and *18.33*).

A less abrasive carborundum-impregnated rubber tool can be used in the first stage of finishing the edge, as in *Figure 18.34*. A high polish can be achieved using the bench motor with a firm rag wheel, as in *Figure 18.35*. Although the bench motor is slower than the suspension motor, the surface velocity is far greater than with the smaller tools mounted on mandrels. This, and the greater surface area,

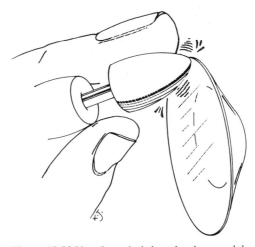

Figure 18.32 Use of a conical-shaped tool to round the inside surface of the edge

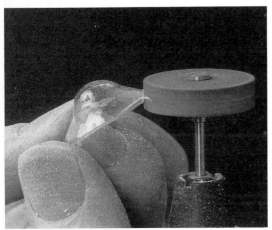

Figure 18.30 Photograph to show the same action, as in *Figure 18.29*

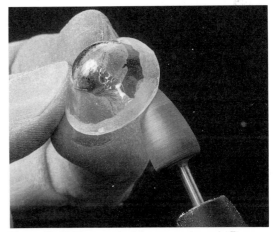

Figure 18.33 Photograph of the same action as in *Figure 18.32*

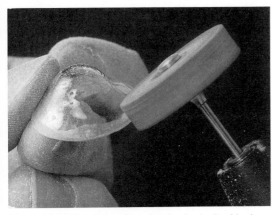

Figure 18.31 Use of disc-shaped tool to begin the thinning down and final profiling of the edge

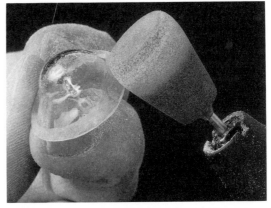

Figure 18.34 A carborundum-impregnated rubber tool with mild abrasive quality used to continue the edge shaping and commence the polishing process

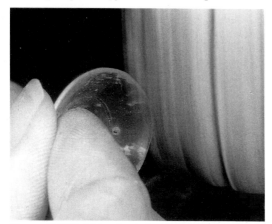

Figure 18.35 Polishing the surface and edge using a polishing mop mounted on a bench motor. This gives a faster and more even polish than if rag wheels are mounted into a flexible drive of the suspension motor

gives a much more even polish. Care must be taken using bench motors or dental lathes because substance is removed quite quickly, and there is a risk of breakage of more delicate shells.

The surface and edge must be well polished before the shell can be put in the eye for inspection of the fit. This applies at all stages of fitting the shell and lens. A final polish of both the back and front surfaces of the shell can be achieved using polish-laden rag wheels mounted in the flexible drive (*Figures 18.36* and *18.37*). Both surfaces can be given a final buff using a loose rag wheel mounted in the flexible drive (*Figures 18.38* and *18.39*).

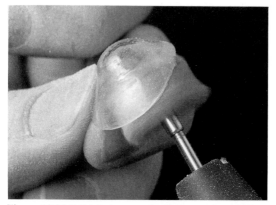

Figure 18.36 Polish-laden rag wheel being used to polish the back (inside) surface of the lens

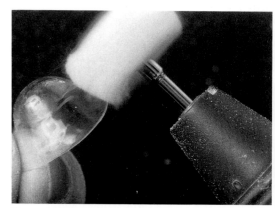

Figure 18.38 Loose rag wheel being used to give a final buff to the front (outside) surface

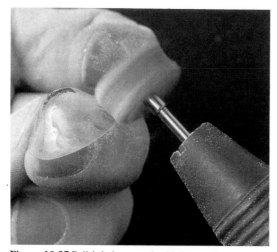

Figure 18.37 Polish-laden rag wheel being used to polish the front (outside) surface

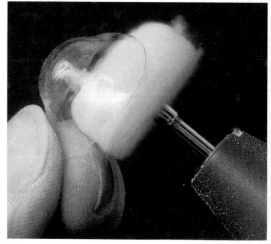

Figure 18.39 Loose rag wheel being used to give a final buff to the back (inside) surface

Inspection of the basic shell on the eye

At this point the fit of the scleral zone only is being checked. Tight areas give rise to blanching due to compression of the conjunctival and scleral blood vessels. Loose areas are easily seen after instillation of fluorescein, or may entrap air. If the inferior scleral zone is too small, the lower lid catches on the edge of the shell. If the shell is too large, it lifts off during nasal and inferior gaze as the lens impinges upon the inner canthus and lower fornix, respectively. If the scleral zone is fitting satisfactorily, the next step can be embarked upon. This is the establishment of physiologically acceptable corneal and limbal clearance.

Cutting the primary optic zone

This phase of manufacture commences the process which is best considered as fitting the fluid lens to the cornea. The primary optic zone is structured on the basis of the contours of the cast or measurements of the corneal topography. The shell with the primary optic clearance is referred to in this text as the primary shell. The usual method for establishing corneal vertex clearance and limbal clearance is by using lapping tools on a vertical spindle. Subsequent modifications are made after observation of the fluid coverage with a shell *in situ*.

Choice of the primary back optic curvature

Empirical selection

Observation of the contours of the cast and offering up the chosen lapping tool to the corneal portion of the shell is the ideal way to select the primary back optic zone radius. The correct tool is the one that cuts at first in the midperiphery, and then simultaneously towards the centre and the outer periphery. More than one may have to be tried before the optimum radius is found, and sometimes the best construction may be a bi-curve or even a multi-curve. More substance needs to be removed from the limbal area than from the central corneal area, the difference depending upon the contours of the eye. The normal corneal curvature is flatter towards the periphery, so a back optic zone curve which is

flat relative to the central cornea will tend towards concentricity nearer the periphery, as in *Figure 18.40*.

A steeper tool cuts more towards the centre and a flatter tool more towards the periphery. *Figure 18.41* represents steep and flat cuts into the back surface of the primary shell. The optimum tool is selected by the process described, and placed onto the vertical bench spindle. To grind the back optic zone radius, a rider is attached to the front of the shell with double-sided adhesive tape. The spindle is set in motion, the diamond surface moistened and the shell held against it using a pencil point placed in the rider as in *Figure 18.42*. When the tool is cutting evenly, the shell spins freely in the same direction as the spindle. The shell should be rotated in the opposite direction with a circular movement of the pencil.

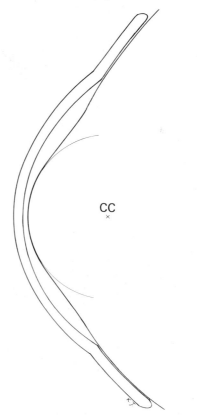

Figure 18.40 Illustration of the effect of the peripheral flattening of the cornea. The back optic zone radius of the shell is flatter than the central corneal curvature, but further towards the periphery of the optic zone the back of the shell and the cornea are nearly parallel. CC = centre of curvature of cornea; fine line = continuation of spherical central corneal curvature

(a)

(b)

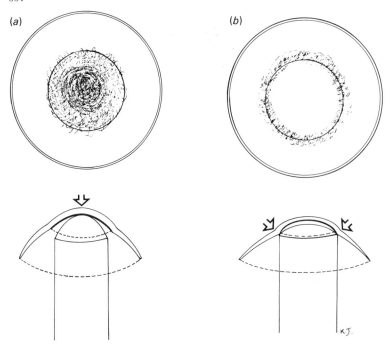

Figure 18.41 Diagrammatic representation of (a) steep and (b) flat lapping tools in use, showing the comparative areas where they cut into the substance of the shell. The arrows show the points of contact during the process of working the back optic zone radius, and the upper diagrams show this as viewed through the shell

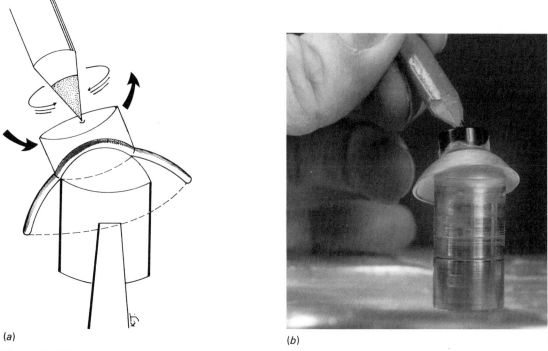

(a)

(b)

Figure 18.42 (a) Illustration of a shell mounted on a rider spinning on a lapping stone. It is held down using a pencil point in the hole in the rider. The graphite assists lubrication. (b) Photograph of same action

Prior measurement of the central and peripheral thickness is necessary so that the amount of substance removed can be accurately monitored. The primary shell for a normal eye should have about 0.15 mm and 0.20 mm removed from the central portion and limbal region, respectively. More can always be removed later when the shell has been inspected on the eye. For normal corneal contours a single curve may suffice for the primary optic clearance. Structuring the primary optic zone for an irregular eye is described later in this chapter on pp. 666–667 and 685–686.

Finally, the surface is polished using cloth-covered tools, wax tools or a combination of both. This is done by the same method as grinding the back optic zone, but polishing tools are substituted for the diamond-coated tools. Lighter pressure is required than for grinding.

Fenestrated lenses for optic measurement (FLOMs)

The use of FLOMs has been suggested as a guide to selection of the back optic zone radius. This is a possibility, but there are problems which should be borne in mind:

(1) When grinding out the back optic zone of a shell made from a cast, the primary optic diameter may not be the same as the FLOM.
(2) The narrow supporting band of the FLOM bears little similarity to the much wider scleral zone of the finished lens. The settling back effect cannot be adequately simulated by a FLOM.
(3) FLOMs have a flat edge curve and are very uncomfortable. The interaction between lens and lid is quite different for a FLOM than for a finished scleral lens.

Keratometry

Keratometry may be used as a guide to the selection of the back optic zone radius (BOZR), but only if the cornea is normal and has a predictable peripheral flattening factor. The assumption that this is the same for steep and flat corneas is not valid. Kiely, Smith and Carney (1982) analysed the corneal topography and confirmed that steeper corneas have a greater flattening factor, so a rule of thumb indicating the BOZR from keratometry readings cannot always be applied. If the anterior topography is irregular, keratometry can hardly be used at all (see Chapter 21, under Keratoconus, p. 755).

Lewis (1969) suggested a bi-curve construction with a back optic zone radius matching the flattest keratometry reading and a BOZD of 7.00 mm, initially removing 0.1 mm of substance. If lapping tools in 0.25 mm steps only were available, the nearest flatter one would be recommended. The optimum back peripheral radius was specified as 1.25 mm flatter than the BOZR, with a diameter of 14.00 mm plus however much was necessary to blend into the scleral zone. This construction produced an even central tear film between lens and cornea with a large annular air space surrounding the limbus.

Marriott (1972) favoured a mono-curve BOZR 0.2 mm flatter than the flatter keratometry reading, ground out to a depth of 0.15–0.20 mm to allow for settling back.

Ordering lenses from outside laboratories

These two techniques have been shown to satisfactory methods of selecting the BOZR if it is not possible for practitioners to produce their own lenses. The order should be enclosed with the cast and should indicate the following details:

(1) Back optic zone radius (BOZR).
(2) Back optic zone diameter (BOZD).
(3) Amount of substance to be removed.
(4) Back peripheral radius (BPR) if appropriate.
(5) Back peripheral diameter.
(6) Whether the BOZR should be blended into the scleral zone, and degree of blending.
(7) Back vertex power (BVP).
(8) Final central substance if this should be different from the optimum for production of the required BVP.
(9) Thickness of scleral zone.
(10) Edge form.
(11) Position and diameter of fenestration.
(12) Any engravings, e.g. R or L, or one or two dots, and where these should be located.

The cast should be marked with the following details:

(1) The patient's name.
(2) Whether the right or left eye.

(3) The top, and the nasal and temporal, positions along the equator.
(4) The limbal margin.
(5) The position of the optical centre.
(6) The desired total diameter and shape of the lens.

The balance between the corneal topography and the curvature of the lens can be quite critical, and this is best evaluated during the process of manufacturing the primary shell. If a good relationship exists between the practitioner and the laboratory, an experienced scleral lens technician should be able to make a primary shell given a cast and just the details of the amount of substance to be removed and the approximate final power. Information of a refraction over a contact lens of known specifications can be supplied at a later stage when the power is to be worked onto the final fitted shell.

clamped to a PMMA backing sheet and both are heated. When soft enough, both are pulled down over the cast, as in *Figure 18.44*. The laminate thins slightly to about 0.18 mm centrally and 0.22 at the limbal diameter. It is removed from the backing sheet and cut to a diameter about 1.5 mm larger than the limbal diameter, chamfered to a thin edge and stuck to the cast, as in *Figure 18.45*. A PMMA sheet is heated and pressed over the combined cast and laminate, as in *Figure 18.46*.

If the vertex clearance is not enough when the shell is inspected *in situ*, either the back optic surface can be ground out or another shell can be pressed using a thicker laminate. If the clearance is too great, it is possible to remove substance from the scleral zone, but probably more constructive to remake the shell using a thinner laminate. A fully settled scleral lens

Alternative methods of constructing the primary optic zone clearance

Two alternative methods have been documented: use of laminates, and a modification of the impression procedure — which is to take the impression with a hydrogel lens of the appropriate thickness *in situ*.

Laminates

Marriott (1970, 1972) described the use of acrylic laminates which are stuck over the corneal portion of the cast to provide the necessary vertex clearance when a sheet of PMMA is pulled over the cast.

The laminate is produced in sheet form, most commonly 0.20 mm thick in the centre and 0.24 mm at the edge, as in *Figure 18.43*. It is

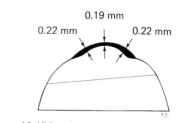

Figure 18.44 Laminate (shown in black) and backing sheet pressed over a cast. (Not to scale)

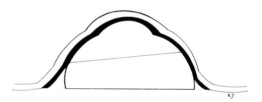

Figure 18.45 Laminate trimmed to a knife edge, diameter just greater than the limbal diameter, and stuck onto the corneal portion of the cast. (Not to scale)

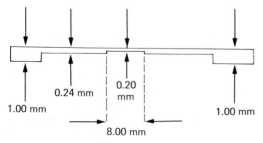

Figure 18.43 Diagrammatic representation of the cross-section of a laminate

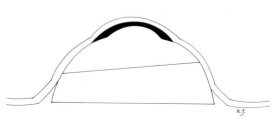

Figure 18.46 PMMA sheet pressed over the cast which has been built up using the laminate to provide automatically for the required corneal and limbal clearance. (Not to scale)

made by the laminate technique is shown in *Plate 76a,b*.

It has been suggested that the use of laminates can reduce the time spent grinding the optic, but this is debatable. Sharp diamond stones can cut sufficient material in a matter of minutes. Pressing and trimming the laminate takes as long or longer. The back surface is wavy and gives poor focimeter images with finished lenses, so there is always a degree of inaccuracy. However, if the visual potential is not too high, the poor back surface quality may not reduce the visual acuity too much. This is because there is a refractive index change of only 0.154 at the tear lens/plastic interface compared to 0.490 in air, so it is much more important that the front surface is of high quality. If a high quality optic zone is needed, the BOZR should be trued up. If this is not done, the front surface radius can only be calculated on the basis of an estimated BOZR. It is usually necessary to re-work the front curve after an over-refraction, calculating the new FOZR according to the change in power.

Another problem is that laminates are not easy to produce. They cannot be made using normal scleral lens manufacturing equipment, so their use creates a reliance upon an outside manufacturer who has to specially prepare them. It is also difficult to control precisely the final clearance. There is no guarantee that the laminate thins evenly as it is pulled over the cast.

A modified version of the laminate method may also be worth trying. A malleable material such as metal foil may be used to give part of the vertex clearance. The remainder is ground using lapping stones in the usual way. A further adaptation of this technique is to build up an area of the cast to make a channel (*see* p. 668 and *see also* Chapter 23).

Taking the impression over a soft lens

Westerhout (1975) first described the method of establishing the optic zone clearance by taking the impression over a soft lens *in situ* (*see* p. 816). A low minus lens (−3.00 D to −4.00 D) of 0.15 mm centre thickness provides for both apical and limbal clearance (*see Plate 82*).

The same problem of lack of control of the corneal clearance applies as with laminates, especially if flexure of the soft lens occurs while the eye is being moulded. In addition, there is the drawback that the soft lens may dislodge completely, which would spoil the impression. Using a steep fitting soft lens or presoaking in hypotonic saline may increase its adherence to the cornea during the moulding process (*Plate 81*). When the moulding has been completed, irrigation with physiological saline will permit its removal. It is also necessary to true up the back optic zone for the same reasons as described when using laminates. An advantage is that there is less trauma to the cornea as a consequence of the moulding procedure. *Plate 80* shows casts of both successful and unsuccessful eye impressions taken in this way.

Both systems have been shown to work well and are worth keeping in mind, but lack the flexibility and precision of the diamond lapping tool method which remains the procedure of first choice for the fully equipped scleral lens practitioner.

The shell fitting

Adjustments to the primary shell are made according to the appearance of the fluid coverage and tear flow, and are not based on measurements of the eye or even on the contours of the cast. Tools of various shapes and grades of abrasiveness can be mounted into the handpiece of the motor to carry out any modifications. These are more difficult to describe because it may be quite different in each individual case, particularly as abnormal eyes now account for the majority of scleral lens fittings. Total flexibility on the part of the practitioner is required.

There are four key processes involved in shell fitting: establishing tear exchange (ventilating); blending the transition; modifying the primary shell after settling back; modifying the scleral zone.

Establishing tear exchange (ventilating)

Before insertion, the primary shell is filled with saline and a drop of fluorescein. To avoid spilling the fluid, the shell must be inserted with the patient leaning forward and facing the floor. This avoids trapping a bubble and, when observed under ultraviolet light, it can be seen how the primary optic zone relates to the corneal topography. All methods of ventilation disrupt the static fluid reservoir, so this should be done before any further modifications are made.

Channels

There is some misconception about channelled lenses which in the past have been confused with sealed lenses. To clarify, a channel is a groove worked on the back of the scleral zone creating an additional clearance linking the limbal region to the edge, as shown in *Figures 18.47* and *18.48*. A channel is a feasible method of creating a degree of ventilation provided that it remains patent throughout any period of wear. The depth is quite critical. If too deep, air bubbles may be admitted and collect under the central area. If too shallow, it occludes when the lens settles back. In the days when many channelled scleral lenses were fitted, there was much discussion about the optimum siting, and lenses were fitted with channels in a variety of positions. Advocates of one style or another had strong views, but the author's observation of the long-term results is that a channel may be

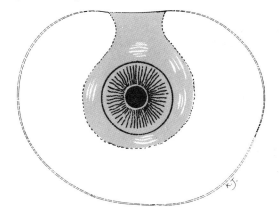

Figure 18.48 Front view of a broad superior channel. The shaded area represents clearance from the eye over the cornea and limbus and in the channel itself

acceptable wherever placed provided the lens has been well made and the depth of the channel correctly structured. The author's preference is for a broad superior channel blended into the space overlying the limbus.

Production of channels Small spherical or disc-shaped tools mounted into the hand-piece attachment to the motor can be used to work a channel. To polish, felt and rag wheels are substituted. An extra 0.5 mm thickness of the PMMA sheet is required to make a channelled shell, and this must be thinned down to the correct thickness before the lens is finally issued. It is not always possible to create a channel that is effectively patent by modifying a finished lens because there may not be sufficient substance.

An alternative method is to stick metal foil over the area of the cast where the channel is to be placed, and to press another shell. Whichever method is selected, care must be taken to ensure that the channel is fully blended into the space overlying the limbal sulcus. MacKay Taylor (1969) described various designs and uses of channels. (*See also* Chapter 23.)

Fenestrations

Fenestrations have been much more commonly used in recent years, and most of the literature relating to scleral lenses describes their fitting. Bier (1948) first described their use in scleral lens fitting (*see* Chapter 1). They are usually placed so that they are in the middle of the

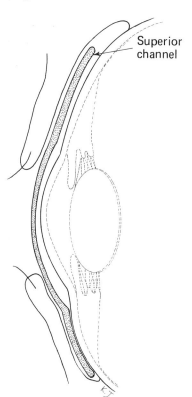

Superior channel

Figure 18.47 Cross-section of a superior channel *in situ*

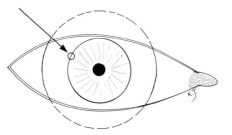

Figure 18.49 Siting the fenestration

palpebral aperture on the temporal side, as in *Figure 18.49*. For maximum effect, the precise siting should be over the limbal sulcus where there is the greatest depth of fluid coverage. The usual size is between 0.5 mm and 0.7 mm in diameter. Fenestrations smaller than 0.5 mm block with mucus too easily, and some practitioners have reported that, if larger than 0.7 mm, there is a tendency for frothing to occur. Countersinking and polishing, diagrammatically illustrated in *Figures 18.50* and *23.14*, gives a final funnelled shape to a fenestration and ensures that no trauma to the epithelium results. Multiple fenestrations may be an aid to some extra tear flow in some instances.

Tear exchange via fenestrations and channels

The intention of fenestrating or channelling is to facilitate a flow of fresh tears to the corneal surface. Tear exchange is usually faster behind a fenestrated lens because there is direct passage of tears from the meniscus along the lid margin into the space over the limbus. With channelled lenses, lacrimal fluid has to percolate to the back optic zone, and this takes longer. However, the faster fluid exchange does not always make a fenestrated lens preferable. If inserted correctly, i.e. fluid filled, and provided that the channel is not too deep, movement of fresh tears along the channel is slower but much more continuous and air is less likely to be admitted. Therefore, channelled lenses can be made with a far greater limbal clearance while retaining full liquid coverage of the cornea. The slow fill rate of a lens with an inferior channel is depicted in the photographs in *Plate 78a,b*.

By contrast, it is rare to see a fenestrated lens without a peripheral air bubble, and the size and shape is used partly to describe the fit of fenestrated lenses. Ideally, there should be clearance over the whole corneal area extending to about 2 mm beyond the visible iris diameter,

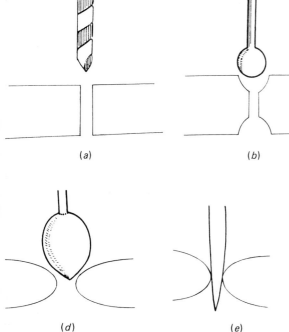

(a) (b) (c)

(d) (e)

Figure 18.50 The stages of fenestrating: (*a*) drilling with a fine drill. A 0.3 mm rose burr can also be used satisfactorily; (*b,c*) countersinking with larger diameter rose burrs; (*d*) blending with a more pointed burr; (*e*) final polishing with a fine pointed wooden stick dipped in liquid polish. (*See also Figures 17.18, 17.19 and 23.14*)

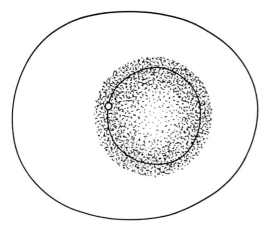

Figure 18.51 Diagrammatic representation of the depth of tear fluid behind a scleral lens

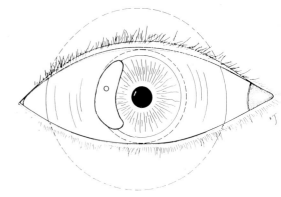

Figure 18.52 Characteristic bubble behind a fenestrated scleral lens

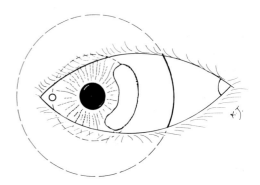

Figure 18.53 Bubble traversing to nasal side during excursions of gaze to the temporal side

with the depth increasing from the corneal apex to the limbus. Marriott and Woodward (1964) found the optimum central clearance to be 0.06–0.08 mm. A bubble often enters via the fenestration, but this is acceptable as long as it is mobile and remains small and crescent shaped. *Figure 18.51* illustrates diagrammatically the desired depth of the tear layer under the lens, and *Figure 18.52* an acceptable bubble shape and size. On gaze to the temporal side the bubble may traverse completely round the limbus to the nasal side, as in *Figure 18.53*. Further assessment of the fit of a fenestrated lens follows the same rationale as for a FLOM. This has been described previously in Chapter 17.

Development of slotted scleral lenses

In 1971 T. C. Trodd described a method of fitting ptosis props (*see* p. 693) whereby the shelf is produced by cutting through the full thickness of a 2–3 mm thick shell, as in *Figure 18.78*, rather than the traditional cemented ledge.

In addition to supporting the lid, enhanced tear exchange resulted from the wide opening, and a superior limbal slot for ventilating was applied to other scleral lenses. *Figure 18.54* shows a front and side view. In the following years Trodd developed this technique of scleral lens production and fitting at the Contact Lens and Prosthesis Department of Moorfields Eye Hospital.

Slots for ventilation enable construction of lenses with far greater limbal clearance because

of the improved tear catchment, maximizing the free-flowing fluid reservoir. The liquid dynamics are more like a channelled than a fenestrated lens, but there is immediate tear exchange. To function, the slot should be cut into the annulus of clearance circumjacent to the limbus. Peripheral air bubbles are more mobile because of the greater depth of fluid overlying the limbal sulcus. They freely enter and escape, sometimes after passing right round the limbus.

The importance of a high quality finish cannot be over-emphasized. A lens with the best possible tear flow is not tolerated if flaws or jagged edges irritate or cause trauma. In particular, the profile of the slot must be made such that there is no lid sensation, as in *Figure 18.55*. Without the deep extralimbal clearance, cutting a slot is ineffective and may be counterproductive because the conjunctiva may herniate into the slot, as in *Figure 18.56*.

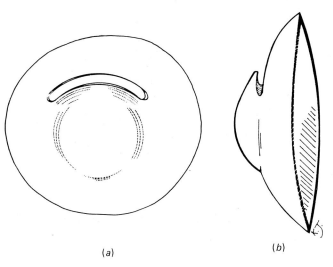

(a)   (b)

Figure 18.54 (*a*) Front view and (*b*) cross-section of a slotted scleral lens

The slot can be cut using thin fissure burrs or sharpened abrasive discs. Conical carborundum points are used for widening and removal of the very rough edges. Finally, the profile is shaped and polished with specially shaped carborundum tools of various grades of abrasiveness, and polish-laden felt or rag wheels. *Figure 18.57a–e* illustrates the process. Pullum and Trodd (1984a) described the development and some methods of fabrication.

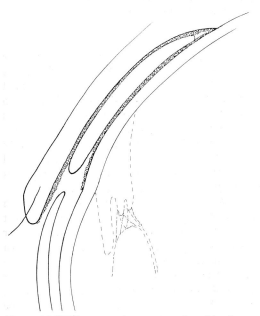

Figure 18.55 Diagrammatic representation of the slot profile in greater detail. (Conjunctiva shown shaded)

Blending the transition

The nature of the transition between the back optic and the scleral zone depends upon the peripheral back optic zone curvature. The junction is less pronounced and further out from the limbus when the peripheral back optic zone is flatter, so less blending into the scleral zone is needed. *Figure 18.58* illustrates the difference between flat and steep peripheral curves. Blending the transition is most effective using round or disc-shaped abrasive tools mounted into the hand-piece of the flexible drive motor. Lapping stones always leave a distinct junction. Felt or rag wheels are used for final polishing. *Figure 18.59a–e* illustrates the stages involved in blending the transition.

The ability of the shell to retain a full liquid coverage limits how flat the peripheral curve can be made. Channelled and slotted lenses give a greater potential for creating limbal clearance and, with this, a more continuous transition. Fenestrated lenses require the back optic zone to conform more to the corneal curvature with less peripheral clearance to retain liquid coverage. When the shell is initially inserted, the limbal clearance can never be too deep as long as the space is filled with tears and not air.

Total elimination of air is not always possible because the balance between excessive and inadequate limbal clearance can be a very delicate one. Air bubbles are acceptable provided that they are mobile and do not encroach into the central region where they would cause troublesome visual disruptions. If they are

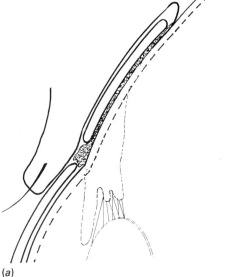

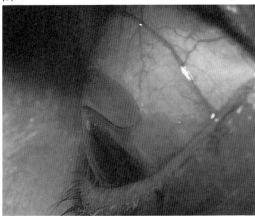

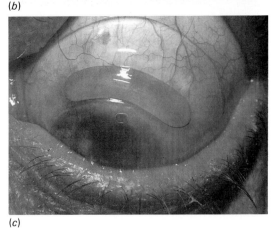

Figure 18.56 (*a*) Herniation of the conjunctiva (shaded) into a slot with inadequate limbal clearance; (*b*) photograph of this occurring, seen from the side; (*c*) the same eye as (*b*) seen from in front and slightly above

static, localized areas of corneal dehydration are the inevitable result. Later, such dehydrated areas can lead to formation of dellen and neovascularization.

Modifying the primary shell after settling back

One of the principal problems with scleral lens fitting is that there is a time-related variation. Even after working the transition and ventilating the primary shell, it is usually still necessary to make further modifications. These are determined by judgement of the fluid coverage immediately after the initial insertion and at various times afterwards while the shell is settling back. A back surface construction must be acceptable at all stages, so a period of trial wear is essential. If there are obstructions to the fluid flow immediately after the initial insertion, these must be dealt with first.

Forces affecting settling back

Settling back is the result of forces acting upon the lens. These are the attraction of the back surface of the lens and the bulbar conjunctiva, the weight of the lens and the pressure exerted by the lids. The resisting forces are the rigidity of the sclera and cornea if there is significant corneal touch. There is a third force, which is the pressure of the tear pool retained behind the lens. This may be positive, i.e. repelling the forces effecting settling back, or negative, which has the opposite effect. *Figure 18.60* illustrates these forces diagrammatically.

All scleral lenses settle back to some degree, but this varies with different lens designs and types of eye. The author's impression is that lenses having a more rapid tear exchange also reach the end-point of settling back more quickly. When there is a rapid exchange of tears, the positive pressure is brought to equilibrium leaving less force to resist settling back. Sealed or channelled lenses with a slow percolation of tears sometimes do not settle back much at all because the positive pressure of the tear pool remains constant. However, the reverse may apply if fluid is expelled under pressure from behind a sealed lens, e.g. during forced lid closure. As the free-flowing tear exchange is minimal, it must be sucked back if the status quo is to be restored. This is likely to be

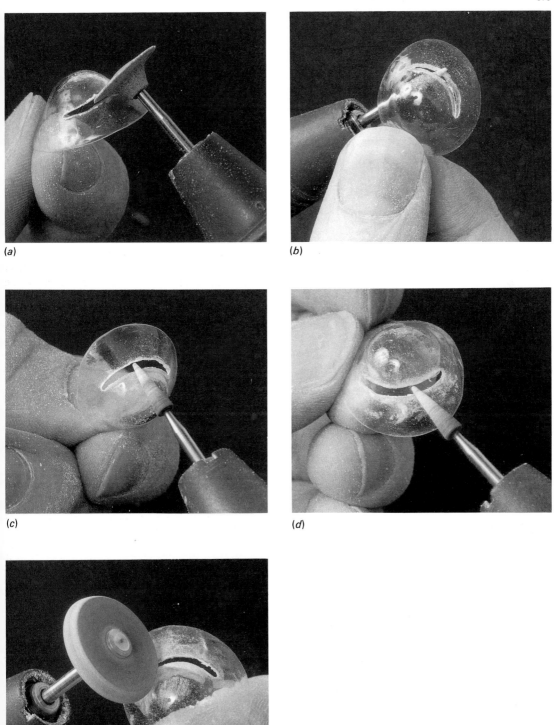

(a)

(b)

(c)

(d)

(e)

Figure 18.57 (a–e) The successive stages of cutting and profiling the slot using specially shaped abrasive tools mounted into the flexible drive of a suspension motor

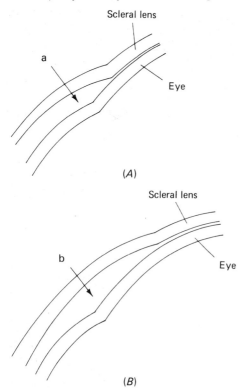

Figure 18.58 Limbal clearance with steep (*A*) and flat (*B*) peripheral back optic zone curvatures. Note the increased depth of the limbal clearance at b when a flatter peripheral back optic radius is used, as compared to a

incomplete, so there may be some negative pressure as the suction acts to draw the lens further onto the globe. When a lens settles back, both the central apical and the limbal clearances are reduced, as depicted in *Figure 18.61* and *Plate 74a,b*.

The effect of altering the back optic zone curvature

Modifications to the central curvature are made using the vertical bench spindle and diamond lapping tools in exactly the same way as the original primary optic zone is cut. Steepening the curve removes substance from the central region so it would be expected to increase the apical clearance. Flattening the curve removes substance from the periphery, increasing the limbal clearance, but the central region may remain effectively untouched. *Figure 18.62* illustrates flattening and steepening the BOZR.

The description of FLOM fitting in Chapter 17 may help to clarify this phenomenon. The effects on central corneal and limbal clearance when the BOZRs of FLOMs are flattened or steepened are well described, and the reader is advised to study these pages again. However, it is emphasized that this is only to assist in understanding the situation. It is not suggested that FLOMs can aid the selection of the BOZR of an impression lens in the same way that they are used to select the BOZR of a preformed lens.

Steepening the BOZR should be undertaken with caution, particularly with the steeper corneas encountered in keratoconus and some grafts. The outcome is not always predictable because apical touch is a factor that may limit settling back. If so, more takes place after steepening the BOZR with the result that a previously patent limbal annulus is occluded. The apical touch remains unchanged or may even cover a larger area because the new contour of the shell is more aligned with the apical corneal curvature. This is illustrated in *Figure 18.73*, p. 687. It may be a good idea to make a new shell from a cast of the original beforehand because adverse changes, as described above, are not easily rectified. This is not to say that no attempt should be made to eliminate apical touch, but some may be inevitable and is less undesirable than an occluded limbus. Cutting a flatter BOZR may also have an unexpected result because it extends further into the scleral zone and may precipitate further settling back as the bearing surface is reduced.

Modifying the scleral zone

In theory, if the impression precisely recorded the contours of the globe, modifications ought not to be necessary. In practice, it may be found that adjustments to the scleral zone are needed, but never to the same extent as with preformed lenses. (*See also* Chapter 23.)

Tight and loose areas

Tight peripheral areas may occur as a result of pressure of the impression tray on the sclera. The nasal sector may be loose if the impression was taken with the eye turned too far to the nasal side. A tight or a loose area may be due to an area of the sclera that was not covered when

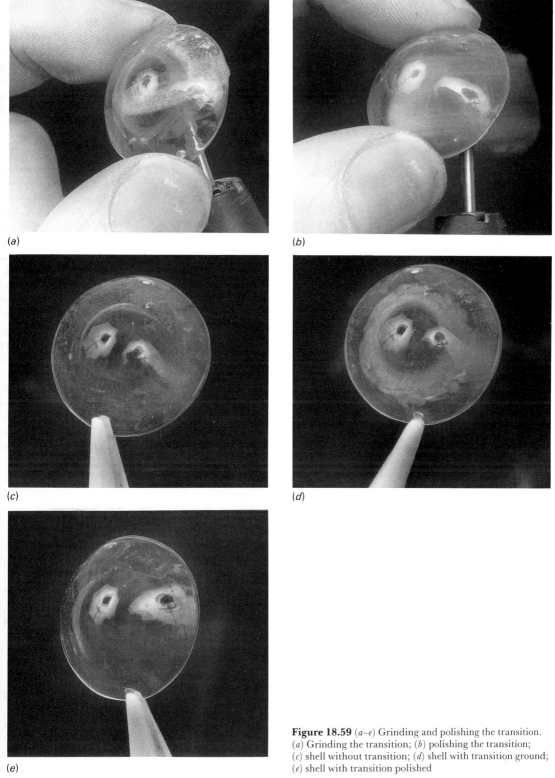

Figure 18.59 (*a–e*) Grinding and polishing the transition.
(*a*) Grinding the transition; (*b*) polishing the transition;
(*c*) shell without transition; (*d*) shell with transition ground;
(*e*) shell with transition polished

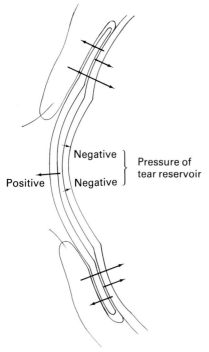

Figure 18.60 Vector representation of the forces involved during settling back of a scleral lens or shell (*see* p. 672)

the impression was taken, and the cast built up with plaster incorrectly. As previously mentioned, if an area of unsupported impression collapsed under the weight of the setting stone, this would result in a loose area bordered on both sides by a tight area. Sometimes, one tight or loose area may be enough to precipitate rotation which may make it necessary to modify other areas of the scleral zone. Hence, it can be seen that there are some potential sources of error which affect the accuracy of this zone.

Tight areas are easily seen because the blood flow through the underlying conjunctival vessels is blocked, causing a blanching of the conjunctiva (*Plate 77*). These should be marked with waterproof fibre pens and can be eased by removing substance using disc, spherical or inverted conical-shaped abrasive tools mounted into the flexible drive motor. Practitioners usually have their individual preferences, so it is not appropriate to be more specific than this. Using a hand-piece attachment gives much more control than using tools mounted onto a horizontal spindle or dental lathe. Polish-impregnated felt wheels and loose rag wheels are

substituted to give the final finish to the surface prior to re-insertion. Transitional grind-out modifications are carried out in the same way.

Loose areas stand off the surface and are easily seen after instillation of fluorescein. They are not always a problem, and this is just as well because modifications can only remove substance. The relatively tight areas in the remainder of the scleral zone can be eased to even out the fit of the shell as a whole. Bier (1957) described spatulation as a method of tightening a loose area. A cast is made of the lens or shell and material scraped away from this cast in the area corresponding to the loose fitting area. The lens is placed on the cast, and the loose area pressed with a spatula heated to 60°C until the plastic softens and conforms to the shape of the modified cast.

If a loose fitting scleral zone causes major difficulties, it is better to start again from a new impression. The only time it is worth removing substance from a large area of the scleral zone is when there is too much corneal clearance. It can

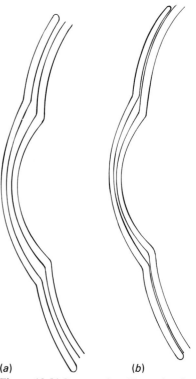

Figure 18.61 Cross-sections illustrating the settling back of a scleral lens or shell showing the reduction of apical corneal and limbal clearance: (*a*) prior to settling; (*b*) after settling has taken place

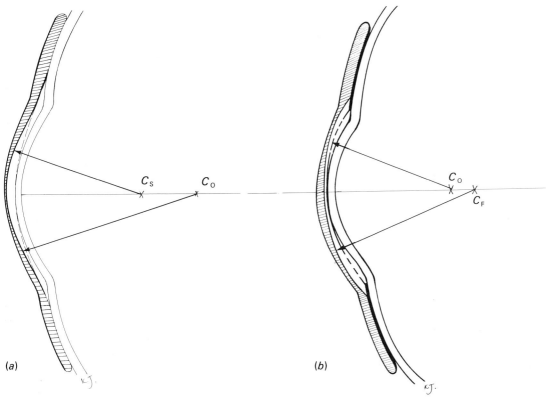

Figure 18.62 Illustration of the effect of steepening and flattening the back optic zone radius (BOZR). (*a*) C_O = centre of curvature of original BOZR; C_S = centre of curvature of steeper BOZR. (*b*) C_O = centre of curvature of original BOZR; C_F = centre of curvature of flatter BOZR

be reduced by removal of substance from the scleral zone to make the shell settle back. Sometimes a lens can be tilted to reduce back

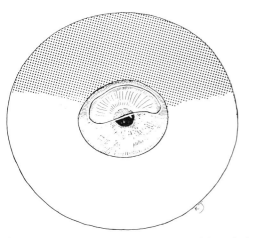

Figure 18.63 Removal of substance (shaded) from the back scleral zone to effect a preferential settling back in the area from which the substance has been removed

optic zone clearance preferentially in one area. This is done by removing substance uniformly from the half of the scleral zone adjacent to that area, as in *Figure 18.63*.

The results of removal of scleral zone substance are not always predictable. It is worth a try, but not a sustained effort. Remaking the shell with less vertex clearance is again probably a better prospect as it is rather difficult to remove material evenly over a large area and it must be a large area to have the desired effect. Removal of substance from a small area merely creates a clearance channel in the scleral bearing surface.

Total diameter reductions

These can be classed as a scleral zone adjustment. Local reductions in diameter should be made if the shell impinges against the inferior fornix or the inner canthus. The latter situation is shown in both photographs of *Plate 72*. The superior scleral zone may be reduced if it is too large, causing difficulty in removing the lens. When deciding upon the final diameter, it is worth remembering that the only function of the scleral zone is to ensure stability on the globe. There is no reason for making the total diameter as large as the original cast if a smaller one achieves the intended objective. The new perimeter of the shell is marked with a waterproof marking pen and the unwanted area is removed using a carborundum disc of about 25 mm in diameter and 5 mm thick. The edge is reworked and polished as previously described. Cosmetically, a larger lens is usually preferable, but the majority of scleral lens wearers are not worried at all by this, especially if a smaller one is more comfortable or easier to handle.

Manufacture of the finished lens

The same principles apply to scleral lenses as to corneal lenses for calculating and cutting the front surface radius, and these are described in Chapter 22. Some points relating specifically to scleral lenses should be briefly mentioned.

Specifying the power

The required power is calculated by refracting over a rigid lens of known BOZR and power. A scleral lens is ideal, but a corneal can be used if sufficiently stable. Otherwise an Apex lens or, if a set is available, a suitable FLOM, can be used. An important criterion for selection of a trial lens is that the power should be such that the over-refraction is not much more than ±5.00 D. It is less important that the BOZRs of the trial and final lenses are similar, because the power allowance for a different BOZR is easily calculated. The shell can be sent to a comprehensive contact lens laboratory for powering, and the resultant work can be easily verified by the practitioner. This is the only aspect of impression scleral lens production where this applies. However, generating the front surfaces within the confines of the clinic is also recommended if possible. Sometimes, the only way to establish the final power is to cut an FOZR onto the final fitting shell and carry out a refraction using the known data of the lens just made. The front surface may also need to be re-cut after modifications to the BOZR. There is

extra delay if the lens has to be sent away for these alterations.

The front optic zone can be placed as desired. The chosen position of the optical centre should be marked with a dot on the front of the shell. Placing this at the geometric centre of the back optic zone is usually satisfactory because the optic zones are relatively large compared to corneal lenses. However, it is sometimes necessary to centre the front optic zone over the visual axis of the eye which is not necessarily coincident with the geometric axis, for example, if the pupil is eccentric.

Front optic zone/scleral zone junction

After the FOZR is cut a distinct junction remains between this curve and the scleral zone. This is a downward step with a high negative lens, i.e. such that the cut FOZR is flatter than the uncut front curve, and an upward step with a low negative or a positive lens, as in *Figure 18.64*. The uncut front curve is approximately equal to the corneal curvature (keratometry reading) plus the thickness of the original flush shell.

Care is required when cutting an FOZR that leaves an upward step because it is possible to cut through the full thickness of the shell. Furthermore, when the step is blended out, yet more substance has to be removed from the

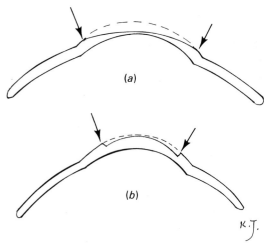

Figure 18.64 Cross-section of (*a*) high negative and (*b*) positive scleral lenses. Dotted line indicates original front surface of shell before lathe-cutting the front. → indicates the limits of the powered front surface. The positive lens is yet to be lenticulated

areas both just inside and just outside the junction. If this is left too thin, there is a risk of distortion or subsequent breakage.

A downward step may not need any blending, depending on how sharp and where it is. The FOZR for a moderate minus power, i.e. between −1.00 and −10.00 D leaves a step somewhere near the limbus, and this can be blended if necessary without affecting the optical quality. The step formed when a higher powered minus lens is produced is closer to the centre of the optic zone, depending on the thickness of the shell and the centre thickness of the final lens and blending may then affect vision.

Power adjustments during the front surface generating process

If the lens is mounted on a hollow chuck, the front vertex power can be checked after the lens has been removed from the lathe without unblocking. Therefore, adjustments can be made to the lens at this stage. Polishing for a little longer is sufficient to add small amounts of minus power and retain a high quality optic zone. Adding a similar amount of positive power requires re-cutting a steeper front curve with the lathe, so it is always better to err on the positive side.

High positive powers on scleral lenses

High positive lenses are more difficult to cut than negative, requiring much more care during the lathing process. This is for the following reasons:

(1) The negative liquid lens behind the scleral lens *in situ* can be up to −3 D or −4 D. Extra positive power in the lens is needed to compensate for this, so an aphakic scleral lens is often of the order of +18.0 D or +19.0 D. A relatively flatter BOZR may be necessary with a steeper cornea, giving a still greater negative liquid lens. Negative scleral lenses need less power because of the liquid lens. In addition, the power of the finished lens is better if it errs on the plus side to improve intermediate vision.

(2) As the FOZR is steeper than the BOZR, more substance must be removed from the periphery than from the centre. Careless lathe work results in a fully penetrating cut

if the optic zone diameter is too large. The latitude for error is further reduced because more substance is removed from the periphery during the shell fitting stage. *Figure 18.65* illustrates the process of lenticulating a scleral lens mounted on a chuck on a lathe.

(3) An error in calculating or setting the steeper FOZR of the positive lens produces a much greater difference in the power. There is also a greater change in the vergence of light at the air–lens interface compared to a flatter fronted minus lens, so there is a greater increase in vergence during its passage through the lens. Thus there is a greater positive power addition per unit thickness of a positive lens (which also has more centre substance). There is nearly a three-fold difference in the change in the power resulting from similar alterations to the front surface radius or the thickness of +18.0 D and −18.0 D scleral lenses.

(4) The front vertex power of the lens blocked on a hollow chuck can be checked during the process of lathe-cutting. There is hardly any difference between this and the back vertex power of a minus lens, but the difference can be over 2 D with a high plus lens (*see* Appendix D). This introduces another source of error.

Thinning down the finished lens

Thinning is one of the last manufacturing procedures that may be carried out. The final thinning down can only be done after the final FOZR has been cut. Too thin a lens rules out further alterations, so thinning should only be done when it is clear that no more changes are necessary. Substance is removed from the front scleral zone with broad flat-edged discs mounted into the hand-piece until the lens is as thin as required, and is given a high polish. All front surface ridges and flaws must be removed before the lens can be issued.

Modifying the finished lens

During the course of after-care visits, further adjustments may be necessary. Any modification carries a risk of upsetting a previously satisfactory result. If there is any risk that this

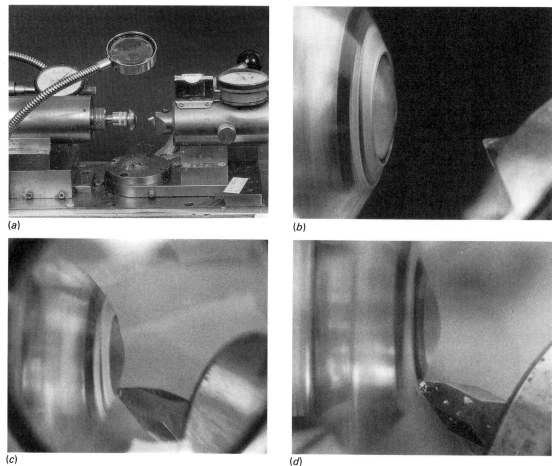

(a)   (b)   (c)   (d)

Figure 18.65 The process of lenticulating a positive lens. (a) The lens mounted on a lathe. (b) After the central front surface has been cut. The central front curve is steeper than the front radius of the shell, therefore there is a well-defined groove at the extremities of the front surface. The diamond point is withdrawn from the surface of the lens and set to a flatter radius. (c) The diamond point is replaced back into the groove. (d) The carrier curve is cut using a much flatter radius, perhaps as much as 3–4 mm flatter than the central curve

may happen, it is advisable to make a cast of the lens before proceeding. As previously discussed, alterations to the BOZR are especially precarious because the outcome is not always predictable. Changing the BOZR of a finished lens also alters the BVP. Approximate rules and examples are given in Chapter 5. However, scleral lenses are made with a large range of BOZRs, so there is a difference depending upon whether the BOZR is at the steep or the flat end of the range. Four factors affect the power of a scleral lens *in situ* after BOZR modification:

(1) Change in BOZR of the lens.
(2) Change in front radius of the liquid lens.
(3) Reduction of thickness of the lens.
(4) Increase in thickness of the liquid lens.

Effect of steepening BOZR

(1) Increase in negative power of back surface of lens.
(2) Increase in positive power of front surface of liquid lens.
(3) Reduction of thickness of lens, therefore reduction of positive power, or increase in negative power.
(4) Increase in thickness of liquid lens, therefore increase in positive power or reduction of negative power.

Effect of removal of substance using an unchanged BOZR

(1) No effect on surface powers of lens or liquid lens.
(2) Reduction of thickness of lens, therefore reduction of positive power.
(3) Possible increase of thickness of liquid lens, therefore possible increase in positive power.

Effect of flattening BOZR

(1) Reverse effects on powers of lens and liquid lens to steepening BOZR.
(2) Usually no alteration to paraxial thicknesses of lens and liquid lens.

The intricacies are best illustrated by examples. Using the surface power formula

$$F = \frac{1000(n' - n)}{r}$$

where F = surface power $\pm$ surface radius, n' = 1.336 (tears), n = 1.490 (PMMA); approximate rule (3) (*see* Chapter 5, p. 218) gives a $-0.12\,D$ power addition for every 0.10 mm of substance removed, allowing for a comparable increase in the thickness of the liquid lens.

BOZR steepened from 6.00 mm to 5.70 mm — thickness of lens reduced by 0.1 mm

$F = -25.667\,D$ when $r = 6.00$ mm and $-27.018\,D$ when $r = 5.70$ mm

Power change due to alteration of BOZR	-1.351
Power change due to reduction in thickness of lens	-0.12
Total power change	-1.471

BOZR steepened from 9.00 mm to 8.70 mm — thickness of lens reduced by 0.1 mm

$F = -17.111\,D$ when $r = 9.00$ mm, and $-17.701\,D$ when $r = 8.70$ mm

Power change due to alteration of BOZR	-0.590
Power change due to reduction in thickness of lens	-0.12
Total power change	-0.71

Flattening the BOZR is usually carried out to increase the limbal clearance, only skimming the centre of the back optic zone, so the allowance for the change in thickness is not normally applicable. The opposite power changes apply, therefore flattening the BOZR from 5.70 mm to 6.00 mm would give rise to a power change of $+1.351\,D$ and flattening from 8.70 mm to 9.00 mm a power change of $+0.59\,D$.

When substance is removed from the back optic zone using an unchanged radius, the only variable is the thickness difference of the lens and liquid lens with no change to either surface power. Therefore the only change is to add $-0.12\,D$ for every 0.10 mm removed, and this is constant across the range of BOZRs. However, as previously mentioned, it is not constant across the range of powers, with positive lenses affected more by a change in thickness.

The reduction in thickness of the lens is not necessarily equal to the increase in thickness of the liquid lens because central corneal touch may remain after a back optic grind-out. If so, $-0.25\,D$ is added for each 0.10 mm removed. This adds significantly to the total minus power if a steep BOZR is further steepened. Up to 0.30 mm can be removed from lenses fitted to advanced keratoconus without relieving the apical touch after further progression of the condition.

In addition, the interface may not be PMMA/tears (refractive indices 1.49 and 1.336), but PMMA/cornea (1.49 and 1.376), depending on the area of contact and the pupil size. The latter regularizes the corneal surface, eliminating any loss in acuity due to a refractive index difference. A small contact zone and a large pupil would have a functional tear lens, but a large contact zone and a small pupil would give rise to a PMMA/cornea interface. If the modification eliminates central touch, the original PMMA/cornea interface is replaced by PMMA/tears. As previously suggested, it is also possible that steepening the BOZR may increase the area of central touch. If so, there could be an effective tear lens before modification, and a PMMA/cornea interface afterwards.

One final consequence of corneal contact is that the axial length may be reduced when a scleral lens is *in situ*. If so, more minus power may have to be added to the contact lens if the globe resumes its original shape when the central touch is eased. Corneal lenses fitted with apical touch probably would not have a comparable effect as the pressure on the cornea is much less.

Figures 18.66–18.71 Cross-sections of various different types of keratoconus. The arrows mark the limbal margins. The scleral sections are marked superior (Sup) or nasal appropriately

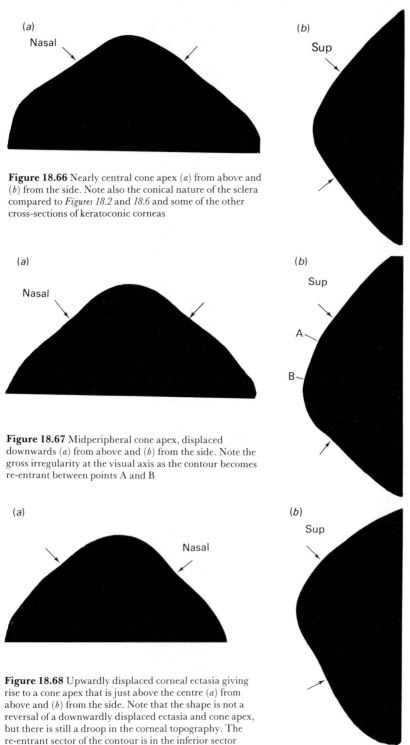

(a)

Nasal

(b)

Sup

Figure 18.66 Nearly central cone apex (*a*) from above and (*b*) from the side. Note also the conical nature of the sclera compared to *Figures 18.2* and *18.6* and some of the other cross-sections of keratoconic corneas

(a)

Nasal

(b)

Sup

A

B

Figure 18.67 Midperipheral cone apex, displaced downwards (*a*) from above and (*b*) from the side. Note the gross irregularity at the visual axis as the contour becomes re-entrant between points A and B

(a)

Nasal

(b)

Sup

Figure 18.68 Upwardly displaced corneal ectasia giving rise to a cone apex that is just above the centre (*a*) from above and (*b*) from the side. Note that the shape is not a reversal of a downwardly displaced ectasia and cone apex, but there is still a droop in the corneal topography. The re-entrant sector of the contour is in the inferior sector

(a)

Nasal

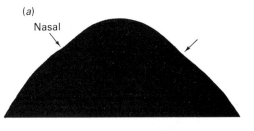

(b)

Sup

Figure 18.69 Terrien's marginal dystrophy (a) from above and (b) from the side, illustrating the high regular astigmatism in the central region. In this instance there was 15.00 D of astigmatism, negative cylinder axis 90°

(a)

Nasal

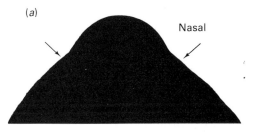

(b)

Sup

Figure 18.70 Keratoglobus (a) from above and (b) from the side. Note the remarkable sphericity and symmetry in both meridians, not present with the other kinds of keratoconus. This gave rise to 30.0 D of myopia

(a)

Nasal

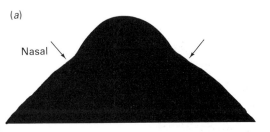

(b)

Sup

Figure 18.71 Another example of keratoglobus (a) from above and (b) from the side, but lacking the symmetry of the previous example. The limbus for both keratoglobus examples is not at the apparently obvious position, but about 1.5 mm more peripheral. The true limbus is not well defined in a cross-section

The application of impression scleral lenses in pathological conditions

A number of pathological conditions may benefit from application of scleral lenses.

Keratoconus and other primary corneal distortions

Topographical classification of keratoconus using casts of eyes

The implication of the name of this condition is that the corneal topography resembles a cone. In reality, 'keratoconus' is the term often loosely used to describe a number of different related conditions, but sometimes with markedly varying topography. The common feature is corneal ectasia (*see* Chapter 21). *Figures 18.66–18.71*, photographs of keratoconus casts, illustrate some examples of the variety of the contours.

An area of thinning in the central third of the cornea gives rise to a relatively symmetrical protrusion of the affected cornea, similar to *Figure 18.66*. This is the only example of the cornea bearing any resemblance to a cone. The sclera is also rather conical compared to some of the others, to a normal eye with spherical K readings, 8.25 mm (*Figure 18.2*, p. 647). *Figure 18.67* illustrates the topography when the ectasia is midperipheral and displaced downwards. An upwardly displaced ectasia with less eccentricity is shown in *Figure 18.68*. The topography is not simply inverted, but retains its own typical shape. Terrien's marginal dystrophy (*Plate 97*) is an ectasia affecting the very periphery of the cornea in the inferior sector, as in *Figure 18.69*. It results in very high but quite regular against-the-rule astigmatism, sometimes in excess of 15 D. Keratoglobus (*Figures 18.70* and *18.71*) is consequent to a larger area of thinning in the central region. It is characterized by a sphericity not present in any of the other forms. The resultant refraction can be over 30 D of myopia. All are subject to the effect of the forces exerted by the intraocular pressure and gravity, but are affected differently.

Indications for scleral lenses

Irregular topography

It may not be possible to fit corneal lenses or they may frequently dislodge.

Lid sensation of corneal lenses restricts tolerance

Use of both corneal and scleral lenses can maximize total daily wearing time. Normally, it would be advisable to wear the corneal lens first. Irritation of the lids may not necessarily rule out an immediate switch to a scleral lens, but scleral lens-induced corneal hypoxia takes longer to resolve and may prevent further contact lens wear of any kind for quite long periods.

The alternative to keratoplasty

Davies, Ruben and Woodward (1977) showed that the prognosis for keratoplasty is favourable when keratoconus is the underlying indication. There remains a 5% failure rate, so it is still necessary that all contact lens management options, including scleral lenses, are available and fully investigated. Keratoplasty may be contra-indicated or not advised when:

(1) The patient does not wish to undergo surgery or wishes to postpone a graft. A scleral lens may be an acceptable temporizing procedure. If successful, the operation could be put off indefinitely.
(2) The cone is steep with few opacities and there is good visual potential with a contact lens.
(3) There is an increased chance of rejection due to pre-existing corneal neovascularization, or because a very eccentric cone apex requires a large diameter graft which increases the proximity to the limbal vascular arcades.
(4) There has been a previous failed graft in the other eye.

Keratoconus patient management with scleral lenses

Keratoconus patients are highly motivated contact lens wearers because the unaided vision or spectacle visual acuity is usually poor, especially in the advanced stages when scleral lens wear is indicated. Notwithstanding a high incidence of Down's syndrome, Woodward (1981) demonstrated that the keratoconics presenting at Moorfields Eye Hospital are generally of above average intelligence and their occupations carry more responsibility. Onset is at a time when they are trying to develop a career. The visual disabilities can be a major hindrance, as can the frequent and time-consuming follow-up visits. They usually respond well if they can see that effort is being made to make scleral lens wear as tolerable as possible, although too many ineffective modifications can easily generate the feeling that progress is not being made.

Wearing schedules

Long-term prospects must not be jeopardized by problems caused by over-wear in the early stages. Selective rather than all day wear is often a more realistic target.

Individuals cope quite differently with all the visual problems that can arise. Some wear one lens at a time to make up nearly a full day. Others cannot tolerate the loss of binocular function and prefer part-time wear in both eyes simultaneously. Scar tissue is common as the condition advances, reducing the contact lens visual acuity. If progression is unequal, contact lens wear in the more affected eye may not improve the binocular acuity. However, there may be a worthwhile degree of binocular vision even if the visual acuities are as different as 6/6 and 6/18. Flare from point sources of light with uncorrected advanced keratoconus can be very troublesome, rendering activities such as night driving impossible. If only worn when necessary, scleral lenses may be the optimum contact lens type to reduce these problems.

Low to moderate grade keratoconus

Most moderate grade keratoconics manage well with corneal lenses, but some are unable to tolerate the lid sensation. Scleral lenses usually cause discomfort to these sensitive patients for other reasons, but some are able to wear them quite well.

Advanced keratoconus

Scleral lenses are required for advanced keratoconus when corneal lens fitting has become impossible or very difficult. It is usually possible to fit with some kind of scleral lens, but they still remain very difficult cases and the practitioner must be prepared to provide supervision of scleral lens wear for as long as this remains necessary. A successfully fitted slotted lens is shown in *Plate 76*.

Special considerations in the fitting of scleral lenses in keratoconus

An entirely satisfactory end-point is not always possible. Modifications can only reduce the thickness and total diameter, so it is periodically necessary to produce a new lens. As the patient may be highly dependent on continued wear of some kind of functional lens, it is not unusual to have one lens that is being worn while the next one is being constructed.

Impression procedure

The impression procedure is not substantially different than for any other eye, but use of a more conical-shaped impression tray is advisable in order to avoid abrasion of the apex of the cornea. There may be less corneal rigidity than normal, so particular care should be exercised to avoid compression of the cornea.

Constructing the back optic zone curvature

The objective is an uninterrupted fluid coverage without apical touch, occlusion of the limbus or intrusion of air bubbles. In practice, these criteria are rarely met to complete satisfaction. More important is to distinguish between acceptable and unacceptable departures from this ideal.

Low to moderate grade keratoconus   If the back surface is constructed in the same way as for a non-keratoconic eye having a similar peripheral curvature, there is almost invariably some apical touch. A blended bi-curve with the steeper curve clearing the corneal apex may give an acceptable result, as in *Figure 18.72*.

Advanced keratoconus   The selection of the primary back optic zone radius is always best made empirically from the individual cast. In advanced cases, no useful information can be gleaned from keratometry and, even with a moderately advanced form, it is of limited value. The peripheral corneal contour is of just as much significance as the radius of the central 3 mm. It is often better to start by establishing a limbal clearance, as this is not affected so much by the central irregularities. Because the difference between the central and peripheral radii is greater than normal, heavier blending with the central curves is required.

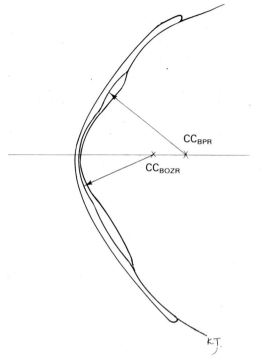

Figure 18.72 Bi-curve back optic surface for moderate keratoconus. CC$_{BOZR}$ = centre of curvature BOZR; CC$_{BPR}$ = centre of curvature BPR

The steepest of a number of lapping stones may just skim the centre of the flush-fitting shell if the cone apex is nearly central. Up to 0.20 mm must be removed from the limbal region. The aim is to create a primary back optic zone curve with the most even reduction in the clearance between the periphery and the apex by monitoring the thickness and comparing it to that of the original shell. The final blending of the transitions may have to be done using abrasive tools and polish-laden rag wheels mounted on mandrels driven by the suspension motor. Care is necessary here to avoid touching the central back optic zone.

The primary shell should have some apical contact but be clear at the limbus, giving a starting point for the shell fitting. Further adjustments depend upon the area and weight of the apical touch, the depth of the midperipheral clearance, the width and depth of the limbal clearance and, finally, on how much settling back takes place. There are so many variables that it is only possible to describe the general principles in a contact lens textbook. Elimination of apical touch may not be possible, but, as

previously discussed, this may be a factor limiting the settling back. *Figure 18.73* illustrates the possible effect of removal of central substance in an attempt to alleviate settling back. The author's view is that light apical touch does not appear to be a major source of intolerance unless the cornea is particularly sensitive or fragile. Any corneal touch should be minimized, but total elimination need not be the paramount goal as it is usually far less of a drawback than an occluded limbus, provided that most of the weight of the lens is borne by the sclera.

Eccentric cone apices   A greater eccentricity of the cone apex gives rise to more irregular peripheral corneal flattening as well as irregular central topography. Curves cut coaxially about the geometric (visual) axis do not end up in a concentric configuration until so much substance is removed that there is no longer any resemblance to the original corneal shape. While substance is removed from the portion of the optic most distant from the cone apex, little or none is removed from the sector in which the apex is located. If the central region is cut with steep radius tools, the evolute tends to be symmetrical about the cone apex rather than the geometric axis, and substance is not removed evenly from all regions of the optic. This results in excessive clearance, with possible intrusion of air bubbles, between the apex and the furthermost limbal margin, which embraces the geometric axis. To avoid this, the back optic zone curve must be flat enough so that the BOZD encompasses both the geometric axis and the cone apex. This may lead to excessive clearance between the apex and the proximal limbal margin with a consequent bubble there, but this causes less of a visual problem as it is displaced away from the geometric axis. *Figure 18.74* illustrates the incompatibility of the two resultant curves cut about the cone apex and the geometric axis.

It may still be possible to fashion the back surface shape using diamond-coated spherical tools, but preferential lapping may be necessary. To do this, the shell must be held against the lapping tool and tilted so that the tool only touches a particular area. Alternatively, part of the back surface may be shaped using abrasive tools driven by the suspension motor, and given a final polish with rag wheels. These methods demand greater manual skills because it is difficult to control how much substance is being removed. It is also necessary to true up the back optic zone before the correct power is put on. The aim, by whichever means, is to achieve the most uniform possible removal of substance over the whole of the central area while retaining a good quality back optic zone.

Use of channelled scleral lenses in keratoconus

The more rapid tear exchange provided by fenestrations or slots would usually be preferred, but the slower and steadier liquid movement afforded by a channel may help to maintain an air-free space between the cornea and lens when the corneal contour is excessively steep or re-entrant. However, channels are not without their problems. The less direct tear exchange may cause more long-term hypoxic corneal changes, especially if patency of the channel is reduced after full settling back. In the short term, this may reduce tolerance after a period of wear. Handling is more difficult because the lenses have to be inserted filled with fluid, which can only be done facing the floor. If it is not done properly, large bubbles are trapped behind the optic. Wearing schedules may have to be broken into short periods during the day in order to make up a useful total number of hours. These problems are not insurmountable, and the motivation to succeed can be very high when there is no better option.

Sealed lenses

Sealed lenses for limited periods of wear may be considered, but only if all systems of ventilation disrupt the fluid coverage unacceptably. They may solve the problem of incomplete liquid coverage, but great care must be taken to ensure that hypoxic corneal changes do not ensue.

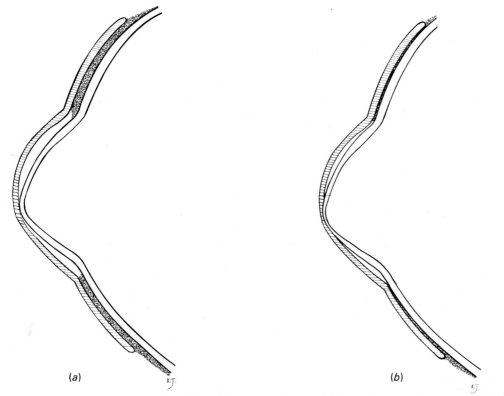

(a)   (b)

Figure 18.73 Diagrammatic representation of a possible outcome of removal of centre substance using a steeper back optic zone radius. If the corneal contact is a factor limiting settling back, the result may be further settling with no reduction of apical touch and an unwanted reduction of the limbal clearance. (a) Apex of cone tangentially in contact with the back surface of the lens. (b) The back optic zone of the lens has been steepened in an attempt to reduce apical touch. Apical touch now covers a larger area and the limbal clearance has been obliterated following further settling back

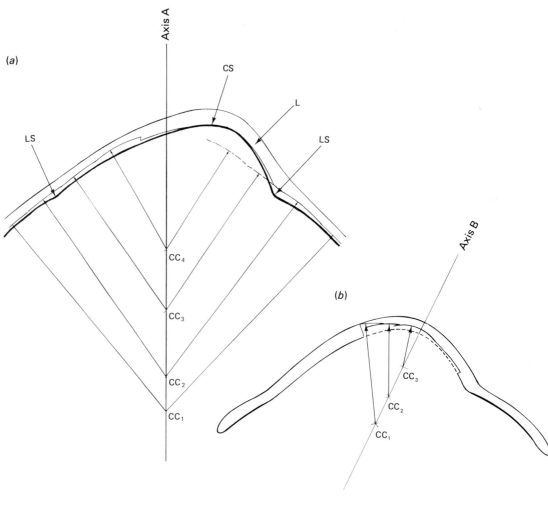

(a)

(c)

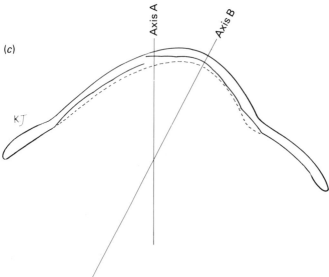

Figure 18.74 Diagrammatic representation of cutting the back optic zone surface shape using diamond lapping tools when the cone apex is more eccentric than in *Figure 18.73*. (*a*) Coaxially cut curves about the geometric or visual axis. (The suffix numbers below indicate the order in which the curves are cut.) CC_1 = centre of curvature of most peripheral curves; CC_2, CC_3 = centres of curvature of midperipheral curves; CC_4 = centre of curvature of central back optic zone curve; CS = corneal surface; LS = limbal sulcus; L = substance of scleral lens. Dashed line shows imaginary continuation of the flatter peripheral curves. (*b*) Coaxially cut curves about the cone apex. CC_1, CC_2, CC_3 = centres of curvature of each curve. Dashed line shows back surface contour of original shell. (*c*) Illustrates the non-compatibility of the two curves cut in this manner. Axis A: geometric axis of eye; axis B: axis of maximum symmetry of cone. Dashed line shows original flush fitting shell

Results of scleral lens fitting in keratoconus

The criteria for success are that the visual advantages enable the patient to conduct his normal occupation, and that any scleral lens-induced ocular changes are within acceptable limits. Pullum and Trodd (1984b) showed that keratoconus patients constitute about a third of the total number referred for continuing management or new fitting of scleral lenses. The results showed that the majority were partially successful to various degrees, evenly spread between those patients who totally succeeded, those who totally failed and four grades of success between these extremes. The authors' impression was that they took up much more than a third of the allocated time, putting a strain on the resources available but reflecting the greater occupational needs of this group.

Aphakia

The optical advantages of contact lenses in the correction of aphakia are well documented in Chapter 5. Some superior corneal scarring may be present after a corneal section and gaping of a postoperative wound induces a degree of against-the-rule astigmatism (Reading, 1984); but apart from traumatic aphakia, abnormal corneal topography is usually not expected. Shell fitting is consequently simpler and quicker than for other groups.

Management of aphakia with scleral lenses

Corneal or hydrogel lenses would normally be preferred, but most patients are elderly and there are many management problems. There are some advantages of scleral lenses (see pp. 645–646 and Chapter 21) for aphakia, especially the comparative ease of handling and maintenance. Extended wear hydrogel lenses often work well when handling is not possible, but frequent supervision is required. Graham, Dart and Buckley (1986) have shown that aphakes are at a higher risk of incurring sight-threatening infections than other extended wear groups. Spoilation of hydrogel lenses may be worsened by the thicker substance and the likelihood of age-related tear dysfunction. Surface deposits rarely adhere to scleral lenses made from PMMA. Corneal lenses for aphakia can be quite mobile and tend to drop so that the periphery may lie over the visual axis. The greater stability of scleral lenses is often preferable, and the optic zone can be specifically sited if necessary, perhaps over a postoperatively updrawn pupil Plate 83 shows an example of an eye with a small updrawn pupil fitted successfully with a scleral lens and worn for many years.

Tolerance of scleral lenses

Aphakes generally appear to tolerate scleral lenses very well. The age-related reduction in sensory nerve function and looseness of eyelids as well as the severing of nerve fibres during the operation contribute towards this. There is some evidence that the cornea of an aphakic eye exhibits less hypoxic change than the cornea of a phakic eye when presented with the same physiological challenge, i.e. a contact lens (Holden, Mertz and Guillon, 1980), which may also be a factor.

Motivation and wearing programmes in aphakia management

Aphakes usually see quite well with spectacles if visual acuity is the only criterion, but they can still feel very handicapped due to the aberrations and ring scotoma experienced with spectacle lenses. Thus, their motivation is often quite high. However, there is not the same total dependency on contact lenses for visual function compared to keratoconus. Many lead a comparatively sedentary existence. Reading and watching television is as good with aphakic spectacles as contact lenses, so selective use of contact lenses when mobility is required may be entirely adequate. Sometimes a few hours' wear a week is all that an elderly person needs to carry out everyday tasks, and this may go a long way to giving independence and peace of mind. Scleral lenses may be preferred if used in this manner for the reasons previously discussed, and because they are usually comfortable for short periods if not for longer durations of wear.

On the other hand, some aphakes may demand all day wear. Many achieve this with scleral lenses provided that the tear exchange is acceptable. Such a case is illustrated in Plate 75 fitted with a slotted scleral lens. For elderly patients having perhaps a 5- to 10-year life expectancy, long-term contact lens-induced ocular changes do not pose anything like the same threat that exists for the younger patient.

Postoperative divergence

A divergent squint with diplopia is a common complication of aphakia. Correction of a unilateral aphakic eye with a contact lens brings the quality of a disparate image nearer to that of the fellow eye, making any diplopia more noticeable. In spite of this, some patients prefer to wear a lens because the binocular field is increased. A scleral lens may be indicated because of topographical irregularities or because it is more static. If for short periods of wear only, a scleral lens may be preferred because adaptation may be easier.

Incorporating prisms

Some prism may be incorporated into a scleral lens and, provided that the lens does not rotate, the base can be oriented as desired. However, not much more than 5Δ can be worked on the lens, and the effectivity may be reduced *in situ* to about three because of a reverse prism in the liquid lens. Spectacle lenses worn in conjunction with scleral lenses are much better for correcting prisms of this order.

Aphakia after traumatic cataract

Traumatic cataract may result from impact of a blunt object or a penetrating injury puncturing the lens capsule. Both may cause other ocular injuries, but the latter is of greater consequence to the contact lens practitioner. Scleral lenses may be indicated if contact lens fitting is complicated by corneal irregularity or scar tissue, or if there has been eyelid injury or loss. Iris loss or pupil displacement may need a scleral lens so that the optic can be positioned over the visual axis.

Traumatic corneal irregularities

The optimum shell construction can only be arrived at empirically, as with abnormal topographies of other aetiology. The limbus must not be closed up, and central touch minimized, but contact on scar tissue is not likely to be a cause for concern. Any attempt to match the contours generates too much clearance adjacent to the scar tissue. Proud scars tend to conform more to the original contours after a while, so it may be necessary to review the fitting periodically.

Iris loss or injury

Photophobia and glare after iris loss can be reduced in two ways.

Stopped down optic zones

A painted iris can be incorporated into the lens. This may have the desired effect of reducing the flare, but the visual field is restricted because the entrance pupil is displaced forwards. Partial stopping down to cover localized iris loss may be better.

Full diameter optic zone

Sometimes glare may be significantly reduced with use of a full diameter front optic zone. This reduces the peripheral scattering caused by zone lenticulation of the front optic. To be effective, the front optic zone must be placed accurately over the pupil and should be at least as large. If there is complete iris loss, the front optic zone diameter must be 12 mm. With high positive power, this requires use of a thick shell to give sufficient peripheral substance to the optic zone.

Results with scleral lenses

Pullum and Trodd (1984b) demonstrated a polarization of the results with aphakes who, as a group, tend to do quite well or they find scleral lenses are no improvement and give up. The authors' opinion was that the patients who were successfully fitted required less subsequent follow-up than any other group and it was also technically easier and quicker to fit the lenses. With the exception of the traumatic cases, there were relatively few partially successful cases which are the ones that require maximum follow-up.

High myopia

High myopia is normally adequately catered for by corneal or soft lenses, so it has become uncommon to resort to scleral lenses. Age-related handling problems are rarely encountered because the patients are either younger or have been wearing lenses for many years. The optical distortions are less pronounced with negative spectacle lenses compared to positive, and corneal irregularities are not usually present. However, there remain problems with prescriptions of over −20 to −25 D and it is worth remembering the potential advantages of scleral lenses in relation to myopia of this magnitude:

(1) They are more easily found when patients have poor unaided vision.
(2) There is not the problem of lid traction.
(3) There is a significant negative liquid lens which reduces the power necessary to work onto the lens.
(4) Any power up to about −40 D can be worked onto a scleral lens.

In the early 1950s, scleral lenses were the only lenses available, and some people who were fitted at this time are still successfully wearing them now — sometimes the original lenses. By comparison, corneal lenses may be uncomfortable because of the increased mobility and lid sensation. The more complex and expensive maintenance of soft lenses compares unfavourably with the simplicity of looking after scleral lenses. Also, the visual acuity is usually better with scleral lenses. For these reasons, it may be quite impossible to persuade such patients that corneal or hydrogel lenses are an advantage, so continued supervision of scleral lens wear is needed. From a clinical standpoint, there is no reason to change if there are no significant scleral lens-induced ocular changes.

Corneal grafts

The techniques of keratoplasty and postoperative care have improved enormously in recent years, with the result that there are now far fewer instances of high corneal astigmatism following surgery. Refractive surgery, after the primary procedure, has reduced this still further. The call for scleral lenses after grafting is consequently much reduced compared to that of the 1960s and 1970s. However, there still remain a number of cases where sclerals are the lenses of choice because of the irregularity of the corneal surface or for any of the other general indications previously covered. In addition, there is a significant number of patients who had corneal grafts up to 20 years ago and who have managed well with scleral lenses. It is necessary to see them from time to time, preferably annually, for routine after-care appointments.

The same manufacturing principles apply as for an irregular eye of other aetiology. Selection of the back optic zone curvature must be on the basis of each individual shape. Sometimes, the graft springs forward at the time of removal of the sutures because an area of the donor cornea has failed to knit in place. This can happen even if the sutures are left in place for over a year. There is often a pronounced step to contend with, as in *Figure 18.75*. In other cases, the donor corneal profile is depressed compared to the host, as in *Figure 18.76*. These shapes are all technically possible to fit with scleral lenses, but entrapped bubbles are a particular problem. It is quite often necessary to use channelled lenses to ensure coverage of tears. *Plate 84* is a good example of such an eye.

Use of shells as splints following grafts

Ruben (1975) described the use of scleral lens splints used immediately postoperatively to re-shape grafts that had sprung forward, but re-suturing or refractive surgery is now preferred by most corneal surgeons. Soft therapeutic

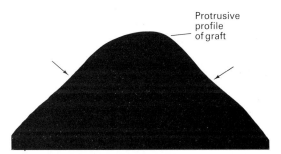

Figure 18.75 Photograph of the outline of a cast made from an impression of an eye with protruding contours following corneal graft surgery. ↓ indicates limbus

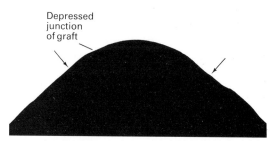

Figure 18.76 Photograph of the outline of a cast made from an impression of a grafted eye where the donor cornea formed a trough. ↓ indicates limbus

lenses are used under some circumstances (*see* Chapter 21), but it is rare for scleral lenses to be fitted.

Analysis of results of graft patients fitted with scleral lenses

Results of fitting grafted corneas in a sample analysed by Pullum and Trodd (1984b) showed that successful wearers were spread in a similar fashion to the keratoconus sample. Corneal oedema was highlighted as the principal reason for failure or a reduced wearing time. It occurred more frequently in the corneal graft group than any other, and it was often in the absence of discomfort. This was presumed to be due to endothelial cell loss during and soon after the operative procedure (Bron and Brown, 1974; Olsen, 1981). It was not a universal feature of scleral lens fitting in graft cases and, when the cornea remained clear, the result was usually a good one.

Therapeutic applications of scleral lenses*

A number of pathological conditions may benefit from the fitting of therapeutic contact lenses. Prior to the advent of hydrophilic materials, these were almost entirely the preserve of scleral lenses, but they are used less frequently now. Scleral lenses are usually less comfortable and rarely can be used on an extended wear basis. Fitting from an inventory is another attraction of hydrogel lenses. Chapter 21 covers therapeutic applications of contact lenses, but this section describes the use of scleral lenses in comparison to hydrogels.

Limitations of hydrogel therapeutic lenses

Dehydration and surface spoilation

If hydrogels are not kept continually moist, dehydration of the surface and polymer matrix follows. The lens may become uncomfortable, dislodge, or tighten on the eye as partial shrinkage takes place. In addition, the formation of deposits is common with hydrogels.

---

* For a fuller account of the abnormal conditions discussed in this section, readers are referred to *Contact Lens Practice, Visual, Therapeutic and Prosthetic* (1975) By M. Ruben, Chapter 13, London, Ballière Tindall.

Visual acuity

If visual acuity is an important factor, a hydrophilic lens may not give sufficiently clear vision when the topography is irregular.

Mobility

If the lens dislodges or comes out completely, therapeutic uses are limited.

Corneal exposure

If lid closure is impaired, the precorneal tear film is disrupted and exposure keratitis results. The aetiology may be ectropion, coloboma of the lid, loss of lid tissue, lid retraction after surgery or neurological, e.g. seventh nerve lesions. Exophthalmos is a common cause of precorneal tear film disruption and, although it would not usually part the lids permanently, it may cause serious epithelial lesions. A contact lens helps to provide fluid coverage and prevent evaporation. Hydrogels are subject to dehydration under these conditions, but this problem does not exist with scleral lenses. On rare occasions, e.g. in cases of major lid loss, a scleral lens may be worn continuously for severe exposure keratitis if it can be demonstrated that this is preferable to continuous exposure. However, if the lens is removed and the lids can be held closed at night by secure padding, this is a better management option. Woodward (1984) described the use of silicone rubber lenses in some cases of exposure. They do not dehydrate, but there are problems of surface deterioration.

Ptosis

Ptosis may follow lid trauma or third nerve palsy. It may be present as part of general myasthenia gravis or in ocular myopathy, when the condition is specific to the levator muscle, or it may be congenital. Scleral lens ptosis props can be offered, but their fitting is not necessarily an easy task. Other options may be simpler and preferable. Thoughtful selection of the right types of patient who stand a reasonable chance of success with ptosis props can avoid unnecessary and misplaced effort.

Construction of ptosis props

There are four possible methods of constructing a functional ptosis prop.

With cemented ledge A scleral lens is produced in the usual manner, but a ledge is cemented onto the front. If positioned correctly, this should hold the upper lid open. Sometimes another ledge, placed to open the lower lid and to prevent lens depression and rotation, may also be added. *Figure 18.77* illustrates such a lens.

Cutting through full thickness of shell Trodd (1971) described the production of a ptosis prop constructed by cutting through a thick shell, leaving a shelf as in *Figure 18.78*. The extra thickness is required only at the optic zone, so the remainder must be thinned down to normal thickness. The shelf only needs to be about 2.5 mm wide in order to support the lid.

Cutting through part of a thick shell This is a variation of the second example, and entails partially cutting through the shell to create the shelf, as in *Figure 18.79*. This enables use of fenestrated or channelled shell fitting. To allow

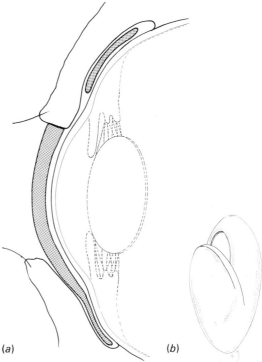

(a)   (b)

Figure 18.78 Fully penetrating shelf (T. C. Trodd type). A 2.5 mm wide shelf is sufficient to support the ptosed lid in most cases. (*a*) In section on the eye; (*b*) appearance of complete shell

for the thickness of the superior scleral zone, a PMMA sheet of thickness of about 3.5 mm is necessary.

Thick finished lenses An alternative to props is a thick finished shell to force the lids apart. This removes any problem of the upper lid forcing the lens down. The lens is easier to make as the only difference from any other scleral lens is that a thicker sheet is needed and that some substance has to be removed from the scleral zone, as in *Figure 18.80*. If unsuccessful, the same lens can be converted to a solid prop as previously described, so the original shell work is not wasted. The extra bulk is a major drawback. When the lids are forced forwards, there is considerable force exerted on the globe. Unless the lids are very flaccid, it is not a recommended procedure.

The second (Trodd type) is preferred by the author. Lowering the shelf is easily carried out by cutting more of the shell away without affecting the optic zone. It is also easier to

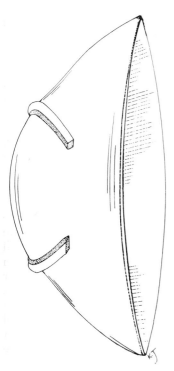

Figure 18.77 Double-ledged ptosis prop

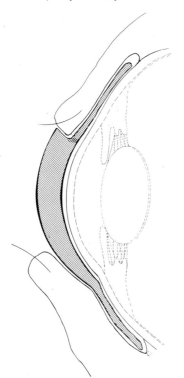

Figure 18.79 Partially penetrating shelf

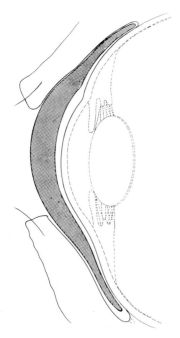

Figure 18.80 Thick shell used for ptosis prop. A very thick shell must be used to have any significant effect as the lid is being stretched rather than lifted up

construct a shelf that is highly polished and free from imperfections. Repositioning a cemented ledge is more difficult, and the optic zone has to be cut before a ledge can be cemented on. With the Trodd type, the optic zone can be cut at the end of the fitting procedure and can be re-cut without affecting the shelf. Being a solid single piece, there is less risk of breakage and, as previously discussed, the tear exchange is very good.

Problems with ptosis props

Apart from the usual problems inherent with scleral lens fitting, there is extra discomfort caused by the ledge or shelf. In addition, because the lid is forced open, closure becomes impossible, so blinking to clean the front surface of the lens is not possible. Frequent wiping of the front surface with a damp tissue may be necessary.

The positioning of the shelf or ledge is very critical. It is tempting to place it in what may be thought of as the normal position for the upper lid, i.e. at the approximate level of the upper limbus. Unfortunately, any raising of the ptosed lid tends to increase the weight exerted on the shelf. The higher it is raised, the greater the pressure on the shelf, and the more it is pushed down, which is contrary to the desired effect. The correct height is the lowest whereby the lid is sufficiently raised to enable unobstructed vision.

One effect of the lens being pushed down is to introduce a bubble over the inferior part of the cornea, with a corresponding area of contact in the upper half, as in *Figure 18.81*. The bulk of the lens and the unusual lid action help to keep this bubble mobile, so it may not be a major problem. If necessary, it may be possible to reduce this by remaking the lens with the optic zone displaced upwards using preferential lapping.

Alternative methods of management

Sometimes the vision is not impaired in ptosis, or all that is required is an occasional manual lifting of the lid with a finger. If the cosmetic appearance is the main complaint, scleral lens ptosis props are not often successful. If vision is restricted, spectacle frame-mounted props can be quite effective. Another possibility is to lift

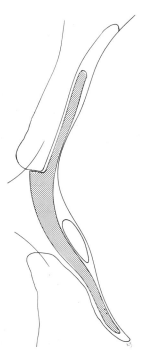

Figure 18.81 Ptosis prop (partially penetrating shelf in this diagram) with the shelf placed too high. It is pushed down by the upper lid and causes an inferior bubble

the lid by attaching one end of a small piece of surgical tape to the eyelid just above the lashes and the other end to the smooth skin below the eyebrow.

Spectacle props and protective shells   Because spectacle props and surgical tape cause forced opening of the eye leading to corneal exposure, a protective contact lens may be indicated. For the reasons previously discussed, this may have to be a scleral lens. The suggestion that, if a scleral lens is needed, it may as well be a ptosis prop is not valid. A ptosis prop is much more likely to be uncomfortable and is more difficult and time consuming to construct.

Bullous keratopathy

Bullous keratopathy is a late stage of chronic corneal oedema. It may be secondary to long-standing glaucoma, a complication of cataract or other anterior ocular surgery, or due to advanced endothelial dysfunction such as

Fuchs' dystrophy. It is characterized by epithelial bullae associated with pain which may be increased by contact with the eyelids. Contact lenses may be prescribed to separate the bullae from the lids. Hydrogel lenses are almost universally preferred nowadays, but there may be a theoretical indication for scleral lenses if the visual acuity is an important factor. However, this is not generally so as the corneal transparency is lost.

Ruben (1975) described how compression of a large area of the cornea with the back surface of a scleral shell acts as an anterior water barrier to reduce oedema. He recommended that at least three-quarters of the corneal surface be constantly compressed, but there should be interchange of tears via a nasal channel. Frequent changes of the fit during the first few weeks may be necessary to maintain these requirements. He emphasized that corneal vascularization, if present, may be increased by this mode of treatment. He also pointed out that it is usually more important to alleviate the pain rather than to reduce the oedema, so if there is a choice of contact lens type, the one which performs this function most effectively is better.

Fluid retention in dry eye conditions

If there is a deficiency in volume of the tear fluid, a contact lens helps to maximize wetting of the corneal epithelium. A hydrogel lens may help, but maintenance of its own hydration is a prerequisite in keeping the cornea moist. Frequent instillation of artificial tears is usually needed for this.

A scleral lens may be indicated because it can be constructed to retain a substantial amount of fluid with which to bathe the cornea. Instillation of artificial tears may be necessary to replenish this reservoir, but if so, not to the extent required with a hydrogel. What may be preferable, so that the reduced volume of tears is put to maximum effect, is to give optimal clearance consistent with the minimum exchange of tears. All types of scleral lenses can be investigated, including channelled or even sealed. A full day's wearing time without breaks may be required, even if there is a preference for a lens with reduced tear exchange. For this reason, follow-up appointments to monitor any neovascularization or other hypoxic changes must be carried out regularly. However, cessation of contact lens wear would almost certainly result in more serious and more rapid damage as a consequence of the dry eye condition. Scleral lenses may be used in conjunction with continuous perfusion apparatus to provide a constant supply of fluid or drugs to the cornea (Ruben, 1975).

Prevention of fornix shrinkage and symblepharon

Ocular pemphigoid (essential conjunctival mucoid atrophy) is a progressive atrophy of the mucous membrane. The adenoid layer is affected and has secondary effects on the secretory cells causing drying of the cornea. The adenoid layer becomes fibrous and, as the fornices are involved in the early stages, shrinkage results. The acute phase of Stevens–Johnson syndrome involves a severe mucopurulent conjunctivitis. This leaves areas of scarring and symblepharon, with ultimate loss of the fornix and acute tear dysfunction. The condition is caused by drug sensitivity, especially associated with sulphonamides. Symblepharon may also be the result of burns, particularly from alkaline chemicals. Normal blinking is affected with consequent corneal damage due to exposure or entropion and trichiasis.

Shells or scleral rings help to prevent symblepharon re-forming after surgical separation. A ring, i.e. an annulus, may be preferable to a complete shell because there is no occlusion of the cornea. Their fitting may prevent the loss of the fornix in ocular pemphigoid, but the results are not encouraging unless the disease progress can be arrested by medical treatment (Ruben, 1975). However, shells may still be indicated to minimize the effects of the drying and trichiasis. New vessel growth may be a serious complication of scleral shells, but if the deterioration caused by the disease process is more rapid, this may not be a sufficient cause for discontinuing scleral lens wear. Close liaison with the ophthalmologist who is responsible for the patient is required under these circumstances.

Trichiasis and entropion

Trichiasis does not usually cause the same intensive pain as bullous keratopathy, but there is a constant irritation. A contact lens may be used as a protective barrier to alleviate the discomfort and reduce the threat of long-term erosion of the corneal epithelium. The lashes may be pushed under the edge of hydrogel lenses, or the rubbing on the surface may cause rapid deterioration. Scleral lenses are not subject to these drawbacks and are usually a better prospect. Trichiasis may be treated by removal of the lashes, e.g. by repeated epilation or electrolysis, which is a more permanent remedy. However, if the lid is inverted so that keratinized tissue instead of the mucous membrane of the lid margin is in contact with the cornea, persistent abrasion can still occur. A scleral lens provides the most effective protection.

Recurrent erosions

Therapeutic lenses may be indicated to alleviate the pain when the exposed deeper layers of the cornea are in contact with the lid and to prevent dislodgement of freshly regenerated epithelial cells. Hydrogel lenses are nearly always the lens of choice under these circumstances. Scleral lenses are rarely, if ever, indicated because they carry too much of a risk of further abrasion of the fragile epithelium. This may happen on insertion, if there is corneal contact when the lens settles back on the globe or if movement of the lens takes place when it impinges on the inferior fornix or inner canthus.

Anaesthetic cornea

An anesthetic cornea may be at risk of injury through foreign bodies lodging in the epithelium or because of abrasions caused by tarsal plate foreign bodies. Scleral lenses can afford excellent protection in these circumstances. The anaesthetic eye is very tolerant, so the patient may not report the early manifestations of the complications of scleral lens wear. The practitioner must therefore be especially alert to their onset.

Cosmetic shells

Chapter 21 covers the various types of cosmetic contact lenses available to mask scarred or disfigured eyes. It is beyond the scope of this chapter to describe the fitting and manufacturing principles of cosmetic shells, but their mention here in a comparative sense is appropriate.

Shells are more difficult and time consuming to fit and are generally immediately less comfortable than cosmetic hydrogel lenses, but for purely cosmetic reasons are usually preferable. The whole anterior eye is covered, and any iris and scleral combination can be chosen for the best possible match with the fellow eye. Very fine detail can be included, such as conjunctival blood vessels and pingeculae. Because the painting is incorporated quite deeply into the substance of the shell, there is a very good three-dimensional effect which is not possible with hydrogel lenses. A competent specialist artist should be able to produce a cosmetic scleral shell that is virtually undetectable in room illumination at a distance normally separating two people holding a conversation. Any space can be built up by a cosmetic shell, so unsightly phthisical eyes can be satisfactorily masked. The same applies to empty sockets, except that artificial eyes are static in the orbit. The exception to the general rule that shells are the best cosmetic option is if the eye is protrusive, when the extra bulk may be unfavourable. The main advantage of cosmetic shells is in the masking of disfigured eyes that have also become strabismic.

Complications and problems with scleral lens wear

Minor problems of scleral lens wear

There are a few difficulties commonly described by scleral lens wearers which are a nuisance, but could not truly be called complications warranting cessation or reduction of wearing times.

Frothing

The depth of limbal clearance reduces during the process of settling back, but the volume of any entrapped air does not decrease. The bubble breaks up into smaller units each with a more spherical shape. Small frothy bubbles are more troublesome because they may encroach under the optic zone. Frothing is not a problem if air is excluded in the first place or if bubbles freely escape. However, this is not always possible, especially with irregular corneal topography causing variations in the depth of the fluid coverage.

Fenestrating into any area retaining a permanent bubble may help to reduce its size. However, like many other scleral lens modifications, the result is far from predictable, and it is quite possible that the opposite may happen. Instillation of a drop of saline directly into the space behind the lens may have the desired effect for a short while, but the air is almost certain to return. A more viscous eye drop may have a somewhat more sustained effect. Removal of the lens and re-inserting with the addition of more wetting solution can be tried. If adjusting or refitting is necessary to rectify the complaint, removal of substance from the whole of the scleral zone helps to reduce the corneal clearance. This is not an easy adjustment because there is no way of ensuring that it is done evenly. If too much is taken off, the eventual corneal clearance may be inadequate. If remaking is preferred, the optic should be ground with less clearance. This can only be done accurately if a record is kept of the amount of substance originally removed. One way of solving the problem may be to fit a high water content soft lens under the scleral lens (Westerhout, 1975) (see Plate 85). This may also have some protective application if the cornea is especially susceptible to abrasions. However, the situation would have to be monitored very closely indeed. If there is insufficient oxygenation due to the scleral lens the added presence of the soft lens would reduce still further the oxygen available to the cornea, and could seriously compromise the corneal metabolism. If pathogens were introduced because of poor soft lens hygiene procedures, and this were in conjunction with an increased oxygen deficit, the result could be a very high infection risk.

Clicking sounds

Clicking sounds are caused by air bubbles entering the space behind the lens. They can be very annoying, but there is not much that can be suggested to eliminate them other than refitting with reduced limbal clearance or with a lens design that promotes better fluid filling.

Collection of mucus beneath a lens

Scleral lenses sometimes seem to generate over-secretion of mucus. This is presumably due to contact over a large area with the tarsal conjunctiva. A deep clearance with a full and free-flowing tear exchange that looks very encouraging can be spoilt by collection of mucus in this space. This is more of a problem when slotted lenses are fitted because of the wider opening and deeper space behind the lens. Occasional flushing out with copious amounts of saline may be the best solution, or removal and re-insertion with fresh saline in the lens. Mucolytic drops such as acetylcysteine may be considered.

Conjunctival hyperaemia

Some degree of conjunctival hyperaemia may accompany scleral lens wear. If this is localized, it may indicate an area of tight scleral fitting. The limbus should be watched carefully for early signs of limbal arcade vessel engorgement which may be the precursor of corneal neovascularization.

Discomfort

It is difficult to fit scleral lenses that are entirely free from any discomfort. They may become uncomfortable after a period of wear, possibly in the absence of specific aetiology. However, discomfort may also be an early sign of more serious complications.

Settling back

This phenomenon has been discussed at length earlier in this chapter. Further elaboration is not necessary, but it should be remembered that the fitting of scleral lenses should always be assessed immediately after insertion and after a period of settling back.

Complications of scleral lens wear

Abrasions

Abrasions may be caused by clumsy insertion or due to heavy central touch on a fragile corneal apex. Unusual discomfort after a period of wear is an early symptom. This should be watched for carefully in keratoconus when corneal touch cannot always be eliminated. An abrasion may be exacerbated if lens wear is continued in the mistaken belief that the discomfort is something to be put up with as a normal part of scleral lens wear. As a scleral lens is the only means by which some keratoconus patients see adequately, there is a tendency among this group to soldier on until the lens becomes absolutely unbearable. The result is almost certain worsening of the abrasion and forced cessation of all contact lens wear until the cornea is fully healed. This emphasizes the importance of ensuring good communications, and explanation of the reasons for not over-wearing from the outset of fitting.

Exposure keratitis

Static bubbles behind the lens cause localized drying leading to epithelial erosions because the liquid coverage is absent. Dealing with unwanted bubbles has been discussed previously in this chapter.

Exacerbation of corneal scarring

Corneal scarring is part of the disease process of keratoconus. Persistent central contact may make this worse, although there is no way of being sure that the scarring would not have progressed to the same extent in the absence of a lens. If the lens is indicated for visual purposes, it may be necessary to proceed in any case.

Compression of blebs

Care should be taken to avoid affecting blebs which may be necessary for drainage of aqueous, for example, if secondary glaucoma is a complication of cataract surgery. This is not necessarily a contra-indication for scleral lens fitting, but there is a risk of intraocular infection if the bleb is ruptured as pathogens would have direct access into the globe. The shape of the bleb registers on the impression and cast, so the shell is initially flush over the bleb. Some substance should be removed from the area of the shell overlying the bleb to allow for settling back. The bleb is often located at the superior limbus, which is just the position where a lens may be slotted. It may be necessary to relocate the slot to avoid the spongy conjunctiva being squeezed into the slot, which would obstruct the tear flow and cause possible damage to the bleb or restrict the aqueous outflow.

Pressure on the anterior chamber

If the anterior chamber is shallow, scleral lens fitting should be undertaken with caution, as extra pressure on the iris root when the lens settles back could conceivably precipitate angle closure. The same precautions apply following anterior segment surgery such as trabeculectomy. The fluid coverage should be assessed after something approaching a full day's wearing time, when maximum settling back should have taken place. The optic zone/scleral zone transition should err on the deep and wide side if there is any risk.

Giant papillary conjunctivitis

This is a possible complication of any kind of contact lens wear. There is no evidence that it is more likely with scleral lens wear, and it does not appear to cause any of the typical subjective problems that are described when the condition develops in association with hydrophilic lenses. The comparative lack of severity is presumably explained by the fact that there is no contact between the tarsal conjunctiva and a lens edge or spoiled surface during blinks or saccadic eye movements. Also PMMA material does not attract a protein build-up. The issue is rather clouded in any case when one considers the relatively high percentage of scleral lens wearers, i.e. keratoconus patients, who have atopic lid changes as part of the condition.

Hypoxic changes

Oxygen deprivation accounts for the most common complications of scleral lens wear. In the short term, corneal oedema with attendant discomfort and misty vision may cause reduction of wearing time. As the wearer becomes more tolerant of the lens, the onset of oedema and misty vision may occur after longer wearing spells, but there may be a chronic subclinical oedema.

It is quite possible that misty vision consequent on scleral lens-induced oedema may not be obvious to the patient because of the presence of other ocular pathology that may also reduce the visual acuity or cause hazy vision. Opacities which are part of the underlying disease process, or other media opacities such as lenticular changes, can easily cause this confusion. Under these circumstances, the cornea must be carefully observed and insidious scleral lens-induced corneal changes carefully monitored. Permanent reduction of transparency and corneal neovascularization are the long-term complications of chronic corneal oedema, and it is desirable to minimize these.

The rate of new vessel growth is variable. If there is a high visual indication for a lens, a small amount may not represent a serious threat. When myopia is the indication for scleral lenses, if it can be shown that, with a continuation of the same rate of new vessel growth, they will not cross the pupil margin in the patient's lifetime, it is hardly improving the quality of life to withdraw the visual advantages provided by the lens. In addition, as new vessels grow to compensate for a corneal oxygen deficit, it is possible that once this is sufficiently met, the rate may slow down. In the absence of evidence to support or refute this, clinical judgements should be made in the light of observations. Aphakia is a more common indication for scleral lenses. The patient's average life expectancy is much less, which makes slow neovascularization a less serious problem.

A rather different and more substantiated set of criteria applies to new vessel encroachment into keratoconic corneas fitted with scleral lenses. There is a very real risk associated with only very slight neovascularization because a graft must never be ruled out as a future treatment. The risk of subsequent rejection is greatly increased by the presence of corneal blood vessels. The more the cone apex is decentred, the larger the graft may have to be, so this risk is particularly applicable to more eccentric cone apices. Most cones are decentred downwards, and the author's impression is that a common origin of major fronds of new vessels seen in keratoconic eyes fitted with scleral lenses is from the inferior sector of the cornea. This could be due to drying of the lower cornea following entrapment of an immobile bubble below the cone apex. For these reasons, it is essential that regular liaison with the ophthalmologist who may carry out a future graft is an essential part of scleral lens after-care in keratoconus.

Rigid gas permeable impression scleral lenses

Development of rigid gas permeable (RGP) materials could be a major help in the reduction of hypoxic corneal changes consequent to scleral lens wear. Production of RGP pre-formed scleral lenses has been described by Ezekiel (1983), and an evaluation of the corneal oxygen uptake *in situ* with RGP pre-formed scleral lenses of various thicknesses made from materials available at the time has been carried out by Ruben and Benjamin (1985). The limitations of pre-formed scleral lenses have already been discussed, and these apply whether the lenses are made from PMMA or RGP materials.

RGP materials do not lend themselves readily to making impression scleral lenses in the traditional manner, because the materials tend to break down when heated and are not available in sheet form. In addition, the normal thickness of scleral lenses would negate any improvement afforded by the gas permeability of the material. This second problem applies to both pre-formed and impression lenses.

Production of RGP impression scleral lenses

A hybrid mould casting and lathe-cutting system for production of rigid gas permeable impression scleral lenses was investigated by Pullum (1987). In this study, rough rigid gas permeable blanks were produced by using a specially designed mould with a cast of a PMMA shell or lens for the basic back surface shape, and a spherical surface for the front. The specific radius of the front surface was not important, except that it had to be flatter than the average scleral radius, so that there would always be a space between the surface of the cast and the front surface. *Figure 18.82* is a simplified diagram of the mould box used for this purpose.

Liquid monomers in the correct proportions were poured into the mould and the cast lowered into the mixture. Polymerization was effected by curing in an oven for 2 days at 110°C. The cast of a finished PMMA shell or lens was preferred to a cast of an eye because the liquid coverage could be created in the usual manner using PMMA shells, which were relatively expendable items by comparison to the rough RGP blanks. The handwork on the finished

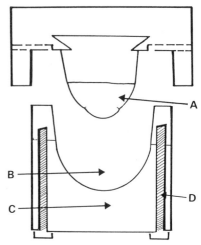

Figure 18.82 Design for the mould box used to produce rigid gas permeable impression scleral lenses. A: cast of PMMA lens made in Panasil material; B: space into which cast is lowered. This is filled with the monomer mix. C: body of mould box; D: bolts to facilitate easy separation of the two halves of the mould box for release of the shell when polymerized

RGP shells is also minimized if a cast of a lens is used.

Adherence between dental stone and the polymer was a problem which was resolved by use of rubber moulding material for the cast of the lens. Panasil was readily available and proved to be satisfactory. The rough blanks produced were at least 2 mm thick all over with a minimum thickness at the corneal apex. Surplus material was removed from the scleral zone using various abrasive tools to leave a uniform thickness of 0.6–0.8 mm. This was intentionally left as thick as a normal PMMA lens to give rigidity. The optic zone was lathe-cut to a thickness of 0.11 mm to permit oxygen permeability over the central area.

It was reported that the surface wetting of the lenses was inadequate. There were a number of factors involved, including the possibility of this being partly due to the increased surface area as compared to corneal lenses. Coating or re-formulation of the polymer was suggested as possible remedies. Apart from this, it was shown that impression scleral lenses could be produced thin enough to allow a significant transmission of gas while retaining acceptable optical standards.

Bleshoy and Pullum (1988) produced an impression sealed scleral PMMA lens and made a cast of this lens, from which a rigid gas permeable lens was produced in the manner described. This RGP lens was made with a uniform optic zone thickness of 0.50 mm. The increase in corneal thickness after 5 hours wear of these two lenses was compared. The thickness of the RGP lens was then reduced to 0.40 mm, 0.30 mm and finally to 0.18 mm. The corneal thickness increase was measured when each of these lenses was worn. When the RGP lens was worn, a central corneal swelling of between 3.6% and 4.8% was demonstrated, compared to 9.4% with the PMMA lens, which was highly significant. The percentage increase showed a downward trend as the thickness of the RGP lens was reduced, but the difference between any of the RGP lenses was not statistically significant. At the time of writing this study is being extended (Pullum and Parker, 1989). It has been shown that scleral lenses made from a material with a nominal Dk value of 160 can be produced using the same manufacturing technique. This development could represent a major improvement in the long-term prospects for scleral lens wear in the future.

An alternative method of production of gas permeable scleral lenses is described by Sapp (Lyons *et al.*, 1989), where a lathe-cut rigid gas permeable optic zone is fused into a PMMA scleral zone. The optic zone of a fitted PMMA shell is cut out and an RGP blank is reduced to the same diameter as the hole. The back optic zone surface is lathed to the spherical equivalent curve of the original PMMA scleral lens and cemented into the PMMA scleral zone. The front optic zone is lathed to the appropriate power and polished.

The role of scleral lenses within the field of contact lens practice

Today's requirement for scleral lenses constitutes the smallest of all lens types. However, there is generally a strong visual or clinical indication, and so it is necessary to continue to preserve the art of scleral lens practice in an effective way. Scleral lens practice offers important support to comprehensive ophthalmology, but, because of the nature of the cases where scleral lenses are applied, it needs the back-up provided by ophthalmology. In addition, the

labour intensiveness inevitably makes production an expensive proposition which may put the service out of reach for some of the most needy cases. For these reasons, hospital clinics are the ideal environment for scleral lens units. Because of the necessity of individual tailoring, production techniques can only be learned by experience.

While there is such a small demand for the service, it is particularly important that it is carried out as efficiently as possible, and that the treatment is not discredited because it takes too long and does not yield satisfactory results. There is a need for a small number of practitioners to be prepared to develop skills in manufacturing and fitting, but dabbling in contact lenses is a practice that should be discouraged, and this is especially so as far as scleral lenses are concerned. However, it is important that contact lens practitioners are familiar with the theory and application of all aspects of contact lens practice and scleral lenses should not be an exception to this.

Acknowledgements

Acknowledgements are due to colleagues who read the manuscripts and made helpful comments in the preparation of this chapter, namely, Miss C. Astin, Mr R. J. Buckley, Mrs S. Halliday, Dr J. Kempster, Miss J. Stone and Professor E. G. Woodward. Assistance with diagrams was provided by Miss K. Johnstone and, with black and white photographs, Mr K. Sehmi and Mr M. McHale, all from the Medical Illustrations Department of Moorfields Eye Hospital. A special acknowledgement is due to Mr T. C. Trodd who worked for many years fitting and designing scleral lenses and ocular prosthetic appliances at Moorfields Eye Hospital. His experience and guidance have been invaluable to the author in learning the skills of scleral lens practice.

References

BIER, N. (1948). The practice of ventilated contact lenses. *Optician* **116**, 497–501

BIER, N. (1957). *Contact Lens Routine and Practice*, 2nd edn. London: Butterworths

BLESHOY, H. and PULLUM, K. W. (1988). Corneal response to gas permeable impression scleral lenses. *J. Br. Contact Lens Ass.* **11**(2), 31–34

BRON, A. J. and BROWN, N. A. P. (1974). Endothelium of the corneal graft. *Trans. ophthal. Soc. UK* **94**, 863–873

DAVIES, P. D., RUBEN, M. and WOODWARD, E. G. (1977). Keratoconus: An analysis of the factors which affect the optical results of keratoplasty. *Transactions of the European Contact Lens Society of Ophthalmologists, Ghent*, pp. 97–99

EZEKIEL, D. (1983). Gas permeable haptic lenses. *J. Br. Contact Lens Ass.* **6**(4), 158–161

GRAHAM, C. M., DART, J. K. G. and BUCKLEY, R. J. (1986). Extended wear hydrogels and daily wear hard contact lenses for aphakia. Success and complications compared on a longitudinal study. *Ophthalmology* **93**, 1489–1494

HOLDEN, B. A., MERTZ, G. W. and GUILLON, M. (1980). Corneal swelling response of the aphakic eye. *J. Invest. Ophthal. vis. Sci.* **19**, 1394–1397

KIELY, P. M., SMITH, G. and CARNEY, L. G. (1982). The mean shape of the human cornea. *Opt. Acta* **29**, 1027–1040

LEWIS, E. M. T. (1969). Some aspects of haptic lens technique. *Contact Lens* **2**(4), 35–36

LYONS, C. J., BUCKLEY, R. J., PULLUM, K. W. and SAPP, N. (1989) Development of the gas-permeable impression-moulded scleral contact lens: a preliminary report. *Acta ophthal.* **67** (in press)

MARRIOTT, P. J. (1966). An analysis of the global contours and haptic lens fitting. *Br. J. physiol. Optics* **23**, 3–40

MARRIOTT, P. J. (1970). The use of acrylic laminates in fitting haptic lenses. *Br. J. physiol. Optics* **25**, 29–43

MARRIOTT, P. J. (1972). *Contact Lenses*, 1st edn. London: Barrie and Jenkins

MARRIOTT, P. J. and WOODWARD, E. G. (1964). A method of measuring the clearance of a haptic lens. *Br. J. physiol. Optics* **21**, 61–83

OLSEN, T. (1981). Post-operative changes in the endothelial cell density of corneal grafts. *Acta ophthal.* **59**, 863–869

PULLUM, K. W. (1987). Feasibility study for the production of gas permeable scleral lenses using ocular impression techniques. *Transactions of the British Contact Lens Association Annual Clinical Conference* (1987)

PULLUM, K. W. and PARKER, J. H. (1989). Development of gas permeable scleral lenses produced from impressions of the eye. Dallos lecture 1989, awaiting publication in *J. Br. Contact Lens Ass.*

PULLUM, K. W. and TRODD, T. C. (1984a). Development of slotted scleral lenses. *J. Br. Contact Lens Ass.* **7**, 28–38; 92–97

PULLUM, K. W. and TRODD, T. C. (1984b). The modern concept of scleral lens practice. *J. Br. Contact Lens. Ass.* **7**, 169–178

READING, V. M. (1984). Astigmatism following cataract surgery. *Br. J. Ophthal.* **68**, 97–104

RUBEN, M. (1975). *Contact Lens Practice*. London: Baillière Tindall

RUBEN, M. and BENJAMIN, W. J. (1985). Scleral contact lenses: preliminary report on oxygen-permeable materials. *Contact Lens* **13**(2), 5–10

STOREY, J. K. (1987). The use of Panasil C silicone rubber impression material in contact lens work. *Optom. Today* **27**, 711–714

STOREY, J. K. and VALE, M. J. (1970). A rubber moulding material for ocular impressions in contact lens work. *Ophthal. Optician* **10**, 948–949

TAYLOR, C. M. (1969). The S-bend and other channelled lenses. *Ophthal. Optician* **9**, 1256–1258

TRODD, T. C. (1971). Ptosis props in ocular myopathy. *Contact Lens* **3**(4), 3–5

WESTERHOUT, D. (1975). The use of soft lenses in the fitting of haptic lenses. *Optician* **169**(4363), 13, 16

WOODWARD, E. G. (1981). Keratoconus: Maternal age and social class. *Br. J. Ophthal.* **65**, 104–107

WOODWARD, E. G. (1984). Therapeutic silicone rubber lenses. *J. Br. Contact Lens Ass.* **7**, 39–40

Erratum

Plate 73, first two lines of the caption to read: 'The FLOM 8.25/13.00 on an eye with keratometer readings of 7.91 mm along 180, 7.81 mm along 90.'

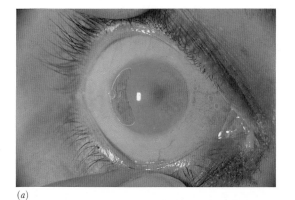

(a)

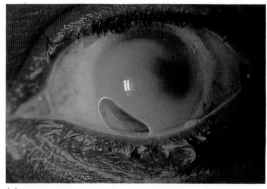

(a)

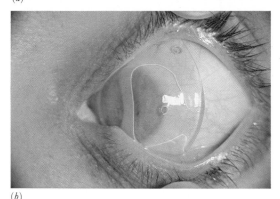

(b)

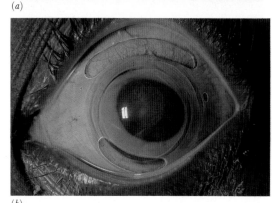

(b)

Plate 72 Well-fitting scleral lenses but with a slightly over-large nasal scleral portion. The patient's right lens is shown in (a) with glancing nasal touch of the back optic zone and a slightly large bubble. The left lens is shown on dextroversion in (b). The immediate contact with the nasal canthus pushes the lens temporally creating a larger temporal bubble. For both lenses the remedy lies in reduction of the nasal scleral portion. (Copyright Moorfields Eye Hospital)

Plate 74 The effect of scleral lens settling. The fluorescein picture in (a) was taken within a few minutes of lens insertion. It shows a slotted scleral lens with light corneal contact in the superior optic zone area and a small lower nasal limbal bubble. One and a half hours later the picture shown in (b) is that of extensive corneal contact necessitating an optic zone grind-out. While settling to this degree does not always take place, these pictures serve to show the need to wait at least one hour before an accurate assessment of a scleral lens fitting can be made. (Copyright Moorfields Eye Hospital)

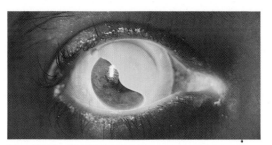

Plate 73 The FLOM 8.25/13.00 on an eye with keratometer readings of 7.91 mm along 180, 7.18 mm along 90. The fluorescein picture shows too large and slightly too round a bubble with condensation on the back optic zone of the lens. Limbal clearance is insufficient as shown by the touch at the top. The next FLOM to try would be 8.50/13.25 which would give slightly less apical clearance and more limbal clearance. The 0.25 mm increase in diameter would give more apical and limbal clearance, but the extra apical clearance would be more than offset by flattening the radius by 0.25 mm which would also increase the limbal clearance. (Courtesy of E. G. Woodward)

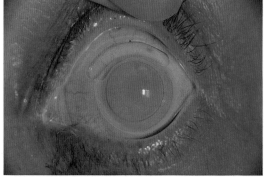

Plate 75 A well-fitted aphakic slotted scleral lens. (Copyright Moorfields Eye Hospital)

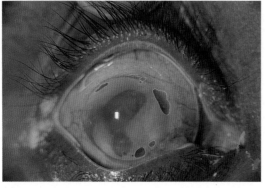

(a)

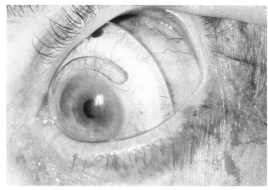

Plate 77 Slotted scleral lens causing blanching of conjunctival blood vessels necessitating a mid-rim scleral zone grind-out to relieve the pressure. (Copyright Moorfields Eye Hospital)

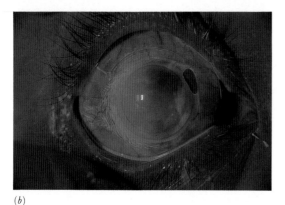

(b)

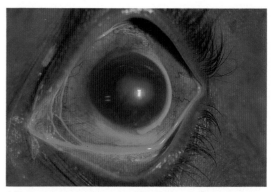

(a)

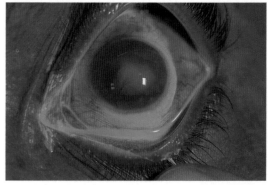

(c)

(b)

Plate 76 Advanced keratoconus fitted with a slotted scleral lens. (a) Heavy central touch; (b) after 0.2 mm back optic zone grind-out. The central touch is now much lighter. Superior sealing between the channel and optic zone can be seen; (c) after a further 0.2 mm grind-out of optic and transition zones. There is now light cone apex contact only and clearance around the limbus. (Copyright Moorfields Eye Hospital)

Plate 78 This illustrates the slow 'fill rate', i.e. tear interchange, of an inferior channelled scleral lens. (a) Fluorescein was instilled at the upper temporal fornix simulating the lacrimal fluid origin point. (b) Approximately 10 minutes elapsed between the two pictures. No fluorescein circulation is apparent in the central optic zone area due to central corneal touch. (Copyright Moorfields Eye Hospital)

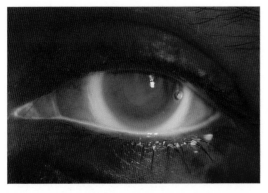

(a)

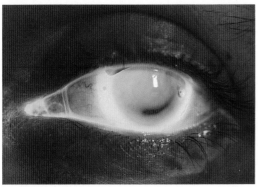

(b)

Plate 79 (a) A fully settled impression scleral lens made by the laminate method. The transition region extends well beyond the limbus giving adequate clearance. The patient is looking down slightly and there is a 'glancing' touch in the midperiphery of the cornea. (b) The same lens showing the introduction of a bubble following an extreme movement of the eye down and to the temporal side. The eye is still looking slightly in that direction and the 'glancing' corneal touch has moved to the lower, midtemporal cornea. (Courtesy of P. J. Marriott)

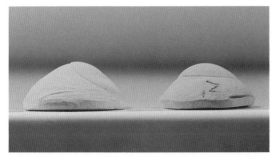

Plate 80 Side view of casts taken from impressions made with a soft lens *in situ* on the eye. Both successful (right) and unsuccessful (left) impressions are illustrated. The scleral lens is made by pressing the plastic sheet directly onto the cast. (Courtesy of D. Westerhout)

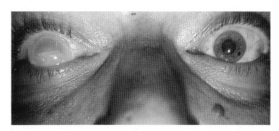

Plate 81 By putting a steeply fitting soft lens on an eye and staining it with fluorescein its correct location can be checked once the injection method impression tray has been inserted. The impression material can then be injected knowing that the lens is central rather than slipped (*see Plate 80*). (Courtesy of D. Westerhout)

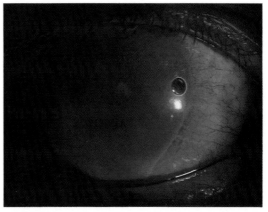

Plate 82 Scleral shell made by fitting from an impression taken over a soft lens. (Courtesy of D. Westerhout)

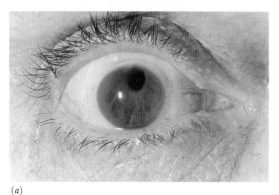

(a)

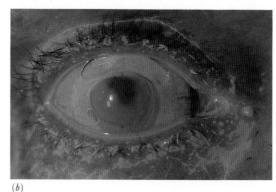

(b)

Plate 83 One eye of a bilateral aphake following congenital cataract. The small upswept pupil makes corneal or soft lens wear effectively impossible. (a) The eye without a lens; (b) slotted scleral lens showing light corneal touch just below the slot. Copious clearance and tear exchange made this fitting perfectly acceptable and acuity of 6/9 was achieved. (Copyright Moorfields Eye Hospital)

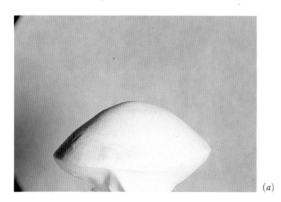

(a)

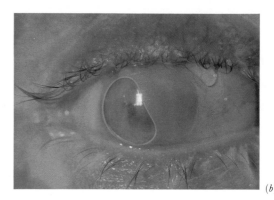

(b)

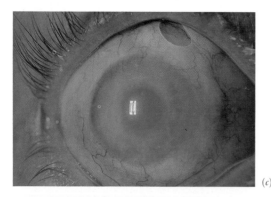

(c)

Plate 84 Flat or depressed corneal graft. Corneal topography made corneal and soft lens fitting difficult or impossible. (a) Cast of eye showing the relatively flat corneal shape; (b) when fitted with a slotted scleral lens there is a large centrotemporal bubble due to the flat graft; (c) superior channelled scleral lens subsequently fitted providing even central fluid coverage. Partial occlusion of the limbus in the temporal area and a small bubble in the channel are visible. (Copyright Moorfields Eye Hospital)

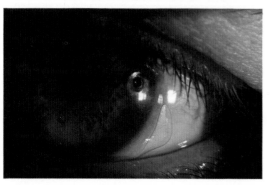

Plate 85 Soft lens worn beneath a scleral lens. In this case a scleral lens could not be produced in a fenestrated form without troublesome bubbles. A high water content soft lens of 12.5 mm total diameter was worn under the scleral lens without discomfort and removed all troublesome bubbles. (Courtesy of D. Westerhout)

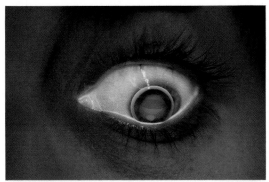

Plate 86 A crescent fluorescent fused bifocal in a truncated, prism ballasted, corneal lens. The segment half covers the pupil area as the wearer begins to look downward. There is some fluorescein on the front of the lens opposite the centre of the segment. (Courtesy of D. C. Campbell-Burns)

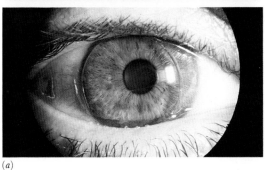

(a)

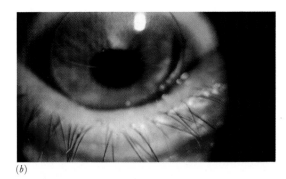

(b)

Plate 87 (a) A straight top fused bifocal corneal lens correctly positioned for distance vision with the top of the segment slightly overlapping the lower margin of the pupil. (b) Fused bifocal moving up as the patient looks down to read. (Courtesy of D. Westerhout)

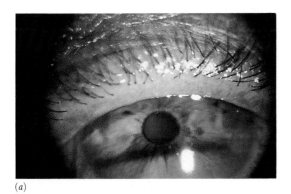

(a)

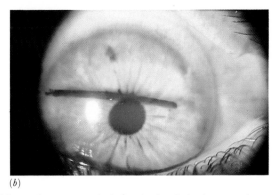

(b)

Plate 88 (a) Soft R seg bifocal (Madden & Layman, England) with top of segment marked, showing it to be in the correct position at the lower pupil margin with the eye in the primary position. (b) The segment has moved up as the wearer looks down to read. (Courtesy of D. Westerhout)

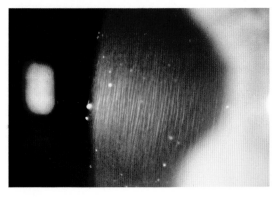

Plate 89 Striae form one of the diagnostic signs in keratoconus. They are almost invariably located orientated vertically at the apex of the cone. They occur in the posterior stroma. (Courtesy of A. J. Phillips)

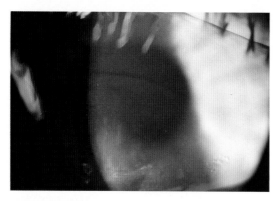

Plate 90 Fleischer's ring is the faint brown ring, probably of ferrous deposits, sometimes found around the base of the cone in keratoconus. The deposits probably arise from stagnation of tear liquid in a zone not fully wiped by normal lid action since similar lines are seen in other conditions of corneal irregularity, e.g. Hudson Stahle lines. (Courtesy of A. J. Phillips)

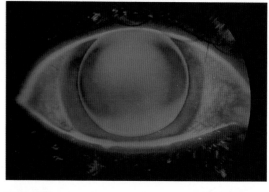

Plate 92 Keratoconic corneas frequently show marked with-the-rule toricity. The above fluorescein fit shows minimal cone contact just below the lens centre with peripheral curves aligning (to borderline tight) in the horizontal meridian but with marked edge standoff vertically. The use of a toroidal periphery increases the area of alignment and often avoids the optical complications of a fully toric lens. (Courtesy of A. J. Phillips)

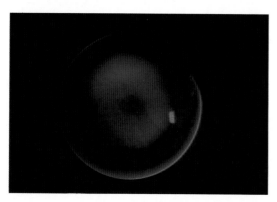

Plate 91 A classic 'three point touch' alignment fit in keratoconus, i.e. alignment of the majority of the peripheral curve and capillary contact with the cone apex by the central back optic zone. (Courtesy of A. J. Phillips)

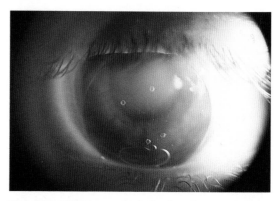

Plate 93 A PMMA corneal lens fitted to a keratoconic cornea. Four fenestration holes have been used in an attempt to relieve the central oedema – visible as the haze in the pupil region. Bubbles have collected below the cone apex. (Courtesy of J. Mountford)

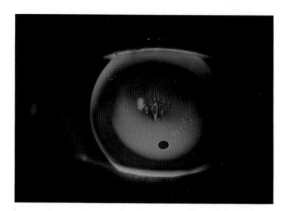

Plate 94 As keratoconus advances the cornea becomes so steep centrally that the sharp change in curvature between the back optic zone and aligning periphery becomes so great that bubbles under the optic zone area cannot escape. These break up to form froth centrally. Dimple 'staining' is shown under the lens here and dimple veiling usually results. Fenestrating the lens may help but often worsens the situation. Utilizing a flatter BOZR may reduce the frothing but at the risk of causing increased cone pressure and possible subsequent central scarring. Just above the cone apex can be seen vertical epithelial wrinkling due to pressure on the cone apex (*see Plate 70*). Fluorescein collects in the channels with the lens *in situ* but runs out on lens removal. The wrinkles can then only be seen by indirect illumination. Epithelial wrinkling can also occur after wearing thin hydrogel lenses. (Courtesy of A. J. Phillips)

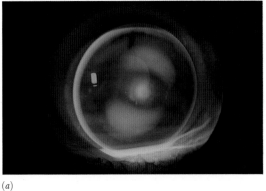
(a)

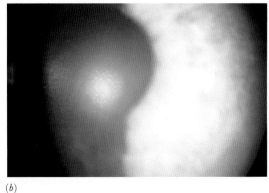
(b)

Plate 95 As keratoconus progresses the cone increasingly presses against the back surface of the lens. If regular monitoring and re-fitting (where necessary) is not undertaken either central scarring or epithelial erosion may result. In (a) is shown a case of central erosion visible through the lens at the cone apex. In (b) is shown the staining with sodium fluorescein at higher magnification. The dense but diffuse nature of the staining indicates that Bowman's layer has been eroded and that the fluorescein is diffusing into the surrounding stroma. (Courtesy of A. J. Phillips)

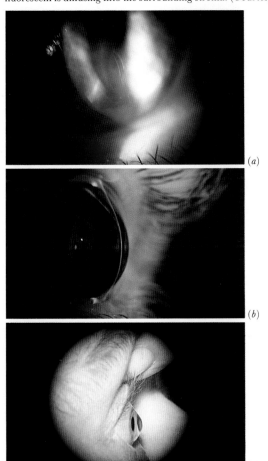
(a)

(b)

(c)

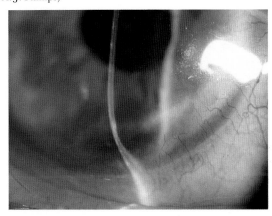

Plate 97 Terriens marginal ulcer shown in cross-section by optical section slit-lamp viewing. The thin lower area of the cornea can sometimes produce a major effect on vision in much the same way as keratoconus. Contact lenses represent the only way of restoring useful vision other than keratoplasty. (Courtesy of A. J. Phillips)

Plate 96 Advanced cases of keratoconus may develop endothelial splitting (a). Gross oedema of the stroma occurs and the cornea bulges forward demonstrating hydrops (b, c). (Courtesy of D. J. Coster)

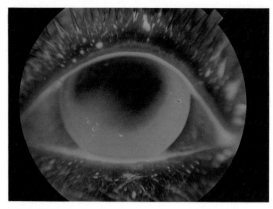

Plate 98 Corneal grafts commonly stand slightly proud of the host tissue. This is illustrated here by using a conventional tri-curve lens to align the graft. The clearance around the graft area is easily visible. (Courtesy of A. J. Phillips)

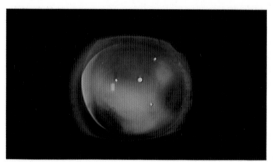

Plate 99 In some cases of corneal grafting a grossly irregular surface is produced such that whilst a contact lens is the only means of producing reasonable vision it is equally impossible to provide a normally fitting lens. The fluorescein fit shown above is an example of the bizarre fitting sometimes necessary. Four fenestrations have been provided to prevent tear liquid stagnation in the gutter zones. (Courtesy of A. J. Phillips)

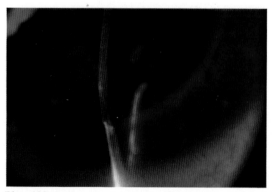

Plate 100 'Optic section' viewing by slit-lamp microscopy of the graft–host junction in keratoplasty. The raised nature of the graft in this instance can be clearly seen. (Courtesy of A. J. Phillips)

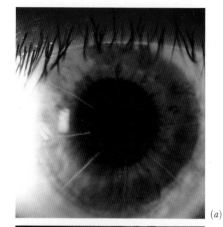

(a)

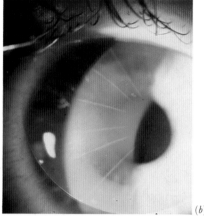

(b)

Plate 101 Radial keratotomy: shown in (a) by sclerotic scatter illumination are the incision scars. In (b) is shown the fitting of a typical corrective RGP lens with central and peripheral clearance and midperipheral alignment. (Courtesy of C. Astin)

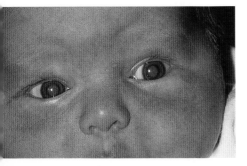

Plate 102 A neonatal child with bilateral congenital cataract. The white pupils, often visible to the parent give the first clue. Immediate referral for ophthalmological treatment is essential. (Courtesy of G. A. Gole)

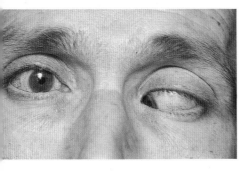

(a)

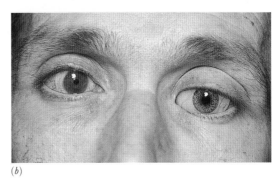

(b)

103 *(a)* Congenital monocular cataract covered effectively; *(b)* with a black pupil soft lens. (Courtesy of M. J. A. Port)

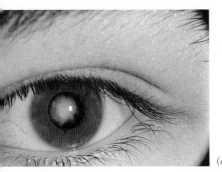

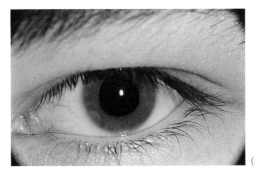

(b)

104 *(a)* A large angle left convergent squint greatly enhanced; in *(b)* using a scleral shell with opaque optic and scleral (Courtesy of M. J. A. Port)

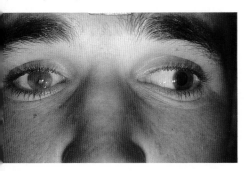

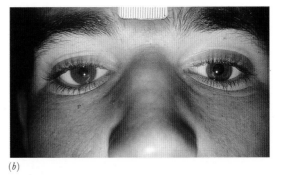

(b)

105 *(a)* A disfigured right eye with permanent divergent strabismus (the left eye is looking temporally to show the red eye clearly); *(b)* a cosmetic shell made by impression taking over a soft lens and incorporating an off-centre painted pattern to make the eye look straight. (Courtesy of D. Westerhout)

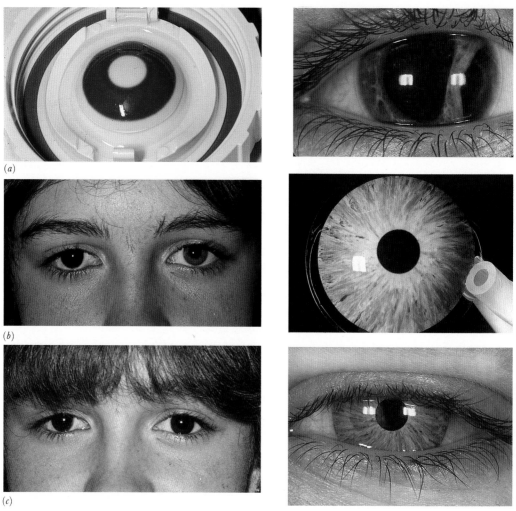

Plate 106 (*a*) A simple tinted soft lens used for heterochromia iridis (*b*) to darken the lighter coloured iris (*c*). (Courtesy of A. J. Phillips)

Plate 108 (*a*) Trauma due to an airgun pellet produced damaged iris giving monocular diplopia and severe photophobia; (*b*) a hand-painted Weicon cosmetic soft (CIBA Vision Titmus) made with back surface opaque black plastic; (*c*) the lens *in situ*. (Courtesy of G. Lowther

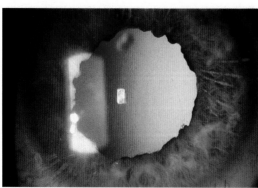

Plate 107 Iris atrophy shown by retroillumination through the pupil. (Courtesy of A. J. Phillips)

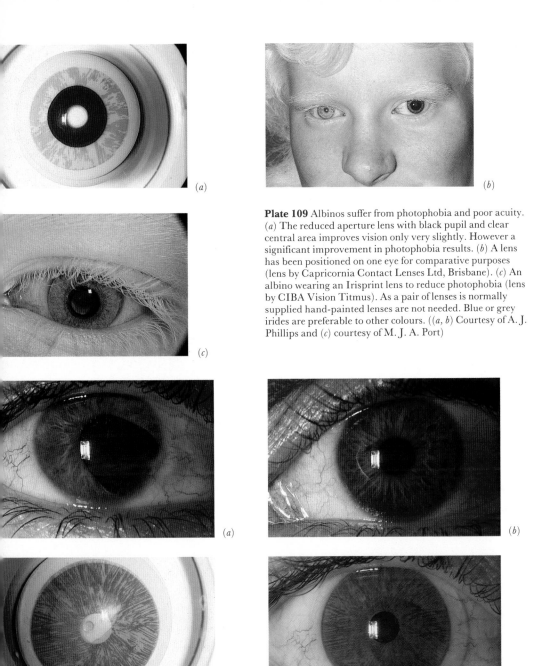

(a)

(b)

Plate 109 Albinos suffer from photophobia and poor acuity. (a) The reduced aperture lens with black pupil and clear central area improves vision only very slightly. However a significant improvement in photophobia results. (b) A lens has been positioned on one eye for comparative purposes (lens by Capricornia Contact Lenses Ltd, Brisbane). (c) An albino wearing an Irisprint lens to reduce photophobia (lens by CIBA Vision Titmus). As a pair of lenses is normally supplied hand-painted lenses are not needed. Blue or grey irides are preferable to other colours. ((a, b) Courtesy of A. J. Phillips and (c) courtesy of M. J. A. Port)

(c)

(a)

(b)

(c)

(d)

110 In cases of severe iris trauma the patient experiences both loss of visual quality and marked photophobia. The lens ~~illus~~rated is semi-opaque and incorporates an iris pattern. Too opaque a lens produces an unreal 'painted' eye effect even ~~thou~~gh better in terms of reducing the photophobia. The 'trade-off' must be carefully discussed with each patient (lens by ~~Came~~ron (Australia) Ltd). (a) Traumatized eye; (b) normal eye; (c) cosmetic lens; (d) cosmetic lens on the eye. (Courtesy of A. ~~Ph~~illips)

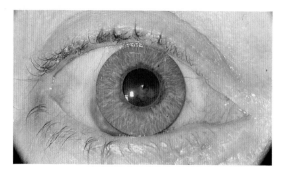

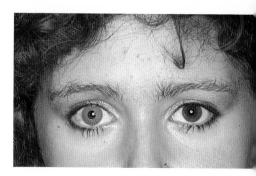

Plate 111 A poorly centring painted hard corneal lens. A soft or scleral lens might be preferable. (Courtesy of M. J. A. Port)

Plate 112 A 'homogeneous' iris pattern lens fitted to ch the eye colour – seen here in the right eye (lens by Conta Lenses Manufacturing Ltd). (Courtesy of D. Westerhou

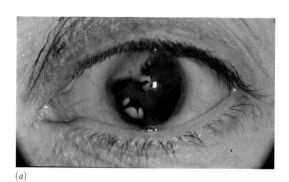

(a)

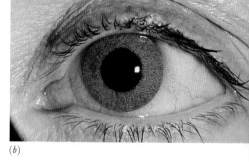

(b)

Plate 113 (a) An eye with corneal opacity, disorganized iris and cataract following trauma; covered in (b) by a CIBA Visio Titmus Irisprint soft lens with opaque black pupil. (Courtesy of M. J. A. Port)

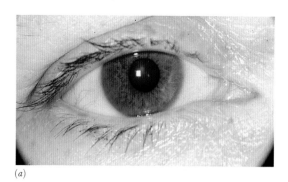

(a)

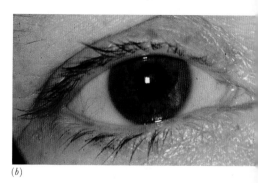

(b)

Plate 114 This illustrates the apparent difference in iris colour at two different aperture stops (a) f16 and (b) f22. For matcl a hand-painted cosmetic lens these are significantly different and such photographs should be backed up with another matching sample such as an ocular prosthesis or iris colour card. (Courtesy of M. J. A. Port)

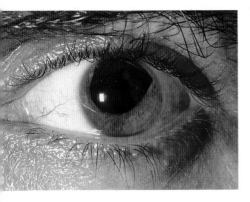
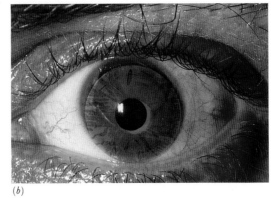

(b)

115 (a) A case of traumatic iridectomy with marked photophobia. (b) The fully opaque cosmetic soft lens with clear used to disguise it. The colour and iris pattern are applied to the front lens surface and the opacification to the back e. The two tinting processes are clearly visible in the temporal pupil area where there has been slightly imperfect overlap clear pupil area (lens by Hydron (Australia) Ltd). (Courtesy of A. J. Phillips)

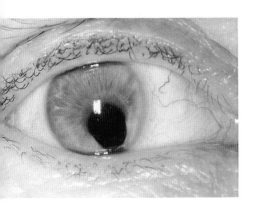
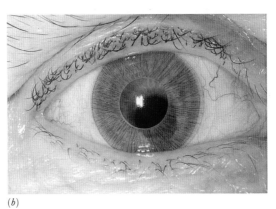

(b)

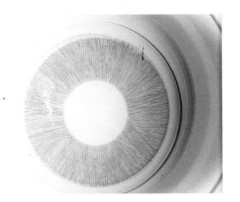

Plate 116 In iris coloboma (a) there are two subjective problems – cosmesis and photophobia. In (b) the patient has been fitted with a semi-opaque lens (c) incorporating an iris pattern similar to that in *Plate 110c*. A moderately large clear pupil area is necessary to allow overlap of the natural pupillary area. From a metre or so distance the coloboma is almost unnoticeable (lenses by Hydron (Australia) Ltd). (Courtesy of A. J. Phillips)

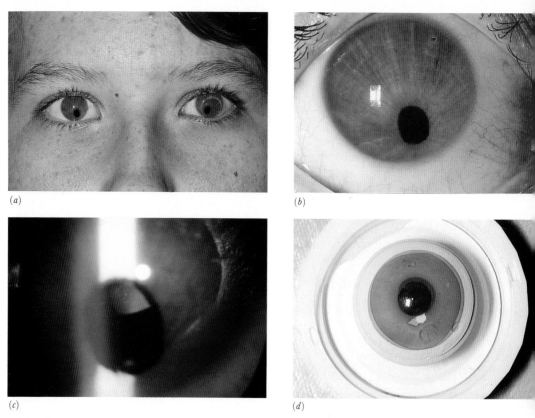

(a)

(b)

(c)

(d)

Plate 117 Congenital displacement of the pupil (*a, b*) can result in a peculiar situation for the patient (similar to that occur with subluxation of the crystalline lens). In the case illustrated the patient had two refractive results for the same eye. With −26.00 D she achieved 6/24 (through her own crystalline lens – *see c*), whilst with +10.00 D she achieved 6/12 but with monocular diplopia. In order to gain the benefit of the higher acuity she was fitted with the lens shown in (*d*) which utilize black pupillary area for both better cosmesis and also to occlude the upper half of the displaced pupil. The clear sighted zo was located by superior and inferior zonal thinning of the front surface (lens by Hydron (Australia) Ltd). (Courtesy of A. J Phillips)

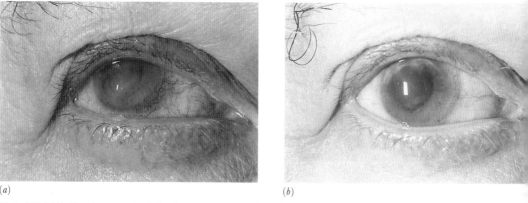

(a)

(b)

Plate 118 (*a*) Bullous keratopathy following cataract extraction. The cornea is irregular and staining with fluorescein. (*b*) T cornea after 1 week of wear of a bandage soft lens (removed at the time) showing a much smoother surface and less oedema (Courtesy of D. Westerhout)

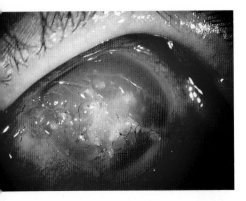

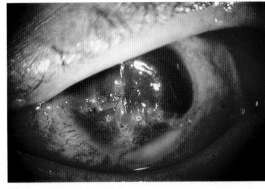

(b)

Plate 119 Primary care of this corneal wound was done in a remote hospital. The corneal surface was grossly irregular and the suture ends exposed as shown in (a). A bandage lens was used for comfort. When the cornea had healed and the inflammation settled (shown in b) keratoplasty was performed with good visual results as shown in (c). (Courtesy of D. J. Coster)

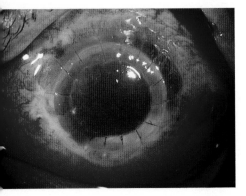

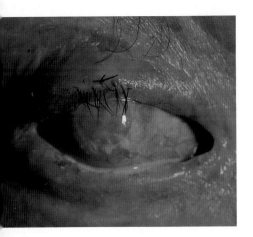

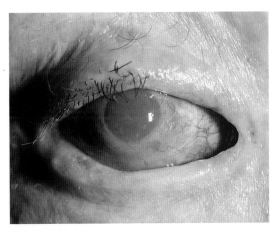
(b)

120 (a) The third keratoplasty of a severely burned eye and eyelids, showing gross staining with fluorescein due to the ɡ out of a standard sized bandage soft lens because of incomplete lid closure leading to exposure keratitis. (b) A steeply extended wear soft bandage lens custom-made in an extra large size provided the same eye as in (a) with protection ᵗ exposure keratitis. (Courtesy of D. Westerhout)

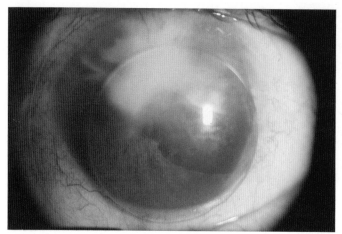

Plate 121 A combination of hard on soft lens on a severely damaged eye incapable of obtaining good vision with any other device. (Courtesy of D. Westerhout)

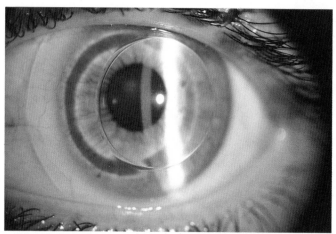

Plate 122 Sunken piggy-back lens. In cases of gross corneal irregularity and high sensitivity, e.g. advanced keratoconus, an RGP lens may have to be fitted over a soft carrier lens. In order to prevent lens decentration the RGP lens has been inset into a recess cut into the soft lens (lenses by Hydron (Australia) Ltd). (Courtesy of A. J. Phillips)

Chapter 19

After-care symptoms, signs and management

C. W. McMonnies

Contact lens after-care is the key to developing and sustaining good lens performance. During this period of intermittent patient contact, the initial prescribing of lenses and maintenance methods can be modified according to individual patient experience so that optimum results are achieved and sustained. For this reason, it is sometimes referred to as *continuing care*. After-care is the most time-consuming and demanding challenge for contact lens practitioners. The task can be difficult and draws, at various times, on all aspects of contact lens and eye-care knowledge. Training in optometry or ophthalmology is an essential prerequisite for this form of patient care, especially as all symptoms and signs require differential diagnosis from ocular pathology that is unrelated to contact lens wear. Successful practice depends on a thorough and responsible approach to after-care that results in correctly identifying or predicting problems, so that appropriate management and remedial steps are taken. An after-care examination should be based on the following structure:

(1) History of contact lens use including hours per day, days per week, and any limitations on wearing that are experienced.
(2) Symptom analysis in regard to prevalence, onset, duration and associated provocative circumstances.
(3) Evaluation of vision performance including visual acuity and over-refraction using retinoscopy and subjective methods.
(4) Examination of lens fitting in regard to centring, movement, tear circulation and appropriate lens/cornea alignment.
(5) Examination for signs under white light, with low magnification using a Burton, or similar, contact lens lamp and with higher magnification using a biomicroscope. Lens

and tissue changes should be noted including the use of stains. Further examination of lenses off the eye may be indicated including additional microscopic examination for signs of degradation, and re-assessment of lens parameters.
(6) Non-routine tests and measurements such as keratometry, Schirmer tests, corneal sensitivity and assessment of ocular health.

This structure is not intended to imply a rigid examination sequence. Usually symptom analysis continues throughout the examination when additional information is sought from the patient in the search for a conclusive diagnostic assessment. Skilled interviewing and observation techniques need to be supported by a thorough base of pre-fitting assessment, and a knowledge of normal and abnormal tissue appearances including the pathological and physiological responses to contact lens wear. An observer who is unaware of particular tissue or lens changes is unlikely to look for them, and is even less likely to appreciate their significance if they are observed. Under these circumstances, the correct basis for good management will be absent.

An analysis of 600 contact lens consultations and examinations (McMonnies, 1987) showed how after-care consumes the greater proportion of contact lens fitting time. It was found that, within the first year of prescribing contact lenses, after-care visits subsequent to initial prescribing and delivery of lenses occurred at the rate of at least 4.2 per fitting in the case of hard lenses, and 4.4 per fitting in the case of soft lenses. A detailed analysis of a second series restricted to 600 after-care visits, indicated the wide range of problems encountered (126 subtypes), and remedial strategies employed (64 subtypes). At 32% of after-care visits, there were no significant symptoms and yet adverse signs (conjunctival hyperaemia, surface deposits, oedema, epitheliopathy etc.), were recorded at 81% of those symptom-free visits and resulted in remedial action being taken. This finding indicates a significant problem-preventing mode of practice which was further indicated by the finding that 32% of the management procedures recorded were found to involve some aspect of controlling lens surface deposits or some other feature of maintenance technique, even though surface deposits were recorded as a problem at only 10% of visits. Within the first year of prescribing, 74% of remedial action was *not concerned* with lens modification through changes in fit, design, material, prescription or quality of manufacture. In the years beyond the first year of prescribing, 67% of after-care management is concerned with areas *other than* the technical aspects of lens and fit modification. For example, additional instruction and counselling were major areas of management, accounting for 36% of all remedial and prophylactic actions.

The findings revealed numerous insights into current contact lens practice showing that, for example, significant corneal oedema accounted for only 2% of after-care problems and severe over-wear oedema was not encountered at all during the period of survey. Overall, the findings provide a basis for determining how teaching emphasis should be distributed among the many facets of this complex subject and serve as a guide to developing practice management techniques that are appropriate for particular types of problem, according to their prevalence. In undergraduate teaching, for example, there is a need to reduce reliance on symptoms in regard to the evaluation of lens performance and a need to reduce emphasis on remediation through modification of lens fittings. There needs to be an increased emphasis on other methods of management of problems, especially in regard to problem prevention. The findings indicated the potential to improve after-care management in many areas, but especially surface deposit control and methods used for patient instruction and re-instruction.

This chapter is as much concerned with describing methods for adapting and organizing contact lens and eye-care knowledge in the interests of effective after-care as it is about particular problems and optimum management.

The problem areas dealt with here-in are not exhaustive and there is no way of anticipating the problems that face us in the future. A systematic approach to the after-care examination sequence, as described in this chapter, will provide a firmly based pool of information for correct identification of problems and their causes even beyond present knowledge. In the early stages of fittings, the concern is to determine how adaptation can be facilitated and tolerance improved. The practitioner can usefully analyse findings with the objective of separating the patient's limitations from those of the lens and how and where it is used. When problems develop in adapted patients the same analysis structure is equally productive. Is lost tolerance due to changes in the eye's receptivity, changes in the lenses' wearability or changes in the circumstances under which the lenses are worn? Deductive analysis leads to remedial strategies being sought along lines previously found to be successful and based on the art and science of established contact lens knowledge, but limited by the practitioner's experience and familiarity with that knowledge base. In a field of constantly evolving technology, inductive analysis of after-care findings is also employed and leads to remedial strategies being discovered from accumulated personal experiences. Contact lens practitioners have a long history of sharing these discoveries through publication and seminar contributions. After-care problems and their prevention and remediation form the bulk of interest at seminars and in the literature because they constitute the greatest challenge to a practitioner's skill and knowledge.

Interviewing and history taking

Patient interviewing is one of the key skills of after-care and the efficiency of this process should derive in part from the trust, confidence and rapport developed between practitioner and patient at prescribing visits (Enelow and Swisher, 1972). Interview technique will vary depending on whether the visit is prompted by an emergency, a particular problem, or is in the nature of a scheduled re-evaluation with or without symptoms.

Open-ended questions are appropriate at the initial stages, but questions should become increasingly more direct as specific details are sought later in the interview. 'What kind of troubles have you been having?' is not open ended enough to start, because it assumes that there have been some difficulties. A preferred start is 'How have you been getting on with your lenses?' and, as will be necessary with the reticent patient, a follow-up may be employed along the lines, 'Do you wear your lenses routinely?', and then, if necessary, 'Are there any restrictions on wear?'. If reduced or occasional wear is reported, the more direct, 'Could you wear them longer or more often if you needed to?', which allows for reports of the practice of casual use that is available with soft and gas permeable hard lenses.

According to the patient's personality or mood (cooperative, angry, paranoid, evasive, embarrassed, shy, guilty etc.), an interviewer should vary approaches across the range between an active authoritarianism, through a guiding and cooperative mode, to one of mutual participation between patient and practitioner as the clues are sought that lead to a solution to a particular problem. Mutual participation is of most value when discussing a patient's compliance with handling and maintenance instructions. A patient's embarrassed attitude may correctly indicate problems in not following instructions and an aura of shared responsibility needs to be engendered as, through mutual participation in discussion, the reasons for non-compliance will become apparent. Some humour may help combined with an acknowledgment that lack of strict discipline is a common failing, and the use of euphemistic 'casual approach' rather than 'incorrect' may help expose the need for changes in the patient's attitude. Conversely, when changes are needed, stronger authoritarian terms such as 'dangerous procedures' may be required in the case of a high risk of infection when negligence prevails. Thus the tone of the interview is adjusted between excessive authority at the risk of prompting an unproductive defensive patient attitude, and excessively passive at the risk of promoting a non-problem-solving ambience. It may help to acknowledge that the nature of a patient's tears may be responsible for excess deposits but that only through increased patient effort will further problems be avoided. Blaming tear quality may not be valid if patient negligence is suspected, but if the outcome is desirable (greater maintenance effort and compliance), then making such an assumption is justified, even if incorrect.

Interviewing is time consuming but there is no completely satisfactory alternative. Despite limitations of language, intelligence and literacy, questionnaires may be useful (McMonnies, 1978, 1986a; McMonnies and Ho, 1987a,b) especially when they can be completed without supervision. However, the precision of a questionnaire increases with the narrowness of the area of enquiry, and may be best suited to pre-fitting visits. Problem-orientated interviews frequently need great skill in handling so that, from a broadly based beginning, progress to appropriate emphasis on the nature of the problem can be achieved rapidly.

Symptom analysis

Although symptoms related to vision and comfort may occur together, it is instructive to consider them separately.

Vision symptoms

A report of poor vision requires careful analysis and consideration of numerous possibilities. Is the problem a blur that suggests incorrect lens power, or a distortion that suggests faulty optical quality or residual astigmatism? Is the problem a ghost image that suggests incomplete pupil coverage or faulty optical quality? Does the problem only occur at near distances because the patient is a presbyope, or because of the nature of the near vision task, such as typing or using a visual display unit, that leads to inefficient blinking? Do vision symptoms occur intermittently because of flexure of a thin lens or rotation of an unstable toric lens? Do vision difficulties increase during the day as surface deposits accumulate, and is the problem relieved by removing the lenses for cleaning? Does increased blinking improve vision because the lenses are soiled or unwettable? Does the difficulty only occur with reduced illumination because of a myopic shift under these conditions? Reference to established findings may help identify causal factors. For example, what are the patient's age, occupation and hobbies? Have poor blinking habits previously been noted? Was the lens found to have doubtful optical quality or power when checked prior to delivery? Is the lens too thin, and easily flexed by lid pressure? Did the lens previously give good vision and has it become accidentally warped in handling?

Tests, such as retinoscopy or front surface keratometry, may be needed to detect lens flexure. Is the lens inside out or have right and left or old and new lenses been mixed? Ophthalmoscopy may indicate cataract development, retinal changes or other pathology. Further questions may be needed. Does the vision problem become more apparent when reverting to spectacles after lens wear? Have there been systemic health changes and possible ocular side effects of medications or general anaesthesia? Has there been an increase in near vision due to examinations or a change in work demands on vision?

Symptom analysis should proceed as tests of vision performance are conducted. In most cases, a systematic approach to vision symptoms and associated tests of vision performance, lead to the identification of the important factors in each case. Simple explanations should always be sought first and, if over-refraction indicates antimetropia, the possibility of lenses being reversed between right and left eyes should be considered. Variations from expected acuity should be noted and the difference between quantitative and qualitative vision performance should be recognized when good letter reading acuity is achieved but complaints of poor vision persist. Contrast sensitivity or low contrast acuity tests may be useful. Retinoscopy may indicate an irregular residual astigmatism that could be due to a distorted lens or one with poor optics. Biomicroscopy may reveal a soiled and/or non-wetting lens surface. Before ordering a power change there should be confidence in the cleanliness and parameters of the lens used for over-refraction because assumptions about the lens being worn can lead to false conclusions. Even when a patient presents a copy of their lens prescription issued by their previous practitioner, it is wise to remember that the prescription only tells you what the lenses are supposed to be, whereas their actual parameters are determined by measurement, and are often found to be different from expected. Your own patients may present wearing a lens or lenses from an earlier fitting, forgetting or not realizing that they are not wearing the pair most recently prescribed.

Symptoms of discomfort

When some degree of discomfort is reported, further questioning and consideration of numerous possibilities is again required to discriminate between multiple possible causes. Is it a chemical sting or a gritty, foreign body sensation? How is it rated in intensity: 1 — lens awareness; 2 — irritation, 3 — pain? Is there associated headache and/or visual phenomena suggesting migraine? Is the discomfort an itch (allergy)? Does it occur after lens removal (giant papillary conjunctivitis)? Is discomfort present prior to lens insertion and eliminated when lenses are inserted (suggesting trichiasis, retained foreign body or extruding concretion of the upper palpebral conjunctiva)? Is the lens damaged or ill fitting, and does localized limbal hyperaemia or epitheliopathy give a clue to the cause? Is the lens inside out or mixed (left with right or old with new)? Is the cornea significantly oedematous and does the discomfort occur some hours after lens removal (over-wear (3 a.m.) syndrome)? Is the discomfort constant — only on insertion, only after several hours wear, only when reading, only in glare situations? Are hard lens back surface transitions smooth? Is the edge shape satisfactory? Is the lens too thick? Was this lens previously comfortable? Has a duplicate lens been incorrectly made with or without lenticulation, fenestration, truncation etc.? Are different maintenance products being used? Are the lenses being over-worn? Are the lenses being worn in a harsh environment? Is the discomfort associated with the use of certain cosmetics? Does lens insertion require multiple attempts that cause irritation? Are there 'psychological' reasons for the patient to exaggerate or fabricate discomfort symptoms? For example, is the patient trying to justify not paying his or her account? Is the patient unhappy with the choice of tint? Is this a case of an industrial compensation claim that is yet to be settled? Has the patient lost the motivation for wearing contact lenses? Has the patient been subjected to adverse comments about his or her appearance without spectacles?

Again a systematic examination sequence combined with symptom analysis provides an effective base of information from which the correct cause(s) of discomfort can be identified. Examination may reveal hyperaemia, lacrimation, lid oedema, photophobia and other generalized responses to discomfort. However, localized hyperaemia or epitheliopathy are strong clues, as is a degraded or damaged lens condition. Stereomicroscopic examination of the lens off the eye may reveal defects not evident with on-eye inspection. Fit evaluation may reveal excess looseness, tightness, heavy or harsh bearing areas or truncated edges that cause abrasion. Fenestrations may be blocked with a solid mucus plug. The lens surface may be excessively soiled or seen to dry rapidly, suggesting inefficient blinks or an unwettable surface. Other evidence of tear deficiency may be present and blepharitis, chalazion, hordeolum, acne rosacea, or other external eye condition, may be present.

Summary and conclusions

The analysis of lens-wearing history and symptoms should continue during the examination of vision performance, evaluation of lens fitting, and the examination for signs of problems. For example, changes in refraction may prompt questions regarding general health, use of medications and recent alteration to vision demands. When a degraded lens condition is encountered prematurely, it will be necessary to ask questions about maintenance procedures. When the symptoms are not specific and the cause of problems remains uncertain, caution regarding alterations to an apparently successful fitting is advised. The after-care study discussed previously (McMonnies, 1987), found that two-thirds of after-care management was unrelated to the technical aspects of lens fitting and design and unnecessary lens changes may compound the difficulties associated with the ultimate resolution of the problems of a difficult case. The patient does not need another pair of lenses that cannot be worn successfully. When the cause of problems remains uncertain, and both eyes have the same or similar prescriptions, it is frequently useful to switch lenses, left with right where appropriate, or old with new, as the outcome is often very useful. If the problem of discomfort occurs in the same eye, even when the comfortable lens from the other eye or the old pair is worn, then the eye appears to be the problem, not the lens. If the problem of discomfort transfers to the other eye, now wearing the suspect lens, then the lens appears to be the problem, not the eye. Sometimes vision problems associated with suspected inferior quality optics can be resolved by switching the lenses, left with right, as poor results with the suspect lens on both eyes help to confirm suspicions of poor optical quality.

Whether after-care visits are complicated or not, it is not possible to understate the value of biomicroscopic examination. The after-care glossary that completes this chapter cites numerous examples of the need for a comprehensive biomicroscopic technique. However, the most important lesson to be gained from the following glossary concerns the need for a wide ranging and thorough approach to after-care. It is apparent that all aspects of vision care and contact lens practice can be relevant at different times when dealing with after-care problems. Usefully organizing such a multifaceted subject into an accessible form is difficult, and it is hoped that the glossary presented in this chapter, combined with the remainder of this book, proves to be a practical guide to meeting the challenge of effective after-care.

After-care glossary

The entries in this glossary are chosen according to their relevance to after-care consultations rather than contact lens fitting in general, and reference to other chapters of this book is made where appropriate. Cross-referencing within this glossary is used to limit repetition, and to broaden the usefulness of individual entries. The distinction between gas permeable hard and PMMA hard lenses is only made when necessary and other references to hard lenses include both types. Similarly, entries in this glossary refer to hard and soft lenses unless otherwise stated.

Variations in terminology used may cause some problem in locating information in this glossary. It is suggested to the reader that reference to the major index should facilitate the search for particular after-care glossary entries.

Advice

Advice regarding the use of contact lenses in a variety of sport, work and leisure situations is frequently required at after-care visits so that problems can be avoided by inexperienced wearers (*see* Flying, Travelling, Toxic fumes and Swimming).

After-care examination sequence and structure

For this *see* the introduction to this chapter.

Allergies

These may be a complicating factor of contact lens wear (*see also* Chapters 4 and 8). Although sensitivity to lens material is difficult to confirm, circumstantial evidence for it is strong in those uncommon instances when a change of lens material results in a resolution of symptoms and signs of sensitivity. Similarly, sensitivity to cosmetics occurs occasionally (*see* Cosmetics), the complication being unsuspected after long periods of successful use of a particular product in cases of delayed reactions. The evidence for solution hypersensitivity (*see* Preservative), is convincing and, like other allergies, is managed by recognition and elimination of suspected products. If a history of allergies (atopy) predisposes patients towards contact lens-related allergies, it may be only in cases when the eye has been the shock organ in previous episodes of hypersensitivity (McMonnies, 1978).

Signs of ocular allergy

These include: oedematous lids, watery discharge, conjunctival hyperaemia and oedema (*see* Fit evaluation and Vascularization and *Plate 55*).

Symptoms of ocular allergy

These include: burning, itch and irritation.

Management of ocular allergy

This requires trial and error elimination of suspected antigenic factors such as maintenance solution preservatives, cosmetics, soaps and the contact lens material. Antigens encountered independently of contact lens wear should also be considered, especially in Spring, when treatment with systemic or topically administered antihistamines may be indicated.

Aphakia

For aphakia and associated after-care considerations, *see* Chapters 5, 15, 18 and 21.

Bacterial conjunctivitis

This is more likely to occur in contact lens wearers who are negligent regarding hygienic lens handling and maintenance.

Risk factors

These are failure to wash hands effectively prior to insertion and removal (*see* Hand washing and *Plate 1*), failure to prevent case and storage solution contamination (*see* Case contamination), and a predisposition towards chronic external eye conditions such as tear deficiency or blepharitis (*see* Reactive eye, and Chapter 8 and *Plates 6* and *8*).

Signs

Signs of bacterial conjunctivitis may include watery, mucoid or purulent discharge, crusted exudate on lid margins, conjunctival hyperaemia and oedema, and lid oedema.

Symptoms

These include an irritative/foreign body sensation (monocular initially) and photophobia (Wilson, 1979a). Often the cornea becomes involved, when, for example, discrete punctate epithelial keratitis involving the inferior cornea may develop. Patients need advice regarding the earliest removal of their lenses and abstinence until medical treatment is completed and the patient can be given a careful follow-up examination that confirms recovery has taken place. Even though symptoms resolve, the patient may require further advice to abstain from lens wear when the cornea shows symptomless lesions. For example, the corneal infiltrates associated with viral keratoconjunctivitis do not develop until about 10 days after onset of the conjunctivitis, even when treated as a presumed bacterial infection. Premature resumption of lens wear will result in a new inflammatory response and irritative symptoms (*see* Corneal infiltrate).

Bacterial corneal ulcers

These can be a consequence of contact lens wear. Extended wear is a predisposing factor additional to those described for bacterial conjunctivitis (Lippman, 1986; Stenson, 1986; *see* Bacterial conjunctivitis). Microbial infection is suggested when there is rapid development of a necrotic, greyish, stromal infiltrate in the bed of an epithelial injury, attended by surrounding epithelial oedema, radiating posterior corneal folds, endothelial plaque (fibrin), and severe anterior chamber reaction. An abundant mucopurulent discharge may also be present. In pseudomonas keratitis it is often yellowish green in colour (Wilson,

1979b). Prompt medical treatment is indicated and often hospitalization of the patient is required for effective treatment (*see under* Infection).

Bifocal and multifocal

For after-care considerations, *see* Chapters 5, 11 and 16.

Biomicroscopy

During after-care, biomicroscopy is directed towards lens condition and fit, as well as tissue changes, compared with a baseline record of pre-fitting observations. (*See also* Chapters 6, 7 and 8.)

After-care biomicroscopy is the key to determining the cause of symptoms but must be broadly based so that signs indicating the need for prophylactic management are also detected. Biomicroscopy is more efficient if preceded by a lens-wearing history and an analysis of symptoms, especially as this interview period allows for general observations of the patient's response to contact lenses to be made, including blink pattern, head position, hyperaemia and lacrimation. General room illumination sources that favour natural skin tone appearance, for example a Philips fluorescent tube number TLD 36/84, is recommended. An examination of lens centration and movement with low magnification and white light before tear volume and lens movement is altered by the instillation of fluorescein (*see* Burton lamp), can usefully precede biomicroscopy especially as changes to the adnexa or lid margins, or localized hyperaemia, can be detected at the same time. The combination of symptoms and preliminary observations help to identify areas of special interest with the biomicroscope. Essential areas for detailed inspection are tear quality, lens condition and fit, and corneal integrity. Corneal integrity is further assessed after lens removal, especially as removal affords an opportunity to use stains in the case of soft lens wear.

Blinking efficiency

This may be found to be reduced at after-care visits, the most common problem being an excess of partial blinks compared with full, complete blinks (Korb, 1974). Both partial and complete blinks are normal, but the unadapted wearer may be seen to produce an excessive number of the partial, hesitant, incomplete type. *Signs* of inefficient blinking are the observation of an interrupted tear layer (prowline) across the pupil region of the lens front surface, excess tear debris under lenses and superficial punctate epitheliopathy on the inferior area of the cornea exposed by partial blinks in soft lens wearers. Another important clue is the observation of excess drying and deposits on the inferior, exposed area of lenses. These deposits are particularly noticeable on lenses that do not rotate

(toric and/or prism ballast etc.). It is likely that contact lenses increase the blink frequency during adaptation or when discomfort is present but, when lenses are worn comfortably by adapted patients, the frequency of blinks is determined by factors such as the patient's personality, mood, fatigue level, visual task, state of alertness and ambient atmosphere conditions etc. Thus frequency of blinking is predetermined by prevailing conditions and the quality of blinks (the ratio of complete to partial) is the area in which efficiency can be improved. Efficient, complete blinks help to position lenses correctly, promote tear circulation, help to eliminate debris from under lenses, and help to prevent deposits from forming. Helping the patient understand these various blink functions, and the nature of their problem, is a key factor in motivating them to make the effort required to develop more efficient blinks. An instruction period is needed for the patient's appreciation of a full or complete blink (when the top lid lightly touches the bottom lid) which is also relaxed (does not involve facial muscles). Facial muscles become involved in blinking to either increase the force of closure (blepharospasm) and/or to increase the widening of the palpebral aperture. Thus facial muscle involvement will cause blinks to appear forced and unnatural and cannot be justified, irrespective of how much such blinks might help contact lens performance. Patients should be asked to practise relaxed complete blinks that do not involve the facial muscles but should only involve the 'muscles of the lid' (the levator and only the palpebral portion of the orbicularis). They should be warned against developing slow blinks while practising, as these will look unnatural, reduce efficiency, and attract the wrong kind of comments from friends. Thus, an efficient blink is complete, relaxed and rapid and the ratio of these to incomplete blinks can be increased by frequent periods of practising voluntary blinks with these characteristics. Sessions of 20 blinks, 20 times per day for a week should be sufficient, but patient motivation to achieve this is of paramount importance. A full explanation of the problems associated with inefficient blinking should be given using any aids such as photographs, to help establish understanding. Further motivation can be gained with an account of the advantages associated with inefficient blinking. Without these explanations, it is not possible to motivate the patient to do the exercises both properly, and often enough, to achieve the required changes. The matter is crucial sometimes as inefficient blinking may be the only barrier to complete success with contact lenses. (*See also* Chapter 8.)

Bubbles of air

When trapped under lenses, bubbles may form a froth. An excessively steep hard lens fitting may trap a bubble of air at the time of insertion (*Plate 14*), or during lens displacement with eye movements, and successive blinks cause the bubble to break up into a froth. In the case of hard lenses a flatter fitting is indicated. However, in some keratoconus fittings, excess para-apical or inferior peripheral clearance will lead to froth formation (*Plate 93*) and, although a fenestration can relieve the problem, it should be noted that, in some cases, the fenestration allows the bubble to form. Repeated fluorescein observation during blinking and eye movements will reveal whether a fenestration is desirable. Bubbles under soft lenses (*Plate 34*) can form a finer froth that is usually observed in association with excessive stationary tear debris. These findings may indicate a fitting with insufficient lens movement. Centrally located froth is likely to reduce vision only slightly, if at all, but can cause increased glare due to light scattering. Froth may cause epithelial indentation that disappears within 0.5–1 hour of lens removal. Such 'dimple stains' fill with fluorescein (*Plate 22*) but the corneal surface may not actually be stained unless the epithelial cells are damaged. The areas of fluorescence are typically larger, brighter and have sharply defined edges compared to punctate keratitis staining. The long-term effects of froth indentation on epithelial integrity have not been recorded. However minor, non-central froth in keratoconus fittings does not appear to harm the cornea and may be acceptable in advanced cases, if attempts to eliminate the froth by fitting modification are not successful (*Plate 94*). (*See also* Chapters 10, 11, 17, 18 and 21.)

Burton lamp

Evaluation of lens fittings with white and ultraviolet light has several advantages not available with the biomicroscope. It is convenient to make rapid evaluation with the Burton or similar contact lens fitting lamp prior to trial lens refraction, more complete evaluation being made after trial lenses have settled because *both* eyes are visible within the field of the magnifier. This type of lamp permits rapid alternation between fittings on each eye so that repeated comparisons of movement and centration can be made over a period of several successive blinks. The patient's head can be maintained in a natural position during these observations and, when required, lid control can be used to compare fit characteristics for both static and dynamic blinking situations. The biomicroscope can be used for more detailed examination, although without the convenience of the Burton lamp and without freedom of patient head position. The Burton lamp is also ideal for low magnification bright white light illumination observations of adnexal skin, lid margin, lower palpebral and bulbar conjunctival conditions. (*See also* Chapters 8 and 10.)

Case contamination

This is a common suspicion at after-care visits when the external and internal appearance indicates lack of attention to routine cleaning. Cases with white or light-coloured lens wells are essential because dark colours conceal accumulated dirt and are more likely to lead to high levels of contamination. Re-instruction on this aspect of lens care is frequently needed and many patients benefit from having a clear plastic pouch as a case retainer for their pocket or bag, so that dust and dirt is prevented from soiling the case exterior. Soiled cases provide a nutrient for colonies of microorganisms that may cause infection or other problems. Case contamination is presumed or suspected when infection occurs (*see* Infection and *see also* Chapters 4 and 9).

Case design problems

For these, *see* Scratches.

Chronic hyperaemia

This may be evident at after-care visits, especially in soft lens wearers (McMonnies, Chapman-Davies and Holden, 1982; McMonnies and Chapman-Davies, 1987a). Some patients will have been noted to present with chronically hyperaemic eyes at pre-fitting visits (*see* Reactive eyes and *Plate 3*), and contact lens wear can be expected to have increased the hyperaemia depending on many factors, including the quality of the fitting, the suitability of, and compliance with, procedures used for maintenance and the frequency with which the lenses are over-worn. Wearing history may reveal patterns of lens wear under harsh conditions of smoke, smog, wind, dust or glare. Systemic conditions such as hay fever may be relevant. Frequently, little can be done about atmospheric or systemic factors that are unrelated to contact lenses, although they should be identified to enable valid assessment of the contact lens contribution to hyperaemia. The main factors are likely to be over-wear, surface deposits, degraded or damaged lenses and adverse reactions to preservatives (*Plate 56*). In the case of soft lenses, tight fittings that restrict blood flow in limbal vessels to cause passive 'limbal flush' hyperaemia should be improved. However, hyperaemia is a very common response to all kinds of contact lens trauma and looking for multiple causes is necessary if improvements in chronic levels are to be achieved. (*See also* Chapters 11 and 15.)

Compliance with instructions

Lens care and maintenance compliance cannot be assumed during after-care examinations. For example, soiled lenses serve as a prompt for having the patient recount their usual maintenance routine. Despite good initial instruction (*see* Chapter 9) that recognizes optimum teaching conditions (McMonnies, 1974a), departures from recommended techniques are common (Collin and Carney, 1986), sometimes because of a lazy, indifferent attitude, but sometimes because of misunderstanding or incorrect advice from other sources. In the latter case simply eliminating the confusion is all that is required but a defensive patient may wish to deny having been taught correctly and/or having been negligent (*see* Informed patient). Motivating the patient towards the development of a responsible attitude will necessitate a discussion of infection risk and consequences. Also the risk of increased hyperaemia and discomfort, reduced quality of vision and shortened lens life can be described as consequences of poor compliance. Repeated or additional hand-out literature may be helpful but, depending on the patient's attitude, it may have to be read and discussed with the patient for it to have the desired effect. (*See also* Chapters 4, 8 and 9.)

Concretions

These develop from retention cysts in goblet cells or accessory lacrimal glands in the palpebral conjunctiva, resulting in the formation of discrete white aggregates of sebaceous material and crystals. The formation stage is characterized by a clear vesicle that traps the gland production. The accumulated secretions form a hardened core that is gradually extruded onto the conjunctival surface. Concretions are benign and associated with chronic hyperaemia, but at the stage of extrusion they may cause symptoms of a foreign body sensation (*see* Foreign body sensation) that could be attributed to a contact lens. Alternatively, an extruding concretion in the superior palpebral conjunctiva may cause symptoms when the cornea is exposed on lens removal, but which are not present when the contact lens is worn and serves to protect the cornea from irritation. The same finding may occur in the case of a foreign body retained under the upper lid or in the case of trichiasis-related lash irritation. (*See also* Chapter 8 and *Plate 7*.)

Corneal fatigue/exhaustion

This is a non-specific term which is used to describe the phenomenon of lost tolerance to contact lens wear. Often the mechanism of lost tolerance is not evident, especially when the patient is examined after some period of forced abstinence from lens wear. Usually there are no symptoms until contact lenses are re-worn but then the findings can be hyperaemia, lacrimation, sting and discomfort. The patient is frustrated because of the previous record of satisfactory tolerance, and the practitioner finds attempts to

relieve symptoms, at best, only moderately successful. Sometimes there is a history of chronic over-wear and sometimes fittings that provide barely adequate oxygen transmission and tear circulation are associated with the corneal fatigue/exhaustion syndrome. On occasion, there is a history of conjunctivitis and careful biomicroscopy reveals residual infiltrates in the cornea which suggest that a viral infection had been the initial problem (*see* Corneal infiltration). Other signs that may be evident include endothelial bedewing (*Plate 63*), epithelial basement membrane dystrophy, endothelial guttata (*Plates 65* and *66*), fine pigmentary keratic precipitates and tear deficiency. There may be systemic factors associated with corneal fatigue, such as chronic fluid retention and hormonal imbalance or emotional and physical stress (e.g. over-work).

Corneal infiltration

Infiltration of the cornea with inflammatory cells, may occur in response to solution preservatives or another immune stimulus associated with contact lenses. Such infiltrates should dissipate on removal of the contact lenses and differential diagnosis with the chronic phase of a viral infection needs to be made for effective management. A history of a recent red eye episode, that cleared with or without treatment, is a clue to a viral aetiology for infiltrates that do not disperse with lens removal. In some cases many weeks may be needed for contact lens wear to be possible. Premature resumption of lens wear may result in no symptoms on day 1, but on day 2 or 3, the patient will be very disappointed to experience a red eye episode that indicates the need for an additional and greater period of abstinence from lens wear. Subepithelial infiltrates do not stain and it may require careful marginal retroillumination or sclerotic scatter for them to be detected. In nummular keratitis, corneal scarring that is apparent in direct focal illumination may remain after infiltrates have cleared. Cautious resumption of contact lens wear is possible in these cases. In all cases of resumption following infection or immune response, lens purging (*see* Purging) or lens replacement is indicated as toxic contamination with staphyloccus toxins, viral extract or inflammatory by-products should be suspected (*Plate 57*).

Corneal oedema

This is a common response to contact lens wear, leading to symptoms of photophobia, spectacle blur, coloured haloes seen around lights, and even irritation after lens removal (*see* Over-wear syndrome). For some patients low levels of corneal oedema are a normal response to sleep, and this factor needs to be taken into account when evaluating contact lens oedema symptoms that are exaggerated in the first hours of waking, especially for extended wear patients (*see* Chapter 15). Biomicroscopy permits objective evaluation of epithelial oedema when loss of corneal transparency is evident using sclerotic scatter (*see Figure 6.15* and *Plate 23*) or marginal retroillumination. Epithelial oedema is also evident by slit lamp examination with an optic section whereby disturbance to the epithelium can be distinguished from the normal transparency of the stroma (Schoessler and Lowther, 1970). Epithelial oedema will be observed when hypotonic tears are provoked by contact lenses that cause a foreign body sensation (*see* Foreign body sensation), especially in the early stages of adaptation to hard lenses when corneal and lid margin sensitivity have not reduced significantly. A similar epithelial oedema can be induced by prolonged emotional tearing or exposure to hypotonic water when swimming. Stromal oedema is a common response to contact lens-induced hypoxia and increased corneal thickness is evident using a pachometer. The first sign of stromal oedema is the appearance of vertical striae in direct observation of a parallelepiped slit lamp beam (*Plate 67*). These wispy white lines lie in the posterior stroma and do not have the discrete appearance of lines of Vogt seen in keratoconus, or more anterior nerve fibres observed in normal corneas. Higher levels of stromal oedema cause folds in Descemet's membrane to appear as dark lines that traverse the specular reflection from the endothelium (*see* Chapter 15 and *Plate 68*). Very high levels of stromal oedema result in loss of corneal transparency (*Plate 93*). In summary, corneal oedema *symptoms* are photophobia, haloes, spectacle blur, stinging, burning and pain. *Signs* of corneal oedema include loss of transparency of the epithelium evident with an optic section or marginal retroillumination. In the case of stromal oedema, stromal striae, Descemet's membrane folds and loss of transparency are observed as well as some limbal and conjunctival hyperaemia. *Management* of contact lens-induced corneal oedema includes reduction in lens awareness (*see* Chapters 10 and 11), increase in oxygen supply (*see* Chapters 10 and 11) and reduction of wearing times. (*See also* Chapters 6, 10, 11, 14–18, 20, 21.)

Cosmetics

Cosmetics need not cause problems for contact lens wearers if used sensibly, but sometimes advice is required when, at after-care visits, problems are noted. The main difficulties are accidental soiling of lens surfaces (*see Plate 26*) and chronic irritation associated with cosmetic contamination of lashes, lid margins and tears, that leads to physical and/or allergic reactions. In regard to careful application, myopes may benefit from the suggestion of applying cosmetics before inserting their lenses which must then be placed on the eye with greater care. Hyperopes will find application easier with their lenses on the eye, but greater care is required to avoid accidental application onto the lens. For presbyopic hyperopes, special cosmetic application spectacles with hinged lenses may be necessary to ensure accurate application, and good illumination and a magnifying mirror also help increase the precision of application. Mascara that releases particles onto the conjunctiva should be avoided in favour of non-particulate types, and preferably a type that is not water based, so that lacrimation associated with contact lens wear (e.g. dust under a hard lens) does not become an embarrassment. Having lashes tinted is a safer and satisfactory alternative to mascara for some contact lens wearers. A cream eye shadow that smudges easily should be avoided if lid manipulation is required. Hypoallergenic brands are preferred, especially for the atopic patient, as sensitivities can develop, particularly because cosmetics and cosmetic containers become increasingly contaminated with use. Additionally, cosmetics should be regarded as a possible source of infection or as potential causal factors in a chronically infected and irritated eye, especially when applied excessively. Eye liner applied to the lid margin can easily be a source of irritation and interference with meibomian gland function. Hyperaemia and irritation may also develop from agents used to remove cosmetics or from false eyelash glue, skin conditions and soaps. Trials by elimination of suspected factors may lead to a cause of irritation or reaction being identified. Over-frequent application of suntan lotions and anti-wrinkle creams to the lids and adnexa is sometimes associated with tear lipid that is excessive and/or contaminated. Careful counselling will be required when a desire to wear inappropriate cosmetics outweighs a common-sense approach from the patient. (*See also* Chapters 8 and 9.)

Counselling

Counselling patients at after-care visits may be an important component in contact lens management. The most common circumstances requiring counselling involve patients with chronic tolerance problems (chronic hyperaemia and symptoms) associated with a lifestyle that creates high demands on time and causes excessive stress. Common factors in this syndrome are over-work complicated by study and/or frequent and demanding social activities that lead to a chronic pattern of insufficient sleep and contact lens over-wear. Advising such patients to reduce demands on their eyes and contact lenses is not usually productive without an examination of the underlying causes of their high stress levels. To this end, careful counselling is required (*see* Interviewing and history taking). (*See also* Chapters 8 and 9.)

Dermatological conditions

These can be associated with reduced contact lens tolerance reported at after-care visits. Any evidence of a deteriorated adnexal or facial skin condition should be considered as a potential causal factor in symptom analysis. Medical treatment may be indicated and reduction in, or cessation of, lens wear could be necessary until elimination or control of the dermatological condition is re-established. Signs of these conditions include erythema and pustules of acne rosacea, oiliness, scales or crusts of seborrhea, erythema and various localized eruptions, including exudative lesions associated with eczema and dermatitis (*Plates 5* and *6*). (*See also* Chapter 8.)

Diabetics

Such patients may be predisposed to contact lens intolerance, although published studies provide conflicting evidence (*see also* Chapter 8). The corneal endothelium in diabetes has been found to be both morphologically abnormal (Schultz *et al.*, 1984), and not abnormal (Pardos and Krachmer, 1980). Healing rates for the epithelium were found to be the same for diabetics and non-diabetics (Snip, Thoft and Tolentino, 1980), although the same study found a tendency towards recurrent epithelial defects in diabetics, a finding that is supported by a study that showed that diabetic corneas have increased epithelial fragility (O'Leary and Millodot, 1981). Diabetic corneas have also been shown to have depressed touch sensitivity (O'Leary and Millodot, 1981). Variation in sampling criteria in these studies may explain the different results found (Snip, Thoft and Tolentino, 1980). Some diabetics show good tolerance to contact lenses and individual response to contact lens trauma may depend on age of onset of diabetes, whether there is insulin dependency and whether response to insulin is satisfactory. A diabetic patient may be predisposed to epithelial fragility or other form of contact lens intolerance, and this possibility should be considered at after-care examinations, even if the patient has not been previously diagnosed as diabetic.

Dimple veil

For this *see* Bubbles of air.

Diplopia

This may present as a symptom of unstable binocular vision, for example, during the adaptation phase of a fitting for an intermittent strabismus or aphakia (especially monocular). Vision training to develop binocularity may be needed to aid adaptation to the new relationship between retinal image sizes, accommodation and convergence that prevails with the change from spectacles to contact lenses. However, a complaint of double vision may be a monocular symptom in the case of poor pupil coverage, especially in the case of bifocals, occurring when secondary ghost images are seen (*see* Ghost images) and are described as double vision. (*See also* Chapters 5, 10 and 16.)

Discolouration

This usually occurs as soft lenses degrade with use, although the reasons for these changes are not completely understood. Possibly the selective adsorption of amino acids or other by-products of the protein-denaturing process on the lens surface, leads to gradual loss of transparency over many months and years (Wardlaw and Sarver, 1986). Perhaps lenses adsorb substances from the skin of the hands during surfactant use and it is possible that some patients have tear chemistry that causes increased discolouration in association with particular systemic medication (*see* Chapter 4). Sometimes maintenance methods lead to discolouration as in the case of heat applied to some high water content materials or the case of certain preservatives, such as sorbic acid, causing discolouration of higher water content lenses (Wardlaw and Sarver, 1986). However, mild to moderate degrees of discolouration do not seem to have clinical consequences, although in some cases patients demonstrate a capacity to cause severe lens discolouration over short periods of time, leading to a need for replacement because lenses are cosmetically unsatisfactory (*Plate 35*). (*See also* Chapters 11 and 13.)

Discomfort symptoms

For details, *see* the beginning of the chapter and also under Irritation, Itch, Stinging, Lid twitch sensation, and Concretions.

Distortion

Distortion or warpage of hard lenses may occur due to lens ageing or accidental stress in handling, and can lead to alterations in lens performance. When a lens flattens, steepens or develops toricity, there will be effects at both front and back surfaces, as well as in the shape of the tear lens. For this reason over-refraction results through a patient's lens should not be used for re-prescribing without checking lens parameters. Distortion of soft lenses is apparent if they do not show a regular edge contour when placed on a finger tip and when focimeter readings show distortion. Retinoscopy is a superior means of examining for lens distortion and/or poor optical quality, especially in the case of soft lenses (*see* Chapter 11). When the quality of visual acuity is reduced, the retinoscopic reflex may show evidence of a refractile disturbance that is not detectable by any other objective means (clinical or laboratory). (*See also* Chapters 5, 10 and 12.)

Dry eyes

For dry eyes *see* Tear deficiency, Tear deficiency management and Three and nine o'clock peripheral stain.

Duplicate lenses

These can be the source of many problems, especially when manufacturing tolerances result in a lens that is significantly different from the one it replaces. This problem may occur when the same laboratory is involved, but is more likely if a second laboratory attempts to duplicate the original prescription (*see also* Chapters 12 and 13). Apart from variations in quantifiable parameters, problems arise with features of lens manufacture (peripheral flattening of the back surface, front optic zone diameter, edge shape etc.) that cannot always be quantified. The older the prescription, the greater the chance of problems arising from attempts to produce a duplicate, especially if the original lens was modified to improve performance, or has undergone age-related changes, such as a flattening of curvature, prior to its loss. The potential for problems with duplicate soft lenses is not as great as found with hard lenses because BOZR variations are not as critical.

Emergency examinations

These are not usually true emergencies as the drama may be more in the patient's mind than real, but the patient's problem must still be handled sympathetically. For example, depending on the patient's personality, a lost lens can be a greater crisis for the low ametrope than for one with a very high refractive error. A lens that cannot be retrieved from under the lid is a greater problem if there is fear of the lens 'lodging in the brain'. True emergencies are not common. Severe over-wear oedema occurs with PMMA lenses (*see* Over-wear), but is seldom encountered with increasing use of gas permeable hard materials. Patients should be instructed to report marked symptoms of photophobia and irritation, especially when associated with conjunctival injection and increased lacrimation or exudative secretions. The pathology may not be contact lens related and care should be taken to differentiate the signs and symptoms from those of other ocular emergencies, for example acute glaucoma or retinal detachment, but often a patient needs to be reminded to remove the contact lens and some might resist this advice. The earliest re-examination should be arranged and medical treatment given when appropriate. (*See also* Chapter 9.)

Endothelial bedewing

This appears as a cluster of drop-like particles, usually located near to the inferior pupil margin, and is normally only visible using marginal retroillumination (*see* Chapter 6) and at least ×25 magnification. This finding may occur in association with marked contact lens-induced corneal oedema and represents cellular keratic precipitates without obvious exudate (McMonnies and Zantos, 1979). After the oedema subsides and the cornea has regained transparency, the observation of endothelial bedewing may indicate that a limited uveal response occurred in association with the corneal oedema. It has been reported that chronic contact lens intolerance can be associated with endothelial bedewing in a cornea that otherwise appears to be normal (McMonnies and Zantos, 1979). Physiological endothelial bedewing will show amoeboid movement of particles and this observation may be an important indication of recovery when attempting to re-establish contact lens tolerance following a severe oedema response (*see* Over-wear) (*Plate 63*).

Endothelial response

This response to contact lens wear consists of dark areas of non-reflecting individual cells (blebs) when observed by specular reflection (*Plate 64*). A normal finding is characterized by bleb formation that peaks approximately 30 minutes after insertion, and then falls back towards a normal continuous endothelial reflection and appearance (Williams and Holden, 1986). For daily wear patients, care should be taken not to confuse these changes with corneal guttata (*see* Guttata), and observations after at least 1 hour of wear may be more reliable. However, in the adapting stage of extended wear, bleb responses show peaks at eye opening and 6 hours later. These responses are not detected after about 5 days of extended wear (Williams and Holden, 1986). (*See also* Chapters 6, 7 and 15.)

Epithelial basement membrane dystrophy

For this *see* Recurrent corneal erosion syndrome.

Epithelial dimpling

For this *see* Bubbles of air.

Epithelial splitting

This is characterized by a horizontal lesion, usually adjacent to the superior limbus and occurring in soft lens wearers (*Plates 48–52*; *see also* Chapters 11 and 15). Depending on the stage of repair or splitting, the split will show diffuse stain into the surrounding cornea. The cause of this response is not known but may be related to predisposing epithelial fragility factors. Precipitating factors may include tightening of lens fittings through tear hypotonicity, localized drying associated with the upper lid tear meniscus or overall lens dehydration. The split may occur during lens removal or during blinking when lid shear forces may be increased by surface deposits, palpebral conjunctival thickening or tear deficiency. Any combination of these proposed causal factors may be associated with prolonged periods of reading as an additional factor. The finding is sometimes symptomless, but usually is associated with irritation leading to intolerance. In mild cases, superficial healing can occur overnight and cautious wear can be resumed if there are no obvious fitting problems. However, in some cases, healing takes longer and care should be taken to ensure that the various risk factors are eliminated to avoid recurrence.

Epithelial staining

For this *see* Superficial punctate epitheliopathy.

Extended wear

For extended wear, *see* Chapter 15.

Fenestrations

These should have polished bevels to avoid epithelial abrasion. Sometimes they become plugged with a solid core of mucus and tear debris that requires removal with sharpened/splintered soft match wood or a brush bristle, because use of a metal pin or needle will risk lens damage. Fenestrations in hard lenses, that provide good tear circulation, may result in watery vision, especially if located superiorly and, in the case of non-rotating lenses, re-ordering with the fenestration not positioned above the pupil may be necessary. The fenestration of soft lenses does not offer as much potential for improving fittings compared with hard lenses. The value of placing fenestrations 3 mm from the edge of soft lenses is minimal in regard to central corneal oedema, although there appears to be an advantage gained in reducing peripheral oedema (Brennan, Efron and Carney, 1986). However, there is a greater risk of damaging soft lenses when clearing a mucus plug, even when using the methods described above. (*See also* Chapters 10, 17, 18, 22 and 23.)

Finger nails

These may be a source of eye and soft lens damage depending on their length, condition and the technique for lens removal employed. Jagged nicks and gouge marks should be suspected of being caused by accidental finger nail contact. Occasionally, a patient with long nails will accept advice that the finger nails of at least one index finger and thumb need to be kept shorter to allow for safe removal. Otherwise a technique that recognizes the possible danger to lens or eye tissue should be taught. However, the problem may recur intermittently when nails grow beyond manageable length. (*See also* Chapter 9.)

Fit evaluation

This is valid at after-care visits provided that lenses are fully settled and lacrimation and blepharospasm that can occur at insertion are not influencing lens performance. Patients should wear their lenses for after-care examinations, even in the presence of symptoms, because useful evaluation will depend on seeing lens position, axis location and movement when lacrimation and blinking have stabilized. Soft lenses appear tight when bound to the ocular surface by osmotic forces in the presence of hypotonic excess tears. Tight soft lenses show little or no movement with upward gaze blinks and can cause limbal conjunctival indentation. However, limbal indentation can occur with a well-fitted lens that shows good movement with upward gaze blinks, when the conjunctiva is oedematous and susceptible to indentation. Movement and centring of hard lenses maybe best assessed with white light because the instillation of fluorescein can invalidate the evaluation by significantly altering tear volume. Fluorescein assessment should follow to allow for evaluation of the lens/cornea relationship and tear circulation. (*See also* Chapters 10, 11, 14–18 and 21.)

Flare

This occurs with inadequate pupil coverage by the optic zone of the lens. Large pupils, hard lenses, small optic zone diameters on either front or back surface and lenses that decentre are all factors likely to induce flare. Bifocal designs with small central optic zones are commonly associated with flare. Flare is most apparent when light sources are seen against a dark field and at night with dilated pupils. This problem may be insurmountable with bifocal lenses but reasonable flare levels apparently become progressively acceptable because new patients report the symptom less frequently, presumably as lacrimation reduces, blink efficiency improves, and lens centration is maintained more effectively. Altering fit to a larger optic zone diameter, and/or a lens that centres better over the pupil, helps relieve the problem of flare (*see* Chapter 10).

Alternatively, soft lenses can be used to avoid the problem. The reduced front optic zone in toric soft lenses can also cause occasional flare problems. The answer again lies in re-ordering the lens with a

0.5 mm larger front optic zone diameter. (*See also* Chapters 5, 10, 11, 14 and 16.)

Flexure

This is seldom a problem with soft lenses that are fitted to align completely with corneal shape, but hard lenses, that are less than a critical thickness, flex with lid pressure during blinks, depending on corneal astigmatism and the material used (*see* Chapter 3). The cornea/BOZR fitting relationship is also important. Steep lenses flex more and the least flexure is found with lenses fitted in alignment (about 0.08 mm flatter than the flattest corneal meridian) (Herman, 1983). The critical centre thickness for PMMA lenses is about 0.12 mm, but gas permeable hard materials may vary from this guideline figure and usually need to be much thicker to reduce flexure. Changes in residual astigmatism due to lens flexure should be considered as a possible cause of reduced acuity noted at after-care visits (*see* Chapters 5 and 10).

Fluorescein

Use of fluorescein is limited by lens materials that absorb ultraviolet so that the appearance of fitting patterns is not evident when a hand ultraviolet lamp is used. For these types of materials, it is necessary to use a cobalt blue filter on a biomicroscope or appropriate filters over a white hand Burton lamp to obtain a satisfactory evaluation of fit (Pearson, 1986) (*see* Chapters 4, 10 and 24). Fluorescein should be used to examine soft lens patients after lens removal with the precaution of irrigating the eyes with a tear supplement or physiological saline prior to re-insertion, especially for patients with reduced tear flow. Residual discolouration of soft lenses is not usually permanent, but is undesirable because of the slight additional risk of pseudomonas growth and infection.

Flying

In contact lenses, flying can create problems when reduced oxygen levels become critical in cases of borderline tolerance, especially when systemic oedema develops during a long flight. Window glare is frequently excessive and contact lens-induced oedema exacerbates the discomfort. However, even for short flights in pressurized cabins, the principal difficulty is likely to be the dehumidified air, and tear supplements may be necessary. Contact lenses should be removed before boarding for long flights, especially if there is a long period of wear during the day prior to boarding for an evening flight. Even for extended wear lenses, sleep will be complicated by the adverse conditions on board and the very unsatisfactory circumstances for handling contact lenses in flight.

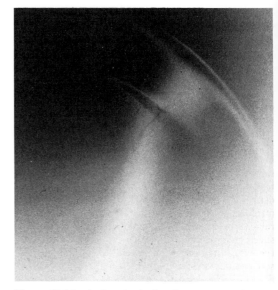

Figure 19.1 Lack of continuity in a fluorescent tube image formed by reflection from the back surface of a hard lens, indicates a poor transition between optic zone and periphery. Additionally, the non-paraboloidal shape of that image towards the edge indicates unsatisfactory formation of the most peripheral curve and its transition to the posterior edge. This image can be viewed using a × 7 to × 10 hand-held magnifier (*see Figure 19.2*)

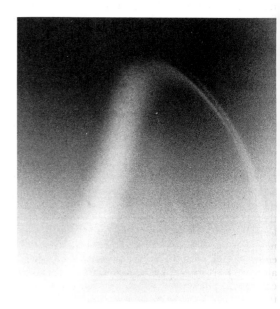

Figure 19.2 The fluorescent tube image from the back surface of this hard lens has a satisfactory shape. Smooth transition between optic zone and periphery is evident. Also the paraboloidal shape of the peripheral part of the image indicates a well-formed transition between flattening peripheral curves and posterior edge (*see Figure 19.1*)

The use of contact lenses by aircrew is covered in Chapter 8. (*See also* Chapter 8.)

Foreign body sensation

This may be otherwise described as a gritty or 'lash in the eye' sensation. A real foreign body sensation occurs when solid matter is trapped under a lens (soft or hard) and causes epithelial abrasion. Instantaneous lacrimation should wash the foreign matter away in the case of hard lenses but a soft lens needs to be deliberately displaced with an index finger, side to side, across the face of the cornea, to allow the foreign body to be displaced from under the lens. Voluntary eye movements in the opposite direction to the lens displacement will exaggerate the lens excursion relative to the cornea, and increase the chance of success. If the foreign body sensation persists, lens removal and rinsing is indicated. The 'lash in the eye' sensation associated with adaptation to hard lenses is also sometimes called a foreign body sensation (in this case the lens is the foreign body). As adaptation proceeds, lid and corneal sensitivity reduce, together with lens awareness, until the lens causes either no sensation or only a mild awareness that is easily ignored. Any lens that causes persistent awareness in an adapting patient may be found to have a poorly formed edge, even in the case of a soft lens (especially if fitted very loosely and/or too small and/or with truncation so that limbal irritation occurs). Apart from poor edge shape, hard lenses cause a foreign body type of sensation when the back surface is made with harsh/unblended transitions. The difference between a lens with sharp transitions and one with blended transitions is depicted in *Figures 19.1* and *19.2*, respectively (*see also* Chapter 12). A foreign body sensation that occurs with a previously comfortable lens may be due to a lens split, chip or other form of damage or deposit (*Plates 12, 24–27* and *59*). A foreign body sensation can occur in eyes that develop a variety of external eye conditions and recognition of this possibility may help avoid unnecessary and unproductive lens alterations (*see* Dermatological conditions, Tear deficiencies and Concretions). If doubt exists regarding the origin of lens awareness (is the cause the eye or the lens?) it is useful to switch lenses (right with left where appropriate, or old with new), as a problem lens will cause awareness on either eye, whereas a problem eye will be uncomfortable even when wearing a lens known to be previously comfortable, or which is comfortable when worn on the other eye. (*See also* Chapters 8, 9, 10 and 11.)

Front surface keratometry

This may be used to assess the image-forming properties of the major optical component of the eye/lens system. However, with some lens powers, supplementary lenses are needed to extend the effective range of the keratometer (*see* Chapters 6, 12 and 13). Frequently, surface deposits degrade the mire image quality so that reliable readings are not possible. Excess lens movement with blinks also reduces the reliability of measurements. Mire image quality improves with blinks and readings are more reliable when voluntary blinks are encouraged. Complete voluntary blinks help to stabilize lens position for more reliable readings, but it should be noted that readings derived from repeated blinks, measure maximum lens flexure. Usually the type of information yielded by front surface keratometry can be derived with other methods of assessment (such as retinoscopy and biomicroscopy), which are more convenient and are adequate for most clinical purposes.

Ghost images

These are secondary images adjacent to the primary image. Ghosting may occur momentarily due to tears, poor lens wetting and lens displacement, but will occur more consistently when due to incomplete pupil coverage, a distorted lens or one with faulty optics. Ghosting is a monocular symptom, although it can occur simultaneously in both eyes and will be most obvious when a bright image is viewed in a relatively dark field. It is a common symptom with bifocal contact lenses. (*See also* Chapter 16.)

Giant papillary conjunctivitis (GPC) or contact lens-induced papillary conjunctivitis (CLPC)

This is an extreme form of a range of palpebral conjunctival responses to contact lens wear (Allansmith *et al.*, 1977). The first (pre-clinical) stage is characterized by a mild increase in mucus that accumulates at the inner canthus during sleep (morning mucus), and mild symptoms of itchiness on lens removal. The second stage involves a moderate increase in morning mucus discharge, mild blurring, increased lens awareness and mild itch late in the day, that increases on lens removal. The third stage includes moderate to severe mucus discharge in the morning, increased lens awareness throughout the day, increased mucus accumulation on lens surfaces; lens wearing time begins to decrease, there is mild to moderate itch during wear and moderate to severe itch on lens removal. Additionally, there is some increase in lens movement (the fitting appears to loosen). The fourth (or terminal) stage is characterized by morning mucus discharge being sufficient to cause the lids to stick together; lenses are uncomfortable, surface deposits are excessive, mucus production during wear accumulates excessively at the inner canthus, wearing times are very restricted, itch is mild to severe and lens movement is excessive.

Conjunctival signs associated with GPC show progressive stages that correspond approximately with the four stages just described (Allansmith *et al.*, 1977). In the pre-clinical stage there are no signs associated with the mild symptoms. In the second stage, normal papillae show some elevation and the thickened conjunctiva shows a hyperaemic appearance. Stage three includes loss of translucency of the conjunctiva and the giant papillae begin to form from a combination of several smaller papillae, producing a clover-like appearance. Stage four involves giant papillae of increased size and elevation with flattening of the top surfaces that show fluorescein stain during active development. At later stages, scar tissue at the top of papillae obscures the characteristic papillary blood vessel stalk (glomerulus). The observation of papillae on the non-tarsal palpebral conjunctiva is not relevant to contact lens-induced changes which are restricted to the tarsal area (Allansmith *et al.*, 1977). Frequently, signs of papillary conjunctivitis exist without significant symptoms and prophylactic management is usefully applied at any stage and includes reducing wearing time, changing to lenses of different polymer and design (especially from soft to hard), and maximum effort on preventing deposits (*see* Surface deposits) and eliminating preservative from storage solutions. Sodium cromoglycate 2% (*see* Chapter 4) may help relieve symptoms and some practitioners will use steroid drops to control the conjunctivitis. However, the main thrust should be aimed at the reduction in symptoms as an indication of successful management rather than dependence on medication. The same management principles apply to cases with symptoms and signs, but, regrettably, in some cases cessation of wear is necessary when all efforts do not yield the desired improvement. Cases that do not respond to remedial measures require a period of complete abstinence from lens wear, possibly for 6 months. Even very occasional social use of lenses may be sufficient to re-activate the immune processes involved. Aetiologies such as vernal conjunctivitis or chlamydial infection should always be considered in cases of giant papillary conjunctivitis, especially when no progress is made with contact lens management methods. (*See Plate 71; see also* Chapters 4 and 15.)

Glare

Glare or photophobia was once a universal symptom of contact lens wear but occurs less frequently with the use of gas permeable hard lenses. The principal types are discomfort glare and, to a lesser extent, disability glare. Depending on climate and oedema levels that develop, sunglasses are needed by contact lens wearers, especially during periods of adaptation. Increasing the contact lens tint is not indicated as reduced transmission is a disadvantage at night. The problem is exacerbated if the patient's habit had been to wear tinted prescription spectacles excessively (constantly?) prior to starting with contact lenses. Glare is worse in the mornings and evenings, when higher levels of oedema may be present and when sunlight is oblique to the earth's surface. Glare symptoms in adapted patients may signal loss of tolerance or corneal pathology associated with ciliary injection. The possibility of cataract development or other changes in the transparency of ocular media should be considered when glare is a presenting symptom at after-care. (*See also* Chapters 9 and 10.)

Glaucoma treatment

This can usually continue without interruption of contact lens wear. Morning and evening instillations of drops can be performed before and after lens wear so that associated lacrimation does not influence lens performance. A mid-day instillation may necessitate lens removal, depending on a balance between patient convenience and consideration of the possibility of soft lens discolouration. Soft lenses can be used as a means of achieving greater anterior segment penetration for protracted periods, when the lens acts as a constant reservoir for slow release of the therapeutic agent. However, except in some cases of secondary glaucoma, the practical approach to soft lens glaucoma therapy is limited by cost and annoyances that are far greater than the general need for such systems (Galin, 1978). (*See also* Chapters 4, 21 and 24.)

Guttata

These are usually observed in the corneas of middle-to-older age groups and are wart-like excrescences on Descemet's membrane. On specular reflection, guttata are seen as dark spots and are regarded as a normal finding in the peripheral cornea, even in young individuals, when they are called Hassall–Henle bodies. When located in the central cornea in sufficient numbers, endothelial function may be compromised. Stromal oedema develops followed by epithelial oedema and bullous keratopathy as found in Fuchs' endothelial dystrophy (Grayson, 1979). The significance of corneal guttata in contact lens wearers is greater when seen in the central cornea (usually older female patients). In these cases, contact lens tolerance may be limited by significant oedema developing over short wearing times. Corneal guttata need to be distinguished from the transient endothelial bleb response to contact lens wear (*see* Endothelial response) (*Plates 64–66*). (*See also* Chapters 6 and 15.)

Hand ultraviolet lamp

For this *see* Burton lamp.

Hand washing

This needs to be stressed when a negligent approach to lens maintenance is evident from case contamination and poor lens condition. If previous advice regarding hygienic lens handling appears to have been disregarded, compliance can be improved by anecdotal discussions of the potential for undesirable consequences of negligence and by providing information regarding the prevalence of contact lens-related infection (Lippman, 1986; *see* Infection). Patients at risk may also benefit from advice given to people who work in occupations that lead to greater amounts of hand soiling. Car mechanics, for example, need to wash their hands two or three times (lather/rinse cycles) before lenses can be handled safely. Telling the negligent patient that repeated washing is necessary when hands are more than normally soiled, might help increase compliance under routine conditions. Another approach to increasing compliance is to discuss the potential for natural skin secretions or hand creams to disturb contact lens surfaces and the need to thoroughly rinse hands after washing to avoid stinging on insertion. The negligent patient may be impressed by the fact that the practitioner takes hand washing seriously. (*See Plate 1; see also* Chapters 4, 8 and 9.)

Hard lens verification

For hard lens verification, *see* Chapter 12 and Lens parameters and Quality control.

History taking technique for after-care

For this, *see* Interviewing and history taking at the beginning of this chapter.

Infection

This is sometimes encountered in association with contact lens wear (*see* Bacterial conjunctivitis, Bacterial corneal ulcer and Corneal infiltrate). Apart from medical treatment, resumption of contact lens wear should be conditional on a complete re-assessment of patient hygiene. Case disinfection or replacement is a fundamental step followed by changes to disinfection methods, especially in regard to compliance. That extended wear patients are at greater risk is indicated by the finding that corneal ulcers reported to the US Food and Drug Administration (FDA) occur at a seven to one ratio in extended wear compared with daily wear (Lippman, 1986). (*See also* Chapter 4.)

Inferior front surface deposits

These form on the area of lens exposed by inefficient blinking and/or lagophthalmos. The problem is less apparent on lenses that rotate, because the deposits occur around the entire annulus of lens periphery. However, non-rotating lenses show these deposits more obviously because they are concentrated in the area of lens surface that is, depending on the frequency of incomplete blinks, more or less constantly exposed by the lower half of the palpebral aperture. Improved blink efficiency is required to help prevent the problem but a special cleaning technique is indicated for non-rotating lenses. Patients can be taught to identify the lower half of their lenses by the truncation or the thicker edge of the prism ballast. In the case of prism ballast soft lenses that do not have engraved axis markings, the thicker edge can be identified as the portion that does not fold as easily when the lens is buckled gently between finger and thumb. The more soiled lower half of the convex surface can then be given special emphasis when using a surfactant cleaner (*see Plate 32*).

Informed patients

Those patients with a complete understanding of contact lens wear and management are the exception rather than the rule, even when optimum conditions for instruction, advice and counselling are observed (*see* Re-instruction, Advice, Compliance and Counselling). Priluck, Robertson and Buettner (1979) found that, although 97% of patients presenting for retinal detachment surgery acknowledged the thorough preoperative discussion that they were given, overall retention of disclosures was only 57%. When patients failed to remember particular aspects of the preoperative discussion, more than half the time there was denial of having discussed that particular aspect previously. Written confirmation of advice was not used in the study of retinal surgery patients but, even then, judging by experience in contact lens practice, the issue of handouts would not guarantee that they would be read or that receipt would be acknowledged at a later time. (*See also* Chapters 8 and 9.)

Departures from recommended maintenance methods are commonly found in contact lens fitting (Collins and Carney, 1986). A major problem in contact lens practice is the large amount of information that needs to be taught at the initial stage of lens use. Balance should be attempted by spacing the delivery of instruction and new information throughout the after-care period, according to need. For example, instruction regarding the use of protein-removing enzyme tablets need not be given at the initial delivery visit, but can be given at a subsequent examination when the individual patient's deposit experience can be assessed, and the expected rate of use of enzyme tablets can be appropriately recommended.

Inside out lenses

These may be unwearable in higher powered soft lenses (especially plus), but, in low powers, only small degrees of reduced vision performance and/or increased lens movement and/or lens awareness may occur (*see* Chapter 11). The more difficult it is to judge whether a soft lens is inside out or not when off the eye, the smaller the effect of wearing it inside out. Mild symptoms of sudden onset, in a previously comfortable low power lens, warrant suspicion that the lens is inside out. In the case of very thin hard lenses, inversion may occur and this results in irreversible changes in parameters.

Instructions at delivery

For these, *see* Chapter 9.

Interviewing technique for after-care history taking

See Interviewing and history taking at the beginning of this chapter.

Irritation

This is a general term that is used for symptoms that are reported in response to a range of problems. It is helpful to ask the patient reporting irritation to discriminate between a chemical sting (*see* Sting) and a foreign body sensation (*see* Foreign body). If the irritation only occurs at the time of insertion, it may be due to clumsy insertion technique or lens contamination from unwashed hands. If the irritation develops as the lenses are worn, it may be due to the onset of oedema, the increase in surface deposition during wear or the progressive drying of the lenses. If the irritation occurs intermittently, it may be due to a damaged lens that only causes abrasion when located in particular positions. Adverse responses to maintenance solutions can cause an acute irritation on insertion or a lower intensity chronic hotness and burning. When irritation occurs monocularly, switching lenses (right with left where appropriate and old with new) may help demonstrate whether the lens or the eye is the problem.

Itch symptoms

These may be associated with allergic conditions but need not be derived necessarily from contact lenses or lens solutions. A day without contact lens wear may be necessary to determine if the itch occurs independently of lens wear. Often itch symptoms are mild but prompt a vigorous eye rubbing episode immediately on lens removal. Patients should be persuaded to avoid eye rubbing, especially those with keratoconus, but simply advising them to not rub their eyes is poor management. An alternative means of relieving the itch symptoms is required and, when convenient, hot and/or cold compresses offer the best alternative, especially as suspected or potentially antigenic matter can be removed from the lids and lashes at the same time (*see* Lid hygiene). Itch symptoms that develop after lens removal are a possible indication of giant papillary conjunctivitis (*see* Giant papillary conjunctivitis).

Keratoconus

See Chapters 8, 18 and 21.

Keratometry

See Chapters 6, 8–18 and 20.

Lens condition

This is best assessed after lens removal because re-wetting by blink action masks the appearance of deposits during biomicroscopy. The deposits become increasingly apparent when the lens surface is allowed to dry and is illuminated with an external spot source. Additionally, lens damage is more easily detected with intense transillumination that can be achieved with off-the-eye inspection, as a background of even light-coloured irides may obscure small splits or nicks during biomicroscopy. Off-eye examination is possible with a slit lamp, but a stereomicroscope with transillumination facilities is preferable and will allow for accurate estimation of depth of lens changes. Even a monocular microscope with transillumination facilities is superior to on-eye inspection. The advantage of transillumination is that refractile changes in the lens material, including most forms of damage, will become evident with this method. The microscope transillumination mirror can be rotated to achieve useful dark-field effects for the examination of surface deposits but, again, direct illumination with an oblique external spot source is ideal for assessing surface scratches and deposits as the lens dries. Magnification between ×20 and ×40 is adequate for clinical purposes. (*See also Plates 24–27, 30–33* and *35–40; see* Chapters 12 and 13.)

Lens insertion

Insertion sometimes remains a problem during after-care and recourse to the fundamentals of lid and eye control through fixation control is required (*see* Chapter 9). The most common problems associated with insertion are poor fixation control, inaccurate lens positioning (aim) and failure to maintain a wide palpebral aperture due to lack of lid control. It is often useful to teach patients with insertion problems to place the lens on their eye by approaching along the visual axis. If a target is fixed carefully and head position controlled so that the cornea is centred in the palpebral aperture, patients with binocular vision can learn to appreciate that correct lens placement can be achieved by maintaining fixation *through* the finger tip on which the lens has been placed for insertion. The patient will experience an apparent 'X-ray vision' providing both eyes are kept open and, with this form of control, accuracy of placement can be achieved. An additional advantage of this method is that the need to keep the contralateral eye open helps reduce the muscle tonus and blepharospasm of the lid of the eye receiving the lens. Additional lid control is usually needed and patients with strong blepharospasm can be taught to restrain the lashes of the upper lid against the supraorbital margin, so that a non-traumatic, effective control can be maintained. A finger of the hand holding the lens can be usefully placed on the lower lid to steady the control of placement and to increase the palpebral aperture. When eye position, lid separation and placement accuracy are controlled, there is a good chance of successful placement (*see* Patient management and instruction, Chapter 9).

Lens parameters

These require re-assessment when there is suspicion of change. Usually, soft lenses do not require inspection for parameter changes because significant loss of shape or change in optical quality can be detected on the eye from fit and retinoscopy observations. Hard lenses should be re-measured when over-refraction results are used for re-prescribing or when parameters considered to be just within tolerance at pre-delivery checks are suspected of being the cause of after-care problems. Pre-delivery findings can be recorded in pencil on record cards, adjacent to the ink record, and question marks used to indicate doubtful readings. For example, a power reading that is correct quantitatively can be given a pencilled question mark if focimeter image quality is doubtful and, during after-care, attention will be drawn to this factor if vision results are poor. The same approach is useful for all quantitative and qualitative assessment but it is vital that re-assessment should be convenient and rapid so that after-care consultation time is not wasted. By far the most suitable method for consulting room assessment of edge shape and other qualitative features is obtained with hand magnifiers (McMonnies, 1986c). It should be remembered that laboratories may have difficulty in maintaining objectivity when re-assessing doubtful quality lenses at the request of a practitioner. Skill in the assessment of lens parameters and quality are a vital asset to a practitioner throughout

after-care (*see* Verification of hard and soft lenses in Chapters 12 and 13). (*See also* Chapters 10–23.)

Lid hygiene

This may need to be recommended to contact lens wearers with chronic blepharitis and/or meibomian gland dysfunction and/or palpebral conjunctivitis (*see* Reactive eye, Tear deficiency). Apart from normal ablutions, about which nothing should be assumed, recommending hot compresses on waking and before retiring will frequently improve lid condition and contact lens performance. A steaming hot face cloth, as hot as the hands can accept, should be held against closed lids so that gentle massage and manipulation of the lashes can remove the dust that has collected during the day (evenings), and remove the discharge that accumulates during sleep (mornings). A recommendation of two applications of the hot face cloth each night and morning is appropriate in most cases. This simple hygiene measure will be all that is required to improve cases of mild meibomian gland dysfunction and will be appropriate as a maintenance regimen for more serious cases that have initially responded to stronger measures (*see* Tear deficiency management). Chronic blepharitis is improved by removing the crusts that form at the base of the lashes and by providing a cleaner environment that is less conducive to the proliferation of *Staphylococcus* sp. (Catania, 1987). Additionally, hordeola will resolve more rapidly with this form of lid hygiene and the chances of recurrence are reduced. To avoid patient embarrassment it may be more acceptable to refer to lid hygiene euphemistically as lid management when instruction is given (*Plates 5* and *6*). (*See also* Chapter 8.)

Lid twitch sensation

This is a minor but annoying symptom that may be attributed to contact lenses. The innervation to lid muscle fibres (of Riolan) discharges haphazardly to cause minor flexing of the surrounding tissue including the skin of the lid margin. It has been suggested that twitching eyelid symptoms are related to diet, for example, lowered concentration of calcium ions at myoneural junctions (Hall and Cusack, 1972). Under conditions of fatigue, stress and/or debility, haphazard discharge causes a nuisance symptom. Reassurance should be given to the patient that the symptom is probably unrelated to contact lenses and that it will pass, perhaps especially if eyestrain and stress levels are reduced (*see* Counselling).

Limbal indentation

For limbal indentation, *see* Fit evaluation and Vascularization.

Lost lenses

These may be retained on the eye without the patient's awareness or with minimal symptoms. Hard lenses may be displaced and retained in the superior fornix as can ultrathin soft lenses that crumple into a folded shape. Large eyes and lids with loose tonus may complicate finding and retrieval procedures. Eversion of the upper lid is usually sufficient to disclose the lens position, if combined with extreme downward gaze lateral eye movements. Fluorescein may aid discovery and is useful if pieces of a soft lens are suspected to be retained after a broken lens is removed. Biologically inert contact lens materials have been unwittingly retained for months and a concerned patient will require careful management (*see* Emergency examinations). (*See also* Chapter 9.)

Low vision

When encountered in contact lens practice, low vision is frequently associated with myopic retinal degeneration. In advanced cases, the need for power changes should be based on subjective assessment rather than the number of additional letters read with over-correction, because it is not uncommon for a highly valued improvement to be realized in the dominant eye with a power change that does not alter measured acuity significantly. In the case of the non-dominant eye having much lower acuity than the dominant eye, the possibility of wearing a lens of the same power as the dominant eye on the non-dominant (low vision) eye should be considered as that lens would then serve as a useful spare for the dominant eye in the case of lens loss. Many low vision myopes would prefer to read unaided rather than with a contact lens and high positive powered spectacle lens combination (a form of microscope). The reading distance may be similar, but preference for reading without cosmetically disabling spectacles will be shown. Filing a tactile groove in the storage case, or marking one end with clearly visible nail polish, will aid low vision patients in keeping their lenses on the correct eyes. Tinted lenses aid handling and lens location. Using different colours to identify left and right lenses should be employed when cosmetically acceptable (patients with moderate to dark iris colours). (*See also* Chapters 18, 21 and 24.)

Maintenance of contact lenses

For maintenance, *see* Surface deposits, Compliance, Case contamination, Discolouration, Fenestration, Finger nails, Hand washing, Inferior surface deposits, Informed patients, Lens condition, Paper tissue, Polishing, Preservative, Purging, Reconditioning, Re-instruction and Scratches.

Maintenance solutions

For maintenance solutions, *see* Chapter 4.

Medication

Medication taken for systemic conditions may induce ocular side effects that interfere with contact lens performance or are mistaken for contact lens symptoms. Usually these effects only occur in susceptible individuals on high and/or prolonged dosage treatment. For example, tear production may be reduced by antihistamines, diuretics, sleeping tablets, tranquillizers and oral contraceptives (*see* Oral contraceptives) and medication for duodenal ulcer, digestive problems or high blood pressure. Current medication use should be considered when signs and symptoms of tear deficiency are encountered. Some systemic medications may alter accommodation function and lead to near vision difficulties (loss of accommodation) or to transient myopia (spasm of accommodation). Conditions for which medication may induce accommodative disorders include psychiatric disorders, depression, insomnia, anxiety, tension headaches, hypertension, cardiac and vascular conditions, malaria, rheumatic disorders, epilepsy, diabetes, fluid retention, painful muscular conditions, cramps, torticollis and infections (O'Connor Davies, 1972). Thus, unusual changes in refraction, especially loss of near vision, should prompt consideration of medication side effects as a contributing cause. Additionally soft lenses may discolour in response to systemic medication (*see* Chapter 4). Finally, some patients may experience a delayed recovery to normal accommodation function after general anaesthesia, and this change may be confused with medication side effects (*see* Chapter 4).

Microcysts

For microcysts, *see* Chapters 6 and 15 and *Plates 61* and *62.*.

Meibomian gland dysfunction

For meibomian gland dysfunction, *see* Tear deficiency and Tear deficiency management and *Plate 5.*

Mixed lenses

Mixed lenses (left on right eye and vice versa, or old with new) are frequently encountered at after-care visits (McMonnies, 1987). Usually lens prescriptions are either identical or very similar so that wearing them on the wrong eyes is of little or no consequence. For some patients, the only reason that their lenses are not mixed is because they have unwittingly switched them an even number of times. However, when prescription differences are significant, an induced antimetropia will be evident from over-refraction results, when one eye accepts plus and the other eye requires an identical (or similar) amount of minus, indicating that lenses are mixed. Greater care by the patient in not switching lenses may be possible, but, depending on iris colour, coding lenses with different tints may solve the problem without inducing significant cosmetic disadvantage.

Modifications

Those that can be made to hard lenses during the course of an after-care visit greatly facilitate management. Simple procedures such as polishing surfaces or fenestration bevels, re-shaping edges, adding posterior edge curves, creating a ski lift, or making small power changes can be completed within a few minutes (*see* Chapters 22 and 23). Sending lenses to a laboratory causes inconvenience to the patient and removes the advantage of being able to assess the influence of a modification immediately on its completion, so that further change can be made instantly if needed. Modifying gas permeable hard lenses requires caution as these materials are more susceptible to heat-induced distortion. All operations should be kept as wet as possible to minimize heat production. The solvent in some polishing compounds (e.g. ammonia) may cause a gas permeable hard material to lose transparency. Caution with unidentified materials is required. Soft lens modification is extremely difficult and unreliable (*see* Chapters 14 and 23) and best avoided.

No symptoms

No symptoms reported at after-care visits allows for an emphasis on the detection of signs of short- or long-term impending difficulties. Findings such as hyperaemia, surface deposits, oedema etc. may be symptomless in early stages, but improvement in lens fitting and advice regarding better lens management and maintenance are warranted in order that future problems can be prevented.

Ophthalmoscopy

This may be aided by not removing contact lenses in cases of high myopia, astigmatism or corneal irregularity. However, compared with soft lenses, the smaller optic zone diameter and instability of hard lenses may restrict the patient's eye movements so that viewing the peripheral fundus is restricted. Ophthalmoscopy through contact lenses may be disturbed by contact lens surface conditions and the lenses may need to be cleaned and/or the patient may need to be reminded to blink so that a clean, wet surface is maintained during the examination.

Oral contraceptives

These have been reported to be associated with contact lens intolerance, but the evidence for a causal relationship is circumstantial and not very strong. Studies that compared contact lens tolerance in groups of users and non-users of oral contraceptives did not detect any significant differences (Ruben *et al.*, 1976; de Vries Reilingh, Reiners and van Bijsterveld, 1978). However, while those results showed there was no general effect, they do not discount the possibility of individual adverse reactions to oral contraceptives, a view supported by anecdotal case reports of relief from symptoms after abandoning this medication. The prevalence of oral contraceptive-related contact lens symptoms may have reduced with increasing use of low dosage formulations and current experience supports that view. A readiness to blame oral contraceptives may delay the identification of the real cause of after-care symptoms (*see* Chapter 4). (*See also* Chapter 8.)

Over-refraction

This is performed with contact lenses on the eye. If the expected visual acuity and binocular balance are achieved, then the only interest may be to determine if any additional plus will be accepted. A hand-held +0.50 D spectacle trial set lens should blur distance acuity slightly if the contact lens power is correct. This procedure is adequate over-refraction in many cases and confirms that the contact lens power is correct. If expected acuity is not achieved and plus blurs and minus does not give any improvement, retinoscopy may indicate excess surface deposits, poor wetting, residual astigmatism and/or poor lens optical quality. Lenses may be on the wrong eyes or a lens may be distorted by handling or have been supplied to give a monocular near vision correction, and these alternatives should be explored before a decision is made to alter lens power. Additionally, it is always necessary to consider the possibility of ocular pathology being the cause of reduced acuity noted at after-care visits. (*See also* Chapters 5, 10, 11 and 14–18.)

Over-spectacles

For over-spectacles, *see* Supplementary spectacles.

Over-wear

This syndrome, involving significant oedema and symptoms that develop a few hours after hard lens removal, is becoming an increasingly less frequent occurrence with greater use of gas permeable hard lenses. This syndrome is also known as the '3 a.m. syndrome' because onset of the severe symptoms is often around that time in the morning after the patient has been sleeping for a few hours (perhaps cumulative oedema or the rapid eye movement phase of sleep are provocative factors). Intense pain may be experienced depending on the degree of oedema and disturbance to the epithelium. The morning brings intense photophobia and continued pain and lacrimation. Examination is difficult because of photophobia, but symptoms and the history of lens use, together with the obvious gross signs, permit the syndrome to be diagnosed without detailed biomicroscopic examination. If necessary, a local anaesthetic will allow a more detailed examination. Usually lenses have been over-worn, or worn all day after a period of abstinence. Even well-adapted patients can experience this response when lens wear is resumed after a period of abstinence or when reverting to a spare non-gas permeable lens. There may be systemic factors, such as fluid retention, that help predispose towards the over-wear syndrome. The presumed mechanism is greater than usual corneal swelling due to increased oxygen deprivation associated with over-wear. The thickened cornea then becomes mechanically abraded. Apparently sufficient corneal anaesthesia develops for symptoms to be non-existent or minimal at the time of lens removal. However, as the corneal sensitivity returns, the rapid eye movement phase of sleep results in intense irritation through lid movements over a swollen cornea. The patient requires maximum reassurance that vision is not permanently impaired and that the symptoms will dissipate slowly during the course of the following day. Oral analgesics may help as well as avoiding the light. Prophylactic drops may be used to minimize risk of secondary infection. Apart from avoiding the circumstances that lead to this response, re-fitting lenses with increased oxygen supply may be indicated. Cautious lens wear can be resumed within a few days in most instances, but a clear biomicroscopic appearance of the cornea is not sufficient evidence that the cornea has completely recovered. The abraded epithelium may require several weeks for complete recovery. When the corneal oedema and epithelial damage have cleared, endothelial bedewing may be detected, indicating that an anterior uveal response may have occurred in association with the corneal insult (*see* Endothelial bedewing and *Plate 63*). (*See also* Chapter 10.)

Paediatric fitting factors

For these factors, *see* Chapters 8, 9 and 21.

Paper tissue

This can be recommended for use with hard lenses under certain circumstances and can give significant advantages. Provided that a lens is wet first, and then wiped dry with tissue, the mildly abrasive effect of wet tissue will remove almost all unbound deposits. When used in this way, the surface is not scratched and a surfactant cleaner can be much more effective when used to remove the residual deposits that remain after tissue use. An added advantage of tissue use accrues because fenestrations are prevented from becoming occluded by mucus and tear debris because the tissue absorbs these tear residues before they form a solid plug. It is essential that paper tissue is not used on a dry lens, because scratching may result, and static electricity that builds up on the surface of the dry lens can attract dust particles.

The more abrasive 'wet-strength' or 'extra-strength' tissues should be avoided.

Pervaporation

For pervaporation, *see* Silicone rubber lens.

Phone calls (during office hours)

These may contribute to better management by avoiding unnecessary consultations. A progress report by telephone may allow for action, such as the manufacture of lenses to a modified prescription, that can be evaluated at the next visit. However, the longer the interval since the previous examination, the greater the need for re-examination so that problems are correctly identified.

Phone calls (out of office hours)

These are an essential means of patient management, especially if a patient reacts adversely to a crisis. Difficulty removing a lens, a lost or broken lens, or a lens displaced (or suspected of being displaced) under the upper lid, can be emergencies depending on the patient's reaction to each situation. Reassurance is required in large measure. It is important to realize that the patient would not telephone if he or she did not think the predicament was a crisis. Telling a patient not to worry is not an adequate response. A thorough analysis of his or her predicament is required with explanations phrased to reduce anxiety, for example, 'the lens cannot be lost behind the eye. Even if under the lid the lens will not cause any harm. A loan lens can be used while a new lens is manufactured etc.'.

Photography

For photography, *see* Chapters 6, 7 and 24.

Photophobia

For photophobia, *see* Glare.

Polishing

Polishing of hard lenses may be required more than once per year in some cases, but usually annual repolishing is sufficient. Convex surfaces show the greatest need because they attract the larger quantity of deposits and scratches, but polishing the inside surface can be important as a degraded surface may cause discomfort. Although it is not possible to completely remove significant scratches by polishing, it is an advantage to reduce them so that their capacity to collect mucus is lessened. Thus, polished lenses are cleaner, stay cleaner longer and are easier to clean, but if lenses show advanced degradation, polishing is of little value and replacement is necessary. (*See also* Chapters 18, 22 and 23.)

Postkeratoplasty fitting

For this, *see* Chapters 18 and 21.

Postradial keratotomy fitting

For this, *see* Chapter 21.

Presbyopia

This may take up a large amount of after-care consultation time (McMonnies, 1987), especially as patients cannot be expected to know in advance which method of presbyopic correction will be most appropriate. The simplest solution of an over-correction for near work is often as appropriate as the sophisticated approach of bifocal contact lens fitting (*see* Chapters 5 and 16). Between these two extremes of difficulty, other solutions such as monovision or near contact lenses and distance over-spectacles may be found to be more appropriate. All these techniques involve some compromise of visual efficiency, and the most careful pre-prescribing consultation may not lead to the most suitable method of correction being prescribed initially. Once presbyopes start to use their new correction, they may become aware of previously unsuspected visual requirements that necessitate an alteration in method of correction. For example, in theory it is possible to determine the most appropriate eye to be corrected for near when monovision is prescribed (McMonnies, 1974b). However, in practice, it is often only when this has been experienced in a variety of circumstances that the choice of dominant eye and the success or otherwise of this form of correction is determined. Trials with alternate eyes corrected for near are sometimes needed to determine the most suitable combination, if monovision is acceptable at all.

Understanding the presbyope's complex needs and variable capacity to accept vision compromise is the cornerstone to success, even if sometimes laboriously achieved. Power changes, that increase distance vision at the expense of near, are a step that should not be taken without a full discussion of the consequences. A signed consent form would not assure that a change of mind will not be encountered.

Preservatives

These may be suspected if symptoms of stinging and burning occur (*see* Chapter 4). In chronic responses, however, symptoms may be mild and only increased lens awareness may be reported. Signs may include hyperaemia of the limbal, bulbar and palpebral conjunctiva, conjunctival oedema, punctate epithelial stain and corneal infiltration with inflammatory cells. Evidence of hypersensitivity may be obtained from a positive ocular reaction to a provocative test with the suspected preservative or from a skin patch test, or if cytology results show eosinophils. However, management can proceed on the basis of a presumed diagnosis, by a trial elimination of suspected preservative from storage, cleaning and 'in eye' solutions. Usually lenses can be purged successfully (*see* Purging) and wear resumed. However, corneal infiltrates should be given time to disperse because earlier resumption may cause symptoms to recur (*see* Corneal infiltrates). Careful examination using marginal retroillumination and sclerotic scatter may be necessary to detect residual infiltration. Because of their capacity to bind preservatives, soft lenses are more likely to be associated with adverse preservative responses and a greater level of limbal hyperaemia has been found in soft lens wearers who use preserved storage solutions compared with those who use unpreserved storage solution (McMonnies and Chapman-Davies, 1987a). (*See Plates 53–57.*)

Prosthetic lenses

For prosthetic lenses, *see* Chapters 8 and 21.

Pseudopterygia

These appear to be a sequel to chronic epithelial erosion (*see* Three and nine o'clock peripheral stain) occurring in hard lens wearers (Stainer *et al.*, 1981). The temporal and/or nasal limbal cornea can become scarred and vascularized superficially, leading to subepithelial opacities that give the appearance of corneal involvement from a pterygium, except for a diffuse leading edge. Initially, there are no symptoms but later increased lens awareness, burning and stinging occur. Predisposing factors are over-wear, inferiorly locating lenses, superiorly locating lenses with low lower lids, tear deficiency, lenses with excess peripheral clearance, lenses with thick edges and inefficient blinking. Remedial approaches with hard lenses include re-fitting lenses to locate more centrally, reducing excess edge clearance, relieving tear deficiency with tear supplements, improving blink efficiency, encouraging lateral eye movements, thinning the lens edge and reducing wearing times. Re-fitting with soft lenses may be indicated if the vascularized scars continue to progress. (*See Plates 20, 21, 53* and *54.*)

Pterygia and pingueculae

These may become injected (*Plates 2* and *3*) during contact lens wear. Because these lesions are highly vascularized, any stimulus to conjunctival injection will result in a greater concentration of redness in these exposed scar tissues. Contact lenses add to the list of potential causes of injection but, when well cleaned and fitted, do not appear to cause significant problems. However, a contact lens may be incorrectly regarded as the cause of pterygium growth activity when other factors, such as exposure to excessive sunlight, are more significant. It is possible that soft lenses help by acting as a bandage for the head of the pterygium and preventing epithelial drying that is associated with increased growth and corneal involvement. Changes in corneal astigmatism may be caused by a pterygium requiring surgical treatment and could be confused with contact lens-induced changes. (*See* Chapters 8, 11 and 21.)

Purging

Purging lenses suspected of being contaminated with toxic materials may be required when stinging, hyperaemia and lacrimation develop with lenses that were previously comfortable. Soft lenses especially are susceptible to adsorbing irritant substances from storage solutions and toxic gases, vapours or sprays (*see* Toxic fumes). Purging of these substances is slow and requires multiple cycles of soaking in unpreserved saline or distilled water. Purging efficiency is improved with use of larger volumes of fluid (a lens vial is better than a lens case), and with agitation to circulate the purging fluid. If acceptable to the lens, heating the saline will help speed up the process. The suspected toxic contamination is confirmed if $4 \times$ 12-hour soaking cycles with heat and occasional agitation result in a significant reduction in symptoms. (*See also* Chapter 4.)

Quality control

For lens manufacture, quality control depends on the laboratory observing satisfactory tolerances for accurate radii, power, edge shape, back surface transitions etc. (McMonnies, 1986c).

Urgent manufacturing schedules create pressure for lenses to be supplied that do not meet normal standards. Practitioner time spent in assessing lenses prior to delivery is easily justified when significant errors can be corrected before delivery and when after-care problems are encountered. A difference in acuity between the two eyes, for example, might be explained by one lens being 0.12 D strong and the other being 0.12 D weak. The powers read at the pre-delivery check can be recorded in pencil next to the record card prescription, so that the probable cause of the difference in acuity is immediately apparent when unequal acuity results are encountered. Questionable quality of optics could be indicated on the record card by a question mark over the lens power, and this information would again shorten the problem-solving process when the eyes yield different acuity results (*see* Chapters 12 and 13).

Reactive eye

This is a general term for those eyes that have a greater propensity to react to many ordinary, everyday stimuli, and contact lenses in particular (McMonnies, 1978). These eyes show chronic conjunctival hyperaemia and injection of episcleral vessels and may have pterygia or pingueculae. Other signs and findings associated with the reactive eye syndrome include lid conditions such as blepharitis, skin conditions such as acne rosacea, tear deficiency, chronic follicular or papillary changes in the palpebral conjunctiva and meibomian gland dysfunction. There may be a history of allergies such as hay fever, as well as a propensity for reactive eyes to respond adversely to normal stimuli such as wind, dust, glare, smoke, smog, lack of sleep, eye strain and food allergies such as an ocular hyperaemia response to alcohol consumption. The reactive eye syndrome, and associated chronic hyperaemia, are usefully noted at pre-fitting examinations because levels of ocular hyperaemia observed at after-care visits need to be assessed in relation to expected or normal levels of vascular response that prevail independently of contact lens wear. Steps that are not taken to prevent adverse responses in patients with reactive eyes when prescribing should be accounted for at after-care visits. These steps include advice not to over-wear lenses, to avoid exposure to maintenance solution preservatives and to make a maximum effort to restrict the development of surface deposits. Additionally, steps taken to control associated conditions such as meibomian gland dysfunction and blepharitis help to reduce the response to the physical, chemical, physiological and immunological stimuli provided by a contact lens. After-care visits are the opportunity to re-emphasize the key management factors for these patients. *Plates 3–9* and *46–58* illustrate many of the above-mentioned conditions.

Reconditioning

Reconditioning of lenses may be performed for patients whose lenses have become degraded, but do not necessarily need replacing. Patients should be encouraged to accept responsibility for maintaining their lenses in satisfactory condition. If patients think that their poor compliance with maintenance instructions can be absolved by occasional recovery operations performed by the practitioner, there is reduced incentive for them to look after their lenses. However, when considered appropriate, more powerful cleaning measures can be performed 'in office' (*see* Chapter 4), but care should be taken to avoid accepting responsibility for the outcome. The more degraded the lenses are the stronger the measure required for improvement and the greater the chance of a less than satisfactory result, and the stronger the indication for replacement rather than reconditioning. (*see also* Polishing.)

Record keeping

This requires a balance between filling cards with unnecessary details of after-care visits and not recording sufficient information for effective problem solving. For example, it is unnecessary to record that the patient *is* complying with maintenance instructions although any departure from recommended technique should be noted so that future visits can include a follow-up discussion. Again, if a trial with lenses reversed, right switched with left, is not recorded, confusing results may be obtained at the subsequent visit. Economy of detailing findings is achieved through the use of abbreviations. An uncomplicated soft lens visit might show the record: WT 12, No S, R&L 6/6, No O/R, R&L (o,o)M1, B-ve, Rep 12/12 indicating that wearing time is 12 hours average each day, there are no symptoms, both eyes read 6/6 with neither eye having significant over-refraction, both lenses centre and move 1 mm on upward gaze blink, biomicroscopy results are unremarkable, and the patient is to report for the next after-care visit in 12 months. Many observations are readily rated on nominal or ordinal scales that can be described economically. For example, hard lens/corneal curvature relationships can be described by the following short hand system: AL− for borderline flat, AL for alignment, AL+ for slight clearance, AL++ for definite clearance etc. (A. J. Phillips, 1987, personal communication). The recording of conjunctival hyperaemia is another example, where a photographic reference scale allows six grades of hyperaemia to be determined (McMonnies and Chapman-Davies, 1987b) and these can be recorded as H0 through to H5 so that time and record card space is conserved.

Recurrent corneal erosions

These are associated with an abnormal epithelial basement membrane and symptoms of sharp pain, lacrimation and photophobia that usually occur upon waking (Brown and Bron, 1976). Evidence of the abnormal basement membrane is found when refractile changes such as maps, dots, fingerprints, blebs, nets etc. are observed using marginal retroillumination. In mild cases, the epithelial disturbance has healed superficially at the time of examination later in the day and changes are difficult to detect. In marked cases, a frank epithelial defect is observed. Mild cases may be complicated by contact lens wear, but the problem can be reduced by patching or taping the lid during sleep to eliminate nocturnal lagophthalmos and by using tear supplements or lid lubricants prior to sleep. Severe cases require medical treatment including the use of hypertonic preparations, epithelial debridement and the use of bandage soft lenses (Kenyon, Fogue, and Grayson, 1982). In some cases of epithelial basement membrane dystrophy, the response to contact lens wear is the rapid formation of microcysts (McMonnies, 1981) (*see Figure 15.7* and *Plates 61 and 62*). If spectacles are prescribed for a period of enforced contact lens abstinence in these cases, difficulty may be encountered with variable astigmatic power and axis and associated spectacle blur (*see* Chapter 20).

Re-fitting contact lenses

Re-fitting contact lenses to an existing wearer is indicated when changes in refraction and/or a degraded lens condition indicate a potential for significant improvement with new lens prescription, design or material. Degraded hard lenses show accumulated surface scratches and/or significant changes to the back optic radius, including warpage. Degraded soft lenses also show surface scratches and deposits, as well as loss of shape and discolouration. Depending on the date of the previous prescription, accidental lens damage in the form of splits or nicks may precipitate a decision to re-fit rather than obtain a duplicate lens. A gradual loss of lens performance (comfort and vision) over a number of years is often not appreciated by patients with good tolerance until the change is made to a new fitting. It is part of the responsibility of after-care to advise that re-fitting is required when sufficient indicators are encountered. (*See also* Chapters 10, 11 and 14–21.)

Refractive changes after wearing contact lenses

For these, *see* Chapters 5 and 20.

Re-instruction

Re-instruction of handling and maintenance techniques that were taught at the time of lens delivery are sometimes needed at after-care. Occasionally, amazing departures from recommended methods are encountered, but not necessarily due to ineffective instruction, because sometimes patients have taken incorrect advice from other sources. In either case, re-instruction is needed. Apart from re-instruction, additional instruction is needed at after-care that cannot be anticipated at the delivery visit. For example, after-care patients may require instruction regarding blink efficiency, lid hygiene, cleaning the inferior portion of non-rotating lenses, tear supplement use, tissue use on the removal of hard lenses etc. The principles of optimum conditions for effective instruction also apply to these situations (McMonnies, 1974a) including the use of supporting visual display during instruction, and written hand-outs that can be issued for home reference in support of the consulting room discussion.

Reports

These are needed by patients who require after-care from another practice when travelling or after transferring their home to a new location. A copy of the latest keratometry findings, spectacle prescription and contact lens prescription, including recommended maintenance products, are the most useful basic information. Other significant details can be added if needed to facilitate the transfer of after-care responsibility.

Residual astigmatism

This is suspected when expected acuity is not obtained with spherical over-refraction, and can be most conveniently confirmed with retinoscopy. Retinoscopy allows for the influence of varying lid postures and changing lens position to be assessed. A decentred lens, especially with high power, will induce an astigmatic effect and variations in lens flexure may be induced with changes in palpebral aperture width and lid tonus. These factors cannot be accounted for without multiple readings using an automatic refractor, and the dynamic assessment offered by the retinoscope offers the advantage of allowing observation of the effects induced by successive blinks. After retinoscopy, the degree and axis of residual astigmatism can be refined with subjective refraction, but allowance should be made for variation in subjective responses that occur from blink to blink. Reliability of responses during subjective astigmatism analysis can be increased for contact lens wearers by removing any surface deposits and ensuring an even wetness of the front surface. In addition, greater viewing time of the alternatives should be allowed during subjective refraction so that blinking can clear vision and stabilize lens position. Even with these precautions, retinoscopy should be regarded as the principal finding. In the case of hard lenses, residual astigmatism induced by flexure can sometimes be eliminated by varying centre thickness and lens/cornea fitting relationship (see Flexure and rigid gas permeable lenses).

Sometimes lens flexure fortuitously compensates for residual astigmatism that would occur if a non-flexing lens was fitted and this phenomenon may explain some of the differences in vision performance found with lenses of the same prescription made with different centre thickness or in a different material. For either hard or soft lenses, front and/or back toroidal surfaces can be used to compensate for residual astigmatism, or supplementary spectacles can be prescribed for occasional use. (See also Chapters 5, 10 and 11 and 14.)

Rigid gas permeable lenses

Rigid gas permeable or gas permeable hard lenses may be associated with particular after-care problems at a greater rate than that encountered with PMMA lenses (Bennet and Egan, 1986). They may need to be re-ordered with greater centre thickness and flatter in curvature when flexure results in unacceptable levels of residual astigmatism (Herman, 1983; see Flexure and Chapters 5 and 10). Greater care in avoiding stress that increases lens warpage (see Distortion) may be needed in lens handling. Cleaning or removal techniques (see Chapters 4 and 9) may need to be modified for rigid gas permeable (RGP) lenses and case designs that avoid stress are indicated. Very flexible (high Dk) materials used for extended wear may have to be fitted flatter if they tend to adhere and embed into corneal epithelium during sleep (see Chapter 15). These lenses can also turn inside out accidentally. Maintenance may have to be intensified with RGP materials that soil more readily (see Chapters 3, 4 and 10), with the use of emulsion cleaners and enzyme tablets. Case design is more critical to avoid scratching RGP lenses that have reduced surface hardness (see Scratches). Difficulties in manufacture of RGP lenses (see Chapter 22) may result in 'burnt' unwettable surfaces, inferior edge quality, unstable (flattening) base curves and inferior quality optics (Schwartz, 1986). Lenses which develop marked surface cracking (Plate 27) should be replaced.

Scleral lenses

For scleral lenses, see Chapters 17, 18 and 21.

Scratches

Scratches that develop in advance of expected normal rates of lens ageing should be noted at after-care visits, and are usually due to faulty case design. Incorrect retrieval of a dropped lens is an occasional factor in lens scratching, but case-induced scratches can be a daily event. When the lens convex surface matches a smooth or basket-type case surface, the lens will usually be removed by sliding. Wet or dry, the daily opportunity for dust or the degraded plastic surfaces to scratch the lens leads to excess scratches. Soft lens case wells should be ribbed and/or flat bottomed to minimize this problem. The best hard lens case design allows for the lens to be suspended, free from flexure stress, by soft plastic holders that project from the case ends into the storage fluid. However, a large diameter lens may be warped if lens flexure is induced by this method. Chapter 23 describes the technique for polishing out scratches on hard lenses (*See also* Chapters 12 and 13.)

Sequential stain

This occurs with multiple instillation of fluorescein and is associated with contact lens intolerance, but can be observed in mild forms in successful wearers (Korb and Herman, 1979). Several instillations of 2% liquid fluorescein at 5-minute intervals may be necessary to identify at-risk patients, or to detect signs consistent with poor contact lens tolerance. Absence of fluorescein stain upon sequential instillation suggests normal epithelial integrity.

Silicone rubber lenses

These may be found to adhere tightly to the ocular surface because of pervaporation (the evaporation of tears through the lens; Refojo and Leong, 1981). Attempted removal may lead to corneal abrasion unless the depleted tear layer under the lens is supplemented with isotonic saline. Frequent instillation with head tilted back, or the patient lying in a supine position, so that the palpebral aperture acts as a reservoir for excess fluid, is required. When lens movement is restored, removal can be completed safely. (*See also* Chapter 11 and *Plates 41–45.*)

Slit lamp biomicroscopy

For this, *see* Biomicroscopy and Chapters 6, 7 and 8.

Soft lens verification

For this, *see* Chapter 13.

Spectacles

For contact lens wearers, spectacles are usually most appropriately prescribed after a 12-hour break overnight from lens wear providing the lenses have not been over-worn the previous day. Prescribing spectacles immediately after lens removal will often give less reliable results (especially for astigmatism) and a myopic over-correction (or hypermetropic under-correction). Some practitioners like to obtain a mid-afternoon refraction, immediately after lens removal and another first thing in the morning, after no contact lens wear overnight. The correction given is a compromise between the two results. Waiting days or weeks for keratometry findings to stabilize is not practical as the patient does not wait days or weeks before wearing spectacles (*see* Chapter 20). If poor results are obtained after a 12-hour break from lens wear, keratometry will indicate corneal changes that necessitate improvement in the contact lens fitting and management. Keratometry changes and spectacle blur are greatest with PMMA lenses and changing to gas permeable hard materials and reducing wearing times are key factors in recovery of a regular corneal shape that allows a reliable refraction. For the patient who has no spectacles, wearing times cannot be reduced without some form of correction for the non-contact lens periods. In these cases an initial prescription of approximate spectacles is needed, which allows for reduced contact lens wearing times and, together with lenses of increased gas permeability, lays the foundations for corneal recovery and an improved spectacle prescription in the future.

Striae

For striae, *see* Corneal oedema.

Stinging

This is usually reported on lens insertion or soon after. Possible causes include an adverse reaction to the pH, buffering, tonicity or preservative in a storage or rinsing solution, including hydrogen peroxide that has not been effectively neutralized. The sensation and associated hyperaemia and lacrimation should pass after a few minutes if the stimulus is mild. Other possible causes include lens contamination from unwashed hands or misapplied cosmetics. New lenses may sting if not completely leached of toxic substances introduced during manufacture, and in mild cases a few minutes immersion of the lens in fresh saline will allow for comfortable re-insertion. (*See also* Chapter 4.)

Suction holders

Suction holders intended for contact lens removal should not be recommended. If after-care visits reveal continuing problems with lens removal (loose lids that do not dislodge a hard lens, or long finger nails that inhibit soft lens removal), further instruction should be given rather than allowing the use of a suction cup. These devices always become contaminated and are potential sources of corneal abrasion if removal is attempted after a lens has become displaced onto the conjunctiva. Perhaps most importantly, a patient who is dependent on a suction holder is in an awkward predicament if it is lost. Nevertheless, a suction holder may provide a feeling of security for a patient who lacks confidence in lens removal techniques, even if it is never used. (*See also* Chapter 9.)

Superficial punctate epitheliopathy (SPE)

SPE is a common corneal finding in contact lens wearers, being caused by many factors including surface deposit abrasion, incomplete tear distribution, tear deficiency, lens damage abrasion and toxic or sensitivity reactions to solution preservatives etc. (*see* Chapters 4, 6, 10, 11, 14–18 and 21). Additionally, corneal pathologies that are not contact lens related can cause changes that must be correctly identified (*see* Corneal infiltrates). Increased visibility of punctate epithelial lesions suggests associated infiltration with inflammatory cells that reduce transparency rendering them visible with direct focal illumination. Infiltrative lesions may stain better with rose bengal than fluorescein, but will not stain at all when superficial healing takes place and the infiltrates become subepithelial. However, abrasive and dessication aetiologies result in lesions that stain better with fluorescein and these are translucent when viewed with marginal retroillumination. Haphazard linear distributions of SPE suggest a foreign body abrasion whereas a damaged lens, especially a non-rotating fitting, will cause a localized or arcuate lesion. When only the lower (exposed) area of cornea is involved, inefficient blinking and tear deficiency are indicated as causal factors. Sensitivity and toxic reactions lead to generalized SPE in contact lens wearers, as may the lesions due to multiple causes. Superiorly located SPE suggests superior limbic keratitis. (*See Plates* 9, 11, 12, 19, 20, 48–52, 55 and 58–60.)

Superior limbic keratitis (SLK)

SLK is characterized by localized bulbar conjunctival injection beneath the upper lid and, as a contact lens-related condition, usually occurs unilaterally in soft lens wearers (*see* Chapters 11 and 15). Symptoms vary with severity and include irritation, photophobia and lacrimation. Apart from localized injection, the superior limbal epithelium shows various combinations of dulling, infiltration and opacities, and the palpebral conjunctiva shows hyperaemia. Abstinence from contact lens wear is the principal factor in management, and successful resumption can occur when signs have resolved in most cases, although sometimes recovery takes several months. However, because thimersal (thimerosal) toxicity has been a common factor in some reports (Stenson, 1986), resumption with new or thoroughly purged lenses is indicated together with, when necessary, a change of maintenance products to avoid thiomersal (thimerosal). If soft lens intolerance recurs, re-fitting with hard lenses is indicated. SLK may occur independently of contact lens wear, sometimes in association with thyroid disease. In some of these cases, treatment with bandage soft lenses is required to reduce abnormal lid friction (shear forces) on the superior bulbar conjunctiva. In contact lens wearers, routine examination under the top lid allows for early signs to be detected, and localized hyperaemia should prompt the use of rose bengal stain. (*See Plates 48–52.*)

Supplementary spectacles

These are usually required as a reading correction (*see* Presbyopia), but there are other indications. When residual astigmatism is encountered, but a toric lens is an unwanted complication to the fitting (for example in keratoconus), a supplementary pair of spectacles worn over the contact lenses is indicated. These may be prescribed with photochromic lenses so that their usefulness is increased. Patients, usually myopes, who report difficulty seeing at dusk and at night, may benefit from minus supplementary spectacles if their contact lens powers are correct for day use. The spectacles provide greater confidence for driving at night, for example. Additionally, 'monovision' patients may require supplementary spectacles for concentrated distance or close work purposes that require maximum binocular vision (*see* Chapter 16). (*See also* Chapters 10, 11, 14–18 and 21.)

Surface deposits

These form on some types of lenses more than others and develop excessively for some patients despite their best efforts in following maintenance instructions. The reasons for susceptibility of particular materials and particular patients to have deposits are not known with certainty, but the numerous associated problems must be dealt with at after-care visits. A simple remedial approach is to recommend an increase in lens cleaning time so that if 10 seconds per lens surfactant cleaning was recommended, an increase to 20 seconds is suggested. Another technique is to simply repeat the surfactant–rinse cycle. Increased frequency of use of enzyme tablets may help as will the use of a surfactant cleaner prior to using the enzyme tablets, so that unbound deposits (the most recently formed) are removed. This procedure exposes the bound (older) deposits to a greater concentration of enzyme because the unbound deposits, if not removed, would have first contact with the enzyme action. Use of surfactant cleaner immediately after enzyme tablet exposure will help to remove deposits partly broken down by enzyme action (as well as helping to remove the residual enzyme itself, so that the risk of an adverse reaction to the enzyme is reduced). Problem levels of deposits observed at after-care visits may be due to inappropriate product recommendations. Changes to more powerful surfactants that contain particulate matter for more effective cleaning (emulsion cleaners) may be indicated. For the worst deposit problems, the addition of sodium bicarbonate granules to the surfactant increases cleaning performance. Risk of surface damage from this potent technique should be avoided by ensuring that the mixture is very wet (not a paste). Because enzyme action is specific to certain types of protein, it may be found that a different type of enzyme (for example, animal *vs* vegetable derived) is indicated. The comparative performance of enzyme cleaners can sometimes be determined by suggesting that two different types are used on alternate weeks, so that the patient can assess, by estimation of relative comfort levels, which product is the most effective. By a similar process, it may be found that a patient is better off to continue alternating brands of enzyme weekly, as this procedure will expose deposits to a greater range of enzymes, and may result in cleaner lenses. Dealing with a deposit problem effectively may require consideration of factors other than maintenance procedures. When tear deficiency leads to increased lens soiling, any step to improve tear function will help relieve the deposit problem. Use of tear supplements may be indicated along with improvement in blink efficiency for example. Excessively oily deposits may be noted at after-care visits indicating abnormal meibomian gland function that requires attention to lid hygiene (*see* Lid hygiene and Tear deficiency management). Non-rotating lenses show greater deposits on the inferior convex surface in patients with inefficient blink patterns. These patients need to be taught special methods that emphasize more efficient cleaning of this area (*see* Inferior surface deposits). Most importantly, compliance with recommended techniques is essential for achieving a sustained optimum level of lens maintenance (*see* Compliance with instructions). Chapter 4 should be consulted for additional information on lens maintenance. (*See Plates 24–26, 31, 32, 35, 36, 38* and *39; see also* Chapters 3 and 4.)

Swimming

In hard lenses swimming may lead to lens loss (J. Josephson and B. Caffery, 1987, personal communication). Goggles can be worn over hard lenses but are seldom effective enough to be completely safe. For snorkelling and diving, a face mask offers satisfactory protection as water that leaks in can usually be eliminated by an experienced diver/hard lens wearer, without lens loss. Although the risk of losing soft lenses is very much less, patients should still be warned of the possibility. Splashing the eyes with water (hypo- or hypertonic) with a narrowed palpebral aperture before entering the water is a good precaution, because osmotic forces will help secure the lenses onto the eye. Protective 'squinting' on entering the water with a dive, or when a wave is anticipated or being ridden, is also recommended. Excess water in the eye should be removed by blinking, as wiping the eyes may displace the lens or cause it to fall out (J. Josephson and B. Caffery, 1987, personal communication). Swimming pools that are chlorinated may cause ocular irritation and epithelial changes because of non-physiological tonicity and pH levels. Additionally, chlorine irritation and water contamination may also contribute to ocular symptoms and precautions against lens loss should also help to minimize these irritations. After swimming, care should be taken to delay removal of lenses that may have become osmotically bound to the ocular surface, but thorough rinsing with sterile saline is advisable to remove contaminants from the lenses, as soon as is feasible. (*See also* Chapters 8 and 24.)

Tear circulation

Tear circulation, which is a critical source of oxygen exchange when non-gas permeable lenses are worn, is most effectively evaluated at after-care visits when lenses have fully settled. Indications of poor circulation include delayed movement of fluorescein-stained tears under a hard lens, or the accumulation of stationary tear debris under either hard or soft lenses. Lack of lens movements with blinks is another clue to this potential problem which may predispose towards red eye responses, especially with extended wear (*see* Chapter 15). The observation of poor tear circulation indicates the need to reduce the possibility of oedema with any type of fitting. (*See also* Chapters 10, 11, 14–18 and 21.)

Tear deficiency

This may cause contact lens intolerance. The most common symptoms are dryness and grittiness for hard lens wearers, and dryness and soreness for soft lens wearers. Soft lens wearers report these symptoms significantly more than hard lens wearers (McMonnies and Ho, 1986). The prevalence of established dry eye conditions is low for populations wearing contact lenses for the correction of refractive error (McMonnies and Ho, 1986). However, patients with marginal dry eye conditions may be susceptible to tear deficiency problems when contact lenses are worn, and it has been shown that a dry eye questionnaire and biomicroscopy can be used to identify these patients (McMonnies and Ho, 1987a,b). At after-care visits, a principal sign of this problem is contact lens surface drying and associated surface deposits. Other signs of tear deficiency include:

(1) Conjunctival hyperaemia.
(2) Reduced height, irregular or excessively viscous marginal tear strips.
(3) Excessive precorneal tear debris (*Plate 8*).
(4) Dull specular reflection from a dessicated bulbar conjunctiva.
(5) Meibomian gland secretion that is excessive and indicated by oily lid margins (and that may be exacerbated by frequent application of suntan oil or cosmetic preparations) (*Plate 5*).
(6) Meibomian secretion that is contaminated and deficient in association with blockage of the gland orifices with waxy plugs of abnormal secretion (Henriquez and Korb, 1981). The interference pattern caused by the lipid layer with corneal specular reflection will be disturbed or not present when meibomian gland secretions are deficient (Josephson, 1983). Sometimes the deficient meibomian glands are obviously infected with *Staphylococcus* sp., when purulent plugs occlude the orifices in meibomitis, or hordeola are present that lead to contaminated tears and symptoms. Also, meibomian gland dysfunction may be indicated by a froth formation at the canthi and along the lid margins.
(7) Fluorescein and rose bengal stains may facilitate the observation of excess blobs and strands of mucus, and will reveal epitheliopathy, although rose bengal stain of devitalized cells is often not seen until dry eye pathology has advanced past the marginal stage (*Plate 9*). Reduced aqueous volume is indicated by dull fluorescein appearance (hypofluorescence) and by delayed elimination of the stained tears (necessitating irrigation before soft lenses can be re-inserted).
(8) Superficial punctate epitheliopathy may be apparent, especially in the inferior areas of the cornea exposed by inefficient blinking, nocturnal lagophthalmos, or exophthalmos.
(9) Tear instability may be indicated by rapid break-up time that suggests mucin deficiency and/or poor lid apposition to the globe during blinks. Tear break-up observed during normal

interblink intervals is more significant than that induced by having the patient refrain from blinking.
(10) Stain at 3 and 9 o'clock with hard lenses (*see* Three and nine o'clock peripheral stain), and superficial punctate epitheliopathy in the exposed area of the cornea with soft lenses (especially torics) are probably both manifestations of tear deficiency.

See Plate 20 and *see also* Chapters 4, 8 and 9.

Tear deficiency management

This can be crucial to maintaining satisfactory levels of contact lens tolerance. The principles of prescribing tear supplements depend on the correct identification of the type of tear deficiency detected during biomicroscopy. If aqueous deficiency is apparent then a bulk aqueous supplement is required, e.g. Liquifilm (Allergan), and a hypotonic formulation may be better suited to compensating for hypertonicity expected in these cases, e.g. Hypotears (CooperVision) or TearGard (Bio Products). If mucin deficiency is diagnosed, a mucomimetic supplement is indicated, e.g. Tears Naturale (Alcon), Adapette (Alcon), Neo-Tears (Barnes–Hind/Hydrocurve). However, for many cases of marginal tear deficiency the distinction between classes of deficiency is not certain. Trials of a variety of tear supplement types are recommended, including right *vs* left eye comparisons, so that the patient can choose the most suitable product. If excess stinging is experienced then an alternative preservative and/or unbuffered formulation is indicated, e.g. Liquifilm (Allergan), Hypotears (CooperVision), Tears Naturale (Alcon). When surface deposits are predominantly mucoid or lipid, then an 'in eye' lens cleaning product that is appropriately mucolytic, e.g. Clerz (CooperVision), or lipolytic, e.g. Blink-n-Clean (Allergan), is indicated. Ordinarily tear supplements cannot be overused, but products with a lysis function could cause problems if used indiscriminately, because their action is on tissue as well as the lens surface. A mucin-deficient condition may be exacerbated by over-use of a mucolytic product for example. In the case of lipid abnormality, a deficient or absent superficial lipid layer may benefit from a lipid-containing (lipopheric) tear substitute, e.g. TearGard (Bio Products).

Meibomian gland dysfunction in which the orifices become plugged with waxy secretion can be treated with expression of the blocked gland, hot compresses, lid massage and the scrubbing of the lid margins with a cotton bud, using either a shampoo that is not irritant to the eyes, or mineral oil (paraffin) (Henriquez and Korb, 1981). Scrubbing and expression are required when the orifices are plugged but, as the gland condition improves, simple lid hygiene involving hot compresses and massage should be sufficient to maintain the improved function. Treatment for blepharitis and seborrhoea control helps to maintain the improved meibomian gland condition. When meibomian gland secretion is excessive and causes lens surface oiliness and non-wetting, lid hygiene measures (*see* Lid hygiene) assist, but advice to reduce the application of suntan oil or cosmetic creams such as skin conditioning and anti-wrinkle preparations may be necessary. Tear deficiency associated with exposure (partial blinks and inferior location of deposits etc.) is managed through improvement in blink efficiency and by avoiding wearing lenses in provocative drying conditions whenever possible. For example, removal should be recommended during prolonged periods of intense vision (reading or visual display unit activity etc.), especially when the patient is fatigued and/or exposed to heating systems that dehumidify the air (*see also* Chapters 4 and 21).

Three and nine o'clock peripheral stain

This occurs in hard lens wearers, presenting as a chronic condition for many patients and progressing to scarring and vascularization of the cornea in some cases (*see* Pseudopterygium). Possible causes include inadequate tear spreading due to lid-bridging over the contact lens edge, and abrasion due to lens movement. These factors may combine with predisposing conditions such as a hot dry climate, tear deficiency and inefficient blinking (Sarver, Nelson and Polse, 1969). Treatment and prevention include reducing edge clearance, thinning of thick edges, improving the quality of lens surfaces, treating tear deficiency, encouraging lateral eye movements and improving blink efficiency. Inefficient blinking may be induced by an uncomfortable lens and improving quality of manufacture and design may be a key factor in treatment. In severe cases, soft lenses are indicated (*see* Pseudopterygium). (*See Plates 20* and *21; see also* Chapter 10.)

Tonometry

Tonometry using the non-contact tonometer has been shown to be reliable and valid when performed through soft contact lenses with a centre thickness of 0.15 mm or less (McMonnies, 1986b). Soft lenses of greater thickness will increase readings significantly. It is possible that these conditions of measurement apply with other types of tonometer such as the Mackay–Marg, Schiötz and Alcon pneumotonometer, but readings with the Goldmann applanation tonometer have been found to be unreliable due to inadequate mire pattern quality (DeLuca, Forgacs and Skolnick, 1974).

Toric lenses

These may not give expected vision results because of incorrect prescribing of power or axis, inaccurate manufacture, poor fit, or meridional mislocation that is either constant or variable. In the case of toric soft lenses, it is useful to rotate the lens in 2.5° steps to find the axis of maximum acuity. A cotton bud provides a hygienic and convenient method of altering axis location in a controlled manner for this purpose. If satisfactory acuity cannot be achieved by this technique, and the correct prescription has been confirmed, then it can be concluded that the lens is incorrectly made in regard to power or quality of optics. A lens that gives good acuity intermittently or when rotated to the correct axis, is probably a correctly prescribed and accurately made lens that requires a tighter fit and/or increased prism or truncation to stabilize axis location (*see also* Chapter 14).

Toxic fumes

These may contaminate soft lenses and lead to symptoms and loss of tolerance. Industrial sites that expose workers to fumes and vapours from paint, glue, plastic, solvents, cleaning agents or any other source of air-borne contamination, need to be identified so that the patient can be advised accordingly. Anti-splash protective goggles worn when toxic liquids are handled are not enough protection against adsorption from the air. Goggles need to be air-tight for adequate protection. Apart from vocational risk, it is necessary to remember that hobbyists (e.g. model makers) and home renovators may also be exposed to toxic fumes intermittently. Such exposure may be forgotten when a cause for symptoms is sought at an after-care visit. Purging may be successful in reducing contamination (*see* Purging), but sometimes suspect lenses must be replaced and advice given about avoiding future exposure. (*See also* Chapters 4, 8, 9, 11 and 15.)

Travelling

Travelling in contact lenses may be complicated by restrictions on the amount of baggage that can be carried so that contact lens accessories must be limited. Unit dose and other small quantity containers, such as sample bottle sizes, are preferred. Multidose unpreserved salines should not be used for travel as they cannot be refrigerated. Contact lens wearers may encounter hygiene problems in some countries, depending on the availability and quality of water supply. Spectacles should be worn under these circumstances as the availability or standard of contact lens after-care in these countries may be limited. Heat disinfecting units may not be operable on voltages available overseas and conversion plugs that give access to different outlet configurations are often required, even when there is no voltage difference. For additional information concerned with travelling, *see* Flying. (*See also* Chapter 8.)

Vascularization

Vascularization of the cornea may occur in contact lens wear in cases of both acute and chronic injection of limbal vessels (McMonnies, 1983). Factors that may predispose towards this complication include over-wear, especially of soiled or degraded lenses, adverse reactions to preservatives, high levels of oedema, loss of epithelial integrity, such as 3 and 9 o'clock stain, tight lenses which trap debris and metabolic waste and which cause passive hyperaemia by restriction of limbal blood flow, poorly finished edges, and any environmental cause of ocular irritation and injection. These risk factors occur more frequently in soft lens fittings (McMonnies, 1984). Criteria for the assessment of suspected corneal vascularization include the following:

(1) Terminal limbal capillaries should be at least partly empty and should be seen to lie in translucent conjunctival tissue no more than 1 mm beyond the limit of visible iris (2 mm superiorly where the transitional conjunctiva encroaches over the transparent stroma to a greater extent). A biomicroscopic eyepiece scale can be used to measure the degree of incursion of vessels beyond the limit of visible iris.
(2) New vessel growth is indicated by spike vessel development projecting from normal limbal loops (*Plate 54*). During development these will be blind-end capillaries surrounded by inflammatory exudate, but, once established, new spikes can be seen to consist of arterial and venous portions when viewed under high magnification. Adjacent spikes may be seen to join to form a new arcade. Stromal vessels are not continuous with the conjunctival vessels and their growth should be regarded as a more serious complication as they indicate a deeper pathology.

See Plates 3 and *48–56; see also* Chapters 6 and 15.

Vasoconstrictors

These may be self-prescribed and their use can obscure clinical appearances observed at after-care visits. Some brands contain a fluorescent component that is evident on lid margins and lids during ultraviolet examination. Whereas occasional use of vasoconstrictors is not potentially harmful, and helps to relieve intermittent periods of hyperaemia, patients should understand that redness is a sign of ocular stress and, if contact lens induced, vasoconstrictors do

not remove the underlying cause. It is preferable that the cause of increased hyperaemia is treated rather than attempting to mask the problem with a vasoconstrictor, especially as frequent vasoconstrictor use may lead to rebound hyperaemia. (*See also* Chapter 4.)

Verification of lens parameters

For this, *see* Chapters 12 and 13.

Vision symptoms

For visual symptoms, *see* the beginning of this chapter and *see also under* Diplopia, Flare, Ghost images, Glare, Over-refraction, Presbyopia, Residual astigmatism and Spectacles.

Visual field examination

This may have reduced validity when contact lenses are worn. The intense concentration required of the patient induces prolonged inter-blink intervals that allow the lens surface to dry in some cases. Subsequent irritation and lacrimation can interfere with the patient's vision and fixation so that target awareness is reduced. A spectacle trial set lens held close to the eye is usually a more successful means of correcting refractive error during examination of the visual fields of contact lens wearers. (*See also* Chapter 5.)

Wearing schedules

For wearing schedules, *see* Chapter 9.

Conclusion

A special class of tissue responses is encountered in contact lens after-care for which the classification pathophysiological seems appropriate. There is a critical need to monitor these responses so that prophylactic management procedures can be employed to control adverse responses. Compared with earlier stages of contact lens fitting, the current approach to after-care appears to be very sophisticated. However, as observation techniques have evolved to reveal contact lens responses in much greater detail, so has come the realization that many gaps exist in after-care knowledge. The need for optometrists and ophthalmologists to continue searching for a greater understanding of contact lens adaptation is clear, and those involved can look forward to the fascination of a complex mystery that unravels on many fronts.

References

ALLANSMITH, M. R., KORB, D. R., GREINER, J. V., HENRIQUEZ, A. S., SIMON, M. A. and FINNEMORE, V. M. (1977). Giant papillary conjunctivitis in contact lens wearers. *Am. J. Ophthal.* **83**, 697–708

BENNET, E. S. and EGAN, D. J. (1986). Rigid gas permeable lens problem solving. *J. Am. optom. Ass.* **57**, 504–511

BRENNAN, N. A., EFRON, N. and CARNEY, L. G. (1986). The effects of fenestrating soft contact lenses on corneal swelling: a re-examination. *Clin. expl Optom.* **69**, 120–123

BROWN, N. A. and BRON, A. J. (1976). Recurrent erosion of the cornea. *Br. J. Ophthal.* **60**, 84–96

CATANIA, L. J. (1987). Contact lenses, staphylococcus and 'Crocodile O.D.'. *Int. Contact Lens Clin.* **14**, 113–115

COLLINS, M. J. and CARNEY, L. G. (1986). Compliance with care and maintenance procedures amongst contact lens wearers. *Clin. expl Optom.* **69**, 174–177

DELUCA, T. J., FORGACS, L. S. and SKOLNICK, S. D. (1974). The use of the Bausch and Lomb Soflens in tonometry. *J. Am. optom. Ass.* **45**, 1028–1038

ENELOW, A. J. and SWISHER, S. N. (1972). The problem-oriented medical record. In *Interviewing and Patient Care*, Chap. 5, pp. 66–101. London: Oxford University Press

GALIN, M. A. (1978). Therapy of glaucoma with hydrophilic lenses. In *Soft Contact Lenses*, edited by M. Ruben, Chap. 18, pp. 281–284. London: Baillière Tindall

GRAYSON, M. (1979). *Diseases of the Cornea*, pp. 240–248. St Louis: C. V. Mosby

HALL, R. J. and CUSACK, B. L. (1972). The measurement of eye behaviour: critical and selected reviews of voluntary eye movements and blinking. *Technical Memorandum 18–72*, pp. 67–69. Human Engineering Laboratory, US Army Aberdeen Research & Development Center, Maryland AMCMS code 501B.11.84100

HENRIQUEZ, A. S. and KORB, D. R. (1981). Meibomian glands and contact lens wear. *Br. J. Ophthal.* **65**, 108–111

HERMAN, J. P. (1983). Flexure of rigid contact lenses on toric corneas as a function of base curve fitting relationship. *J. Am. optom. Ass.* **54**, 209–214

JOSEPHSON, J. E. (1983). Appearance of the pre-ocular tear film lipid layer. *Am. J. Optom. physiol. Optics.* **60**, 883–887

KENYON, K. R., FOGUE, J. A. and GRAYSON, M. (1982). Dysgenes, dystrophies and degenerations of the cornea. In *Clinical Ophthalmology*, edited by T. D. Duane, Chap. 16, pp. 15–20. Hagerstown, NY: Harper and Row

KORB, D. (1974). The role of blinking in successful contact lens wear. *Int. Contact Lens Clin.* **1**, 59–71

KORB, D. R. and HERMAN, J. P. (1979). Corneal staining subsequent to sequential fluorescein instillation. *J. Am. optom. Ass.* **50**, 361–367

LIPPMAN, R. E. (1986). FDA awaits results of acanthamoeba extended wear studies. *Contact Lens Forum* **11**, 32–33

McMONNIES, C. W. (1974a). Optimum conditions for contact lens patient instruction. *Aust. J. Optom.* **57**, 381–386

McMONNIES, C. W. (1974b). Monocular fogging in contact lens practice. *Aust. J. Optom.* **57**, 28–32

McMONNIES, C. W. (1978). Allergic complications in contact lens wear. *Int. Contact Lens Clin.* **5**, 182–189

McMONNIES, C. W. (1981). Contact lens intolerance in association with epithelial dystrophy. *Am. J. Optom. physiol. Optics* **58**, 414–418

McMONNIES, C. W. (1983). Contact lens-induced corneal vascularisation. *Int. Contact Lens Clin.* **10**, 12–21

McMONNIES, C. W. (1984). Risk factors in the aetiology of contact lens-induced corneal vascularisation. *Int. Contact Lens Clin.* **11**, 286–293

McMONNIES, C. W. (1986a). Key questions in a dry eye history. *J. Am. optom. Ass.* **57**, 512–517

McMONNIES, C. W. (1986b). Non-contact tonometry through soft contact lenses. *Am. J. Optom. physiol. Optics* **63**, 948–951

McMONNIES, C. W. (1986c). Assessment of hard lens edges. *Int. Eyecare* **2**, 532–538

McMONNIES, C. W. (1987). Contact lens after-care: a detailed analysis. *Clin. expl. Optom.* **70**, 121–127

McMONNIES, C. W. and CHAPMAN-DAVIES, A. (1987a). Assessment of conjunctival hyperaemia in contact lens wearers: Part II preserved versus unpreserved storage of soft lenses. *Am. J. Optom. physiol. Optics* **64**, 251–255

McMONNIES, C. W. and CHAPMAN-DAVIES, A. (1987b). Assessment of conjunctival hyperaemia in contact lens wearers: Part I. *Am. J. Optom. physiol. Optics* **64**, 246–250

McMONNIES, C. W. and HO, A. (1986). Marginal dry eye diagnosis: history versus biomicroscopy. Part one. In *The Pre-ocular Tear Film*, edited by F. J. Holly, pp. 32–40. Lubbock, Texas: The Dry Eye Institute

McMONNIES, C. W. and HO, A. (1987a). Patient history in screening for dry eye conditions. *J. Am. optom. Ass.* **58**, 296–301

McMONNIES, C. W. and HO, A. (1987b). Responses to a dry eye questionnaire from a normal population. *J. Am. optom. Ass.* **58**, 588–591

McMONNIES, C. W. and ZANTOS, S. (1979). Endothelial bedewing of the cornea in association with contact lens wear. *Br. J. Ophthal.* **63**, 478–481

McMONNIES, C. W., CHAPMAN-DAVIES, A. and HOLDEN, B. A. (1982). Vascular response to contact lens wear. *Am. J. Optom. physiol. Optics* **59**, 795–799

O'CONNOR DAVIES, P. H. (1972). *The Actions and Uses of Ophthalmic Drugs*, pp. 237–262. London: Barrie & Jenkins

O'LEARY, D. J. and MILLODOT, M. (1981). Abnormal epithelial fragility in diabetes and in contact lens wear. *Acta ophthal.* **59**, 827–833

PARDOS, G. J. and KRACHMER, J. H. (1980). Comparison of endothelial cell density in diabetes and a control population. *Am. J. Ophthal.* **90**, 172–174

PEARSON, R. M. (1986). The mystery of missing fluorescein — a postscript. *J. Br. Contact Lens Ass.* **9**, 36–37

PRILUCK, I. A., ROBERTSON, D. M. and BUETTNER, H. (1979). What patients recall of the pre-operative discussion after retinal detachment surgery. *Am. J. Ophthal.* **87**, 620–623

REFOJO, M. F. and LEONG, FEE-LAI (1981). Water pervaporation through silicone rubber contact lenses: a possible cause of complications. *Contact Intraoc. Lens med. J.* **7**, 226–233

RUBEN, M., BROWN, N., LOBASCHER, D., CHASTON, J. and MORRIS, J. (1976). Clinical manifestations secondary to soft contact lens wear. *Br. J. Ophthal.* **60**, 529–531

SARVER, M. D., NELSON, J. L. and POLSE, K. A. (1969). Peripheral corneal staining accompanying contact lens wear. *J. Am. optom. Ass.* **40**, 310–315

SCHOESSLER, J. P. and LOWTHER, G. E. (1970). Slit lamp observations of corneal oedema. *Am. J. Optom. Archs. Am. Acad. Optom.* **48**, 666–670

SCHULTZ, R. O., MATSUDA, M., YEE, R. W., EDELHAUSER, H. F. and SCHULTZ, K. J. (1984). Corneal endothelial changes in type I and type II diabetes mellitus. *Am. J. Ophthal.* **98**, 401–410

SCHWARTZ, C. A. (1986). Radical flattening and RGP lenses. *Contact Lens Forum* **11**, 49–52

SNIP, R. C., THOFT, R. A. and TOLENTINO, F. I. (1980). Similar epithelial healing rates of the corneas of diabetic and non-diabetic patients. *Am. J. Ophthal.* **90**, 463–468

STAINER, G. A., BRIGHTBILL, F. S., HOLM, P. and LAUX, D. (1981). The development of pseudo-pterygia in hard contact lens wearers. *Contact Intraoc. Lens med. J.* **7**, 1–4

STENSON, S. (1986). Ocular surface disease complicating hydrophilic lens wear. *Contact Lens Ass. Ophthal.* **12**, 158–164

de VRIES REILINGH, A., REINERS, H. and VAN BIJSTERVELD, D. P. (1978). Contact lens tolerance and oral contraceptives. *Am. J. Ophthal.* **10**, 947–952

WARDLAW, J. L. and SARVER, M. D. (1986). Discoloration of hydrogel contact lenses under standard care regimens. *Am. J. Optom. physiol. Opt.* **63**, 403–408

WILLIAMS, L. and HOLDEN, B. A. (1986). The bleb response of the endothelium decreases with extended wear of contact lenses. *Clin. expl Optom.* **69**, 90–92

WILSON, L. A. (1979a). Bacterial conjunctivitis. In *External Diseases of the Eye*, edited by L. A. Wilson, Chap. 4, p. 31. Maryland: Harper & Row

WILSON, L. A. (1979b). Bacterial corneal ulcers. In *External Diseases of the Eye*, edited by L. A. Wilson, Chap. 17, p. 220. Maryland: Harper & Row

Chapter 20

Refractive changes after wearing contact lenses

R. H. Rengstorff

Contact lenses are capable of causing both temporary and permanent refractive changes. This is of considerable significance particularly when it is necessary to prescribe spectacle lenses for patients who are wearing or have worn contact lenses. Polymethyl methacrylate contact lenses, fitted to millions of people during 1950 to 1970, are still happily worn by many of them and the understanding of the refractive and corneal curvature changes associated with their long-term wear is still an important aspect of contact lens practice. Hydrogel and rigid gas permeable lenses may not cause refractive changes of similar magnitude and duration, but the long-term effects from these lenses are not yet known. This chapter is a review of various aspects which affect the refractive changes from lenses made of these different materials.

Polymethyl methacrylate lenses

Many studies and clinical observations have provided a great deal of information about the ocular effects associated with wearing polymethyl methacrylate (PMMA) contact lenses since they came into common use over 30 years ago.

What is known about refractive changes after wearing PMMA contact lenses will be reviewed from the following aspects:

(1) Temporal variables.
(2) Changes in corneal curvature.
(3) Relationship between changes in refraction and changes in corneal curvature.

Temporal variables

Some contact lens wearers experience blurred vision when they temporarily remove their lenses and wear spectacles. According to many early reports in the 1950s, the blur generally lasts from minutes to hours. This is particularly common during the adaptation period and can be attributed to temporary corneal distortion and epithelial oedema. Another type of blurred and variable vision occurs among persons adapted to contact lenses when they resort to wearing their spectacles. This may persist for many weeks and is caused by refractive changes (Rengstorff, 1965a). Knowledge of these changes is important. From a practical point of view, refractive changes affect the practitioner's ability to prescribe satisfactory spectacle lenses. From a theoretical point of view, refractive changes may be controlled for therapeutic purposes such as reducing or eliminating certain refractive conditions.

The most significant refractive changes occur after the first year of wearing lenses. During adaptation to contact lenses the most common refractive change is an increase of about 0.50 D more myopia (Carney, 1975a; Hovding, 1983b). At 6 months, the initial myopic increase is lessened and, after wearing lenses 1 year, the tendency is towards about 0.50 D less myopia (Rengstorff, 1965b; Hovding, 1983b).

After lenses have been worn 1 year, refractive changes have been found to follow orderly and specific patterns of change. One such pattern refers to short-term changes (circadian variations), occurring from day to day as the individual normally wears contact lenses. Another pattern refers to long-term changes (withdrawal variations), occurring for days and weeks after wearing is discontinued.

Both short-term and long-term changes occur after wearing contact lenses for at least 1 year. Another consideration is the method of determining refractive error. After removal of contact lenses, many long-term habitual wearers respond poorly to subjective testing, and they cannot discriminate lens changes as can persons who do not wear contact lenses. This may persist for many days after they remove their contact lenses (Rengstorff, 1965a, 1966). Arner (1970) likened the subjective testing of some of these individuals 'to examining a bilateral amblyope with metamorphopsia and low intelligence'. The best method to determine refractive error is by careful subjective testing and not by retinoscopic measurements which are in many cases unreliable when corneal distortion is present (Rengstorff, 1965a). A recommended procedure to determine refractive error is to monocularly blur vision with a lens $+2.00\,D$ over the retinoscopic or other objective measurement and reduce the lens power in $0.50\,D$ steps until the subject can read 6/12 (20/40) letters. Additional reductions in $0.25\,D$ steps are made until the best visual acuity with the minimum negative or maximum positive powered lens is attained. Cross-cylinder and astigmatic chart testing are used to measure astigmatism.

Short-term changes (circadian variations)

The circadian rhythm of habitual PMMA contact lens wearers is characterized by steepening of corneal curvature and increasing myopia after lenses have been worn during the day and flattening of corneal curvature and decreasing myopia after lenses have been removed overnight (Rengstorff, 1978b).

Overnight: myopia decreases while lenses are not worn

Contact lens wearers frequently describe improved unaided visual acuity after arising in the morning. Saks (1966) reported this occurrence and other studies (Rengstorff, 1970a,b) confirmed the improvements, showing them to be caused by a measurable decrease in myopia. The improvements occurred among myopic

men, aged 20–27 years, who had worn contact lenses 12 hours or more daily for at least 1 year. All individuals showed consistent overnight decreases in myopia ranging from $0.25\,D$ to $1.50\,D$. Changes were smaller when contact lenses were not worn all waking hours.

Astigmatism increases slightly overnight while lenses are not worn

Subjective tests for astigmatism on 10 habitual contact lens wearers at 11 p.m. and 7 a.m. revealed a slight trend towards increased with-the-rule astigmatism overnight. This occurred in about two-thirds of the tests (Rengstorff, 1971c).

Sleeping with contact lenses increases myopia

Wearing lenses during sleep did not consistently decrease myopia; in fact, there was a slight trend towards increased myopia (Rengstorff, 1970b). After wearing lenses overnight, 6 of 10 eyes had increased myopia. When these men did not wear lenses overnight all had decreased myopia. Similar findings occurred in another study of two habitual contact lens wearers who slept overnight with a contact lens on only one eye (Rengstorff, 1978a).

Diurnal: myopia increases during the first 8 hours that lenses are worn

Individuals who do not wear contact lenses show no evidence of daily (diurnal) variations in refractive error. However, there is a specific diurnal pattern of changes among individuals who wear contact lenses (Rengstorff, 1970c). This pattern of changes is illustrated in *Figure 20.1* based on habitual wearers, men between the ages of 19 and 26 years, who removed their lenses at specific times during the day for refractive tests. Myopia can be seen to increase from 0 to 8 hours and decrease slightly from 8 to 16 hours, followed by further overnight decreases in myopia when lenses are not worn. The mean change from 0 to 8 hours was almost $1.00\,D$; the decrease in myopia from 8 to 16 hours was approximately $0.25\,D$.

Measurements of myopia at the same time on different days showed considerable variation. This lack of consistency, i.e. over $0.50\,D$, is not

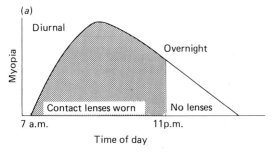

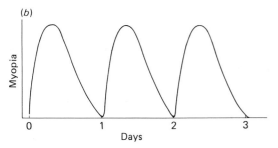

Figure 20.1 (*a*) Circadian changes in ametropia when contact lenses are worn during the day and removed overnight during sleep. (*b*) Circadian changes in ametropia for 3 consecutive days

Astigmatism varies during the hours that lenses are worn

Repeated diurnal measurements of eight habitual wearers of contact lenses have failed to reveal any conclusive pattern of changes in astigmatism such as those found for myopia. The responses of the subjects were not as critical as those of non-wearers, but some of the variance may be attributed to irregular astigmatism and the difficulties these subjects had in discriminating small lens changes (Rengstorff, 1971c).

Long-term changes (withdrawal variations)

Days after removing contact lenses: myopia decreases for about 3 days (1–14 days), and then begins to increase

There is considerable evidence of refractive variations for many days after contact lenses are removed (Rengstorff, 1965a), and these variations follow a specific pattern. Measurements for myopia in 68 habitual wearers of contact lenses revealed a transitory reduction in myopia (Rengstorff, 1967). These results are illustrated in *Figure 20.2*. The average individual had

remarkable because contact lens wearers frequently lack discrimination in subjective tests following the removal of their lenses. The reliability problem was common to all subjects; nevertheless, a diurnal pattern was obvious. The pattern was evident in both averages and in single measurements.

Diurnal increases in myopia appear to be directly related to the daily wearing time and the number of years that contact lenses have been worn. The average diurnal increase in myopia for individuals who wore lenses for 6 months was less than 0.75 D, compared to about a 1.50 D increase for those who wore lenses for more than 3 years. Wearing lenses all the waking hours was associated with diurnal increases in myopia of over 1.00 D, but individuals who wore contact lenses only 12–14 hours a day had diurnal increases of less than 1.00 D. Testing habitual wearers before insertion of lenses and after wearing lenses for 8 hours provided a good indication of the magnitude of diurnal changes that occur (McLean and Rengstorff, 1978).

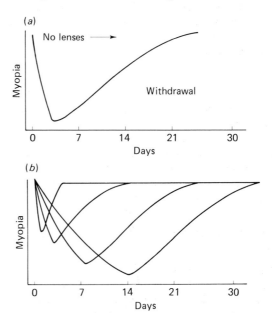

Figure 20.2 (*a*) Withdrawal changes in ametropia at specific times after the removal of contact lenses. (*b*) Individual examples of myopia changes between test days

decreases in myopia up to 1.32 D for 3 days, followed by increases until 21 days. Some individuals showed progressive decreases in myopia for 1, 3, 7 or 14 days. A 7.50 D decrease in myopia is described in an individual case. The extent and duration of the after-effects were found to be directly related to the daily wearing time and the number of years that contact lenses had been worn (Rengstorff, 1968b).

Myopia measurements are relatively stable 3 weeks after removing contact lenses

Variations in myopia stop or become very small in most cases after 3 weeks without contact lenses (Rengstorff, 1965a; Harris, Blevins and Heiden, 1973).

Astigmatism increases after removing contact lenses

There is a strong trend towards increased with-the-rule astigmatism associated with the withdrawal pattern (Pratt-Johnson and Warner, 1965; Rengstorff, 1965c). The average increase was 0.45 D for 64 subjects who had worn lenses for 6 months to 6 years. The astigmatism increased from 0 to 3 days after removing the lenses. From the third to the forty-eighth day, no significant variation was apparent (Rengstorff, 1968b). Hartstein (1965, 1967) found 2.50–6.00 D of with-the-rule astigmatism in 27 patients who had worn their contact lenses from 2 to 6 years without difficulties.

Corneal rigidity is an important factor in the development of astigmatism after wearing contact lenses. Eyes with low corneal rigidity have developed higher amounts of with-the-rule astigmatism; rigidity has been related to the length of time lenses were worn: rigidity was high for individuals who had worn lenses for an average of 3.5 years and low for those who had worn lenses for an average of 5.5 years (Ing, 1976). Low corneal rigidity associated with the wearing of lenses for many years and the mechanical effects of the eyelids against the cornea very probably induce with-the-rule astigmatism during the first few days after the abrupt discontinuance of contact lenses. Reducing wearing time gradually over a period of many weeks increases corneal rigidity and minimizes, but does not completely eliminate,

the astigmatism induced by long-term wearing of contact lenses (Rengstorff, 1977b).

Prescribing spectacle lenses

How to determine a satisfactory spectacle lens prescription for an habitual wearer of contact lenses is a difficult clinical problem. Results from the studies cited should be helpful in making this determination. It can be seen in *Figures 20.1* and *20.2* that a considerable range of possible spectacle prescriptions depends on when measurements are taken. Arner (1970) and Barradell (1972) have considered the diurnal and long-term refractive variations in their recommendations for prescribing spectacles to contact lens wearers. The relative stability of ametropia measurements after 21 days has, unfortunately, led some practitioners to insist that their patients stop wearing contact lenses for 21 days or more before they prescribe spectacles. Such treatment is rarely necessary; it can be very inconvenient for the patient to experience these withdrawal effects, often without any suitable spectacles. It is also recommended not to advise patients with severe corneal distortion to stop wearing contact lenses suddenly after many years because of a potential exacerbating effect (Rengstorff, 1975).

Corneal damage can be minimized and refractive variations can be reduced to obtain a suitable spectacle lens prescription by recommending that patients gradually reduce their wearing time.

The practical requirement to provide the best possible all-round spectacle prescription is probably best accomplished by prescribing for the maximum amount of myopia, which is found after contact lenses have been worn for 8 hours (*see Figure 20.1*). The least satisfactory approach occurs when prescriptions are based on measurements taken hours or days after removing the lenses (*see Figure 20.2*) because this is when myopia is temporarily decreased.

Myopia control

The literature contains several suggestions that myopia may be controlled by the wearing of contact lenses. Neill (1962), reporting on cases since 1946, found that while contact lenses were worn the development of myopia was inhibited. Rengstorff (1967) has reviewed the period

1956–66 when there were many conflicting reports of the subject of myopia control (Bier, 1956; Morrison, 1956, 1958; Dickinson, 1957; Steele, 1959; Barksdale, 1960; Black, 1960; Treissman, 1960; Boyd, 1962; Fonda, 1962; Black-Kelly and Butler, 1964; Jessen, 1964; Nolan, 1964; de Carle, 1965; Enoch, 1965; Hodd, 1965; Mandell, 1965; Saks, 1966). There are still conflicting views on this subject but now more reports acknowledge the short-term and long-term effects and the unstable state of myopia during the 3-week period following the removal of contact lenses (Black-Kelly and Butler, 1971; Grosvenor, 1972; Stone, 1973). After removing contact lenses for more than 3 weeks, Rengstorff (1965b) reported that the average change was 0.60 D less myopia in a study of 55 eyes. Kemmetmuller (1972) found that patients wearing contact lenses show a significantly slower progress of their refraction than those of the same age group who wear spectacles. Stone (1973) conducted a longitudinal study to determine how contact lenses affect changes in myopia in children. Her tentative conclusions from reviewing data gathered on over 100 children suggested that, after wearing contact lenses for 2 years, myopia in growing children appears to stabilize, although it increases up to that time. Over a period of 4 years the rate of increase of myopia may be expected to be slowed down by 0.75–1.00 D (Stone and Powell-Cullingford, 1974). Black-Kelly (1975) has described myopia control using atropine in conjunction with wearing contact lenses.

There have been some publications on the subject of using contact lenses to reduce myopia by a technique called orthokeratology. This subject will not be reviewed here because careful analysis of these reports fails to report or control the most important variable in any such study, namely, when the refractive measurements were made or the time course of these changes in refraction. Temporary reduction of myopia and the pattern of refractive changes after lenses have been removed varies considerably both in duration and magnitude. However, there are orderly patterns for these changes. These details have been summarized in the previous pages and should be a well-known occurrence. Reports which claim a procedure to change the refractive errors have ignored or failed to consider the facts of short- and long-term changes in refraction after wearing contact lenses. They have not resulted in any new information on the subject of refractive changes or an effective procedure to change refractive error.

Changes in corneal curvature

The anterior corneal surface is the predominant refracting surface of the eye and it has been reported frequently that corneal contact lenses cause a change in corneal curvature. Because of this close association between corneal curvature and refractive changes, a brief discussion of changes in corneal curvature is included in this chapter. Similar to the preceding discussion on refractive changes, both short-term and long-term changes in corneal curvature apply to individuals who usually wear lenses all waking hours for at least 1 year (Rengstorff, 1971a). When lenses are worn less than all waking hours, the magnitude of the changes is reduced significantly. Furthermore, the effects appear directly related to the number of years contact lenses are worn. This information has proved useful to optometrists in the management of patients who wear contact lenses.

During adaptation to contact lenses the corneal curvature steepens about 0.50–1.00 D* (Pratt-Johnson and Warner, 1965; Miller, 1968; Hazlett, 1969; Manchester, 1970; Farris *et al.*, 1971; Masnick, 1971; Westerhout, 1971; Berman, 1972; Carney, 1975b) and this steepening gradually decreases during the first year (Rengstorff, 1969b; Grosvenor, 1972; Hill, 1975).

Short-term changes (circadian variations)

Overnight corneal curvature flattens while the lenses are not worn

A conspicuous finding in testing habitual wearers for consecutive days was a flattening of the cornea (about 0.75 D), which occurred overnight when the contact lenses were not worn (Rengstorff, 1968a, 1971b). The horizontal curvature was consistently flatter in the morning than on the previous evening, but when the vertical curvature was measured only a slight trend towards flattening was evident.

---

*Curvature changes are expressed in approximately equivalent dioptre effects for convenience in relating changes to ametropia. Further elaboration on curvature/refractive power appears on p. 744.

Sleeping with contact lenses steepens corneal curvature

Tests of habitual wearers showed that wearing contact lenses during sleep causes steepened curvature (about 0.50 D) of both the horizontal and vertical principal meridians of the cornea (Rengstorff, 1971d).

When contact lenses are prescribed, patients are usually advised not to wear them during sleep because of possible corneal damage. However, there have been many reports describing patients who have worn their lenses not only during sleep but continuously for months and even many years without ever removing them (Levey, 1964; Rengstorff, 1965a; Allen, 1968). How these individuals can do this without experiencing any harm to the eyes, or discomfort, is not completely understood, but evidence indicates that tolerance must be built up gradually. A frequent consequence of wearing contact lenses during sleep, particularly with new wearers, is superficial corneal damage and considerable discomfort. Some months after wearing contact lenses every day, these individuals can often tolerate the lenses during and after short naps and sleeping. However, such tolerance is rapidly lost when the lenses are not worn for a few days. It appears, therefore, that the more completely the patient adapts to wearing contact lenses and the more consistently they are worn, the smaller the risk of corneal damage will be from wearing the lenses when sleeping.

Diurnal: corneal curvature steepens during the first 8 hours that lenses are worn

The measurements of corneal curvature at the same time on different days showed some variations; nevertheless, a diurnal pattern was obvious in both averages and single measurements found in five habitual wearers who were tested before inserting their lenses and at intervals after wearing them. Mean horizontal curvature steepened an equivalent 0.71 D, 0.84 D and 0.55 D after 4, 8 and 16 hours of wear; mean vertical curvature steepened an equivalent 0.52 D, 0.50 D and 0.38 D at the same time (Rengstorff, 1971b). These findings suggest that the fit of contact lenses changes during the day. The magnitude of this pattern appears to be directly related to the number of years

contact lenses have been worn and the amount of daily wearing time. Similar tests on non-wearers confirmed the generally held assumption that the corneal curvature of non-wearers is stable (Rengstorff, 1972), or any variation in curvature is so small that it challenges the reliability of keratometer measurements (Grosvenor, 1972).

Consistent astigmatic changes are not a part of the circadian pattern. Meridional differences in corneal curvature may vary considerably and even appear as irregular astigmatism.

Long-term changes (withdrawal variations)
Days after removing contact lenses

Some individuals showed progressive flattening for 1, 3 or 7 days.

A specific pattern of variations in corneal curvature occurs following the withdrawal of contact lenses from individuals who have habitually worn lenses for at least 1 year (Rengstorff, 1969a). Group data on over 100 eyes of men aged 18–26 years showed progressive corneal flattening (about 0.75 D) of both the vertical and horizontal meridians for 1 and 3 days, respectively, followed by corneal steepening to the forty-eighth day of the test period. Some individuals showed progressive flattening for 1, 3 or 7 days. The most common changes in astigmatism were increases in with-the-rule astigmatism for 0–3 days.

Insertion of contact lenses, after not wearing them for 2 or more weeks, caused corneal steepening (Rengstorff, 1969a; Ong and Bowling, 1972). After wearing lenses again for 60–90 days, removing lenses for many days caused less corneal curvature variations than they did the first time they were removed, after wearing them at least 1 year.

The extent and duration of changes in corneal curvature were found to be directly related to the number of years contact lenses had been worn. The variations were less for individuals with reduced wearing time than for subjects who wore lenses all their waking hours.

Corneal curvature is relatively stable 3 weeks after removing contact lenses

Many of the early observations in the 1960s suggested that the cornea reverted to its former curvature after lenses were removed for varying periods of time. However, a study of 64 subjects

(Rengstorff, 1969a) indicated that the cornea did not revert to its former curvature after lenses had been removed for more than 30 days. In most cases, variations in corneal curvature have stopped or become very small after 3 weeks without contact lenses. At that time the cornea is somewhat flatter (0.50–0.75 D) than before wearing contact lenses and there is an increase in with-the-rule astigmatism.

Although information has been obtained by studying certain time variables, the whole field of corneal changes still remains tremendously complex. The problem may be approached by eliminating other variables, specifically, physical factors such as contact lens specifications and physiological mechanisms which may affect corneal curvature.

Contact lens design

From the preceding discussion, it is obvious that there are number of significant time variables which influence changes in corneal curvature. Failure to eliminate these variables is likely to invalidate research in this area. Such is the case in many conflicting reports that attribute changes in corneal curvature to the design of the contact lens. A review of these changes (Rengstorff, 1969a) did not confirm that flattening of the cornea is associated with flat-fitting lenses and steepening of the cornea is associated with steep-fitting lenses. Either fitting technique can cause the cornea to steepen or flatten and astigmatism to increase or decrease (Mobilia and Kenyon, 1986). Goldberg (1965) did not find changes in corneal curvature related to the fitting technique or to the design of the contact lens. In the study carried out by Sarver and Harris (1967), no significant difference in changes in corneal curvature was found between one group of subjects fitted with small lenses 0.37 D 'steeper than K' and another group fitted with large lenses 'on K'. Rengstorff (1973) measured the corneas of 81 long-term wearers immediately after removal of their contact lenses and only one cornea had steepened in curvature. In that study, most lenses were fitted 'flat' or 'on K' and only 10 eyes were fitted 'steep'. Another study was made to determine whether steep fitting lenses cause steeper corneal curvature (Hill and Rengstorff, 1974). Since only slightly more than half the corneas became steeper, one cannot conclude that steep-fitting back optic zone radii will steepen the corneal curvature.

Both studies eliminated the withdrawal variable, because measurements were taken immediately after removal; however, the diurnal variable was not eliminated and it probably influenced the results. In another study, 17 subjects wore lenses with back optic zone radii fitted parallel to the flattest corneal meridian, steeper by up to 6.00 D or flatter by up to 3.50 D. The short-term effect was a trend towards corneal curvature steepening in all cases and no apparent relationship between the design of the back optic zone curve and the resulting corneal curvature change (Rengstorff, 1977a).

Finally, there are physiological mechanisms which may affect corneal curvature (Rengstorff et al., 1974). It has been shown that structural changes in the cornea can have circadian and long-term effects. The mechanism for these changes is unknown; however, every anatomical change has a chemical basis and it is possible that a return to a normal environment may play a role in the corneal curvature and refractive variation.

Relationship between changes in refraction and changes in corneal curvature

Studies have shown that refractive changes after wearing contact lenses are not solely attributable to changes in corneal curvature, as measured with an ophthalmometer.

Changes in myopia and corneal curvature for more than 100 eyes during a period of weeks after the removal of contact lenses were analysed (Rengstorff, 1969c). Group data showed some agreement between myopia and changes in corneal curvature, i.e. there were myopia decreases with corneal flattening and myopia increases with corneal steepening. This also occurred in some individual cases either throughout the test period, after the first day or after the third day. However, in many individual cases, there were contradictory results, e.g. myopia decreases with corneal steepening and vice versa. Changes between test days were also frequently in opposite direction, showing differences of up to 4.00 D. These contradictory findings restrict the generality suggested by group similarities and point out that the process of changes in refraction following the removal of contact lenses cannot be attributed solely to the refractive changes caused by flattening or steepening of the anterior corneal curvature. It is more likely that refractive changes are functionally related to a number of variables besides anterior corneal curvature.

Throughout this chapter, the corneal curvature is expressed in dioptres rather than in radius of curvature. Conversion is shown on most instruments by manufacturers who assign each corneal radius a specific refractive power based on an average refractive index. There is some error when different instruments are compared. Stone (1973), for example, found the discrepancy between Gambs and the Bausch & Lomb ophthalmometers was about 0.15 D.

The quantitative differences between refractive and corneal curvature changes, however, are often considerable and cannot be attributed to the conversion of radii to dioptres. The effects of changes in parameters other than anterior corneal curvature are more likely to explain these differences. Determination of the actual corneal refractive power requires precise knowledge of the refractive index, corneal thickness and curvature of the anterior and posterior corneal surfaces. Also any alteration in the cornea which increases or decreases the anterior chamber length changes the total refractive power of the eye. An analysis has shown how refractive changes may be influenced by changes in each corneal parameter as well as a change in anterior chamber length (Rengstorff and Arner, 1971).

For example, a reduction of refractive power (less myopia) may be brought about by any or all of the following changes: flattening of anterior corneal curvature; steepening of posterior corneal curvature; increased index of refraction; decreased corneal thickness; and depressing the cornea and reducing axial length. Conversely an increase of refractive power (more myopia) results with opposite changes in each of the preceding variables.

Each corneal component may have an increasing or decreasing effect on the total

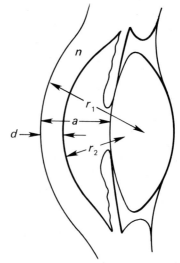

$$\Delta F_s = \Delta a + \Delta r_1 + \Delta r_2 + \Delta n + \Delta d$$

Figure 20.3 The change in spectacle refraction following contact lens wear is brought about by dioptric changes (Δ) in each of the corneal parameters, where F_s = spectacle refraction; a = anterior chamber depth; r_1 = radius of front central surface of cornea; r_2 = radius of back central surface of cornea; n = refractive index of cornea; d = central corneal thickness

refractive change and the net effect is the algebraic sum of the individual variations. *Figure 20.3* illustrates that refractive changes are the result of increases and decreases of each component and the total effect is the sum of the individual changes in each component. The relative significance of each corneal component was determined mathematically. In order of magnitude, the effect of a 10% change in each component was as follows: anterior corneal curvature (4.87 D), index of refraction (1.87 D), depth of anterior chamber (1.20 D), posterior corneal curvature (0.62 D) and corneal thickness (0.01 D) (Rengstorff, 1985).

Chapter 5 should also be consulted about changes in corneal curvature and refraction (*see* Optical changes of the eye caused by contact lenses, p. 224).

Hydrogel and rigid gas permeable lenses

In comparison with PMMA lenses, far less information is available about refractive changes after wearing the relatively newer lenses made from hydrogel, cellulose acetate butyrate (CAB), silicone and silicone–acrylate materials, especially those effects that may occur after wearing such lenses more than 1 year.

Hydrogel lenses do cause refractive changes

during the adaptation period. Grosvenor (1975) studied 23 wearers of hydrogel (HEMA) lenses and found decreases of about 0.50 D in myopia occurring during the first 6 weeks followed by increases to about 0.50 D more myopia during the next 6 weeks. He also reported the most common corneal change was an initial flattening of approximately 0.25 D in one or both meridians of the cornea during the first few weeks followed by a steepening of curvature which began after wearing lenses for 6 weeks. Hill (1975) has also described similar results on 36 eyes; likewise, Harris and co-workers (Harris, Sarver and Polse, 1975) found 0.23 D corneal steepening on 4–30 eyes after 30 days and Baldone (1975) described increased myopia and corneal steepening that was reversible. Astigmatic changes with hydrophilic lens wear was also resolved on discontinuing the lenses (Morgan, 1975). In a 3-month study (Barnett and Rengstorff, 1977) of 40 hydrogel lens wearers, there was a gradual increase in myopia from 0.12 D at 1 month to 0.50 D more myopia at 3 months. The mean corneal curvature flattened during the first 3 weeks, but steepened by about 0.37 D at 3 months. Similar corneal changes and increases in myopia have been reported during the first year of hydrogel lens wear (Hovding, 1983a,b).

'Creeping myopia' after wearing hydrogel lenses has been frequently observed, in some cases more than 2.0 D (unpublished studies). It has been reported that some hydrogel lenses may cause greater increases in myopia than other hydrogel lenses (Saks, personal communication). There is a report of high water content, non-HEMA extended wear lenses causing insignificant refractive and keratometric variations (Rengstorff and Nilsson, 1985). Nineteen patients had worn non-HEMA lenses monocularly, on an extended wear basis, for an average of 5.4 years. Measurements were made after lens removal and again 2 days and 7 days later. They caused no significant difference in refraction or keratometry in comparison with the non-contact lens eye. Refractive changes on the lens-wearing eye averaged less than 0.37 D, astigmatism and keratometric changes averaged 0.25 D. Factors which very likely can be attributed to maintaining the stability of these measurements were the lens material and quality, extensive practitioner experience with extended wear lenses, and patient management which emphasized regular

after-care, including lens replacement at least annually.

Silicone lens wearers had very little change in refraction during the first year of lens wear (Hovding, 1983b). This may also occur with silicone–acrylate lenses. After wearing the Boston Lens, a silicone–acrylate lens, about 17% of patients described a slight amount of spectacle blur in the evening after removing their lenses, most frequently during adaptation or changing from other hard lens wear, but no detailed study of refractive changes was reported (Odby and Rengstorff, 1985). In another study (de Ruebeis and Shily, 1985), these lenses fitted on 132 eyes did not cause significant changes in corneal curvature during the first 3 months of wear.

Orderly patterns of refractive changes, such as those demonstrated to occur with PMMA lenses, have not been documented for hydrogel and other newer lenses, including the rigid gas permeable lenses. Until there are more definitive and long-term studies of refractive changes after wearing these newer lenses, it will be difficult to come to conclusions or make comparisons about the magnitude and duration of refractive changes after wearing these lenses. Nevertheless, it does appear that the problem of refractive changes following daily contact lens wear with newer materials is, at least in the short term, considerably less than with PMMA.

References

ALLEN, M. J. (1968). Contact lenses, six months continuous wear. *J. Am. optom. Ass.* **39**, 231–233

ARNER, R. S. (1970). Prescribing new contact lenses or spectacles for the existing contact lens wearer. *J. Am. optom. Ass.* **41**, 253–256

BALDONE, J. A. (1975). Corneal curvature changes secondary to the wearing of hydrophilic gel contact lenses. *Contact Intraoc. Lens med. J.* **1**, 175–176

BARKSDALE, C. B. (1960). The attrition and control of myopia in some selected cases. *Contacto* **4**, 349–366

BARNETT, W. A. and RENGSTORFF, R. H. (1977). Adaptation to hydrogel contact lenses: variations in myopia and corneal curvature measurements. *J. Am. optom. Ass.* **48**, 363–366

BARRADELL, M. J. (1972). Spectacles for contact lens wearers. *Ophthal. Optician* **12**, 763–768

BERMAN, M. R. (1972). Central corneal curvature and wearing time during contact lens adaptation. *Optom. Wkly* **63**(6), 27–30

BIER, N. (1956). A study of the cornea in relation to contact lens practice. *Am. J. Optom.* **33**, 291–304

BLACK, C. J. (1960). Ocular, anatomical and physiological changes due to contact lenses. *Ill. med. J.* **118**, 279–281

BLACK-KELLY, T. S. B. (1975). The clinical arrest of myopia. *Optician* (i) **169**(4387), 13–23; (ii) **169**(4388), 8–11; (iii) **170**(4389), 4–8, 35

BLACK-KELLY, T. S. B. and BUTLER, D. (1964). Preliminary report on corneal lenses in relation to myopia. *Br. J. physiol. Optics* **21**, 175–186

BLACK-KELLY, T. S. B. and BUTLER, D. (1971). The present position of contact lenses in relation to myopia. *Br. J. physiol. Optics* **26**, 33–48

BOYD, H. H. (1962). One thousand consecutive contact lens cases. *Northwest med. J.* **61**, 933–936

de CARLE, J. (1965). In an abstract of a lecture on contact lenses and myopia. *Optician* **150**, 467

CARNEY, L. G. (1975a). Refractive error and visual acuity changes during contact lens wear. *Contact Lens* **5**(3,4), 28–34

CARNEY, L. G. (1975b). The basis for corneal shape change during contact lens wear. *Am. J. Optom.* **52**, 445–454

DICKINSON, F. (1957). The value of microlenses in progressive myopia. *Optician* **133**, 263–264

ENOCH, J. M. (1965). Discussion of papers dealing with plans for contact lens research in myopia; lecture delivered at First International Conference on Myopia. Printed as a separate publication. Chicago: Professional Press

FARRIS, R., LINSY, KUBOTA, Z. and MISHIMA, S. (1971). Epithelial decompensation with corneal contact lens wear. *Archs Ophthal.* **85**, 651–660

FONDA, D. (1962). Complications of contact lens wearing. *Southern med. J.* **55**, 126–128

GOLDBERG, J. B. (1965). A commentary on corneal curvature and refraction changes observed among twenty contact lens patients. Paper read at American Academy of Optometry, Section of Contact Lenses, Chicago, Dec. 1965

GROSVENOR, T. P. (1972). *Contact Lens Theory and Practice.* Chicago: Professional Press

GROSVENOR, T. P. (1975). Changes in corneal curvature and subjective refraction of soft contact lens wearers. *Am. J. Optom. physiol. Optics* **52**, 405–413

HARRIS, M. G., BLEVINS, R. J. and HEIDEN, S. (1973). Evaluation of procedures for the management of spectacle blur. *Am. J. Optom.* **50**, 293–298

HARRIS, M. G., SARVER, M. D. and POLSE, K. A. (1975). Corneal curvature and refractive error changes associated with wearing hydrogel contact lenses. *Am. J. Optom. physiol. Optics* **52**(5), 313–319

HARTSTEIN, J. (1965). Corneal warping due to contact lenses. *Am. J. Ophthal.* **60**, 1103–1104

HARTSTEIN, J. (1967). Astigmatism induced by corneal contact lenses. In *Current Concepts in Ophthalmology*, edited by B. Becker *et al.*, pp. 207–210. St Louis, Missouri: C. V. Mosby

HAZLETT, R. D. (1969). Central circular clouding. *J. Am. optom. Ass.* **40**, 268–275

HILL, J. F. (1975). A comparison of refractive and keratometric changes during adaptation to flexible and non-flexible contact lenses. *J. Am. optom. Ass.* **46**, 290–294

HILL, J. F. and RENGSTORFF, R. H. (1974). Relationship between steeply fitted contact lens base curve and corneal curvature changes. *Am. J. Optom.* **51**, 340–342

HODD, F. A. B. (1965). Changes in corneal shape induced by the use of alignment fitted corneal lenses. *Contacto* **9**(3), 18–24

HOVDING, G. (1983a). Variations of central corneal curvature the first year of contact lens wear. *Acta ophthal.* **61**, 117–128

HOVDING, G. (1983b). Variations of refractive error during the first year of contact lens wear. *Acta ophthal.* **61**, 129–140

ING, M. R. (1976). The development of corneal astigmatism in contact lens wearers. *Ann. Ophthal.* **8**, 309

JESSEN, G. N. (1964). Contact lenses as a therapeutic device. *Am. J. Optom.* **41**, 429–435

KEMMETMULLER, H. (1972). Results of contact lens correction in myopia compared with spectacle correction. *Klin. Mbl. Augenheilk.* **160**(1), 75–83

LEVEY, E. M. (1964). A case history of two years continuous wearing of contact lenses, followed by six months of non-continuous wearing. *Am. J. Optom.* **41**, 703–718

McLEAN, W. A. and RENGSTORFF, R. H. (1978). Evaluating the effects of wearing contact lenses. *J. Am. optom. Ass.* **49**, 443–444

MANCHESTER, P. T. (1970). Hydration of the cornea. *Trans. Am. Ophthal. Soc.* **68**, 425–461

MANDELL, R. B. (1965). *Contact Lens Practice: Basic and Advanced.* Springfield, Illinois: C. C. Thomas

MASNICK, K. (1971). A preliminary investigation into the effects of corneal lenses on central corneal thickness and curvature. *Aust. J. Optom.* **54**, 87–98

MILLER, D. (1968). Contact-lens-induced corneal curvature and thickness changes. *Archs Ophthal.* **80**, 420–432

MOBILIA, E. F. and KENYON, K. R. (1986). Contact lens-induced corneal warpage. *Int. Ophthal. Clins* **26**(1), 43–53

MORGAN, J. F. (1975). Induced corneal astigmatism with hydrophilic contact lenses. *Can. J. Ophthal.* **10**, 207–213

MORRISON, R. J. (1956). Contact lenses and the progression of myopia. *J. Am. optom. Ass.* **28**, 711–713

MORRISON, R. J. (1958). Observations on contact lenses and the progression of myopia. *Contacto* **2**(1), 20–25

NEILL, J. C. (1962). Contact lenses and myopia. In *Transactions of the International Ophthalmic Optical Congress*, 1961, pp. 191–198. New York: Hafner

NOLAN, J. (1964). Progress of myopia and contact lenses. *Contacto* **8**(1), 25–26

ODBY, A. and RENGSTORFF, R. H. (1985). The Boston lens: clinical study in Sweden. *Int. Contact Lens Clin.* **12**(2), 104–109

ONG, J. and BOWLING, R. (1972). Effect of contact lens on cornea and lid on a 10-year wearer. *Am. J. Optom.* **49**, 932–935

PRATT-JOHNSON, J. A. and WARNER, D. M. (1965). Contact lenses and corneal curvature changes. *Am. J. Ophthal.* **60**, 852–855

RENGSTORFF, R. H. (1965a). The Fort Dix report. *Am. J. Optom.* **42**, 156–163

RENGSTORFF, R. H. (1965b). Contact lens application and myopia research in the US Army. *Optom. Wkly* **56**(10), 34–35

RENGSTORFF, R. H. (1965c). Corneal curvature and astigmatic changes subsequent to contact lens wear. *J. Am. optom. Ass.* **36**, 996–1000

RENGSTORFF, R. H. (1966). A study of the visual acuity loss after contact lens wear. *Am. J. optom.* **43**, 431–440

RENGSTORFF, R. H. (1967). Variations in myopia measurements: an after-effect observed with habitual wearers of contact lenses. *Am. J. Optom.* **44**, 149–161

RENGSTORFF, R. H. (1968a). An investigation of overnight changes in corneal curvature. *J. Am. optom. Ass.* **39**, 262–265

RENGSTORFF, R. H. (1968b). Contact lenses and after effects: some temporal factors which influence myopia and astigmatism variations. *Am. J. optom.* **45**, 364–373

RENGSTORFF, R. H. (1969a). Variations in corneal curvature measurements: An after-effect observed with habitual wearers of contact lenses. *Am. J. Optom.* **46**, 45–51

RENGSTORFF, R. H. (1969b). Studies of corneal curvature changes after wearing contact lenses. *J. Am. optom. Ass.* **40**, 298–299

RENGSTORFF, R. H. (1969c). Relationship between myopia and corneal curvature changes after wearing contact lenses. *Am. J. Optom.* **46**, 357–362

RENGSTORFF, R. H. (1970a). Overnight decreases in myopia. *S. Afr. Optometrist* **27**(16), 18–22

RENGSTORFF, R. H. (1970b). Overnight myopia changes induced by contact lenses. *J. Am. optom. Ass.* **41**(3), 249–252

RENGSTORFF, R. H. (1970c). Diurnal variations in myopia measurements after wearing contact lenses. *Am. J. Optom.* **47**, 812–815

RENGSTORFF, R. H. (1971a). Corneal curvature: patterns of change after wearing contact lenses. *J. Am. optom. Ass.* **42**, 264

RENGSTORFF, R. H. (1971b). Diurnal variations in corneal curvature after wearing of contact lenses. *Am. J. Optom.* **48**, 239–244

RENGSTORFF, R. H. (1971c). Variations in astigmatism overnight and during the day after wearing contact lenses. *Am. J. Optom.* **48**, 810–813

RENGSTORFF, R. H. (1971d). Wearing contact lenses during sleep; corneal curvature changes. *Am. J. Optom.* **48**, 1034–1037

RENGSTORFF, R. H. (1972). Diurnal constancy of corneal curvature. *Am. J. Optom.* **49**, 1002–1005

RENGSTORFF, R. H. (1973). The relationship between contact lens base curve and corneal curvature. *J. Am. optom. Ass.* **44**, 291–293

RENGSTORFF, R. H. (1975). Prevention and treatment of corneal damage after wearing contact lenses. *J. Am. optom. Ass.* **46**, 277–278

RENGSTORFF, R. H. (1977a). How different base curves affect corneal curvature. *Contact Lens Forum*, August, 25–27

RENGSTORFF, R. H. (1977b). Astigmatism after contact lens wear. *Am. J. Opt. physiol. Optics* **54**(11), 787–791

RENGSTORFF, R. H. (1978a). Wearing one contact lens overnight: corneal curvature and refractive changes. *Rev. Opt.* **115**(4), 67–69

RENGSTORFF, R. H. (1978b). Circadian rhythm: Corneal curvature and refractive changes after wearing contact lenses. *J. Am. optom. Ass.* **49**, 443–444

RENGSTORFF, R. H. (1985). Corneal refraction: relative effects of each corneal component. *J. Am. optom. Ass.* **56**, 218–219

RENGSTORFF, R. H. and ARNER, R. S. (1971). Refractive changes in the cornea: mathematical considerations. *Am. J. Optom.* **48**, 913–918

RENGSTORFF, R. H. and NILSSON, K. T. (1985). Long-term effects of extended wear lenses: changes in refraction, corneal curvature and visual acuity. *Am. J. Opt. physiol. Optics* **62**(1), 66–68

RENGSTORFF, R. H., HILL, R. M., PETRALI, J. P. and SIM, V. M. (1974). Critical oxygen requirement of the corneal epithelium as indicated by succinic dehydrogenase reactivity. *Am. J. Optom.* **51**, 331–339

de RUBEIS, M. J. and SHILY, B. G. (1985). The effects of the Boston II gas-permeable contact lens on central corneal curvature. *Am. J. Optom.* **62**, 497–500

SAKS, S. J. (1966). Fluctuations in refractive state in adapting and long-term contact lens wearers. *J. Am. optom. Ass.* **37**, 229–238

SARVER, M. D. and HARRIS, M. G. (1967). Corneal lenses and 'spectacle blur'. *Am. J. Optom.* **44**, 316–318

STEELE, E. (1959). Observations on the fitting of corneal contact lenses. *Am. J. Optom.* **36**, 194–199

STONE, J. (1973). Contact lens wear in the young myope. *Br. J. physiol. Optics* **28**, 90–134

STONE, J. and POWELL-CULLINGFORD, G. (1974). Myopia control after contact lens wear. *Br. J. physiol. Optics* **29**, 93–108

TREISSMAN, H. (1960). The role of corneal microlenses in ophthalmic practice. *Trans. Ophthal. Soc. UK* **80**, 25–37

WESTERHOUT, D. (1971). A clinical survey of oedema, its signs, symptoms and incidence. *Contact Lens* **3**(2), 3–25

Chapter 21

Contact lenses in abnormal ocular conditions

Keratoconus
E. G. Woodward

Although keratoconus has been recognized as a clinical entity for more than two millenia, the first monograph which adequately described the condition and fully differentiated it from other abnormalities of the cornea did not appear until 1854 (Nottingham). Nottingham was the first to appreciate that keratoconus is essentially a disease producing corneal thinning and then protrusion, the initial corneal thinning not having previously been noticed or if noticed not associated with the disease process. This is not so surprising when it is remembered that the first measurement of corneal thickness in the living eye was not carried out until 1880 by Blix. Nottingham describes fully the degradation of vision produced by the irregular keratoconic cornea. The management of the condition as described by Nottingham is mainly surgical, all the techniques being designed to produce, in a controlled manner, scarring to strengthen the cornea. Cauterization, using silver nitrate and mercury, is described and the passing of a seton (a fine thread or bristle) vertically through the cornea to produce scarring, but he concluded the most simple and least dangerous technique was a straightforward puncturing of the cornea. Nottingham also mentioned using glass shells filled with gelatin, but the first report of a powered contact lens used in connection with keratoconus was by Fick (1888).

Contact lenses have become the management of choice in the majority of patients with keratoconus. In some patients the condition does not progress very far and they retain a reasonable level of visual acuity with spectacles or unaided. This group, usually lacking motivation, are notoriously unsuccessful with contact lenses, as is also the case where the patient has the condition only very mildly in one eye and retains normal vision with the better eye. A very high proportion of keratoconus patients have a personal or family history of atopic disease (Cox, 1984) and if they were able to obtain normal vision with spectacles, contact lens fitting would not be recommended. In early keratoconus it is usually desirable to delay fitting until there is a significant difference between the best spectacle and contact lens acuity thus increasing motivation.

Incidence of keratoconus

Although keratoconus is usually described as a rare disease it is very difficult to obtain exact figures as to its frequency. Jonkers (1950) found the incidence in Holland to be 1 in 40 000 of the general population, whereas other authors had given figures as high as 1 in 286 by Catsch (1938) in Germany and 1 in 703 by Cambiaggi (1955) in Italy; Franceschetti and Carones (1960) in Italy and Jaensch (1929) in Switzerland considered the incidence to be approximately 1 in 3000 and Forrest (1929) in England 1 in 7000.

Ruben (1978a) in England, basing his figures upon the number of keratoconus patients treated at Moorfields Eye Hospital for a catchment area which is approximately 5.5 million, arrived at a figure of 1 in 10 000 who must be affected by this condition.

This large variation in the quoted frequency of the disease may be explained in two ways: first owing to the genetic nature of the condition there are pockets of the disease, i.e. areas where it is considerably more common (Nottingham, 1854; Woodward, 1980a; Ihalainen, 1986). Secondly, there is substantial variability in the diagnosis of the abortive forms of the condition. For example, Kornerup and Lodin (1959) showed that there is a significantly higher incidence of 'bi-oblique corneal astigmatism' among atopic dermatitis patients and some authors would classify these cases as keratoconus. Amsler (1961) using a classification based on subjective impression of mire distortion found that of 600 cases 52% were of the rudimentary type and might often not be diagnosed. At the time of writing there is no doubt that cases are being diagnosed much earlier including many mild cases who will still always retain a reasonable level of visual acuity with spectacles.

There is an interesting variation in the reported sex ratio in the incidence of the disease, all writers prior to 1955 reporting a preponderance of women sufferers — Thomas (1955), Barth (1948), Fox (1910), Nuel (1900), Hansell and Sweet (1903) and Wood and Woodruff (1907) who wrote 'Particularly females of a feeble or debilitated constitution', which may represent the prevailing view of the condition at the time of writing.

Since 1958 all writers have reported a preponderance of male sufferers with an average ratio of 60:40 (Obrig and Salvatori, 1958; Amsler, 1961; Arias, 1962; Karseras and Ruben, 1976; Woodward, 1981; Ihalainen, 1986).

A high incidence of keratoconus in patients with Down's syndrome has been reported by many authors including Hofman (1956), Zajacz (1963), and Stucchi and Erpelding (1966). Cullen and Butler (1963) who examined 143 patients suffering from Down's syndrome found an incidence of keratoconus of 5.5%.

Symptoms and signs

The primary symptom of keratoconus is usually deteriorating vision more marked in one eye than the other. Occasionally patients first notice monocular diplopia in the form of a superior ghost image while retaining visual acuity as good as 6/5. Refraction reveals an against-the-rule astigmatism becoming increasingly irregular, but in the early stages keratometry is not necessarily steep. Sometimes the mean keratometry readings are at the flatter end of the normal range, corneal thinning preceding ectasia by some considerable time (Woodward, 1980a).

In patients who have already been wearing contact lenses, the differential diagnosis from contact lens-induced corneal warping can sometimes be difficult. In such cases early keratoconus can best be diagnosed by topographical pachometry. A central or paracentral corneal thickness of less than 0.48 mm is almost certainly keratoconus, or where the thinnest part of the cornea can be shown to be off its central axis.

As the condition progresses the characteristic swirling retinoscopy reflex appears and the near visual acuity is found to be better than would be anticipated from the distance visual acuity.

One of the most common early signs of keratoconus is enhanced visibility of the corneal nerves. The next finding is usually that of vertical striae (*Plate 89*), first described by Elschnig (1894). In 1906 Fleischer first described the iron pigment ring which bears his name. This ring (*Plate 90*), often only partial, is thought to be caused by some modification of the normal epithelial slide process. In its early stages it is more easily detected by the use of blue light. Most keratoconus patients eventually show some corneal scarring, quite unrelated to contact lens wear. These scars may be small focal opacities, sub-Bowman's or pre-Descemet's, or Bowman's reticular scarring (*Plate 95*). A certain percentage of patients will develop corneal hydrops or acute keratoconus. Here (*Plate 96*) a sudden gross corneal oedema occurs following a rupture of Descemet's membrane (*Plate 69*), usually in a vertical or vertically oblique direction. Most of these cases resolve spontaneously by Descemet's membrane resurfacing over the gap, but there is often some reduction in vision due to the increased scarring. No relationship between contact lens wear or type of lens worn with the incidence of corneal hydrops has ever been demonstrated although it has been suggested it occurs more frequently in patients with Down's syndrome.

Management of keratoconus

A long-term study of keratoconus patients presenting at Moorfields Eye Hospital (Cox, 1984) showed that over 70% retained a visual acuity of 6/9 or better over a 5-year period with contact lens wear and 88.6% were able to see well enough with contact lenses to drive. A proportion of patients either become unable to wear any form of contact lens or have insufficiently good vision with them; the only remaining option then is keratoplasty (*see* pp. 764–772). The criteria for grafting will vary from one clinic to another but typical indications would be:

(1) Visual acuity 6/18 or less.
(2) Intolerance to contact lenses.
(3) Unresolved corneal hydrops.

Typical figures for patients requiring keratoplasty are 8% (Marechal-Courtois and Prijat, 1972) and 11.4% (Cox, 1984). In terms of a clear graft success rates are very high (Pouliquen *et al.*, 1972; Davies, Ruben and Woodward, 1977). In the Moorfields series (Cox, 1984), of the grafted patients 70% achieved a best acuity of 6/6 or better and 95% achieved 6/12 or better.

It has been suggested that scleral contact lenses can have a direct therapeutic effect on the keratoconic eye (Voss and Liberatore, 1962; Clifford Hall, 1963), in that progressive deterioration may be halted but Ruben and Trodd (1976) showed no recession of the rate of progress of keratoconus, irrespective of the type of fitting. Kemmetmuller (1962) had no doubt that large corneal lenses had a direct therapeutic effect on keratoconus but Woodward (1980a) showed no difference in the rate of progression between lens wearing and non-lens wearing groups. The claims for retardation, remission or reversal being produced by contact lens wear have all been based on keratometry. This is misleading because contact lens wear can produce a temporary flattening of the cornea. However, as keratoconus is essentially a disease of corneal thinning it can only be monitored by serial topographical pachometry. When this is done contact lenses are found to have no effect on the progression of the condition. In some cases the disease progresses very little but in most cases tends eventually to stabilize at a corneal thickness 60% of normal (Woodward,

1980b). Some patients arrive for fitting with the impression that contact lens fitting will control the disease and that this is an indication for fitting as early as possible. It should be explained to them that the only purpose of fitting is visual rehabilitation. Most keratoconic patients fitted with contact lenses are of above average intelligence (Woodward, 1981; Ihalainen, 1986), demanding a clear explanation of the rationale of their treatment.

Conversely, it has also been suggested that contact lens wear can precipitate keratoconus. Gasset, Haude and Garcia-Bengochia (1978) compared the number of patients in their clinics who developed keratoconus after having worn hard and soft contact lenses and went on to claim an association between hard contact lens wear and the risk of keratoconus. However, the soft lens wearers were analysed prospectively whilst they were compared with a retrospective analysis of a group of patients already wearing hard contact lenses for some time. Although the refractive errors of the two groups were said to be similar in terms of spherical equivalents, it seems unlikely that the proportion of cases with irregular or high degrees of astigmatism were equal since these conditions would suggest the use of hard lenses. In the early stages of keratoconus before diagnosis most cases will show irregular or high regular astigmatism. A population of hard lens wearers is thus much more likely to contain undiagnosed keratoconic patients than a population of soft lens wearers.

However, the possibility should not be completely ruled out. It has been shown that contact lens wear over a period of years does produce slight corneal thinning. Also it has been recently shown that atopic patients with normal vision have an abnormal distribution of corneal thickness skewed to the thinner end of the range (Kerr-Muir, Woodward and Leonard, 1987). Thus it is perhaps possible that prolonged contact lens wear in atopic patients could precipitate latent keratoconus.

Contact lens options
Soft hydrogel lenses

Hydrogel lenses are rarely fitted in keratoconus as the optical results are always inferior, but occasionally they are the only lenses tolerated and give better vision when used in conjunction with a spectacle overcorrection than spectacles alone. Keratoconus patients with abnormal lids and palpebral conjunctivas through atopic eczema and vernal conjunctivitis (*Plate 71c*) are in this group. Corneal sensitivity is reduced in keratoconus (Bleshoy, 1986), but the sensitivity of the inner lid margins is not affected and in these patients their stiffened thickened lids make hard lens wear extremely difficult.

In the early stages of the disease it may be possible to use a low water content lens (35% water or less) without overcorrection but these patients will probably still have reasonable vision with spectacles. The more usual system is a medium water content lens of positive power, to give a significant centre thickness (at least 0.35 mm), with a negative astigmatic spectacle overcorrection. It must be remembered that these patients are very susceptible to solution toxicity and it is desirable that they use a heat disinfection system and non-preserved saline.

Hydrogel lenses manufactured from HEMA material with a trapezoidal cross-section were first described by Ruben (1978b). These lenses are fenestrated and fit rather in the fashion of the optic zone of a fenestrated scleral lens. *Figure 21.1* shows such a lens in section and on an eye. With a centre thickness of 0.60 mm good vision is often obtained without the use of an astigmatic overcorrection. The difficulty with these lenses is that of reproducibility in manufacture — small variations in the midperipheral thickness of the lens producing large changes in the lens flexure effect on the eye. As this design is the only hydrogel lens trapping an optically effective liquid lens, discrepancies in the refractive power on the eye thus often occur when a lens is replaced. In view of this stock fittings are recommended, the three basic lenses being:

C3/12.00:8.50/8.00:14.00/9.00:15.00, BVP +5.00, t_c 0.60
C3/12.00:8.50/8.50:14.00/9.50:15.00, BVP +5.00, t_c 0.60
C3/12.00:8.50/9.00:14.50/9.75:16.75, BVP +5.00, t_c 0.60

Front optic zone diameters: 8.00 mm.

A correctly fitting trapezoid lens should have a small peripheral circulating bubble, very much akin to the appearance of a FLOM

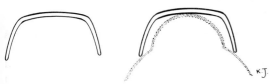

Figure 21.1 Trapezoid hydrogel lens (after Ruben)

(fenestrated lens for optical measurement) (*see* Chapter 17).

It might be thought there was a role for toric hydrophilic lenses in the fitting of keratoconus. Except in the odd *forme fruste* (where corneal thinning and irregular astigmatism do not proceed to complete keratoconus and can be managed with spectacle correction), this is not the case. In order to obtain satisfactory visual results with materials of a relatively low refractive index, large meridional differences in curvature are necessary. The consequential large differences in lens thickness are prone to cause localized corneal oedema. Thus although the lens may be tolerated, areas of corneal neovascularization are often produced to the detriment of any future keratoplasty. Blood vessels in the cornea provide easy access between donor antigen and host lymphocytes thus removing most of the immunological privilege normally enjoyed by the cornea.

The rarity of hydrogel lens fitting in keratoconus is shown by the fact that at 5-year follow-up less than 1% of patients were using hydrogel lenses (Cox, 1984).

Combination lenses and systems

The concept of a lens system which combines the visual result of a rigid lens with the comfort of a soft lens is a very attractive one. This can be done with two separate lenses or a single lens fabricated from two different materials (*see also* pp. 815–817).

The two lens system usually consists of an extra limbal negative powered hydrophilic lens of medium to low water content, in conjunction with a rigid corneal lens of between 9 and 10 mm total diameter (Westerhout, 1973, 1985; Baldone, 1985; *see Plate 121*). In keratoconus this combination can be well tolerated but the problem is that the rigid lens usually rides low on the hydrophilic lens with little or no movement. To avoid this Phillips (A. J., 1987, personal communication) reports the use of a centrally lenticulated low positive soft lens on to which the corneal lens is fitted, the lenticulation aiding the centration of the corneal lens. Corneal lenses have also been fitted into a recessed portion on the front centre of a soft lens (*Plate 122*). Even if the corneal lens is fenestrated or manufactured from a gas permeable material there is always a risk of localized corneal hypoxia (Fatt, 1977). Corneal neovascularization is the reason that most of these lens systems have to be discontinued, but some patients find the handling and upkeep of two different types of lens too much of a nuisance.

At the time of writing the only lens that has been commercially available, manufactured from two different materials is the Saturn II lens (Astin, 1985; Westerhout, 1985). This lens consists of a rigid optical portion of 6.5 mm diameter made from gas permeable pentasilicon P material with a soft peripheral flange of 13.0 mm total diameter of 25% water content HEMA hydrophilic material, polymerized in manufacture. The problem with using this lens on keratoconic eyes is that the chord width of the rigid portion is fixed as is the relationship between the radii of curvature of the rigid and flexible portions. Because the lens is designed for the topography of the normal eye it is rare to find the lens fitting satisfactorily on both the corneal portion and peripheral flange. Usually if the corneal portion fits well the peripheral flange is too tight and the patient shows corneal oedema. Also at the time of writing the steepest BOZR available is 7.2 mm. However, if the lens could be fabricated with differing chord widths and radii combinations, it could be very useful for keratoconus.

Scleral lenses

Although the use of scleral lenses is not high — 4–5% (Cox, 1984) — it is of significance, because for many patients the fitting of such a lens is the only alternative to keratoplasty. Invariably such lenses have to be fitted by the impression technique (*Plate 76*). The chances of fitting with a preformed lens, without hours of modification, are nil; this is because of the eccentricity of the cone in relation to the corneal axis and its asymmetry. Impression taking and the fabrication of scleral lenses is fully described in Chapter 18 and will not be repeated here.

The main candidates for scleral lens fitting are those whose corneas have steepened so that a corneal lens of back optic zone radius 5.5 mm is still too flat, yet with minimal corneal scarring and hence the possibility of a reasonable level of vision. If the apex of the cone is decentred down more than usual, again a corneal lens may not centre sufficiently near the visual axis, whereas a scleral lens affords the opportunity for good vision. There is a high incidence of keratoconus in Down's syndrome: 5.5% is quoted by Cullen and Butler (1963) and 5% by Ihalainen (1986), and these patients usually find scleral lenses easier to cope with.

There is a significant number of patients who have been wearing scleral lenses for many years often fitted prior to the availability of corneal lens fitting sets designed for keratoconus. These patients may present considerable management problems. Usually they wear their lenses most of their waking hours and the inevitable consequence is a low grade but chronic hypoxia and the attendant neovascularization. Furthermore the patients may show good contact lens tolerance and be asymptomatic, only complaining of a reduced level of vision when the vessels and infiltrates reach the central corneal area. Generally scleral lenses give a higher quality of vision than the equivalent corneal lens because of their flatter back optic zone radii and larger back optic zone diameters. It is thus often difficult to wean scleral lens wearers off their lenses when they are beginning to exhibit undesirable contact lens-induced corneal changes but have relatively minor symptoms. A clear explanation that they are putting at risk any future keratoplasty by increasing the possibility of rejection must be given.

The use of gas permeable materials for scleral lenses has an obvious attraction in that they might reduce adverse corneal changes (Ezekiel, 1983; Ruben and Benjamin, 1985). However at the time of writing the only available form of scleral lens made from these materials is a lathe-cut preformed lens unsuitable for the vast majority of keratoconic scleral-lens wearing patients. A more promising option currently being developed is that of a PMMA scleral zone with the optic zone made from a gas permeable material (Sapp, N., 1987, personal communication). Chapter 18, pp. 700–701, describes these options in more detail.

Corneal lenses

As this type of lens is by far the most commonly fitted it is not surprising that the question of the most expedient fitting philosophy has been the subject of much discussion, the variations in approach being both historical and geographical.

In the early days of contact lenses, large relatively flat fitting lenses were advocated and

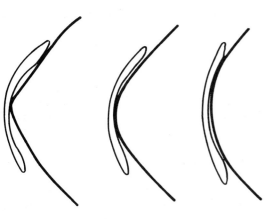

Figure 21.2 A flat-fitting corneal lens, shown from left to right, gradually making a keratoconic cornea more spherical

in a modified form this approach still has its proponents in Scandinavia and the German-speaking countries. As originally described there was a specific intention to reshape the cornea with a large flat lens, the curvature of which bore no relationship to the corneal contour, depending entirely on the plasticity of the cornea (Clifford Hall, 1963). The lenses had total diameters between 9.50 mm and 11.50 mm and had a single back curve apart from a well blended edge bevel 0.50–1.00 mm wide. Initially these lenses rode high with the lower edge often standing away from the cornea. The weight of the lens then tended to push back the cone and 'sphericize' the cornea as shown in *Figure 21.2*; the next lens to try was then an even flatter one.

The fit was also evaluated by repeated refractions, the flattening of the cone reducing both its refractive power and the axial length of the eye. The definitive lens is described as the one requiring the least minus power.

Although not taken to these extremes flat fitting lenses are still currently fitted and this philosophy does have some advantages, the Persecon E Keratoconus lens being an example of this approach (Achatz *et al.*, 1985). The advantages of this type of fitting are mainly optical, flatter fitting lenses giving significant visual improvement. In addition the patient's vision may be enhanced for some time after the removal of the lens due to the cornea remaining relatively flattened. Reservations concerning the use of this approach relate to its possible effect on the natural history of the disease. The majority of patients with keratoconus exhibit

corneal scarring whether or not they have worn contact lenses (Bron *et al.*, 1978), but several writers have suggested that the wearing of a flat fitting corneal lens hastens the rate of scarring in sub-Bowman's stroma as in *Plate 95* (Ruben, 1975; Korb, Finnemore and Herman, 1982). The design of a controlled clinical trial to test the hypothesis that flat fitting corneal lenses exacerbate corneal scarring in keratoconus, would be logistically difficult and ethically dubious. The progression of the condition is so unpredictable and the location of scarring so random that large groups of patients would be needed. Nevertheless many practitioners working in the field have the clinical impression that the relationship does exist.

While the large flat fitting philosophy was being propagated in Europe, in South America and the USA an alternative approach was favoured. This was to fit small thin lenses from 6.00 mm to 8.80 mm in total diameter, with BOZR values between 5.00 mm and 7.50 mm combined with two flatter curves at the periphery (Arias, 1963). The disadvantages with this philosophy are optical. The lenses have an effective optic zone of only 4 mm, they centre on the cone itself which is rarely near the visual axis and monocular diplopia is a common patient complaint. Furthermore in all but the earliest cases the lenses need to be of high negative power with attendant edge thickness problems. This causes especial difficulty if the patient also suffers from atopic eye disease, as is often the case in keratoconus. Generally this group of keratoconic patients is less intolerant to larger corneal lenses.

The most widely accepted corneal lens fitting philosophy, at the time of writing, is one in which the intention is to distribute the weight of the lens between the cone and the more normal peripheral cornea (*Figure 21.3a*). The peripheral cornea does thin in keratoconus but at only half the rate of the centre (Woodward, 1980b). In cases where the cone is well established this philosophy would result in a lens showing an apical contact area of 2–3 mm, an intermediate clearance zone and a midperipheral contact annulus with conventional edge clearance at the periphery (*Plate 91*). In the earlier stages of the condition, owing to the vertical asymmetry of the cone, the intermediate zone forms a crescent rather than an annulus, as shown in *Figure 21.3b* and *Plates 94* and *95a*. With the exception of the

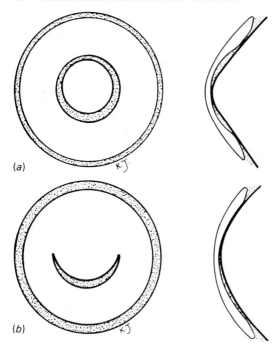

Figure 21.3 Fitting with the weight of the lens distributed (*a*) in developed keratoconus, (*b*) in early keratoconus. The left-hand-side diagrams show a representation of the fit where the dotted areas indicate corneal clearance. The right-hand-side diagrams show the same fit (exaggerated) in cross-section

Table 21.1 Dimensions of offset lenses (Ruben)

Offset lens	BOZD (mm)	TD (mm)	BOZR (range) (mm)
1	6.00	9.00	6.60–8.50
2	7.00	10.00	7.00–8.50
3	5.50	8.50	5.50–7.00

very early case it is necessary to use specifically designed lenses to achieve this type of fit. If conventional design lenses are used, the lens with the desired central fit usually has insufficient edge clearance.

Lens designs which may be used with this fitting philosophy include lenses with peripheral, continuous, contralateral offset curves which simulate a true conicoid surface (Bennett, 1968), and have obvious advantages for fitting keratoconus (Ruben, 1975). The Ruben Offset design is of this type and is widely used in fitting keratoconus; three different combinations being available (*Table 21.1*).

The numbering of these offset lenses seems rather anomalous in that in earlier cases Offset 2 lenses would be used, then as the condition progressed Offset 1 and finally Offset 3. A special lathe is required for the production of these lenses (Ruben, 1975). An offset lathe differs from a normal lathe because the central axis (the lathe spindle) can be moved laterally, or offset, up to 8 mm on either side of the central position. If the trial fitting lens does not give the

desired fluorescein picture, the only variations from the trial lens which can be ordered by the practitioner are additional offset or spherical peripheral curves. Astin (1987) has, however, reported good results with bi-elliptical lenses which have a flatter elliptical periphery than the elliptical back optic zone. Full toroidal back surface corneal lenses are rarely used in fitting keratoconus. Although the cornea is highly astigmatic, the irregularity of the astigmatism is such that it has asymmetry in any one meridian, and centrally a toroidal back surface fits no better than a spherical one. However toroidal back peripheral surfaces can often be used to enhance lens centration. A common problem is where the lens shows reasonable edge clearance except in the inferior quadrant where it is excessive (*Plate 92*), sometimes to the degree of having air under the lens edge (*Figure 21.4a*). Such lenses are unstable and often blinked out by the patient. Here a lens with toroidal periphery can improve the situation, although the inferior clearance always exceeds the superior because of the meridional asymmetry. As this is less peripherally than centrally a compromise fit can often be arrived at, as seen in *Figure 21.4b*.

A toroidal peripheral zone keratoconus fitting set is not a feasible proposition owing to the enormous number of variables, so usually a lens

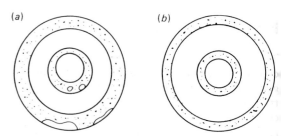

Figure 21.4 Keratoconic cornea fitted with (*a*) a spherical or 'offset' corneal lens, showing bubbles under the lower edge, the dotted areas indicating corneal clearance, (*b*) a corneal lens with a toroidal periphery showing much more uniform clearance at the edge

Table 21.2 Tri-curve keratoconus fitting set (Woodward)

BOZR (mm)	BOZD (mm)	BPR₁ (mm)	BPD₁ (mm)	BPR₂ (mm)	TD (mm)	BVP (D)
5.50	5.60	6.50	7.60	8.50	8.60	−11.00
5.60	5.60	6.60	7.60	8.60	8.60	−10.00
5.70	5.70	6.70	7.80	8.70	8.80	−9.50
5.80	5.70	6.80	7.80	8.80	8.80	−9.00
5.90	5.80	6.90	7.80	8.90	8.80	−8.50
6.00	5.80	7.00	8.00	9.00	9.00	−8.00
6.10	5.90	7.10	8.00	9.10	9.00	−7.50
6.20	5.90	7.20	8.00	9.20	9.00	−7.00
6.30	6.00	7.30	8.00	9.30	9.00	−6.50
6.40	6.00	7.40	8.00	9.40	9.00	−6.00
6.50	6.00	7.50	8.00	9.50	9.00	−5.50
6.60	6.00	7.60	8.00	9.60	9.00	−5.00
6.70	6.00	7.70	8.00	9.70	9.00	−4.50
6.80	6.00	7.80	8.20	9.80	9.20	−4.00
6.90	6.00	7.90	8.20	9.90	9.20	−3.50
7.00	6.00	8.00	8.20	10.00	9.20	−3.00

is estimated from a spherical tri-curve set with the two peripheral curves being toroidal (*Table 21.2*). Such a set allows all the usual variation in ordering by the practitioner for this design (*see* Chapter 10).

In this fitting set the steeper lenses have greater edge clearance than the flatter ones, thus to a certain extent mimicking an increasingly keratonic cornea. A 12.25 mm radius, 0.2 mm wide, may usefully be added as a final peripheral curve if there is any tendency of the lens periphery to fit too tightly around the upper circumference. Additional fitting sets with greater and lesser differences between BOZR and BPR₁ are also useful. The higher negative power on the steeper lenses also represents the actual situation and reduces the power of any supplementary lenses in the trial frame when lens power is determined.

Fitting procedures

The procedure for trial lens fitting in keratoconus is essentially pragmatic. Keratometry gives only minimal help in deciding on the first trial lens to insert. In the earlier stages of the condition the lens closest to the flatter corneal radius is the first trial lens of choice. But as the condition progresses keratometry readings become increasingly meaningless as the irregularity of the cornea increases. Keratometers are calibrated on the assumption that the areas from which the mire images are reflected lie on a spherical surface. If they have a curvature different from each other the measurement will be incorrect and this is invariably the case in keratoconus. Although keratometry is a useful indicator of corneal topographical change in keratoconus, results must be considered in a qualitative rather than quantitative fashion. However, as a means of selecting the first trial fitting set lens, where K readings are possible, the BOZR of the optimum fitting lens is often found in the range corresponding to a value between the K readings of the two 'principal' meridians to slightly steeper than K readings.

More information may be gained from fluorescein pictures with trial lenses and here the use of specifically designed fitting sets is essential. Offset lenses as described earlier may be used or the tri-curve set, but the classic keratoconic fit as shown in *Figure 21.3* and *Plates 91, 92* and *95a* may not always be achievable. Bubble formation and retention below the apex of the cone is common (*Plates 93* and *94*). Ordering of lenses in gas permeable material is obviously desirable in a group of patients who will probably be wearing lenses for most of their lives. When considering materials, however, a low wetting angle and dimensional stability is of more importance than the maximum permeability to oxygen. The steep high minus lens usually necessary in keratoconus is very prone to distortion if made from materials with a high percentage of siloxane.

The ordering of lenses by computer analysis of photokeratograms is only of use in the very early case. Contemporary photokeratoscopes such as the Wesley–Jessen PEK System 2000 make use of an ellipsoidal configuration of the illuminated rings. Despite this configuration, all the rings can only be perfectly in focus for one given corneal radius, the radius usually chosen being 7.90. Within the normal range of corneal radii the fact that any other radius produces a slightly out-of-focus image is of little significance. In progressing keratoconus the image of the reflected rings becomes increasingly blurred, significantly reducing the accuracy. The instrument is useful however in the differential diagnosis of early keratoconus from high naturally occurring astigmatism; a high shape factor $(1-p$, see p. 336) in one or both meridians together with a minimum corneal thickness of less than 0.48 mm confirming keratoconus.

Patient management

If contact lens fitting has been initiated at an appropriate time, i.e. when there is a significant visual gain, patients are usually enthusiastic wearers. It is often counterproductive however to attempt to fit patients if their spectacle visual acuity is reasonable or they retain good unaided vision in one eye.

During an active phase of the condition re-fitting as frequently as every 3 months may be necessary, the patient usually complaining of an unstable lens which easily falls out of the eye and fluorescein demonstrating heavy pressure on the cone with no peripheral support. If corneal hydrops occurs contact lens wear has to be discontinued until all the stromal oedema has resolved (*Plates 69* and *96*). Re-fitting is not always necessary following an episode of hydrops but the visual acuity is usually reduced due to Descemet's scarring.

Where contact lens-induced disease occurs, such as giant papillary conjunctivitis, it is often impossible to persuade patients to cease lens wear. This is understandable in view of the large visual loss. All that can be done is to initiate the appropriate management and try to persuade the patient to reduce wear as much as possible. Where corneal neovascularization is occurring it must be explained to patients that they are placing future surgical options in jeopardy. Seasonal allergic conjunctivitis and less commonly vernal conjunctivitis are often found in conjunction with keratoconus. Such patients may require treatment with sodium cromoglycate, under ophthalmological supervision, during the summer months.

Keratoconic patients have gained the reputation with many eye-care professionals of being awkward and difficult. This has been shown not to be due to any psychoneurotic traits (Karseras and Ruben, 1976), but that compared with the typical ophthalmic patient they are much better educated, more articulate, younger and more willing to voice their doubts and fears concerning the management of their condition. These characteristics must not be forgotten by the contact lens practitioner.

References

ACHATZ, M., ESCHMANN, R., ROCKERT, H., WILKENS, B. and GRANT, R. (1985). Keratoconus: a new approach using bi-elliptical contact lenses. *Contactologia* **7**, 17–21

AMSLER, M. (1961). Quelques donnees du Probleme du Keratocone. *Bull. Soc. Belg. Opthal.* **129**, 331–334

ARIAS, V. C. (1962). El Queratocono su correcion per media de Lentes de Contacto. *Arch. Soc. Oftal Optom.* **4**, 41–44

ARIAS, V. C. (1963). The correction of keratoconus with contact lenses. *Optician* **146**, 447–451, 474–477, 501–505, 527–530, 553–559

ASTIN, C. (1985). Saturn II lenses and penetrating keratoplasty. *Transactions of the British Contact Lens Association Conference*, May 1985, pp. 2–6

ASTIN, C. (1987). Bi-elliptical contact lenses for keratoconus. *J. Br. Contact Lens Ass.* **10**(1), 24–28

BALDONE, J. A. (1985). Piggy-back fitting of contact lenses. *Contact Lens Ass. Ophthal. J.* **11**(2), 130–134

BARTH, J. (1948). Statisk uben 300 Keratoconusfalle mit 557 befallenen Augen. *MD Thesis*, University of Zurich

BENNETT, A. G. (1968). Aspherical surfaces. *Ophthal. Optician* **4**, 1033–1039

BLESHOY, H. (1986). Corneal sensitivity in keratoconus. *Transactions of the British Contact Lens Association Conference*, Jersey, May 1986, pp. 9–13

BLIX, M. (1880). Oftalmometriska studier. *Uppsala Lakareforenigs Farhandiglingar* (15), 349–420

BRON, A. J., TRIPATHI, R. C., HARDING, J. J. and CRABBE, M. J. C. (1978). Stromal loss in keratoconus. *Trans. Ophthal. Soc. UK* **98**, 393–396

CAMBIAGGI, A. (1955). Evidenza Statistica della Associazone della Degenerozione Pigmentoza della Retina con il Cheratocono. *G. Ital. Oftal.* **8**, 13–17

CATSCH, A. (1938). Korrelationspathologische Untersuchunger I. *Albrecht von Graefes Arch. Ophthal.* **138**, 866–892

CLIFFORD HALL, K. G. (1963). A comprehensive study of keratoconus. *Br. J. physiol. Optics* **20**, 215–256

COX, S. N. (1984). Management of keratoconus. *J. Br. Contact Lens Ass.* **7**(2), 86–92

CULLEN, J. F. and BUTLER, H. J. (1963). Mongolism (Down's syndrome) and keratoconus. *Br. J. Ophthal.* **47**(6), 321–330

DAVIES, P. D., RUBEN, M. and WOODWARD, E. G. (1977). Keratoconus: An analysis of the factors which affect the optical results of keratoplasty. *Transactions of the European Contact Lens Society of Ophthalmologists Ghent*. Published by General Secretariat, European Society of Ophthalmologists, Orange Nassaulau 18, (N-L), Warmond, Holland, pp. 97–99

ELSCHNIG, A. (1894). Uber den Keratoconus. *Klin. Mbl. Augenheilk.* **32**, 25–56

EZEKIEL, D. (1983). Gas permeable haptic lenses. *J. Br. Contact Lens Ass.* **6**(4), 158–161

FATT, I. (1977). Oxygen transmissibility considerations for a hard–soft contact lens combination. *Am. J. Optom.* **54**, 666–672

FLEISCHER, H. (1906). Uber Keratokonus unt eigenartige pimentbildung in der kornea. *Münch. med Wochenschr.* **53**, 625–627

FICK, A. E. (1888). Eine Contactbrille. *Arch. Augenheilk.* **18**, 279–288

FORREST, J. (1929). *The Recognition of Ocular Disease*, p. 77. London: J. H. Taylor

FRANCESCHETTI, A. and CARONES, H. V. (1960). Cheratocono. *G. Ital Oftal.* **13**, 143–160

FOX, L. W. (1910). *A Practical Treatise on Ophthalmology*, p. 231. London: Appletons

GASSET, A. R., HAUDE, W. L. and GARCIA-BENGOCHIA, M. (1978). Hard contact lens wear an environmental risk in keratoconus. *Am. J. Ophthal.* **85**(3), 39–41

HANSELL, H. F. and SWEET, W. M. (1903). *Diseases of the Eye*, p. 229. London: Redman

HOFMAN, H. (1956). Keratoconus. *Klin. Mbl. Augenheilk.* **129**, 756–758

IHALAINEN, A. (1986). Clinical and epidemiological features of keratoconus. *Acta ophthal. Suppl. 178* **64**, 1–64

JAENSCH, P. A. (1929). Keratoconus die Engebrisse de Forschung de Cetzen 20 Jahre. *Zbl. ges Ophthal.* **21**, 305–307

KARSERAS, A. G. and RUBEN, M. (1976). Aetiology of keratoconus. *Br. J. Ophthal.* **60**, 522–525

KEMMETMULLER, H. (1962). Corneal lenses and keratoconus. *Transactions of the International Society of Contact Lens Specialists.* 7th Congress, Philadelphia. *Contacto* **6**, 17–21

KERR-MUIR, M., WOODWARD, E. G. and LEONARD, T. (1987). Corneal thickness, astigmatism and atopy. *Br. J. Ophthal.* **71**, 207–211

KORB, D. R., FINNEMORE, D. M. and HERMAN, J. P. (1982). Apical changes and scarring in keratoconus, as related to contact lens fitting techniques. *J. Am. optom. Ass.* **53**, 199–205

KORNERUP, T. and LODIN, A. (1959). Ocular changes in 100 cases of Besnier's Prurigo Atopic Dermatitis. *Acta ophthal.* **37**, 508–521

MARECHAL-COURTOIS, C. and PRIJAT, E. (1972). Relative values of contact lenses and keratoplasty in the treatment of keratoconus. *Contact Lens J.* **3**(6), 36–37

NOTTINGHAM, J. (1854). *Practical Observations on Conical Cornea.* London: Churchill

NUEL, J. P. (1900). In *System of Diseases of the Eye*, Vol. IV, edited by E. Norris and J. Oliver, pp. 249–253. London: Lewin

OBRIG, T. E. and SALVATORI, P. (1958). *Contact Lenses*, pp. 145–146. New York: The Chilton Co.

POULIQUEN, Y., BELLIVET, J., LECOQ, J. and CLAY, C. (1972). Keratoplastic transfixante dans le traitment du keratocone. A propos de 60 cas. *Arch. ophtal. (Paris)* **32**, 735–744

RUBEN, M. (1975). *Contact Lens Practice*, pp. 171 and 283–284. London: Ballière-Tindall

RUBEN, M. (1978a). Treatment of keratoconus. *Ophthal. Optician* **3**(18), 64–72

RUBEN, M. (1978b). *Soft Contact Lenses*, pp. 256–260. London: Baillière-Tindall

RUBEN, M. and BENJAMIN, W. J. (1985). Gas permeable scleral lenses. *Contact Lens J.* **13**(2), 5–10

RUBEN, M. and TRODD, C. (1976). Scleral lenses in keratoconus. *Contact Intraoc. Lens Med. J.* **2**(1), 18–20

STUCCHI, J. and ERPELDING, I. (1966). Down's syndrome. *Confin neurol.* **20**, 376–378

THOMAS, C. I. (1955). *The Cornea*, pp. 233–244. Springfield, Illinois: C. C. Thomas

VOSS, E. H. and LIBERATORE, J. C. (1962). Fitting the apex of keratoconus. *Transactions of the International Society of Contact Lens Specialists.* 7th Congress, Philadelphia. *Contacto* **6**, 33–37

WESTERHOUT, D. (1973). The combination lens and therapeutic uses of soft lenses. *Contact Lens J.* **4**(5), 3–10

WESTERHOUT, D. (1985). Combination and piggy-back lenses — a valuable clinical technique especially in abnormal cases. *Transactions of the British Contact Lens Association Conference*, May 1985, pp. 49–51

WOOD, C. A. and WOODRUFF, T. A. (1907). *Commoner Diseases of the Eye*, pp. 306–307. London: W. T. Keane

WOODWARD, E. G. (1980a). Keratoconus: the disease and its progression. *Doctoral thesis*, The City University, London

WOODWARD, E. G. (1980b). The cornea in health and disease. In *Transactions of the 16th Congress of the European Society of Ophthalmologists, Brighton*, edited by P. Trevor-Roper, Vol. 40, pp. 531–536. London: BMJ Press

WOODWARD, E. G. (1981). Keratoconus: maternal age and social class. *Br. J. Ophthal.* **65**(2), 104–107

ZAJACZ, J. (1963). Keratoconus. *Klin. Mbl. Augenheilk.* **143**, 503–504

Aphakia
M. J. A. Port

The number of contact lenses routinely fitted for the correction of aphakia has declined since the advent of intraocular lenses, but contact lenses still have a place (Stark *et al.*, 1979).

The average aphakic eye has several physiological features of note. These are as follows:

(1) The eye is usually of someone 60 years of age, or greater. When comparison is made with a younger person the implications here are:

(a) the basal metabolic rate (BMR) is lower;

(b) there is less tear production;
(c) the lids may be more flaccid;
(d) more of the cornea may be covered by the upper lids;
(e) there may be incomplete blinking.
(2) the absence of the crystalline lens means that the partial pressure of oxygen at the corneal endothelium is higher than that of a phakic eye, which is advantageous for contact lens fitting.
(3) If the cataract extraction has been performed by a scleral or corneal section then up to half of the corneal nerves will have been severed and corneal sensitivity will be poorer than normal (Guillon, 1985).
(4) The surgery involved may also cause a change in the degree of corneal astigmatism (Kersley and Kerr, 1983) and a tendency towards 'against-the-rule' astigmatism (Reading, 1984; Van Rij and Waring, 1984), a change in the position of the corneal apex (Port, 1983, unpublished data), and some corneal endothelial loss. There may be changes in the posterior segment, e.g. macular oedema, retinal detachment and capsule opacity. These sequelae, together with any pupil changes, affect the standard of vision obtained with an optical correction (Koetting and Von Gunten, 1969).

It is also important to realize that an eye without its crystalline lens is without the retina's ultraviolet protective filter. The effects of ultraviolet light on the retinal tissues are now beginning to be understood. It would seem appropriate that contact lenses incorporate some ultraviolet filter in order to protect the retina from higher levels of this radiation (Port, 1986).

A contact lens for a unilateral aphake can provide binocular vision where the fellow eye has useful acuity. Even so Guillon and Warland (1980) found that most unilateral aphakes only achieved 140 seconds of arc on the Titmus stereopsis test and 80% had intermittent suppression. This may be because the retinal image size difference is often outside normal fusion limits (*see* Chapter 5 and *Figure 5.13*). The quality of vision with contact lenses is very good for aphakes. In comparison spectacles tend to give distortion of vision and this can be upsetting to the wearer. Most aphakes will gladly sacrifice a line or two of Snellen acuity in exchange for the better quality of vision that contact lenses provide. Astigmatism is often around 2 D in an aphakic eye. The simplest solution is to correct this with a hard lens but if such a lens cannot be tolerated then a soft lens may have to be used. In this case, if the astigmatism needs to be corrected it will probably have to be provided in the form of a spectacle correction as the basic power required is often outside the range of available toric soft lenses. In any case the aphakic patient requires a near addition so that bifocal spectacles can be used to correct the astigmatism as well as to provide the near addition. This has the virtue of keeping the contact lens part of the correction as simple as possible. Overall, the practitioner needs a flexible approach to the fitting of aphakes (Cox, 1982; Dube, 1985).

General procedure

(1) A postsurgical period of 6–10 weeks is allowed to elapse in order to permit healing and settling to occur. If inflammation has not subsided by then, the patient has to be rejected for fitting (Astin, 1984).
(2) An ophthalmological examination is carried out to ensure the eye is in a fit state to receive and wear contact lenses. For example, the ophthalmologist will check that there is no aqueous leakage from wounds and that sutures are not causing problems.
(3) An accurate spectacle refraction is performed.
(4) Keratometry is carried out.
(5) Assessment of pupil size, shape and position is made.
(6) Eyelids are assessed.
(7) Contact lens fitting is then undertaken.
(8) Refraction, to include correction of any remaining astigmatism and near addition, as well as oculomotor balance tests are carried out.
(9) After-care is arranged.

Points (3) to (9) above are now discussed in greater detail.

Spectacle refraction

For retinoscopy, some people prefer to use spheres only, whilst others prefer to use spheres and cylinders. The use of positive cylinders permits reduction of the plus sphere before the eye. With sphere powers commonly in the order of +12.00 to +18.00 D it is essential that the back vertex distance is noted accurately. The ocular refraction can then be calculated later.

When a cataractous crystalline lens has been removed it is often assumed that the refraction is going to be straightforward. However, pupil size and position (*Plate 83*), vitreous movement and lens capsule presence may all conspire to make refraction very difficult. Inconsistency of results should be anticipated — the prescription and visual acuity may well vary on a day-to-day, or week-to-week basis. It is important to establish if the eyes are straight. If an eye has been subjected to a blur of the order of 15 D for 2 months, a squint may have resulted. If this has been the case it is worth while fitting a contact lens as soon as it is practical in order to re-establish binocular vision. For example, if it is going to take a long time to get a special rigid lens for the eye it may be useful to fit an extended wear soft lens on a short-term basis.

Keratometry

Keratometry permits measurement of the corneal astigmatism which should correspond to the total ocular astigmatism provided the pupil is reasonably central. To some extent the degree of astigmatism depends on the preoperative degree and the changes induced during the surgical procedure. The keratometer mire images may show some distortion and the principal meridians may not be perpendicular indicating some corneal irregularity. Any type of keratometer is suitable for this measurement.

Pupil size, shape and position

If the eye has been subjected to trauma an abnormal pupil may be present. There may even be some degree of 'aniridia' (*Plate 110*). Modern surgical procedures tend to produce only small pupil changes but the contact lens fitter should take particular account of this important optical aperture. The design of lens chosen must take account of pupil characteristics.

It is pertinent to mention iridectomy apertures. These are usually found in the 12 o'clock position (*Plate 2*) and the size varies. If they are not well covered by the upper lid there may be monocular diplopia problems.

Lid position

Low flaccid upper lids may cover much of the cornea and even without a contact lens a large percentage of the cornea may be relatively hypoxic. There may be some degree of incomplete blinking but the use of vital stains and a slit lamp should identify this problem if it causes epithelial drying. If there is some degree of lagophthalmos then hard lenses may not centre well and hydrogel lenses may dry out.

Lens fitting

The majority of aphakes needing contact lenses are adequately served with either a rigid lens or a daily wear soft lens. The minority need either extended wear lenses, large diameter corneal lenses or scleral lenses. In choosing the best lens form many factors have to be taken into account and some of these factors are initially unknown. The factors fall into two categories — patient factors and ocular factors. As far as patient factors are concerned the following aspects must be assessed: Can they handle various types of lens? Can they understand and remember the hygiene regimen involved? Do they live alone? Are there any friends or relatives available to help out if a lens is lost or cannot be removed? These factors should be assessed as far as possible before fitting proceeds. If there are no indications for a particular type of lens it is worth while trying some form of rigid lens first. Rigid lenses are more robust than hydrogels and are a little more tolerant to poorer hygiene compliance. If there is corneal astigmatism present then this may be corrected simply with a rigid lens. The second option of a daily wear soft lens should be considered if the hard lens fails for some reason. If a hard lens invariably centres poorly on an eye then normally a soft lens centres better because it has a large optic zone which assists centring and is useful for slightly eccentric pupils.

If handling of hard and soft lenses proves to be poor then extended wear lenses should be considered. If patients live alone and perhaps have poor comprehension then extended wear may well be the best option (Kracher, Stark and Hirst, 1981).

In cases of corneal irregularity and astigmatism where centration is poor the use of rigid lenses whose total diameter is in the 10.5–13 mm region should be considered.

Scleral lenses have a place in aphakic fitting (Pullum and Trodd, 1984). The lenses are almost indestructible; they preserve a tear layer behind the lens and so are excellent for dry eyed patients; they are large (*Plate 75*) and therefore can be handled more easily than corneal or soft lenses. Again, the correction of high degrees of astigmatism is not difficult with a scleral lens form. Chapter 18 deals with their fitting for aphakes.

Corneal lens fitting (daily wear)

The criteria used for fitting aphakic eyes are very little different from those used for normal eyes (*see* Chapter 10). Most lenses for aphakia have a relatively large centre thickness which defeats the purpose of using high *Dk* materials for these lenses, because the oxygen transmissibility in the centre is poor. Most of the oxygen required by the epithelium is transported in the tear film and the fitter should ensure that there is an adequate tear pump. Although gas permeable materials are used for aphakics and the small amount of oxygen transmitted through the lens may be advantageous, it is probably the comfort and surface characteristics of the material that make it successful rather than the *Dk* value alone.

Lens diameters tend to be larger for high plus lenses although small PMMA lenses have been advocated (Polse, 1969). For low and medium myopes, total diameters of 9.0–9.6 mm meet most needs, whereas for aphakics the total diameter more commonly falls in the range 9.5–10.0 mm. The larger diameter helps to stabilize the lens and give better centration.

Fitting should be done with lenses from a high plus fitting set so that the effect of lens weight can be seen and also how the lids affect a relatively thick lens. With a good fitting lens the habitual position should be noted especially in conjunction with the pupil characteristics. The BOZD and FOZD should cover the pupil area at all times. If this does not occur, flare and diplopia will almost certainly occur. A decentred corneal apex may consistently cause lenses to decentre. The effect of the lids on a thick lens tends to accentuate this decentration. Larger and/or steeper lenses may be tried to get better centration. If multi-curve lenses have been used it is useful to try some form of aspheric lens, e.g.

Persecon E* as centration may be improved. If it is possible to design a lens with a small front optic zone then a negative carrier may hitch the lens to the top lid (*see* Chapter 10).

Large diameter corneal lenses

If a normal size corneal lens decentres badly and perhaps there are pupil anomalies and corneal astigmatism then a large diameter lens may be useful. It is also simpler to prescribe than scleral lenses. Lens total diameters between 10.5 and 13 mm are usually used for this type of construction. The 'Apex' lens (Bagshaw, Gordon and Stanworth, 1966) uses a bi-curve design. The author has found it preferable to use a tri-curve design for these diameters. BOZD values of 8.5–9.5 mm seem to produce the best results. A small, four lens trial set powered at about +17.00 D with BOZR values of 7.5, 7.8, 8.1 and 8.4 mm should prove useful. Most of the lenses have to be individually designed due to the variation of corneal topography at these larger diameters, so a large trial set may be of limited value. It is better to make a prototype PMMA lens and modify the curves to achieve a good fit. The first lens should have enough thickness to enable such modifications to be done. A gas permeable lens may then be made to the modified specification.

Soft lenses (daily wear)

For aphakics daily wear and extended wear lenses are both practical possibilities. If possible a daily wear lens should be tried in the first instance. It should be possible for the patient to handle the lenses and be competent in lens cleaning, insertion and removal. The hygiene regimen should be understood.

For a patient where a rigid lens is not well tolerated or decentres badly a soft lens can be of help. It also has the advantage of a large optic zone diameter so there is unlikely to be a flare problem. If there is significant residual astigmatism present with the lens *in situ* then some form of spectacle correction may be required to obtain the best acuity, unless a toric soft lens can be fitted, although the latter are very expensive and yet another source of possible variations in vision.

*Persecon E — CIBA Vision (Titmus).

HEMA lenses are recommended as a first choice daily wear lens. They tend not to dry out as much as a higher water content lens on relatively dry eyes. Total diameters of soft lenses, in common with rigid lenses, tend to be about 0.5 mm larger than for normal low power soft lenses. This will keep the lens well centred but should not make the fit tight.

Where a very thin lens is needed the practitioner should consider a lens design such as the Hydron Z-Aphakic which has a hyperbolic front surface. This design (Guillon and Bleshoy, 1983) has a very uniform thickness and hence the transmissibility will be fairly even across the lens. The lens has a thickness of about 0.21 mm which is about half the thickness of a conventional lens with spherical surfaces. However, the disadvantage is that the lens may not perform well if it is not centred about the pupil and it was found that if the thickness was further reduced then the visual performance (especially using contrast sensitivity tests) began to decline. The acuity obtained may also be a little lower than with a conventional lens. Because the lens is uniformly thin it may be torn more easily than a thicker lens.

Regular hydrogel lenses for aphakia are thick, implying that their oxygen transmissibilities are low. Polse, Sarver and Harris (1978), in a provocative 5-hour test, found that corneal thickness increased by 7%. This was 3% better than phakic eyes (used for controls) but it is still a significant amount. The use of thinner designed lenses can reduce this corneal swelling. Bleshoy and Guillon (1983) found that the Hydron Z-Aphakic lenses gave rise to corneal swelling of 2% ± 3% while in use.

Extended wear lenses

The vast majority of extended wear (EW) soft lenses prescribed for aphakics are hydrogel lenses. Generally this is a costly exercise and the general management can be very different from the phakic patient using extended wear lenses (Janoff, 1983). The lenses tend to form deposits quickly and need more frequent replacement. The after-care is also time consuming. For the person living alone who cannot handle contact lenses or look after them properly the EW lens is a boon. Many elderly people are reluctant to seek help if they have a contact lens problem —

they take the view that they are being enough trouble as it is without causing more. As a result serious infections can result (Carpel and Parker, 1985; Mondino et al., 1986; Ormerod and Smith, 1986).

Hydrogels of 60–80% water content can be used for aphakic lenses. Again the total diameters are usually a little larger than for low power lenses. It is most important to give patients an adequate tolerance test as the older eye, being relatively dry, can cause severe lens tightening. In extreme cases all lenses tighten and therefore this type of lens cannot be used. Some practitioners may consider using a silicone elastomer lens with this condition. Certainly the corneas stay exceptionally clear and oedema free but deposits can still be a problem (see Plates 44 and 45).

Gas permeable hard lenses can also be used for extended wear (Benjamin and Simons, 1984). The highest Dk materials available should be used. Elie (1986) reported good results with the Menicon EX material; Muir-Taylor and Levi (1985) have similarly reported success with the Paraperm EW material and Sigband (1986) claimed an 85% success rate using Boston IV material. With high plus lenses parameters should be stable. For normal eyes, lens diameters of 9.3–9.8 mm suffice but in aphakia a larger total diameter is required in order to prevent the lenses slipping off the cornea during sleep. The design of the lens should aim at minimum thickness and if a small front optic zone diameter is feasible this should be used. The main advantages of the rigid lenses are:

(1) Strength.
(2) Debris and excreta behind the lens are removed by blinking on waking.
(3) Higher gas transmissibilities are available compared to hydrogels.
(4) Better correction of corneal astigmatism.
(5) Easier to clean.
(6) Less corneal vascularization, microcysts, and infiltrates.
(7) Fewer red eyes.
(8) Fewer serious infections.

Refraction

If the presurgical ametropia was low then a trial contact lens powered at about +14.00 D is suitable for refraction. The contact lens prescription is found by taking the over-refraction and its vertex distance into account (*see* Chapter 5, *Figure 5.19*). With high powered soft lenses there are some bending effects on the eye so that the power may not always be exactly as anticipated (Chaston, 1979; Chaston and Fatt, 1980; Patel, 1980; Fatt and Chaston, 1982; Weissman and Gardner, 1984). Chapter 5, pp. 209–216, gives further details.

The main characteristic of the aphakic patient wearing contact lenses compared to the patient with normal eyes is the variability of refraction and visual acuity. Even without a contact lens, factors such as pupil size, pupil position, vitreous variation and macular condition can all affect refraction and acuity. With a contact lens *in situ* another high powered element is placed in the optical system. The contact lens is probably not static and lacrimation then affects lens position. It is as well for patients to be told that their vision with a contact lens is likely to be variable and that they will get good days and bad days. It is the function of the practitioner to give as good a correction as possible. Having said that, the correction may well be a compromise. One of the advantages of fitting from an inventory of lenses is that power changes are easily made, but the power of the lens should not be changed at every after-care visit. Certainly over-refraction should be carried out and recorded, and perhaps some months later a power change may be made in light of this information to provide a better spherical correction, once a consistent over-refraction is obtained.

If, for example, the spectacle *Rx* is as follows:

RE −4.00/−2.00 × 105 6/12
LE +14.50/−1.25 × 135 6/6

the practitioner should consider the spherical balance when the contact lens has been fitted. If the normal correction was applied to the contact lens for the left eye the spectacles would be:

RE −4.00/−2.00 × 105
LE   Plano

The spherical imbalance might cause binocular problems. The practitioner has several options:

(1) If the second eye were due for a cataract extraction fairly soon then a normal full correction to the contact lens would be reasonable.

(2) If the patient can handle contact lenses, then a contact lens on the phakic eye might be accepted by the patient.
(3) Overcorrection of the aphakic eye's contact lens (using the above example) by about +4.00 DS would result in a spectacle correction that would be:

RE −4.00/−2.00 × 105 LE −4.00 DS.

Cosmetically, the spectacle lenses would be balanced and there would be less likelihood of binocular problems.

In the case of soft lenses similar arguments apply. In addition, there is the likelihood that some correction of astigmatism will be required and this is best done with additional spectacles:

RE Plano/−1.75 × 55
LE +0.50/−1.25 × 115

A near prescription for close work is usually needed for unilateral and always for bilateral aphakics. The practitioner should ensure that the near prescription is balanced. The patient should be told that the range of clear near vision may well be less in the aphakic eye compared with the normal eye. The choice of single vision or bifocal spectacles is determined by the individual's needs or preferences. In some cases varifocal lenses are appreciated (Koetting, 1969).

Use of tinted lenses

Tinted lenses have two advantages to the aphakic patient. First the lens is more easily seen both on and off the eye and secondly a measure of ultraviolet protection can be given if the tint is chosen carefully.

Fitting babies and infants

Although there are various reasons for contemplating the use of contact lenses for children (Kersley, 1978) the principal reason is for the correction of aphakia after congenital cataracts (*Plate 102*) have been extracted. Fitting of contact lenses must always be considered in conjunction with an ophthalmologist (Morris *et al.*, 1979). Probably the most common lenses are either hydrogel or silicone rubber lenses used for extended wear. With youngsters this may be the only practical solution but the practitioner should aim to move to daily wear lenses as soon as possible (Moore, 1985).

Silicone rubber lenses are very strong and fewer lenses are lost from the eye when compared with hydrogels (Nelson *et al.*, 1985; Hales, 1986; Matsumoto and Murphree, 1986). Pratt-Johnson and Tillson (1985) report the use of PMMA lenses and good tolerance using them. In some cases scleral lenses can be used (*see* Chapter 18).

With hydrogel lenses the breakage and loss from the eye are more common than with silicone rubber lenses but certainly deposition on the lens surfaces is rarely a problem when compared with elderly aphakic patients.

Paediatric contact lens fitting is covered in more detail on pp. 782–789.

After-care

After-care for aphakic patients is very important. The elderly patients may not be mobile and they may forget about appointments. Their eyes, being less sensitive than normal, tolerate chipped and cracked lenses, lenses with bad deposits and early signs of infections. Having said that, it should be remembered that the average life expectancy after a cataract extraction is around 5 years so that long-term problems are less relevant than in normal younger eyes.

It is useful for the contact lens practitioner to ask patients if they have been seen by an ophthalmologist. Patients may get the idea that having been sent for contact lens fitting they do not need ophthalmological follow-ups.

The practitioner should be even more careful than normal in asking about hygiene regimens, not only enquiring about what preparations are used but when and how they are used.

Rigid lenses often need polishing due to poor handling. Surfactant cleaning by the patient may not have been very efficacious.

Soft lenses may have bad deposits on them and with hard lipid/calcium deposits a new lens is recommended once the deposits reach a size that could give rise to corneal or eyelid reactions.

Soft lens wearers — especially those on extended wear — may develop corneal vascularization (*see* Chapters 15 and 19). This can be considerably worse than with normal eyes wearing relatively thin lenses. The vessels may grow 3 mm or more in from the limbus. They may then stabilize at this level of invasion, which, although undesirable, is probably acceptable because the practitioner should consider the patient as a whole. In many cases it may be better to give the patients a better quality of life with contact lenses which give rise to some corneal neovascularization than condemn them to spectacles where the distortion may be intolerable. Obviously some discussion with the patient's ophthalmologist is useful when considering the management of corneal vascularization.

References

ASTIN, C. (1984). Aphakia contact lens fitting in a hospital department. *J. Br. Contact Lens Ass.* **7**, 164–168

BAGSHAW, J., GORDON, S. P. and STANWORTH, A. (1966). A modified corneal contact lens: binocular single vision in unilateral aphakia. *Br. orthopt J.* **23**, 19–30

BENJAMIN, W. and SIMONS, M. (1984). Extended wear of rigid contact lenses in aphakia: a preliminary report. *Int. Contact Lens Clin.* **11**, 44–54

BLESHOY, H. and GUILLON, M. (1984). Soft lens design — clinical results. *J. Br. Contact Lens Ass.* **7**(1), 41–47

CARPEL, E. and PARKER, P. (1985). Extended wear aphakic contact lens fitting in high risk patients. *Contact Lens Ass. Ophthal. J.* **11**, 231–233

CHASTON, J. (1979). Soft contact lenses for aphakia. *J. Br. Contact Lens Ass.* **2**(2), 20–27

CHASTON, J. and FATT, I. (1980). The change in power of soft lenses. *Optician* **180**, 12–21

COX, N. (1982). A flexible approach to aphakia. *J. Br. Contact Lens Ass.* **5**(4), 152–154

DUBE, D. (1985). Contact lenses in pediatric aphakia. *Contact Lens Forum* **10**(12), 23–25

ELIE, G. (1986). Gas permeable extended wear lenses: an excellent solution for aphakic patients. *Contact Lens Ass. Ophthal. J.* **12**, 51–53

FATT, I. and CHASTON, J. (1982). Swelling factors of hydrogels and the effect of deswelling in the eye on the power of a soft contact lens. *Int. Contact Lens Clin.* **9**, 146–153

GUILLON, M. (1985). The corneal physiology of the aphakic eye and its relevance to contact lens wear. *Contact Lens J.* **13**(3), 8

GUILLON, M., BLESHOY, H. (1983). Comparative study of the visual performance of various aphakic corrections. *Acta ophthal.* **61**, 851–859

GUILLON, M. and WARLAND, J. (1980). Aniseikonia and binocular function in unilateral aphakes wearing contact lenses. *J. Br. Contact Lens Ass.* **3**(1), 36–38

HALES, R. (1986). Unilateral pediatric aphakia: current treatments and lens choices. *Contact Lens Forum* **11**(11), 34–35

JANOFF, L. (1983). A comparison of clinical results during extended wear between phakic and aphakic subjects. *J. Br. Contact Lens Ass.* **6**(4), 141–149

KERSLEY, H. (1978). Considerations of the medical use of extended wear lenses in children. *J. Br. Contact Lens Ass.* **1**(3), 2–4

KERSLEY, H. and KERR, C. (1983). Astigmatism and extended wear in aphakia. *J. Br. Contact Lens Ass.* **6**(4), 150–152

KOETTING, R. (1969). Progressive addition spectacles over contact lenses in aphakia. *Am. J. Optom. physiol. Optics* **46**, 470–475

KOETTING, R. and VON GUNTEN, T. (1969). Glare flare with contact lenses in aphakia. *Am. J. Optom. physiol. Optics* **46**, 730–734

KRACHER, G. P., STARK, W. J. and HIRST, L. W. (1981). Extended wear contact lenses for aphakia. *Am. J. Optom. physiol. Optics* **58**, 467–471

MATSUMOTO, E. and MURPHREE, A. (1986). The use of silicone elastomer lenses in aphakic pediatric patients. *Int. Eyecare* **2**, 214–217

MONDINO, B., WEISSMAN, B. A., FARB, M. D. and PETTIT, T. H. (1986). Corneal ulcers associated with daily wear and extended wear contact lenses. *Am. J. Ophthal.* **102**, 58–65

MOORE, B. (1985). The fitting of contact lenses in aphakic infants. *J. Am. Optom. Ass.* **56**, 180–183

MORRIS, J., TAYLOR, D., ROGER, J. E. and WARLAND, V. J. (1979). Contact lens treatment of aphakic infants and children. *J. Br. Contact Lens Ass.* **2**(3), 22–30

MUIR-TAYLOR, D. and LEVI, I. (1985). The correction of aphakia with gas permeable extended wear contact lenses. *Optom. Today* **25**, 808–809

NELSON, L. B., CUTLER, S. I., CALHOUN, J. H. *et al.* (1985).

Silsoft extended wear contact lenses: pediatric aphakia. *Ophthalmology* **92**, 1529–1531

ORMEROD, L. and SMITH, R. (1986). Contact lens associated microbial keratitis. *Arch. Ophthal.* **104**, 79–83

PATEL, S. (1980). A theoretical model for predicting parameter changes in soft lenses due to bending. *Am. J. Optom. physiol. Optics* **57**, 697–710

POLSE, K. (1969). Contact lens fitting in aphakia. *Am. J. Optom. physiol. Optics* **46**, 213–219

POLSE, K. A., SARVER, M. D. and HARRIS, M. G. (1978). Corneal effects of high plus hydrogel lenses. *Am. J. Optom. physiol. Optics* **55**, 234–237

PORT, M. J. A. (1986). The spectral transmission of contact lenses. *Contax*, September, 13–16

PRATT-JOHNSON, J. and TILLSON, G. (1985). Hard contact lenses in the management of congenital cataracts. *J. Ped. Ophthal. Strab.* **22**(3), 94–96

PULLUM, K. and TRODD, T. (1984). Development of slotted scleral lenses. *J. Br. Contact Lens Ass.* **7**(1), 28–38

READING, V. (1984). Astigmatism following cataract surgery. *Br. J. Ophthal.* **68**, 97–104

SIGBAND, D. (1986). RGPs for extended wear: still far off? *Contact Lens Forum* **11**(6), 24–27

STARK, W. J., KRACHER, G. P., COWAN, C. L. *et al.* (1979). Extended wear contact lenses and intraocular lenses for aphakic corrections. *Am. J. Ophthal.* **88**, 535–542

VAN RIJ, G. and WARING, G. (1984). Changes in corneal curvature induced by sutures and incisions. *Am. J. Ophthal.* **98**, 773–783

WEISSMAN, B. and GARDNER, K. (1984). Power and radius changes induced in soft contact lens systems by flexure. *Am. J. Optom. physiol. Optics* **61**, 239–245

Postkeratoplasty
E. G. Woodward

It is just over 100 years since the first successful lamellar corneal graft was performed by von Hippel (1888). The surgery took place in 1886 and 2 years later von Hippel reported that the patient's vision had improved from counting fingers to 6/60. In 1905 the first penetrating keratoplasty which remained clear and transparent was carried out by Edward Zirm on a patient who was blind as a result of lime burns.

Currently about 1400 corneal transplants are carried out each year in the UK and 12500 in the USA (Casey and Mayer, 1984). The number of procedures is steadily increasing all over the world, but in many countries religious beliefs inhibit or prohibit donation of eyes.

Indications for keratoplasty

The indications for keratoplasty may be considered as any or all of the following: optical; tectonic; therapeutic; cosmetic.

Patients in all of these groups may have worn contact lenses prior to surgery and may, in fact, have failed with contact lens wear.

In the first group the most common indication, in the Western World, is keratoconus and it also has the best prognosis (Polack, 1977). Other frequent indications in the other groups are: stromal scarring following herpetic keratitis, corneal dystrophies, interstitial keratitis and trauma. In the Middle East, Africa and the Far East, trachoma, pterygium and measles keratitis are major indications for keratoplasty. The least successful outcome is usually considered to be with chemical burns, particularly alkaline burns. Despite repeated grafting long-term results are poor (Brown, Bloomfield and Pearce, 1974).

The term 'tectonic' is used in grafting in its 'building' sense. For example, if a cornea is very thin a large lamellar graft (tectonic) may be performed so that subsequently a smaller optical penetrating graft will have a reasonably thick corneal host to suture into. In other words it is building up the cornea for later further surgery. A tectonic graft yields no immediate visual gain; in fact in the short term it may render the cornea more opaque.

Following keratoplasty for an optical indication contact lenses may be used to maximize the visual improvement and for any indication they can have a role as a therapeutic device. Since chronologically contact lenses are more likely to be used initially in a therapeutic mode, this application will now be considered.

Postkeratoplasty therapeutic lenses

Where an existing graft has perforated, a silicone rubber therapeutic lens may be used to re-form the anterior chamber (Woodward, 1984). This can be a useful temporizing device, before regrafting, if theatre time or suitable donor material is not immediately available. The flattest available silicone rubber plano lens is inserted, this usually having a back surface radius of 8.40 mm. As the perforation seals and the anterior chamber re-forms the lens becomes too flat and needs to be fitted more steeply. The relative rigidity of a silicone rubber lens is necessary for successful sealing of a perforation. If such a lens is not available a low water content hydrogel may be tried but is rarely successful. In some countries, corneal perforations have been treated by plugging the hole with cyanoacrylate glue and then applying a bandage soft lens to protect the lid from the rough glue surface.

It is not usual to fit therapeutic lenses routinely, following keratoplasty, but this management is advised in certain circumstances: after lamellar or penetrating grafts for chemical burns where the donor epithelium has been retained (Casey and Mayer, 1984), also follow-

Table 21.3 Therapeutic lenses: stock forms

Lens type	Back optic zone radii (mm)	Total diameter (mm)
Bausch & Lomb lenses		
Plano T	8.10	14.70
O4	8.10	14.50
B4	8.10	14.50
Permalens	8.00, 9.00	15.00
Weicon 72	8.00–9.40	14.00
Hoya	8.10, 8.70	14.10, 14.50
Lunelle	7.70, 8.00, 8.30, 8.60, 8.90	13.00, 14.00

ing corneoscleral grafting where failure to re-epithelialize is anticipated.

The decision to fit a therapeutic lens is usually occasioned by one of the following situations:

(1) Where there are protruding sutures which cannot or must not be removed. These cause discomfort to the patient and attract mucus. This may act as a nidus for infection and also stimulate vessel growth.
(2) If there is a leak due to faulty suturing, demonstrated by a positive Seidel's sign.
(3) Failure to re-epithelialize, or epithelial ulceration.
(4) Where a shallow anterior chamber follows grafting combined with surgery for glaucoma.
(5) Where graft dehiscence has followed premature removal of sutures.

The choice of therapeutic lens is crucial and a number of different lens designs and materials is necessary.

Therapeutic plano hydrogel lenses are manufactured as stock lenses by several companies and the more popular ones are given in *Table 21.3*.

Unfortunately in the early stages after grafting, where a lens is most likely to be needed, the majority of these forms are too small or too steep. It is absolutely essential to obtain good cover with therapeutic lenses on grafted eyes. Most grafts at this stage, even when not leaking, are flatter than the surrounding host cornea. Because of this, in order to obtain good cover and good centration, larger, flatter lenses are necessary. At Moorfields Eye Hospital the most frequently used lens forms for therapeutic use on grafted eyes are 9.00/15.00 and 9.50/16.50. Ruben (1978) has suggested the use of a thin

Table 21.4 Therapeutic lens materials

	Fully hydrated water content (%)	Swell factor	Oxygen permeability (Dk value at 21°C)
Hoya	35	1.16	7.0
Bausch & Lomb			
HEMA	38	1.20	8.9
Duragel 75	75	1.64	40.0
Sauflon 85	78	1.75	41.0
Sauflon 70	62	1.50	26.0
Weicon 72	72	1.62	36.6
Permalens	72	1.43	39.0

trapezoid lens on recently grafted eyes, this lens having a peripheral curve which is steeper than the central one.

Some of the hydrogel materials commonly used for therapeutic lenses are listed in *Table 21.4*.

As might be anticipated, materials with a high oxygen permeability are usually indicated, thus causing minimum metabolic embarrassment to a physiologically fragile new graft. The advantage of a high swell factor is that, for a given blank size, a larger lens can be manufactured, allowing more scope in lens ordering. Lower water content materials are indicated where there are leaks or graft dehiscence as they form a firmer seal.

Lenses should be made as thin as possible, compatible with reasonable handling. Insertion of lenses should be as aseptic and atraumatic as possible; very thin plano lenses can be extremely difficult to manipulate particularly on a painful and tender eye.

Postkeratoplasty optical lenses

It is usual to wait for the removal of sutures before optically powered contact lenses are fitted, but this sequence is not inviolate. If there are pressing social reasons, such as the retention of employment, lenses are sometimes fitted before suture removal. The grafted eye may be the only seeing eye, but if it has poor vision with spectacles the patient is thus unable to function adequately. Keratoconic patients may be at a crucial time in their career or training, or responsible for young children.

Fitting with sutures *in situ* is not considered likely to increase the risk of graft rejection but

any contact lens-induced corneal oedema can cause vessel entry along the suture tracks (Steele, A. D. McG., 1987, personal communication). In view of this, patients should be instructed to wear their lenses in 4- or 5-hour stretches only, with a break of at least 1 hour in between. When the sutures are eventually removed the eye invariably needs re-fitting and this should be explained to the patient in advance.

A corneal graft is an attempt to simulate a normal cornea in a normal eye, and in fitting contact lenses it is necessary to consider how successful that simulation has been (Woodward, 1981). Basic measurements demonstrate that both its physiology and topography cannot be considered normal and that a grafted eye lacks many of the inbuilt safety margins of the normal eye, and must be regarded with particular caution.

The variations from the normal will now be considered.

Keratoplasty thickness

Immediately following transplantation the donor button is extremely oedematous; its thickness then gradually returns to normal levels. In the first year postgraft, while steroids are still being used and sutures *in situ*, the grafted cornea may be thinner than normal (Bourne, 1983). However, if corneal thickness is measured when all treatment has ceased and the sutures removed, the vast majority of grafts are thicker than normal. Ruben, Colebrook and Guillon (1979) in a study on 51 successfully grafted eyes showed an average graft thickness of 0.60 mm and only 15% were within the normal limits of thickness. There was no correlation between the age of the graft and thickness but there was correlation between visual acuity and graft thickness, visual acuity falling significantly when the cornea was thicker than 0.62 mm. The implication of these findings is that, even with successful clear grafts, the majority are slightly oedematous even before the application of a contact lens.

Graft endothelial morphology

Brown and Bron (1974) first showed that in many successful clear grafts, individual endothelial cells are very much enlarged. It is now thought that most endothelial cell damage occurs at the time of keratoplasty, with more cells lost from the peripheral graft and recipient cornea nearer the junction than from the central graft. Cells are 'lost' from the central graft as they gradually move towards peripheral areas with larger cells, this slow process of cellular realignment lasting for approximately 3 years (Bourne, 1983). Ruben, Colebrook and Guillon (1979), on the same group of patients whose corneal thickness was measured, showed a mean cell count of 1226.02 ± 393.84 cells for their graft group as against 3233.62 ± 328.38 for a matched control group.

Although corneal thickness near to normal limits may be maintained with endothelial cell counts less than a third of normal, clinical experience indicates that a cornea with a low endothelial cell density is more vulnerable to extraneous conditions which might induce corneal oedema. Thus the occlusive action of a contact lens to oxygen may be just too much for the cornea to cope with.

Graft sensitivity

Ruben and Colebrook (1979b) measured the corneal sensitivity of 50 successfully grafted eyes using the Cochet and Bonnet aesthesiometer. Their findings are shown in *Table 21.5*.

On a normal cornea, central sensitivity is considerably higher than peripheral, but on a typical grafted eye, the reverse applies. Other findings by these workers showed that 14.6% of the grafted eyes had no measurable central sensation at all and that no instances of normal corneal sensation were found until at least 3 years after surgery. The last finding is significant in that most patients who are fitted with contact lenses tend to be fitted fairly soon after sutures are removed, which may be anything from 6 to 18 months after keratoplasty. This means that the majority of patients are fitted

Table 21.5 Results of Ruben and Colebrook (1979b) on corneal sensitivity of successfully grafted eyes

Corneal position	Maximum mean length of monofilament just felt (cm)
Graft centre	1.80
Peripheral cornea	2.66

(A normal reading is 4 cm centrally)

when their central corneal sensation is significantly reduced, if not absent. Furthermore, Millodot (1971) has shown that contact lens wear depresses corneal sensation even further.

This reduction in central sensitivity does not seem to make contact lens fitting any easier. Probably this is because there is no concurrent reduction in lid margin sensitivity; indeed the recent presence of corneal sutures seems sometimes to have increased lid sensitivity, although this is not mentioned in the literature. Nevertheless the patients do not experience the normal discomfort produced by a corneal abrasion or corneal oedema. The symptoms, denoting corneal oedema, about which grafted patients complain, are nearly always visual ones.

Graft topography

When grafts are examined by photokeratoscopy it is found that there are no regular corneal grafts. Ruben and Colebrook (1979a) demonstrated that even the clearest corneal graft giving 6/5 unaided vision has only a small area (2–3 mm) of sphericity. Their results also confirmed the clinical impression of many contact lens practitioners concerning postgraft astigmatism, namely a decrease in postgraft astigmatism in a group wearing contact lenses as compared with those who did not, suggesting an advantageous moulding effect on the graft, particularly if sutures have been removed.

The irregularities of corneal grafts militate against successful contact lens fitting in several ways.

Nipple-like protrusion

Most grafts are steeper than the host cornea and protrude slightly in a nipple-like manner (*Figure 21.5*).

This protuberance has been attributed to the second anchor zone of collagen produced by scarring at the donor–host junction coupled with the lower rigidity of the graft itself, due to its increased thickness or higher water content, or both. Some grafts are also oversized by 0.2–0.3 mm in order to provide a better donor–host junction seal. This oversizing also exacerbates graft protruberance (*Plates 98* and *100*). Whatever the cause, guttering formed by the abrupt change in curvature at the donor–host junction can cause problems to the

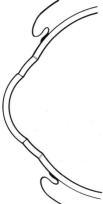

Figure 21.5 Corneal graft in section; seen to be steeper than the host cornea, giving the effect of a nipple-like protrusion

Table 21.6 Keratoconus: method of correction after keratoplasty

Method	No. of cases
Unaided	4
Spectacles	31
Corneal lenses	46
Scleral lenses	18
Hydrogel lenses	1
Hydrogel lenses plus spectacles	4
Total	104

contact lens practitioner. If the lens covers this area there is a likelihood of bubbles collecting. If the edge of the lens is near this sudden change of curvature, excessive stand-off occurs and the lens is unstable.

Graft toricity

As indicated previously there are no completely regular corneal grafts and all are toroidal to some degree. Ruben (M., 1980, personal communication) has reported that elliptical grafts with 1 mm difference between the major and minor axes produce less astigmatism, but these are technically difficult to perform. The astigmatism produced by a corneal graft, usually irregular, is one of the main reasons why contact lens correction gives superior visual acuity to that with spectacles in the majority of cases.

Davies, Ruben and Woodward (1977) gave the method of optical correction following 100 grafts for keratoconus as shown in *Table 21.6*.

As can be seen 65% of patients needed some form of contact lens correction because of unacceptable visual distortion produced by significant degrees of corneal astigmatism. In this sample 65% of the patients had more than 2 D of astigmatism, 23% between 4 D and 7 D and some were as high as 12 D (*Figure 21.6*).

Currently it is likely that the higher degrees of postgraft corneal astigmatism would be corrected surgically, the two favoured techniques being a relaxing incision or a wedge resection.

A toroidal graft in a spherical host cornea produces guttering in one meridian only. In *Figure 21.7* the vertical meridian shows this.

Graft tilting

A graft may register only a low or moderate degree of astigmatism when measured with the keratometer, yet when a corneal contact lens is

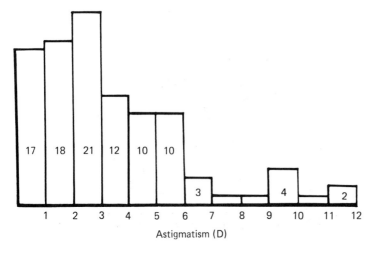

Figure 21.6 Distribution of postoperative astigmatism in keratoplasty following keratoconus (Davies, Ruben and Woodward, 1977). The figures given in the histogram are percentages

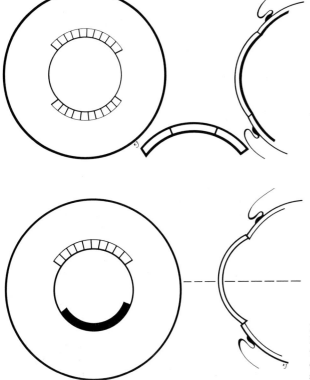

Figure 21.7 Guttering (shown hatched on the left-hand diagram) at the upper and lower graft–host junctions due to the host cornea being spherical whereas the graft is toroidal. The cross-sectional diagrams show the guttering in the vertical meridian (right hand side) and the smooth graft–host junction in the horizontal meridian (lower diagram)

Figure 21.8 Tilted graft. The hatched area on the left-hand diagram shows where the graft tissue is proud whilst the black area shows where it is recessed. This can be seen more clearly in the right-hand cross-sectional diagram

fitted it will not centre and shows excessive stand-off in one area. This is usually due to the graft being tilted in relation to the host cornea (*Figure 21.8*).

If the lens is large enough to bridge the graft there will also be a localized guttering effect. In *Figure 21.8* this would be outside the graft superiorly but within the graft inferiorly. Tilted grafts present a severe problem to the contact lens practitioner and it is difficult to avoid persistent bubbles over a recessed area. However a stationary bubble can soon induce neovascularization and must be avoided.

Graft eccentricity

When grafting a keratoconic eye most surgeons centre their graft on the thinnest part of the cornea which is rarely, if ever, on the visual axis of the eye. In the case of scarring produced by keratitis the graft is usually centred on what was the most densely scarred area. The implications of this are that a lens designed to centre on the graft may be well off the eye's visual axis (*Figure 21.9*).

Furthermore, although the postoperative complication of a dilated pupil, shallow anterior chamber and raised intraocular pressure (Uretts–Zavalia syndrome) is now considered rare, a partially dilated or sluggishly reacting pupil is not an uncommon sequel to keratoplasty.

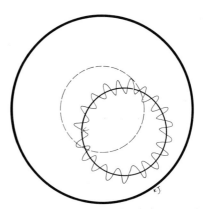

Figure 21.9 An eccentric graft shown relative to pupil position, making contact lens centring relative to the visual axis extremely difficult to achieve

Fitting procedures

Generally the fitting of grafted eyes follows conventional practice for irregular eyes. However the physiological limitations of the grafted cornea must never be forgotten and due awareness maintained for any signs of distress in the graft. Toric lenses are not commonly necessary. Although high graft astigmatism is one of the main indications for fitting, the remaining host cornea is usually regular and the necessity for the prescribing of toroidal back surface lenses is no more than on normal eyes. Toroidal front surface lenses are sometimes necessary for visual reasons.

The majority of grafts become more regular with time after suture removal and it is usual for the eye to require re-fitting at least once in the first 3 years. It is also extremely difficult to design a suitable fitting set for grafted eyes. This is especially so for recently grafted eyes and most are fitted by a combination of an eclectic fitting set and serendipity (*Plate 99*).

Hydrogel lenses

As might be anticipated from the optical indications, hydrogel lenses are rarely fitted for visual reasons. In addition this type of lens may have a greater occlusive effect than a smaller gas permeable lens. As can be seen from *Table 21.6*, patients fitted with hydrogel lenses usually require additional spectacles to obtain optimum visual acuity. A situation where they may perform satisfactorily on their own occurs when combined or separate surgical procedures have rendered the patient aphakic. Here the greater central thickness of the lens reduces any residual astigmatism. Even in this circumstance the lens material needs to be of low or medium water content. Extended wear, with the exception of thin plano therapeutic lenses, is definitely contra-indicated with present generation materials.

Scleral lenses

The necessity for the use of scleral lenses has declined in recent years. This is mainly due to the refinement of surgical techniques for the reduction of graft astigmatism. Relieving incisions and wedge resections are both more effective and more predictable than earlier techniques. Nevertheless there are occasions where a scleral lens is the only possible form of optical correction. On such irregular eyes the impression technique is the only feasible one (*Plate 84*) and this is fully described in Chapter 18. The best results seem to be obtained with minimum clearance over the graft itself. A fluorescein picture which, on an ungrafted eye, would suggest the need for more central clearance, is often satisfactory. Bubbles impinging on the graft itself must be avoided as they can be a stimulus to graft vascularization. However, adequate limbal clearance is most important. A sequence of obtaining good limbal clearance, first by hand grinding the transitional region of the lens and subsequently achieving central clearance by grinding with a diamond tool, is the most successful approach.

Corneal lenses

The majority of lenses currently fitted following corneal grafting are corneal lenses manufactured from gas permeable materials. On grafts of long standing, where corneal topography begins to approximate to the normal, it may be possible to fit lenses of conventional design. But on more recently grafted eyes, aggregation of the various corneal irregularities described earlier, often produces a surface on which conventional design lenses will not centre on or near the visual axis. In order to obtain centration it is usually necessary to fit a larger lens.

When the only rigid lens material available was polymethyl methacrylate (PMMA), fitting a larger lens usually produced graft oedema even where fenestrations were incorporated to improve tear exchange. The advent of rigid lens materials designed to have significant permeability to gases suggested their use for the larger lenses required on grafted eyes and these have been used from 1977 (Woodward, 1981).

The first material used was one of the cellulose acetate butyrates (CABs), which by contemporary standards has a low oxygen permeability. Notwithstanding this, lens designs which produced graft oedema when manufactured from PMMA often did not do so when produced from CAB. It is unlikely that the relatively small increase in oxygen permeability was solely responsible for this, the lower wetting angle of CAB probably also having a beneficial effect. Possibly this lower wetting angle combined with some gas transmissibility alters the frictional forces between the posterior lens surface and tears in such a manner that there is better tear exchange beneath a lens manufactured from CAB than the same design in PMMA. Even with the highly permeable lenses available today a reasonably low wetting angle is still necessary for fitting grafted eyes.

These larger lenses vary between 10.0 mm and 12.0 mm and are of a simple bi-curve or tri-curve construction. As the intention is essentially to span both the graft and the irregular host–donor junction, it is essential that the back optic zone diameter be larger than the diameter of the graft itself (*Figure 21.10*).

Currently the majority of grafts performed have diameters between 7.0 and 8.0 mm. Hence the BOZDs of lenses prescribed vary between 8.0 mm and 10.0 mm. With a BOZD of 8.0 mm or 9.0 mm for a bi-curve lens of 10.0 mm total diameter, the BPR usually needs to be approximately 1.00 mm flatter than the BOZR, for example:

C2/8.30:8.00/9.30:10.00.

With larger lenses the flattening needs to be greater, for example:

C2/8.30:9.50/10.00:11.00

or

C2/8.30:10.00/11.50:12.00.

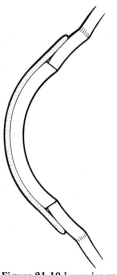

Figure 21.10 Irregular graft–host junction being spanned by the back optic zone of a corneal lens

As suggested earlier it is almost impossible to design a dedicated fitting set for postkeratoplasty fitting. Most practitioners build one up from unsuccessful lenses! It should be explained to the patient that the definitive lens will probably not be achieved with the first fitting and this lens may have to serve as a subsequent fitting lens.

Keratometry represents curvature measurements taken near the centre of the graft so is not of great value in fitting. For these relatively large lenses, however, the flatter keratometry reading can be considered as an indication of an appropriate BOZR for a first lens. Fenestrations are often employed, usually two or three 0.30 mm diameter holes 2 mm from the lens edge. Their function is not so much to enhance tear ingress, but to avoid the trapping of static bubbles (*Plate 99*). These frequently occur where the graft is slightly raised from the host cornea producing a gutter (*Plate 100*).

Over a period of years the graft–host interface tends to become less irregular and it may be possible to fit lenses of a more conventional size. Where this is possible the Ruben Offset 2 design (described under Keratoconus, p. 753) will usually centre more satisfactorily than symmetrical multi-curve designs. Even at this stage it is most unusual to obtain the same clearance all around the lens periphery.

In essence the fitting of grafted eyes demands ingenuity in lens design and the thoughtful use of materials. Furthermore, whatever type of lens is fitted the intrinsic vulnerability of the grafted cornea must not be forgotten.

References

BOURNE, W. M. (1983). Morphologic and functional evaluation of the transplanted human cornea. *Trans. Am. ophthal. Soc.* **81**, 403–450

BROWN, N. A. P. and BRON, A. J. (1974). Endothelium of the corneal graft. *Trans ophthal. Soc. UK* **94**, 863–870

BROWN, S. I., BLOOMFIELD, S. E. and PEARCE, D. B. (1974). A follow up on transplantation of the alkali burned cornea. *Am. J. Ophthal.* **77**, 538–541

CASEY, T. A. and MAYER, D. J. (1984). *Corneal Grafting.* Philadelphia: W. B. Saunders

DAVIES, P. D., RUBEN, M. and WOODWARD, E. G. (1977). Keratoconus: an analysis of the factors which affect the optical results of keratoplasty. *Transactions of the European Contact Lens Society of Ophthalmologists*, Ghent, pp. 97–99

MILLODOT, M. (1971). Corneal sensitivity and contact lenses. *Optician* **162**, 23–24

POLACK, F. M. (1977). *Corneal Transplantation*. New York Grune & Stratton

RUBEN, M. (1978). *Soft Contact Lenses*. London: Baillière Tindall

RUBEN, M. and COLEBROOK, E. (1979a). Keratoconus, keratoplasty curvatures and lens wear. *Br. J. Ophthal.* **63**, 268–273

RUBEN, M. and COLEBROOK, E. (1979b). Keratoplasty sensitivity. *Br. J. Ophthal.* **63**, 256–257

RUBEN, M., COLEBROOK, E. and GUILLON, M. (1979). Keratoconus, keratoplasty thickness and endothelial morphology. *Br. J. Ophthal.* **63**, 790–793

VON HIPPEL, A. (1888). *Albrecht van Graefes Arch. Ophthal.* **34**, 108–110

WOODWARD, E. G. (1981). Contact lens fitting after keratoplasy. *J. Br. Contact Lens Ass.* **4**(2), 42–49

WOODWARD, E. G. (1984). Therapeutic silicone rubber lenses. *J. Br. Contact Lens Ass.* **7**(1), 39–41

Postradial keratotomy
Christine Astin

Radial keratotomy (RK) is a surgical procedure for reduction of myopia by incision into the anterior portion of the cornea, avoiding a central zone of 3–4 mm diameter (*Figure 21.11* and *Plate 101a*). No sutures or other supports are involved. The procedure and effect of the number of incisions (usually 8 or 16 equally spaced) have been described in several papers (Fyodorov and Durnev, 1979; Reddy and Reddy, 1980; Nirankani *et al.*, 1982). The incision depth is usually 90–95% of the previously measured central corneal thickness. Some surgeons cut to a depth equal to central thickness, but in so doing risk perforations of Descemet's membrane. The rigidity of the cornea is decreased such that intraocular forces act on the cornea, causing midperipheral regions to 'bulge' forwards (*Figure 21.12*), effectively giving an apical cap of longer radius of curvature than measured preoperatively. This flatter central curvature has less refractive power and results in a hypermetropic shift, hence reducing the original myopia. The extent of this and its relation to the curvature changes have been investigated by a number of researchers: Yenaliev (1979), Binder (1981), Bores, Myers and Cowden (1981), Cowden and Cichocki (1981), Gonzalez (1981), Hoffer *et al.* (1981), Jester *et al.* (1981), Yamaguchi *et al.* (1981), Arrowsmith, Sanders and Marks (1983), Waring *et al.* (1983), Steele (1984) and Astin (1989). The corneal power change is usually greatest within the first few days postoperatively. During the following months (in some cases 12 months), the incisions heal with scar tissue or new collagen, the corneal rigidity increases and induces a change in the corneal shape returning towards the original shape and power, with variability in healing in each case. Central keratometry readings at intervals show the radius of curvature gradually decreasing from the postoperative value, but still tending to remain greater than the preoperative value. Current studies indicate stabilization by 1–2 years.

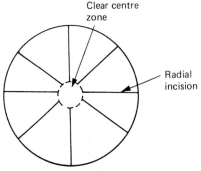

Figure 21.11 Incision pattern in radial keratotomy

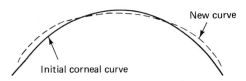

Figure 21.12 Midperipheral corneal region presses forwards, postradial keratotomy

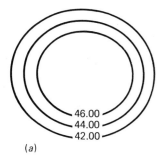

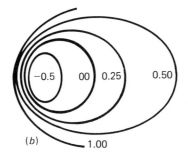

(a)

(b)

46.00
44.00
42.00

−0.5   00   0.25   0.50

1.00

Figure 21.13 (a) Ellipses of identical shape factors (0.25) but different central curvatures. (b) Ellipses of identical central curvatures but different shape factors. (After Bibby, 1976)

Example

Patient H	Pre-operative	Post-operative	1 year later
Keratometry (mm)	7.42 al 180	7.90 al 180	7.88 al 180
	7.29 al 90	7.75 al 90	7.73 al 90

It has been found (Townsley, 1970) that the shape of a high percentage of human corneas is similar to part of an ellipse or parabola, or hyperbola or circle. These are all examples of conic sections, and require two independent parameters to define them: central curvature to define size (*Figure 21.13a*); 'shape factor' (*SF*)* which defines shape or asphericity (*Figure 21.13b*). The latter is a convenient way of describing e, the eccentricity of a conic section, since $SF = e^2$.

Positive 'shape factors' (usual for normal corneas) imply the more pointed (prolate) end of an ellipse, i.e. the radius of curvature of the corneal surface, increases as one proceeds towards the limbus. The 'shape factor' of a circle is zero. As the 'shape factor' value increases, the contour appears less circular and more elliptical (*see also* Chapter 10, p. 336).

After radial keratotomy, the 'shape factor' drastically alters showing a progression towards negative values. Even after the eye reverts towards its original shape during the postoperative months, there is usually a permanent negative 'shape factor' value.

Example

Patient H	Pre-operative	Post-operative	1 year later
Horizontal *SF*	+0.28	−0.32	−0.26
Vertical *SF*	+0.05	−0.35	−0.24

* Not to be confused with the more common use of the term 'shape factor' as one component of spectacle magnification (*see* Chapter 5).

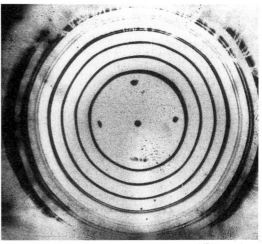

(a)

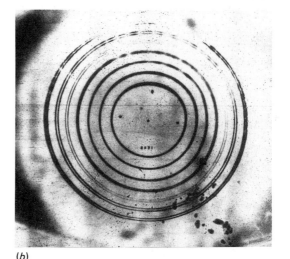

(b)

Figure 21.14 (a) PEK photograph showing octagonal shaped reflected mires, postradial keratotomy. (b) PEK photograph showing smaller reflected mires, preradial keratotomy

This may be shown on the analysis of photo-graphs with a photo-electronic keratograph (PEK) taken at intervals. After an eight-incision operation, the PEK photographs show octagon-al-shaped reflected mires (*Figure 21.14a*). These gradually settle over the following months to a smooth set of concentric ring mire images, although the central rings have a wider diameter than those of the preoperative photographs (*Figure 21.14b*), since they are reflected by a flatter corneal surface (Astin, 1986).

Problems with radial keratotomy

Optical changes

Radial keratotomy may give a good result as measured by visual acuity assessment on the Snellen chart, but there may be visual impair-ment still residual from the operation. Examples are given below.

Anisometropia

There may be up to 9 D difference between the ocular refraction of each eye, possibly leading to diplopia and disturbed binocular fusion. In quite a number of patients, even if *both* eyes undergo the operation, one eye may revert in power nearer to its preoperative value than does the other eye. This residual anisometropia can be very disturbing in respect of the retinal image sizes and to the relative prismatic effects of corrective spectacles.

Diurnal fluctuation of vision

Cowden and Bores (1981) found with two-thirds of their 20 study cases, that this can give problems. Some patients have best vision in the morning, others are best in the evening, but many find difficulty during the day when spectacles are insufficient. Generally, a central steepening of anterior corneal curvature occurs in these patients as the day progresses, necessi-tating evening use of spectacles or contact lenses for some patients. This can be very inconven-ient. Rowsey and Balyeat (1982) noted that most patients eventually stabilized at a point close to their evening refractive status, but were unable to determine what relation the problem had to the number of incisions.

The 'prospective evaluation of radial kerato-tomy' (PERK) study led by Waring *et al.* (1983), indicated that approximately one-third of the subjects experienced this fluctuation and that the refractive variation was greater for cases with diamond knife incisions than with razor blades. It has been speculated that corneal hydration and lid squeezing play a role in this problem.

Astigmatism

This may increase and still result in unsatisfac-tory vision, even if the degree of myopia is diminished. The amount of astigmatism can also vary during the day, and so be impossible to correct with spectacles. Persistent irregular astigmatism may result from combined patterns or erroneous incisions near the visual axis. An example of postoperative astigmatism is given below.

Patient E	Preoperative measurements:	2 years' postoperative measurements:
Refraction	$-1.25/-4.00 \times 15$	$-0.50/-5.00 \times 20$
VA	6/6	6/9
Keratometry (mm)	8.63 al 10	9.20 al 15
	7.99 al 100	8.45 al 105

Fitted with HEMA soft toric lens: 9.00: 14.0 × 12.5
$-0.50/-4.00 \times 15$
VA   6/7.5

Post-lens wear measurements:
Vision   6/24
Refraction $+0.50/-3.50 \times 20$
VA   6/6
Keratometry (mm)   9.32 al 15
8.56 al 105

Increased sensitivity to glare

This and difficulty with detailed vision in dim illumination seem to correlate with the size of the optical zone and the width of the incisional scars. Tests carried out using the clinical glare tester developed by Miller and Miller (1981) indicated that for pupil dilatation above 5 mm, 40% of their 80 patients experienced disturbing glare sensitivity above the 20% level. Glare gradually diminishes as the scar density de-creases up to 5 months, but in some patients the complaint persists.

Residual ametropia

This may not be as minor as the patient hoped. Patients may complain that their unaided vision is unsatisfactory and demand a repeat operation, although this gives an even less predictable result than the first attempt and increases the risk of endothelial damage. Regression of the corneal contour towards its preoperative shape is more likely if the incisions have been less deep than intended, either related to surgical blade problems or decreased intraocular pressure.

Physiological changes

The 4-year study on radial keratotomy changes, led by Steele (1984) revealed minimal physiological side effects and no measurable rate of endothelial cell loss. What is still unknown is the extent to which radial keratotomy will affect the remaining endothelial cell population in future, including corneal surgery with risk of delayed wound healing.

Bores, Myers and Cowden (1981) noted several small corneal changes seen by slit lamp biomicroscopy, and commented on difficulties with contact lens fitting. They noted vessel ingrowth along incision scars after extended wear of soft contact lenses within 4–6 weeks postoperatively. In the incisions was noted the occasional appearance of the following: epithelial inclusion cysts, epithelial ferrous lines, degenerative blood products, foreign bodies, blood vessels, focal thickening of Descemet's membrane, small dense scars. Less myopia reduction was exhibited when such features were present. Perforations have become rarer since more accurate pachometry and calibrated operating knives became available, although some cases of recurrent epithelial erosions or map–dot–fingerprint changes in the basement membrane have been reported (*see* p. 803).

Waring (1984) has enumerated the following *serious physiological risks*:

(1) Cataract.
(2) Endophthalmitis.
(3) Bacterial keratitis.
(4) Endothelial damage and persistent corneal oedema.

In the 1930s, Sato made the radial incisions in the *posterior* cornea but these resulted in permanent oedema 10 years later (Akiyama, 1984). Modern techniques seem to give little endothelial damage although there is increased permeability.

Traumatic globe rupture

Several laboratory studies have shown that the globe ruptures more easily through the keratotomy wounds (Larsen *et al.*, 1983). Cases involving humans are as yet rare (John and Schmitt, 1983).

Why contact lens fitting may still be necessary

(1) Residual astigmatism.
(2) Residual ametropia.
(3) Anisometropia.
(4) To stabilize vision either by 'supporting' the cornea, or providing a corrective tear liquid lens between the rigid contact lens and the fluctuating corneal shape.
(5) To make glare less noticeable.

Postradial keratotomy contact lens fitting and problems

Soft (hydrophilic) contact lenses (Astin, 1986)

Where possible, corneal thickness and topography should be measured at after-care visits to assess whether the contact lens is affecting the eye, and also repeated at different times during the day to measure diurnal variation despite contact lens wear.

For soft lens fitting, the diameter of the first choice lens should be at least 1–2 mm greater than the horizontal visible iris diameter. For 38% water content HEMA lenses of standard thickness range (0.15–0.30 mm), the back optic zone radius (BOZR) of the first lens chosen should be 0.50–0.80 mm flatter than the flattest central keratometry reading. For high water content lenses (e.g. 60–75%) and for ultrathin lenses (e.g. 0.06–0.12 mm thickness) the BOZR could be chosen as 0.20–0.40 mm flatter than the flattest central keratometer reading. Close observation of the lens centration and movement after 20–30 minutes settling time should be made. The lens should centre correctly on the cornea but give 1–2 mm movement on full blinks. There should be neither conjunctival indentation nor vessel blanching. Some practitioners prefer to fit soft lenses since the lenses 'wrap round' the cornea and seem a simpler fit on an unusual shaped eye. There is also less edge sensation, and flexible lenses are often less mobile and less inclined to decentre than corneal lenses. Easier adaptation and the large BOZD are advantages. Some patients prefer them as the lenses seem easier to handle and give less spectacle blur than corneal lenses may have done during previous wear before radial keratotomy. Careful over-refraction should be carried out and the patient warned that visual variability may still occur even though the large BOZD should give good pupil coverage.

Some practitioners may choose standard thickness soft contact lenses to 'mask' some residual astigmatism, ignoring the reduction in oxygen transmissibility, and the increased pressure on the cornea leading to greater corneal curvature changes, and increased risk of vessel ingrowth.

Problems which may arise with soft hydrophilic contact lens fitting

In unoperated eyes, the soft lens fit can vary with hydration of the lens and between individuals with differing peripheral corneal contours even if central keratometry is similar. Hence, on a radial keratotomy patient, there is the added difficulty of the diurnal variation in corneal contour and power. It is best to wait until the cornea has stabilized before attempting fitting and in any case a tight fit should be avoided.

Shivitz et al. (1986) outline the increased incidence of corneal stromal vessel growth following soft contact lens fitting. It is questioned whether the operation alters the oxygen requirements of the cornea or the mode of oxygen flow through the stroma. The factor of endothelial cell loss was revealed by a number of studies of radial keratotomy on non-human primates, carried out by Binder et al. (1984). A study on human endothelium was made by Cowden and Sultana (1982). Steele's (1984) study did not reveal any measurable loss of endothelial cells.

Even if a lens of high oxygen transmissibility is fitted, there may be pressure at the limbus (or negative fluid pressure between the lens and the eye) which could affect corneal curvature and other changes.

Another possibility is that the flexing of imperfectly healed corneal segments acts as a stimulus to neovascularization. Therefore extended or prolonged wear of contact lenses is not recommended and some evidence of vessel growth along the scar lines was reported by Bores, Myers and Cowden (1981). Soft lenses can retain deposits and foreign bodies more easily and so give an increased risk of epithelial erosions and infection, particularly in some cases where there is poor healing of the epithelium over the incisions. Gelender, Flynn and Mendelbaum (1982) and Karr, Grutzmacher and Reeh (1985) have discussed complications in radial keratotomy cases, such as infection and epithelial healing problems.

An example of a soft lens fitting is given below.

Patient H	2 years' postoperative measurements:
Vision	6/18
Refraction	$-1.00/-1.00 \times 170$
VA	6/6
Keratometry (mm)	7.70 al 5
	7.60 al 110
HEMA soft lens fitted	8.70:13.50 -1.00 VA 6/5

This lens was more stable than a rigid lens and suited to a variety of wearing times for work. Wearing time was kept low to avoid vessel hyperaemia or ingrowth. Post-lens wear results were surprisingly good:

	Post-lens wear measurements:
Vision	6/4
Keratometry (mm)	7.97 al 180
	7.84 al 90

Rigid contact lenses

A gas permeable material is recommended because the use of PMMA may lead to corneal oedema, which may not recover as quickly in a radial keratotomy patient, particularly if there has been endothelial cell loss. Oedema may then lead to disturbances in vision and steepening of the corneal curvature, and encourage neovascularization.

Irregular corneal astigmatism may develop after many years of wearing PMMA lenses and reduces if the ametrope is re-fitted with gas permeable lenses. A radial keratotomy patient may be more susceptible to induced corneal warping, which is a further reason for avoiding PMMA lenses.

The negative shape factor of the peripheral cornea makes the eye awkward to fit with a contact lens (*Figure 21.15* and *Plate 101b*). The

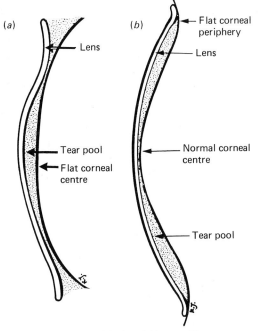

Figure 21.15 Standard design rigid corneal lens on (*a*) postradial keratotomy cornea and (*b*) normal cornea (diagrammatic)

steep 'knee' in the peripheral cornea and the fluctuation of the corneal topography may preclude adequate contact lens fitting.

Most fitting set lenses show excessive edge clearance and mobility on such an eye, since they are designed for the usual positive shape factor contours. Rather than fit steep and have the problem of excess central tear pooling with trapped bubbles and reduced tear flow, it is better to fit with a minimum edge clearance

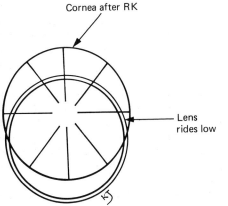

Figure 21.16 Standard design rigid corneal lens may ride low on postradial keratotomy cornea

design lens, e.g. Menicon O$_2$*, or elliptical back surface such as Persecon E† or Klaver‡, or redesign the peripheral curves of a tri-curve lens (*see* p. 778). The fitting takes longer but is necessary to avoid discomfort or decentred lenses. There is an increased risk of the lens either riding very low (*Figure 21.16*) or being held high by the upper eyelid due to the reduced area of corneal alignment.

Example

Patient B	2 years' postoperative measurements:
Vision	6/60
Refraction	$-3.00/-1.25 \times 40$
VA	6/6
Keratometry (mm)	8.54 al 5
	8.53 al 95

Fitted with gas permeable elliptical lens	Post-corneal lens wear measurements:
Vision	6/60
Refraction	$-3.00/-1.25 \times 40$
VA	6/6
Keratometry	8.52 al 15
	8.56 al 105

If the lens is held high, its lower edge projects, irritating the inferior lid margin on blinks, giving rise to frothing, dimpling, increased grease production and in some cases being decentred by the lid. Even if the lens power is adequate, the pupil may not be correctly covered by the optic zone, hence flare is experienced, particularly with pupil dilatation in dim illumination or when the patient looks down to read. Spherical aberration is also increased. After radial keratotomy the central corneal apical 'cap' is wider and needs a larger back optic zone diameter to cover it and give lens stability. Together with a steeper than usual peripheral curve, a large BOZD can be incorporated into a redesigned tri-curve lens to give a more stable fit with better pupil coverage, even if the lid tends to hold the lens high.

Such a lens may be more difficult to remove or recentre than lenses of conventional design.

A more steady fit and visual acuity can be obtained by fitting a larger rigid gas permeable lens with many features similar to those

*Menicon O$_2$ (*CooperVision Ltd*).
†Persecon E (*CIBA Vision, Titmus Eurocon Ltd*).
‡Klaver Elliptical (*Jack Allen Contact Lenses*).

involved when fitting an eye following kerato-plasty (*see* pp. 770–771). Care must be taken that the lens edge is not tight fitting and that there is not undue pressure on the midperi-pheral 'bulge' of the cornea. Good tear flow under the lens is essential. There may be slight central fluorescein pooling, which gives a positive liquid lens contribution so necessitating extra negative power in the contact lens to counteract it. Some practitioners fit steep lenses then fenestrate them to aid tear flow and release of bubbles. Fenestrations may be unnecessary if excessive central pooling is avoided and lens centration controlled by closer fitting peripheral curves which still allow good edge clearance.

Example

Patient L	5 years' postoperative measurement:
Vision	6/36
Refraction	$-1.25/-3.00 \times 170$
VA	6/5
Keratometry	9.16 al 170
	8.71 al 80
Fitted with gas permeable large lens	9.00:8.00/10.00:10.00/ 11.00:12.50 -2.00
VA	6/5 part
	Post-lens wear measurements:
Vision	6/24
Refraction	$-0.751/-2.50 \times 175$
VA	6/5
Keratometry (mm)	9.11 al 165
	8.70 al 75

Examples of corneal lens fitting sets for postradial keratotomy cases

Elliptical back surface rigid gas permeable lenses

(1) Persecon Elliptical*
BOZD 8.00 mm; TD 9.3, 9.8 and 10.3 mm;
BOZR 7.3–8.5 mm in 0.1-mm steps.
Materials: cellulose acetate butyrate; silicone-based copolymer of *Dk* value 54.
(2) Klaver Elliptical 'P'†
BOZD 8.00 mm; TD 9.3, 9.8 and 10.3 mm;
BOZR 7.3–8.5 mm in 0.1-mm steps.
Materials: wide variety of gas permeable types.

*Manufactured by CIBA Vision (Titmus Eurocon) in W. Germany.
†Manufactured by Jack Allen Ltd, England.

'Apex'-type tri-curve rigid gas permeable lenses

(1) Large size: TD 11.5 mm;
BOZR 7.5–8.5 mm in 0.1-mm steps;
BOZD 9.5 mm.
Examples of lens specifications:

(a) C3/7.5:9.5/9.5:10.5/10.5:11.5 BVP Plano
Axial lift at BPD_1 0.14 mm; AEL 0.37 mm;
FOZD 9.00 mm; FOZR 7.57 mm
Front carrier radius 9.30 mm;
t_c 0.20 mm; t_e 0.20 mm
(b) C3/8.0:9.5/10.0:10.5/11.0:11.5 BVP Plano
Axial lift at BPD_1 0.11 mm; AEL 0.30 mm;
FOZD 9.0 mm; FOZR 8.07 mm
Front carrier radius 9.81 mm;
t_c 0.20 mm; t_e 0.20 mm
(c) C3/8.5:9.5/10.5:10.5/11.5:11.5 BVP Plano
Axial lift at BPD_1 0.09 mm; AEL 0.25 mm;
FOZD 9.0 mm; FOZR 8.57 mm
Front carrier radius 10.32 mm;
t_c 0.20 mm; t_e 0.20 mm

(2) Medium size: TD 10.0 mm;
BOZR 7.5–8.5 mm in 0.1-mm steps;
BOZD 8.0 mm.
Examples of lens specifications:

(a) C3/7.5:8.0/8.5:9.0/9.5:10.0 BVP Plano
Axial lift at BPD_1 0.06 mm; AEL 0.18 mm;
FOZD 8.0 mm; FOZR 7.57 mm
Front carrier radius 8.88 mm;
t_c 0.20 mm; t_e 0.20 mm
(b) C3/8.0:8.0/9.0:9.0/10.0:10.0 BVP Plano
Axial lift at BPD_1 0.05 mm; AEL 0.15 mm;
FOZD 8.0 mm; FOZR 8.07 mm
Front carrier radius 9.38 mm;
t_c 0.20 mm; t_e 0.20 mm
(c) C3/8.5:8.0/9.5:9.0/10.5:10.0 BVP Plano
Axial lift at BPD_1 0.04 mm; AEL 0.12 mm;
FOZD 8.0 mm; FOZR 8.57 mm
Front carrier radius 9.88 mm;
t_c 0.20 mm; t_e 0.20 mm

Other methods of contact lens fitting for postradial keratotomy

In the USA methods of fitting the postkerato-tomy patient vary. Some practitioners prefer to fit with steep peripheral curves to assist centration of RGP lenses, and in some cases attempt controlled keratoreformation. Shivitz *et al.* (1986) found excessive lens movement when using standard fitting set lenses based on postoperative keratometry. To combat this they advised a steep fit, often with a large total diameter. The BOZRs were fitted steeper than the flattest postoperative keratometer reading by between 1.75 D (0.26 mm) and 11.38 D (2.05 mm), with an average of 5.91 D (1.09 mm)*. Due to the large pool of tears between the lens and the central cornea, the final refractive power of the contact lens was more negative than the spectacle refraction. To mitigate discomfort due to trapped air bubbles or excess tear pooling, the lenses were fenestrated.

Hydrophilic lenses fitted were steeper than those usually chosen for eyes with flat keratometer readings. Although used only for daily wear, neovascularization was noted after a mean of 7.5 months in 14 of the 21 cases with hydrophilic lenses.

Janes and Reichie (1986) suggested a steep fitting rigid lens and a large tear pool with BOZR of lens related to preoperative keratometry readings, and total diameter of 9.0–9.5 mm to assist centration. The first choice lens would be slightly flatter than mean preoperative keratometry, at a power midway between preoperative and postoperative refraction. Reichert (cited by Greco, 1986) advised using photokeratoscopy but choosing an initial lens based only on peripheral corneal measurements. He found that the central pool of tears led to corneal oedema but this was less significant with gas permeable lenses. For fitting hydrophilic lenses, he recommended a slightly flatter lens than would usually be fitted for the peripheral corneal measurements involved, to avoid reduced visual acuity due to excessive central vaulting of the cornea. Extended wear was not advised, due to increased risk of vascularization.

El Hage and Baker (1986) reported many irregularities in the corneal topography additional to the postradial keratotomy shape. They preferred to attempt controlled keratoreformation by fitting with a specially made lens, which was fitted flat with a steep periphery. Their recommended initial lens had a BOZD of 7.00 mm, TD of 9.00–10.50 mm to bridge the central cornea, with a back peripheral curve 0.75 mm steeper than the BOZR. Particularly for the myope who had become hypermetropic as a result of radial keratotomy, their aim was to steepen the cornea by applying controllable pressure on the corneal periphery to result in an overall quasispherical corneal shape.

Although it may be possible to re-form the cornea to some extent, there is increased risk of oedema and vascularization. A more physiologically acceptable fit was recommended by Goldberg (cited by Greco, 1986) who fitted specially designed contact lenses with toroidal, spherical or aspherical back optic zones to give apical bearing and peripheral clearance. Even if these lenses appeared rather mobile, he felt that they were better than compromising the cornea.

For fitting hydrophilic 55% water content soft lenses, Vickery (1986) advocated using a large total diameter, e.g. 15 mm, and fitting to avoid limbal compression so as to give less stimulus to vascularization. This gave a flatter central fit in close alignment with a large back optic zone diameter.

General problems arising with contact lens wear

Contact lens fitting does not always solve the problems of corneal curvature steepening and vision changes during the day. Patients may still complain of this, particularly if involved in detailed work. If the radial keratotomy was performed on only one eye, then the odd behaviour of the postoperative contact lens compared to that of the other eye may increase binocular fusion difficulties.

Some patients are rendered hypermetropic by the operation, hence they notice presbyopia earlier and have to wear their lenses for prolonged near vision. This may lead to increased corneal disturbance if their blink rate reduces. Previously, as myopes, they could see near vision detail with minimal accommodation, often without any optical correction, and became used to a particular accommodative convergence to accommodation ratio. On becoming hypermetropic, even if corrected with contact lenses, they have to adapt to a new ratio and may experience strain, fatigue and possible binocular fusion disturbance.

If a patient has difficulty handling a contact lens and scrapes the cornea or has a trapped foreign body, there may be increased risk of abrasion and epithelial erosion. There could also be distortion produced on removal of the lenses. Flexing of a weakened cornea may cause loss of endothelial cells.

*In the USA it is common to refer to steepness or flatness dioptrically without quoting the refractive index on which this is based. Because of the confusion so caused, the equivalent in mm is given here in brackets.

Patients demanding radial keratotomy tend to be those who dislike the idea of contact lenses, or have had poor tolerance of lenses in the past. Even if they have not tried contact lenses previously, they believed that the operation would remove their ametropia and so, if left with a residual error requiring correction, are disappointed and poorly motivated to contact lens wear. As Bourque *et al.* (1984) mentioned as part of the PERK study, patients should be fully warned of possible complications.

In both radial keratotomy and in contact lens fitting there is physical intervention to a healthy ametropic eye. Both require good assessment and measurements before the procedure, then accurate operation followed by conscientious after-care. Patients must also comprehend and comply with this. They must accept in each case, and in combination, that there may be disturbances to their quality of vision even if their visual acuity seems reasonable according to the Snellen chart.

Future developments

In future it is likely that there will be a marked increase in the number of radial keratotomy procedures and also more elaborate refractive surgery such as keratophakia, keratokyphosis, keratomileusis and intrastromal corneal implants. Although operations are more costly than contact lens fitting, a significant number of patients would prefer to pay a larger initial fee to avoid time taken up in caring for lenses and attending for regular after-care. Radial keratotomy is not fully penetrating, nor does it involve suturing or difficulty for the surgeon in matching up incision margins, nor is there implantation of any substance which may lead to rejection or allergic reaction. It is carried out on a healthy eye, so there should be fewer risks than operations on abnormal or inflamed eyes.

The continual improvements of operating instruments and techniques, e.g. the use of diamond knives and laser 'knives' will allow more accurate procedures in all corneal surgery including corneal 'grinding'.

Smoother incisions may not heal in the same way as those with rougher margins and more scar tissue, so may have different elasticity and resistance to pressures. This may allow increased response to the wearing of a contact lens to flatten the corneal curvature and decrease myopia further. Future radial keratotomy patients may be fitted with a contact lens aimed to do this, some requiring two or three differently powered contact lenses to wear over the course of a day as their myopia is decreased by the corneal curvature changes induced by each contact lens.

A postrefractive surgery patient presents a definite challenge to the contact lens fitter with respect to clinical skills, interpretation of fluorescein patterns, and designing lenses to minimize variations in visual acuity and in symptoms.

References

AKERS, P. H. and BINDER, P. S. (1981). Laboratory evaluation of radial keratotomy (RK). *Invest. Ophthal. vis. Sci.* **20** (ARVO abstracts Supplement), 160

AKIYAMA, K. (1984). Problems arising from Sato's radial keratotomy procedure from Japan. *Contact Lens Ass. Ophthal. J.* **10**, 179–184

ARROWSMITH, P. N., SANDERS, D. R. and MARKS, R. G. (1983). Visual, refractive, and keratometric results of radial keratotomy. *Archs Ophthal.* **101**, 873–888

ASTIN, C. L. K. (1986). Considerations in fitting contact lenses to patients who have undergone radial keratotomy. *Transactions of the British Contact Lens Association Annual Clinical Conference*, May 1986, 2–7

ASTIN, C. L. K. (1989). Corneal parameter changes following radial keratotomy. (in press)

BIBBY, M. M. (1976). Computer assisted photokeratoscopy and contact lens design. *Optician* **171** (4423), 37–44; **171** (4424) 11–17; **171** (4426), 15–17

BINDER, P. S., ZAVALA, E. Y., BAUMGARTNER, S. *et al.* (1984). Radial keratotomy and keratophakia in a non-human primate. *Archs Ophthal.* **102**, 1671–1675

BORES, L. D., MYERS, W. and COWDEN, J. (1981). Radial keratotomy — an analysis of the American experience. *Ann. Ophthal.* **13**, 941–948

BOURQUE, L. S., RUBENSTEIN, R., COSAND, B. *et al.* (1984). Psychosocial characteristics of candidates for the prospective evaluation of radial keratotomy (PERK) study. *Archs Ophthal.* **102**, 1187–1192

COWDEN, J. W. and BORES, L. D. (1981). A clinical investigation of the surgical correction of myopia by the method of Fyodorov. *Ophthalmology* **88**, 737–741

COWDEN, J. W. and CICHOCKI, J. (1981). Radial keratotomy in monkeys. *Invest. Ophthal. vis. Sci.* **20** (3) (ARVO Abstracts Supplement), 69

COWDEN, J. W. and SULTANA, M. (1982). Corneal endothelial cell density following radial keratotomy. *Invest. Ophthal. vis. Sci. Suppl.* **63**, 22–30

EL HAGE, S. and BAKER, R. N. (1986). Controlled keratoreformation for postoperative radial keratotomy patients. *Int. Eyecare* **2**, 49–53

FYODOROV, S. N. and DURNEV, V. V. (1979). Operation of dosaged dissection of corneal circular ligament in cases of myopia of mild degree. *Ann. Ophthal.* **11**, 1885–1890

GELENDER, H., FLYNN, H. W. and MENDELBAUM, S. (1982). Bacterial endophthalmitis resulting from radial keratotomy. *Am. J. Ophthal.* **93**, 323–326

GONZALEZ, E. R. (1981). Eight centers to assess radial keratotomy. *J. Am. med. Ass.* **245**, 899

GRECO, A. (1986). Fitting the post-operative keratotomy patient. *Int. Eyecare* **2**, 188–190

HOFFER, K. J., DARIN, J. J., PETTIT, T. H. *et al.* (1981). UCLA Clinical trial of radial keratotomy — preliminary report. *Ophthalmology* **88**, 729–736

JANES, J. A. and REICHIE, R. N. (1986). Refractive surgery and contact lenses. *Contact Lens Forum* October, 28–32

JESTER, J. V., STEEL, D., SALZ, J. *et al.* (1981). Radial keratotomy in non-human primate eyes. *Am. J. Ophthal.* **92**, 153–171

JOHN, M. E. and SCHMITT, T. E. (1983). Traumatic hyphaema after radial keratotomy. *Ann. Ophthal.* **150**, 930–932

KARR, D. J., GRUTZMACHER, R. D. and REEH, M. J. (1985). Radial keratotomy complicated by sterile keratitis and corneal perforation. *Ophthalmology* **92**, 1244–1248

LARSEN, B. C., KREMER, F. B., ELLER, A. W. and BERNARDINO, V. B. (1983). Quantitative trauma following radial keratotomy in rabbits. *Ophthalmology* **90**, 660–667

MILLER, D. and MILLER, R. (1981). Glare sensitivity in simulated radial keratotomy. *Archs Ophthal.* **99**, 1961–1962

NIRANKARI, V. S., KATZEN, L. E., RICHARDS, R. D. *et al.* (1982). Prospective clinical study of radial keratotomy. *Ophthalmology* **89**, 677–683

REDDY, P. S. and REDDY, P. R. (1980). Anterior keratotomy. *Ophthal. Surg.* **11**, 765–767

ROWSEY, J. J. and BALYEAT, H. D. (1982). Radial keratotomy — a preliminary report of complications. *Ophthal. Surg.* **13**, 27–35

SHIVITZ, I. A., RUSSELL, B. M., ARROWSMITH, P. N. and MARKS, R. G. (1986). Optical correction of post-operative radial keratotomy patients with contact lenses. *Contact Lens Ass. Ophthal. J.* **12**, 59–62

STEELE, A. D. McG. (1984). An introductory review of refractive keratoplasty. *Trans. Ophthal. Soc. UK* **104**, 26–27

TOWNSLEY, M. G. (1970). New knowledge of the corneal contour. *Contacto* **14**(3), 38–43

VICKERY, J. A. (1986). Post-RK and the soft lens. *Contact Lens Forum*, October, 34–35

WARING, G. O. (1984). Evolution of radial keratotomy for myopia. *Trans. Ophthal. Soc. UK* **104**, 28–42

WARING, G. O., MOFFITT, S. D., GELENDER, H. *et al.* (1983). Rationale for and design of National Eye Institute for prospective evaluation of radial keratotomy (PERK) study. *Ophthalmology* **90**, 40–58

YAMAGUCHI, T., KAUFMAN, H. E., FUKUSHIMA, M. S. *et al.* (1981). Histologic and electron microscopic assessment of endothelial damage produced by anterior radial keratotomy in the monkey cornea. *Am. J. Ophthal.* **92**, 313–327

YENALIEV, F. S. (1979). Experience in the surgical treatment of myopia. *Vestn. Oftalmol.* **3**, 52–55

Further reading

BINDER, P. S. (1984). The status of radial keratotomy in 1984. *Archs Ophthal.* **102**, 1601–1603

DEITZ, M. R. and SANDERS, D. R. (1985). Progressive hyperopia with long-term follow-up of radial keratotomy. *Archs Ophthal.* **103**, 782–784

HOFFER, K. J., DARIN, J. J., PETTIT, T. H. *et al.* (1983). Three years experience with radial keratotomy — the UCLA study. *Ophthalmology* **90**, 627–636

HOFFMANN, F. (1984). Keratomileusis, keratophakia and keratokyphosis. *Trans. Ophthal. Soc. UK* **104**, 48–51

JESTER, J. V., VENET, T., LEE, J. *et al.* (1981). A statistical analysis of radial keratotomy in human cadaver eyes. *Am. J. Ophthal.* **92**, 172–177

KAUFMAN, H. E. and McDONALD, M. B. (1984). Refractive surgery for aphakia and myopia. *Trans. Ophthal. Soc. UK* **104**, 43–47

NEUMANN, A. C., OSHER, R. H. and FENZL, R. E. (1984). Radial keratotomy: a clinical and statistical analysis. *Cornea* **2**, 47–55

NIRANKARI, V. S., KATZEN, L. E., KARESH, J. W. *et al.* (1983). Ongoing prospective clinical study of radial keratotomy. *J. Am. Acad. Ophthal.* **90**, 637–640

ROWSEY, J. J. and BALYEAT, H. D. (1982). Preliminary results and complications of radial keratotomy. *Am. J. Ophthal.* **93**, 437–455

ROWSEY, J. J., BALYEAT, H. D., RABINOVITCH, B. *et al.* (1983). Predicting the results of radial keratotomy. *Ophthalmology* **90**, 642–654

SALZ, J. J., LEE, J. S., JESTER, J. V. *et al.* (1981). Radial keratotomy in fresh human cadaver eyes. *Ophthalmology* **88**, 742–746

SALZ, J. J., LEE, T., JESTER, J. V. *et al.* (1983). Analysis of incision depth following experimental radial keratotomy. *Ophthalmology* **90**, 655–659

SANDERS, D. R., DEITZ, M. R. and GALLAGHER, D. (1985). Factors affecting predictability of radial keratotomy. *Ophthalmology* **92**, 1237–1243

SCHANZLIN, D. J., SANTOS, V. R., WARING, G. O. *et al.* (1986). Diurnal change in refraction, corneal curvature, visual acuity, and intraocular pressure after radial keratotomy in the PERK Study. *Ophthalmology* **93**, 167–175

STEEL, D., JESTER, J. V., SALZ, J. *et al.* (1981). Modification of corneal curvature following radial keratotomy in primates. *Ophthalmology* **88**, 747–754

WARING, G. O. (1985). Making sense of keratospeak. *Archs Ophthal.* **103**, 1472–1477

WARING, G. O., BOURQUE, L., CARTWRIGHT, C. S. *et al.* (1985). Summary of initial results of the prospective evaluation of radial keratotomy (PERK) Study. *Ophthal. Forum* **3**, 177–185

Infants and pre-school children
Lynne Speedwell

Most infants and very young children needing contact lenses are seen in hospital or similar clinics. Older children requiring lenses mainly for refractive purposes are more likely to be seen in private practice. However, the need to cope with both the patient and the parents remains the same. Numerous short visits may be preferable to one long session but there is always a need to be adaptable whenever a child is fitted.

Indications for contact lenses

Contact lenses are only fitted in cases where spectacles would prove inadequate and visual or cosmetic improvements can be achieved in no other way. Fitting falls into three categories: (1) refractive, (2) cosmetic, (3) therapeutic.

Refractive

By far the largest group is the refractive group and of these the aphakes make up the greatest number. These are either congenital or traumatic, unilateral or bilateral.

Other refractive conditions include: high myopia; high hypermetropia; anisometropia; unilateral ametropia; strabismus with a high refractive error, particularly where the good eye is emmetropic.

Cosmetic

The most common conditions which need cosmetic lenses are: aniridia; microphthalmos; iris coloboma; scars; albinism; opacities.

Therapeutic

Very occasionally therapeutic lenses are fitted in cases of corneal epithelial dystrophy or after a corneal graft.

Corneal topography and physiology

The infant has a large eye/head ratio. The length of the eyeball is approximately 17 mm

compared to 24 mm in the adult. The average corneal diameter at birth is 10 mm; by the age of 1 year it has grown to 11.7 mm which is almost adult size. The corneal radius is around 7.1 mm which gradually flattens to an adult average of 7.86 mm. Many figures have been quoted for the refractive error in babies, ranging from slightly myopic in the premature infant to moderately hypermetropic and astigmatic in many normal neonates (Molnar, 1970; Marshall and Grindle, 1978; Weale, 1982).

The corneal physiology differs little from that of the adult except that there are a greater number of endothelial cells. This may account for the apparent ability of the infant to recover rapidly from an hypoxic reaction. The corneal topography of the infant aphake is only slightly altered by surgery since lensectomy and aspiration are the most common procedures and the small scars which remain near the nasal and temporal limbus induce a minimal degree of astigmatism.

Practicalities and types of lenses
Refractive conditions
Aphakia

Infants born with bilateral congenital cataracts (*Plate 102*) or developing them in the first few months of life should have surgery as early as possible to reduce amblyopia (Taylor *et al.*, 1979). Ideally contact lenses should be fitted as soon as the inflammation has settled in the second eye, i.e. about 3 days after the second operation.

Contact lenses provide a more normal visual environment for the aphake as well as overcoming the mechanical difficulties of providing and wearing spectacles (*Figure 21.17*). However a back-up pair of glasses should also be prescribed for periods when the contact lenses cannot be worn, or are lost, thereby ensuring continuous visual stimulation.

It is usual for extended wear lenses to be fitted both for comfort and convenience as it is

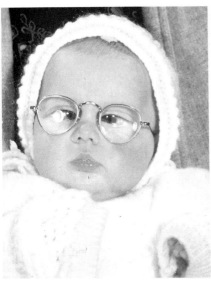

Figure 21.17 Infant in aphakic spectacles — note difficulty in lens centration

impractical to expect that the lenses be removed every time the child has a daytime nap. High water content soft lenses are most common but silicone rubber and high *Dk* gas permeable hard lenses may be used. The parents should be encouraged to start removing the lenses as often as possible from the beginning. When the infant is older and has stopped the daytime sleep, the water content of the soft lenses can be reduced in order to prevent epithelial damage due to lens dehydration and also to reduce lens turnover.

The prescription must be checked by retinoscopy: it is important that the visual pathway remains clear so that the prescription can be as accurate as possible while visual acuity is developing. Mydriatic drops are rarely necessary unless the pupil is very small. No trial frame is used as it is impractical on a baby's small features. Care must therefore be taken not to produce a large back vertex distance (BVD) behind the lens being held as a small increase in BVD induces a large increase in effective power; a +20.00 D spectacle trial lens at a BVD of 16 mm becomes +29.41 D at the cornea.

The back vertex power (BVP) of the aphakic lens at the cornea is usually in the region of +30.00–+32.00 D although BVPs of up to +45.00 D are not unknown. Infants are motivated and attracted by objects which are close to them such as their mother's face, feeding bottle or toys, so that being unable to accommodate

themselves they are focused at a third to a half a metre, i.e. an overcorrection of 2.00–3.00 D. The final prescription, then, is typically between +32.00 D and +35.00 D. These lenses are very thick; a centre thickness of 1 mm is not uncommon, and hence overnight wear can result in corneal hypoxia. A small FOZD is essential to minimize this potential problem. The overcorrection for near is gradually slightly reduced during the first two years of life as the child's visual area of interest increases.

Astigmatism need not be corrected until the child is older, except where gas permeable hard lenses are fitted, but it is usually only of a small degree induced by lensectomy or aspiration (note scars in *Figure 21.18*). It is not practical to fit these infants with anything other than spherical lenses, and as many emmetropic adults start life with varying degrees of astigmatism (Atkinson, Braddick and French, 1980) there is some justification for leaving a small degree of astigmatism uncorrected.

The total diameter (TD) of the lenses usually depends on the corneal diameter, which, as previously mentioned, is around 10 mm at birth growing to 11.7 mm by 1 year of age. Ideally the lens should be 2 mm larger than the visible corneal diameter, so the first soft lens of choice is 12.00–12.50 mm TD, depending on age and corneal appearance. In some cases this may not settle centrally over the cornea. Many congenital cataracts occur in microphthalmic eyes, having a corneal diameter of 9 mm or less, whilst others are fitted when the infant is a few weeks or months old by which time the cornea has grown. A larger or smaller TD may be necessary, depending on the peripheral corneal and scleral topography, in order to achieve

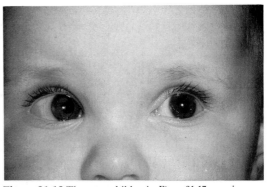

Figure 21.18 The same child as in *Figure 21.17*, wearing lenses — note scars from surgery

adequate centration. This may be further complicated by the action of tight lids on the thick lens and the final lens may need to be as much as 3 mm or even 3.5 mm larger than the corneal diameter.

Actual keratometry measurements are rarely taken. Instead the BOZR of the first lenses are fitted according to age, i.e. on known average 'K' reading, which for a neonate is 7.10 mm. Some of the infant aphakes have marked nystagmus and it may be difficult to maintain reasonable lens centration on the eye; trial and error is then the only way to achieve good results (*Figure 21.18*).

The ideal *minimum* number of trial lenses is 40 (*Table 21.7*), but if infant aphakes are only rarely seen the number can be reduced to 24 (figures in bold type). It is important to keep two of each set of parameters in stock so that lenses can be issued at the first visit. Where possible the parents should always have a spare pair of lenses to keep at home against loss or breakage.

The lenses frequently need changing after they have been allowed to settle. It is not possible to assess the fit conventionally; instead time must be spent watching the eye/lens movement while the baby is shown toys or lights to attract its attention. Many babies allow their eyes to be looked at on the slit lamp as long as it is only for a short period, and the practitioner can thus gain a reasonable view of lens edge indentation, superficial punctate keratitis, new blood vessels and any other contact lens-induced changes.

Where problems are encountered with soft lenses, such as too many lenses lost or broken, or

corneal hypoxia or lid irritation, then silicone rubber lenses may be substituted. These lenses have the advantage that they are not easily rubbed out but they may be very difficult to remove if the eye is sore and also the surface degrades rapidly. They can be obtained from Zeiss–Wöhlk in Europe, and Bausch & Lomb and Danker in the USA.

The initial BOZR of silicone lenses fitted is again age dependent, the steepest radii of 7.60 mm with the smallest TD of 11.20 mm or 11.70 mm being used for the youngest children (note: different parameters are available in the USA). The fit of the lenses can be assessed using fluorescein and the picture should be of minimal apical clearance and moderate peripheral clearance (*Plate 41*). Even with the steepest BOZR the lenses may be flat giving central touch and peripheral stand-off (*Plate 43*). Although not ideal, such a lens is well tolerated and appears to cause no corneal damage (Cutler, Nelson and Calhoun, 1985) and it is better to err towards a flat fit than a tight one. Very few trial lenses are needed: BOZRs of 7.60 mm and of 7.80 mm, and TDs of 11.20 mm, 11.70 mm and 12.20 mm in BVP of +30.00 D.

Since gas permeable lenses for babies need to be fitted under general anaesthetic and keratometry readings taken with the fitting assessed using fluorescein and a hand ultraviolet lamp, to ensure a good fit they are not usually a lens of choice for infants. They are more easily fitted, however, to the slightly older, more cooperative child, when more conventional fitting methods can be used. However, keratometry can be undertaken on babies, preferably with a vertically mounted keratometer, or, if necessary, with the infant lying on its side and the horizontal and vertical reading positions interchanged.

For rigid gas permeable (RGP) lenses similar parameters as are used for adults apply, with BOZR values of 7.00–7.80 mm and TDs of 9.00–9.50 mm for the neonate, increasing to BOZRs of 7.50–8.50 mm and TDs of 9.50–10.00 mm by 1 year of age. The relatively large total diameters aid comfort and minimize the risk of rubbing lenses from the eye.

As the child gets older and the eye grows, the BVP reduces, the corneal diameter increases, and the corneal radius flattens. The lens needed for a 2-year-old aphake may be very similar to that of an adult, though still probably slightly steeper, the parameters being around 7.80/

Table 21.7 Back vertex powers (in D) and appropriate BOZR and TD values for an infant aphakic soft lens fitting set

BOZR (mm)	BVP (D) for TD (mm) of				
	12.00	12.50	13.00	13.50	14.00
7.00	**+34.00** +30.00	**+32.00** +28.00	**+30.00**		
7.20	**+32.00**	**+30.00** +26.00	**+28.00** +24.00	**+22.00**	
7.40		**+28.00**	**+26.00** +22.00	**+24.00** +20.00	**+22.00**
7.60			**+24.00**	**+22.00**	**+18.00**

13.50/+18.00 for a high water content soft lens. The prescription is changed to a distance correction and bifocal spectacles are prescribed for reading and close work as soon as the children need to see clearly further away — often when starting nursery school but sometimes as soon as they start to walk. Any astigmatic error can be corrected at the same time. Soft lens wearers may be changed to gas permeable lenses before school age to improve the vision or if the cornea is showing new peripheral vessels, or if giant papillary conjunctivitis (GPC) is apparent.

Unilateral aphakes are treated similarly except that extensive patching, of up to three-quarters of the waking hours, needs to be carried out to the good, phakic eye in conjunction with contact lens wear in the aphakic eye. Without effective patching the aphakic eye always remains densely amblyopic. However, it is important not to overdo the patching of the good eye, otherwise the vision in that eye may fail to develop normally. Where patching is difficult, an occlusive black tinted contact lens (*Plate 103b*) or a high-powered lens may be used in the good eye. Unfortunately these are rarely successful as the child soon learns to move the lens into the upper fornix or rub it out altogether.

The same applies to traumatic aphakes; dense amblyopia is common as a result of the injury but whilst visual results are usually poor, a contact lens may help in reducing the amplitude of a secondary strabismus. Extra care must be taken to watch for any corneal reaction, especially neovascularization which is more likely in the presence of scar tissue.

Manufacture of aphakic soft lenses for infants is difficult. On hydration the parameters are likely to steepen more than for lenses of lower power. The refractive index of the xerogel is 1.595 giving a BVP of around +60.00 D in the dry state which is very difficult to measure, hence the hydrated BVP is likely to be less accurate and more difficult to check on the focimeter. The carrier zone and junction need to be thicker than in an adult's lens in order to make for reasonable handling.

High myopia

The highly myopic child can develop his vision unaided by holding objects close to his eyes, provided that there is no further disease or

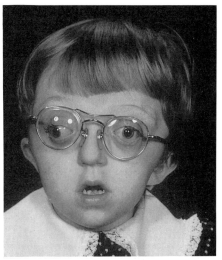

Figure 21.19 Child with clover-leaf skull and high myopia

anomaly along the visual pathway. High minus lenses are very thin in the centre which makes handling difficult. It is, therefore, not a particularly good idea to fit contact lenses with all their inherent problems to the very young myope unless there is some other reason why they cannot wear spectacles, for example certain syndromes produce a misshapen skull which makes the wearing of glasses difficult (*Figure 21.19*).

In these children and also the slightly older child who refuses to wear spectacles, extended wear soft lenses are the first lens of choice and as soon as the lenses can be removed daily, they are changed to lower water content daily wear lenses. The axially myopic eye is larger and the cornea flatter than normal. Infants may start with lenses of 8.00 mm BOZR and as large as 13.50 or even 14.00 mm total diameter in the under 1 year olds.

It has been suggested that PMMA contact lenses have a retarding effect on the progression of myopia (Kelly and Butler, 1971; Stone, 1976) but the adverse effects that this can induce in the cornea are not worth risking in the very young. RGP lenses are satisfactory provided that the child can adapt to the initial foreign body sensation.

High hypermetropia, strabismus and anisometropia

High hypermetropes manage quite well with contact lenses, but they are rarely discovered until they reach school age unless a strabismus is also present. Unilateral ametropes who are discovered early, be they myopes or hypermetropes, are reluctant to wear spectacles with their resultant aniseikonia, as they derive no visual benefit from wearing from; contact lenses are then the only solution. In these children as in the unilateral aphakes, extensive patching needs to be done to the good eye to reduce the amblyopia in the ametropic eye. Again extended wear lenses are initially fitted, progressing to daily wear as soon as their parents are able to manage them.

The visual results obtained with unilateral myopes have been found to be more successful than with unilateral hypermetropes (Morris, 1979) and since aniseikonia has been shown to be less for both axial and refractive anisometropia when contact lenses are employed (Winn *et al.*, 1986), better stereopsis may develop if contact lenses can be prescribed early.

It is always important to keep the patient's interest in mind. There are occasions when the parents bring pressure to bear on the practitioner either to fit lenses initially or to maintain the child in contact lenses when the practitioner advises otherwise. A willingness to discuss with the parents the reason for any decisions made is ultimately in the child's best interest and where possible another appointment should be given so that the situation can be reassessed. If lens handling is the problem they should be shown how to deal with the lenses and by the next visit the decision may be reviewed.

Cosmetic conditions

Conditions requiring cosmetic lenses are similar in both adults and children, although the distribution of the pathology for which they are necessary is different. Soft lenses are the most common lenses fitted, although occasionally corneal lenses are used. Cosmetic shells fall into a different category which is dealt with in another section (*see* p. 789).

Aniridia, iris coloboma and albinism

Photophobia-inducing conditions are sometimes worth fitting in children. Although the visual acuity rarely improves with contact lenses, parents report that the babies seem more

content, and the older children maintain that they can see better.

Aniridia and iris coloboma need an opaque iris lens to partially occlude the light (*Plate 116*). In the case of albinos (*Plate 109*), tinted lenses and even scleral lenses with an opaque scleral zone have been tried in an effort to improve the visual acuity, all to no avail (Ruben, 1967). The lack of pigment epithelium in the retina together with the abnormal percentage of fibres partially decussating at the optic chiasma precludes any recordable visual improvement. Many albinos are hypermetropic and often have a moderate degree of astigmatism, possibly induced by screwing up their eyelids against the light. It is worth correcting their refractive errors where possible, but many find that subjectively, correction of the cylinder provides little or no benefit, so the young albino is typically fitted with spherical soft tinted lenses.

Microphthalmos

Microphthalmic eyes have corneas with steep radii of curvature. The eyes are highly hypermetropic with a correction of up to $+25.00\,D$ or even greater. The eyes are treated, therefore, similarly to those of the infant aphakes, except that they are prescribed contact lenses to the distance prescription as the child still has the ability to accommodate.

Scars and opacities

Scars and opacities can be caused by a variety of conditions, among them penetrating injuries, some keratopathies and removal of dermoid cysts. An eye that has been disfigured in such a way as to cause loss of vision is usually unsightly. In the first months and years of life, these eyes may be fitted more for the parents' sake than any other reason. However, once the child starts playing with other children and going to school, he may develop worries and complexes about his disfigurement; a cosmetic lens helps to prevent this. In fact many children refuse to go to school on days when they are unable to wear their cosmetic lens (*Plates 103, 106, 108* and *110*).

Initially an iris tint lens is prescribed even if it is not an exact match to the good eye. These lenses can be made in a high water content material and can therefore be worn during sleep.

There is an extensive range of colours available and usually an acceptable match can be obtained. It is impractical to try to achieve perfection at this age as the lenses are frequently lost or broken. When the child is older, a hand-painted lens may be ordered.

In cases where some vision has been retained, great care must be taken to ensure that the cosmetic lens does not compromise the cornea. Initially a clear soft lens is fitted to rule out any corneal reaction, and only when that has been established is a cosmetic lens ordered.

Therapeutic lenses

Cases of corneal epithelial dystrophy and postkeratoplasty are occasionally fitted with therapeutic soft or silicone rubber lenses. Because of the difficulties of inserting a thin lens on an often painful eye, they may initially be inserted under general anaesthetic but subsequent handling is when the child is awake. These lenses do not always prove successful More detailed discussion of their fitting is covered elsewhere in this chapter.

Handling of lenses

At the first visit the lenses are inserted by the practitioner while the parent holds the child prone on a couch. The upper lid is held up, making sure that enough pressure is applied, and the lens is slotted underneath (*Figure 21.20*). Removal is as for a corneal lens to avoid any possible damage caused by conventional removal (*Figure 21.21*). Silicone rubber lenses may need to be removed by using a rubber suction holder.

Most parents, once they have been told of the potential dangers of extended wear, are willing to attempt to remove their children's lenses. Time spent in explaining and demonstrating lens insertion and removal at the beginning can save many emergency visits later on, and it is important to stress that the lenses do not cause any pain to the child. However, the regimen must not become too big an event in the family's life. The parents need to be fairly relaxed when the lenses are to be handled; if the parent is tense, the child senses it and also tenses up, making lens insertion or removal much more difficult. The actual handling of the lenses

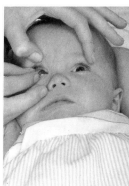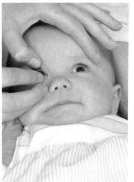

Figure 21.20 Inserting lenses

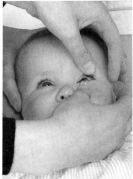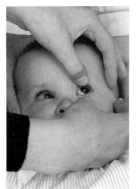

Figure 21.21 Removing lenses

should not automatically be done by one parent; it is better if they can share the task, one holding the child while the other deals with the lenses. The child can be wrapped in a blanket to make lens handling easier or, if the parents are still having difficulty, the lenses may be inserted and removed while the child is asleep. They can be advised to start removing and cleaning the lenses weekly and gradually build up to daily removal.

Those children who have had contact lenses since infancy are often able to remove their own soft lenses by the age of 3 or 4, and by the age of 5 some are able to insert them. Of those who are not as adept, the large majority are very cooperative when their parents deal with their lenses.

Children aged 2–5 years who have not worn lenses previously are less cooperative and where spectacle wear is adequate at this stage, it may be advisable for them to remain thus corrected.

The cleaning regimen of choice must be relatively easy, and must avoid any potential danger to the child's eyes. Chemical disinfection can lead to an allergic reaction which might be confused with an infection when brought back to the clinic. Treatment may then inadvertently be with drops containing the very same preservative which caused the reaction in the first place. Hydrogen peroxide and chlorine-based systems may lead to discomfort or corneal damage if not used correctly. Soft lenses (apart from cosmetic lenses) should therefore be cleaned using heat disinfection and unpreserved saline. Young children tend to require changes to their lenses, or lose or damage them, before many of the deposits associated with this method of cleaning become troublesome. Once the parents have become adept at handling the lenses and the prescription has stopped changing, peroxide or chlorine systems may be used together with protein removal tablets, where necessary. Silicone rubber lenses and rigid lenses should be cleaned using the practitioner's preferred method.

After-care problems

Thick lenses worn continuously or even on a daily basis can lead to changes in the ocular environment. Also many infants have a low blink rate and thus a keratitis may develop. A baby cannot tell the parent of a mild discomfort and so it is not until the eye becomes red or sticky that the parent discovers the problem. By then the child probably needs to have the lens removed for a few days and be given topical antibiotics. Most medical and nursing personnel have no training in contact lens removal for adults let alone children, therefore the parents are advised to remove the lenses themselves before taking the child to the local ophthalmologist for treatment.

In infant bilateral aphakes up to 18 months old, where one lens needs to be removed, it is a good idea to remove both; the eye without the contact lens can quickly become amblyopic even within a few days of lens removal. While the infection is being treated, the back-up spectacles should be worn.

In some syndromes, most notably Down's, the sufferers appear to have reduced tear flow, and in these children it may be advisable to instil physiological saline drops (without preser-

vative) every few hours during the day, even with daily wear lenses.

Corneal anoxia and neovascularization are frequently a problem. In cases where the parents cannot handle the lenses or where the child is too young to be re-fitted with RGP lenses it may be necessary to change to spectacle wear for a time. Another problem for the young lens wearer is GPC. It is not always possible to re-fit a child with rigid gas permeable lenses at the first sign of GPC and it may be another reason for changing to spectacles. Occasionally a child who has been wearing lenses successfully starts to rebel against them at around 2 years old. Again, spectacle wear will solve the problem until such a time as they are themselves keen to revert to contact lenses. The parents of a child who has been wearing lenses successfully (or even unsuccessfully) are usually reluctant to see them revert to spectacle wear. It is therefore expedient to warn them of the possibility when they first bring the child for fitting. It must also be stressed that the visual acuity should develop just as well in glasses as in contact lenses in spite of the possible reduction in visual field.

The number of soft lenses lost or broken especially in the first few months of wear can be very high. It is not uncommon for a pair of soft lenses to be lost or broken every month until both child and parents become used to the routine. It is important to have lenses ready in stock against such events, and it is a good idea to give the parents spare lenses if there is likely to be any delay in replacing the losses. Silicone rubber lenses generally need to be replaced less often, usually only when the surface degrades.

Infants and young children need to be reviewed much more frequently than adults. Their lenses need changing more often and objective refraction checks are more important, as subjective information is less reliable even if available. After the initial fitting and assessment consultations, 3-monthly appointments are standard with open access to the practitioner and medical staff for emergencies.

During follow-up visits, care must always be taken to exclude any developing eye disease. The prescription of the infant aphake is expected to reduce with time, but if too much of a reduction in plus power is needed it may indicate the development of buphthalmos. Likewise a red or watery eye may not be contact lens induced but due to an increase in intraocular pressure. The young contact lens wearer should regularly have fundus and intraocular pressure checks in conjunction with contact lens assessment.

Although most of the problems of contact lens fitting and wear can be overcome and parents' questions answered, the answer to the most frequently asked question 'What will my child see?' still remains elusive. Results differ in every case. Many children with congenital visual handicaps improve beyond expectation whilst others, unfortunately, do not. Even with the sophisticated checking equipment now available, such as VERs, ERGs and preferential looking techniques, it is still not possible to answer with anything other than a calculated guess. An important factor affecting visual prognosis is how quickly contact lens fitting is commenced. For the baby born with cataracts, if surgery and contact lens fitting are delayed beyond 3–4 months after birth, significant visual acuity loss results. For this reason early referral and rapid commencement of lens fitting is vital.

Implants and epikeratophakias are not performed on infant aphakes because the eye is still growing and the prescription of the intraocular lens or epikeratophakia button cannot easily be changed. For the older child implants, explants and keratotomies will no doubt remove the need for many of the current lenses fitted for the children of the future, but until they become the first procedures of choice there will still be the need for the contact lens practitioner in paediatric fitting.

Acknowledgements

The photographs in this section are reproduced by courtesy of Mr D. S. I. Taylor, FRCS and the Department of Medical Illustration Great Ormond Street Hospital for Sick Children, London.

References

ATKINSON, J., BRADDICK, D. and FRENCH, J. (1980). Infant astigmatism: its disappearance with age. *Vision Res.* **20**, 891–893

CUTLER, S. I., NELSON, L. B. and CALHOUN, J. H. (1985). Extended wear contact lenses in pediatric aphakia. *J. Pediatr. Ophthal. Strab.* **22**, 85–91

KELLY, T. S-B. and BUTLER, D. (1971). The present position of contact lenses in relation to myopia. *Br. J. physiol. Optics* **26**, 33–34

MARSHALL, J. and GRINDLE, C. F. J. (1978). Fine structure of the cornea and its development. *Trans. Ophthal. Soc. UK* **98**, 320–328

MOLNAR, L. (1970). Refraktionsanderung des Auges im Laufe des Lebens. *Klin. Monatsbl. Augenheilkd.* **156**, 326–339

MORRIS, J. (1979). Contact lenses in infancy and childhood. *Contact Lens J.* **8**, 15–18

RUBEN, M. (1967). Albinism and contact lenses. *Contact Lens J.* **1**(2), 5–8

STONE, J. (1976). The possible influence of contact lenses on myopia. *Br. J. physiol. Optics,* **31**, 89–114

TAYLOR, D., MORRIS, J., ROGERS, J. E. and WARLAND, J. (1979). Amblyopia in bilateral infantile and juvenile cataract. *Trans. Ophthal. Soc. UK* **99**, 170–176

WEALE, R. A. (1982). *A Biography of the Eye. Development, Growth, Age.* London: H. K. Lewis & Co.

WINN, B., ACKERLEY, R. G., BROWN, C. A. *et al.* (1986). The superiority of contact lenses in correction of all anisometropia. *Transactions of the British Contact Lens Association Conference*, pp. 95–100

Cosmetic and prosthetic contact lenses
M. J. A. Port

Cosmetic contact lenses are sometimes termed 'prosthetic' contact lenses. International Standard ISO 8320–1986 refers to a *cosmetic lens* or *cosmetic shell* being specifically designed to change the appearance of the eye, the former having a refractive effect and the latter not having a refractive effect. In either case the function of the lens or shell is to alter the appearance of the eye such that a disfigurement is covered by an artefact in order to restore the appearance of normality. In some cases, e.g. albinism and iris trauma, the lens may be functioning to reduce the amount of light entering the eye. Such lenses may be used on seeing and non-seeing eyes. In the latter case a plano lens is conventionally employed.

Uses

(1) Covering opaque hypermature cataracts (*Plates 103* and *113*).
(2) Covering a high squint angle where operation is impossible (*Plates 104* and *105*).
(3) Restoration of the iris and pupil to normal size, appearance and colour (*Plates 106, 110, 113, 115* and *116*).
(4) Microphthalmos.
(5) Covering iris holes that give diplopia and polyopia (*Plates 107, 108* and *117*).
(6) Albinism (*Plate 109*).
(7) Eliminating intractable diplopia.

Lenses are not always used for a single purpose, for example, someone may have been in a car accident where broken glass has damaged the eye. The ocular complications which then need correction may be aniridia, aphakia and corneal scars.

Types of lenses

Scleral lenses and shells, corneal lenses and soft lenses are all used and necessary if all types of work are to be undertaken. In the last 10 years the use of scleral and corneal types has decreased due to the larger variety of soft lens tints and tint patterns which have been introduced.

Implications of cosmetic lenses

Perhaps the most important thing to remember with these lenses is that the lens is on the anterior surface of the globe. Thus any artificial pupil or iris is placed in this forward position whereas in the normal eye it is in a relatively flat plane some 4 mm behind the cornea. The appearance is therefore always something of a compromise even if the colour match is good, unless a sufficiently translucent lens is used that allows at least partial visibility of the natural eye through the cosmetic lens. If the general appearance is good the casual observer will not notice the lens and in some respects this aspect is of little consequence. Where the patient is very critical and has fairly exophthalmic eyes then this factor can be apparent but if the eyes are enophthalmic the effect is not so obvious. Perhaps one disadvantage of a scleral lens is that

its thickness may give a proptosed look to an eye (*Plate 104*).

Patients who need these lenses have often had a disfigured eye for a long time and therefore they are extremely aware of the abnormality. In fact they often magnify its appearance in their own minds and think that it is very noticeable because they have looked at themselves close up in a mirror, whereas to the casual observer at 1 metre it may not be noticeable at all. When considering the general appearance of these contact lenses the patient should be encouraged to look at the lens on the eye from a reasonable distance, not from really close up. An obvious aspect is the size and position of the pupil. With either a cosmetic lens or shell, the artificial 'pupil' is of fixed size but may appear to move as the lens moves, and the fitter has to decide on the best compromise in fitting which will permit minimal lens movement. If not warned about pupil size, the patient may comment that it is not large enough in low illumination, or perhaps that it is not small enough in very bright light.

An eye that has suffered trauma and/or surgery may well look a little red compared to the fellow eye. Even if the iris colour of a cosmetic lens is perfectly matched the contrast between the iris and sclera may still be different for both eyes. This may affect the decision on the choice of iris colour itself, for the final cosmetic lens.

Friends and relatives usually have a certain attitude to the patient with a cosmetic lens. If someone has been used to seeing a person they know well with a 'disfigurement', then when it is corrected, the correction is obvious. The patient should be made aware of this. If a normal encounter does not produce a stare or a question such as 'Is there anything wrong with your eye?' then the cosmetic lens is having the desired effect.

With a seeing eye refraction may be irregular. Due to such effects as poor lens centration, an artificial pupil or pathological changes, the visual acuity with the contact lens may be disappointing to the patient after having seen better with a spectacle correction. Of course, the reverse may be true and a contact lens correction may improve upon the spectacle visual acuity. Such possibilities should be discussed with the patient and, if applicable, it should be pointed out that different levels of vision can arise with different types of lens and a compromise between vision, appearance and comfort may be the best personal solution.

Scleral lenses and shells

These are needed when an opaque scleral zone is required as in the case of covering a badly squinting eye (*Plates 104* and *105*). They may be needed when all other types of lens do not centre well on the eye. In cases of trauma the sclera and conjunctiva may be very irregular and chemosed and other lens types may be uncomfortable. The scleral lens is strong and should last a considerable time. The fitting is tedious and the painting of iris and pupil is a very skilled process. As the lens is stable it is possible to incorporate cylinders and prisms. The lens or shell can easily be adjusted for thickness so that if an eye is enophthalmic compared to a fellow eye, thicker than average material can help to equalize the appearance. Often a lens thickness of 1.5 mm or 2 mm will suffice but if it is envisaged that a thicker lens or shell is required then PMMA sheet of 2–3 mm can be used.

A scleral shell is made and fitted in the normal way (*see* Chapters 17 and 18). The necessary painting and construction is carried out for iris and pupil, and blood vessels on the scleral zone if it is opaque. Blood vessels are simulated by fine strands of cotton and/or painting. The iris colours are painted over a fine layer of opaque black PMMA (with or without a central clear pupil, as appropriate), which is stuck to the thinned-down optic zone of the scleral shell. A layer of clear PMMA is then polymerized over all the prosthetic components to form a smooth anterior surface to the shell. It is at this stage that the thickness of the whole shell can be adjusted. If a powered contact lens is required this can be achieved by the correct power being added to the front surface. When the lens is on the eye an over-refraction may indicate that a change in lens power is indicated, which is achieved by re-working the front surface.

A relatively new method of rendering a scleral shell more lifelike is the use of an actual photograph of the patient's unaffected eye. This photograph must be reduced to actual size, i.e. 1:1 and taken in the most natural light possible. It can then be glued to the cosmetic/prosthetic shell and subsequently covered by a clear layer of PMMA.

Corneal lenses

In common with scleral lenses, cosmetic corneal lenses are normally made from PMMA. With both types there is no problem with solution sensitivity or complicated hygiene regimens. Corneal types are sized between 11 and 13 mm in order to cover the cornea (*Plate 111*). The advantage of a rigid lens is in the correction of corneal astigmatism and distortion.

The lens is made in several stages:

(1) A clear PMMA lens is first made and adjusted to give good centration but maintaining good tear exchange. If good tear circulation is not achieved then corneal oedema is likely to lead to poor wearing times for many patients, although for others where the cornea is already vascularized the lack of oxygen available with these lenses does not give rise to problems. Careful monitoring of the results of anoxia is necessary and it may be appropriate to advise only limited wearing of the final lens to avoid long-term problems. The lens design can be the same as indicated in the section on aphakia, and ideally as thick as the final lens (*see below*).

(2) Refraction should be carried out with a trial lens using a similar power and pupil size to that envisaged for the final lens.

(3) A cosmetic lens is ordered taking the above two aspects into account and remembering that with a painted iris it is not possible to check the fit of the lens with fluorescein and blue light.

The iris colours are painted on a black background as for scleral lenses, and after that process an additional layer of PMMA is polymerized over the pigments. The front surface is then cut to give the correct power. If a high power lens is to be produced then the front surface lenticulation can be reduced to approximately that of the pupil size. It is always worth considering the use of a lenticular form in order to reduce the thickness of the lens. The laminate construction implies that the lens thickness is likely to be greater than the clear lens used initially. A thick lens may be less comfortable and may not centre as well, hence the importance of considering this at the fitting stage (*see* point (1)).

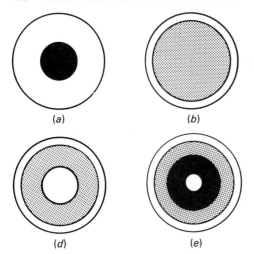

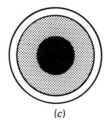

Figure 21.22 Different varieties of tinted or dyed cosmetic soft lenses. (*a*) A black pupil lens; (*b*) a lens with a tinted iris portion; (*c*) a lens with a tinted iris portion and a black pupil; (*d*) a lens with a tinted iris portion and a clear pupil; (*e*) a black pupil with clear small central zone, with or without a tinted periphery

Soft lenses

As mentioned previously, soft lens types are used increasingly and it is always worth while to consider first if the problem can be solved using a soft lens especially as these types of lenses can now be manufactured in both spherical and toric forms. However, if the eye is dry, or irregular corneal astigmatism needs to be corrected, then some form of rigid lens is best. Soft cosmetic lenses can be either of two types:

(1) Homogeneous construction.
(2) Heterogeneous construction.

The first type can be considered as a normal soft lens which has been modified by one or more dyeing processes. The second type has a laminated construction.

Homogeneous types

Five possibilities are usually available as shown in *Figure 21.22*.

Homogeneous construction lenses

The most widely used method of tinting soft lenses for both normal and cosmetic purposes is to introduce a form of water-soluble dye to masked-off areas of the anterior surface of the lens. Demarcation of pupil and iris zones is accomplished by anterior clamping (*Figure 21.23*). This can be achieved with various types of masks within the tinting apparatus. In this manner a variety of iris and pupil sizes (or no pupil at all) can be tinted. By utilizing specialized masks, lifelike striations and iris patterns can be successfully produced. Using a range of tint combinations allows the laboratory to match unusual eye colours. Recent research into this area of cosmetic tinting has allowed laboratories to pre-tint the lenses with a neutral, opaque emulsion and then apply the required colours and patterns to match the patient's sound eye.

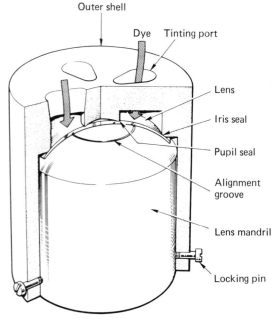

Figure 21.23 Clamp used to dye localized areas of a soft cosmetic contact lens

Both these types of tint are usually fixed by various chemical methods in order to render the tint permanent. Methods of getting the lens to appear opaque include instilling various non-hydrophilic media into the liquid monomer before polymerization. This particulate matter is usually of a non-reactive nature, i.e. mica, titanium dioxide etc.

Occasionally the clamping process used can alter the shape (and hence fit) of the lens.

Advantages

(1) Thin lenses — good comfort.
(2) Oxygen permeability not affected by the tint.
(3) Relatively cheap.
(4) Delivery good.
(5) Some iris texture may be seen through lighter tints.
(6) A wide variety of lens sizes, radii and thicknesses are available.
(7) A large range of colours is obtainable.

Disadvantages

(1) In the main, only a darkening effect is possible.
(2) Unusual iris patterns cannot be matched.
(3) A new pupil aperture is not created with most types.
(4) Complete occlusion is difficult to obtain.

While dealing with homogeneous lenses it is worth mentioning lenses which use more than one dyeing process. For example, in the Hydron Trucolour lens, a white iris tint is applied to a conventional hydrogel lens — the pupil area being excluded. On top of this a colour is applied. With this arrangement a wearer's dark iris can be 'changed' to a light coloured one. At present the colours are limited and a natural appearance is difficult to obtain (*Plate 110*), but the technique is in its infancy. Other manufacturers are experimenting with this type of lens

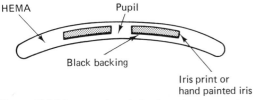

Figure 21.24 Cross-section of a laminated soft cosmetic contact lens

and there are some which have an iris pattern incorporated (e.g. the Aquarius (*Plate 112*) by Contact Lenses (Manufacturing) Ltd). If tinted lenses become desirable as a fashion accessory then the industry will certainly develop more sophisticated designs.

Heterogeneous construction lenses

These soft lenses are of laminate construction (*Figure 21.24*). The most widely used lenses of this type are made by Titmus Eurocon (now CIBA Vision) of West Germany. The lenses have a coloured iris pattern which is sandwiched between two HEMA sections. The iris pattern can then be either painted by hand or printed by machine ('Irisprint lenses' — *Plates 108* and *113*). In both types the iris pattern is put on an opaque black substratum. The machine printed lenses come in brown, green, blue and grey. Each colour may be ordered in a dark, medium or light shade.

The iris texture appearance is fairly good considering the process and it is reasonably consistent. This is helpful when ordering replacements. Where two lenses are required for right and left eyes they are very good, e.g. in cases of albinism, as shown in *Plate 109c*. They are also less expensive than the hand-painted versions. Due to the heterogeneous construction the lenses are rarely spherical in form. The final shape of the lens is affected by its artificial iris size, pupil size, lens power and lens thickness. It is difficult to predict how some lenses will fit. Nothing is more frustrating than waiting 3 months for a lens, finding the colour matches well but the lens fit is poor. However, the lenses are very useful, particularly for unusual iris colours and textures, where complete occlusion is necessary and where there is a requirement for a new pupil aperture to be created. *Plates 109c* and *113* show some examples.

When ordering a hand-painted lens there are several ways of specifying the colour. The numbered paper colour samples supplied by Titmus Eurocon (CIBA Vision) can be used or a colour slide or artificial eye sample may be sent to the manufacturer. The problem with colour film is that the colour rendering is different for different films; the exposure can affect the colour (*Plate 114*), and the artist may not be illuminating the slide with a 'daylight' source. The author's experience has shown that it is better to use at least two of the three methods when trying to arrive at the correct colour and sending the results of both with the lens order. The lens order should specify back optic zone radius (BOZR), total diameter (TD), BVP, iris diameter, pupil diameter, and state if a clear or black pupil is required.

The oxygen transmissibility of these lenses is very poor and the resulting hypoxia is expected to give rise to corneal oedema. There may well be limits on the wearing time because of this. The colours are generally stable provided that chemical disinfection is employed. Hydrogen peroxide has been tried but there may be some effect on lens shape and the chance of some pigment bleaching. Heat disinfection should be avoided as the lamination may break down and cause some bubbling of the lens surface with subsequent discomfort.

When calculating the power of lenses with an opaque iris great care should be exercised. This is especially so in the case of high power lenses. It should be remembered that a new component has been added to the optical system, i.e. an aperture on the most powerful refracting surface. In some cases there may be a normal pupil plane as well, but in others there may be no pupil or a displaced pupil. An example of this effect is: an eye requiring a lens power of +17.00 D with a transparent contact lens may actually need a power of +22.00 D with a cosmetic lens.

The main disadvantages of the hand-painted lenses are the cost, long delivery time and poor physiology.

Ordering cosmetic lenses

When ordering cosmetic lenses from a laboratory, the following guide can be useful:

(1) Lens parameters: ensure that the laboratory is supplied with a comprehensive list of the desired lens parameters. It is preferable to fit using trial lenses as with some compromised eyes it is impossible to achieve accurate K readings. Calcified and phthisical eyes are typical of such a situation. If ordering lenses of higher water content material make sure that any fitting differences due to lens shrinkage on the eye are allowed for.

(2) Let the laboratory know whether the eye is sighted or unsighted as the latter case will give the laboratory some latitude in manufacture. If the eye is sighted and the power is greater than +4.00 D the correct back vertex distance should be given to the laboratory unless this has already been taken into account.

(3) Make sure that the correct material is used for the particular application. If the eye is severely compromised from injury, for example, vascularization may be prominent and corneal infiltration may occur. In these situations the maximum oxygen transmissibility is desirable. It is therefore wise to check with the laboratory to see if the lens can be made in a high water content material.

(4) Specify to the laboratory whether or not a black, clear or tinted pupil is required. If the eye is unsighted and the cornea or lens is opaque then a black pupil can restore a normal appearance (*Plates 103* and *113*). If the patient can tolerate a slight loss of light transmission a tinted pupil is usually far more natural looking than an untinted pupil. It tends to break up the demarcation between the opaque iris and pupil areas. A small clear pupil with a sharply defined, high contrast edge can often give a very artificial appearance.

(5) Iris colour and texture should be specified by colour, depth of pigment and whether the iris area should be patterned or plain.

(6) The total diameter of the tinted area should be specified. It is usually advisable to order the tint either the same as the natural iris size or just less than this (*Plates 110* and *115*). If the lens decentres slightly when blinking it will look more natural if the coloured area does not encroach onto the sclera.

(7) The opaque area can be ordered as either a generalized iris area or as a localized area in order to cover up a coloboma etc. Lens location techniques, as used for astigmatic lenses, will be necessary to correctly locate a localized opaque area.

(8) If possible a colour photograph should be sent to the laboratory, as it can be invaluable. The photograph should be taken in the most natural light and should be taken close enough to show up any iris striations, patterning etc. Due to various differences in photographic developing the finished colours may not be exactly true to

Table 21.8 Some currently available tinted and cosmetic lenses

Manufacturer	Lens type	Water (%)	Fitting parameters	Colours	No. of patterns
Allergan-Hydron	Soft colour (opaque)	38	Z6, Z4, H67, Mini, SC	Aqua Sapphire Emerald Quartz	1
	Soft tint (transparent with clear pupil)	38	Same	Same + Amber	1
Bausch & Lomb	Natural tint	38	U3, U4 B3, Optima	Blue Aqua Green Brown	1
CIBA Vision (Titmus Eurocon)	Ellipticolour	38	38E range	Green Blue Aqua Amber	1
	Irisprint (1150 WIP)	38	8.4–9.6 radius	Green Grey Brown	1 1
	Hand painted	38	8.4–9.6	Custom made	
CooperVision	Mystique (opaque)	38	One	2 Blues 2 Greens	2 pupil sizes
	Permaflex (transparent)	74	8.7 or 8.9 radius	Spring green Sky blue Turquoise Violet blue Gold	1
Focus	Corneal	PMMA		Range of solid tints	
Igel	Hi Tint (transparent) Hi-Colour (opaque)	37, 67, 77	IGEL CD. 67, 77 ranges	Green Blue Aqua Brown All 5% and 10% + specials	4
Lunelle	ES70	70	ES range	Lemon Lagon (blue) Menthe (green)	1
Nissel	Hypa 2	37	One	Blue Aqua Green Yellow Brown	1
	Corneal	PMMA		Hand painted Range of solid tints	
	Scleral	PMMA		Hand painted Solid tinted optic	
Pilkington Barnes–Hind	Soft Mate	45	One	Green Blue Aqua Topaz	1
Sauflon	Aquarius Iris tint Transparent or opaque	77	As Sci-Fi 8.1:13.7 8.4:13.7, 14.4	Blue Green Aqua Yellow All in dark, medium or light patterns	2 pupils 3 iris 7 patterns
	Aquarius Prosthetic	77	Same	Hand-painted version	
Wesley–Jessen	Durasoft 3 allows some normal iris pattern to be seen	55			1, opaque dot pattern

life. In this case indicate any discrepancies between the photography and the patient's eye colour to the laboratory. The technician can then modify the colour to get as close as possible to the practitioner's description.

In some cases more than one lens is necessary before a satisfactory match is obtained. It is best to send the original lens back to the laboratory with a full description of any changes required. This helps the laboratory to produce a new lens to suit the patient's needs.

General approach with cosmetic lenses

As in most spheres, the simplest solution is often the best as well as being easiest to reproduce when a replacement lens is needed. An example is the masking of a white cataract. A scleral lens could be made but it would take longer to make and possibly the extra thickness would not give such a good result, whereas a soft lens with a black pupil area is simpler, and less expensive and time consuming (*Plate 103*). On the other hand there may be an eye where the corneal and scleral topography are extremely irregular and it would then be obvious that only a scleral lens or shell would be useful.

Patience is required when fitting this type of lens. There are many failures. Disfigured eyes are very non-standard. Every eye poses a different problem and there are no set solutions. As experience is gained a collection of lenses is acquired and these become very useful. Some very flat and very steep lenses, large and small lenses can be most valuable when fitting irregular eyes. Patients are frequently disappointed with the final appearance and this should be expected — they are looking for a miracle and generally it is not forthcoming.

Hence the education of the patient is all important. He or she must realize the limitations of the lenses, and time explaining these is often well spent. If some compromises are expected the resulting cosmetic lens is often better accepted.

Additional spectacles may be used if need be to help mask the appearance of a cosmetic lens (Kumar and Krishna, 1981); a negative spectacle lens appears to reduce the size of an enlarged palpebral aperture and a positive lens to increase that of a shrunken eye. Where an increase or reduction in apparent size is required in one meridian only a cylindrical spectacle lens may be used. The type of spectacle frame chosen can also help the general cosmetic appearance as can a slightly tinted pair of spectacle lenses. The practitioner who fits the cosmetic contact lens is in a good position and has a duty to point out the advantages of additional spectacles and to prescribe them with any suitable magnification effect and/or tint.

This form of prosthesis work is still at a relatively new stage but with the input of new research it will not be long before good, reproducible lenses are available. *Table 21.8* lists many of the commercially available tinted and cosmetic patterned lenses and their suppliers. Although challenging and time consuming much can be achieved and patients are frequently delighted with their new appearance and resulting self-confidence.

Reference

KUMAR, D. and KRISHNA, G. (1981). *Cosmetic Contact Lenses and Artificial Eyes*. Contact Lens Research and Training Institute, Aligarh, India

Further reading

RUBEN, M. (1982). *A Colour Atlas of Contact Lenses*. London: Wolfe

---

Soft lenses in other abnormal conditions
D. Westerhout

Contact lenses have been used for therapeutic purposes for over 100 years and, to this day, the well-fitted scleral lens or scleral ring still offers

adequate therapy for a variety of pathological ocular conditions.

Unfortunately, although scleral lens fitting is

still practised in an expert manner in some countries, the same cannot be said of others and in these countries in particular the advent of the soft, hydrogel lens in the 1960s permitted a simpler way of providing therapy with contact lenses.

Early therapeutic soft lens work was unfortunately carried out with thick, low water content, large lenses which proved helpful in some cases but disappointing in others. Certainly the therapeutic soft contact lens has not proved to be the panacea that many practitioners had hoped for.

Today, we have at our disposal more sophisticated technology in the form of new materials, better designs, better lens care pharmaceuticals, more knowledge resulting from research in the field of corneal physiology and the ability of certain designs and materials to permit normal corneal metabolism and integrity to be maintained.

Certainly, therapeutic soft contact lenses (also sometimes called bandage lenses) are now viewed rather differently and their use, for example, in many dry eye conditions is not now always recommended.

In a chapter such as this, it is not possible to cover all the permutations and combinations of lens designs and materials and every condition for which they are indicated or contra-indicated, but the methods of dealing with the conditions included give a sound guide for treating all others. Nor is it intended that this section should present a great deal of detail of ocular pathology. As, however, knowledge of first principles is helpful in any scientific or clinical approach, a brief description of conditions is included where appropriate.

Some duplication is unavoidable in a book such as this and inevitably there is some overlap with other sections and chapters.

The principal aims of therapeutic soft contact lens use

Therapeutic soft contact lenses are mainly fitted with the aim of attempting to maintain or restore the integrity of ocular tissues. Regrettably, despite this aim, many conditions progress although deterioration may, in some cases, be slowed.

Relief of pain

This is perhaps the best known aim of therapeutic soft lenses. In a variety of epithelial disorders, such as bullous keratopathy, relief of pain is often dramatic. This is usually due to preventing painful contact between the eyelid and the exposed nerve endings of the abnormal cornea.

Splinting of epithelium

In many superficial corneal conditions the migrating epithelial cells adhere poorly to their underlying basement membrane. As it can take at least 2 months for full regrowth of epithelium, the use of a therapeutic soft lens as an extended wear bandage for at least this period often provides the protection from the lids needed to allow the epithelium to develop proper adherence to the supporting structures, and thus stabilize.

Mechanical protection from lids, lashes and palpebral conjunctiva

Corneas frequently suffer from being in contact with rough palpebral conjunctival surfaces or ingrowing eyelashes. A therapeutic soft contact lens can provide mechanical protection against such potential trauma.

Maintenance of conjunctival fornices

Obliteration of the conjunctival fornices may occur in several scarring diseases of the mucosa, as for example, erythema multiforme, ocular pemphigoid and chemical burns. Although a scleral lens is commonly used to separate the tissue surfaces (see Chapter 18), a very large and reasonably rigid soft lens can be used for the same purpose.

The maintenance of corneal hydration

The use of therapeutic soft lenses for keratoconjunctivitis sicca is often discouraged as there is a greatly increased risk of infection, exacerbated by the lower levels of lysozyme in the tears. However, they can be useful when cicatrizing conjunctival diseases create problems of abnormal lid position or blinking, resulting in dry eyes.

Reducing the effect of aqueous leaks

Perforations in the anterior segment which lead to loss of aqueous fluid can often be controlled by a tightly fitting soft contact lens which partially seals the perforation, whether it be created by trauma or surgery.

As the anterior chamber refills, however, the eye shape alters and the lens fitting may need to be changed quickly, often more than once.

Improvement of vision

In many diseases and injuries of the cornea, the resultant corneal surface is left irregular, and cannot therefore provide good vision, even with spectacles. Contact lenses, especially rigid lenses such as hard gas permeable and scleral lenses, can then provide a regular anterior refracting surface and improve the visual acuity considerably.

In cases of extreme corneal sensitivity or irregularity, where contact of the cornea with a hard surface is inadvisable, a rigid lens can be fitted on top of a soft lens to provide the required, regular refractive surface (see pp. 751 and 815). The psychological benefits to the patient of improving vision in an abnormal, diseased eye should not be under-estimated. This effect is frequently forgotten.

Drug delivery with a therapeutic soft contact lens

It is recognized that only a very small percentage of topically administered drugs usually penetrate the cornea, due to the tear drainage system and other factors.

Soaking a therapeutic soft contact lens in a solution of the appropriate drug enables a 'slow release' effect to take place which is often found to be more effective (see p. 813 and Chapter 8).

Protection of the cornea during tonometry

Patients whose corneas are prejudiced and likely to be damaged by application of a tonometer or even by instillation of local anaesthetic drops, may have intraocular pressure (IOP) measured if a thin soft lens is used to protect the cornea (see p. 814 and Chapter 8).

Existing wearers of therapeutic soft bandage lenses may also have IOP monitored in this way. High-molecular-weight fluorescein is used for these cases.

Similar protection for the cornea may also be required before taking impressions of the eye for the fitting of scleral lenses (see p. 816 and Chapter 18).

Choice of lens material and design

The correct choice of lens material and design is central to the effective use of therapeutic soft lenses. There is often more than one option available and the practitioner must monitor progress frequently and be prepared to change lens design or material as often as necessary to obtain the clinical effect best suited to the interests of the patient.

The subject is often over-simplified and lenses are frequently classified into scleral, scleral ring, hydrogel low water content (below 40%), hydrogel high water content (above 60%) and silicone rubber, without reference to their parameters.

So many other factors need to be taken into consideration that the practitioner must be fully conversant with the technicalities and all other aspects of soft lens design and characteristics (see Chapters 3, 11 and 15). The tendency to utilize a single 'one fit design' therapeutic lens should be avoided.

It is the height of ill-informed optimism to hope that a lens design marketed as a 'one size fits all' will even fit a high proportion of patients with normal corneas. It is even more optimistic to hope that such a design will fit all abnormal or diseased eyes. Indeed so vital are the fitting and the lens characteristics of a therapeutic contact lens fitted to a prejudiced eye, that even more subtlety of design, available parameters and material are required than if a normal, healthy eye were being fitted.

A good illustration of this is the patient blinded by unusual thermal burns and with reconstructed eyelids which did not fully close. His third keratoplasty was almost as unsuccessful as the first two because an extended wear 'one fit' bandage lens was supplied (with two spares which both fell out), whereas his abnormal eye shape required a custom-made lens (Plate 120). In this case, in order to save the graft the lens was obtained by courier service, and within days the graft improved dramatically.

The importance of being able to obtain individually designed lenses is obvious.

Soft lens materials are commonly available in a variety of water contents from 35% to about 80%. All these materials can be made very thin (below 0.07 mm), standard thickness (from about 0.07 to 0.14 mm), or thick (above 0.14 mm) in their plano form.

Many practitioners feel that to avoid hypoxia they have to choose a very thin 38.6% water content lens or a much thicker 75% water content lens. Very often, given the disadvantages of both these, the best design may be a 55–60% water content lens in a thickness of about 0.08 mm.

Information on the comparative advantages of different materials and thicknesses may be found in Chapters 3 and 11, but the following observations are relevant to therapeutic soft lens fittings.

Choice of the best lens design and material will depend on consideration of the physiological requirements of the diseased eye. Normal eyes differ widely in their requirements, but there is even less margin for error when fitting a diseased eye.

The main preoccupation in contact lens practice in recent years has been with the amount of oxygen able to reach the cornea through the lenses. Nevertheless at least as much interest should be taken in the permeability of lenses to tear fluid and in choosing a design to allow the tear secretions, on which the integrity of the cornea also depends, to pass beneath the lens in contact with the corneal epithelium.

It is common to observe the adverse effects of soft lenses drying on the eye (*Plate 58*). This is seen both in dry eye patients and in normal patients in an excessively dry environment. The complex molecular structure of a soft lens material can, to a degree, be engineered to assist in retaining water within the lens matrix, despite a dry eye or dry environment. Thus knowledge of the characteristics of the lens material is vital in selecting the appropriate lens (*see* Chapter 11, p. 399).

Unfortunately there are some contradictions in therapeutic soft contact lens design which can lead to unpredictable results.

Ultrathin lenses have good oxygen transmission proportional to the water content of the material (Hill and Jeppe, 1976; Holden and Mertz, 1984). However, although this is a desirable feature, on dry eyes they rapidly lose their water content, the more so with low water content materials. This results in an undesirable tightening of the fit which is greater with the more fragile high water content lenses, to the extent that epithelial problems frequently occur (Zantos *et al.*, 1986). Additionally all such lenses are difficult for elderly and/or partially sighted patients to handle. Although both low and high water content lenses may, on occasion, be useful, the best compromise appears to be a fairly thin (0.07–0.10 mm) medium water content (55–60%) lens. Latest materials of this type, such as the Weflex 55, retain their water content well (K. Polzhofer, 1987, personal communication), are resistant to protein deposits and are strong enough to make handling fairly easy, as well as being resistant to damage from knots or sutures. Such lenses have a high proportion of 'bound' water as compared to 'free' water in the material.

Resistance to the formation of deposits is a very important characteristic of a successful therapeutic soft lens as there is no doubt that the worst lens deposits encountered occur on and in many therapeutic contact lenses. The ability to clean them effectively is therefore very important (*see* Chapter 4).

Silicone rubber lenses

Flexible silicone rubber therapeutic lenses have an important role to play as the material is very permeable to oxygen but, at the same time, is not hydrated and absorbs the minimum amount of fluid. Not requiring fluid to retain its shape, its fit is unaffected by a dry eye and thus it may be the lens of choice when dryness is a consideration. Unfortunately though, it has several drawbacks. In spite of surface treatment it is one of the worst materials from the viewpoint of deposit formation, especially protein and lipid deposits (*Plates 44* and *45*). Although these may be removable by soaking in hydrogen peroxide or in 5% sodium hyperchlorite for 5 minutes and rinsing in distilled water there is a risk of damaging the surface. Daily surfactant cleaning and the regular use of enzyme cleaners in an ultrasonic bath have proved best.

Another difficulty is that it is hard to predict how a lens will fit after it has been worn for a few hours. Lenses that look a perfect fit, or even a little loose or flat, can appear to tighten unpredictably to the point where the passage of tear fluid beneath the lens is no longer possible. They are not often successful for extended wear partly due to their tendency to tighten and also due to the need for daily cleaning.

Unlike a hydrogel lens the material is very rigid and springy, and apart from tightening its fit holds its shape very well. It can also be fitted using fluorescein. Illustrations of silicone rubber fittings are shown in *Plates 41–43*.

As the majority of readers are most likely to consult a textbook such as this when they are about to fit a patient with diagnosed ocular pathology, it seems most logical to present information under the categories of the pathology.

Bullous keratopathy

This condition of chronic oedema of the cornea can be extremely painful and the main aim of the therapeutic lens is to alleviate the symptoms of pain, epiphora, photophobia and blepharospasm and also attempt to reduce the chronic oedema. There are many possible causes of gross corneal oedema, but endothelial cell malfunction is frequently a common factor.

Malfunction of the endothelium may occur as the result of a dystrophic process such as Fuchs' dystrophy. Most cases of bullous keratopathy, however, are seen as a result of intraocular surgery, usually cataract extraction. More recently, with the popularity of intraocular lens implants, some cases of endothelial malfunction may be attributed to the trauma of an insecure anterior chamber implant interacting with the corneal endothelium.

Fuchs' dystrophy usually begins with guttata of the corneal endothelium (*Plates 65* and *66*. It is thought to be an inherited trait affecting women more than men. It is bilateral but usually asymmetrical. The guttata are initially seen in the central cornea and spread peripherally. Slight stromal oedema occurs and is eventually followed by epithelial oedema and bullous keratopathy.

Whatever the initial cause of oedema, in bullous keratopathy fluid eventually accumulates in the epithelium and forms cystic spaces (bullae). These bullae often rupture causing severe pain which is exacerbated by the exposed nerve endings being rubbed by the lids (*Plates 68* and *118*).

It is usually treated initially with ocular lubricants and hypertonic saline to attempt to draw water from the cornea. In severe cases penetrating keratoplasty is carried out. However, in some situations this may not be possible or feasible and a therapeutic contact lens becomes the next mode of therapy.

In view of the pain involved, it is usually best to fit the therapeutic lenses as soon as possible. Almost immediate relief of pain usually follows. The reduction of oedema is, however, more difficult to achieve. To reduce oedema, Ruben (1975) has described the principle of compressing large areas of the cornea with a contact lens as a means of creating an anterior water barrier. This is most effectively done by using a flush fitting scleral lens with compression over about two-thirds of the central cornea (Marriott, 1981, and *see* Chapter 18).

A soft contact lens relieves the discomfort by the simple expedient of separating the painful bullae from the lid. Some pain may persist due to the epithelial swelling causing a stretching of the nerve endings. The greater reservoir of fluid in a large soft lens permits a rapid rate of evaporation from the new anterior surface, thus possibly decreasing the flow of water into the cornea. A relative dehydration of the cornea can be achieved by the use of 5% saline solution therapy which, giving a reservoir of hypertonic saline solution in the lens, helps to dehydrate the cornea, thereby reducing oedema. Hypertonic saline had been used for many years before the development of soft lenses, but their reservoir effect has made this therapy much more successful. Repeated instillation permits the ion concentration of the fluid in the lens to reach the same level as that of the hypertonic saline used. The resultant osmotic pressure gradient is sufficient to cause the deturgescence of the cornea in many cases.

Some practitioners prefer to prescribe the prophylactic use of chloramphenicol drops, 0.5%, made without preservative, for the first week of bandage wear (Leibowitz and Rosenthal, 1971). The use of acetazolamide (Diamox) and similar diuretic drugs is also helpful with or without the hypertonic saline therapy.

Some of the milder forms of the condition, following cataract surgery often respond so well that a complete cure may be effected by the use of a soft lens bandage.

Occasionally severe oedema of the cornea, diagnosed as bullous keratopathy, disappears after using a soft lens bandage, never to reappear even when the lens is removed within a few weeks. These cases have occurred in the presence of low IOP.

Liebowitz and Rosenthal (1971), in observations using low water content lenses, reported no improvement in the signs observed despite the relief of discomfort. High water content lenses (for example, Sauflon PW and Permalens) are then often considerably more effective and an improvement in some of the signs occurs, especially when combined with the use of hypertonic saline. It appears necessary to instil 5% saline at 1- or 2-hourly intervals to produce a continuous beneficial effect on the oedema.

Unfortunately, the visual acuity is often extremely poor in bullous keratopathy due to the presence of other pathology.

It is very important to attempt to limit the amount of movement of a soft lens on the eye in bullous keratopathy, and this is best done by using a large, semi-scleral soft lens. However, if the lens is to be used for extended wear over a long period it is vital for the lens to be able to move slightly so that debris can be flushed out from behind the lens by the tear fluid. There is otherwise a risk of inflammatory reactions and one of the difficulties of fitting large ultrathin lenses in these cases is achieving the right balance between these two factors.

Since daily removal of a lens by a clumsy patient often makes the eye extremely painful and negates much of the benefit gained, the use of a continuously worn bandage is then preferred. Provided that lenses of low or medium water content are made sufficiently thin (Hill and Jeppe, 1976), or else lenses of very high water content material are used (for example, Sauflon PW, Permalens or similar materials), there appears to be very little risk in extended wear compared with the problems encountered during the daily use of these lenses. Constant insertion and removal of therapeutic soft lenses, with the possibility of using contaminated solutions, considerably increases the risk of infection (Donzis *et al.*, 1987; Hart and Shih, 1987) whereas in normal soft lens practice the reverse is true and more infections are encountered with extended wear than daily wear. Thus,

provided there are no obvious contra-indications, continuous wear, especially in the earlier stages of therapy, may well be the best course of action.

In general, thicker high water content lenses are better than thinner designs as the lid interaction with a thicker lens helps to create sufficient movement to give a healthy tear flow behind the lens. Even with continuous wear lenses, unless biomicroscopic examination of the cornea contra-indicates it, weekly removal for cleaning and sterilizing the lenses is advisable to remove foreign bodies such as mucus or dead cells.

One of the important factors in soft therapeutic lens use is the need to consider changes in lens type as the condition responds to therapy. The majority of cases of bullous keratopathy benefit most from wearing a high water content lens continuously until the appearance of the cornea indicates that the lens can or should be removed for cleaning. At that stage any protein or other deposits adhering to the lens surfaces should be removed. When pain has almost totally gone and the condition of the cornea appears to be improving, it is often desirable to change the lens to one of medium water content and medium thickness, worn on a daily wear basis. This type of lens is much easier to keep clean, which, particularly in private practice, is much appreciated by the patient as it is less expensive.

However, within a health service environment if the patient can be provided with a new lens whenever an extended wear lens appears to require replacement, this may indeed be the best long-term solution. In either case, the risk of infection must be considered for each particular patient. The decision whether to continue extended wear or change to daily wear is one of the professional judgements that practitioners have to make on observing the progress of the patient and based on their knowledge of the characteristics of the disease and the lenses that they are using.The use of disposable extended wear soft lenses such as the Vistakon lenses may well be the best choice in the future if these can be replaced on a weekly basis.

As it is known that the complete epithelialization of disturbed corneal areas can take between 6 weeks and 4 months, it is often a good strategy to continue the use of a therapeutic extended wear lens for up to 4 months provided there are no obvious contra-indications. In particularly severe cases, the continuous wear bandage lens may need to be left in for periods of up to 9 months to produce the desired results. Although normally ill-advised, this is sometimes the only possible alternative. Unfortunately although it is usually extremely effective in reducing pain, the patient almost always becomes totally dependent on the use of the bandage lens and occasionally the initial progress is not maintained. Vascularization is inclined to increase and a drop in visual acuity is often noticed after a period. The eye often becomes infected in the later stages of the condition and the overall prognosis over a long period is not all that good. In such cases penetrating keratoplasty is the only alternative. However, some patients respond very well to therapy and improve sufficiently to be able to cease the use of the bandage for intermittent periods or even completely. Other patients may cease the use of the bandage lens and go on to more conventional therapy such as the use of glycerin or saline drops.

In the early stages of the condition, soft lens bandage treatment sometimes improves visual acuity from as low as 6/60 to 6/9. This is probably due to the restoration of a reasonably smooth regular anterior refracting surface (*Plate 118*). For a patient who can handle the bandage lens skilfully, normal daily wear may be recommended, but if the bullae rupture and cause severe discomfort, then extended wear is essential and may have to be resumed if bullae rupture after changing to daily wear.

The painful rupture of the bullae often occurs at night when the lens has not been worn. Persistant recurrence of painful bullae is a further indication for corneal grafting.

Although improvement in vision with a therapeutic contact lens is sometimes dramatic in the earlier stages of the disease, Dohlman and Hyndiuk (1972) reported an improvement in visual acuity in only about 20% of those with advanced disease whereas in 1983 Hövding found that about 37% of such patients experienced improved visual acuity. Compared with the often-used alternative of tarsorrhaphy, contact lens wear provides the ophthalmologist and optometrist with a clear view of the eye permitting observation over a period.

The fitting of the soft lens bandage is often difficult and it is helpful to take keratometric readings from the non-affected eye to give guidance as to the required fitting. In general, larger lenses perform better than small ones, most lenses used for this condition having a total diameter in the region of 14.0–15.5 mm (*Plate 120b*).

Accuracy of fit is important to avoid excessive movement of the lens but, at the same time, too tight a lens can result in vascularization of the stroma (Ruben, 1971). Vascularization is not always a serious problem in these cases provided it is limited to the peripheral cornea. Extensive neovascularization may increase the risk of graft rejection in any subsequent surgery. In some cases the vascularization produces an improvement in the keratopathy and its symptoms, thus allowing therapy with a soft lens to be discontinued. In other cases subsequent infection and ulceration occur in the later stages. Unfortunately, especially with a continuously worn bandage lens, protein contamination is often a serious problem as the tear secretion is also often abnormal. The lenses may become incapable of being cleaned and need replacement (*Plates 32* and *35*). If weekly (or periodic) removal is feasible, two lenses worn alternately permit regular prophylactic cleaning by the patient, or if needed, more intensive cleaning by the practitioner. Appropriate methods of cleaning are dealt with in Chapter 4. Jacob (1988) recommends 10% hydrogen peroxide, sodium perborate, citric acid and tensides with heat, as effective cleaners for high water content lenses.

As a large number of patients with bullous keratopathy have had cataract extraction, it is very tempting to fit them with aphakic soft contact lenses to correct their refractive error and visual acuity. Unfortunately, even if made in a material designed for extended wear, the lens thickness reduces oxygen transmission with the risk of compromising the cornea and creating oedema which then exacerbates the problem. Continuing to tolerate this situation can lead to extensive neovascularization. It is better, therefore, to use a plano high water content lens in such circumstances, in conjunction with aphakic spectacle lenses.

Corneal dystrophies

In most corneal dystrophies the problems encountered are similar to those in bullous keratopathy, which is commonly classified as a corneal degeneration, but the painful erosions are usually caused by inadequate adhesion of the epithelium to the underlying basement membrane. Conditions in this category, which can frequently be treated successfully with therapeutic soft contact lenses include both primary and secondary anterior membrane dystrophies.

The conditions include the following:

(1) Meesman's epithelial dystrophy.
(2) Reis–Bücklers' dystrophy.
(3) Map–dot–fingerprint dystrophy.
(4) Macular dystrophy.
(5) Lattice dystrophy.
(6) Recurrent erosions.

There are, of course, less common forms of corneal dystrophy, many of which also benefit from the use of a therapeutic soft contact lens.

Meesman's epithelial dystrophy

In this rare autosomal, dominant hereditary condition the epithelial changes can occur in the infant, and always increase with age. Usually there is only mild ocular discomfort and there may be lacrimation, photophobia and a slight loss of visual acuity. The slit lamp appearance is usually of intraepithelial microcysts in a diffuse pattern in the epithelium of both eyes.

Reis–Bücklers' dystrophy

This is an autosomal dominant condition characterized by recurring, prolonged painful attacks of epithelial erosions with the pain lasting for several weeks. These can occur as early as age 5 years. Fine thread-like or ring-like opacities are seen at the level of Bowman's layer. Eventually corneal sensitivity is reduced and visual acuity often deteriorates in the twenties.

Map–dot–fingerprint dystrophy (Cogan's dystrophy)

This condition is thought to be caused by an abnormal basement membrane. The slit lamp appearance of the lesions is a curious mixture of dots (microcysts), lines (resembling finger-prints) and 'geographical' (map) lesions.

The clinical problem is one of recurrent epithelial erosion which is usually painful and is liable to produce the associated symptoms of foreign body sensations and photophobia common to most epithelial dystrophies.

Macular dystrophy

Recurrent epithelial erosion is often a feature of this condition which is transmitted as an autosomal recessive trait. It is usually seen in the first two decades of life. The stroma is usually diffusely cloudy and there are many greyish-white spots seen in the corneal stroma. These spots tend to be deeper in the periphery than in the centre.

Lattice dystrophy

This is an autosomal dominant condition usually occurring in the first decade of life.

The cornea has a characteristic ground-glass appearance which seldom reaches the periphery. There is usually discomfort and photophobia as a result of corneal erosions and vision has usually deteriorated by the age of 30 years.

The recurrent erosion syndrome

In this condition the patients suffer a painful and severe recurring erosion of the epithelium which appears unrelated to any of the other conditions named above, often following trauma to the cornea. It is usually thought to be an acquired defect in the epithelial basement membrane and in hemidesmosome formation resulting in microcysts, bullae and loss of epithelium. Attacks of pain usually occur in the early morning, or on waking.

In a normal cornea, the epithelium is attached to the basement membrane with structures called hemidesmosomes. If damage occurs in the basement membrane, epithelium cannot migrate over the damaged area and attach. It takes at least 6 weeks and as long as several months for hemidesmosomes to be able to attach the epithelium over the underlying membrane. During this period of healing the epithelium is loose and unattached and lid movement over the area will remove the regenerating epithelium.

In all of the above-mentioned conditions the main function of the therapeutic soft lens is to reduce the pain caused by the lids rubbing on the nerve endings and, by splinting the epithelium, to allow it to attach itself firmly to the basement membrane and to create stable epithelialization. Many of these patients have been frustrated by their condition for years and have often found no relief with conventional therapy. Occasionally sufferers from recurrent corneal erosion are given topical ansesthetics for home use when the pain becomes unbearable.

Although almost any therapeutic soft lens will relieve the pain, it is just as important to allow epithelialization to occur. For this reason it is best not to use a daily wear lens as the frequent insertion and removal will probably damage the fragile epithelial bonds. Protection of the healing epithelium, combined with a splinting effect, is very important. For this reason a thick, firm extended wear bandage lens which is thin enough not to compromise the corneal metabolism, but thick enough to splint effectively, is preferable. It may be necessary to wear the lens continuously for up to 6 months (Grayson, 1983). In general it is better to err on the side of prolonged use of the lens rather than remove it too soon. Ultrathin extended wear lenses often buckle or wrinkle on the eye with lid movement and this may not support or splint the epithelium in a stable manner.

Relapses in these conditions are common when lenses have been removed and this phenomenon also occurs when therapeutic soft lenses have been used to aid the healing of indolent ulcers. Hövding (1983) reported on the advisability of continuing lens wear for at least several weeks after epithelialization is achieved.

However, some conflict may exist in the use of extended wear to aid epithelialization. Madigan, Holden and Kwok (1987) concluded that, in cats, extended wear caused a loss of corneal epithelial adhesion to the basement membrane. Extended wear does not, however, appear to adversely affect epithelial healing. Excessive lens movement is undesirable in these cases, but months of continuous wear indicates a need for some lens movement to occur. Too large a lens is inadvisable as the overlap onto the sclera tends to form a seal preventing the flushing out of debris.

High water content lenses such as the Sauflon PW or Permalens lenses are generally the most suitable, as are many other high water content, extended wear lenses, but it is often difficult to obtain them custom-made in the desired parameters. Most extended wear lenses supplied by the bigger laboratories are available only in stock parameters which may not be suitable for all fittings. A stock of lenses in the most commonly used parameters kept in the consulting room in plano form is most useful as there is often no time for a lens to be purchased from a laboratory.

Parameters commonly used are:

TD (mm)	BOZR (mm)
13.7	7.5, 7.8, 8.1
14.4	7.5, 7.8, 8.1, 8.4, 8.7
15.0	7.8, 8.1, 8.4, 8.7, 9.0
15.5	7.8, 8.1, 8.4, 8.7, 9.0, 9.3

Due to the tendency of these high water content extended wear lenses to become contaminated and coated, regular irrigation of the eye with unpreserved sterile saline is very useful. Unfortunately, despite the need for a therapeutic contact lens to be worn continuously for long periods, the lens can become so heavily coated with jelly bumps (lipids), protein or calcium deposits that the lens rapidly becomes an irritant and may even create persistent inflammation or discomfort. Coated therapeutic soft lenses often produce giant papillary conjunctivitis.

Jelly bumps (caused by lipids) are a frequent cause of contamination of extended wear lenses in particular, but can sometimes be removed by melting and emulsification (K. Polzhofer, 1986, personal communication). Hart et al. (1987) have found that patients with low tear potassium are more prone to jelly bumps, as are patients who have a high intake of cholesterol, protein or alcohol. Some medications such as antihistamines, diuretics and anticholinergics also appear associated with jelly bump deposits. Where appropriate, attention to these aspects should be considered (see Chapter 4).

Despite the need to leave the epithelium undisturbed, it may be essential for the practitioner to remove the therapeutic lens very carefully and replace it with a new one. It is a question of balancing the advantages of continuous wear, leaving the epithelium undisturbed, against the risks inherent in allowing a coated, contaminated lens to provide a source of irritation and/or infection. The prognosis for the recurrent erosion conditions is usually considered quite good, particularly in the recurrent epithelial erosion syndrome and Meesman's dystrophy. Naturally a great deal depends on the condition when the lens is first fitted, for if the cornea has deteriorated over a very long period the outlook may obviously be worse than if the condition is caught reasonably early.

In some cases a keratopathy of uncertain classification may be encountered which does not respond to normal therapy. In such cases a bandage lens is worth using for a trial period.

Cicatrizing conjunctival diseases

Many of these diseases can be effectively treated with therapeutic contact lenses as a means of relieving pain, providing protection for the cornea from the formation of conjunctival keratin or trichiasis and maintaining the conjunctival fornices.

In some instances these diseases may result in symblepharon (adhesions between bulbar and palpebral conjunctivas). This may affect blinking and produce secondary effects of exposure keratitis and related complications. Corneal involvement associated with cicatrizing of the conjunctivas occurs with the following conditions:

(1) Stevens–Johnson syndrome (erythema multiforme).
(2) Ocular pemphigoid.
(3) Chemical burns.
(4) Thermal burns.
(5) Trachoma.
(6) Toxic effects of medication.
(7) Pseudomembranous and membranous conjunctivitis.
(8) Exfoliative dermatitis, dermatitis herpetiformis and epidermolysis bullosa.
(9) Atopic keratoconjunctivitis.
(10) Sarcoidosis.

The more commonly encountered conditions in this group are briefly described below.

Stevens–Johnson syndrome (erythema multiforme)

Most but not all of these cases are drug induced. Bilateral conjunctivitis is a feature of this condition which usually leads to scarring of the conjunctivas. Fortunately the ocular aspects of the condition stabilize once the systemic disease has been resolved. Obviously, however, by the time that this has occurred there may already be severe irreversible changes such as scarring, keratoconjunctivitis sicca, symblepharon, entropion and trichiasis.

Perhaps surprisingly, impression cell cytology taken from the affected conjunctivas does not always reveal eosinophils, but usually shows a preponderance of polymorphonuclear cells.

Treatment with a scleral lens or ring is usually helpful although the scleral ring tends to be unstable. A scleral lens does also retain a tear layer in front of the cornea and this helps in reducing corneal keratinization and provides better vision by negating the optical effects of corneal irregularities. Due to the inability to fit scleral lenses in many parts of the world, the use of therapeutic soft contact lenses has become more common. If, despite abnormal conjunctivas and tear film, there is an adequate volume of tears, it is desirable to use a very large (15–20 mm) low or medium water content lens to prevent adhesions forming or re-forming (Westerhout, 1981). Since a thin lens tends to distort and wrinkle, making it less efficacious and uncomfortable, it is better to use a thicker, more rigid lens, and as low water content materials may lead to hypoxia with attendant risks to the abnormal eye and high water content lenses tend to become coated too quickly with deposits, the use of a medium (55%) water content, relatively thick lens seems optimal. Such a lens can be used mainly as a daily wear lens but thinner versions can be used if extended wear is thought essential for a period. Eventually large sophisticated multi-curved flexible silicone lenses may be the lens of choice in these cases.

Ocular pemphigoid

This is an autoimmune scarring disease of the conjunctivas, usually found in patients over the age of 50 years. It is more common in females.

The disease usually starts with mild recurring attacks of conjunctivitis which are often, understandably, wrongly diagnosed as bacterial in origin. In the early stages of the disease, hyperaemia and oedema of the conjunctivas with dysfunction of the tears is usually noted. The worst ocular complications occur later in the disease and comprise symblepharon, ingrowing lashes, keratoconjunctivis sicca, keratinization and scarring of the lids.

Corneal complications are usually the result of dryness and aberrant lid trauma which leave the cornea vulnerable to infection.

Impression cell cytology of the conjunctivas is most likely to reveal the presence of eosinophils, especially with the condition in an acute state.

Lid surgery is often unsatisfactory in pemphigoid whereas it is usually indicated in erythema multiforme. For this reason, in pemphigoid, the use of a therapeutic soft lens is often indicated to protect the cornea against the action of ingrowing lashes and malpositioned lids (*Plate 7*).

As in erythema multiforme, both scleral and therapeutic soft contact lenses can be used with effect and the same approach to soft lens fitting can be used in either case. Thin lenses are to be avoided and thicker lenses are preferred. The lenses must be large enough, however, to extend almost as far as a scleral lens if possible.

Chemical burns

Chemical burns to the eye form a very complex aspect of ophthalmology due to the large variety of chemicals available to inflict ocular damage.

Strong alkaline chemicals inflict the worst damage due to their potential for penetration and continuing effect long after the affected tissues have been irrigated. The commonly used cleaning agent, ammonia, is one of the worst chemicals to inflict damage on the eye as it can penetrate very rapidly through the epithelium. Acids, on the other hand, have less effect as they tend to bind tissue protein, producing coagulation which then limits further penetration. Therapeutic soft lenses cannot be used in the early stages of chemical burns, but assist later treatment which must be carefully managed and continued until the epithelium has completely covered the area of the lesion. A therapeutic soft lens can aid this process by splinting the epithelium and also preventing damage from lids, trichiasis, exposure or insufficient tears. The lens may also prevent symblepharon.

Provided that no contra-indications are seen, continuous wearing is a better alternative than daily wear until the epithelium has healed.

Thermal burns

Fortunately thermal burns rarely cause cicatrizing effects on the bulbar or palpebral conjunctivas. This is thought to be the result of reflex lid closure before prolonged exposure to heat can occur (J. Davey, 1988, personal communication). In unusual cases, however, patients may deliberately keep their eyelids open, despite the danger, in an attempt to help others at risk. The early fitting of a corneal bandage is then advisable to prevent loss of sight. If eyelids are so badly damaged by burns that they are ineffective, then a therapeutic soft lens used with frequent irrigation may enable a relatively undamaged cornea to retain its integrity. It should also be realized that there is almost invariably an abnormal tear film in all these cicatrizing conjunctival conditions. For this reason the therapeutic soft lens, provided that it is of a suitable material and thickness, is also invaluable in attempting to keep the cornea wet (*see under* The dry eye, p. 807).

Ideally, all eye hospitals should have a selection of large, extended wear therapeutic soft lenses for use in the immediate treatment of burns.

Trachoma

This is a chlamydial infection and a common cause of preventable blindness, and is found mainly in unhealthy, dirty, crowded conditions.

In its earliest stage the main characteristic is the presence of soft immature follicles in the upper tarsal conjunctivas. A punctate keratitis and early superior corneal pannus may be seen. At a later stage cicatrization of the lids, symblepharon, trichiasis and distortion of the lids are common.

Corneal opacification and dryness of the cornea and conjunctivas are additional complications.

The condition is usually treated with oral antibiotics, but on occasion, therapeutic contact lenses can be used to separate inflamed tissue to prevent symblepharon and to avoid the effects of ingrowing lashes.

Toxic effect of drugs

Numerous drugs are known to produce toxic effects in the eye and Grayson (1983) lists idoxuridine, pilocarpine, ecothiopate iodide

(Phospholine Iodide) and practolol as sometimes creating cicatrizing effects in ocular tissue. Grayson reports having seen symblepharon and conjunctival cicatrization caused by idoxuridine and pilocarpine.

In these instances, changing or withdrawing chemical therapy is obviously vital, but therapeutic contact lenses can be used if appropriate, especially in the prevention of symblepharon.

Epidermolysis bullosa

This is an inherited dystrophic condition in which there may be pseudomembrane and vesicle formation, epithelial erosions and symblepharon.

Therapeutic soft contact lens use is indicated when appropriate, and the same choice of lenses applies as in the other cicatrizing conditions.

The author is not yet aware of therapeutic soft contact lenses being used for pseudomembranous and membranous conjunctivitis, exfoliative dermatitis, dermatitis herpetiformis, atopic keratoconjunctivitis or sarcoidosis, but if the clinical evidence indicates the use of a therapeutic soft lens it would be logical to use one.

The dry eye

The dry eye, in all its different forms, represents the most controversial condition for the use of a therapeutic soft contact lens.

Some practitioners seem to feel that the therapeutic hydrogel lenses should be used only rarely in keratoconjunctivitis sicca (Dart, 1987), whereas other practitioners advocate their controlled use (Gassett, 1978; Dada and Acharjee, 1982; Hövding, 1983; Phillips, 1986). The different types of 'dry eye' are caused by different abnormalities and may require different approaches in therapy. A knowledge of dry eye problems in general is central to deciding on the likely safety and efficacy of therapy with a therapeutic soft lens, either hydrogel or silicone rubber.

The tear film

The tear film consists of three main layers. The innermost layer, in contact with the epithelium, is the very thin mucous or mucin layer which, by producing hydrophilic coating, is most important in maintaining a stable tear film. The middle layer is mainly aqueous but contains many metabolites such as salts, glucose, urea, enzymes, proteins and glycoproteins. The other layer is mainly lipids. Abnormalities of the tear film may affect any one or more of the three layers. The effects of the disease or abnormality will depend on which layer is most affected.

The lipid layer is affected mainly by chronic blepharitis (*Plates 6* and *8*) and, less often, by radiation. The aqueous layer is commonly affected by keratoconjunctivitis sicca, rheumatoid arthritis, paralytic hyposecretion and seventh nerve paresis. The mucin layer is secreted by the goblet cells of the conjunctiva and to a lesser extent by the epithelial cells (Phelps-Brown, 1988), and thus it is not surprising that this layer is affected by cicatricial conjunctivitis including ocular pemphigoid, Stevens–Johnson syndrome, trachoma, chemical and thermal burns. Additionally, vitamin A deficiency, especially in less developed countries, can lead to disturbances in the mucin output.

The most commonly encountered form of dry eyes is usually found in menopausal and postmenopausal women, but there appears to be an increase in the number of younger women with this condition, especially those with abnormal hormonal balance and those taking oral contraceptives, particularly if they have other side effects.

The minor degrees of dry eye are usually termed 'conjunctivitis sicca', but when the cornea becomes involved the condition is called keratoconjunctivitis sicca (KCS).

There are two forms of tear secretion. The resting or basic tear secretion continues constantly even when the eyes are closed in sleep. When there is a special demand for additional tears such as occurs in ocular irritation due to dust or fumes, then the reflex tear secretion produces additional tears.

It is for this reason that there are different tear function tests, although these are very approximate. More information on tear tests is available in Chapters 2, 8, and 11. Tests for basic secretion and reflex tear secretions are based on Schirmer's test.

Schirmer's test I

This measures total reflex and basic tear secretion with a strip of Whatman filter paper placed so that 5 mm lies within the lower conjunctival sac and 25 mm projects beyond the lower lid. The length of strip wetted after 5 minutes for most people with normal tear output is 10–30 mm.

The basic secretion test

This is carried out in the same way, but on an anaesthetized eye which cannot, therefore, produce a reflex tear secretion. Reflex secretion is determined approximately by subtracting the basic test result from the result of Schirmer's test I.

The basic (resting secretion) comes mainly from the accessory lacrimal glands around the conjunctival fornices, but the reflex secretion comes from the principal lacrimal glands. It can be readily seen that different diseases affecting different tissues may affect the basic and reflex secretions differently.

One of the most important constituents of the tear film is the enzyme lysozyme which has strong antibacterial properties. The tear film also contains the antibacterial lactoferrin, and γ-globulin, also involved in resisting infection.

A dry eye problem is, therefore, not just a question of having an insufficient quantity of tears, but due to the multifunctional nature of tears any disturbance of its delicate balance can have serious adverse effects.

The lysozyme content in dry eyes is usually found to be present in less than half its normal quantity and thus in that sense alone, the dry eye is more vulnerable to infection. Most patients initially complain of 'gritty' eyes, sometimes with an increase in redness. This is worse in dry, centrally heated or similar atmospheres and is not improved by using decongestant drops with which many sufferers self-medicate themselves.

Frequently, intermittent watering accompanies the symptoms of irritated gritty eyes. The reason for this is usually that the resting tear secretion is affected. This leads to a dry eye which becomes progressively irritating. The irritation then produces a reflex tear secretion which may be unaffected by the condition. The patient notices the reflex tears more than the initial dry eye problem and thus finds it hard to accept the diagnosis of a dry eye. Occasionally debris from the dry eye actually blocks the nasolacrimal duct, and the reflex secretion then gives rise to epiphora, seemingly making the dry eye diagnosis even more improbable to the patient.

Examination of the dry eye patient with a slit lamp usually shows a minimal tear meniscus along the lower lid margin, or even none at all. Increased epithelial cell debris is seen in the tear film and there is usually a quantity of mucous threads visible which may accumulate in the lower fornix.

Using fluorescein, the test for tear film break-up time (BUT), when the patient is asked to blink once and then refrain from blinking should reveal a tear film which is intact for 15–45 seconds. Any BUT less than 10 seconds may be considered abnormal. In some instances no complete tear film forms and the cornea shows constant dry areas (see Chapter 8).

An abnormally low tear BUT is usually indicative of a mucin-deficient eye if there is no obvious lack of aqueous volume and no condition, such as chronic blepharitis, to indicate a lipid abnormality.

In KCS, rose bengal stain, which is specific for dead or damaged cells and mucus, often shows up filamentary keratitis, the filaments consisting of mucin threads attached to desquamated epithelial cells and lipids. These threads are usually attached to the corneal epithelium and are thus usually uncomfortable, as blinking pulls on them and thence on the epithelial cells.

The condition of KCS is usually bilateral but often not symmetrical. When unilateral it is usually as a result of surgery, burns, trauma or paresis.

Apart from conditions producing cicatricial conjunctivitis, the most common cause of mucin deficiency is a lack of vitamin A, and in its worst form, the deficiency can lead to xerophthalmia.

If lack of vitamin A is often a cause of mucin-deficient dry eyes then it is reasonable to hope that its use may prevent or reverse some dry eye problems. That this is indeed the case, when topical use of vitamin A is employed, is now well documented (for example Van Horn et al., 1981; Sommer and Green, 1982; Tseng et al., 1985).

Also the author has been using aqueous eye drops containing vitamin A and other free radical scavengers for the treatment of dry eye conditions for over 2 years. This has been used on its own and in conjunction with therapeutic soft contact lenses. In a series of 143 patients with dry eye problems who had not responded to previous therapy, these drops have proved very effective in reducing patients' symptoms in 88% of cases and in increasing tear BUT in 72% of cases. Most interesting has been the fact that other dry eye patients who are not aided by ocular lubricants, but were very much more comfortable with therapeutic soft contact lenses, were eventually able to discard the therapeutic contact lens after 2–3 months of associated use of the topical vitamin A drops. As the drops are compatible with tears and unpreserved they can be used while soft lenses are being worn. (Details of vitamin A drops are given in Chapter 4 and Appendix F.)

Ohashi *et al.* (1988) have reported on successful treatment of superior limbic kerato-conjunctivitis with a vitamin A eye drop.

The use of therapeutic hydrogel contact lenses in dry eye conditions

The complexities of dry eye problems and their different causes indicate that no one approach is effective in every case.

The main point to be considered is the principal cause of the dry eye. If the problem is a deficiency of the middle, aqueous layer of the tear film, due to KCS or other conditions, then the biggest difficulty in using a therapeutic hydrogel contact lens is a lack of fluid to keep the lens hydrated.

Dry eye patients can be divided into those who have an insufficient quantity of tears and those who have poor quality tears. Some indeed may suffer from both abnormalities.

Generally speaking a sufficient quantity of tears with poor wetting quality is easier to treat with therapeutic hydrogel contact lenses especially if the lids are reasonably normal. The highly absorbent lens material soaks up the aqueous layer, rather like a wick, and redistributes it over the corneal epithelium.

Most of these cases are best fitted with a large, medium water content lens of medium thickness. Such lenses retain their shape well even in a dry eye situation, especially if saline or other rehydrating drops are used throughout the day. Due to the greatly increased risk of eye infection in extended wear and the compromised state of a dry eye, it is not desirable to use an extended wear lens if it can be avoided. Most dry eye patients obtain relief at night with their eyes closed and there seems no justification for the increased risk of extended wear. The exception to this is if a serious eruption of the corneal epithelium occurs, when extended wear for a week or two may help the cornea to epithelialize.

It is often worth fitting dry eye patients, especially those with an adequate aqueous volume, with a high water content extended wear lens for 1 or 2 weeks and then changing to medium water content lenses for daily wear. However, low water content lenses such as HEMA lenses, are often as effective for daily wear because they are less affected by drying and absorb less of the available tears than higher water content lenses. Such lenses, however, should not be ultrathin, and medium to thick lenses are needed (0.1–0.16 mm in plano form). Bilton and Guillon (1984) reported that thick HEMA lenses are associated with a more stable tear film than thin lenses of the same material. The author has several filamentary keratitis and dry eye patients still using 0.12 mm thick low water content lenses for daily wear after more than 10 years without complications. One such case is shown in *Plate 8*.

The rapid build-up of coatings on soft lenses used for dry eyes can be reduced by using medium or low water content lenses and by avoiding extended wear. The hydrogen peroxide maintenance systems combined with modern enzymes assist greatly in avoiding therapeutic contact lens problems by keeping the lenses much cleaner.

Gassett (1978) advised changing clean, sterile therapeutic contact lenses every 4 hours in cases of filamentary keratitis seen in KCS. Gassett also reported that, in cases of 'wet' filamentary keratitis, the use of therapeutic contact lenses with corticosteroids and atropine for a short while results in the disappearance of the filaments within 7 days without recurrence. The use of therapeutic soft lenses in filamentary keratitis protects the epithelium from developing tags of mucus with consequent filament development. Acetyl cysteine 10% drops as a mucolytic combined with wetting agents such as polyvinyl alcohol can be most helpful.

Fatt and Di Martino (1983) showed that a soft lens dehydrates on the eye, and concluded that the tear layer underneath the lens contains only the non-aqueous components of the tears such as lipids and mucin. This tendency to hold a layer of mucin and lipids in contact with the epithelium may be of some significance in certain dry eye conditions.

Contact lens-induced dry eyes

Some hard and soft contact lens wearers develop dry eyes after wearing lenses for a period. This can occur despite the fact that no evidence of dry eyes was seen prior to fitting and the lens has satisfied all the usual criteria of successful fitting. In some cases the dry eye symptoms occur as early as 1 week after all day use is commenced. It seems possible that contact lens wear can damage the delicate microvilli on the superficial epithelial cells. The microvilli appear important as a means of retaining mucin in contact with the epithelial surface.

Dry eyes induced by systemic drugs

Some systemic drugs are known to cause dry eyes (*see* Chapters 4 and 8). The commonly used drugs which do so are: β-blockers, e.g. propranolol (Inderal) (Wartman, 1987); steroids; tricyclic antidepressants and those used for treating allergies.

The effects may mimic contact lens-related problems and, without regular application of sterile saline drops, soft lenses used for therapeutic or other reasons are contra-indicated.

Sjögren's syndrome

This condition is a form of KCS. The syndrome may be defined as a combination of any two of the following (Grayson, 1983):

(1) Keratoconjunctivitis sicca.
(2) Dryness of the mouth or other non-ocular mucous membranes.
(3) Rheumatoid arthritis and similar conditions.

It is most commonly found in the middle age group and more commonly in women.

Most patients who suffer from this conditon are postmenopausal women and may be aided by vitamin A eye drops and medium water content bandage lenses.

Unfortunately, this group of patients appears to have a higher risk of complications from infections and ulceration. Daily wear is to be preferred whenever possible, but many of the arthritics find great difficulty in handling a therapeutic contact lens twice daily.

Many ophthalmologists prescribe a broad spectrum topical antibiotic to be used 3 or 4 times daily when therapeutic contact lenses are used for Sjögren's syndrome, keratitis sicca, keratoconjunctivitis sicca and similar conditions. This is because bacterial keratitis is quite common in patients using daily wear therapeutic soft lenses and very much higher in the case of extended wear soft lenses.

Occlusion of the puncta is thought to be helpful in dry eye problems by reducing tear drainage. Phelps-Brown (1988) has suggested a method of using 'miracle glue' to provide a temporary occlusion in order to test the efficacy of the occlusion.

Other conditions requiring therapeutic soft lenses

Neuroparalytic and neurotrophic conditions

Secondary corneal disease frequently results from lesions of the fifth cranial nerve. The fifth nerve has a trophic effect with regard to the cornea, and lesions of this nerve frequently result in loss of corneal sensitivity. This also adversely affects the tear secretion and blink reflex. The epithelium becomes dry and areas of necrosis eventually occur. The corneal state is thus very vulnerable to infection and the areas of necrosis may eventually become infected, with severe corneal ulceration. Many patients previously treated by tarsorraphy, following neurosurgery, can be helped by daily wear of a large medium water content soft lens. If extended wear is preferred as more appropriate, then two or more lenses should be alternated daily in order to keep the lenses clean. The eye should be irrigated with sterile saline, at the time of changing the lenses, to flush away mucus and debris. Irrigation to rehydrate the lens is essential otherwise the lens tends to dry out and become uncomfortable. If, as frequently happens, the patient is hospitalized, the nursing staff can readily irrigate the therapeutic lens at regular intervals to ensure that the lens and thus the cornea is kept wet. If the lens is not irrigated regularly, its periphery begins to dry and often stands away from the conjunctiva, causing irritation and possible fracture of the lens.

Exposure keratitis

In this condition, often the result of lid dysfunction after lesions of the seventh cranial nerve, and cicatricial conjunctivitis, the cornea becomes extremely dry despite normal tear secretion (*see Plate 9*). Many cases are the result of neurosurgery and involve some degree of facial paralysis. As in the last category of cases, the soft contact lens is used purely to provide protection for the eye, but as the tear secretion is usually normal, irrigation is not so vital as in the neurotrophic and neuroparalytic conditions. If these patients are viewed during the hours of sleep a drying of the lens surface through non-closure of the lids is frequently observed, but it is interesting to note that the upward rotation of the eye still appears to take place despite the other complications, and this partially protects the lens and eye from drying. The treatment decided upon by the ophthalmologist greatly depends on the overall general prognosis. The choice of daily or extended wear depends on the degree of coverage of the eye tissues during the hours of sleep.

Indolent corneal ulcers

Patients with indolent corneal ulcers probably constitute one of the largest groups of people treated with soft contact lenses for therapeutic purposes. In most of these cases, a therapeutic contact lens protects the epithelium from lid disturbances and also splints the healing epithelium, as well as reducing pain.

This condition is usually treated for a long period before soft lens therapy is considered, and since herpes simplex keratitis is one of the most common causes of this condition, many patients have undergone some degree of therapy with idoxuridine. It is normally considered appropriate to use soft lens treatment only for cases where the corneal ulcers are sterile. This form of therapy is well known and has been prescribed for many years (Gassett and Kaufman, 1970; Liebowitz and Rosenthal, 1971; Westerhout, 1973; Ruben, 1975). A wide variety of clinical pictures exist, but generally there is an area of chronic erosion exposing Bowman's membrane and often some stroma. Previous medical treatment often indicates that the epithelium appears unable to grow across the crater area. In most cases prior therapy has resulted in intermittent and temporary healing, particularly with herpes infections, when recurrent attacks occur with consequential epithelial loss and further infection. Later in the progress of the condition secondary stroma involvement occurs, further reducing visual acuity.

Treatment is sometimes initiated by the total denudation of the corneal epithelium after topical application of proparacaine (Liebowitz and Rosenthal, 1971), or local débridement of the ulcer at its margins and cleaning of the crater (Ruben, 1975). Often the eroded area then heals. The slit lamp picture usually indicates that the epithelium appears to grow under the bandage from the periphery of the crater inwards.

Liebowitz and Rosenthal (1971) indicated that a soft lens bandage could be fitted without recourse to keratometry. In any case, keratometry is usually impossible on an ulcerated eye but a useful indication of the likely fitting is obtained by keratometry on the other eye. Normally it is necessary, first, to clean the edges of the ulceration to remove the necrotic and hyperplastic tissue, but results have been equally satisfactory on patients where this was not possible, provided that the bandage lens was removed regularly and cleaned thoroughly, and the eye itself irrigated to remove loose debris.

Most of the earlier work involving treatment of corneal ulceration with soft lenses related to the use of large, low water content lenses of medium thickness. Although these produced good results, it is now found that large, high and medium water content lenses such as the Sauflon PW, Permalens, and Hydrocurve lenses, used continuously, produce better results. Generally it seems better to leave the lens *in situ* for the first week, while watching the condition carefully with a slit lamp microscope. Premature removal of the bandage lens disturbs the vulnerable area during early healing and can be dangerous. The preferred method of treatment is a bandage lens used in conjunction with antibiotic drops made up without preservatives (Liebowitz and Rosenthal, 1971; Westerhout, 1973), although it is felt that low strengths of preservatives (Ruben, 1975) may be satisfactory.

It is especially interesting to observe the growth of the epithelium underneath the bandage lens as it appears to grow initially on the posterior surface of the bandage, forming a bridge across the crater. This is not always the case but has been described by Liebowitz and Rosenthal (1971). It is disappointing that so many of these cases are frequently the result of prescribing steroids for viral infections of the cornea which might well have been satisfactorily treated by other means (Westerhout, 1973).

Another fairly common cause of peripheral ulceration is that seen in conditions associated with rheumatoid arthritis. A soft lens used as a bandage appears to produce the desired result by shielding the ulcerated area from irritation, due to blinking, and from a variety of noxious environmental stimuli. Because the regenerating tissue requires a fairly high level of oxygen, it is important that the material used for the bandage lens either has a high water content, adequately permeable to oxygen, or else a thinner, medium water content lens is used, also allowing sufficient oxygen permeability (Hill and Jeppe, 1976). One of the most difficult aspects of this form of treatment is to know when the bandage should be removed from the eye, after healing appears complete. Westerhout (1973) feels that the corneal surface should appear as regular as possible before the use of the bandage is discontinued, and not merely show the absence of staining with fluorescein.

It is not uncommon to find ulceration recurring with severe results, even to the extent of corneal perforation and loss of aqueous, after the bandage has been discontinued for a matter of a few days (Westerhout, 1973; Hövding, 1983). Frequently the corneal surface seems to have healed reasonably well, but the appearance of dry spots, between blinking, and slight irregularity are suspicious signs suggesting that the bandage use should be continued for a longer period.

Despite the complications of this form of treatment, it is found to work extremely well in the majority of patients (Liebowitz and Rosenthal, 1971; Hövding, 1983; Mobilia and Kenyon, 1984), and there is often no other method of treatment available for some of these severe, chronic conditions. At the time when soft lens bandage therapy is commenced, the condition has frequently progressed to the stage where tarsorraphy or even enucleation has been considered (*see*, for example, *Plate 119*), but after several months of soft lens bandage treatment, the cornea has healed giving useful vision.

One serious problem with the use of soft bandage lenses in cases of ulceration is the severe lens contamination which results. It is quite common for the lens to become completely soiled beyond reclamation within 1–2 weeks and this is clearly an economic consideration which cannot be ignored. Although continuous wear bandage lenses are usually desirable in the early stages of treatment, during the later stages, when the cornea has largely healed, a daily wear lens can be substituted. Not only can this be cleaned satisfactorily but it is more economical.

Thygeson's keratitis

This is an interesting condition in which differential diagnosis from herpes simplex keratitis and adenovirus keratitis is important.

The common signs are of punctate epithelial keratitis which stains with fluorescein but is not usually associated with subepithelial infiltrates. The condition is usually improved with corticosteroids but made worse by topical idoxuridine. This is the reverse of herpes simplex keratitis which is usually improved with idoxuridine but exacerbated with corticosteroids.

The condition can often be assisted with soft lenses used with topical corticosteroids. Some patients who, during drug therapy, have continued to wear cosmetic or refractive soft contact lenses despite advice to the contrary from their practitioners have steadily improved. This tends to indicate that soft contact lenses are not contra-indicated in this condition, and usually the patient is much more comfortable wearing a therapeutic soft lens than without one.

Penetrating and leaking corneal wounds

Liebowitz (1972) has described the use of a hydrophilic contact lens as a means of sealing a corneal laceration. Soft lenses appear to be relatively effective as a splint and a temporary seal, provided that cases are selected for the small size of the laceration, good apposition in the alignment of the wound edges and absence of incarceration or prolapse of the uvea and crystalline lens. Since it is a very much simpler procedure than suturing with very fine sutures, or other alternative methods, this technique has been recommended, especially as the outcome is not prejudiced if initially unsuccessful. The lens supporting the laceration may be removed easily and adhesives or direct suturing employed if required. The use of the soft lens bandage in this instance also permits a direct view of the wound edges at the time of repair and afterwards, and requires far less skill than the suturing of the wound by a highly trained ophthalmologist. In cases of collapse of the anterior chamber the lens fitted must be very large in order to overlap the limbus by a large margin. By sealing off the edge of the lens on the more rigid and normal scleral area, the lens is effective as a seal and permits the aqueous to re-form the anterior chamber. Because they are reasonably rigid the best lenses to use are very large, medium thickness, medium water content lenses. As the anterior chamber fills and the corneal shape thus changes, the contact lens parameters may have to be altered to take account of the new corneal shape.

Filariasis

In filariasis, a relatively uncommon condition resulting from nematodes, the eye often becomes extremely painful. This is normally due to corneal involvement so that considerable relief and comfort can be afforded by the wearing of a soft lens bandage. Indeed it is frequently impossible for the patient to manage without such a bandage (Westerhout, 1973). In this instance the bandage probably acts purely as a mechanical protection for the corneal epithelial layer.

The use of drugs with soft lenses

One of the problems of applying topical drugs to the eye is that with the tear flow and drainage system, most of the drug is washed away very quickly. This is made worse by the irritation and reflex lacrimation caused by administration of the drops which wash away the drug even more quickly. The more the drops sting and irritate, the worse the problem.

When soft lenses were first used, practitioners were faced with the dilemma of whether drops or ointment could be used during their wear. Fearful of the risk of preservatives binding to the lens, it was considered safer to remove the lens. This is most inappropriate for patients who have to use an extended wear therapeutic lens to permit the epithelialization of the cornea. In general, ointments are unsatisfactory as the therapeutic lenses rapidly become coated with a greasy film which is often difficult to remove.

It was then thought that the absorbent lens, if soaked in the drug, would act as a steady 'slow release' system with obvious advantages. Rather surprisingly, this technique has not been well developed, but this may be due to the greatly increased costs, and the problems of patient instruction and management. Of greater technical importance is the fact that different drugs are released at different levels and speeds from different contact lens materials. This leads to a dilemma of whether or not to remove the lens frequently and resoak (with the additional risks of frequent insertion and removal) or whether to attempt topical application with the therapeutic lens in place to 'top up' the drug level in the lens.

It is considered unsafe to use commercially prepared drugs with a soft lens on the eye. The preservatives used, such as benzalkonium chloride, become concentrated in some of the lens materials and may possibly reach toxic levels. The drug should thus be made up unpreserved whenever possible.

It is thought that drugs such as cycloplegics, pilocarpine, phenylephrine, idoxuridine, steroids and other high-molecular-weight drugs which are water soluble, may be more effective if administered in a hydrogel lens delivery system (Robinson and Eriksen, 1978). Resoaking the lens for 1–2 hours before insertion is adequate. If these sterile presoaked lenses are stored in a refrigerator they are found to have a shelf life of some 4 months (Hillman, Masters and Broad, 1975).

Usually presoaked lenses are soaked in a lower concentration of the drug than that used topically.

Since liquids can pass more readily through a high water content lens, than one with a low water content, the drug is usually released more quickly from a high water content lens. Thus for acute attacks of glaucoma, a high water content lens presoaked in pilocarpine would be indicated, but a low water content lens would be better for a chronic glaucoma.

The author finds that a low water content lens soaked in pilocarpine for 2 hours will normally control the IOP well for 12 hours of wear. Podos, Becker and Asseff (1972) however, found that IOP is controlled for up to 23 hours after lens insertion.

The drugs used with a lens can cause its discolouration and adrenaline, for example, gives rise to a dark brown stain (*see* Chapter 4).

Despite the apparent lack of enthusiasm for this type of drug release system, it is clearly an appropriate technique if the patient is already wearing a lens for a refractive correction or for therapeutic use. As already stated many ophthalmologists use antibiotics with therapeutic contact lenses. The compatibility of the drug with the lens is, therefore, of relevance. The author finds that idoxuridine can be used with a lens in place, and the lens may be soaked in a solution before application.

In many cases standard collyria have been used with a soft lens in place without any apparent ill-effects. These collyria have included antibiotics, mydriatics, corticosteroids and idoxuridine. It may be that when the drug is instilled 3 or 4 times each day, the tears are able to wash out much of the preservative and reduce its concentration. It would appear that the concern over preservatives in eye drops used with soft lenses may be overstated, especially since most plano therapeutic lenses are thin and do not absorb much preservative. If, however, there is an obvious adverse reaction then the position should be reconsidered.

In cases such as pemphigoid and Stevens–Johnson syndrome, the use of preserved artificial tears every 15–30 minutes may create a risk of an adverse reaction to preservatives. In this case unpreserved saline may be considered better. The pH, however, of unpreserved saline is usually on the acidic side and not well tolerated by some patients, in which case, an unpreserved, isotonic, buffered saline with a pH of about 7.2 should be more satisfactory.

The use of drugs after surgery is very important as these may strongly influence the effects of the contact lens. Many patients initially consult a practitioner fairly soon after surgery while still using local antibiotic cover, or steroid therapy. Premature fitting could then result in fairly severe corneal oedema, far worse than would have been encountered had steroids not been utilized.

In summary the advantages of drug therapy with soft lenses are:

(1) A lower dose may be used to achieve therapeutic effect, allowing the use of drugs which in higher concentrations are toxic.

(2) Better penetration of the drug is achieved than by normal topical use or by injection subconjunctivally, the latter technique carrying more risk.

The disadvantages are:

(1) The expense and difficulty of soft lens fitting with the possible risk of giant papillary conjunctivitis in long-term use.
(2) Corneal neovascularization and ulceration.
(3) The necessity for repeated applications of the drug to maintain effective therapy.

Protection of the cornea during applanation tonometry

Many patients wearing therapeutic soft lenses need to have their IOP monitored regularly.

Although a therapeutic lens can be removed for tonometry this is undesirable in some cases such as extended wear to encourage epithelialization. The use of a topical anaesthetic in such a case is also undesirable as it may reduce the adhesion of epithelium to the basement membrane.

For this reason many practitioners have taken IOP measurements over the soft contact lens, usually using a high-molecular-weight fluorescein which is not absorbed into the lens (e.g. Fluorexon or Fluoresoft). Meyer, Stanifer and Bobb (1978) compared IOP measurements with and without a Bausch & Lomb Plano T bandage lens. Results indicated an error of approximately ±4 mmHg with the bandage in place. Draeger (1980) measured IOP with plano and +12 D, 80% water content lenses and compared the IOP readings with and without the lenses in place. His results showed a remarkable correlation, with the plano lens results being higher than the naked cornea results and the +12 D lens results being lower. Westerhout and Chibert (1988), using a Goldmann applanation tonometer, did not find a good correlation between 'over lens IOP' and naked corneal IOP even with low power plus lenses. Unreliable and unrepeatable results were obtained even with low plus lenses. High plus, high water content lenses gave very high results.

Insler and Robbins (1987) reported that non-contact IOP readings can be taken accurately with a thin lens on the eye but that positive powered hydrogels should be removed.

In general, with plano therapeutic soft contact lenses, the IOP can be measured accurately enough for a useful indication. For accurate results, however, the lens needs to be removed.

Pterygium

It is frequently necessary or desirable to fit contact lenses to a patient with a considerable growth of pterygium onto the cornea. Some patients may have successfully worn corneal lenses for many years before the edge of the lens begins to cause irritation by its contact with the enlarging pterygium.

Surgery is sometimes resorted to before lenses are fitted, or to remove a pterygium which is beginning to cause discomfort in a previously successful wearer. Unfortunately, in addition to the commonly seen regrowth of the pterygium, the tissues often become extraordinarily sensitive after surgery and corneal lenses are often not tolerated, although very small corneal lenses of 8.0 mm total diameter, or less, may be helpful.

Soft lenses are of great value after excision, or if the lens is to be fitted over the pterygium. The use of a small soft lens is, however, of limited application as the edge may irritate the sensitive tissue left postoperatively and if fitted over a pterygium it may lift, thus allowing the edge to dry out, risking damage to the lens and possible irritation. Large lenses of 14–15 mm total diameter are more applicable for both types of case. The edge of the lens should reach well beyond the limbus to cover a large proportion of the affected areas.

Complications of therapeutic soft contact lenses

There is always a risk of complications with therapeutic soft contact lenses. The risk of bacterial keratitis is always present, especially in the dry eye conditions and the risk is much higher with extended wear than with daily wear.

The complications are essentially the same as those occurring with soft contact lenses used for refractive or cosmetic purposes, but the risks are much greater given the diseased state of the eye. Indeed many complications are difficult to distinguish from the effects of the primary disease being treated with the therapeutic soft lens. In some cases the use of a therapeutic lens

immediately appears to produce a deterioration in the condition, but as this is difficult to predict and there may be no other apparently effective therapy available, the risk must be weighed against the likely benefits.

The use of a therapeutic contact lens should only be considered if it is possible to carry out regular and frequent after-care examinations. Adaptive oedema is common in all forms of contact lens use and the more so in abnormal corneas. Long-term hypoxia can lead to neovascularization, but this risk must be weighed against the advantages of therapeutic contact lenses. Hypoxia can in some cases be relieved by selection of a more permeable lens material, and in some instances only silicone rubber lenses can prevent it.

Postoperative aphakia, postkeratoplasty, postradial keratotomy, albinism

The most important aspects of contact lens use in postoperative aphakia, postkeratoplasty, postradial keratotomy and albinism are dealt with earlier in the chapter (see pp. 757–796).

Keratoconus

In the author's practice this represents the most common use of a therapeutic contact lens, living as he does in a country where keratoconus is extremely common.

This condition is covered comprehensively in pp. 748–757 but the use of therapeutic soft contact lenses as a bandage for the support of a rigid contact lens is also covered here.

'Combination or piggy-back lenses'

Corneal pathology or trauma such as is found in advanced keratoconus, or corneal scarring due to penetrating wounds, can cause severe irregular astigmatism which is not correctable by spectacles or orthodox soft lenses. Usually it is possible to use hard lenses for this type of case provided that scarring is not severe. Unfortunately, however, hard contact lenses are often not tolerated by a patient despite the motivation given by the great improvement of visual acuity which they provide.

Westerhout (1973) has described a method by

which the combination lens (often now called a 'piggy-back' lens) may be fitted to such a patient. In this technique the cornea and surrounding tissues are treated in the usual way for the fitting of an orthodox soft lens. The lens is usually fitted relatively large, to achieve stability, and keratometer readings are then taken from the front of the soft lens *in situ*. These findings are then used when fitting the hard corneal lens on top of the soft lens to overcome the effects of the irregular astigmatism. For keratoconus the soft lens is usually supplied as a fairly high negative lens in order to provide a flatter front surface to which a steeper and therefore less mobile corneal lens can be fitted. In other cases a low positive soft lens (of about +4 D) is found to be more suitable. The fact that the combination hard lens is able to fit on the soft contact lens rather than on the naked cornea enables much greater comfort to be achieved and results have been extremely helpful in many cases. Fortunately, as a soft lens still permits the pump action to be maintained, the hard corneal lens may be fitted substantially tighter on the soft lens than it would be on the cornea — a technique which is particularly helpful in cases of advanced keratoconus (*see also* p. 751 and *Plates 121* and *122*). The hard lens is usually best fitted using a gas permeable material and medium water content soft lenses seem to be the most suitable.

A lower rate of success has been achieved when hybrid lenses such as the Saturn lens with rigid centre and soft periphery have been substituted for 'piggy-back' lenses. This may be due to the limited parameters of the Saturn lens and its fragility. 'Piggy-back' fittings are preferred for the majority of complex fittings.

The use of soft lenses with scleral lenses

Scleral lenses are still of great value today both as therapeutic devices and as cosmetic shells to conceal a disfigured eye. Unfortunately few practitioners can fit them well and even those who do fit them do so rarely and thus tend to lose their expertise. The difficulties of fitting scleral lenses (*see* Chapters 17 and 18) deter many practitioners from attempting to fit them and any technique which assists their quick and easy fitting is of value. Westerhout (1975) has described an improved method, simplified by the use of soft lenses. It is based on Marriott's technique (1970) whereby the accurate fitting of a scleral lens to a highly irregular eye is achieved by covering the plaster cast, made from the eye impression, with a laminate. This provides the correct amount of clearance of the final lens over the entire cornea and limbus.

The latter method is usually successful in skilful hands, but is somewhat time consuming and requires a considerable amount of technical skill.

The method Westerhout (1975) has described involves the eye being fitted with a large, tight-fitting, negative powered, soft lens over which the practitioner takes the eye impression. It is helpful to stain the soft lens yellow with fluorescein to make it visible and ensure that it stays in place while the impression shell is being applied (*Plate 81*).

The cast taken from this impression allows the direct pressing of a scleral shell which should provide adequate and gradually increasing corneal clearance from centre to limbus (due to the negative soft lens) (*Plate 82*). This method permits very much more rapid fitting of scleral lenses to irregular eyes and also has the effect of providing protection for the cornea while the impression taking is being carried out. This is of great value if the condition of the cornea makes impression taking risky. It can also be of benefit in areas of the world where optometrists are not permitted to use topical anaesthetics. Certainly very little, if any, subsequent corneal staining is seen when this method is used.

That excellent and rapid fitting can be achieved by this technique is shown in the cosmetic shells illustrated in *Plate 80*.

The control of the bubble in fitting a scleral lens to a highly irregular eye is also found to be extremely difficult on occasions, no matter what fitting technique is used. Westerhout (1975) has described the use of a small (almost corneal diameter) high water content, soft lens fitted underneath the scleral lens which is then ground out to permit a slightly larger than normal corneal clearance. The use of the soft lens underneath the scleral lens can, in some cases, considerably reduce the size of the troublesome bubble and may be found satisfactory, particularly in cases of high or advanced keratoconus (*Plate 85*).

References

BILTON, S. and GUILLON, M. (1984). In vivo hydrogel lens dehydration. Paper presented to N.E. Contact Lens Society

DADA, V. K. and ACHARJEE, S. C. (1982). Soft lenses as therapeutic device. *Ind. J. Ophthal.* **30**, 201–203

DART, J. (1987). Therapeutic contact lenses. *Contax* March, 11–17

DOHLMAN, C. H. and HYNDIUK, R. A. (1972). Subclinical and manifest corneal edema after cataract extraction. In *Symposium on the Cornea: Transactions of the New Orleans Academy of Ophthalmology*, edited by R. Castroviejo *et al.*, pp. 225–232. St Louis: CV Mosby

DONZIS, P. B., MONDINO, B. J., WEISSMAN, B. A. and BRUCKNER, D. A. (1987). Microbial contamination of contact lens care systems. *Am. J. Ophthal.* **104**, 325–333

DRAEGER, J. (1980). Applanationstonometrie auf Kontaklinsen mit hohen Wassergehalt. Probleme, Ergebnisse und Korrekturfaktoren. *Klin. Monatsbl. Augenheilk.* **176**, 38–43

FATT, I. and DI MARTINO, R. B. (1985). Water content of a hydrogel lens on the eye. *Optician* **190** (5011), 19–22

GASSETT, A. R. (1978). Corneal diseases and soft contact lenses. In *Soft Contact Lenses: Clinical and Applied Technology*, edited by M. Ruben, pp. 245–254. London: Baillière-Tindall

GASSETT, A. R. and KAUFMAN, H. E. (1970). Therapeutic uses of soft lenses. *Am. J. Ophthal.* **69**, 252–259

GRAYSON, M. (1983). *Diseases of the Cornea.* St Louis: CV Mosby

HART, D. and SHIH, K. (1987). Surface interactions in hydrogel extended wear contact lenses: microflora and microfauna. *Am. J. Optom. physiol. Optics* **64**, 739–748

HART, D. E., LANE, B. C., JOSEPHSON, J. E. *et al.* (1987). Spoilage of hydrogel contact lenses by lipid deposits. *Ophthalmology* **94**, 1315

HILL, R. M. and JEPPE, W. H. (1976). Hydrogels: is a pump still necessary? *Int. Contact Lens Clin.* **2**(4), 27–29

HILLMAN, J. S., MARSTERS, J. B. and BROAD, A. (1975). Pilocarpine delivery by hydrophilic lens in the management of acute glaucoma. *Trans. Ophthal. Soc. UK* **95**, 75–84

HOLDEN, B. and MERTZ, G. (1984). Critical oxygen levels to avoid corneal oedema for daily and extended-wear contact lenses. *Invest. Ophthal. vis. Sci.* **25**, 1161–1167

HÖVDING, G. (1983). Hydrophilic contact lenses in corneal disorders. *Acta ophthal.* **62**, 566–576

INSLER, M. S. and ROBBINS, R. G. (1987). Intraocular pressure by noncontact tonometry with and without soft contact lenses. *Archs Ophthal.* **105**, 1358–1359

JACOB, R. (1988). Principles of cleaning soft contact lenses. *Int. Contact Lens Clin.* (in press)

LIEBOWITZ, H. M. (1972). Hydrophilic contact lenses in corneal disease: IV. Penetrating corneal wounds. *Archs. Ophthal.* **88**, 602–606

LIEBOWITZ, H. M. and ROSENTHAL, P. (1971). Hydrophilic contact lenses in corneal disease: 1. Superficial, sterile, indolent ulcers. *Archs Ophthal.* **85**, 163–166

MADIGAN, M. C., HOLDEN, B. A. and KWOK, L. S. (1987). Extended wear of contact lenses can compromise corneal epithelial adhesion. *Curr. Eye Res.* **6**, 1257–1260

MARRIOTT, P. (1970). The use of acrylic laminates in fitting haptic lenses. *Br. J. physiol. Optics* **25**, 29–43

MARRIOTT, P. J. (1981). Impression scleral lens fitting for special and pathological conditions. In *Contact Lenses: A Textbook for Practitioner and Student*, 2nd edn, Vol. 2, edited by J. Stone and A. J. Phillips, pp. 592–603. London: Butterworths

MEYER, R. F., STANIFER, R. M. and BOBB, K. C. (1978). MacKay Marg tonometry over therapeutic soft contact lenses. *Am. J. Ophthal.* **86**, 19–23

MOBILIA, E. F. and KENYON, K. R. (1984). A new bandage lens for treatment of corneal disease: Softcon XT. *Contact Lens Ass. Ophthal. J.* **10**(4), 353–355

OHASHI, Y., WATANABE, H., KINOSHITA, S., HOSOTANI, H., UMBMOTO, N. and MANABE, R. (1988). Vitamin A eyedrops for superior limbic keratoconjunctivitis. *Am. J. Ophthal.* **105**, 523–527

PHELPS-BROWN, N. (1988). The dry eye. *Optician* **195**(5139), 26, 28, 30–31, 33

PHILLIPS, A. J. (1986). Contact lenses and the elderly patient. In *Vision and Ageing*, edited by A. A. Rosenbloom and M. W. Morgan, pp. 267–300. New York: Professional Press

PODOS, S. M., BECKER, B. and ASSEFF, C. (1972). Pilocarpine therapy with soft contact lenses. *Am. J. Ophthal.* **73**, 336–341

ROBINSON, J. R. and ERIKSEN, S. P. (1978). Drug delivery from soft lens materials. In *Soft Contact Lenses: Clinical and Applied Technology*, edited by M. Ruben, pp. 265–280. London: Baillière-Tindall

RUBEN, M. (1971). Soft lenses. *Trans. Ophthal. Soc. UK* **91**, 59–74

RUBEN, M. (1975). *Contact Lens Practice: Visual, Therapeutic and Prosthetic.* London: Baillière-Tindall

SOMMER, A. and GREEN, W. R. (1982). Goblet cell response to vitamin A treatment for corneal xerophthalmia. *Am. J. Ophthal.* **94**, 213–215

TSENG, S. C. G., MAUMENEE, A. E., STARK, W. J. *et al.* (1985). Topical retinoid treatment for various dry-eye disorders. *Ophthalmology* **92**, 717–727

VAN HORN, D. L., DECARLO, J. D., SCHATTEN, W. H., HYNDIUK, R. A. and KURZ, P. (1981). Topical retinoic acid in the treatment of experimental xerophthalmia in the rabbit. *Archs Ophthal.* **99**, 317–321

WARTMAN, R. (1987). Contact lens-related side effects of systemic drugs. *Contact Lens Forum* **12**(8), 42–44

WESTERHOUT, D. I. (1973). The combination lens and therapeutic uses of soft lenses. *Contact Lens J.* **4**(5), 3–10, 12, 16–18, 20, 22

WESTERHOUT, D. I. (1975). The use of soft lenses in the fitting of haptic lenses. *Optician* **169**(4363), 13, 16

WESTERHOUT, D. I. (1981). The use of soft lenses in ocular pathology. In *Contact Lenses: A Textbook for Practitioner and Student*, 2nd edn, Vol. 2, edited by J. Stone and A. J. Phillips, pp. 604–616. London: Butterworths

WESTERHOUT, D. I. and CHIBERT, J. (1988). IOP measurement over soft contact lenses. *Contact Lens J.* (in press)

ZANTOS, S., ORSBORN, G. N., WALTER, H. C. and KNOLL, H. A. (1986). Studies on corneal staining with thin hydrogel contact lenses. *J. Br. Contact Lens Ass.* **9**, 61–64

Chapter 22

Contact lens manufacture

E. J. D. Proctor

This chapter aims at giving the clinician and student a brief outline of manufacturing procedures. It in no way claims to be comprehensive for there are now many advanced and sophisticated techniques used in mass production of both hard and soft lenses which herein are mentioned only briefly. Scleral lenses will not be discussed in this chapter because their use is mainly restricted to those cases where pathology has been involved and in such cases the impression technique generally seems to offer better results. This latter procedure, which is mainly carried out by the clinician is dealt with in Chapter 18, which deals fully with the making of the lens from the stage of the eye impression.

The two main methods of manufacturing contact lenses are moulding and generating.

Moulding

Moulding can be by casting, compression or injection. Spin-casting is used for mass production of soft lenses, while compression and injection moulding are largely used for mass production of hard corneal lenses.

Bausch & Lomb in the USA have refined the Czechoslovakian spin-casting technique to produce soft lenses. This procedure involves spinning a mould, at a computer-controlled speed, into which the mixture of monomers is injected. The centripetal force causes the mixture to climb the wall of the mould to form into the required shape, the polymerization and spinning taking place simultaneously. The method is described in Chapter 11, p. 423 and Chapter 13, and *Figures 11.27* and *11.28* show diagrammatically the form of the mould and the resultant shapes of some lens back surfaces.

The formed dehydrated lens has to be edged before being hydrated and released from its mould. This is a technique which is extremely suitable for mass production of soft spherical lenses. Its disadvantages are as follows:

(1) It is extremely expensive to set up the laboratory and therefore a large production is essential for it to be viable. This means that the available lens parameters are very restricted.

(2) The technique cannot be used for individual prescriptions such as soft toric lenses, which are becoming routine fitting for the practitioner.

Further details and other lens properties are discussed in Chapter 11.

The moulding of hard lenses is mainly of interest for historical reasons as the bulk of the rigid lenses fitted present day are gas permeable which are mainly produced by generating.

In a compression moulding technique developed by Kelvin in the UK for production of hard lenses, separate steel tools for front and back surfaces are made. Under controlled conditions of heat and pressure, both front and back curves are produced simultaneously on a disc of PMMA inserted between the tools.

On removal from the pressing jig, the surface finished lens has to be cut to the required total diameter and edged. This procedure requires a very large number of tools to obtain all the various possible combinations of parameters. It has the advantage that lenses can be made both quickly and fairly cheaply because it requires less skilled labour than for lathe-cut lenses. The expense and expertise are introduced when making the steel tools. It is a good technique for producing a continuous curve lens, but it does have the following disadvantages:

(1) Because of the cost of tooling the available range of parameters is limited. For example, only one back optic zone diameter (BOZD)

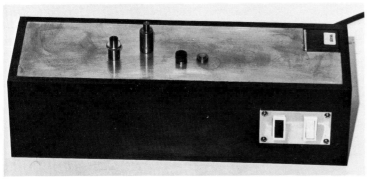

Figure 22.1 Hot plate for heating steel buttons and chucks

can usually be obtained with any one given radial edge lift.

(2) If manufacturing conditions are not carefully controlled, it can introduce stress into the lens material and this can cause the lens curvature to change after manufacture and during use. This is particularly so with thin lenses.

(3) For the same reason as (2) above, poor optics and hence poor power readings are easily produced.

Another moulding technique for hard lens production, developed by Wöhlk (now Zeiss) of West Germany, involves placing powdered PMMA in the concavity of a Pyrosil mould to which is clamped a quartz-glass convex die. This is slowly moved through an oven at 200°C for three-quarters of an hour, after which the surface-finished lens is removed from the separated mould. The lens is then cut to the required size and edged. A similar technique using stainless steel moulds and dies is used by Silor in France. This procedure has one big advantage over the compression technique in that it does not introduce any strain. However, there are disadvantages, as follows:

(1) As with compressed lenses the cost of tooling reduces the available range of parameters.
(2) There are difficulties preventing impurities, such as specks of dust, from entering the powdered PMMA and thus the matrix of the finished lens.

Generating

Generating is the technique favoured by all small to medium laboratories as well as most of the large ones throughout the world. For this reason it is the technique on which the author has concentrated in this chapter. This procedure does not lend itself to mass production as readily as the moulding techniques, the emphasis being on individual prescription work. The method of manufacture is basically the same for soft lenses as it is for hard corneal lenses; in fact, it is the main method of manufacturing soft lenses throughout the world. Any difference between hard and soft lens fabrication will be pointed out as the procedures are described, otherwise it is to be assumed that the same techniques apply to both.

Cutting back surfaces

A PMMA (or RGP or soft lens) blank is mounted on a heated stepped steel button (*Figures 22.1* and *22.2*) with the aid of a thin layer of beeswax to hold it approximately central. When the button is cool it is placed in the collett of a heavy based high precision micro-lathe (*Figure 22.3*) and the diameter of the blank is reduced to 0.10 mm or 0.15 mm above the final

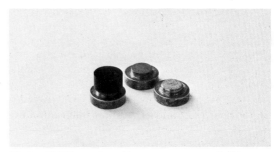

Figure 22.2 Stepped steel buttons, one mounted with a PMMA blank

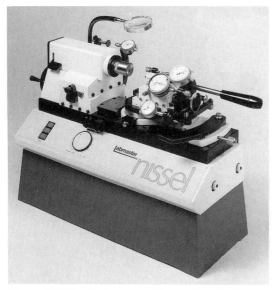

Figure 22.3 Nissel Labmaster: high precision lathe for cutting front and back surfaces

total diameter of the required prescription lens (*Figure 22.4*). The next operation is to cut the required back optic zone radius (BOZR). This is done with a diamond-tipped tool which ensures that an extremely high surface finish is achieved prior to polishing (*Figure 22.5*). Material is first removed from the centre and, in increasingly wider sweeps, eventually from across the entire surface of the blank, thus covering the whole diameter. The last few cuts

remove a thickness of 0.005–0.02 mm; the speed at which the diamond traverses the surface during these final cuts is very much slower in order to produce a smoother finished surface. The cutting finishes in the centre of the lens, the collett holding the blank is wound back from the diamond, and the extreme knife-edge of the blank blunted with a blade or grinding stone. If the last-named procedure is not done the edge of the blank digs into the wax polisher in the next phase of the work.

Polishing back surfaces

The steel button with semi-finished blank attached is removed from the collett and the blank and button separated; this helps to release any strain which has been introduced during cutting. With some techniques the blank is held directly in the collett of the lathe without the need to mount on a stepped steel button. After removing wax from the base of the blank, using an aliphatic hydrocarbon solvent such as Shell Super VM&P Naphtha in an ultrasonic cleaner, it is mounted on a clean steel button using double-sided sticky tape. For hard lenses a wax polisher is then cut on the lathe to the required radius (*Figure 22.6*) and a spiral groove (*Figure 22.7*) or series of circular grooves made in its surface to aid the distribution of the polish. The blank is polished on an automatic polisher (*Figures 22.8* and *22.9*) using a double rotation technique; the movements involved are as

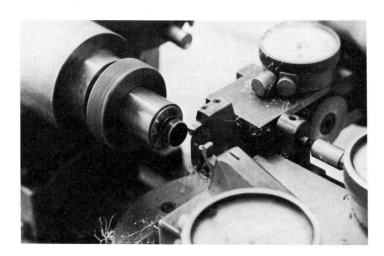

Figure 22.4 Reducing the diameter of the blank

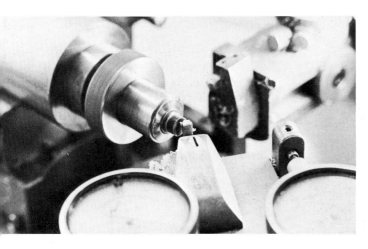

Figure 22.5 Cutting the back optic zone radius. The material removed is termed 'swarf'

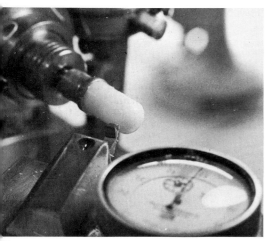

Figure 22.6 Cutting the back surface wax polishing tool

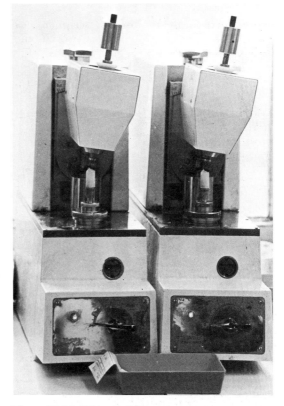

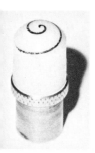

Figure 22.7 Spiral groove in wax polishing tool. Ink has been run into the groove for illustration purposes

Figure 22.8 Polishing the back surface using automatic back surface polishing machines. Detail is shown in *Figure 22.9*

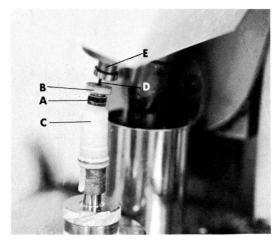

Figure 22.9 Close-up of polishing the back surface. The blank (A) mounted on its steel button (B) being polished on the wax tool (C). The steel button is held and rotated by a steel pin (D) held in the head (E) of the polisher

follows:

(1) The wax polisher rotates clockwise on a vertical spindle.
(2) The angled steel pin describes an anti-clockwise movement.
(3) The head oscillates from side to side.
(4) The blank rotates due to friction.

The polish for hard lenses is concentrated Silvo (Reckitt and Colman), most of the surplus ammonia having been drained off. For gas permeable materials, an ammonia-free polish is used (X-Pal, Alox-PG, Alumina, dissolved in water or silicone oil).

The finish of the surface is checked using a loupe ($\times 10$), and the radius checked on a radiuscope (*Figure 22.10*) to an accuracy exceeding 0.01 mm. The radius can be adjusted by polishing for longer periods and recutting the wax polisher to make any necessary allowances.

Peripheral curves

The next stage is to generate the secondary and peripheral curves using fine diamond-coated tools (*Figure 22.11*, right-hand side) which give a high degree of accuracy. With hard lenses, water or paraffin is used as a lubricant. The BOZD and peripheral diameters are measured using a band measuring magnifier (*Figure 22.12*) and a skilled technician can control the diameters to within ±0.05 mm. These peripheral curves are generated on the semi-finished blank (*Figure 22.13*). This technique ensures that the peripheral curve exactly matches the diamond tool.

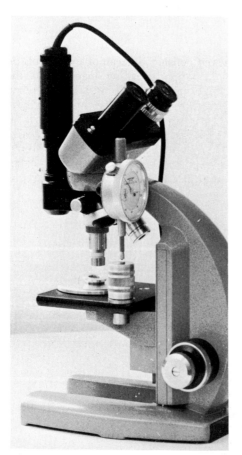

Figure 22.10 Radiuscope set for checking the back optic zone radius

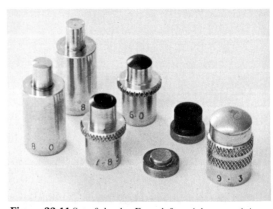

Figure 22.11 Set of chucks. From left to right: two edging chucks (convex and concave tips); hollow and solid front surface chucks; unmounted and mounted stepped buttons; diamond impregnated generating tool. Radius of curvature is engraved on each tool where appropriate

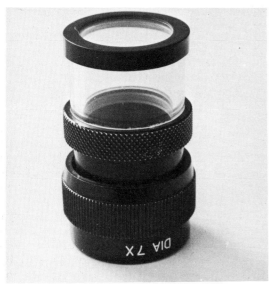

Figure 22.12 Band measuring magnifier. The upper surface has a scale engraved on it in 0.1 mm divisions (*see Figure 12.11*)

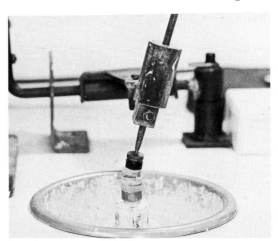

Figure 22.13 Generating back peripheral curves

Some laboratories grind these curves after generating the front curves, using a suction holder to grip the lens. If the lens is to be as thin as it should be, the latter procedure allows it to flex and flatten slightly under the pressure of grinding and polishing, and the result is a peripheral curve that becomes steeper than required once the pressure is removed, and which may also be distorted. On the latest CNC lathes (*Figure 22.14*), the whole of the back surface geometry can be cut in one process, thus five spherical curves or an aspherical design can be readily generated obviating the need to grind on the curves in a separate process.

Once the peripheral curves have been generated many laboratories polish them using a tape-covered polisher (instead of a wax tool) on a double rotation polishing machine. If the practitioner asks for them to be well blended some laboratories merely overrun the polishing, thus blurring the transitions, not, in fact, removing the apices of the transitions. This results in a back surface with relatively sharp transitions which are prone to cause physiological problems because they produce an effectively 'tight' fitting

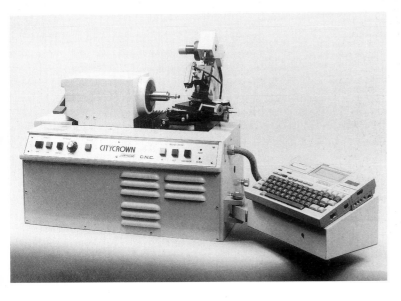

Figure 22.14 CNC lathe

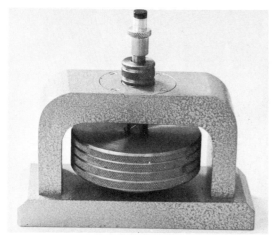

Figure 22.15 Blank mounted on a front surface chuck on a centring device

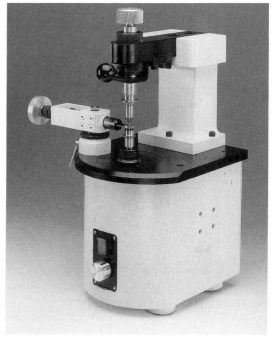

Figure 22.17 Nissel precision blocker

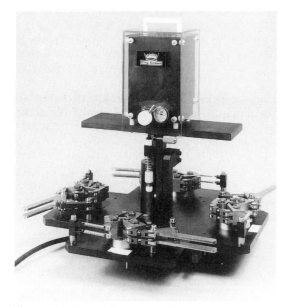

Figure 22.16 Four station precision blocker

periphery to the lens (*see* Chapter 10). Thus, poor tear exchange under the lens may result, and turbulence of the tears resulting in bubbles with consequent dimpling of the corneal epithelium.

The author feels that the correct procedure is to leave the peripheral curves unpolished until the very last stage of production, when polishing, blending and edging can be done accurately in one stage. This has the advantage that the surface of the peripheral zone, which is the bearing surface in the next stage of

production, will not sustain any permanent damage in the following procedures, whereas if it is fully polished and blended, fine scratches may develop during the next stages and such scratches are likely to go unnoticed and hence unrectified by the laboratory.

Cutting front surfaces

The blank is removed from the stepped button, cleaned and the centre thickness recorded. It is then mounted by its back surface on a hot hollow chuck (*see Figure 22.11*) using wax as an adhesive (normally a solid chuck is used for soft and gas permeable materials; this is necessary with softer materials because the forces that are introduced during the cutting and polishing may cause the optic zone of the lens to drop if a hollow chuck is used). The blank is centred on a vertical spindle or special rotating centring device as shown in *Figure 22.15* by watching the reflected image of a strip light seen in the rotating back surface edge adjacent to the chuck, and not the flat top. Two new tools for blocking lenses onto front surface chucks have recently been produced. One by City Crown Ltd (*Figure 22.16*), in the UK, in which the chuck is

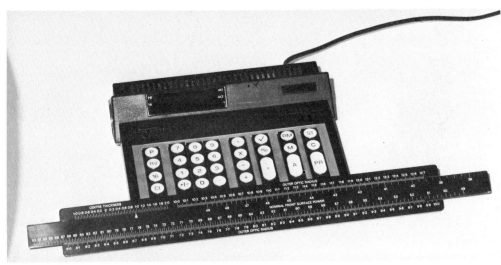

Figure 22.18 Contact lens slide-rule in front of a programmable calculator

held centrally by three finger-like clamps, and hot wax then dispensed onto the chuck from a temperature-controlled bath. The blank, which is held in a vertical acting clamp, is then lowered and guided by the precision-machined clamps so as to fit with perfect symmetry onto the chuck, where it is held until the wax cools. The other blocking tool (*Figure 22.17*) is made by Nissel Ltd, also in the UK. In this second system the hot chuck, with the blank already roughly positioned, is placed on a vertical spindle, a free spinning tool is lowered onto the top of the blank to gently force it onto the chuck, while at the same time a V-gauge is brought in from the side to act against the vertical sides of the blank, thus ensuring centration. Both of these systems seem to work exceptionally well. The front surface power required is calculated using a special slide-rule or a programmable calculator (*Figure 22.18*) and hence the front optic radius determined. The hollow chuck is placed on the taper of the front surface lathe and the front optic radius is cut using a diamond tool, the blank being reduced to the required centre thickness in the process (*Figure 22.19*). At this stage any lenticulation of positive powered lenses has to be carried out. With hard positive lenses it is usual to put on a 'negative' front surface carrier curve such as a $-10.00\,\mathrm{D}$ or $-15.00\,\mathrm{D}$ curve (i.e. to give the peripheral zone this power) which will facilitate lid attachment and thus assist greatly in stabilizing the lens or, alternatively, a front surface carrier curve which is parallel with the back peripheral surface (*see* Chapter 10). The determination of these curves is made easier if a cross-section of the lens is drawn out to scale (*see* Chapter 5).

Polishing front surfaces

Finally, the lenticulation on a positive lens is polished while the lens is still on the lathe. For hard lenses this is done by hand using a chamois leather impregnated with Silvo. The lens and hollow chuck are then removed from the lathe. A front surface wax polisher is cut using steel male gauges to obtain the correct radius (*Figures*

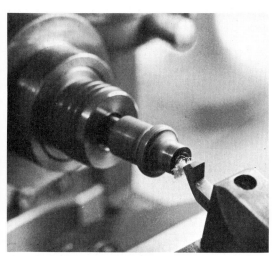

Figure 22.19 Cutting the front surface

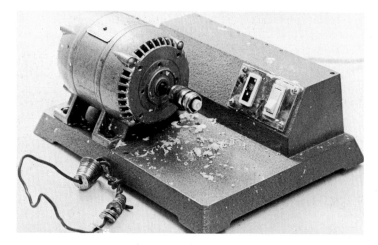

Figure 22.20 Front surface wax polisher mounted for cutting. Also shown are male templates threaded on flex in the foreground

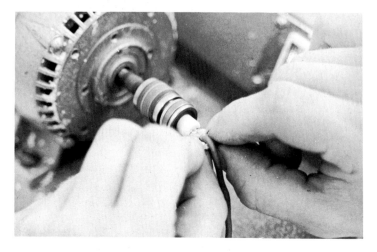

Figure 22.21 Close-up of cutting front surface wax polishing tool using a male template

22.20 and 22.21). The sharp edge of the wax polisher is now removed and a small central recess made to retain the polishing liquid. For hard lenses the front optic is then polished on the double rotation polishing machine (*Figure 22.22*) using this small wax polisher and Silvo (*Figure 22.23*). The movements executed during this polishing process are the same as those for back surface polishing (*see* p. 820).

With negative lenses traditionally the optic was polished before lenticulating; this was because it was difficult to control the power accurately once the front periphery of the lens had been removed (*see* Power adjustments, p. 837). However, with better quality lathes and diamonds, less time is needed to polish these surfaces and frequently the lenticulation is cut at the same time as the optic zone. It is possible to lenticulate negative lenses by hand so that a gradually changing curve can be formed ending in the correct edge thickness. This is done by removing material with a razor blade while the lens, which is still mounted on the hollow chuck, is rotating on the vertical spindle of the edging bench. It requires a skilled and experienced technician to be able to judge the correct thickness across the peripheral surface. This lenticulation is then polished with a felt wheel in a flexible drive (*Figure 22.24*) while the lens rotates on the vertical spindle (*Figure 22.25*).

While polishing the front optic, the power of the lens could, if necessary, be altered by several dioptres, although the greater the shift in power the poorer the focimeter reading is likely to be (*see* Power adjustments, p. 837).

The edge of a soft lens is frequently formed and polished on the lathe while the lens is mounted on the front surface chuck. It is usual

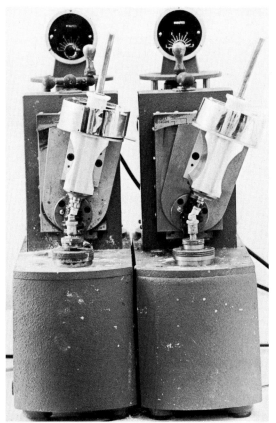

Figure 22.22 Polishing the front surface using automatic front surface polishing machines. Detail is shown in *Figure 22.23*

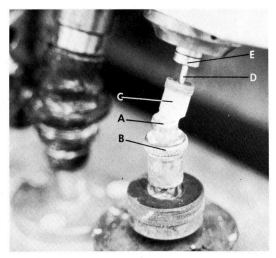

Figure 22.23 Close-up of polishing the front surface. The blank (A) mounted on its steel button (B) being polished on the wax tool (C). The steel button is held and rotated by three steel pins (D) held in the head (E) of the polisher

to do it at this stage because the dehydrated soft lens material is fragile and needs adequate support to stop it chipping.

After polishing the front surface and, while the lens is still on the chuck, any necessary

engraving is carried out (*Figure 22.26*). Engraving is usually confined to hard lenses because of the possibility of weakening the structure of a soft lens and also because the risk of mucoprotein binding to the uneven surface would be increased (although the engraving of a hard lens also attracts mucoproteins and lipids).

The lens is removed from the chuck and the wax cleaned off in an ultrasonic bath containing an aliphatic hydrocarbon solvent. The hard lens is now ready for edging, and polishing and blending of its peripheral curves, while the soft lens has to be hydrated in 0.9% saline solution and later cleaned in a hypertonic wetting

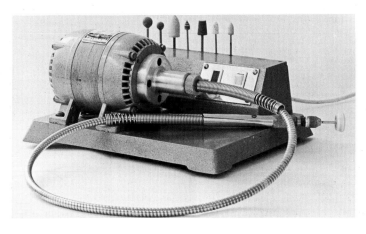

Figure 22.24 A flexible drive unit with a felt wheel mounted in the chuck

828

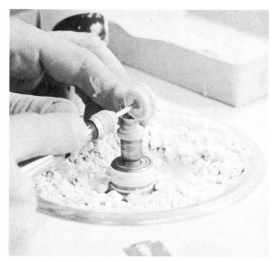

Figure 22.25 Polishing the 'cut-down' on a negative lenticular lens, using the felt wheel in the flexible drive handpiece

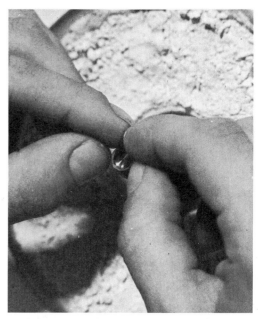

Figure 22.27 Centring a lens on an edging chuck using forefingers and thumbs

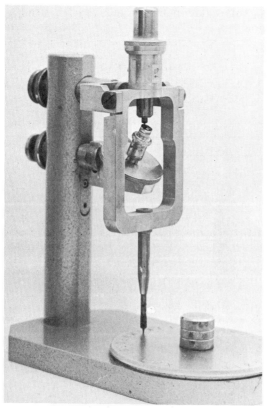

Figure 22.26 Engraving the front surface of a lens using the pantograph system

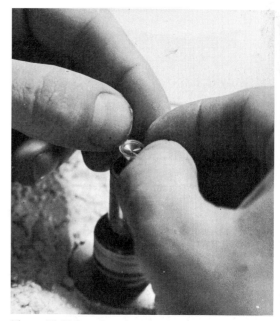

Figure 22.28 Centring a lens on an edging chuck: the reflections from the back surface must remain stationary as the lens rotates

solution to remove any remaining polishing compound.

Edge shaping

Edging, polishing and blending are the most difficult procedures in making a hard lens, and the success or otherwise of the lens is largely decided at this point.

Traditionally, the dry lens is mounted with wax on a hot chuck, the concave surface being uppermost. The hot chuck is then transferred to a rotating vertical spindle, and centring, which should be extremely accurate so as not to offset the lens, is achieved by steadying the rotating lens between the thumb and index finger of both hands (*Figures 22.27* and *22.28*). If the reflection of an overhead spotlight or striplight from the rotating surface is seen to be steady then the lens is centred correctly. It is then left to cool so that the wax sets with the lens correctly centred. With gas permeable materials the addition of hot wax at this stage can cause surface changes and it is therefore usual to mount the unedged lens using double-sided sticky tape. The difficulty with this method is in getting the lens accurately centred. As an alternative it is possible to use a vacuum chuck although this may cause the lens to distort if the vacuum is too strong.

Any reduction of total diameter and shaping of the edge is done by arching a razor blade around the rotating lens, starting on the back surface and working onto the lower front surface (*Figure 22.29a–c*). Care has to be taken not to cut into the peripheral curve on the back surface and to hold the razor blade so that it trails against the edge, i.e. with its edge facing in the direction of travel to avoid nicking the edge. Because of the nature of gas permeable materials, the reduction and shaping of the edge is usually done with an emery board. The shape and thickness are checked by observing the edge with a high powered loupe (×10) and the total diameter is measured using a micrometre gauge (*Figures 22.30* and *22.31*). The edge surface is smoothed off using a conical-shaped carborundum stone which is rolled around the rotating edge of the lens (*Figure 22.32a–e*). The edge surface is again inspected before polishing.

As a practitioner, the author feels the ideal edge shape for a hard lens is as in *Figure 22.33*; this type of edge will not be damaged so easily

from handling as one with its apex towards the back of the lens. The final edge shape will be influenced to a certain extent by the peripheral curves and hence the thickness of material available.

Polishing and blending peripheral curves

The peripheral curves are now ready to be blended and polished. With the lens still mounted on the edging chuck, so that it is held firmly by the wax or double-sided sticky tape so that it will not flex, the apices of the transitions are removed. This is done with wax tools, each cut to the required radius, usually one-third to midway between the two adjacent curves. The wax tool is mounted on the vertical spindle and the lens/edging-chuck combination is allowed to rotate and at the same time is oscillated to and fro on top of the polishing tool (*Figure 22.34*). The lens is periodically inspected using a ×10 loupe and, when all the transitions have been blended (to whatever degree has been requested by the practitioner), all the remaining peripheral curves are polished and blended using a progression of felt tools (*Figure 22.35*) so as to obtain a gradual and continuing flow of curves. Thus, as near as possible, a continuous curve lens is then produced but with the advantage that the original curves are known and can thus be altered at a later stage if modification becomes necessary.

Edge polishing

Finally, the edge has to be polished. With the lens still on the edging chuck and placed back on the taper of a vertical spindle with the concave side uppermost, this is done by wrapping a chamois leather around the index finger and a forwards and backwards movement is made across the top of the lens edge, the chamois leather being soaked in polish (*Figure 22.36*). The ball of the finger is then rolled around and under the edge of the lens as shown in *Figure 22.37a–d*. These two procedures remove material from the inner or more central part of the edge of the lens to the apex of the edge. When the inner or back edge of the lens is fully polished the lens is cleaned and remounted the other way round on a convex edging chuck. The outer or front edge of the lens is polished in a similar manner (*Figure 22.38a–d*). The lens is removed from the edging

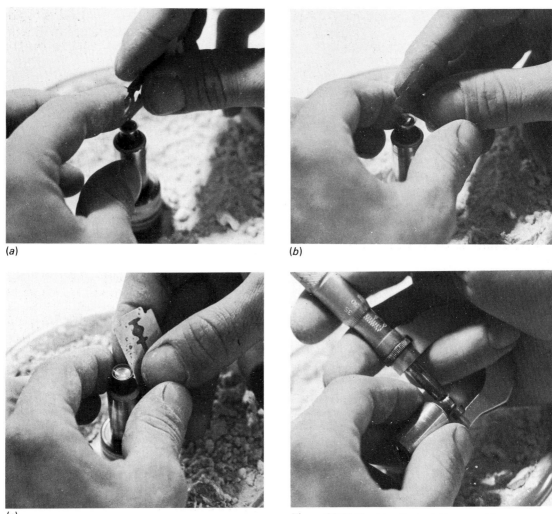

(a)

(b)

(c)

Figure 22.29 Reducing total diameter and edge shaping with a razor blade. (a), (b) and (c) show successive positions of the trailing cutting edge of the blade

Figure 22.30 Checking the total diameter with a micrometer gauge

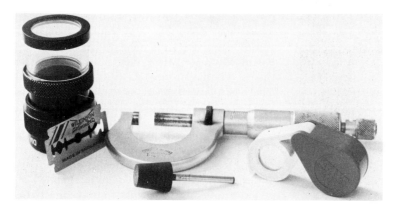

Figure 22.31 Tools for edging and checking. From left to right: band measuring magnifier, razor blade, micrometer gauge, conical carborundum tool, ×10 loupe

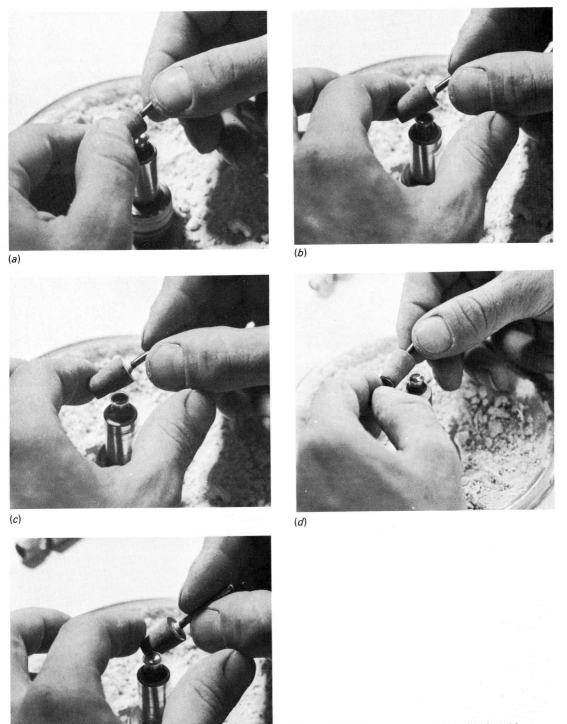

(a)

(b)

(c)

(d)

(e)

Figure 22.32 Shaping and smoothing the edge with a conical carborundum stone. The stone is carefully 'rolled' around the lens edge: (a)–(e) show successive positions of the conical tool

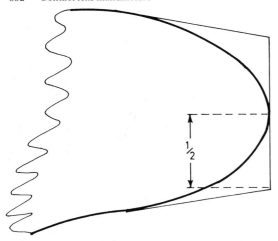

Figure 22.33 The author's ideal edge shape shown in cross-section

chuck and cleaned in an aliphatic hydrocarbon solvent. Some laboratories use a series of hollow cone tools of varying angles to shape and polish the edge (*see* Chapter 23). These rotate on a vertical spindle and the edge shape and polish is produced by running the lens inside each tool for a specific time. This technique does not give very satisfactory results. Alternatively, many laboratories use an automatic edge polisher (*Figure 22.39*). The lens is held by a suction cup and rotated on a revolving sponge containing polish. This latter procedure produces better results provided the edge has already been shaped and it is quite suitable for stock lens production. While neither procedure gives the best results, the latter technique usually means

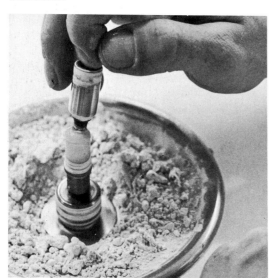

Figure 22.34 Blending transitions by removing their apices on a wax tool

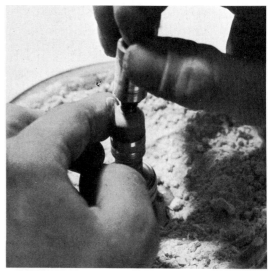

Figure 22.35 Blending of transitions and polishing of peripheral curves may be done with felt tools in this manner

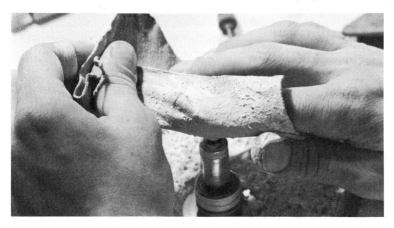

Figure 22.36 Starting to polish the edge of a PMMA corneal lens with a Silvo-soaked chamois leather moving the finger forwards and backwards across the lens edge with its back surface uppermost

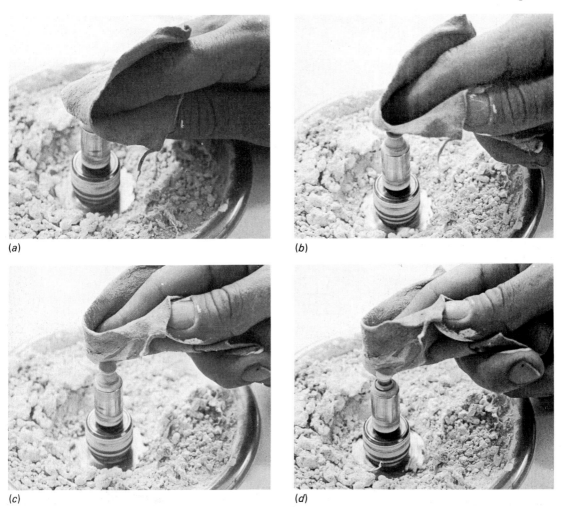

(a)   (b)

(c)   (d)

Figure 22.37 Polishing the edge of a lens — concave surface uppermost. The chamois leather is rolled over the edge of the lens on the ball of the finger as shown in the successive photographs (a)–(d)

that the edge is polished, but not correctly shaped unless this has been done prior to polishing; thus, the lens may have a polished square edge. The edge may also be polished by hand on a rotating chamois or velveteen-covered drum chuck, the lens being held on some type of suction device and rotated by hand with first the concave and then the convex surface facing the direction of rotation of the drum. This is followed by apical polishing of the edge with the lens rotated parallel to the edge of the drum. There seems to be no better way of shaping and polishing the edge of a lens than by the hand of a skilled technician. Unlike a machine, he is able to observe the lens constantly and make allowances for the different thickness of individual prescription lenses.

The finished lens is dried, inspected for surface blemishes and finally its specification is checked. Thickness checking is shown in *Figure 22.40*.

Soft lens fabrication

Lathe-cut soft lenses are produced in an almost identical manner to hard lenses. The variations, other than those already mentioned, are few but important.

Because the lens is formed in the dehydrated state any error in tolerance will be increased by

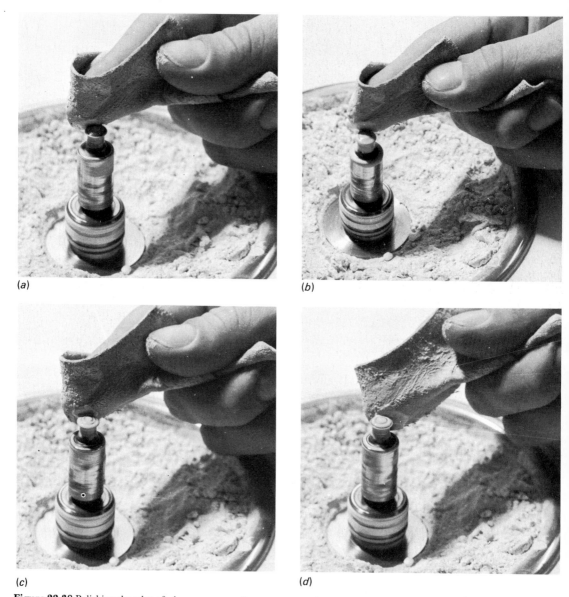

(a)   (b)

(c)   (d)

Figure 22.38 Polishing the edge of a lens, convex surface uppermost. Again the chamois leather is rolled over the edge of the lens as shown in the successive pictures (a)–(d)

a multiple of the linear expansion ratio. Thus, an environment which will cause the lens to start to hydrate before completion of its fabrication has to be avoided. Contrary to popular belief, this does not usually mean excessive environmental humidity control. However, extremes of humidity and temperature will have an effect on manufacture just as they do with hard lens fabrication. Of course, it does mean that all materials that come into

direct contact with the lens must be completely free from moisture, and this is achieved by storing such articles as polish, polishing tape, chamois leathers, cotton wool and so on, in an incubator (*Figure 22.41*), and only removing small quantities at the time they are required for use in the laboratory. The polish has to be free of all water and thus a grease-based medium has been developed. Additionally, if there is a pause in manufacture, the lens blank should be sealed

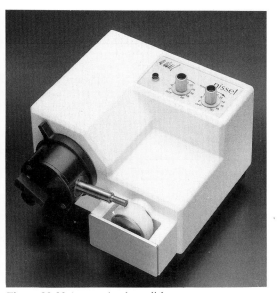

Figure 22.39 Automatic edge polisher

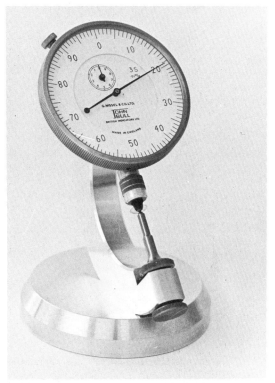

Figure 22.40 Checking centre thickness using a dial gauge marked with 0.01 mm divisions

in an air-tight tube which has previously been stored in the incubator. The technicians must take great care not to breathe over the lens nor to touch the surface with their skin. If any of these precautions are not taken the surface starts to hydrate prematurely and, besides affecting the final hydrated parameters, the surface finish is poor resulting in areas which may be relatively hydrophobic. Equally, dust has to be

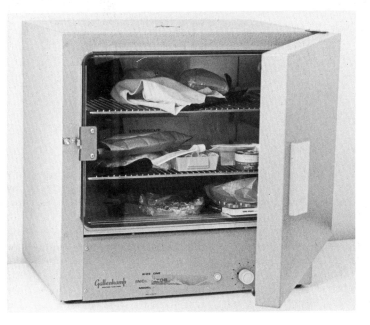

Figure 22.41 An incubator for storing soft lens blanks and related materials

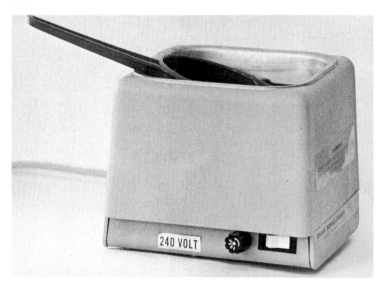

Figure 22.42 An ultrasonic cleaner for removing wax and grease from tools and lenses

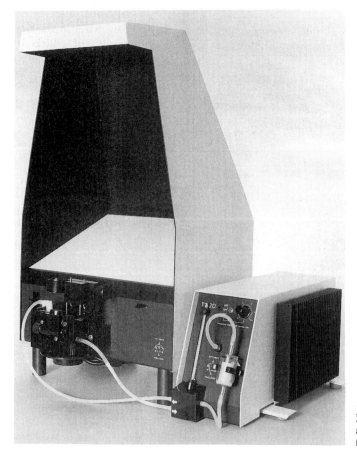

Figure 22.43 A wet-cell analyser, coupled with a saline filtration and temperature control unit for checking soft lens radii (*see also Figure 13.17*)

kept to an absolute minimum so that the surface finish is perfect.

The dehydrated lens has to be cleaned in an ultrasonic bath of solvent (*Figure 22.42*) and is then hydrated in sterile physiological (0.9%) saline solution. The hydration time varies with the type of polymer. Following hydration the lens should be checked. *Figure 22.43* shows a wet cell analyser. Other items used for checking are described in Chapter 13.

Practitioners are also reminded of the effect of *average* lens thickness on oxygen transmissibility and hence corneal metabolism both at the time of lens ordering and checking (*see Figure 13.24*). The determination of average thickness is discussed in Chapter 13, p. 485.

Sterilization

The only satisfactory way of sterilizing a soft lens is by autoclaving (*Figure 22.44*). Asepticization by chemicals or boiling is not, in the present day, an acceptable procedure as there may be a significant time delay before the lens is actually used, and microorganisms may survive simple disinfection by forming spores. Besides being in the patient's best interest it should be remembered that it is also in the practitioner's best interest, for it is he who is in the litigation front line.

The autoclave is thus an essential tool, not only for the laboratory, but also for the practitioner (Litvin, 1977). A few words of advice on its usage are therefore appropriate.

(1) Isotonic saline solution should always be used, never solutions containing preservatives.
(2) Ensure that the bottles are only three-quarters full, thereby avoiding a build-up of excess pressure which might force off the caps.
(3) The caps must be metal crimp type.
(4) The practitioner must ensure that the lens material will not be damaged by the high temperature of autoclaving.

Power adjustments to hard lenses by the laboratory

When the lens is being fabricated the power can be adjusted at the polishing stage, subject to certain requirements. On a lenticulated positive lens it is almost impossible to add plus power without ending up with a double optic, whereas adding minus power is very much easier. The reason for this is the relative difficulty in removing material at varying rates from the different areas of the optic, all of which is necessary to bring about these power changes. *Figure 22.45* shows a lenticulated positive lens in cross-section. In the case of adding positive power, material has to be removed from the periphery of the optic and it can be seen from *Figure 22.45a* that the lenticulation prevents a

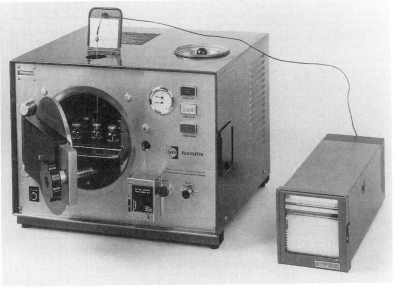

Figure 22.44 A small bottle autoclave with temperature recorder

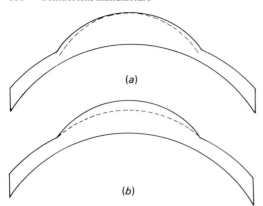

Figure 22.45 Power adjustments to positive lenticulated lenses. The broken lines represent areas where material is removed. (*a*) Adding plus power. (*b*) Adding minus power

proper sweep across the lens surface. This means the polisher cannot even out the bands which are formed when the removal of material from this area has taken place. However, when adding negative power the majority of material is removed from the centre of the lens with hardly any from the periphery of the optic as shown in *Figure 22.45b*. Thus, the bands which have formed can be blended into one another to produce a single optic.

With a negative lens the power can be altered either by adding positive or negative power provided that the lens has not been lenticulated and that there is sufficient thickness of material at the removal regions. *Figure 22.46a,b* shows the areas where material has to be removed. Once a negative lens has been lenticulated it is difficult to adjust its power accurately because the polishing button drops over the edge of the optic

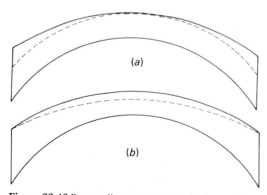

Figure 22.46 Power adjustments to negative lenses. The broken lines represent areas where material is removed. (*a*) Adding plus power. (*b*) Adding minus power

and, again, it becomes difficult to blend the polishing bands into one another.

The alteration of a patient's hard lens involves the above difficulties, but if the lens is thin in the centre, as with negative lenses, it is extremely difficult to re-centre the lens correctly on the hollow chuck. With a lens which is so thin, no pressure can be used to re-centre it on the hollow chuck without causing distortion. If this happens the lens is held in this distorted manner and the distortion or irregularity polished off the front surface, only to find on releasing the lens from the chuck that it relaxes back to an equal but opposite distortion of the front surface and hence a resultant poor power reading. The use of a polishing drum (*see* Chapter 23) for power modification has similar inherent problems and its use frequently results in a poor power reading. The real answer to this problem lies with the practitioner. First and foremost he should have good quality diagnostic fitting lenses with a comprehensive range of powers. Secondly, if the lens requires a power alteration it is usually better to order a new one, the old lens adding to the practitioner's fitting set of prescription lenses. Practitioner modifications are best restricted to altering the total diameter, edge shape, optic diameters and peripheral curves; interfering with the optic, front or back, does not result in a good lens.

Toric lenses

Concave and convex toroidal surfaces can be produced by crimping, polishing or generating.

Crimping

To produce a toroidal back surface, a concave spherical surface is first cut and polished with its radius midway between the required radii. The blank is cut with a central thickness of approximately 0.20 mm and a diameter of 0.20 mm above its final requirement. An outer stepped rim at the base of the blank is formed on which to apply the pressure during crimping. The blank is placed concave surface uppermost in the small crimping tool (*Figure 22.47*) which applies pressure at four points on the stepped rim — two points along the one meridian to flatten the radius and the other two points at right-angles to steepen the radius. The amount of toricity is then produced by altering the

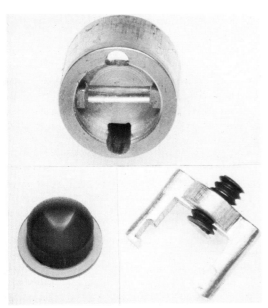

Figure 22.47 A simple crimping tool showing its three component parts, and a lens blank with an outer stepped rim, in place for crimping

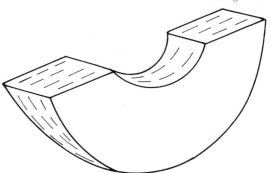

Figure 22.48 Half a felt tool with central cut-out for hand polishing a toroidal front surface

pressure until the required difference between the radii is achieved. The toroidal surface thus produced is then checked on the radiuscope. The blank, still held in the crimping tool, is then re-cut on the lathe to produce a spherical curve midway between the required radii. After polishing, the blank is released from the crimping tool and forms into a toroidal surface.

A similar procedure is used to produce a toroidal front surface. However, it is necessary to cut a curve on the back of the blank before crimping, although this does not require polishing. This back curve is necessary to reduce the amount of pressure required to flex the lens. Once the toroidal front surface is completed the final back surface has to be produced. At the same time any prism necessary for stabilizing the lens has to be incorporated, as well as reducing the blank to the required thickness of the finished lens.

Polishing

This involves creating a toroidal surface by hand polishing and is usually confined to the front surface of the lens. This technique is only possible on PMMA material and then only for relatively low cylindrical powers. The lens has to be finished on both surfaces and mounted on a hollow chuck. A positive cylinder is then polished on using a felt wheel which has been cut across its diameter and a radius cut out of its centre, giving the appearance of a female cutting gauge shown in *Figure 22.48*. An allowance has to be made initially when working the spherical power as some negative sphere is added at the same time as the positive cylinder. It requires an extremely skilled technician to obtain an acceptable result.

Generating

To obtain a toroidal concave surface a spherical curve is first cut on the blank. The toroidal curve is then generated by attaching a toric wheel to the polishing machine by means of a spindle. A fork, which holds the arms on which the blank is mounted, maintains the arms at right-angles to the spindle of the toric wheel. The whole unit then rotates together while the oscillating head of the polisher moves the blank across the axis of the toric wheel (*Figure 22.49*).

The toric wheels are usually cut from brass (*Figure 22.50*), and emery is used as an abrasive. For the more popular toric radii, diamond-coated toric wheels may be used. A wax toric wheel, which is cut in a similar manner to the brass wheel, is used for polishing (*Figure 22.51*).

The cutting of brass and wax toric wheels involves the use of a special toric lathe. The radius is cut at right-angles to the spindle axis which is displaced by the required difference between the two radii (*Figure 22.52*).

Once the central curves have been generated any number of toroidal peripheral curves may be formed.

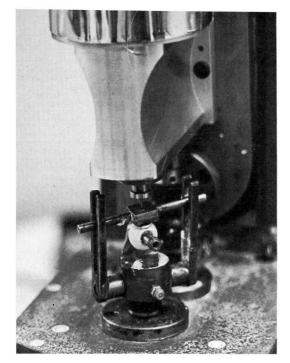

Figure 22.49 Close-up of a back surface toric polisher

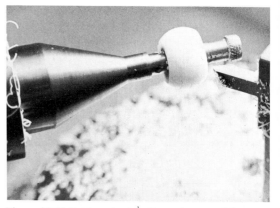

Figure 22.51 Cutting a back surface toric wax polisher

Generating convex toroidal surfaces poses a greater problem. To cut them on the toric lathe requires a special chuck for each lens because of the many possible combinations of power and thickness for each prescription lens. An alternative is to place the blank in the mould used for making the wax wheels. The hot wax is poured around the blank, so that the blank becomes integral with the wax wheel. The wheel/blank combination is then cut to the required toricity on the toric lathe and polished using a small front surface wax polisher. This wax polisher, which is mounted on the rocker arm, has previously been moulded to the cut toroidal surface. In effect the small wax polisher takes the place of the blank on the polishing machine.

In this procedure, as with crimping front surfaces, the back surface has to be cut after the front surface has been completed.

Recently toric lathes which are designed to cut toroidal surfaces directly onto the blank have been introduced. These lathes still have to prove themselves and at present they seem to be falling short of their original expectations. C.L.M. Group Ltd in London grind and then polish front surface cylinders onto high water content soft lenses using the traditional Nissel toric polishing machine, but with the lens mounted on a solid chuck and the grinding and polishing tool held in the dolly on top of the lens. This is the reverse of the conventional Nissel set-up. This system works fairly well but restricts the means of stabilization to truncating only.

Advantages and disadvantages of toric techniques

Crimping has the advantage that a laboratory can produce a wide range of toroidal surfaces without the expense of a toric lathe. It is particularly useful for toric soft lens production where, especially with the high water content materials, very steep radii have to be generated in the dehydrated state. These are usually too steep to cut on the toric lathe and so an

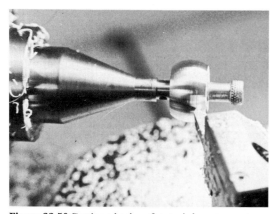

Figure 22.50 Cutting a back surface toric brass generator

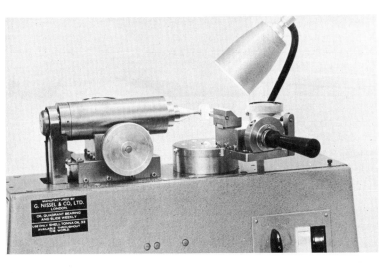

Figure 22.52 A toric lathe with wax tool in place for cutting

extremely wide range of toric wheels, which have to be specially manufactured, are necessary, thus making the procedure very costly. Its one disadvantage is that in hard lens production it introduces strain into the lens. This does not happen with soft lenses as all strain is released on hydration.

Polishing gives varied results because it is very dependent on the skill of the technician and is only satisfactory on PMMA. Its use is generally restricted to negative and low positive powered lenses, for with lenticulated positive lenses, it is difficult to polish the periphery of the optic.

Generating is most definitely the best method of producing toroidal back surface hard lenses.

Prisms

A prism may be incorporated into the lens either to correct a vertical extraocular muscle imbalance or more usually to stabilize the lens, i.e. to stop it rotating on the eye.

The prism is introduced when the last surface, usually the front, is cut. Either a special hollow chuck or a prism adaptor, on which a standard front surface chuck may sit, is used for this purpose (*Figure 22.53*). The prism chuck has its face cut at an angle corresponding to the apical angle of the prism. The prism adaptor has an outer male taper which has a different axial centre line to that of its inner female taper. Thus, any standard chuck which sits on the adaptor is angled by the same amount as the apical angle of the required prism.

It is preferable to use a prism adaptor rather than a prism chuck, for after polishing the front surface, which is done with the standard chuck still mounted on the adaptor, the chuck should be placed back in the lathe without the adaptor. The lens is then re-cut and because it contains a prism, only material from the high spot (i.e. the thickest part of the prism base at the lens edge) is removed. Thus, the thickness of the base of the prism is reduced, producing a lens with a good edge thickness all round but still containing the necessary ballast to stabilize it. The reduced base is then polished on a vertical spindle using a felt wheel in a flexible drive.

Wax polishers

Back and front surface polishers are made with dental or paraffin wax and magnesium carbonate, the latter acting as a very fine abrasive.

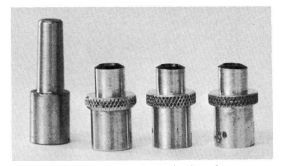

Figure 22.53 From left to right: 1.5 Δ prism adaptor; standard hollow chuck; hollow chuck with 1.5 Δ prism; hollow chuck with 3 Δ prism

Such wax polishers, their chucks, and the blocks in which they are made, are shown in *Figures 22.54* and *22.55*. In hot climates large quantities of magnesium carbonate are required to prevent the wax from softening.

After cleaning the chuck and casting blocks in paraffin, they are heated to approximately 85°C and the molten mixture of wax and magnesium carbonate, which is at approximately 125°C, is poured into the blocks. The blocks are then banged several times on a solid surface to release any air bubbles. After cooling slightly the wax contracts and the blocks need to be topped up with additional wax.

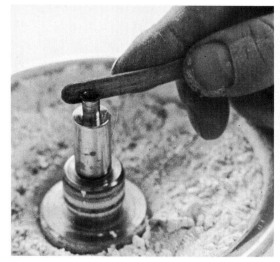

Figure 22.56 Truncating a lens with an emery board using the (stationary) vertical spindle as a base

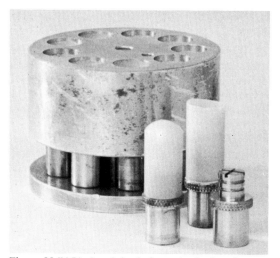

Figure 22.54 Block and chucks for casting back surface wax polishers: from left to right are the block for making nine wax tools, a finished tool with radius cut on, an uncut wax tool and basic chuck for taking a wax polishing tool

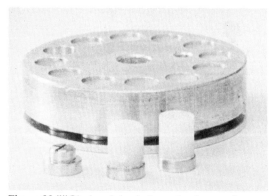

Figure 22.55 Block and chucks for casting front surface wax polishers: a basic chuck and a cut and uncut wax tool are shown in front of the block for making 12 wax tools

When the wax is cold the chucks can be forced out of the casting blocks with the aid of a dowel. The back surface polishers are cut on the lathe while the front surface polishers are cut using steel male gauges.

Truncating

Truncating is usually carried out to help stabilize a toric or bifocal lens and is nearly always combined with prism ballast. Most frequently it involves only the lower edge. The edge is removed using an emery board (*Figure 22.56*) or a diamond impregnated tool. It is polished with a felt wheel rotating in a flexible drive (*Figure 22.57*) or on a rotating velveteen drum-chuck, while the lens is mounted on an edging chuck. The corners of the truncation are rounded to minimize discomfort to the lower lid. With a bifocal, the edge is left fairly square to assist in raising the lens, by support on the lower lid margin, when the gaze is depressed.

Annealing

PMMA blanks are made from cast sheet, cast block or rod turned from cast block. Gas permeable blanks are either individually cast or rod cast. All casting introduces strain which needs to be released from the material to ensure consistent results in hard lens fabrication. This is done by annealing which involves heating the

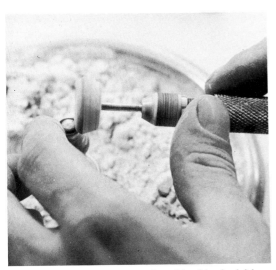

Figure 22.57 Polishing a truncation with a felt wheel driven by a flexible drive

material to a temperature of between 140 and 150°C for a short period and slowly returning it to room temperature. This does not cause any difficulty when done to thin sheet material, but with thick material the temperature has to be low enough to prevent depolymerization of the surface although heated long enough to ensure the centre of the block reaches at least 130°C. Annealing is usually carried out by the supplier of the blanks.

Fenestration

Fenestration involves forming a hole, typically 0.20–0.30 mm diameter, with a vertical drill while the lens is mounted convex surface uppermost on a chuck containing a small depression (or hole) which receives the penetrating drill. Both sides of the fenestration must be countersunk and polished. This is best done with a sharpened boxwood stick which is rotated in a circular fashion in the opposite direction to the vertical spindle on which the chuck and lens is rotating. To polish and countersink the back surface of the fenestration the lens is placed on a concave chuck with the fenestration hole at its centre. The lens may be held in place by wax or double-sided sticky tape, avoiding the central depression (or hole) in the chuck. The central part of the fenestration may be polished by running the lens up and down a length of polish-soaked cotton, threaded through the fenestration hole.

Note. Fenestrating, to aid tear exchange, only works successfully on a steep fitting lens; if the lens is an alignment or flat fit, the fenestration merely creates another tear meniscus between it and the cornea which reduces the mobility of the lens and thus tends to aggravate any corneal oedema. Additionally, if the fenestration is small enough to minimize any interference with vision it usually quickly becomes blocked with mucoproteins — thus losing its usefulness and adding a site in which to harbour pathogens. Conversely, if the fenestration is large enough to prevent blockage then the vision may be greatly interfered with.

The author feels that if a corneal lens requires fenestrating then there is something basically wrong with the fit of that lens or the tear flow and these should be attended to rather than introducing a fenestration. Oedema problems can now be alleviated much more successfully in hard lens-wearing patients by using a gas permeable material, although fenestration of some lenses for keratoconus can be helpful.

Fenestration of corneal and scleral lenses is also dealt with in Chapters 17, 18 and 23.

Bifocals

Bifocals may be fused or solid in the hard lens form, but can only be made solid in a soft lens construction at the present time. Of recent years the most frequently fitted hard lens bifocals have been the D-shaped and, more recently still, the crescent-shaped fused bifocals (*Figure 22.58*). The last few years have seen the appearance of

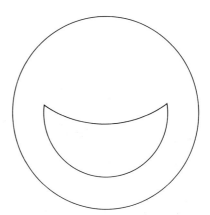

Figure 22.58 Crescent fused bifocal lens

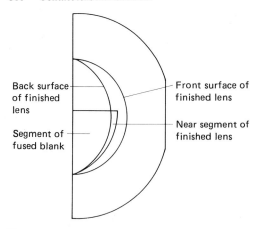

Back surface of finished lens

Front surface of finished lens

Segment of fused blank

Near segment of finished lens

Figure 22.59 Crescent fused bifocal blank in cross-section

soft lens bifocals; these are constructed in the dehydrated state in exactly the same manner as the hard solid bifocals.

Fused bifocals

The fused bifocal blank (*Figure 22.59*) is made by fusing together two pieces of PMMA with different refractive indices, in an oven at high temperature. This is a similar process to constructing a fused bifocal spectacle lens. The segment can be fused on the back surface of the blank or internally fused. With the former the different powers of the near additions are obtained by varying the radius of the segment interface. Thus, for any given BOZR with any given near addition an appropriate segment radius is cut into the blank and the matching segment inserted into this cavity. Therefore, for any given blank there is a fixed BOZR and near addition. Consequently, a comprehensive stock of blanks is required for surface fused bifocals to cover all possible combinations of BOZR and near additions (*see* Chapter 5), as well as the range of tints.

The fabrication of a fused bifocal lens is much the same as for a single vision lens. Greater care has to be taken in centring the lens on its mount, and in calibrating and cutting the thickness in order to avoid the segment breaking through the lens onto the front surface. A prism and truncation are usually needed to stabilize the fit and quite often the optic is displaced upwards. Displacement of the optic requires the initial diameter of the blank to be cut oversize by an amount slightly above the required displace-

ment. The back peripheral curves are then generated. The lens is displaced on its button by the required amount and the diameter re-cut to 0.20 mm above the finally required total diameter to allow for edging. The front surface is then cut in the normal manner.

Internally fused bifocal blanks are frequently used at the present time. These are constructed with an internal segment of a higher refractive index than the outer material and the radii of the segment are adjusted to give the required near addition power. Internally fused bifocal blanks need only to be stocked by their near addition power without any consideration for the front or back curves to be worked. Additionally there is no risk of the segment coming adrift from the main lens. Their disadvantage lies in the restriction in the minimal centre thickness that may be obtained before cutting into the segment.

Solid bifocals

Solid bifocals may be crescent, downcurve or concentric shaped. All of these usually have the segment worked on the front surface.

Crescent or upcurve shaped

This is constructed by cutting a lens incorporating a large prism (*Figure 22.60*). The front surface is polished and then replaced on the lathe with a lower powered prism adaptor. The base of the prism is then removed by cutting a steeper front surface curve corresponding to the near power of the lens. This produces a crescent-shaped segment which is then polished.

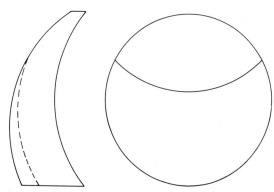

Figure 22.60 Crescent or upcurve solid bifocal lens. The broken lines represent the area where material has been removed to create the near segment on the front surface. Cross-section and front views are shown

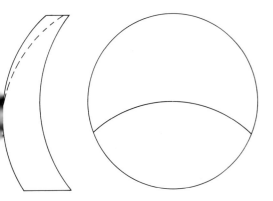

Figure 22.61 Downcurve or arc solid bifocal lens. The broken lines represent the area where material has been removed to create the distance portion on the front surface. Cross-section and front views are shown

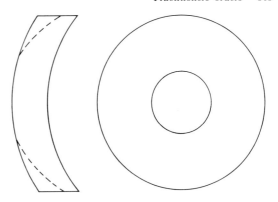

Figure 22.62 Concentric solid bifocal lens. The broken lines represent the area where material has been removed to create the near portion on the front surface. Cross-section and front views are shown

Downcurve or arc shaped

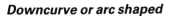

This is constructed by the reverse approach to the crescent-shaped segment (*Figure 22.61*), i.e. the lens is cut to a much thicker substance and with a small prism. The front surface radius is such that it produces the required near portion power. After polishing the front surface, the lens, still mounted, is placed on a higher powered prism adaptor and is re-cut using a flatter radius corresponding to the distance power. This produces an arc-shaped or down-curve segment, ballasted with a prism. The segment is then polished.

Concentric shaped

These do not contain a prism as they are often used for simultaneous vision or 'bivision' through both distance and near portions. If used for successive vision (alternating vision) or simultaneous vision any rotation on the eye is not important unless the lens is in the toric form. The centre is sighted for distance vision and the main outer lens for near. Although it can be reversed, in practice there are difficulties in constructing the junction properly because of the change from steeper to flatter radius; also, with a distance negative prescription the edge of the lens could be unduly thick. The lens is cut, with the front radius for distance vision, and polished; the periphery of the lens is cut down with a steeper radius corresponding to the near prescription (*Figure 22.62*). This cut-down is taken into the centre of the lens far enough to

produce the required central segment diameter, and is then polished.

The difficulty in fabricating a solid bifocal lens is in obtaining a sharp transition between the distance and near segments. During the process of polishing the second radius there is inevitably some blending of the junction of the near and distance portions and hence an area of visual confusion may be produced for the patient, although this blending may be sufficient to provide a progressive power lens.

Practitioners' orders

Laboratories quite frequently have to refer back to a practitioner about an order which has been received with either insufficient or total lack of instructions; for example, a tint is omitted, there may be no instructions as to whether a lenticulation is required with a positive lens, no position given for a fenestration, no amount, angle or location (top or bottom) of a truncation given. Impossible or extremely complex orders may be received. For example, a practitioner may specify, with a positive lens, a centre thickness which is too thin for a given front optic zone diameter or total diameter, or the almost impossible order for an oblique bi-toric lens — almost impossible, that is if a good power reading and accurate axes are wanted.

If a negative lens is requested to be made extremely thin in the centre (less than 0.10 mm), the lens will have to be fabricated on a solid chuck so that the centre of the lens is properly supported and will not drop during the cutting and polishing stages. This means that the power cannot be assessed and adjusted as the polishing proceeds, any adjustments having to be made after the lens has been removed from its initial mounting. Hence, poor power readings may result (*see* Power adjustments, p. 837). Because all gas permeable hard lenses are made on solid chucks to prevent the optic dropping, any adjustment to the power of prescription lenses has to take place after fabrication and consequently the same problem can occur.

Laboratories should soak rigid gas permeable lenses for 24 hours before finally checking the parameters and practitioners should also check the lenses under the same conditions, although there may still be changes to the dimensions occurring many days after the initial hydration (Walker, 1988). There may also be variations in BOZR recorded on different radiuscopes and between different personnel on the same instruments; these possible variations have to be considered when ordering and allowances made so that impossible tolerances are not expected.

Recent work (Walker, 1988) has suggested that the observed radical flattening on hydration, as measured on a radiuscope, in high minus gas permeable hard lenses may be restricted to the central 2 or 3 mm, the midperiphery being somewhat steeper. In the same study it was also suggested that, as a consequence of this variation between central and midperipheral BOZR, any allowances made during manufacture to compensate for this apparent central flattening may, once the lens is on the eye, produce a steeper clinical fit than desired. It was therefore proposed that laboratories should supply graphs of these flattenings to assist practitioners to predict the amount acceptable for a range of powers in a given material and thus a laboratory should only steepen the lens during manufacture by a nominal amount corresponding with the flattening observed in the equivalent lens made from PMMA. The author feels that, while this suggestion is commendable, a more suitable approach would be for the development of a radiuscope that could accurately measure these small variations thus removing the dependency upon arbitrary measurements from tables or graphs.

A little thought by the practitioner before putting pen to paper would save both the practitioner and laboratory a lot of time and annoyance. Chapter 5 and Appendix E cover the calculations and/or drawing to scale necessary to determine adequate thicknesses to permit lenses to be made.

To help in the choice of hard lens thickness, lenticulations and tints the practitioner is referred to *Table 22.1* and to Chapter 10. Chapter 24 also includes some information on tints.

Conclusion

Good manufacturing practice is the sure way to produce good quality lenses. The key to good manufacturing practice is quality assurance. The Food and Drugs Administration (FDA) in the USA has laid down a minimum of nine key-quality assurance activities (Ratkowski, 1984). They are as follows:

(1) Button inspection.
(2) Acceptance/rejection criteria at each manufacturing step.
(3) Identity and specifications for each processing compound, such as mounting waxes and polishing compounds.
(4) Cleaning instructions, and specifications for cleaning compounds.
(5) Final product acceptance criteria and test methods.
(6) Identity and specification for packaging and labelling materials.
(7) Disinfection instructions (or sterilization instructions if labelled as sterile), process validation, and product release procedures.
(8) Records maintenance, including but not limited to maintenance of batch records and complaint files.
(9) Continuing audit procedures to be employed by the laboratory's personnel.

Production of good lenses will partly be dependent upon a good surface finish; this in turn will only be obtained if the surface has been cut with the minimum amount of damage. To minimize surface stress and 'burning', good quality machinery and skilled operators are needed. To achieve a quality surface, lathes must have minimum vibration and high mechanical stiffness (Dent, 1986). Ideally spindle speeds should be above 8000 rev./min. Depth of cut should be minimal as bulk removal

Table 22.1 Hard PMMA lens tints

Code number	Description	Code number	Description
★200	Light yellow	★2092	Bright green
★300	Amber	2219-1	Pale amber
★400	Bright red	2240-1	Dark green
★401	Bright cherry red	2240-2	Light green
★512	Light brownish-grey	2240-3	Medium green
★600	Bright medium green	2241-1	Ruby red
★603	Bright green	2241-2	Medium pale pink
★700	Pale blue	2241-3	Pale pink
★703	Medium blue	2241-4	Very dark ruby red
★911	Very pale grey	2241-5	Dark pink
★912	Pale grey	2242-2	Pale lavender
★962	Very dark grey	2285	Dark brown
★999	Dark grey	2285-1	Light brown
1077	Very dark blue	2285-2	Medium brown
1077-1	Light blue	6077	Dark grey
1077-2	Dark blue	6610-1	Medium grey
1077-3	Medium blue	6610-2	Extreme pale grey
★2002	Bright light green	★★9042	Very light brownish-grey
★2045	Bright light blue	★★9043	Light brownish-grey
★2069	Very light blue	★10910	Violet
★2082	Very pale green		

Commercial grade polymethyl methacrylate (ICI) is available in those tints marked with an asterisk. Other tints are the American 'De Luxe' material. Double asterisk indicates CQ or clinical quality material.

of material rapidly produces damage by chipping and fracture to the lens surface and destruction of the cutting edge of the diamond. It is preferable to remove the bulk of the material and profile the lens on a roughing lathe to within 0.20 mm of its finished surface in order to extend the life of the finishing diamond and minimize heat-induced stress in the material. The rate at which the cutting tool is fed across the surface is of extreme importance as this decides the rate of removal of material for any given spindle speed. Changes in surface finish have been evident with feed rates as low as 2°/s (Dent, 1986). To this end, CNC lathes remove the operator variables in cutting and, when combined with top quality diamonds which are regularly inspected after a given number of passes, should ensure a good surface which can be polished in the minimum of time. With the latest CNC lathes, aspherical surfaces can be readily generated but unfortunately there is still no accurate means of polishing the surface. Most machinery manufacturers suggest holding a chamois leather, soaked in polish and placed over the finger tip, against the surface of the lens while it is still rotating in the lathe. This leads to a less than satisfactory result with a curve that is difficult to reproduce.

British and American approved names for contact lens materials

Any new 'drug' licensed in the UK must have a British Approved Name (BAN). There is a high degree of international cooperation in establishing approved names and the BAN is usually the same as the US Approved Name (USAN) and the International Non-proprietary Name (INN).

The US approved names are already adopted for contact lens materials. Names employ a characteristic suffix of which two are currently in use:

(1) Filcon, applied to soft type materials.
(2) Focon, applied to gas permeable hard materials.

Names also have a letter suffix A, B, C etc., which is used to indicate the same polymer from different manufacturers. It has also been used in the case of Lidofilcon (Sauflon) to indicate different content of two materials from the same manufacturer. Sauflon 70 is Lidofilcon A and Sauflon 85 is Lidofilcon B. No direct reference is made to water content in any USAN. A new letter suffix would be applied to a new formulation of an existing material.

The naming system is not totally consistent because the first material in the hydrophilic group (the Hydron/Bausch & Lomb material) has the name Polymacon omitting the suffix and letter, and the Danker–Wöhlk CAB material has a USAN (Cabufocon A) different from the two other named CAB materials (Porofocon A and B). The reason for these anomalies is unknown.

Table 22.2 is based on information extracted from the US Pharmacopeia and, although not exhaustive, it refers to the main lenses currently marketed and listed in the USAN directory up to 1982. The terms 'filcon' and 'focon' refer, respectively, to soft and gas permeable hard materials.

Although there is a claimed difference in chemical composition it can be assumed that the materials in each group, once made into contact lenses, will be effective in identical ways. It is on this basis that the Association of Contact Lens Manufacturers Ltd (ACLM) in the UK has proposed generic identities rather than specific labels as in the USAN system. The ACLM proposals are that the suffixes 'filcon' and 'focon' be retained as applied to soft and hard

Table 22.2 Contact lens material terminology in the USA

USAN	Main user	Main component	Monomers		Cross-linker
Hard					
Cabufocon	Danker/Paragon	CAB			
Dimefocon	Danker	Polysiloxane			
Porofocon	Rynco	CAB			
Silafocon	Polycon	Silicone MA	MMA	MA	TEGDMA
Soft					
Group I (36–38% water content)					
Crofilcon	Syntex	Dihydroxypropyl MA	MMA		?
Dimelfilcon	Dow	PHEMA			Ethyl bis(oxyethyl) DMA
Phemfilcon	WJ	PHEMA	Ethoxyethyl	MA	?
Polmacon	Bausch & Lomb/ Hydron	PHEMA			EGDMA
Tefilcon	Ciba	PHEMA			?
Group II (40+% water content)					
Bufilcon	Hydrocurve	HEMA	-acrylamide		TriMA
Deltafilcon	BP/Alcon	HEMA	MA	iBMA	TriMA
Droxifilcon	Strieter	HEMA	NVP		Ethyl bis(oxyethyl) DMA
Etafilcon	Frontier	HEMA	MA(Na)		TriMA
Hefilcon	Flexlens/ Bausch & Lomb	HEMA	NVP		EGDMA
Ocufilcon	Alcon	HEMA	MA		EGDMA
Perfilcon	Cooper	HEMA	NVP	MA	?
Tetrafilcon	AO	HEMA	NVP	MMA	DVB
Vifilcon	AO	HEMA	NVP	MA	EGDMA
Group III (40+% water content, non-HEMA)					
Hydrofilcon	Parke Davis	NVP	Phenylethyl MA		AOEMA
Lidofilcon	Sauflon	NVP	MMA		AMA/EGDMA
Others (hydrophilic surface)					
Elastafilcon	Dow	Polysiloxane			
Silafilcon	Dow	Polysiloxane			

Note. Chapters 3, 10 and 11 give details of properties of materials used for contact lenses.
See also Tables 3.2–3.5, pp. 101–102 and 117.

Abbreviations:

AMA	allyl methacrylate	iBMA	isobutyl methacrylate
AOEMA	2-allyl-oxyethyl methacrylate	MA	methacrylic acid
CAB	cellulose acetate butyrate	MMA	methyl methacrylate
DMA	dimethacrylate	NVP	*N*-vinyl pyrrolidone
DVB	divinyl benzene	PHEMA	2-hydroxyethyl methacrylate
EGDMA	ethylene glycol dimethacrylate	TEGDMA	tetra-EGDMA

materials, respectively, but that this is then followed by an integer and letter suffix denoting the chemical composition, and then a number suffix in parentheses to denote the saline content for soft lenses and the oxygen permeability for gas permeable hard lenses. This would enable easy classification of lens materials into different groups. Examples might be:

(1) Filcon 4a (75) for a soft lens.
(2) Focon 2b (6) for a hard lens.

The first example would indicate a 75% water content soft lens of a particular chemical composition denoted by the '4a' group, and the second example a gas permeable hard lens of *Dk* value of 6 in the group whose chemical composition falls in the category '2b'. This should also help overcome some of the difficulties of patents and so on.

Once the proposed framework for the naming of contact lens polymers is accepted the full details of the chemical classification groupings and other related information will be available from the ACLM.

References

DENT, M. (1986). Life at the cutting edge. *Optical World* **6**, 16–23

LITVIN, M. W. (1977). The incidence of eye infections with contact lenses. *Optician* **174**(4496), 11–14

RATKOWSKI, D. (1984). Good manufacturing practice. G.M.P. highlights. *Contact Lens J.* **12**(12), 11–22

WALKER, J. (1988). Radical flattening — a laboratory enigma. *Optician* **195**(5142), 21–23

Further reading

BRYANT, P. G. (1973). Construction and manufacture of a fused bifocal lens. *Ophthal. Optician* **13**, 1052–1056

CORDREY, P. (1973). Technical and economic effects of contact lens production methods. *Ophthal. Optician* **13**, 230–236

CRUNDALL, E. J. (1977). Spun to curve. *Optician* **173**(4483), 15–16, 19–20, 23, 28

HAYNES, P. R. (1965). Modification procedures. In *Contact Lens Practice: Basic and Advanced*, 1st edn, edited by R. B. Mandell, pp. 252–280. Springfield, Illinois: Thomas

HICKS, M. (1975). More than a million. *Optician* **170**(4407), 18–26

HODD, F. A. B. (1974). Bifocal contact lens practice. *Ophthal. Optician* **13**, 315–320, 325–326, 378–380, 385–388

INMAN, D. R. (1974). Peripheral design of toric corneal lenses. *Optician* **167**(4318), 13–17

NISSEL, G. (1975). Manufacturing techniques. In *Contact Lens Practice: Visual, Therapeutic and Prosthetic*, edited by M. Ruben, pp. 314–342. London: Baillière Tindall

PHILLIPS, A. J. (1970). Alterations in curvature of the finished corneal lens. *Ophthal. Optician* **9**, 980–986, 1043–1054, 1100–1110

SHANKS, K. R. (1966). Subjective comparison of corneal lens edges. *Br. J. physiol. Optics* **23**, 55–58

Chapter 23

Modification procedures

A. J. Phillips

The importance of the practitioner being able to carry out modifications

Nowadays, when modifications can be carried out relatively quickly and cheaply by laboratories, it is often difficult to impress on students, and even qualified practitioners, the following reasons why the contact lens practitioner should be able to carry out his own modifications:

(1) There is no interruption to the patient's wearing schedule and no necessity for extra visits.
(2) Often only the practitioner knows exactly what is desired and it may be difficult to describe to the laboratory just what is required. (This is particularly so with scleral lenses.)
(3) Modifications can be done in increasing stages, with the effect of the modifications on the patient noted at each stage. Laboratories either have to do the full modifications in one step, or the patient is required to make many unnecessary visits and to be without lenses for several days.
(4) Subsequent modifications may become apparent and can be done immediately.
(5) Practitioners who carry out modifications are better able to evaluate lenses which have been made or which have to be modified by a laboratory.

Against these advantages must be set the cost of the equipment involved. However, much of this cost can be redeemed, not only from tax relief but also on the savings of doing the modification oneself. It is important to remember also that patients are more satisfied because they do not have to be without their lenses. Further, most of the equipment, especially the more expensive items, will last a lifetime.

The advent of a whole range of new rigid gas permeable (RGP) materials has complicated practitioner modification of lenses but has not prevented it, except for the surface-treated and moulded groups which should not be modified, and the very high permeable materials, such as the fluorosilicone acrylates, which warp and burn easily and should only be modified by a skilled technician.

The following section lists the equipment which can be used for contact lens modification. It should be emphasized that many of these are alternatives and are discussed as such.

Modification equipment for corneal lenses

Corneal lens holders

Glass tube and double-sided adhesive tape

This is one of the simplest and cheapest forms of corneal lens holder.

A glass tube of about 6 mm in diameter, with rounded ends, has a small strip of double-sided adhesive tape stretched over one end on to which the lens is lightly pressed. An inverted glass tube from a dropper bottle is ideal.

This holder has the disadvantages that tape adhesive may stick to the lens when removed for checking and that the tape may need replacing if polishing liquid gets between the lens and tape.

Modified scleral lens holder

The simplest form of corneal lens holder consists of an ordinary scleral lens suction holder which has been cut down and thinned on a rotating rough grinding stone to an internal diameter of about 7.5 mm and an edge thickness of about 0.5 mm (*Figures 23.1* and *23.2*). A corneal lens

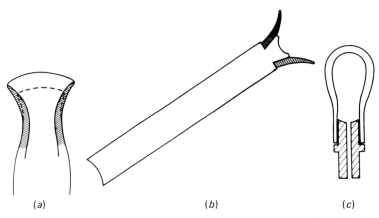

Figure 23.1 Corneal lens holders. (*a*) Cross-section of a scleral lens suction holder with the dotted line indicating the reduced size suitable for holding corneal lenses. (*b*) Cross-section of the end of a corneal lens suction holder mounted on a Perspex or nylon rod. (*c*) Cross-section of a double-ended suction holder. The lower shaded portion is removable and reversible having a flat end and a concave end for holding back and front surfaces of corneal lenses, respectively

holder may also be used with a hollow plastic tube in the stem to give support (Haynes, 1965). These holders are best used filled with water.

They have the disadvantage that they cannot be allowed to rotate between the fingers and may therefore occasionally cause oval optic

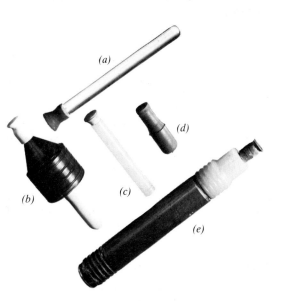

Figure 23.2 Corneal lens holders. (*a*) Corneal lens suction holder cup mounted on a Perspex handle; (*b*) spinner (Madden & Layman Ltd); (*c*) corneal lens suction holder cup mounted on a nylon handle; (*d*) modified scleral lens suction holder; (*e*) spinner

zones — when polishing peripheral curves, for instance — or possibly occasional lens scratches. They can, however, be rotated manually.

Modified corneal suction holder

This design, as used by Shick in America and sometimes known by his name, is shown in *Figures 23.1b* and *23.2c*. The end of a corneal lens suction holder is placed over a short nylon or Perspex rod cut as shown. Again, best used with the open end full of water, this type gives good control and spins easily with one finger resting lightly on the upper end.

Spinner

A more efficient version of the previous holder, the spinner consists of a rotatable spindle with a corneal lens suction holder at the end, mounted in a handle (*Figure 23.2b,e*). The lens can rotate freely on the end of the spindle while the handle is held still.

Double-ended suction holder

This type of suction holder has a reversible end, one end for attachment to convex surfaces and the other for concave surfaces. As this is the only type of lens holder, apart from those using adhesive tape, which will attach to the back surface of a corneal lens, it finds particular application in the alteration of lens power and removal of front surface abrasions (*see* p. 860). A cross-section is shown in *Figure 23.1c*. All suction holder ends have the disadvantage that the lens may flex, particularly with thinner lenses, so that the curves will be produced slightly steeper than desired, or slightly distorted.

Double-sided adhesive tape

Double-sided adhesive tape, of about 7 mm in width, is ideal for attaching corneal lenses to non-suction types of holder.

Vertical spindle or Office Modification Unit (*Figure 23.3*)

A speed of between 500 and 1500 rev./min is required — ideally, variable over this range, especially in the slower region. Models with clockwise or anti-clockwise rotation may be obtained, as preferred.

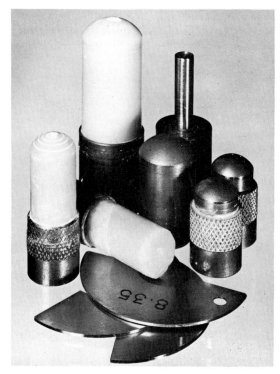

Figure 23.4 From left to right. Rear: large wax tool and spindle lens holder (or edging chuck). Centre: small wax tools, cut and uncut, and large and small diamond impregnated brass tools. Front: female gauges. (*See also Figures 22.11, 18.21 and 18.22*)

This is the most expensive single item of all modification equipment.

Ideally, the unit should be mounted in a bench with the taper slightly above the level of the bench (*see Figure 18.21*). This enables the operator: to rest his elbows on the table top and thus to steady his hands, and to roll the cutting blade and smoothing tools around the edge of the lens when shaping the edge or reducing the total diameter.

Spindle lens chuck or edging chuck

This lens chuck (*Figure 23.4*), used for edge and total diameter modifications, should be carefully chosen so that its taper fits the practitioner's own vertical spindle (for example, standard or 0-morse tapers). It is preferable to have a chuck the stem of which is not too short or too thick; approximately 6 mm wide and 2 cm long enables easy holding by the stem.

The same chuck may also be used for holding

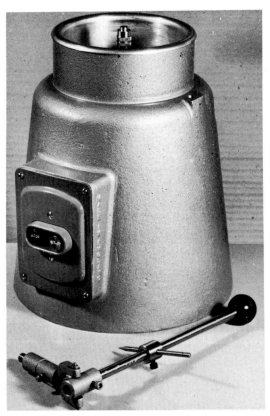

Figure 23.3 Vertical spindle or Office Modification Unit (G. Nissel & Co.)

lenses for peripheral curve modification of the back surface. The lens is stuck on to the chuck with wax or double-sided adhesive tape. As the lens is held rigid on the tool there should be no flexing of the lens during polishing, although if the stem is very narrow the periphery of a large corneal lens may still flex.

Adhesive wax and bunsen burner

Adhesive wax, obtainable in stick form, is one way of attaching the lens to the spindle lens chuck. A bunsen burner is used to melt the wax. Alternatively, a compressed butane burner may be used or even a spirit burner. More sophisticated electric heaters are also available to heat the metal chucks (*see Figure 22.1*). Low melting point wax should be used for RGP materials.

Centring devices

Centring devices are used where double-sided adhesive tape is used on the spindle lens chuck instead of beeswax, and where the lens must be accurately centred when it is placed on the chuck.

The lens is placed in the well of the device. The centring part is carefully lowered on to the lens and slowly rotated to centre the lens within the well and is then withdrawn.

These devices do not, in general, give such accurate lens centration as that carried out by hand, as described below.

Wax polishing tools

These tools are made up by the practitioner with molten wax poured into moulds and allowed to set hard. They are used for accurate polishing to a specific radius (*Figure 23.4*). Instructions for the manufacture of the tools are given by the laboratory supplying them. Alternatively, the tools may be made up by the laboratory. Further details are given in Chapter 22 on pp. 841–842 and *Figures 22.54* and *22.55* show the blocks and chucks used for making back and front surface wax polishers, together with cut and uncut finished wax tools. Normally, only convex curves are cut on these tools by practitioners doing their own modifications. Front surface wax polishers (concave) are used almost exclusively by laboratories.

Female gauges

Female gauges are necessary to cut the wax tools to the required radius (*Figure 23.4*). Stainless steel gauges are the most accurate and long lasting. Ideally, a razor blade should be used to cut the wax cylinder to approximately the correct radius, and the female gauge should be used only for final 'truing up' in order to prevent excessive wear on the gauge.

Metal or plastic tools and adhesive tape

Adhesive cloth tape 'sticking plaster' of the 'zinc oxide' type is stretched over a suitable tool, and this cloth surface is used for polishing lens peripheries — an allowance of approximately 0.2 mm (depending on the tape used) being made for the thickness of the tape. This can be used as an alternative to the wax polishing tools mentioned above. The practitioner using brass or plastic tools of this type must check with the manufacturing laboratory whether or not an allowance for an average tape thickness has been made when constructing the tool.

This method has the advantage that it is not normally necessary to put on a separate transitional curve as with the wax tools. For this reason, it is the one favoured by most laboratories for peripheral curves. 'Cloth polishing' has the one serious drawback that the accuracy of curves polished by this method cannot be guaranteed.

Wax tools may be used instead of the metal or plastic tools, the tape being stretched over the suitably cut wax curve.

Tools may also be covered in muslin, stretched taut and held in place with a rubber band.

Polishing liquids

The polishing liquid used most frequently for PMMA lenses is the metal polish Silvo. The container should be allowed to stand for 2 or 3 days, after which most of the excess clear fluid is poured off. This is in order to give a more suitable, slightly thicker polishing fluid.

For most rigid gas permeable lens materials the ammonia in Silvo acts as a solvent and this polish should not therefore be used.

As a general rule, solvents or polishing compounds containing alcohol, esters, chlorinated hydrocarbons, ammonia etc., should not be used. Suitable polishes* are X-Pal, Linde A, SPI, Hyprez, Boston, Silo₂ Care polish etc., but ideally individual material manufacturers should first be consulted.

For soft lenses a good standard polish which will give an excellent surface finish is CCPI* polishing compound mixed with silicone oil.

Paraffin oil

Ordinary paraffin oil (kerosene) is used to remove any wax that remains attached to a lens after removal from a chuck. It may also be used as a lubricant with diamond impregnated tools when putting on the major part of a corneal lens peripheral curve prior to final polishing, or grinding out the back optic surface of a scleral lens. Being slightly more viscous than water, it prevents such deep scratches (though grinding is slightly slower), enabling the final polishing to be done more quickly.

Paraffin oil, water, and polishing liquids are best used in 250 ml wash bottles with jet dispensers or 'sprays'. They may possibly be more economically applied with a large artist's paint brush from a bowl, especially where they are being used frequently and evaporation causes no problems — though, where applicable, fire hazards must be considered.

Razor and scalpel blades

Single-edge ('safety') razor blades and scalpel blades, straight and curved, are useful for certain modifications (see p. 858). Alternatively, a thicker square-edged cutter may be used.

Carborundum tool for total diameter reduction

This consists of an internally tapering cone, which is held in a Jacob's chuck (Figure 23.5). It is used for reduction in lens size. It has the disadvantage that, if the lens is not placed centrally in the hollow, stock will be removed unequally (Haynes, 1959). Also, with lenses

*X-Pal polish (Davison Chemicals, Tennessee, USA, imported by Cerium Chemical Co., Tonbridge, Kent); Linde A polish (Union Carbide); SPI polish (Sauflon); CCPI polish (City Crown); Hyprez polish (Engis Ltd); Boston polish (Bausch & Lomb); Silo₂ Care polish (Chase Precision International Ltd).

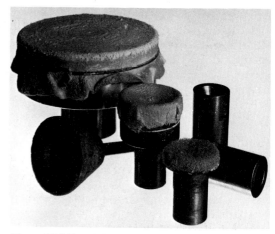

Figure 23.5 From left to right. Rear: large polishing drum. Centre: carborundum tool for reduction of total diameter, small polishing drum, and Conlish tools. Front: flat plate sponge chuck

incorporating prism, there is a tendency for more material to be removed from the thinner lens edge than the thicker edge.

Before use, the tool should be soaked well in water.

Assorted carborundum or diamond impregnated burrs

These (Figure 23.6) are used for final edge shaping. Very fine emery paper may also be used.

Polishing cloth

This very soft cloth (for example, 'Selvyt' cloth) is used for adding small amounts of power to lenses. Suitable cloth may be obtained from any contact lens laboratory at little cost, or ordinary velveteen material may be purchased.

Flat plate and sponge or drum chucks

These chucks (see Figure 23.5) are used on a vertical spindle for adding positive and negative power to lenses, removing surface scratches, and for edge polishing. The drum chuck consists of a hollow chuck over which a piece of chamois leather or similar material has been stretched and held in place with a rubber band or wire. The flat plate chuck consists of a chuck with an upper flat portion to which is attached a thin piece of sponge rubber or moleskin.

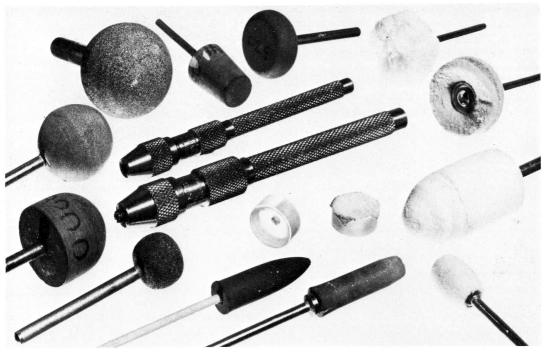

Figure 23.6 Assorted grinding tools and polishing buffs. Top centre: large and small pin-vice holders for drills. Lower centre: corneal lens buttons with one surface cut for use as scleral lens runners. Left button shows guide hole on rear surface and right button has double-sided adhesive tape on concave surface

Chamois leather

A large piece of chamois leather 15 × 15 cm often forms a useful backing to the polishing cloth mentioned above, and is sometimes used as an alternative.

A smaller piece of thinner chamois leather may be used for edge polishing while the lens is still mounted on the spindle lens chuck as shown in *Figures 22.36–22.38*. Alternatively, a small piece of sponge rubber may be used.

Conlish tools (from *con*ical and po*lish*)

These are a series of hollow cone tools of varying angles (*see Figure 23.5*) which are used on a vertical spindle.

Lined with adhesive cloth tape, they are used for shaping lens edges. The lens is mounted, for instance, on a glass tube and the edge is polished for a specific number of seconds on each tool. Generally, a slower speed vertical spindle appears preferable (100–500 rev./min). Although used successfully by certain laboratories, often as diamond impregnated tools, they are not very popular with practitioners in the UK.

Further details can be found in most American textbooks on this subject and in the original paper on this method by Cepero (1959).

Drills

Drills of diameters from 0.10 to 0.30 mm mounted in hand drill (or pin-vice) holders are used to fenestrate corneal lenses. *Figure 23.6* shows pin-vice holders.

A dental countersink rose, as fine as possible (size 0 or 1), is necessary for countersinking fenestrations. Several finely sharpened boxwood sticks are also needed for hand polishing the countersink, or may be used for complete countersinking if the lens is mounted on a suitable chuck on a vertical spindle.

For scleral lenses the following additional tools are required.

Scleral lens runners

Scleral lens runners are attached to the front optic surface of lenses by means of broad (12 mm) double-sided sticky tape on the concave runner surface. They are used with a pencil or ball-point pen tip in the guide hole on the upper flat surface (*see Figure 23.6*) to control the lens on wax or diamond tools.

Runners can be obtained from laboratories; or a corneal lens blank may be used, with the concave surface cut but not polished and a small central guide hole drilled a short way into the flat surface.

Rough grinding stone and buff

These (*Figure 23.7*) are used respectively for reducing lens total diameters and edge polishing. The grinding stone is not an essential since a file and emery paper serve the same function, though more slowly, or a 25 mm carborundum ball may be used (*see Figure 23.6*, top left).

Horizontal spindle with Jacob's chuck fitting or flexible drive (*Figure 23.7*)

This is necessary for holding many of the tools used for back scleral zone surface modifications and in fenestrating. A Jacob's chuck attachment may also be obtained for the vertical spindle. Alternatively, some practitioners prefer to use a small motor with flexible drive attachment, which should have a foot operated speed control to allow both hands freedom for lens and tool manipulation (*see Figure 22.24*).

Grinding balls and polishing buffs

A selection of grinding balls and polishing buffs of various sizes and shapes are necessary (*see Figure 23.6*).

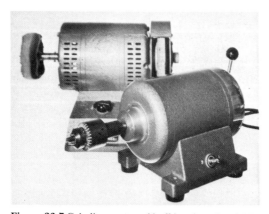

Figure 23.7 Grinding stone and buff (rear), and variable speed horizontal spindle with Jacob's chuck fitting (front). A flexible drive may be attached to the right-hand end of the grinding stone and buff motor

Tripoli or Buffite polishing compound

One or more polishing compounds are preferred by many practitioners for use with polishing buffs. The initial polishing after grinding is carried out more quickly with these compounds, but with some danger of burning the plastic. Final polishing is best carried out with Silvo or similar compounds.

Diamond impregnated brass tools

Used with or without a runner, back optic zone and spherical transition grind-outs are performed by means of these tools (*see Figure 23.4*). Tools of radii commonly used by the practitioner for transitional curves are usefully obtained. A basic set includes the radii 7.80, 8.00, 8.20, 8.40, 8.60, 8.90, 10.00 and 11.00 mm but a more comprehensive range would include tools of radii from 5.00 mm to 15.00 mm.

Large wax tools

These (*see Figure 23.4*) are used for polishing spherical transitions.

Drills and dental burrs

Drills of 0.50 mm, 0.75 mm and 1.00 mm in diameter may be required for making fenestration holes in scleral lenses. Slightly larger round or flame-shaped dental burrs may be used for countersinking, or even a larger drill may be used.

Corneal lens modifications

Reducing the total diameter of a lens

Reduction of the total diameter of a lens may be carried out for any of the following reasons:

(1) To relieve corneal oedema by exposing more of the cornea to a normal atmosphere.
(2) To reduce excessive edge clearance which may be causing discomfort, or causing visual interference due to bubbles getting under the edge during blinking. These bubbles frequently get under the lower edge of a high riding lens and can readily be seen with the slit lamp. They cause reflections and may result in dimpling of the corneal epithelium (*Plates 22* and *94*). Excessive edge clearance (*Plates 11* and *12*) can also cause the lens to become misplaced easily or even

ejected from the eye. It may also be partially responsible for drying of the 3 and 9 o'clock areas of the cornea which then stain with fluorescein when this is applied (*Plate 20*).

(3) To reduce edge thickness of a high negative lens, which can cause discomfort, and if the upper lid is tight and grips the lens after a blink, the lens may ride too high. Alternatively, a thick edge may cause a loose lid to knock the lens down after each blink. Thick edges also encourage 3 and 9 o'clock staining as does excess edge clearance by holding the eyelids away from these areas of the eye during blinking, thereby preventing proper wetting.

(4) To reduce the weight of a lens, thereby encouraging it not to ride so low on the cornea.

The lens total diameter is first checked on a magnifying gauge or V-gauge (*see Figures 12.11, 12.12 and 22.12*), and the amount to be removed is noted. A spindle lens holder is now heated at its upper end with a bunsen burner for a few seconds, old wax polishing compound being removed with a tissue.

Directing the bunsen flame on to the top of the chuck, the end of the adhesive wax stick is touched on the upper end of the chuck stem so that one small drop of the wax is left in the concavity. Too much wax here causes it to spread over the underside of the lens when placed on the stem, often making the edge difficult to modify as well as making it difficult to check and clean.

While the wax is still soft (reheat for a second, if necessary), the lens with convex side down is placed on the chuck as near centrally as possible. Setting the spindle in motion will show that the lens is not yet exactly centred about the spindle axis of rotation. Cutting it now would give a non-circular lens. The next step, therefore, is to centre the lens.

For this, the wax on the chuck, if not still soft, must be softened without burning the lens. The safest way of doing this is shown in *Figure 23.8*. Holding the inverted chuck by the stem, the base of the chuck is held in the lower part of the bunsen burner flame until the stem begins to get too hot to hold. It is now placed firmly on the spindle, and the spindle is set in motion. One finger of each hand is immediately but very carefully touched on the lens — one on the side,

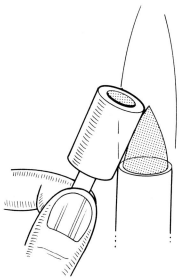

Figure 23.8 Heating the spindle lens chuck. The chuck is held by the stem and the base placed in the lower part of the bunsen burner flame

and the other on the opposite top edge (*Figure 23.9*). This is done until an object (such as a strip light) mirrored by the concave surface of the lens appears perfectly stationary as the lens rotates. Two smooth round wooden rods may be used as an alternative to the fingers. The lens is now perfectly centred. (Centration will be difficult in those lenses incorporating a prism.)

Carefully holding the chuck as near vertically as possible, the base is held under running cold water to cool it. Care should be taken not to

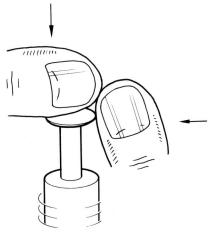

Figure 23.9 Centring the lens. While the adhesive wax is still soft, the lens is centred on the edging chuck by gently touching the top edge with one thumb and the side edge with the other (compare *Figures 22.27* and *22.28*)

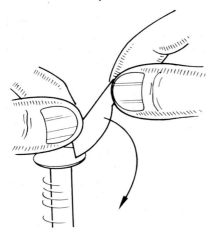

Figure 23.10 Shaping the edge. The blade or cutter is arching around the lens working from the back surface to just over the mid-edge, and then again from the front surface to slightly over the mid-edge position (compare *Figure 22.29*)

allow water to enter the spindle recess in the base and not to knock the lens off the chuck.

The lens is then replaced on the spindle, which is set in motion. A single-edge razor blade or hard, carborundum impregnated rubber tool is carefully brought into contact with the lens edge in line with the centre, with its cutting edge vertical and very slightly trailing to the direction of rotation of the lens edge. The total diameter is now reduced (*see Figures 23.10* and *22.29*).

Every few seconds, the total diameter of the lens is checked, and cutting is ceased about 0.20–0.30 mm above the final required total diameter to allow for the edging.

The lens is now edged as described below.

Edging and re-edging

When the total diameter is reduced a lens must be re-edged. Otherwise it may be done if a small chip has accidentally been removed from a lens. Then re-rounding that portion of the edge, although making the lens slightly 'truncated', saves having to order a new lens. This is an easy remedy for such slightly damaged lenses. Lenses with thin edges are easily damaged at the edge, for example, positive lenses (unless made lenticular) and the upper edge of a prism ballasted lens and, in all these cases, re-edging may become necessary to restore a comfortable fit. Occasionally, a replacement lens has a different edge shape from the original and from

the lens in the other eye, and it needs reshaping to make it comfortable to wear. Edges which indent the cornea or conjunctiva and cause epithelial damage should always be well rounded.

Unfortunately, many laboratories — even those using automated edging techniques — only produce good edges on about two-thirds of their lenses. Edging and re-edging therefore becomes the most desirable modification to be able to carry out oneself at the present time.

The lens is mounted on a spindle lens chuck, as described above. The edge of the lens is then examined by the Plasticine and binocular microscope (or slit lamp) method described in Chapter 12, and the points to be altered are noted.

A thick square-edged cutter or large curved scalpel blade with the tip removed (*Figure 23.10*) is used for cutting and shaping, though some practitioners prefer a single straight-edged razor blade. This is preferably held gently against the rotating lens by the first finger and thumb of both hands, as shown. A little practice and regular checking of the edge profile soon shows how much to remove from the lens, but the following points may be of assistance.

First, cutting should start either on the back or front surface of the lens, working round the outside of the edge and slightly over to the opposite surface.

Secondly, when cutting on the front surface, care should be taken not to cut more than 0.5–1.0 mm in from the lens edge as scratches caused by the blade can be difficult to remove. Similarly, when cutting on the back surface edge, care should be taken not to scratch any peripheral curve.

Thirdly, if the lens has yet to have a peripheral curve put on, the edge must be shaped as in *Figure 23.11a*, with a very rounded rear edge to allow for the material which will be removed when polishing on the peripheral curve (*Figure 23.11b*).

Farnum (1959) has stressed the importance of matching left and right lens edge thicknesses for optimum patient comfort.

These points having been carried out and the edge shaped to the practitioner's satisfaction, any sharp points, for example, those at the junction between the peripheral curve and edge curve, and scratches must be removed. This is carried out by means of a hard rubber burr,

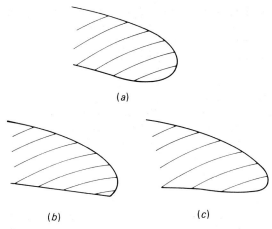

Figure 23.11 Corneal lens edge profiles. (*a*) Profile of initial mono-curve lens prior to the addition of peripheral curves. (*b*) The same lens after the addition of a small peripheral curve (no edge treatment). (*c*) The final edge profile (compare *Figure 22.33*)

preferably cylindrical or conical in shape and impregnated with carborundum or diamond. The burr is carefully rolled around the edge a few times in the same manner as the cutting blade (*see Figure 22.32a–e*).

Inspection should show the lens edge now ready for polishing and with a profile as in *Figure 23.11c*.

This is most easily done by means of a piece of thin chamois leather and Silvo polish, the leather either being wrapped around a finger or folded double and the folded edge used. Polishing should be done for several minutes until a high polish is obtained (*see* p. 834 in Chapter 22 and *see Figures 22.37* and *22.38*).

To remove the lens from the chuck, it is given a light flick with the finger on the front surface and it comes away easily. Any adhesive wax remaining on the front lens surface can be removed by wetting the surface with paraffin and rubbing gently with the finger, when the wax will slowly dissolve.

Some manufacturers produce edge contours by means of a rag wheel buff. While this is not so easily variable for each lens, it does have the advantage of speed and can be usefully employed when razor-cutting the edge. For preference, a sewn rag wheel buff should be used, because this has plenty of body, and it should be only lightly applied with buffing compound. Ideally, the lens should be mounted on a spinner-type holder for regular polishing, as recommended by Haynes (1959), and held lightly against the edge of the rotating buff, hardly penetrating the fibres and, if not mounted on a spinner, slowly and evenly rotated, arching the holder and lens round the full edge curve. A final minute or so is spent polishing with Silvo, using a piece of chamois leather. This gives a highly polished well-shaped edge curve.

The edge may also be polished (or the total diameter reduced) on a drum tool or flat sponge pad. The lens, mounted by its front surface, is first pressed lightly into the drum surface perpendicular to the direction of rotation. It is then arched around the edge profile, parallel to the direction of drum travel, the lens being rotated all the while. This is then repeated with the lens mounted on its back surface.

Reduction of the back optic zone diameter, alteration of peripheral radii, addition of new curves and transition blending

All these modifications are normally carried out to improve tear flow under the lens, as a remedy for corneal oedema. Transition blending may be necessary to remove sharp transitions causing arcuate epithelial damage seen with fluorescein staining. Flattening of peripheral curves can remedy the epithelial damage caused by too steep a peripheral curve which digs into the cornea as the lens moves. All sharp transitions can cause breaking up of any bubbles which may get beneath a lens, thereby causing dimpling.

A wax tool, free from cracks and air bubbles, is first cut to the required radius by means of a razor blade and a female gauge of the correct radius (*see Figure 18.24*). This is held vertically and stationary on the centre of the wax tool rotating on a spindle. If stainless steel tools are used, it is best to incline them very slightly towards the operator initially and gradually approach the true vertical as the wax tool is cut to the correct radius. This avoids the gauge 'skidding' and damaging the wax tool.

Two or three small circular grooves are then cut in the surface of the wax with a pin point while the tool is rotating (*see Figures 23.4* and *22.7*). These grooves aid in retaining the polish on the tool surface and in preventing the lens adhering to the tool by suction. They also prevent surface waves forming, due to build-up of polish on the tool, during polishing. One small indentation cut in the very centre of the tool aids positioning of the female gauge during final cutting. The female gauge is then retouched on the wax tool to smooth off the surface of the grooves. Alternatively, tape or cloth-covered tools may be used.

The lens is then placed on one of the corneal holders or an edging chuck as described earlier. A few drops of polishing liquid are applied to the rotating wax tool and the lens is slowly oscillated either backwards and forwards from near the edge to near the centre of the tool or across one side of the tool, being slowly rotated at the same time. Too fast a movement results in the periphery being scratched. Polishing liquid should be applied to the tool every 5–10 seconds to prevent the surface drying and scratching the lens.

Depending on the adjustment being done, the lens should be taken off its holder every so often to see the effect of the polishing. Blending transitions and alteration of a peripheral curve by a small amount may only take 2 or 3 seconds; a small peripheral curve or reduction of the back optic zone diameter takes a little longer; and putting on a complete peripheral curve may take several minutes.

Measurement of the back optic zone diameter is best carried out by means of a scale and magnifier. With a very narrow peripheral curve, however, the width may be impossible to measure. Such curves are best judged by means of a slit lamp or other high-powered magnifier, or by optical projection. The degree of blending may also be judged by inspecting the reflection of a strip light from the back of the lens surface using a ×8 loupe (see Chapters 12 and 19 and Figures 19.1 and 19.2).

Approximate measurement of curves is facilitated by coating the lens back surface with a waterproof 'instant drying' ink. This is removed in the areas where the lens is being polished and makes the curve easily seen, though it is not necessarily sufficiently accurate for measurements to be made from it. When blending transitions, this becomes extremely useful. It may also be used as a gross test for checking the accuracy of a peripheral curve. The periphery is marked with ink and the lens is touched briefly on a wax tool of the correct radius. If the peripheral radius is accurate, ink will be removed over the whole width of the curve.

Alteration of power

Addition of negative power

Addition of negative power becomes necessary as the refractive error changes, particularly in children, keratoconic patients and those with senile nuclear sclerosis of the crystalline lens. Any other marked change in refraction should lead to further investigation in case of lens warpage, gross changes in the corneal curvature occasioned by the fit of the lens, gross changes in the crystalline lens due to pathological conditions, or changes in the retina also due to pathological conditions. It should be noted that lens warpage often occurs when patients accidentally squeeze their lenses in the screw cap of the soaking case. The power on a focimeter may then appear satisfactory, but this distortion of the surfaces can be seen with a radiuscope or keratometer. Usually, an irregular, hazy line where the lens has been bent is visible if it is held up to the light.

This is considered by some practitioners to be a much easier modification than increasing positive power. For this reason, most practitioners tend to err on the positive side when ordering lenses.

The simplest method of carrying out this modification is by means of a 15 cm square of soft, clean, moistened polishing cloth spread over a similar-sized piece of chamois leather or moleskin laid on a smooth flat surface. A small amount of polishing fluid is spread in a circle on the cloth, using a finger. The dry back surface of the lens is then positioned, preferably, on a suitable lens holder, or on the tip of either the first or second finger. This is then placed on the polishing cloth in the circle of polish. Circular movements of about 5–8 cm in diameter are then described by the hand, exerting only a light pressure on the lens and taking great care not to tilt the lens holder or finger. After every six complete circular movements, the direction of rotation should be reversed to counteract the effect of any slight tilting, which will either cause distortion or give cylindrical power. Depending on the pressure on the lens, approximately 12 rotations are needed for every $-0.25\,D$ increase, and when nearing the end of a power alteration, the pressure on the lens must be gradually lessened to almost zero. Even when adding more than $-0.25\,D$, the power must be checked frequently, not only to check on the progress of

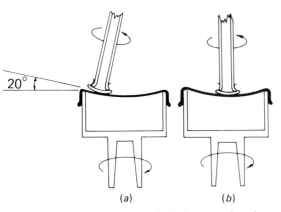

20°

(a)　　　　(b)

Figure 23.12 The use of a drum chuck for power alterations (cross-sections). (*a*) Addition of negative power. The lens is held near the drum edge at approximately 20° to the horizontal. The lens is slowly rotated in either the same or the opposite direction to drum movement. (*b*) Addition of positive power. The lens is held vertically close to the drum centre and again slowly rotated

the power alteration but also because this will ensure that the lens is rotated to a different position on the finger, again to counter any distortion effects.

A more accurate method of adding negative power is by the use of a 10 cm drum chuck as described by Isen (1959). The lens is mounted on a holder by its back surface and placed near the edge of the rotating chuck, normally being tilted to about 20° to the horizontal (*Figure 23.12a*). The drum 'skin' should be kept continually moist with polishing fluid and the lens kept slowly rotating, using both hands. Pressure on the lens should be just sufficient to contour the drum material to the lens shape. Excessive pressure will cause vibration of the lens and holder. For RGP materials, which polish faster than PMMA, the lens should be held nearer the drum centre where the rotational speed is less.

Addition of positive power

A drum chuck is also used for this modification, except that the lens is placed at or near the centre of the drum. Since the drum speed of rotation is zero at its centre, more lens material is removed from the lens edge and, consequently, positive power is added. Provided the chamois surface is kept moist with Silvo or other suitable polish, the addition of positive power is

straightforward; and as long as the lens is gently rotated, no cylindrical effect is introduced.

With conditions as for the addition of negative power, the lens is slowly moved in a small circle of about 3 or 4 mm or less around the drum centre, in either the same or opposite direction to that of drum rotation (*Figure 23.12b*). This avoids the small 'pip' sometimes obtained in the centre of the lens if it is held stationary at the drum centre, where there is no polishing action.

In adding positive power, occasionally a 'haze' may appear round the target image of the focimeter when checking the lens power. If this occurs, the diameter of the circle that the lens is being moved in should be increased to about 8 or 9 mm. This gives a more even polishing over the whole front surface and should add neither positive nor negative power. If this does not remove the 'haze', an alternative method is to add about +0.12 D too much positive power and then remove this by adding −0.12 D.

Either of these two latter methods may also be used for removing superficial front surface scratches.

Fenestration

If corneal oedema occurs, central fenestration holes — up to five in number — may help to encourage tear flow, but only if the lens is fitted apically well clear of the cornea; otherwise each hole can provide an additional meniscus of tears between lens and cornea — discouraging tear flow but aiding lens centration and reducing movement. Occasionally, holes may be drilled near the edge in one sector of a lens to lighten the weight there, i.e. the reverse of a prism ballast.

A typical diameter is 0.20–0.30 mm (0.01 inch).

The lens is placed on the tip of the forefinger and, after marking the position of the holes with a waterproof fibre pen, it is drilled from the front by hand, using a pin-vice to hold the drill. This is easier from the front surface and keeps the drill at the correct angle, perpendicular to the convex surface. The pin-vice should be rotated slowly and without pressure as excessive pressure may break the fine drill or crack the lens. To minimize the risk of the drill slipping and scratching the front surface of the lens, it should protrude as little as possible from the pin-vice. Also, the hole can be drilled through sticky tape stuck to the front surface of the lens.

The edges of the hole must now be counter-sunk on both sides. This is achieved by gently rotating a dental burr, size 0 or 1, anti-clockwise in the fenestration. Only a touch is needed, and it is quite easy to see the countersunk effect when using a suitable binocular magnifier.

Finally, the hole is carefully polished by hand using a finely sharpened boxwood stick and a trace of suitable polishing fluid with as rapid a rotation as possible. Several changes of sticks may be needed in order to maintain a sharpened point. For larger fenestrations, a fine-pointed felt buff in a spindle may be used for a few seconds. Final careful inspection is a necessity.

Alternatively (*see* Chapter 22), the lens may be mounted, using double-sided adhesive tape, on to first a convex chuck, and then a concave chuck so that the fenestration hole is positioned over a small central depression in each chuck. As the chuck rotates on the vertical spindle, a drop of polish is applied in the hole, and a boxwood stick — sharpened to a suitably angled point — is gently held in the fenestration hole. The boxwood stick is slowly rotated in a small circle in the opposite direction to the spindle rotation. This both countersinks and gives a fine polish (Mackie, 1968). If necessary, the inner part of the fenestration may be polished by running the hole up and down a length of polish-covered cotton sewing thread.

A fenestrating machine available to the practitioner is shown in *Figure 23.13*.

Truncation

Truncation may be necessary if an existing truncation does not line up correctly with the eyelid margin, or if the edge of a lens is slightly damaged in one place. Sometimes a round, prism ballast lens must be truncated to assist it to locate correctly if a front surface cylinder is present, or an already truncated bifocal lens must be truncated more to lower the segment height when the latter interferes with distance vision.

The most important factor to bear in mind before truncating a lens is the final edge thickness of the truncation (Haynes, 1959, 1965). For instance, it is useless to truncate a high-powered negative lens with minimal centre thickness as the edge thickness of the truncated portion may be too thin for easy modification and will be easily damaged.

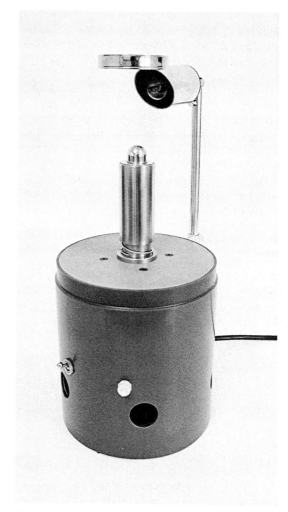

Figure 23.13 Fenestrating machine developed for the practitioner and suitable for both corneal and scleral lenses. (Photograph by courtesy of Focus Contact Lens Laboratory Ltd)

The desired portion is first marked with a suitable marking agent, such as one of the 'instant drying' inks. Lens stock is then removed with either a pin-file, a hand manipulated abrasive stone or a rotating fine abrasive wheel, the lens being held between the fingers. The edge is then contoured, using a pin-file or fine emery paper. Polishing should be carried out using a rag-wheel buff, a drum chuck or a foam rubber pad. The part of the lens not being modified may be protected by adhesive tape. The lens may also be truncated by the edge being held firmly against the material of a rotating drum chuck and the edge shape rounded as previously described. It should also be stressed that in some instances the truncated edge may need to be kept relatively flat to align the lid margin. *Figures 22.56* and *22.57* also show lens truncation and polishing.

Truncating a lens can also be a way of rescuing a lens which might otherwise be scrapped because of a small edge defect. By grinding away the defective area and then repolishing the edge the lens may be rendered wearable again. The fact that it is no longer round does not matter if it is comfortable. If successful the patient also gains a quick way of distinguishing right and left lenses!

Modification of rigid gas permeable lenses

As mentioned earlier, rigid gas permeable lenses may be modified in much the same way as PMMA lenses. The following additional points should be considered:

(1) Surface treated or moulded lenses should not be modified, at least until the effect on a spare lens has been tested.

(2) The higher *Dk* materials, e.g. fluorosilicone acrylates, warp and burn easily and are best done by a skilled laboratory technician.

(3) Ammonia-based polishes, such as Silvo, should not be used, and alcohols, esters, ketones and aromatic hydrocarbons will damage most materials. Suitable polishes have been discussed earlier.

(4) Over-heating RGP lenses induces material stress which causes subsequent lens flattening (Schwartz, 1986). All cutting and polishing should therefore be done as slowly and gently as possible and at a relatively slow lathe or spindle speed.

(5) RGP lenses should not be allowed to dry out during polishing. Surface 'burning' caused by drying out may show as poor wetting areas when the lens is dispensed and may also add to stress-induced flattening.

(6) Preheated blocks or high melting point waxes should be avoided. Suction holder attachments should be used where possible.

(7) Newman (S., 1987, personal communication) recommends the use of more than one type of polishing medium for modification

to the optic zone in order to obtain a good surface finish, e.g. CCPI polishing compound in water followed by Boston finishing solution. Another method of maintaining good polishing medium viscosity is to add some dishwashing liquid to the medium. A mixture of dishwashing liquid and water also makes an excellent finishing solution.

(8) In order to prevent burning or 'orange peeling' of the lens surface, abrasive cloth type coverings of tools such as velveteen or pellan pads should be treated with respect. Velvet, cotton, chamois leather and vinyl are all preferable.

(9) Grind and polish lenses with the absolute minimum of pressure.

(10) Never wipe polish off a lens with a dry tissue. Keep a bowl of water and detergent mix next to the work station for washing the lens. Rubbing the lens between fingers while submerged in this solution will clean the lens adequately. The lens can then be gently blotted dry for inspection.

(11) Always store polishing cloths and polishing powders in clean, air-tight containers. This prevents dust and other contamination which may in turn cause lens scratching.

Scleral lens modifications

Indications for carrying out modifications to scleral lenses made from eye impressions are given in Chapter 18. A general reduction in total diameter is indicated when a lens remains stationary as the eye moves behind it, i.e. the lens appears a 'steep fit'. Localized reductions of diameter may be made if, for example, the lower scleral zone is too big for the lower fornix, or if the nasal scleral zone is pushed onto the nasal corneal limbus when the eye looks inwards (*Plate 72*). Sometimes the temporal scleral zone catches at the outer canthus but this is more often because that portion of the scleral zone is too small rather than too large.

A lens may be made horizontally oval if a horizontal oval fluorescein pool shows against-the-rule astigmatism with edge stand off at nasal and temporal edges and edge blanching at upper and lower edges. Making the vertical meridian smaller effectively flattens it in that meridian allowing it to settle but midtemporal (*Plate 77*) and midnasal back scleral zone grinding out may also be necessary. A vertical oval lens for with-the-rule astigmatism is not normally satisfactory cosmetically unless the palpebral aperture is particularly small.

Reducing an equal amount from all round the lens edge, in the case of a regular pre-formed lens, is carried out by simply rubbing the lens against a piece of medium-grade sandpaper placed on a flat surface. Care must be taken to maintain an even pressure around the whole lens edge.

Localized or overall reductions in lens total diameter may be carried out by means of either a rotating grinding stone or an ordinary hand file.

The definition of back scleral size assumes sharp edges to the back lens surface. Thus, when reducing a lens to a specific back scleral size, provided that only minimal material is removed during the final edge shaping, little, if any, allowance need be made for plastic removed during this latter process.

Edging

Edging is necessary when total diameter reductions have been carried out, if the edge has been damaged, or if scleral zone modifications have altered the edge shape.

A stone grinding ball of 1 inch (2.54 cm) in diameter, previously soaked in water and held in a horizontal spindle, may be used for the rounding of both front and back edge surfaces. Alternatively, an ordinary small hand file, followed by fine emery paper, may be used for the front surface. A large rounded rubber tool impregnated with diamond or carborundum may be used for the back surface.

Polishing is easily carried out, using a rag-wheel buff. The lens edge should be held vertically and approximately in line with the rotating buff to polish the back edge surface. The lens should be held lightly and continually rotated during polishing to prevent burning of the plastics. This also prevents a ridge of plastics building up on the back edge. Great care should be taken to check that this does not happen, and final examination must ascertain that there is no such ridge. The final edge should be of a blunt, rounded form.

Alternatively, the lens may be edged and polished by tools held in a flexible drive, as explained on p. 659, Chapter 18 and shown in *Figures 18.29–18.39*.

Back optic zone grind-out

This is done to increase the clearance of the back optic zone from the cornea. A steeper radius may be required if heavy central touch exists with a large annular bubble at the limbus. A flatter back optic zone radius is indicated if central corneal touch and midperipheral corneal or limbal touch occur together. It must be borne in mind that changing the BOZR alters the power of the contact lens and liquid lens (*see* Chapters 5 and 18). Where possible the BOZR should therefore be kept the same.

The optic zone thickness is measured (*see Figure 18.20*) and a central waterproof mark is made on the front surface at this point. A 'runner' is attached to the centre of the front surface of the optic zone with double-sided adhesive tape. A diamond impregnated brass tool of the desired radius is placed on a vertical spindle, which is then set in motion. Using paraffin or water as the lubricating agent, the back optic zone of the lens is ground out, using a pencil point or similar object in the runner guide hole, the lens being moved slowly backwards and forwards across one side of the head of the diamond tool (*see Figures 18.41* and *18.42*). The lens should be allowed to rotate freely and lubricant should be used as necessary to prevent the tool surface drying out. The lens should be removed at frequent intervals to check the rate of reduction in central thickness. Final grinding is best performed with paraffin as the lubricating agent. Being slightly more viscous than water, it allows the tool less possibility of abrading the surface and thereby facilitates final polishing.

The increased viscosity slows the rate of grinding out, however. Paraffin is inconvenient with fenestrated lenses as it tends to leak through the fenestration, occasionally dissolving the adhesive, and causing the runner to become detached from the lens. About 0.02 mm thickness should be allowed for final polishing of the back optic zone. This is carried out in exactly the same way as for corneal lenses — retaining the lens on the runner and using either a wax, tape or cloth covered tool of the correct radius with suitable polish (*see* p. 859).

Transitional grind-out or extension

This is done if the transitions are sharp and cause frothing of the bubble, if limbal touch occurs or where there is insufficient clearance beyond the limbus, as indicated by the extent of the fluorescein pool.

This is carried out as described under Back optic zone grind-out above but using the large-size diamond impregnated tool, the only other difference being that widths of transition are normally taken rather than thickness removed, and the final polishing is carried out using a large wax tool or felt ball.

A transitional grind-out is normally necessary after a back optic zone grind-out owing to the reduction in width of the transitional curve(s) caused by the central grind-out. (A fenestration will similarly need re-countersinking and polishing when such a transitional or optic zone grind-out has been performed.)

A transitional grind-out is best carried out after the back optic zone has been polished to facilitate measurement of the transition width. Alternatively, the area may be marked with ink to show the border between the transition and optic zones during grinding. (Paraffin cannot be used as a lubricant if it dissolves the inks used.)

Polishing the rough ground transition extends its width slightly. This becomes important when extending a transition well into the back optic zone, and especially when making a double curve back optic zone.

Localized scleral zone and transition grind-outs

This is done in regions where the scleral zone or transition touches the eye heavily, as evidenced by blanching of the conjunctival blood vessels. The latter may be seen more easily if a little digital pressure is applied to the lens. Also, if the optic zone gives too much clearance from the cornea the whole back scleral zone surface may be ground out to settle the lens. More substance should be removed from near the transition region to maintain the same curvature and give the most effective settling.

One of the most common modifications needed is a temporal scleral zone grind-out near the transition to permit the lens to settle and move slightly nasally. This is indicated when a large temporal static bubble occurs at the limbus accompanied by nasal corneal touch

from the optic (*Plate 72*). A slight reduction in nasal scleral zone size may also be needed to permit the nasal shift of the lens.

The area to be ground is first marked on the back surface (or front, according to preference) with a suitable quick-drying ink or grease pencil. For the beginner, it is useful to measure the average thickness of the area to be ground out — at several noted points in the area if this is large. This can be checked during the grind-out to determine the amount of material removed and, in a large area, to check that the material is being removed evenly. If necessary, the back optic zone may be protected with a small piece of Plasticine (Bier, 1957) or adhesive tape pressed firmly into it.

The grind-out is performed with a spherical, cigar-shaped or wheel-shaped stone, the size of which depends on the size of the area to be ground out. This is held in a Jacob's chuck on a horizontal spindle, and it should be kept moist throughout the operation. In order to prevent deep scratches in the scleral zone, the lens should be kept continually moving back and forth slightly, until the ink over the area (if on the back surface) is removed. Surplus lens material and polish should be regularly removed with a tissue. The scleral zone thickness should be checked before continuing.

The rough area may now be smoothed, if necessary, with a rotating hard rubber burr. Polishing may be carried out with a felt buff and polishing compound or, more slowly, with a soft mop buff and Silvo (*see Figure 18.59*). Final polishing with a soft mop and Silvo is always preferable as it gives a better finish. To save time, this may be omitted until the lens has been checked on the eye and has been found to fit satisfactorily.

Examination under magnification will show areas which have not been polished completely. Forknall (1953) has shown that for equal scleral zone settling, relatively more plastics must be removed from near the transition than from the periphery.

Fenestration

Most scleral lenses are fenestrated to permit tear flow and oxygen exchange behind the lens. If a fenestration hole becomes covered by the upper lid regularly, or otherwise blocked as by loose conjunctival tissue or mucus, then a further hole

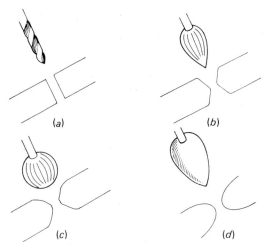

Figure 23.14 The four stages of fenestrating a scleral lens (compare with *Figure 18.50*)

or holes may be required within the palpebral aperture.

The position having been determined, as explained in Chapters 17 and 18, the fenestration hole is made as follows.

With a 0.50 or 0.75 mm drill (typically), a hole is drilled normal to the surface to minimize its length. Care should be taken not to slip with the drill and scratch the optic zone surface. The drill should be held in a pin-vice so that a minimum length of drill protrudes. This gives greater control over exact positioning. Alternatively, the drill may be held in a Jacob's chuck on a horizontal spindle, which lessens the risk of the drill or lens slipping and scratching the optic zone surface, and the lens 'fed' on to the drill.

A flame-shaped dental burr is then turned anti-clockwise (to give a finer cut) in the hole to countersink (*Figure 23.14*). A few turns initially with a 1.50 or 2.00 mm drill can be used to speed up the process of countersinking. Countersinking should be continued equally on both sides of the lens until examination under ×50 magnification shows the two countersinks are almost meeting. Funnel shaping is essential to create an even tear flow and prevent turbulence likely to remove epithelium from the corneal surface.

A slightly larger spherical dental burr is then used, as before, to taper the outer edges of the countersinking.

The countersinks are then polished at low speed, to avoid burning, using a pointed soft felt burr soaked in Silvo, until a high polish is obtained.

Inspection under ×50 magnification should show a fenestration polished all the way through and with tapered edges as shown in *Figure 23.14*. Any remaining polishing residue may be removed with a tapered stick (for example, a toothpick), tissue, or bristle.

Channelling

Channelling is an alternative to fenestration, and may be indicated if the limbal region is very irregular and the introduction of a bubble would lead to frothing, or if the limbal conjunctiva is very loose and blocks the fenestrations. (A loose conjunctiva may also block a channel.)

Although sometimes not so successful as fenestration, it may become a necessity under certain conditions (*see* Chapter 18). Various uses and designs of channel have been discussed by McKay Taylor (1969).

The channel is cut in exactly the same way as a local back surface scleral zone grind-out, along a specific line or curve, and, where possible, using a sharp-edged wheel-shaped grinding tool. This is usually cut from the upper temporal lens edge into the midtransition, though an inferior channel and/or other channels may also become necessary. The channel should occupy about half the lens thickness and have well blended edges to prevent conjunctival abuse (*see Figures 18.47* and *18.48*).

Fluorescein examination should show a clear channel from the lens edge into the back optic zone.

An alternative method, using either the cast of an eye impression or of a preformed lens, is to glue a suitable piece of nylon on to the cast along the desired line of the channel. A shell then made from the cast has a channel pressed into the plastic to the desired depth. The slightly raised area on the front of the finished lens is not noticed subjectively. The advantage of this method is that it enables the shell to be pressed from thinner sheet initially than for a lens where a channel is to be ground into the scleral zone.

Power alterations

Power alterations must be made if the refraction changes or if a change in BOZR is carried out for fitting purposes. Other points to note are mentioned in connection with corneal lens power changes (*see* p. 860).

These are normally carried out by the laboratory as the front surface must be recut each time. Minor front surface alterations may be made on a drum, as for corneal lenses (*see* p. 861).

Practitioners should bear in mind that a back optic zone grind-out, by reducing the thickness of the optic zone, will effectively add a small amount of negative power to the lens. In order to prevent unnecessary modification, +0.25 to +0.50 D should be added to the power required if back optic zone grind-outs are likely to become necessary (*see* Chapters 5 and 18).

Spatulation

Spatulation should rarely be necessary but is indicated if an area of the scleral zone stands clear of the eye, and to settle the rest of the scleral zone by grinding it out would not be feasible due to too thin a lens — or lack of time to carry out the tedious grinding.

Such loose areas may be reshaped by means of spatulation (Obrig, 1942; Bier, 1957). A cast is made of the lens, and the loose area is marked on the back surface of the lens and on the cast. Material is then scraped off the cast in this area. A spatula is heated to approximately 70°C for lenses cut from solid plastic and 60°C for impression lenses (Bier, 1957) and pressed on the front lens surface over the loose area, the cast being held in position against the back surface of the lens.

Tight areas may also be removed in an opposite manner by taking a cast of the front lens surface. Spatulation is best performed on thin lenses, i.e. thinner than approximately 0.75 mm. Too great a rise in temperature of the lens is not desirable as residual monomer may be released, which is toxic to the eye (Estevez, 1967).

Plastic build-up

Again, plastic build-up should not be necessary but it is an alternative to spatulation.

This method of building up the back lens surface, as described by Bier (1957), is no longer recommended as the new material added is likely to be toxic to the eye (Estevez and Ridley, 1966).

Modification of soft contact lenses

While it has been traditional for rigid lenses to be modified for various reasons after the initial fitting, it is perhaps not as well known that soft lenses can be modified in a number of ways to achieve optimum fitting results. These range from simple dotting of lenses to aid identification to complicated cut-outs to circumnavigate pingueculae or fluid drainage blebs (*see* p. 884).

Most modifications are best done by skilled technicians at the laboratory from which the lens was obtained. This ensures that the modifications are performed by those with an intimate knowledge of both the lens material and design.

Lens dotting

Perhaps the simplest and often a very helpful modification the practitioner can do is to dot lenses either to identify left and right, or to enable orientation of a toric lens on the eye by the patient.

The lens should be blotted dry, preferably with lint-free tissue, and then mounted on the dome of a suitable patient soft lens container. A water-proof marking pen with a fine point, e.g. Sanford's Sharpie No.3000 or Nikko Permanent Ink Marker No.150, are then used to apply a single dot (right lens) or two dots (left lens) to the lens edge. The lens is allowed to dry for a further 1–2 minutes before thorough surfactant cleaning and rinsing. Dots applied by this method will gradually fade over several months, faster if the lenses are thermally disinfected, but are easily re-applied at after-care visits (Hallock, 1980).

Lens engraving

Bailey (1975) recommends that all soft lenses entering the practitioner's office be engraved with a suitable code number to aid later identification. Bailey recommends that the lenses are partly dehydrated on a soft lens 'optical gauge' or brass tool, the curvature of which approximates to that of the lens back surface. Because soft lenses become increasingly brittle with extended drying time it is recommended that etching is done no more than 1 hour after dehydration commences. Engraving is performed using a fine-pointed instrument or small high-speed drill and viewed under a stereomicroscope. Bailey reports no increased incidence of lens tearing around the engraving but practitioners must obviously be aware of the increased risk of lens breakage, particularly with higher water content lenses.

Fenestration and truncation

Sellers (1979) and Westerhout (Chapter 14) have described practitioner fenestration and truncation techniques for soft lenses. These are also mentioned below under laboratory modification procedures.

Laboratory modification procedures

While theoretically possible for a practitioner skilled at soft lens modification procedures, the following list shows those modifications possible to a soft contact lens best carried out by an expert laboratory technician:

(1) Adding peripheral curves in order to loosen, i.e. flatten, the lens fit.
(2) Diameter reduction; again to loosen the fit of the lens.
(3) Edge thinning and/or re-shaping to improve comfort or to reduce conjunctival indentation or blanching.
(4) Truncations: to loosen the lens and/or improve axis location in the case of a toric lens.
(5) Cut-outs can be positioned to circumnavigate pingueculae thus improving lens stability and comfort. This is usually performed on a reverse prism toric lens or on a spherical lens with prism ballast. Cut-outs will also have the effect of flattening the lens fit.
(6) Grinding ptosis prop-like shelves into a lens can help position a lens on the eye. This technique can be used to reposition a high riding lens downwards or conversely a low riding lens upwards.
(7) Fenestrations can be added to specific areas of the lens to reduce an oedematous response. This technique is still under review as to its effectiveness. Efron, N. and Ang, J. (1987, personal communication) are currently investigating the optimum size fenestration hole which will provide sufficient oxygen to the cornea and still maintain comfort *in vivo*.
(8) Re-shaping prism facets on a toric lens can be very effective in relocating the lens to its correct axis. Lens mislocations of up to approximately 20° can be corrected in this manner. This technique involves careful measuring of the lens's geometrical thickness profiles, along and across prism faces. Careful assessment of the lens's overall thickness gradients allow the laboratory to change these profiles in order to redirect the upper lids' blink action to other areas of the lens thereby effecting a location change. Due to the complications involved in re-ordering toric lenses with axis allowances incorporated, this method has proved very successful in improving practitioners' fitting success rate. However, it suffers from the disadvantage that lens duplication is difficult if not impossible.
(9) Minor power changes can be made to some types of soft lenses. This is an extremely delicate procedure and is best attempted by skilled technicians only. It requires very careful dehydration procedures and is not always successful. It can, however, be very useful in the tailoring of bifocal contact lenses where one portion of the optic zone is changed only.
(10) The removal of small edge chips, gauges and some surface deposits can also be achieved by careful modification techniques.

The major factor controlling all of these soft lens modifications is the dehydration techniques used. The laboratory must be able to dehydrate the lens completely and still maintain the original surface geometry.

The most common problem encountered with soft lens dehydration is lens buckling. This is especially true of ultrathin lenses and high water content lenses. If the lens dries out to a buckled form it is almost impossible to modify it successfully.

Two of the more successful methods of lens dehydration are:

(1) Slow dehydration in silica gel filled chambers. This technique involves the use of special chambers which contain a small amount of used silica gel suspended in a permeable subchamber. This chamber is placed over the contact lens, which has been dabbed surface dry on lint-free tissue, and will dehydrate the lens over a period of hours. This technique is successful only when used silica gel is placed in the

chamber. Fresh silica gel or a too short drying time will result in a buckled lens.

(2) Microwave ovens are very successful in dehydrating the lens back to a workable hardness. Again the lens is dabbed surface dry on a piece of lint-free tissue before being placed in the microwave oven. It must be accompanied by suitable energy absorbing material to prevent oven damage during the drying cycle. The drying time should be slow in order to maintain the lens shape. This technique will dehydrate the lens more completely than the current traditional methods.

It must be noted that soft lenses will dehydrate closer to their original form if they are soaked in distilled water for some time before drying out. This soaking (preferably in a magnetic stirrer) will remove the sodium chloride from the matrix and prevent crystallization.

The actual modifications to these lenses can be performed by a number of standard laboratory techniques.

Diamond wheels and domes are used for grinding material away. Padded flat wheels and domes can be covered with velvet, velveteen, chamois etc., for polishing the lens back to its original finish.

Different polishing compounds can be used for different requirements just as different polishing materials are used for various applications. A good standard polish which will give an excellent surface is CCPI polishing compound mixed with Silicone Oil.

One of the most important considerations that must be addressed when modifying soft lenses is to keep the material dry. A previously worn dehydrated lens will rehydrate far more quickly than an unworn lens and therefore must be kept dry at all times. It is often an advantage to modify the lens in stages, keeping it stored in silica gel periodically. If a lens starts hydrating while being modified, a good surface finish will be impossible to achieve.

Conclusion

Practitioners are advised to obtain a selection of reject lenses on which to practise modifications.

The majority of modifications may be accurately carried out with only a little practice, but practitioners are urged to maintain their own standards to at least those that they would expect from their laboratory.

Acknowledgement

I am indebted to Stephen Newman of Capricornia Contact Lenses Ltd (Australia) for help with the laboratory section of soft lens modification and for additional help with the modification of rigid gas permeable lenses.

References

BAILEY, N. J. (1975). Soft contact lens identification. *J. Am. optom. Ass.* **46**, 1177–1178

BIER, N. (1957). *Contact Lens Routine and Practice*, 2nd edn. London: Butterworths

CEPERO. G. (1959). Conical and concentric polishing. *Contacto* **3**, 28–34

ESTEVEZ, J. M. J. (1967). Poly(methyl methacrylate) for use in contact lenses. *Contact Lens* **1**(3), 19–21, 26

ESTEVEZ, J. M. J. and RIDLEY, F. (1966). Safety requirements for contact lens materials: and their manipulation and use. *Am. J. Ophthal.* **62**, 132–139

FARNUM, F. E. (1959). Refinements in contact lens adjustments to increase wearing time. *Am. J. Optom.* **36**, 382–384

FORKNALL, A. J. (1953). Conversion of sealed to ventilated contact lenses. *Optician* **125**, 327–330, 356–358

HALLOCK, S. J. (1980). Dotting soft contact lenses. *J. Am. optom. Ass.* **51**(3), 237

HAYNES, P. R. (1959). Modification of contact lenses. In *Encyclopaedia of Contact Lens Practice*, edited by P. R. Haynes, Vol. 22, pp. 1–97. South Bend, Indiana: International Optics Publishing Corporation

HAYNES, P. R. (1965). Modification procedures. In *Contact Lens Practice, Basic and Advanced*, edited by R. B. Mandell, Springfield, Illinois: Thomas

ISEN, A. (1959). Spherical power changes in contact lenses. In *Encyclopaedia of Contact Lens Practice*, edited by P. R. Haynes, Vol. 22, pp. 72–74. South Bend, Indiana: International Optics Publishing Corporation

McKAY TAYLOR, C. (1969). The S-bend and other channelled haptic lenses. *Ophthal. Optician* **9**, 1256–1258

MACKIE, I. A. (1968). Lecture to The Contact Lens Society

OBRIG, T. E. (1942). *Contact Lenses*. Philadelphia: Chilton

SCHWARTZ, C. A. (1986). Radical flattening and RGP lenses. *Contact Lens Forum* **11**(8), 49–52

SELLERS, E. (1979). Adjusting soft contact lenses. *Aust. J. Optom.* **62**(5), 212–213

Chapter 24

Special types of contact lenses and their uses

Janet Stone

Since the first and second editions of this book were written, the role of contact lenses in the treatment and amelioration of many pathological and traumatic ocular conditions has increased world wide. In this third edition, this is reflected in the much larger size of Chapter 21, and in the revised and enlarged chapter on scleral lenses fitted by the impression method (Chapter 18), which now covers two former chapters. Hence these special aspects of contact lens fitting are no longer covered here. However, with the increase in the medical use of contact lenses have come other particular uses for them in ocular diagnosis and in various forms of surgery where they aid observation and simultaneously act as protective devices. Along with other special types of contact lens not covered elsewhere in this book, these lenses are described in this final chapter.

Other contact lenses or aspects of contact lens work which were formerly considered as special, have now become commonplace; such features as tints, surface treatments, materials of different refractive index and oxygen permeability are now taken for granted as part of everyday fitting, and are only touched on in this chapter for the sake of completeness.

Yet other special lenses, mainly varieties of scleral and sports lenses are now of historic interest only and no longer included here, although interested readers may wish to consult the final chapter of the second edition.

Lenses to aid diagnosis and surgery

A number of special contact lenses has been developed to assist observation of the eye in diagnosing eye disease.

Contact lenses for corneal observation

During examination of the corneal endothelium by specular reflection with the slit lamp biomicroscope, the bright reflection from the epithelial/tear layer surface is very intrusive. By employing a thick aplanatic planoconvex lens with the plane face towards the cornea but separated from it by a solution, such as 2% methyl cellulose, the annoying bright reflex is removed and transferred to the front of the contact lens where it is no longer within the field of view of the microscope. Haag–Streit's Eisner Contact Glass is manufactured for this purpose and is shown in *Figure 24.1a,b*. It has been fully described by Eisner, Lotmar and Papritz (1985), who have demonstrated its usefulness in studying the corneal endothelium and epithelium as well as the stroma and Descemet's membrane, and for photographic documentation.

The lens includes an in-built orange filter to remove light scattered by the corneal stroma, and it provides ×2.2 magnification of the corneal endothelium with additional magnification supplied by the microscope itself. It is free from spherical aberration, coma and astigmatism, and any reflections from the plane back surface of the lens are easily removed by slightly tilting the lens. Light transmission is improved by anti-reflection coating of the lens surfaces. It permits observation of the epithelium and endothelium by both specular reflection and indirect illumination. Used with microscope magnification of ×25 a total of ×55 magnification is achieved, and with the McIntyre eyepiece grid (*Figure 24.1c*) it can be used for estimating endothelial cell density. Endothelial cell abnormalities (*see Plates 64–66*) as well as the state of

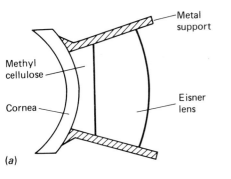

(a)

Metal support

Methyl cellulose

Cornea

Eisner lens

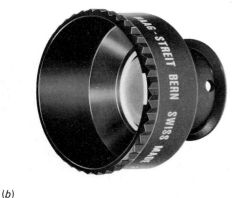

(b)

Number of cells total magnification 40×	cells/mm²	Number of cells total magnification 55×
40x		**2.2x 25x**
250		500
500		1000
1000		2000
2000		4000
4000		8000

(c)

the epithelial cells and other features of the cornea can be studied and photographically recorded to permit, for example, pre- and postsurgical comparison. There is no direct contact of the lens with the cornea, but a suitable solution should be chosen to fill the precorneal space and prevent oedema which would interfere with endothelial observation. A maximum area of specular reflection of about $10 \, mm^2$ can be seen and recorded with this lens.

Diagnosis of corneal abnormalities

Any ordinary sighted contact lens may be used to assist in the diagnosis of suspected keratoconus. If visual acuity during refraction with a contact lens in place is markedly better than visual acuity with the best possible spectacle correction and keratoconus is suspected, its diagnosis may be confirmed. Suspected corneal dystrophies also show a similar improvement in visual acuity with contact lenses, as do many other conditions of corneal irregularity.

The presence of a contact lens also permits abnormal corneal conditions to be studied more easily with the slit lamp, for the contact lens gets rid of unwanted reflections from the irregular corneal surface.

By largely removing the corneal irregularities, a contact lens permits ophthalmoscopic or slit lamp examination of the media and fundus, thereby making easier the diagnosis of internal eye conditions in patients having an irregular cornea. The fundus of the high myope is also

Figure 24.1 The Eisner Contact Glass: (a) cross-section on the cornea showing its planoconvex form which gives a ×2.2 magnification of the corneal endothelium. The bright anterior corneal reflex is removed by its presence and transferred to the front surface of the Eisner lens, out of the field of view of the slit lamp microscope. (After Eisner, Lotmar and Paprita, 1985.) (b) The supporting structure which holds the eyelids apart and permits easy handling of the lens so that it can be tilted *in situ* to get rid of any reflections from its plane back surface separated from the cornea by a solution such as methyl cellulose. (c) The McIntyre eyepiece comparison grid which allows the corneal endothelial cell density, seen by specular reflection, to be estimated. The illustration shows the number of cells per square millimetre for two different magnifications. On the right are the cell density values for a ×55 magnification achieved with ×2.2 from the Eisner lens, and ×25 from the slit lamp microscope. The McIntyre grid is incorporated in a ×12.5 eyepiece which is used with a ×2 objective lens. (b,c) Reproduced by kind permission of Haag–Streit Ag, Switzerland

more easily observed if viewed through a high minus contact lens which reduces the excessively high magnification obtained in direct ophthalmoscopy of these patients.

Assessment of corneal thickness

Friedman (1967) has developed a corneal lens having a stepped front surface to give a central portion 0.8 mm thick, an intermediate portion 0.6 mm thick and an outer portion 0.4 mm thick. Used with a narrow slit beam corneal thickness can be estimated by comparison with the lens, prior to surgery (*see* Measurement of corneal thickness, Chapter 6, and Pachometry, Chapter 8).

Gonioscopy contact lenses

Observation of the angle of the anterior chamber has been made possible by the use of contact lenses which either partially or completely neutralize the power of the cornea, thus enabling observation of the anterior chamber angle directly or by means of mirror devices.

Most modern gonioscopy lenses are based on the designs introduced by Koeppe (1919), Uribe Troncoso (1921) and Goldmann (1938). The Goldmann lens incorporates a mirror and is used in conjunction with a slit lamp biomicroscope (*Figure 24.2*). The angle of the anterior chamber is seen by reflection.

To see the entire angle, the lens must be rotated on the eye and the slit beam rotated with

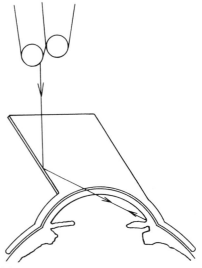

Figure 24.2 Cross-section of a Goldmann gonioscopy lens. Light from a slit lamp is reflected, as shown, into the anterior chamber angle, and returns along the same path to be viewed through the microscope

it but perpendicular to it, a horizontal slit being used when the mirror is vertical and vice versa. Magnification is given by the biomicroscope. The need for all but small amounts of rotation of the lens has been overcome by the use of multiple mirrors, as in the Lovac six-mirror goniolens, the pyramid gonioscope of van Beuningen (1953), and the Zeiss pyramid or four-mirror gonioscope (*Figures 24.3–24.5*). The principle employed by Koeppe and Uribe Troncoso was to use a spherical contact lens and

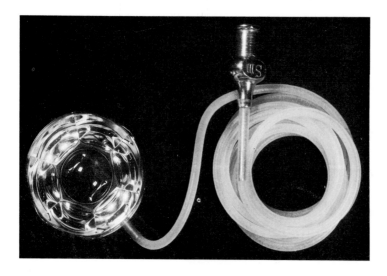

Figure 24.3 Lovac six-mirror goniolens giving a composite image of the entire anterior chamber angle. The central fundus can be viewed through the centre of the lens. (Reproduced by kind permission of Medical Workshop, Holland)

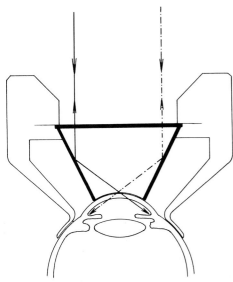

Figure 24.4 The pyramid gonioscope of van Beuningen. The pyramid goniolens is held in place by a support which rests on the sclera

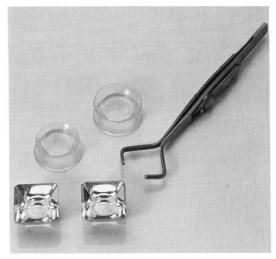

Figure 24.5 The Zeiss four-mirror gonioscope with special forceps, and scleral holders which keep the lids apart. (Reproduced by kind permission of Carl Zeiss, Oberkochen)

observe by looking perpendicular to the anterior lens surface (*Figure 24.6*). This allows observation of the entire angle of the anterior chamber without rotation of the lens. Although the narrow focal beam from a slit lamp is to be preferred, illumination without a slit lamp is possible and may be provided by an opthalmoscope or pen torch. The magnification is about ×2 unaided and may be increased with the aid of a loupe. The disadvantage of this system is the aberration given by the steeply curved spherical front surface of the goniolens.

A modern development of this is the Lovac Double Focus contact lens, which has a small section of convex radius of curvature of 6.00 mm incorporated in the major lens, which has a front surface radius of 8.00 mm (*Figure 24.7*). Magnification of ×15 may be obtained by direct ophthalmoscopy through the steeply curved

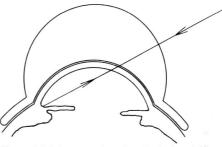

Figure 24.6 Cross-section of a spherical goniolens as used by Koeppe and Uribe Troncoso. Observation and illumination are from the same direction, perpendicular to the front surface. Alternatively, the limbus region may be illuminated by a slit beam from one side

sector. A stereoscopic appearance is obtained if an indirect binocular ophthalmoscope is used, as in *Figure 24.7*.

The Lovac series of lenses adhere readily to the eye by means of negative pressure afforded

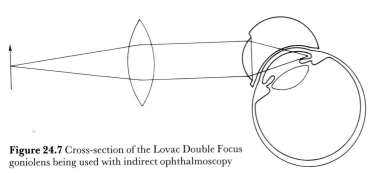

Figure 24.7 Cross-section of the Lovac Double Focus goniolens being used with indirect ophthalmoscopy

by a long cannula running from the back surface of the lens, which is filled with saline prior to insertion. As soon as the lens touches the eye, the end of this cannula is lowered, thereby creating a negative hydrostatic pressure. This prevents the lens dropping out and prevents the

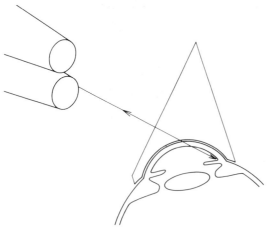

Figure 24.8 Cross-section of the Lovac Direct Goniolens being used with the biomicroscope. The direction of illumination and observation are the same

formation of bubbles behind the lens – problems common with other types of goniolens. However, if left in place for too long (more than about 15 minutes), corneal oedema sufficient to disrupt the observer's view may result (Sabell, 1970).

A further type of goniolens is the Lovac Direct Goniolens as shown in *Figure 24.8*. The anterior chamber angle is viewed directly without reflection through the flat surface of the goniolens, which is angled at about 45° to the patient's visual axis. This allows about half the entire anterior chamber angle to be viewed at one time and readily permits goniophotography.

Lenses employing similar optical principles to the various gonioscopy lenses are also used in the surgical technique known as goniotomy. The Barkan lens, originally developed in 1936 (Barkan, 1936), is shown in *Figure 24.9* and the Medical Workshop prismatic goniotomy lens is shown in *Figure 24.10*.

The anterior chamber angle

Gonioscopy permits observation of the angle of the anterior chamber. The essential features of

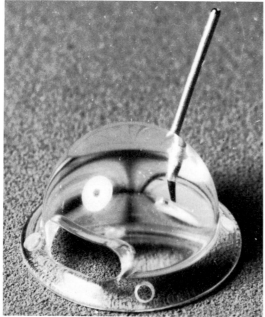

Figure 24.9 The Barkan goniotomy lens giving ×2 magnification. This has a small scleral zone with four perforations, as well as a lateral window and a cannula. (Reproduced by kind permission of Medical Workshop, Holland)

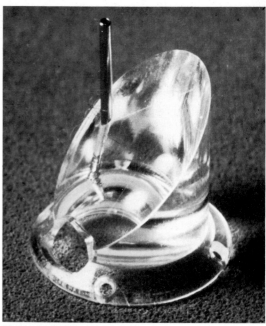

Figure 24.10 The Medical Workshop prismatic goniotomy lens which is used in conjunction with an operating microscope. (Reproduced by kind permission of Medical Workshop, Holland)

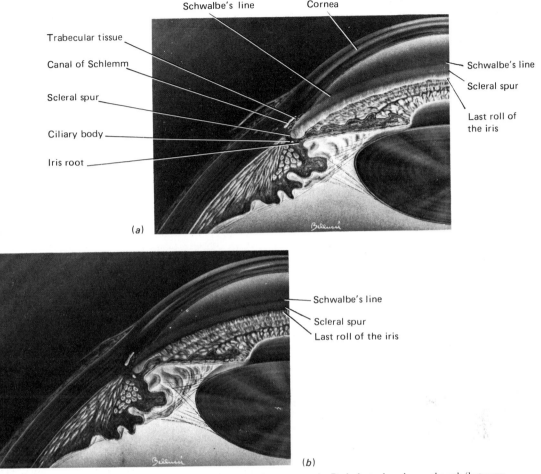

Figure 24.11 (*a*) Cross-section and gonioscopic appearance of an open angle. Both the trabecular meshwork (between Schwalbe's line and the scleral spur) and the ciliary body (between the scleral spur and iris) appear wide, with classification 3-C–*see* text. (*b*) Cross-section and gonioscopic appearance of an angle classified as 3-O. Such an angle might close completely during mydriasis as the last roll of the iris could move forward blocking the aqueous outlet via the trabecular tissue. This could occur with or without pupil block and its resultant iris bombé. (Reproduced from Becker (1972) by kind permission of the author and the publishers, CV Mosby, St Louis, Missouri)

the angle are illustrated in *Figure 24.11a*. On the corneal side of the angle these are as follows.

Schwalbe's line is the termination of the corneal endothelium and Descemet's membrane. Sometimes this is visible using ordinary direct illumination and slit lamp biomicroscopy, because the endothelium may terminate in a small tag of tissue which projects into the aqueous. This is then known as posterior embryotoxon or embryotoxin and if it occurs all round the entire angle it adds to the risk of angle closure glaucoma. It delineates the anterior end of the *corneoscleral trabecular meshwork*. This is the sponge-like tissue separating the aqueous from

the *canal of Schlemm*. The latter becomes visible in gonioscopy if filled with blood. The rear of the corneoscleral trabecular tissue is demarcated by the *scleral spur* which is scleral tissue projecting forward as far as the angle at this point. It can be said to represent the midpoint of the angle as seen by gonioscopy.

Beyond the scleral spur on the iris side of the angle is first the *ciliary body* and then the *root of the iris* at the apex of the angle and just beyond. Then the iris tissue itself takes over and the *last roll of the iris* is seen.

Becker (1972) has devised a goniogram (*Figure 24.12*) to illustrate the state of the

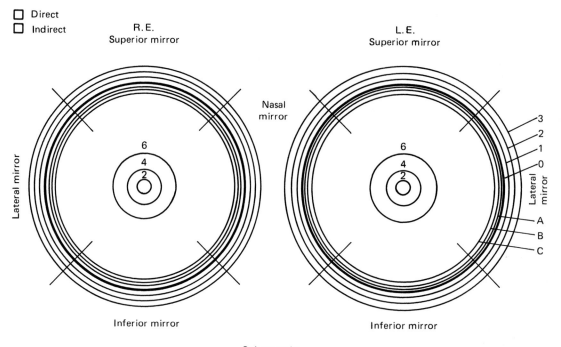

☐ Direct
☐ Indirect

Figure 24.12 Becker's goniogram. The apparent width of the corneoscleral trabeculum is marked in on one of the outer three circles depending on the apparent separation of Schwalbe's line from the scleral spur. The latter is represented by the heavy central circle. Likewise, the width of the ciliary body seen between the scleral spur and iris is marked on the inner three circles. Other features may be drawn in as indicated. The pupil size and characteristics may also be recorded. (Reproduced from Becker (1972) by kind permission of the author and the publishers, CV Mosby, St Louis, Missouri)

anterior chamber angle as seen by gonioscopy, which also relates to his classification of the angle. The goniogram consists of seven concentric circles, the central one denoting the scleral spur. The outer three circles are used to denote the apparent width of the trabecular tissue, i.e. the relative distance of Schwalbe's line from the scleral spur. If the trabecular tissue appears wide (classification 3) then Schwalbe's line is marked in on the outermost circle, if medium (2) on the next circle, and if narrow (1) on the innermost of these three outer circles. The apparent width of this trabecular tissue depends on the angle at which it is viewed. This in itself depends on the narrowness of the anterior chamber angle. If the latter is very narrow, the angle of view to see into it is so tangential to the trabecular meshwork that it appears foreshortened (1).

The three inner circles of the goniogram are used to denote the position of insertion of the iris root into the ciliary body relative to the scleral spur. The iris root is marked on the innermost circle if it is inserted posteriorly (classification C) allowing a good view of the ciliary portion of the angle; on the next circle if the iris is inserted in a midposition (B) and on the third circle in if the iris insertion is anteriorly placed (A) indicating a narrow angle, with hardly any of the ciliary body visible.

Thus, the angle of the anterior chamber is denoted by first a number (0, 1, 2 or 3) and then a letter (O, A, B or C) enabling a description of both 'sides' of the angle. An 0 indicates that the structure is not visible and 0O indicates complete closure. All four quadrants of the angle can be drawn in on the goniogram as indicated, so that variations can be seen and pigmentation and other features such as iris processes can be marked in. The upper quadrant usually has the narrowest portion of the anterior chamber angle, and the angle is at its widest in the lower quadrant.

Other methods of classification include the Shaffer (1962) system which relates the grade to the angle made by the iris with the ciliary body and trabecular tissue. Grade 0 is a closed angle. Grade 1 is 10° or less – an extremely narrow angle. Grade 2 is 20° – a narrow angle. Grade 3 is 20–35° and grade 4 is 35–45° – both wide open angles. Angle closure is thought to be impossible in grades 3 and 4, possible in 2 and probable in 1.

Prior to this, Scheie (1957) used a grading system to denote angle width and pigmentation.

Considerable experience is required for correct interpretation of the anterior chamber angle. *Figure 24.11a* shows an open angle (classification 3-C), and *Figure 24.11b* shows a narrower angle (3-O) with potential for closure if pupil block should occur during mydriasis with resultant iris bombé pushing the last roll of the iris forward to close the angle.

Greater detail of gonioscopy and the appearances seen is available in Becker's work.

Contact lenses for examination of the fundus

Any high-negative-powered contact lens assists observation of the fundus of the high myope

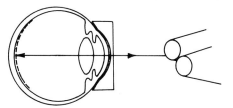

Figure 24.13 Fundus observation with the biomicroscope, by means of a contact lens with a flat front surface

during ophthalmoscopy by reducing the magnification and enlarging the field of view.

Observation of the ocular fundus employing the slit lamp is useful as it allows detection of changes in level of the fundus (by bending and alteration in focus of the slit) and permits a binocular view with magnification. Such observation is aided by the use of special contact lenses having flat front surfaces which eliminate refraction due to the cornea (*Figure 24.13*). The central (macula) region of the fundus may be observed directly with such a high negative lens, and mirrors may be employed to observe the midperiphery and extreme periphery of the fundus. A dilated pupil is necessary. The Zeiss three-mirror contact lens allows all these methods of observation as well as gonioscopy (*Figure 24.14*).

Haag–Streit make a similar lens with mirrors inclined at 73°, 66° and 59° to the plane front surface, the 59° mirror being used for gonioscopy, the 66° mirror for the region around the

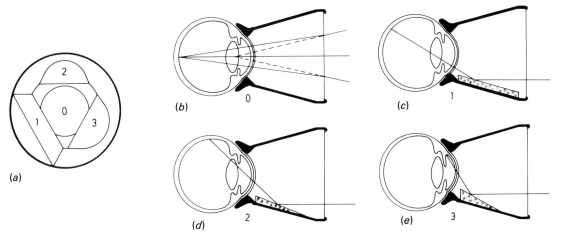

Figure 24.14 (*a*) Location of mirrors in the Zeiss three-mirror goniolens. 0 gives direct viewing as in (*b*). 1, 2 and 3 are mirrors inclined as in (*c*), (*d*) and (*e*). (*b*) The central fundus viewed directly through portion 0, without utilizing a mirror. (*c*) Observation of the midperipheral fundus using mirror 1. (*d*) Observation of the peripheral fundus using mirror 2. (*e*) Observation of the anterior chamber angle using mirror 3

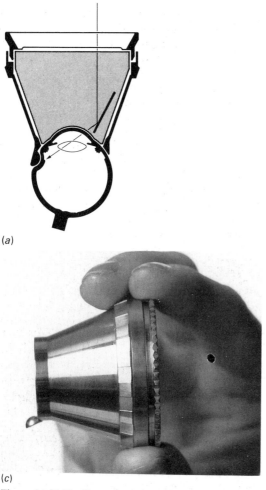

(a)

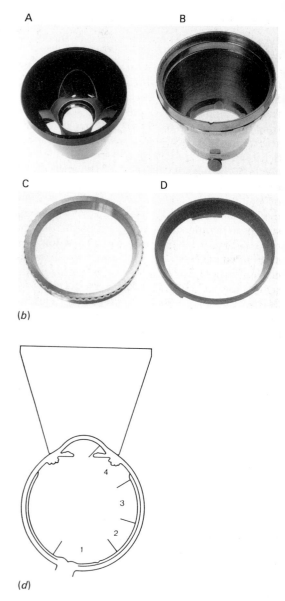

(b)

(c)

(d)

Figure 24.15 The Haag–Streit three-mirror diagnostic lens. (a) Diagram showing observation of the ora serrata using a 6 mm ball scleral depressor attached to the mount opposite the 59° mirror. (b) The three mirrors can be seen in A, the mount with scleral depressor in B, a locking ring C to hold the two together, and a plastic protection ring D, to prevent scratching of the front surface of the lens. (c) Side view showing scleral depressor which is rotated by the middle finger on the milled ring, the lens being held by thumb and forefinger on the notched locking ring or plastic protective ring if in place. (d) Diagram to show areas of the eye seen with the lens. Area 1 is seen through the plane face, 2 via the 73° mirror, 3 via the 66° mirror, and 4 via the 59° mirror. (Reproduced by kind permission of Haag–Streit Ag, Switzerland)

equator, the 73° mirror from there to within 30° of the posterior pole of the eye, and the posterior pole itself being viewed through the plane face of the lens. Slight tilting of the lens is sometimes needed to give complete fundus coverage. The same lens may be used with an ora serrata attachment for depression of the sclera to aid observation just behind the ciliary body (*Figure 24.15a–d*).

Goldmann and Schmidt (1965) have also described a contact lens which allows observation of the ciliary body and ora serrata with the assistance of scleral depression. It is similar to the three-mirror lens shown in *Figure 24.15*, but has one mirror inclined at 62° with the scleral depressor opposite it, as in *Figure 24.15*, allowing the depressed area to be seen in the centre of the mirror.

A paediatric three-mirror lens is also made by Haag–Streit in two sizes, one for the newborn and one for older children.

A lens similar to the Lovac Direct Goniolens (*Figure 24.8*), known as the Lovac Peripheral Fundus contact lens, also allows direct observation of the peripheral fundus. The lens must be rotated to see the entire peripheral fundus and a scleral depressor is used to view the ora serrata. Schirmer (1965) has described a modification of the Troncoso goniolens using either plane or concave facets. These may form part of the lens or may be additions adhering to the lens with methyl cellulose, and thus movable over its surface. The fundus may be inspected through these facets by means of a special gonio slit lamp suspended from above. These facets have enabled observation as far round as the ora serrata and pars plana of the ciliary body (*Figure 24.16*). Better viewing, with a bigger field of view, is obtained if the facet is cut with its surface as near to the pupil as possible (*Figure 24.17*).

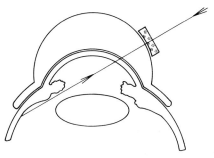

Figure 24.16 Observation of the ora serrata by means of a Troncoso goniolens with negative additional lens

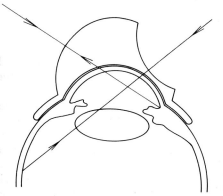

Figure 24.17 A negative facet cut into a Troncoso goniolens to allow observation of the peripheral fundus as well as the anterior chamber angle

An entirely different method of observation of the fundus is employed when using the Panfunduscope, a lens manufactured by Rodenstock (*Figure 24.18*). It allows the entire central fundus beyond the equator to be seen at one time, by means of a two-element optical system. A high positive lens contacts the cornea via a contact fluid such as methyl cellulose, and forms a real inverted image of the fundus, reduced in size by about 30%. To obtain field flatness and an image of adequate size, this real fundus image is formed within a completely spherical lens which then allows it to be viewed by the stereomicroscope of the slit lamp, the latter compensating via its magnification for the image size reduction.

Foreign body locator

Metallic intraocular foreign bodies show up on X-rays, but their relative position is difficult to decide on without adequate reference marks on the X-ray.

These reference marks may be provided by lead pellets incorporated in a scleral contact lens. Typically, four to six lead pellets are used (*Figure 24.19*), and X-rays taken in different planes allow the metallic intraocular foreign body to be located with respect to these. This method has been and is still being used satisfactorily to locate foreign bodies. Their removal is then effected with a strong magnet from the nearest position to the foreign body. A similar lens has a metal ring for X-ray localization (*Figure 24.20*). However these methods of localization are now being superseded by the use of ultrasonic apparatus.

Exophthalmometry

Contact lenses incorporating a metallic insert at the central optic have been used with X-rays to make measurements for both relative and absolute exophthalmometry. Silva (1967) has described these techniques.

Contact lenses for laser surgery

Photocoagulation employing argon, krypton or Nd:YAG (neodymium:yttrium–aluminium–garnet) lasers is used for:

(1) Iridectomy and trabeculotomy, as in the treatment of glaucoma.

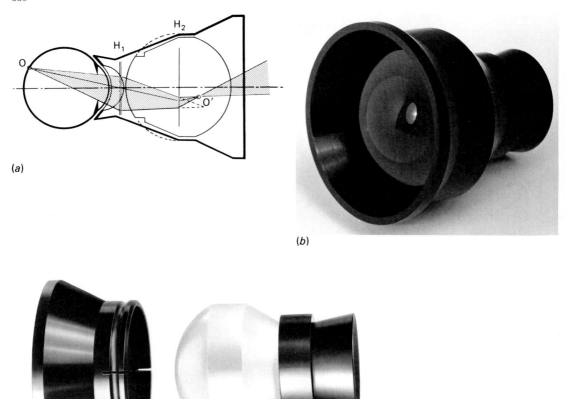

(a)

(b)

(c)

Figure 24.18 The Rodenstock Panfunduscope. (a) Ray diagram showing the high positive lens in contact with the cornea, with its principal planes at H_1, and in front of it the spherical lens with the principal plane H_2 through its centre of curvature. For simplicity the rays showing the fundus point O imaged within the spherical lens at O', are drawn as if refracted at the principal planes rather than at the lens surfaces. The entire fundus beyond the equator is imaged within the spherical lens and viewed by the slit lamp. (b) The lens in its mount which allows it to be supported by the observer's fingers and also acts to hold apart the patient's eyelids. (c) The supporting cone is removed for cleaning, revealing the spherical lens. (Reproduced by kind permission of Rodenstock)

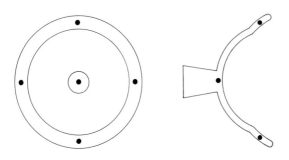

Figure 24.19 A foreign body locator with a handle attached to the front surface, showing lead reference pellets. (a) Direct view; (b) cross-section

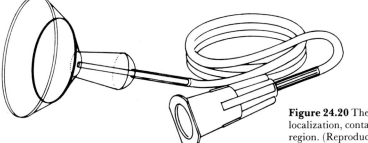

Figure 24.20 The Lovac Comberg contact lens for X-ray localization, containing a metal ring opposite the limbal region. (Reproduced by kind permission of Medical Workshop, Holland)

(2) Capsulotomy and similar treatments to destroy opaque membranes in the pupillary region, often following insertion of intraocular lenses (pseudophakia).

(3) Vitrectomy to break up severe vitreous opacities and posthaemorrhagic conditions in the vitreous likely to result in retinal detachment.

(4) Certain types of retinal detachment, and for sealing new blood vessels in the retina particularly in diabetic patients.

To avoid risk of damage by the laser beam to areas of the eye which are not being treated, a minimal amount of laser energy should be used. To utilize this minimum amount of energy in as efficient a way as possible special contact lenses are often helpful. These are anti-reflection coated to give maximum transmission of the low energy beam. They can aid the surgeon by magnifying the image seen through the slit lamp biomicroscope enabling accurate location of the laser beam focus; they can increase the cone angle of the beam (*Figure 24.21*), thereby dissipating the energy of the beam both in front of and beyond its focus, so avoiding damage to tissues in those areas; and they can, by suitable optical design, form a pinpoint focus rather than a comatic blur.

During laser surgery the eye must be kept wide open and eye movements avoided. This could lead to drying of the cornea disturbing the efficiency of the laser beam and risking corneal damage. The special contact lenses used have the added advantage of keeping the cornea moist, also of neutralizing any corneal irregularities which might otherwise distort the beam, and they keep the eyelids out of the way and steady the eye, as well.

However, there are certain instances where a smaller and therefore more efficient focal spot is formed without the use of a contact lens. For the midvitreous area, 12–15 mm behind the cornea, provided the eye is phakic, then the largest cone angle and smallest spot size is achieved without a contact lens in place (*Figure 24.22*). Beyond this area, and for retinal surgery, a lens with a plane front surface is optimal (*Figure 24.23*), whereas in front of this lenses with convex front surfaces are desirable, as shown in *Figures 24.21,*

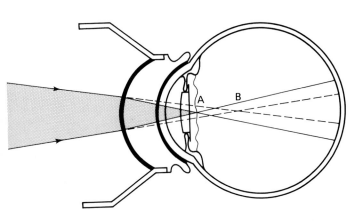

Figure 24.21 Lens used for laser capsulotomy. The spherical front surface refracts the beam to a larger angle at A, thereby diffusing the energy in the surrounding tissues. This gives less risk of damage than with a plane front surface which would give a smaller angle of beam, B, with less spread and more concentration of energy in the surrounding tissues

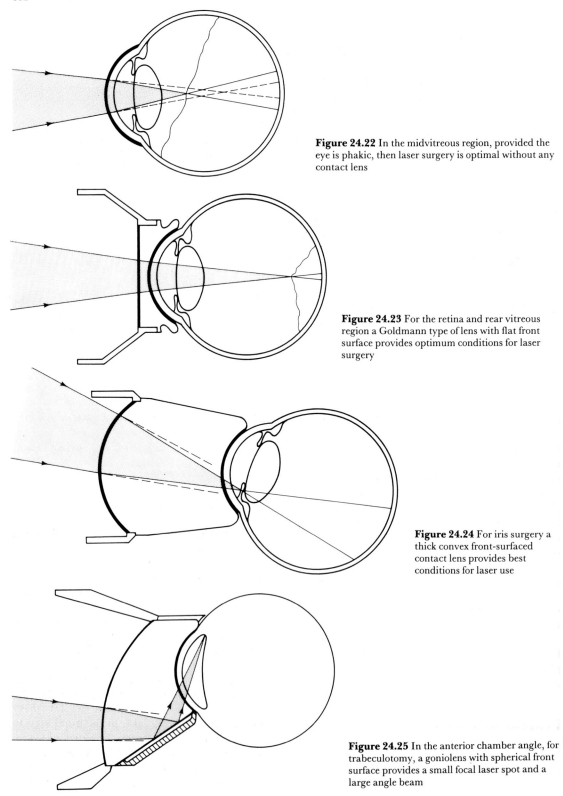

Figure 24.22 In the midvitreous region, provided the eye is phakic, then laser surgery is optimal without any contact lens

Figure 24.23 For the retina and rear vitreous region a Goldmann type of lens with flat front surface provides optimum conditions for laser surgery

Figure 24.24 For iris surgery a thick convex front-surfaced contact lens provides best conditions for laser use

Figure 24.25 In the anterior chamber angle, for trabeculotomy, a goniolens with spherical front surface provides a small focal laser spot and a large angle beam

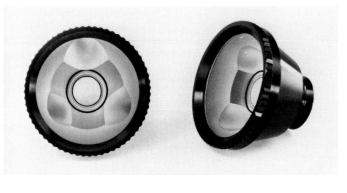

Figure 24.26 Etienne three-mirror laser gonioscope lens with flat front surface. (Reproduced by kind permission of Haag–Streit Ag, Switzerland)

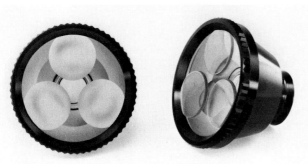

Figure 24.27 Etienne three-mirror laser gonioscope lens with three aplanatic lenses, each giving ×1.5 magnification, which assists observation thereby helping the surgeon, produces a smaller focal spot, and diffuses the energy more rapidly in the surrounding tissues. (Reproduced by kind permission of Haag–Streit Ag, Switzerland)

24.24 and *24.25* illustrating pupil area surgery, iris surgery and trabeculotomy, respectively.

Alternatively laser gonioscopy lenses such as the Etienne lenses made by Haag–Streit may be used. These have three mirrors set at 57°, 59° and 61° inclination, the smallest being at 57°, as seen in *Figure 24.26*. The mirror which renders the laser beam as close to parallel to the iris as possible should be used, i.e. as close to perpendicular to the trabecular tissue to be treated as can be arranged. Greater magnification is afforded by aplanatic lenses on the front surface of the goniolens, as *Figure 24.27* shows. These give ×1.5 magnification and decrease the coagulated spot by two-thirds, as well as reducing the power density at the cornea.

For retinal laser surgery Rodenstock manufacture a special anti-reflection coated, mineral glass version of the Panfunduscope (*see Figure 24.18*).

Protective lenses
Radiation treatment

For malignant tumours of the orbital region, the eye itself may be protected by a plastic-covered lead scleral shell. Where the tumour is ocular, a partial lead shell may be specially constructed to cover all of the anterior eye except the part to be irradiated.

Visible light

During surgery of the anterior segment of the eye, particularly when an operating microscope is used, the intensity of the visible light beam is very high. With the dilated pupil and length of exposure of the eye to this beam, there is risk of damage to the ocular tissues from the visible, infrared and ultraviolet radiations (Kirkness, quoted by Hardy, 1986).

Brown and Parrish (personal communication, 1987) have developed a black PMMA corneal contact lens of total diameter 11.00 mm and back optic radius of 10.00 mm, having a dimple in its front surface to enable it to be moved easily over the cornea with a probe or forceps. The flat curvature and large size also facilitate easy movement, permitting 90% of the pupil area to be covered during surgery. By blocking wavelengths below 500 nm they feel that there is far less risk of damage to the macular area during, for example, cataract surgery and implantation of intraocular lenses. As a result of this simple expedient the number of patients suffering subsequent macular oedema has been reduced.

Protection from visible radiation in normal contact lens wear, for those individuals who are photophobic, is now an easy matter as most contact lens materials are available in a variety of tints. Further comments on tints are to be found in Chapter 21 and later in this chapter on p. 896.

Ultraviolet radiation

As discussed in Chapter 8, ultraviolet radiation is damaging to ocular tissues. Not only may the epithelium, stroma and endothelium of the cornea itself be damaged, but also the crystalline lens may be affected, leading long term to early senile cataract formation. Ultraviolet exposure may also contribute to macular degeneration and loss of retinal sensitivity (Pitts, 1981; Bergmanson quoted by Benjamin, 1987).

Fortunately it is not just spectacle lenses which can be used to block ultraviolet radiation; contact lenses also are now available in all types of material – soft, RGP and PMMA – with varying amounts of ultraviolet absorption. Soft lenses such as the Permaflex UV (Cooper-Vision), available in negative powers of up to −10 D and positive powers of up to +5 D, and Lunelle's aphakic ultraviolet lens, cover between them the major portion of the prescription range, blocking most wavelengths below 400 nm. Other ultraviolet-absorbing soft lenses are the Bausch & Lomb Sofscreen and Vistakon UV-Bloc (Johnson & Johnson), available in the USA.

A number of RGP lenses is also available such as the Boston Equalens and the Optacryl UV range in *Dk* values of 1, 18, 32 and 59, the latter range being also known as UV Asorb.

A study of some of these materials by Chou, Cullen and Dumbleton (1988) has shown that the RGP materials are most effective in blocking UV-B (290–320 nm) and UV-C (200–290 nm) radiations, and all of the materials tested transmitted a significant amount of UV-A (320–400 nm). The soft lens materials, although less effective in blocking UV-B and UV-C are made up in lens forms which cover the entire cornea, whereas RGP lenses, being smaller, do not give complete corneal protection. Of the

materials they tested Chou, Cullen and Dumbleton showed that the material with the best protection factor (PF) was Vistakon UV-Bloc. PF is inversely proportional to the amount of ultraviolet radiation transmitted and therefore depends on lens thickness and power. They concluded that none of the contact lens materials is as effective in blocking ultraviolet light as proper sports and industrial eyewear, but that all these contact lenses probably afford ocular protection against normal lifelong exposure to environmental ultraviolet radiation.

Although rarely fitted now, there are still some PMMA materials in which the molecular structure is altered to improve the wettability of the surface. The method of cross-linking renders them opaque to wavelengths of less than 370 nm – thus cutting out all UV-B and UV-C radiation and a lot of UV-A. They also block the peak wavelength (365 nm) emitted by ultraviolet contact lens fitting lamps. The latter aspect is of importance as it means that the fluorescein pattern cannot be satisfactorily seen using an ultraviolet fitting lamp, but must be viewed with slit lamp biomicroscope and blue filter to obtain an accurate indication of the fit. This also applies to those ultraviolet-absorbing RGP materials mentioned above – the Boston Equalens and Optacryl UV range.

Lasers

During laser photocoagulation special contact lenses are used both to facilitate the surgical technique and to protect the other areas of the eye from the laser beam (*see* pp. 879–883).

Therapeutic lenses

Contact lenses are often helpful in treating certain eye conditions. They fall into several categories.

Bandage and special soft lenses

Hydrophilic contact lenses, of the order of 0.07 mm thickness (for example, the Bausch & Lomb Plano U lens), have been very successfully used as corneal bandage lenses for severe corneal ulceration, following keratoplasty and in the management of bullous keratopathy (Petropoulou, 1975; Aquavella, 1976). In the latter case they are often used in conjunction with hypertonic saline drops. Levinson, Weissman and Sachs (1977) report the successful use of thicker lenses (averaging 0.17 mm, such as the Bausch & Lomb Plano T lens) of HEMA material for cases of bullous keratopathy and following corneal grafts and burns. But in neuroparalytic keratitis and in the dry-eye syndrome difficulty was experienced with lenses drying out and falling off the eye, as well as becoming contaminated with biochemical deposits. They also point out the necessity for in-patient hospital supervision of many of these patients because the risk of infection is so high. The presence of the bandage lens aids regular corneal healing and prevents the eyelid from rubbing the damaged cornea. Aphakic continuous wear hydrophilic lenses have also been successfully applied at the time of operation for cataract extraction, acting as a splint and bandage, as well as permitting immediate good vision postoperatively (Kersley, 1975). Astin (1987) has described fitting specially shaped soft lenses, cut with an upper crescent or upper truncation to avoid intraocular fluid draining blebs beyond the upper limbus, and proud upper scar tissue following cataract surgery. These types of lens are dealt with, in detail, in Chapter 21.

Medical applicators

The use of hydrophilic lenses as medical applicators is now well established (Hillman, 1976). As stated in Chapter 21, p. 813, they have been used in the application to the eye of antibiotics, mydriatics, local anaesthetics and particularly the miotic pilocarpine in the treatment of glaucoma. The lens is soaked in the drug for about 2 hours so that it becomes saturated. When placed on the eye there is a slow release of the drug into the conjunctival sac over the following 2 hours. Hillman reports that high water content material is slightly more efficient than low water content material, and with pilocarpine treatment best results have been obtained using a solution of 1% strength rather than the higher strengths which are usually used in drop form. Hillman also reports the introduction into the UK of the Ocusert which is shaped to be placed in the lower or upper fornix and consists of a hydrophilic core, soaked in pilocarpine, 2% or 4%, surrounded

by a hydrophobic membrane to delay drug release. This provides continuous delivery of the drug for 7 days, at which time it is replaced.

Backman (1983) has reported on the use of a slow-release artificial tear (SRAT) insert known as Lacrisert similar to the Ocusert. Reaction to it varied considerably and in some patients it gave rise to blurred vision, but it is another option worth considering for dry-eyed patients.

Collagen lenses or shields, sufficiently transparent to permit hazy vision through them, can also be used for applying both water-soluble and non-water-soluble drugs to the eye, and to aid postoperative healing. They can be used with any preservative provided the patient is not allergic to it. The shield is placed on the eye by the practitioner, after using a topical anaesthetic if necessary, and does not require removal as it gradually dissolves away. Such a shield is the Bausch & Lomb Bio-Cor Collagen Shield, of total diameter 14.5 mm, back optic radius of 9.0 mm and centre thickness of up to 0.71 mm, based on an idea by Fyodorov of Moscow (Morris, 1988) of using collagen from pig sclera.

Other medical applicators are still sometimes used in intensive drug therapy when it is necessary to keep antibiotic or other drugs in constant contact with the eye. Two examples are the Klein applicator (Klein, 1949) and the Anderson medicator (Anderson, 1952), shown in *Figures 24.28* and *24.29*. Both basically consist

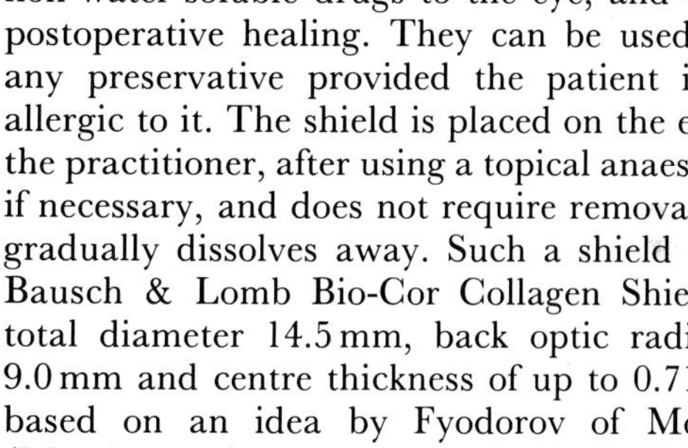

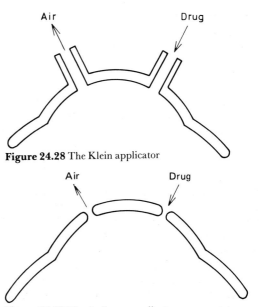

Figure 24.28 The Klein applicator

Figure 24.29 The Anderson medicator

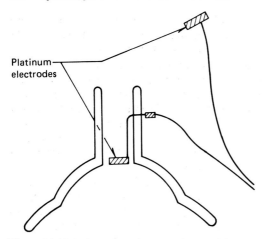

Figure 24.30 An iontophoresis contact lens used for application of drugs to the eye, seen in cross-section

of modified scleral contact lenses. The Anderson medicator has two holes – through one the drug is instilled and out of the other air escapes. The optic zone gives ample corneal clearance, and this acts as a reservoir for the drug. The Klein applicator is similar but has two tubes extending from the optic in place of the holes. This is easier for nurses to handle but a little less comfortable to wear than the Anderson medicator as the lids cannot close over it.

Another, more elaborate, lens is one containing a platinum electrode which almost touches the cornea. Another electrode is attached to the cheek, or elsewhere on the body, and a continuous low voltage electric current is passed. This serves to make the cornea more permeable. Drugs administered via the tube and holes around the electrode gain more rapid entry to the cornea and thence into the aqueous. The lens is illustrated in section in *Figure 24.30*.

Splints

In the emergency departments of hospitals, scleral shells are frequently applied to the eye following facial burns. The shell prevents the lids sticking to the globe (symblepharon). Another type of shell can be used to prevent the lids sticking together (ankyloblepharon). The shells are left in place during the healing process so that the fornices remain formed, otherwise the conjunctival sac might become almost non-existent. As an alternative, large soft lenses

may be used (*see* Chapters 18 and 21). Scleral or soft lenses may have to be worn during attacks of Stevens–Johnson syndrome, when all bodily mucous membranes become severely irritated: in the eye, the bulbar and palpebral conjunctivas may adhere unless a scleral or large soft lens is used to prevent it (*see also* Chapters 18 and 21).

Splints, in the form of large corneal lenses, are also used to hold corneal grafts in place following keratoplasty and to hold the cornea in position following cataract extraction. In both cases, the front surface of the cornea is not held by stitches, which tend to encourage irregular healing, but by the smooth spherical back surface of the contact lens. Good optical results have been achieved with this method of supporting the healing tissue. The splint itself may be held by stitches to the bulbar conjunctiva. When these are cut, the splint is removed by special toothed forceps which fit into small slots on the front surface of the splint (*Figure 24.31*).

Orthoptic uses

A contact lens may be used as a cosmetic occluder in cases of intractable binocular diplopia. Any type of contact lens may be used. Usually, complete occlusion can only be achieved by having an opaque iris pattern and

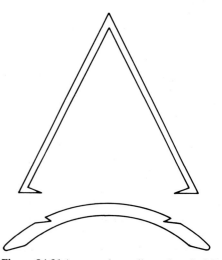

Figure 24.31 A contact lens splint and toothed forceps in cross-section

opaque pupil (*see* Chapter 21), but an opaque pupil in an otherwise clear lens may be sufficient.

In squint treatment, contact lens occluders have been used before the better eye to assist in eliminating amblyopia. Rather than fitting an opaque prosthetic type of shell, adequate occlusion may be achieved with a high negative lens or a very high positive lens (Catford and Mackie, 1968).

Partial occlusion with contact lenses has also been used in the treatment of suppression.

The fitting of anisometropic amblyopes with contact lenses has brought about some dramatic improvements in visual acuity and assisted in the orthoptic treatment of squints in such cases.

Control of refractive errors

It has been suggested that contact lenses prevent the progression of myopia. Most contact lens practitioners have noticed the apparent stabilization of myopia from the time when PMMA contact lenses are first worn, and there are many reports of such instances. Most, such as Dickinson (1957), Morrison (1958), Neill (1962) and Nolan (1964), attributed the stabilization directly to the contact lenses, and stabilization of myopia has been reported where no flattening of the cornea occurs, although the latter can obviously bring about reduction in myopia. On the other hand, Bailey (1966) had shown that the apparent halt in the increase in myopia which occurs when contact lenses are worn can be explained by alterations in corneal curvature being neutralized by the liquid lens, by too much negative power being used to start with to minimize the blur due to residual astigmatism, and by other factors such as flattening of the contact lens itself.

Kelly and Butler (1964, 1971), Baldwin *et al.* (1969), and others, including the author, have investigated this apparent stabilization of myopia. Controlled studies have been undertaken in an attempt to produce positive proof of the therapeutic value of contact lenses on myopia. Results (Stone, 1976) show that conventionally fitted hard corneal lenses, fitted with BOZR just steeper than the flattest keratometer reading, have brought about a slowing down of the rate of progress of myopia in a group of contact-lens-wearing children, as compared to a similar group of spectacle-wearing children.

About half of the reduction in rate of progress could be attributed to corneal flattening by the contact lenses (*see* Chapter 20), but the remainder can only be explained on the basis that wearing corneal lenses has some retarding effect on axial elongation. This aspect is being monitored by Perrigin in a study of 9 to 12 year olds wearing silicone–acrylate RGP lenses which have also been found to retard myopic progression, as she has shown (Perrigin, reported by Morris, 1988).

The technique of orthokeratology is a purposeful attempt to reduce the refractive error of an eye by changing the corneal curvature with hard corneal contact lenses. The change in corneal curvature is normally brought about in gradual stages, by progressively changing the back surface radii of curvature of the lens fitted. The technique has certain uses in helping recruits achieve suitable standards of visual acuity to gain entry to the armed services or other occupations, and it has permitted many ametropes to obtain adequate visual acuity without any form of optical correction for at least part of the time. In some cases myopia is reduced but contact lenses still have to be worn to permit maximum visual acuity; in other cases emmetropia is achieved and may last for a few hours, days, weeks or months but then retainer lenses must be resorted to for varying periods of time. To reduce myopia the aim is to fit lenses which slightly flatten the cornea, but do not cause distortion, oedema or tissue damage. Once a flatter corneal curvature has been achieved and this remains stable, a slightly flatter lens is fitted to flatten the cornea a little more, and again on stabilization a flatter lens still is fitted, and so on. The cost to the patient is obviously high, but for some people the reward justifies the expense. Further details of the methods used have been described by Jessen (1964) and more recently by Nolan (1969) and by Grant and May (1972). Kerns (1977), in a carefully controlled study of orthokeratological procedures, found that whilst the technique is predictable in as far as flattening of corneal curvature and reduction of myopia is concerned, the magnitude of this change is not predictable. He also concluded that changes in the vertical meridian of the cornea could not be predicted and he noted that the corneas of young people are more likely to be flattened than those of older patients.

As an aid to defective colour vision

A red contact lens, of peak transmission 595 nm, worn in one eye only has been recommended by La Bissoniere (1974) in an attempt to overcome certain red–green colour deficiencies, by allowing a comparison of the different contrasts then perceived by the two eyes. Known as the X-Chrom lens, during binocular viewing it gives rise to a different perception of hues, altering their saturation or brightness, or imparting a lustre, and the wearer learns to relate that appearance to a particular colour name. It takes some time to adapt to the situation but it is reported as being very successful. During the initial stages of wear, until adaptation has taken place, there may be some disorientation of depth judgement, which should be pointed out to patients for reasons of safety. Ciuffreda (1980) has reported on the Pulfrich effect elicited when subjects first wore the lens in one eye, being equivalent to the effect of a 0.57 neutral density filter or of 27% light transmission.

Contact lenses used for research into visual function

Contact lenses are a means of holding suitable objects in contact with the eye for research purposes. Such objects may be electrodes, thermistors, oxygen probes, mirrors or telescopic devices, all of which have been incorporated in contact lenses at various times.

Electrodes

An electrode incorporated in a contact lens may be used in iontophoresis for therapeutic purposes, as already mentioned. For research purposes, the most frequent use of electrodes in contact lenses is in ERG (electroretinography) studies. Most electrical activity in the eye region takes place in the retina, and the potential difference in the retina may be measured – as different light stimuli are applied – by means of one electrode attached to the nearby skin and one touching the eye, the two electrodes being connected to a suitable meter, amplifier and pen-recorder. Typical contact lenses for this purpose are illustrated in *Figure 24.32*. The conical front surface projection is to prevent eyelid closure and to prevent any discomfort from the eyelids contacting the electrode. Electrodes are usually of silver or platinum. Small scleral lenses have been most frequently used in the past. A good description of the method of making these lenses has been given by Fletcher (1966) under the pseudonym Haptos.

A flexible glycol methacrylate corneal lens has been described by Bornschein, Wichterle and

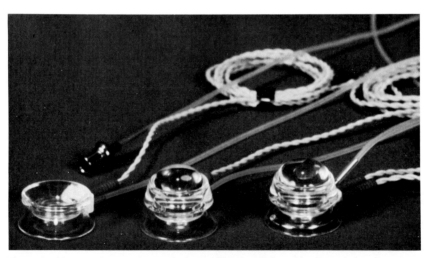

Figure 24.32 Lovac electroretinography lenses. These are lightweight electrode-bearing contact lenses used in ERG studies. Each has a small scleral zone and a blepharostatic cone which takes different colour filters and diaphragms. A circular silver electrode in the limbal region is connected to a tiny permanently attached electric flex leading to the electroretinograph.
(Reproduced by kind permission of Medical Workshop, Holland)

Wündsch (1966). This incorporates a silver spherical electrode in its front surface. The lens itself is electrically conducting. A corneal contact lens using a silver electrode has also been described by Ruedmann and Noell (1961).

ERG studies by Alvis (1966) have suggested that this may, in future, form an additional diagnostic test in glaucoma.

Other more complicated types of electrode are used for measurement of temperature and gas exchange at the eye's surface and are described in the appropriate sections below.

Eye movements

Studies of voluntary and involuntary eye movements have been made by mounting a small mirror on a contact lens and reflecting light from a stationary source. The angular movement of the reflected image is then double the angular movement of the eye. However, the method has been largely superseded by cine-photography of reflections from the anterior surface of the cornea.

Stabilized retinal images

A better understanding of the physiological and psychological aspects of seeing has been achieved by studying what happens when the retinal image of an object remains stationary on the retina, i.e. when small movements of the retinal image, due to saccadic movements of the eye, are prevented. This may be done by flash exposure of short duration or by means of contact lenses, which, because they move with the eye, may be used to overcome the effects of eye movements in the formation of the retinal image.

Two basic systems have been employed. One utilizes a tightly fitting contact lens with a protruding stalk on the end of which is a plane mirror. The mirror is used to reflect light from a target through a compensating optical system into the eye. Such a system was originally devised by Ditchburn and Ginsborg (1952). A more recent system (Millodot, 1965) is depicted in *Figure 24.33*.

Any movement of the eye causes a corresponding movement of the mirror, and the reflected image of the target is moved through twice this angle. To compensate for this doubling of angular movement, lenses S_1 and S_2 give a reduction in magnification of a half. Thus, light passing through the optical system is always imaged on the same portion of the retina, regardless of eye movements.

The other system, used by Evans and Piggins (1963), is to incorporate a small telescopic device into the contact lens itself, as shown in

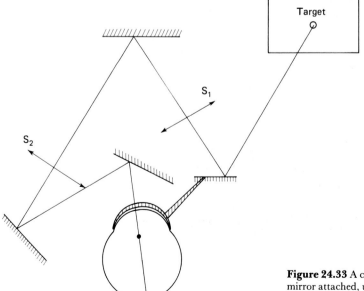

Figure 24.33 A contact lens with projecting stalk and mirror attached, used to produce a stabilized retinal image by means of a mirror and lens system (after Millodot, 1965)

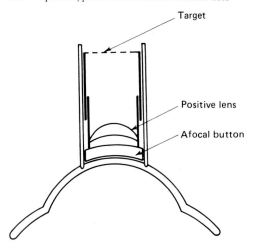

Figure 24.34 A contact lens incorporating a small telescopic device, used in the study of stabilized retinal images. The target is in the focal plane of a positive lens. Sliding supports allow some latitude in focusing. The positive lens is separated from the eye by an afocal button

Figure 24.34 and as described by Evans (1965). A suitably illuminated target is placed approximately in the anterior focal plane of a high positive lens, which is itself separated from the contact lens by an afocal button. The whole optical system is contained in aluminium tubing, and the target and positive lens are movable relative to each other to facilitate accurate focusing on the retina.

In attempts to provide contact lenses which did not lag behind the eye during eye movements, rubber contact lenses with attached pressure bulbs to obtain suction have been used in the past. These were liable to cause damage to the eye. Best results seem to have been achieved with small scleral lenses (17 mm back

scleral diameter) for the telescopic type of device, and a 14 mm total diameter, single curve corneal lens, fitted tightly, for the type incorporating a mirror.

The results obtained with these devices suggest that perception comprises multiple pattern recognition.

Lid pressure

In the first part of a study of the effects of lid pressure on corneal shape, and on deformation or flexure of rigid lenses on the eye, Lydon and Tait (1988) used a scleral lens into which they incorporated a pressure transducer. They showed that the eye retracts 0.5 mm on blinking and 1 mm on forced blinking, and that upper lid tension is compensated for by orbital resistance and should not therefore affect corneal toricity. Possible effects of lid pressure on contact lens flexure have yet to be established.

Temperature measurement

In studying ocular changes due to contact lenses, the effects of lid aperture size, lid closure, eye position and the very presence of the contact lens itself cause temperature changes of the cornea, sometimes to an extent beyond which normal corneal metabolism can no longer continue.

These temperatures changes can be monitored, using a thermistor – a tiny electrical device sensitive to temperature changes. Thermistors can be incorporated in both scleral and corneal lenses. Typical lenses are shown in *Figure 24.35*. Hill and Leighton (1965) have described their findings on temperature changes

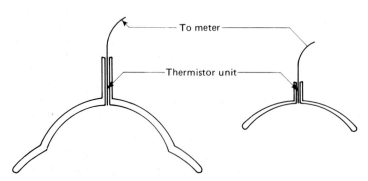

Figure 24.35 A scleral and a corneal lens, each incorporating a thermistor for temperature measurement

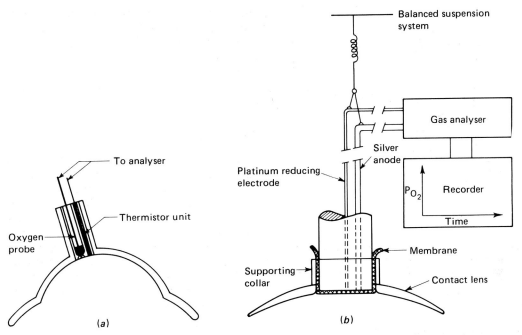

Figure 24.36 (*a*) A scleral contact lens incorporating a probe for recording oxygen tension (after Hill and Fatt, 1966). (*b*) A corneal lens used for measurement of oxygen uptake (after Fatt and Hill, 1970)

of the eye when using a scleral contact lens containing one of these devices, and they have shown how the rise in temperature behind a lens affects the corneal metabolism.

Gas exchange of the cornea during contact lens wear

In order to hold an oxygen probe against the cornea, scleral lenses were used at first. Hill and Fatt (1966) have described such a lens which is depicted in *Figure 24.36a*. The probe is a polarographic oxygen electrode covered by an oxygen-containing membrane. As the oxygen from this is lost to the corneal cells or surrounding liquid, the current in the electrode is lowered. A similar system has since been used in a corneal lens (Fatt and Hill, 1970) as pictured in *Figure 24.36b*.

Similar systems allow the output of carbon dioxide by the corneal epithelium to be recorded.

Lenses for animals

Many experiments are carried out on animals prior to being carried out on humans, and special lenses have been constructed for monkeys, rabbits, cats, squirrels, octopi and other creatures to assess various aspects of visual function.

The contact lens has become a major tool in visual research, both from the physiological and psychological aspects. There is no doubt that it will find further uses in addition to those described above.

Lenses for sports purposes

The criteria to be satisfied if contact lenses are to be worn for sports purposes are: the lens must not be capable of being misplaced on the eye due to accidental foreign pressure; the optic must remain centred; the tear lens must remain completely free of bubbles in front of the pupil area; and corneal metabolism should not be interfered with during the period required for the game.

In the past (*see* second edition of this book), special large corneal lenses, as well as semi-scleral soft lenses and purposely designed scleral lenses have all been employed solely for sports use. With current materials and lens designs, in general a fairly tight fitting RGP corneal lens or a well-fitted soft lens satisfy the above criteria most of the time, although a slight risk of lens displacement remains. To minimize this risk a soft lens of total diameter 14.0 mm or more is desirable, fitted slightly steeper than normal. The same approach to lens stability is also advisable if fitting an RGP lens – as large a lens as possible should be used with a minimum of peripheral corneal clearance, and a large BOZD of 8.0 mm or more.

Saturn II lenses which have an RGP central zone and soft periphery overlapping onto the sclera may prove useful for some people engaged in sports, particularly if corneal astigmatism requires correction and toric soft lenses are unsuccessful but the comfort of a soft lens is needed (Minarik, 1987).

Scleral lenses, although still ideal in that they are unlikely to be dislodged from the eye, are difficult to fit satisfactorily compared to other lenses, and they are now rarely an economic option, particularly as most participators in sporting activities frequently want to wear the same contact lenses on an all day wearing basis.

Climbing and cold weather sports and activities

In a survey of contact lens wearers engaged in cold weather activities outdoors, Socks (1983) found that no significant problems were experienced and that contact lenses had a decided advantage over spectacles, as they do not mist up and do not become brittle and break as spectacles may do when cold. Contact lenses protect the eye from wind-driven ice and snow, and indeed have been successfully worn up to 26 000 feet on an assault on Mount Everest (Clarke, 1975).

Most difficulties occur with the cleaning fluids and procedures, as the liquids may freeze and contact lenses be difficult to handle with cold fingers if camping out in extremely low temperature conditions. In such cases extended wear lenses have a distinct advantage.

Swimming

There is some risk of loss of contact lenses from the eye while swimming, which is much less with soft lenses than with rigid lenses (Lovsund, Nilsson and Oberg, 1980), and with the latter it

is less with RGP than PMMA lenses due to the mode of fitting. Other than this there is the distinct possibility that contact lenses may to a certain extent protect the eye from chlorinated water and reduce the effects of exposing the cornea to swimming pool water which can lead to oedema (Hill, 1985; Solomon, Snyder and Klein, 1987), but this depends on methods of fitting and exposure time to pool water. If hypotonic saline or water is instilled or splashed into the eye prior to swimming, the osmotic effect is to make the lens cling to the cornea so reducing the initial risk of loss (Diefenbach et al., 1988). The longer a soft lens comes into contact with pool water, the more hypotonic its own saline content becomes and the greater the risk of corneal oedema and difficulty of removing the lens from the eye, associated with the hypotonicity. (There may then be a need to bathe the lens and eye with hypertonic saline in order to effect lens removal, and incidentally to reduce oedema.) However, for short exposures, soft lenses have a definite protective function, but should be rinsed thoroughly in fresh sterile saline following any contact with chlorinated water.

Sealed scleral lenses are the ideal form of contact lens correction for swimming, with no risk of loss, and almost complete protection of the eye. However, the use of swimming goggles with normal contact lens wear is probably just as satisfactory. The optical aspects of swimming under water are covered in the following section on lenses for skin diving.

Lenses for skin diving

Under water, the power of the eye is reduced by approximately 42 D. This is due to water replacing air in front of the cornea. If the front surface of the cornea is assumed to have a radius of curvature of 8.0 mm, then the reduction in power is as follows.

$$\frac{\text{Power of front surface}}{\text{of cornea, in air}} - \frac{\text{Power of front surface}}{\text{of cornea, in water}}$$

$$\frac{(1.376 - 1)1000\,\text{D}}{8.0} - \frac{(1.376 - 1.333)1000\,\text{D}}{8.0}$$

$$= 41.5\,\text{D}$$

The emmetropic eye therefore becomes hypermetropic to this extent. This power loss may be replaced in two ways, as follows.

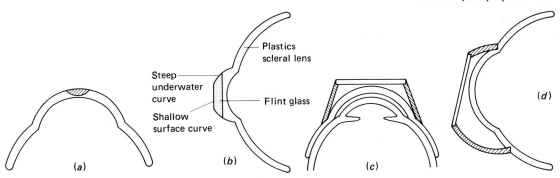

Figure 24.37 Underwater contact lenses. (*a*) Lens containing a high refractive index button to give added power. (*b*) Douthwaite's bifocal flint glass button lens (reproduced by kind permission of W. A. Douthwaite). (*c*) Lens containing an air space. The flat front surface has dark tinted supports to prevent distortion and glare. (*d*) An air space with tilted front surface, which gives added comfort and is supported by the lower lid during wear

A contact lens may be worn which incorporates a steeply curved high refractive index glass button (*Figure 24.37a*). The additional power is achieved by the difference of refractive indices, these being 1.6 and 1.333 at the front surface as compared to 1.49 and 1.333 for the carrier portion, and 1.6 and 1.49 at the interface. It is necessary to incorporate the button in a fairly thick scleral lens.

The button may be made very small so that it only partially covers the pupil. This allows vision through the carrier portion of the lens when in air as the carrier portion can be correctly sighted to allow for the wearer's normal refractive error.

Such a lens has been reported by Ward (B., 1961, personal communication and unpublished report). It suffered from two main disadvantages, namely, that it was extremely difficult to locate the button so that vision both above and below water was possible, and it was difficult to find a suitable cement which did not dissolve in sea water to attach the button to the carrier portion.

These problems appear to have been overcome by Douthwaite (1971) who described a similar type of lens in which a flint glass button was fused by the 'Uniseal' method to a plastics scleral lens, the interface between the two being plane (*Figure 24.37b*). The same concentric principle is employed but the outer steep curve on the front of the flint button permits vision under water where the illumination is low and pupil dilated, and the central flatter front surface curve caters for vision in air when the pupil is likely to be more constricted in daylight.

The type of bifocal lens described is less noticeable than the air-cell type of lens described below, is more comfortable to wear, does not give rise to the magnification effect nor to the distortion encountered with the air-cell lens. It gives a full, unrestricted field of view. Its disadvantages are slight displacement on the eye which can cause a loss of vision above water, and also the out-of-focus image formed by the peripheral zone in air may give rise to a haze which reduces contrast and affects visual acuity.

Douthwaite also suggested a bifocal underwater lens similar to a solid spectacle bifocal lens, the lower part being used for vision above water when the wearer is likely to be looking in a relatively downwards direction while treading water, and the upper part being used for underwater vision when the gaze is usually relatively upwards as the diver swims along in a horizontal direction. He also pointed out that direction of gaze can vary considerably which would then make this type of lens difficult to wear.

The air-cell types of lens is one which has a plane front surface enclosing an air space in front of a conventional scleral lens sighted to correct the wearer's normal refractive error. This type of lens is, as it were, a tiny 'face mask' worn in front of the eye only (*Figure 24.37c*). The optical effect is the same as looking through any plane surface into water.

Refraction of light from water to air causes objects to appear at three-quarters of their real distance, giving a magnification of ×1.333. Due to total internal reflection at the plane face, the visual field is restricted to 97.2° in air and approximately 55–60° in water (Cockell, 1967). If the side supports are left transparent, there is considerable distortion of the peripheral visual field.

Mossé (1964) described a lens in which the front plane face is tilted, as in *Figure 24.37d*, and in which the supports are opaque, eliminating the distortion of the peripheral field. The tilt of the plane face makes upper lid movement more comfortable and prevents the lens from sagging as it is better supported by the lower lid.

The mode of attachment of the plane face to the lens is important so that the air chamber does not collapse in the pressures experienced under water. *Figure 24.37d* shows the system used in France, and *Figure 24.38* shows Cockell's construction in which all but the plane face is made from one solid piece of plastics material.

Attempts have been made to fill the space with air under pressure. The incorporation of a little silica gel in the air space prevents condensation. The plane face should be as close as possible to the front optic surface of the scleral lens, but not sufficiently close to cause interference fringes.

The advantage of such a lens is that it gives adequate vision both above and below water without allowing the diver to be seen from afar, which happens due to reflections when a plane face mask is worn. (This is an important function in times of war, when skin divers need to remain as invisible as possible – especially on surfacing.) This type of lens can be worn satisfactorily for periods of about 4 hours.

Bennett (1985) states that during normal diving procedures where a face mask is worn, soft lenses with their greater adhesion to the eye are preferable to hard lenses particularly for highly ametropic wearers. In the unlikely event

of the loss of the face mask the diver would then be able to surface and see his support vessel. This becomes important for police and military divers who might lose a face mask during a skirmish.

Where deep diving is undertaken PMMA lenses are contra-indicated (Simon and Bradley, 1980; Molinari and Socks, 1986) due to bubble formation under the lenses and oedema, and for commercial diving in a chamber or bell, contact lenses should not be worn at all (Bennett, 1985). This is due to the divers living for long periods under high pressure, as well as to the fact that *Pseudomonas aeruginosa*, which can rapidly destroy a damaged cornea, is known to thrive in diving chambers.

Lenses for the partially sighted

Partially sighted people need additional magnification in order to be able to see detail. Such magnification may be provided in the form of a Galilean telescope device, in which a contact lens forms the eyepiece and a conventional spectacle lens the objective. The optical system is depicted in *Figure 24.39*.

Since the eyepiece contacts the cornea, the magnification (for an emmetropic eye) is given directly by

$$\frac{w_2}{w_1} = \frac{f_1'}{f_2'} = \frac{f_1'}{f_1' - d} = \frac{1}{1 - dF_1'} \ (d \text{ in metres})$$

With a typical power for F_1' of $+25\,\text{D}$ and a vertex distance, d, of $12\,\text{mm}$

$$\text{Magnification} = \frac{1}{1 - 3/10} = \frac{1}{0.7} = \times 1.4$$

The powers of the two lenses and their separation must be such as to correct the patient's refractive error, K, where

$$K = \frac{F_1'}{1 - dF_1'} + F_2' \ (d \text{ in metres})$$

This system has been used with soft, scleral and corneal lenses forming the eyepiece, soft and scleral lenses being generally more satisfactory as they are more stable. The advantages over the telescopic type of spectacle aid are the reduction in weight and the psychological benefit of improved cosmetic appearance. The

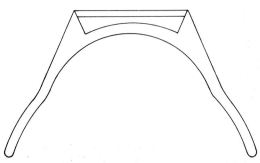

Figure 24.38 Cockell's underwater contact lens (developed at the City University, London)

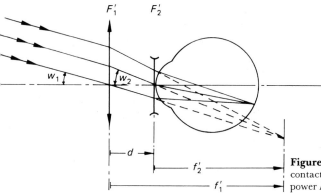

F_1' F_2'

w_1 w_2

d

f_2'

f_1'

Figure 24.39 A Galilean telescope system incorporating a contact lens of power F_2' as eyepiece, and a spectacle lens of power F_1' as objective

weight of the high positive spectacle lens can be further relieved by the use of a Fresnel press-on lens as utilized and recommended by Gerstman and Levene (1974). The disadvantage is that contact lenses cannot be removed as quickly and conveniently as spectacles. This is less of a disadvantage when the system is worn by one eye only, as is often the case. The patient then has a normal visual field with one eye, whilst the other eye receives the magnified image for detailed vision, in a reduced visual field (Moore, 1964). However, this does require the facility of alternate suppression by the patient, or else alternate occlusion of the eyes to avoid confusion. It is surprising how well patients with low visual acuity are able to adapt to such a system so long as it provides an obvious benefit to them.

The magnification reduces the visual field and can cause disorientation, but this may be minimized to some extent by magnifying only a small central portion of the visual field. This may be done by using a carefully fitted contact lens worked to correct the refractive error but with the front central portion made quite flat, giving a high negative power centrally. The diameter of this portion must be about two-thirds of the pupil diameter in normal illumination; and according to Filderman (1964), it is typically between 3.5 and 4.0 mm, and of about $-50\,\mathrm{D}$ power. This is the high negative eyepiece of power F_2' which is used in conjunction with a positive segment of about 10 mm diameter and $+25\,\mathrm{D}$ power, cemented on to the back surface of an afocal spectacle lens of 12 D base. Below this, a near addition may be cemented on to the carrier lens (*Figure 24.40*). Fresnel press-on segments may be used as an alternative to cemented segments.

F_2' depends on the thickness and back optic zone radius of the contact lens. Since

$$K = \frac{F_1'}{1 - dF_1'} + F_2'$$

and since d is known, or can be measured, F_1' may be determined. The magnification may then be computed from

$$\frac{1}{1 - dF_1'}$$

Filderman described a small corneal lens fitted to rest on the lower lid and ballasted to keep it down, with the optic zone displaced to put it in front of the pupil and the upper edge of the lens only just above the upper pupil margin. He also stated that best results were obtained with scleral lenses, but soft lenses may now supersede them (Stone and Breakspear, 1977).

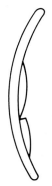

Figure 24.40 A spectacle lens used as the objective for a Galilean telescope system, having separate portions for distance and near vision, cemented on to an afocal carrier lens

Such lenses cannot be fitted to old people. Not only do they have pupils which are too small but also the disorientation is usually too great to be tolerated by them. Young people can usually cope with these difficulties.

An attempt has been made by Feinbloom (1961) to incorporate both positive objective and negative eyepiece in one scleral lens with an air space between the two. While being theoretically possible, lenses so far made have been very thick and heavy, making them uncomfortable to wear and unsightly.

Drasdo (1970) has developed a similar lens to be used in conjunction with a spectacle lens, which he described as a 'feedback corrected' lens system since it gives magnification without altering the angular amount of movement of the eye required to take up fixation of peripheral objects. It therefore overcomes one of the major disadvantages, i.e. disorientation.

A reversed telescope system has been mentioned by Bier (1960) for people with loss of peripheral vision, and the author, with others, has also successfully fitted one for a person with homonymous hemianopia. A high positive scleral lens used with a high negative spectacle lens, suitably designed to give minimum aberrations, gives a reduction in magnification (and, incidentally, a reduced visual acuity) but allows more to be seen in the existing visual field.

Animals' lenses

At various times, contact lenses have been used for animals. Most fall into three categories as follows.

Experimental lenses

Lenses used for research purposes have already been mentioned earlier in this chapter.

Utilitarian lenses

Chickens and turkeys have been provided with opaque and coloured contact lenses to reduce their acuity and so prevent featherpecking (Anon, 1967).

Therapeutic lenses

The use of a specially made 72% water content soft lens of 34 mm total diameter and 18 mm back optic radius for a horse with an injured cornea has been reported by Tammeus, Krall and Rengstorff (1982). Worn continuously for 6 days in a therapeutic capacity the lens permitted corneal healing to take place following corneal perforation. Soft lenses have been used in the same way for treatment of corneal conditions in dogs and cats (Schmidt, Blanchard and Keller, 1977).

Miscellaneous lenses

Certain lenses or types of lens do not fall into any of the above categories, and yet some mention of them should be made.

Tinted lenses

The reasons for prescribing tinted lenses have already been dealt with. Tinted hard lenses are available in a large number of different hues usually denoted by a number (see Table 22.1), their spectral transmission curves being available from the plastics or contact lens manufacturers.

Two main dangers arise in the use of tinted hard lenses. The first, as has been pointed out by Estevez (1967), is their possible toxicity to ocular tissues – particularly if soluble dyes or surface dyeing is used for colouration. In the UK, only Perspex CQ, made by ICI, has been proven by clinical trials to be non-toxic to ocular tissues. This is available in clear and neutral grey tints (9042 and 9043, previously 911 CQ and 912 CQ), the latter tinting being achieved by the use of inert fine carbon particles dispersed in the monomer before polymerization. The pigment is thus locked in the molecular chain. The fine carbon particles are visible in the material when the contact lenses are observed on the eye with the biomicroscope.

Although Estevez states that pigments incorporated in this way are solid particles and therefore may reduce the transparency of the material (except where fine carbon particles are used), contact lenses tinted with such insoluble dyes have proved satisfactory in wear. Capelli (1966) has shown that no dye leached out of 20 different coloured samples boiled for 80 hours. A minute non-coloured residue was obtained after boiling, which was slightly less from tinted lenses (33.5 μg) than from clear lenses (40.0 μg). The fact that these lenses have been worn so satisfactorily by many wearers suggests that the toxicity problem and the transparency problem are both small ones.

No problems have been reported due to the tints used in RGP materials. The stringent testing carried out to satisfy FDA requirements in the USA and similar authorities in other countries has ensured the safety of these lenses.

Soft lenses may be tinted by the use of vegetable dyes. Some of these dyes leach out of the lens during wear and the patient can renew the tint by the application of a few drops of dye to the lens each day. Other dyes are more stable but may be removed from the lens during one of the stringent cleaning processes, such as the Ren-O-Gel (Alcon) system. Ciba Vision tinted lenses are also affected by chlorine disinfection systems, e.g. Alcon's Softabs (Opti-tabs).

The second danger has been outlined by Fletcher and Nisted (1963), who have shown that some tinted lenses raise the light threshold, thereby worsening dark adaptation. Also, by their selective spectral transmission, they can be potentially dangerous when used in certain near monochromatic illumination. For example, certain blue-tinted lenses used in sodium lighting could severely reduce visibility, and green lenses could reduce the visibility of red traffic lights and rear lights.

In some countries there is a legal limit to the density of any tint worn during night driving.

Another hazard, which is not confined to tinted lenses but applies equally to clear lenses, has been suggested by Ball (1964). He postulated that some of the photophobia experienced by new contact lens wearers may be due to increased ultraviolet radiation reaching the cornea (see p. 884). The cornea is most sensitive to a radiation of 288 nm, and most plastics (tinted or otherwise) have a cut-off at 290 nm. An alternative explanation for increased photophobia with contact lenses was given by Fletcher (1964), who showed that significantly more light is admitted to the eye by a clear lens of approximately 0.3 mm thickness and this increase is offset by tinting. He attributes the increase to the optical effect of moving the entrance pupil forward, which increases its size

and thereby admits more light into the eye. However, the entrance pupil size would only be increased by a positive contact lens system. Its size would be decreased by a negative lens (Stone, 1968). This factor would therefore only be of significance in causing photophobia if positive lenses are worn, as in aphakia. In all probability, most photophobia is due to corneal oedema during the adaptation period (see Chapter 19).

Surface coating

Some contact lens wearers have problems because their rigid lenses do not wet properly. The contact angle may be reduced (i.e. surface wetting improved) by coating the surfaces of the lenses chemically or by deposition of a thin metal compound. In either case the surface of the lens is converted from a hydrophobic to a hydrophilic one.

The former method, of chemical coating, was developed by Erb (1961) and is known as the Erb method. The lens is thoroughly cleaned and dipped in a solution of titanium dioxide. This improves the wetting properties of the lens; but if the lens becomes greasy, the effect is spoiled. Eventually, the coating deteriorates due to wear. A thin film of silica, applied by treating the surface with water and silicon tetrachloride vapour, has since proved more reliable (Blue, 1966).

Vacuum coating is the other method, which is also of rather a temporary nature because plastics material, for obvious reasons, has to be coated in a cold state. The method, apart from the difference in temperature, is essentially that used to put an anti-reflection coating on glass lenses.

Both methods must be carried out on a finally finished contact lens, when all modifications to the fit have been made. In both cases, greasing of the lenses is minimized; but if it does occur, the wetting properties are spoiled until the grease is removed.

Another vacuum method of converting the surface to hydrophilic has been described by Gesser, Funt and Warriner (1965). It is claimed that about half the surface molecular groups are changed in chemical composition by removal of hydrogen atoms. Lenses are placed in a vacuum discharge tube in the presence of ammonia but out of the path of the discharge glow. An electrical discharge causes a chemical action to take place on the surface of the plastics material. The altered molecules are hydrophilic instead of hydrophobic. Lenses treated in this way wet well, and there is minimal build-up of grease and oil on their surfaces.

A similar technique, known as plasma modification, using an oxygen plasma glow discharge method has been successful in treating the surfaces of gas permeable hard lenses (Hough and Patel, 1986).

Materials with lowered wetting angle

Besides the special surface coatings and treatments mentioned above, several materials for hard lenses are still available made of polymethyl methacrylate in which the cross-linking agents have been changed to reduce the surface wetting angle (Harris *et al.*, 1973). Such materials are, for example, the Aqua-Lens made by Morgan Optics in the USA, BP-flex made by Burton Parsons which is PMMA with an added methacrylic component, and the Hydro-15 lens marketed by Madden Contact Lenses in England. These materials are very useful for patients who suffer greasing problems with conventional polymethyl methacrylate lenses. Goldberg (1975) found such a material very good for patients having corneal oedema with conventional lenses. He attributes the reduction of oedema with this material to better transport of tears and therefore of gaseous exchange behind the lens, due to less frictional resistance and by allowing more oxygen to be present in the tears at the lens–cornea interface. He also found the same effect with CAB material. The latter material also has a lower wetting angle than polymethyl methacrylate. The fluorescein pattern with a Hydro-15 lens must be viewed with blue light as the material does not transmit the appropriate ultraviolet wavelength. Improved wettability is also claimed for the fluorosilicon–acrylate group of RGP materials.

Lenses of high and low refractive index

Chapter 3 includes details of refractive indices of various contact lens materials. It is sometimes useful to use a lower or higher refractive index to help solve an optical problem, as for example to reduce induced astigmatism with a back toroidal surface on a rigid lens (*see* Chapters 5 and 14).

Lenses of high refractive index have been tried, with varying degrees of success. The higher refractive index allows a thinner lens to be made, which is useful for lenses of high power. Hyfrax, a material produced in the USA, has been described by Morrison (1962). It has a refractive index of 1.568 and is lighter in weight than polymethyl methacrylate. Some difficulties have been experienced with its wetting properties. Although the contact angle is smaller than with polymethyl methacrylate, the material is somewhat lipophilic (fat attracting). It absorbs less water than polymethyl methacrylate and, correspondingly, contact lenses made from Hyfrax have a more constant curvature.

Similar high refractive index plastics are now being used, often with the addition of a fluorescent dye, for the segments of bifocal contact lenses. The addition of the dye, though invisible in normal light, renders fitting more easy when viewed by ultraviolet illumination.

The experimental use of synthetic sapphire material has been reported by Nissel (G., 1969, unpublished report). This has a very high refractive index of about 2.

Lenses incorporating bactericides

The material for such contact lenses has been developed in the USA (Torgerson, 1964). These lenses have a significant effect in inhibiting bacterial growth as compared with normal lenses, the degree of inhibition depending on the contact time (Mote, Schoessler and Hill, 1969; Mote and Hill, 1970). Conversely, Chalkley, Sarnat and Shock (1966) had previously found lenses of this material to be of no apparent value. It should not be forgotten that soft lenses stored in preserved saline effectively incorporate a bactericide, as the solution preservative is slowly released onto the eye during wear. The effect of this on the normal ocular flora has not been ascertained.

This concludes the details of special contact lenses; but it is anticipated that, in the near future, there will be many more special types of lens and special uses for contact lenses in the fields of scientific research, where expansion continues at a phenomenal rate.

References

ALVIS, D. L. (1966). Electroretinographic changes in controlled open angle glaucoma. *Am. J. Ophthal.* **61**, 121–131

ANDERSON, J. M. (1952). *Contact Lenses, Clinical and Other Observations*, p. 33. Brighton: Courtenay Press

ANON (1967). Contact lenses for turkeys – report. *Optician* **154**, 575

AQUAVELLA, J. V. (1976). New aspects of contact lenses in ophthalmology. In *Advances in Ophthalmology*, **32**, pp. 2–34, edited by M. J. Roper-Hall, H. Sauter and E. B. Streiff. Basel:Karger

ASTIN, C. (1987). Case report: three cases of fitting a superiorly truncated hydrophilic lens. *J. Br. Contact Lens Ass.* **10**(2), 27–28

BACKMAN, H. A. (1983). Ocular inserts for contact lens patients with dry eyes. *Int. Contact Lens Clin.* **10**, 43–48

BAILEY, N. J. (1966). Do contact lenses control myopia? *Opt. Int.* **3**, 25–30

BALDWIN, W. R., WEST, D., JOLLEY, J. and REID, W. (1969). Effects of contact lenses on refractive, corneal and axial length changes in young myopes. *Am. J. Optom.* **46**, 903–911

BALL, G. V. (1964). Characteristics of tinted contact lenses. *Br. J. physiol. Optics* **21**, 219–223

BARKAN, O. (1936). New operation for chronic glaucoma: restoration of physiological function by opening Schlemm's canal under direct magnified vision. *Am. J. Ophthal.* **19**, 951

BECKER, S. C. (1972). *Clinical Gonioscopy*. St Louis, Missouri: Mosby

BENJAMIN, W. J. (1987). CL solutions and materials: why prescribe UV-blocking contact lenses? *Int. Contact Lens Clin.* **14**, 164–165

BENNETT, Q. M. (1985). Contact lenses for diving. *Aust. J. Optom.* **68**(1), 25–26

BIER, N. (1960). *Correction of Subnormal Vision*, p. 87. London: Butterworths

BLACKSTONE, M. (1966). Hydrophilic lenses: some practical experiments. *Optician* **151**, 5–6

BLUE, H. D. (1966). Method of producing permanent wettability on plastic contact lenses. *J. Am. optom. Ass.* **37**, 678–681

BORNSCHEIN, H., WICHTERLE, O. and WÜNDSCH, L. (1966). A contact lens electrode for comparative E.R.G. studies. *Vision Res.* **6**, 773–774

CAPELLI, Q. A. (1966). Water extractives from coloured contact lenses – a report. *Opt. J. Rev. Optom.* **103**, 32

CATFORD, G. V. and MACKIE, I. A. (1968). Occlusion with high plus corneal lenses. *Br. J. Ophthal.* **52**, 342–345

CHALKLEY, T., SARNAT, L. and SHOCK, D. (1966). Evaluation of 'bacteriostatic' contact lenses. *Am. J. Ophthal.* **61**, 866–869

CHOU, B. R., CULLEN, A. P. and DUMBLETON, K. A. (1988). Protection factors of ultraviolet-blocking contact lenses. *Int. Contact Lens Clin.* **15**, 244–251

CIUFFREDA, K. J. (1980). Binocular space perception and the X-Chrom lens. *Int. Contact Lens Clin.* **7**, 71–74

CLARKE, C. (1975). Contact lenses at high altitude: experience on Everest south-west face 1975. *Br. J. Ophthal.* **60**, 479–480

COCKELL, R. R. (1967). A survey of underwater visual problems. Paper read to The Contact Lens Society, January, 1967

DICKINSON, F. (1957). The value of microlenses in progressive myopia. *Optician* **133**, 263–264

DIEFENBACH, C. B., SONI, P. S., GILLESPIE, B. J. and PENCE, N. (1988) Extended wear contact lens movement under swimming pool conditions. *Am. J. Optom. physiol. Optics*, **65**, 710–716

DITCHBURN, R. W. and GINSBORG, B. L. (1952). Vision with a stabilized retinal image. *Nature* **170**, 36–37

DOUTHWAITE, W. A. (1971). Bifocal underwater contact lenses. *Ophthal. Optician* **11**, 10–14

DRASDO, N. (1970). The effect of high powered contact lenses on the visual fixation reflex. *Br. J. physiol. Optics* **25**, 14–22

EISNER, G., LOTMAR, W. and PAPRITZ, F. (1985). A new contact glass for slit-lamp examination of the cornea, especially in specular reflection. *Ophthalmology, Instrument and Book Supplement*, Vol. 92, pp. 72–83

ERB, R. A. (1961). *Method for Producing Wettable Surfaces on Contact Lenses by Chemical Formation of Inorganic Films*. US Dept of Commerce, Office of Technical Services, Government Research Report AD-257290

EVANS, C. R. and PIGGINS, D. J. (1963). A comparison of the behaviour of geometrical shapes when viewed under conditions of steady fixation, and with apparatus for producing a stabilized retinal image. *Br. J. physiol. Optics* **20**, 261–273

EVANS, C. R. (1965). A universally fitting contact lens for the study of stabilized retinal images. *Br. J. physiol. Optics* **22**, 39–45

ESTEVEZ, J. M. J. (1967). Poly(methyl methacrylate) for use in contact lenses. *Contact Lens* **1**, 19–26

FATT, I. and HILL, R. M. (1970). Oxygen tension under a contact lens during blinking – a comparison of theory and experimental observation. *Am. J. Optom.* **47**, 50–55

FEINBLOOM, W. (1961). Feinbloom miniscope contact lens. Described by Allan Isen, *Encyclopaedia of Contact Lens Practice III*, Supplement 13, Appendix B, 53–55. South Bend, Indiana: International Optics Publishing Corporation

FILDERMAN, I. P. (1964). The spectacle lens – contact lens system. *Br. J. physiol. Optics* **21**, 195–196

FLETCHER, R. J. (1964). A study of the total light flux admitted to the interior of the eye through contact lenses. *Br. J. physiol. Optics* **21**, 134–146

FLETCHER, R. J. ['Haptos'] (1966). Electrode-bearing contact lenses. *Contact Lens* **1**(1), 19

FLETCHER, R. J. and NISTED, M. (1963). A study of coloured contact lenses and their performance. *Ophthal. Optician* **3**, 1151–1154, 1161–1163, 1203–1206, 1212–1213

FRIEDMAN, B. (1967). A contact lens for estimating corneal thickness. *Eye Ear Nose Throat Mon.* **46**, 344–345

GERSTMAN, D. R. and LEVENE, J. R. (1974). Galilean telescope for the partially sighted. *Br. J. Ophthal.* **58**, 761–765

900   Special types of contact lenses and their uses

GESSER, H. D., FUNT, B. L. and WARRINER, R. E. (1965). A method of improving the wettability of contact lenses by free radical treatment. *Am. J. Optom.* **42**, 321–324

GOLDBERG, J. B. (1975). Must the gas go through? *Optom. Wkly* **66**(34), 15–16

GOLDMANN, H. (1938). Zur Technik der Spaltlampenmikroskopie. *Ophthalmologica* **96**, 90

GOLDMANN, H. and SCHMIDT, T. (1965). Ein Kontaktglas zur Biomikroskopie der Ora Serrata und der Pars Plana. *Ophthalmologica* **149**, 481–483

GRANT, S. C. and MAY, C. H. (1972). Orthokeratology – the control of refractive errors through contact lenses. *Optician* **163**(4214), 8–11

HARDY, S. (1986). Ultraviolet and the eye: report of CooperVision symposium. *Optom. Today* **26**, 841, 844

HARRIS, M. G., OYE, R., HALL, K. and FATT, I. (1973). Contact angle measurements on hard contact lenses. *Am. J. Optom.* **50**, 446–451

HILL, R. M. (1985). The swimming eye. *Int. Contact Lens Clin.* **12**, 175–179

HILL, R. M. and LEIGHTON, A. J. (1965). Temperature changes of human cornea and tears under a contact lens, I, II & III. *Am. J. Optom.* **42**, 9–16, 71–77, 584–588

HILL, R. M. and FATT, I. (1966). Oxygen measurements under a contact lens. *Am. J. Optom.* **43**, 233–237

HILLMAN, J. S. (1976). The use of hydrophilic contact lenses. *Optician* **172**(4458), 9–11

HOUGH, D. A. and PATEL, K. D. (1986). Case report: plasma modification of GPH lenses – an unexpected clinical result. *J. Br. Contact Lens Ass.* **9**(1), 38–40

JESSEN, G. N. (1964). Contact lenses as a therapeutic device. *Am. J. Optom.* **41**, 429–435

KELLY, T. S-B. and BUTLER, D. (1964). Preliminary report on corneal lenses in relation to myopia. *Br. J. physiol. Optics* **21**, 175–186

KELLY, T. S-B. and BUTLER, D. (1971). The present position of contact lenses in relation to myopia. *Br. J. physiol. Optics* **26**, 33–48

KERNS, R. L. (1977). Research in orthokeratology. Part VI: Statistical and clinical analyses. *J. Am. optom. Ass.* **48**, 1134–1147

KERSLEY, H. J. (1975). Continuous wear lenses after aphakic operation. *Optician* **170**(4393), 12–18

KLEIN, M. (1949). Contact shell applicator for use as a corneal bath. *Br. J. Ophthal.* **33**, 716–717

KOEPPE, L. (1919). Die Theorie und Anwendung der Stereomikroskopie des lebenden menschlichen Kammerwinkels in fokalen Lichte der Gullstrandschen Nernstspaltlampe. *Münch. med. Wschr.* **66**, 708

LA BISSONIERRE, P. E. (1974). The x-chrom lens. *Int. Contact Lens Clin.* **1**(4), 48–55

LEVINSON, A., WEISSMAN, H. A. and SACHS, U. (1977). Use of the Bausch & Lomb Soflens™ plano T contact lens as a bandage. *Am. J. Optom.* **54**, 97–103

LOVSUND, P., NILSSON, S. E. G. and OBERG, P. A. (1980). The use of contact lenses in wet or damp environments. *Acta ophthal.* **58**, 794–804

LYDON, D. and TAIT, A. (1988). Lid-pressure: its measurement and probable effects on the shape and form of the cornea-rigid contact lens system. *J. Br. Contact Lens Ass.* **11**(1), 11–22

MILLODOT, M. (1965). Stabilized retinal images and disappearance time. *Br. J. physiol. Optics* **22**, 148–152

MINARIK, K. R. (1987). Using Saturn II lenses to manage toric soft lens 'failures'. *Contact Lens Forum* **12**(9), 80–81

MOLINARI, J. F. and SOCKS, J. F. (1986). Effects of hyperbaric conditions on corneal physiology with hydrogel contact lenses. *J. Br. Contact Lens Ass. Scientific Meetings 1986*, 17–19

MOORE, L. (1964). The contact lens for subnormal visual acuity. *Br. J. physiol. Optics* **21**, 203–204

MORRIS, J. (1988). Into tomorrowland: report on 1988 Bausch & Lomb national research symposium. *Optician* **196**(5169), 37, 40–41, 43

MORRISON, R. J. (1958). Observations on contact lenses and the progression of myopia. *Contacto* **2**, 20–25

MORRISON, R. J. (1962). A new substance for contact lenses. *Am. J. Optom.* **39**, 252–256

MOSSÉ, P. (1964). Underwater contact lenses. *Br. J. physiol. Optics* **21**, 250–255

MOTE, E. M. and HILL, R. M. (1970). Lens incorporated germicides: II. *J. Am. optom. Ass.* **41**, 260–262

MOTE, E. M., SCHOESSLER, J. P. and HILL, R. M. (1969). Lens incorporated germicides: I. *J. Am. optom. Ass.* **40**, 291–293

NEILL, J. C. (1962). Contact lenses and myopia. *Pen. State Alumni Bulletin* **16**, 109–116

NOLAN, J. A. (1964). Progress of myopia and contact lenses. *Contacto* **8**, 25

NOLAN, J. A. (1969). Approach to orthokeratology. *J. Am. optom. Ass.* **40**, 303–305

PETROPOULOU, N. (1975). The soft lens as a therapeutical dressing. *Optician* **169**(4380), 6–11

PITTS, D. G. (1981). Threat of ultraviolet radiation to the eye – how to protect against it. *J. Am. optom. Ass.* **52**, 949–957

RUEDMANN, A. D., Jr. and NOELL, W. K. (1961). The electroretinogram in central retinal degeneration. *Trans. Am. Acad. Ophthal. Otolaryngol.* **65**, 576–594

SABELL, A. G. (1970). Some notes on diagnostic contact lenses. *Ophthal. Optician* **10**, 1160–1162, 1173–1178

SCHEIE, H. G. (1957). Width and pigmentation of the angle of the anterior chamber. *Am. Med. Ass. Archs Ophthal.* **58**, 510–512

SCHIRMER, K. E. (1965). Faceted contact lens with a modified viewing device for fundus examination. *Archs Ophthal.* **74**, 465–469

SCHMIDT, G. M., BLANCHARD, G. L. and KELLER, W. F. (1977). The use of hydrophilic contact lenses in corneal diseases of the dog and cat: a preliminary report. *J. Small Anim. Pract.* **18**, 773–777

SHAFFER, R. N. (1962). *Stereoscopic Manual of Gonioscopy*. St Louis, Missouri: Mosby

SILVA, D. (1967). Radiographic exophthalmometry examination with the use of contact lenses. *Contacto* **11**, 57–60

SIMON, D. R. and BRADLEY, M. E. (1980). Adverse effects of contact lens wear during decompression. *J. Am. med. Ass.* **244**, 1213–1214

SOCKS, J. F. (1983). Use of contact lenses for cold weather

activities: results of a survey. *Int. Contact Lens Clin.* **10**, 82–91

SOLOMON, J., SNYDER, R. P. and KLEIN, P. (1987). Swimming with soft contact lenses. *Contact Lens Forum* **12**(5), 56–57

STONE, J. (1968). The effects of contact lenses on heterophoria and other binocular functions. *Contact Lens* **1**(7), 5–8, 26, 32

STONE, J. (1976). The possible influence of contact lenses on myopia. *Br. J. physiol. Optics* **31**, 89–114

STONE, J. and BREAKSPEAR, H. R. (1977). Two interesting cases of low visual acuity seen at The London Refraction Hospital. *Contact Lens J.* **6**(3), 3–4, 6

TAMMEUS, J., KRALL, C. J. and RENGSTORFF, R. H. (1983). Therapeutic extended wear contact lens for corneal injury in a horse. *J. Am. Vet. Med. Ass.* **182**, 286

TORGERSON, J. T. (1964). Antimicrobial activity of contact lenses incorporating disinfectants through a process of polymerization. National Eye Research Foundation Report. *Contacto* **8**, 9–26

URIBE TRONCOSO, M. (1921). Gonioscopy with the electric ophthalmoscope. New York Academy of Medicine, referred to in *Gonioscopy*, by Troncoso, Davis Company, Philadelphia, 1947

VAN BEUNINGEN, E. G. A. (1953). Das Pyramidengonioskop. *Klin. Mbl. Augenheilk.* **122**, 172–178

Appendices

Appendix A: Spectacle and ocular refraction, or effective power of spectacle lenses in air at various vertex distances: Positive lenses

Body of table shows effective power at stated vertex distance. (*See* Appendix E, program index no. 8)

Spectacle refraction or spectacle lens power (BVP) (D)	Ocular refraction (D) *for vertex distances (mm) of:*														
	6	7	8	9	10	11	12	13	14	15	16	17	18	19	20
+0.25	0.25	0.25	0.25	0.25	0.25	0.25	0.25	0.25	0.25	0.25	0.25	0.25	0.25	0.25	0.25
.50	0.50	0.50	0.50	0.50	0.50	0.50	0.50	0.50	0.50	0.50	0.50	0.50	0.50	0.50	0.51
.75	0.75	0.75	0.75	0.76	0.76	0.76	0.76	0.76	0.76	0.76	0.76	0.76	0.76	0.76	0.76
+1.00	1.01	1.01	1.01	1.01	1.01	1.01	1.01	1.01	1.01	1.02	1.02	1.02	1.01	1.02	1.02
.25	1.26	1.26	1.26	1.26	1.27	1.27	1.27	1.27	1.27	1.27	1.28	1.28	1.28	1.28	1.28
.50	1.51	1.52	1.52	1.52	1.52	1.52	1.53	1.53	1.53	1.53	1.54	1.54	1.54	1.54	1.55
.75	1.77	1.77	1.78	1.78	1.78	1.79	1.79	1.79	1.80	1.80	1.80	1.81	1.81	1.81	1.81
+2.00	2.02	2.03	2.03	2.04	2.04	2.04	2.05	2.05	2.06	2.06	2.07	2.07	2.07	2.08	2.08
.25	2.28	2.29	2.29	2.30	2.30	2.31	2.31	2.32	2.33	2.33	2.34	2.34	2.35	2.35	2.36
.50	2.54	2.54	2.55	2.56	2.56	2.57	2.58	2.58	2.59	2.60	2.60	2.61	2.62	2.62	2.63
.75	2.79	2.80	2.81	2.82	2.82	2.83	2.84	2.85	2.86	2.87	2.87	2.88	2.89	2.90	2.91
+3.00	3.06	3.06	3.07	3.08	3.09	3.10	3.11	3.12	3.13	3.14	3.15	3.16	3.17	3.18	3.19
.25	3.31	3.33	3.34	3.35	3.36	3.37	3.38	3.39	3.40	3.42	3.43	3.44	3.45	3.46	3.48
.50	3.58	3.59	3.60	3.61	3.63	3.64	3.65	3.67	3.68	3.69	3.71	3.72	3.74	3.75	3.76
.75	3.84	3.85	3.87	3.88	3.90	3.91	3.93	3.94	3.96	3.97	3.99	4.00	4.02	4.04	4.05
+4.00	4.10	4.12	4.13	4.15	4.17	4.18	4.20	4.22	4.24	4.26	4.27	4.29	4.31	4.33	4.35
.25	4.36	4.38	4.40	4.42	4.44	4.46	4.48	4.50	4.52	4.54	4.56	4.58	4.60	4.62	4.64
.50	4.63	4.65	4.67	4.69	4.71	4.73	4.76	4.78	4.80	4.83	4.85	4.87	4.90	4.92	4.95
.75	4.89	4.91	4.94	4.96	4.99	5.01	5.04	5.06	5.09	5.12	5.14	5.17	5.19	5.22	5.25
+5.00	5.15	5.18	5.21	5.24	5.26	5.29	5.32	5.35	5.38	5.41	5.43	5.46	5.49	5.52	5.56
.25	5.42	5.45	5.48	5.51	5.54	5.57	5.60	5.63	5.67	5.70	5.73	5.76	5.80	5.83	5.87
.50	5.69	5.72	5.75	5.79	5.82	5.85	5.89	5.92	5.96	6.00	6.03	6.07	6.11	6.14	6.18
.75	5.96	5.99	6.03	6.06	6.10	6.14	6.18	6.22	6.25	6.29	6.33	6.37	6.41	6.46	6.50
+6.00	6.22	6.26	6.30	6.34	6.38	6.42	6.46	6.51	6.55	6.59	6.64	6.68	6.72	6.77	6.82
.25	6.49	6.54	6.58	6.62	6.67	6.71	6.76	6.80	6.85	6.90	6.94	6.99	7.04	7.09	7.14
.50	6.77	6.81	6.86	6.91	6.95	7.00	7.05	7.10	7.15	7.20	7.26	7.31	7.36	7.42	7.47
.75	7.04	7.09	7.14	7.19	7.24	7.29	7.35	7.40	7.46	7.51	7.57	7.63	7.69	7.75	7.82
+7.00	7.30	7.36	7.41	7.47	7.52	7.58	7.64	7.70	7.76	7.82	7.88	7.94	8.01	8.07	8.14
.25	7.58	7.64	7.70	7.76	7.82	7.88	7.94	8.01	8.07	8.14	8.20	8.27	8.34	8.41	8.48
.50	7.86	7.92	7.98	8.05	8.11	8.18	8.24	8.31	8.38	8.45	8.53	8.60	8.67	8.75	8.83
.75	8.13	8.20	8.26	8.33	8.40	8.47	8.55	8.62	8.70	8.77	8.85	8.93	9.01	9.09	9.17
+8.00	8.40	8.47	8.55	8.62	8.70	8.77	8.85	8.93	9.01	9.09	9.17	9.26	9.35	9.43	9.52
.25	8.68	8.76	8.83	8.91	8.99	9.07	9.16	9.24	9.33	9.42	9.51	9.60	9.69	9.78	9.88
.50	8.96	9.04	9.12	9.21	9.29	9.38	9.47	9.56	9.65	9.75	9.84	9.94	10.04	10.14	10.25
.75	9.23	9.32	9.41	9.50	9.59	9.68	9.78	9.87	9.97	10.07	10.17	10.28	10.38	10.49	10.60
+9.00	9.51	9.61	9.70	9.79	9.89	9.98	10.09	10.19	10.30	10.41	10.52	10.63	10.74	10.86	10.98
.25	9.79	9.89	9.99	10.09	10.19	10.30	10.41	10.52	10.63	10.74	10.86	10.98	11.10	11.22	11.35
.50	10.07	10.17	10.28	10.38	10.49	10.60	10.72	10.83	10.95	11.07	11.20	11.33	11.45	11.59	11.72
.75	10.35	10.46	10.57	10.68	10.80	10.92	11.04	11.16	11.29	11.42	11.55	11.68	11.82	11.96	12.11

Appendix A (contd)

Ocular refraction (D) for vertex distances (mm) of:

Spectacle refraction or spectacle lens power (BVP) (D)	6	7	8	9	10	11	12	13	14	15	16	17	18	19	20
+10.00	10.64	10.75	10.87	10.99	11.11	11.24	11.36	11.49	11.63	11.76	11.90	12.05	12.20	12.35	12.50
.25	10.92	11.04	11.17	11.29	11.42	11.55	11.69	11.83	11.97	12.11	12.26	12.41	12.57	12.73	12.89
.50	11.21	11.33	11.46	11.60	11.73	11.87	12.01	12.16	12.31	12.46	12.62	12.78	12.95	13.12	13.29
.75	11.49	11.63	11.76	11.90	12.05	12.19	12.34	12.50	12.66	12.82	12.98	13.15	13.33	13.51	13.69
+11.00	11.78	11.92	12.06	12.21	12.36	12.51	12.67	12.84	13.00	13.17	13.35	13.53	13.72	13.91	14.10
.25	12.06	12.21	12.36	12.52	12.68	12.84	13.01	13.18	13.35	13.53	13.72	13.91	14.11	14.31	14.52
.50	12.35	12.51	12.66	12.83	12.99	13.16	13.34	13.52	13.71	13.90	14.09	14.29	14.50	14.71	14.93
.75	12.64	12.80	12.97	13.14	13.31	13.49	13.68	13.87	14.06	14.26	14.47	14.68	14.90	15.13	15.36
+12.00	12.93	13.10	13.27	13.45	13.64	13.83	14.02	14.22	14.42	14.63	14.85	15.08	15.31	15.54	15.79
.25	13.22	13.40	13.58	13.77	13.96	14.16	14.36	14.57	14.79	15.01	15.24	15.47	15.72	15.97	16.23
.50	13.51	13.70	13.89	14.08	14.29	14.49	14.71	14.93	15.15	15.38	15.62	15.87	16.13	16.39	16.67
.75	13.81	14.00	14.20	14.40	14.61	14.83	15.05	15.28	15.52	15.77	16.02	16.28	16.55	16.83	17.11
+13.00	14.10	14.30	14.51	14.72	14.94	15.17	15.40	15.64	15.89	16.15	16.41	16.69	16.97	17.27	17.57
.25	14.39	14.60	14.82	15.04	15.27	15.51	15.76	16.01	16.27	16.54	16.82	17.10	17.40	17.71	18.03
.50	14.69	14.91	15.14	15.37	15.61	15.86	16.11	16.37	16.65	16.93	17.22	17.52	17.83	18.16	18.49
.75	14.99	15.21	15.45	15.69	15.94	16.20	16.47	16.74	17.03	17.32	17.63	17.94	18.27	18.61	18.96
+14.00	15.28	15.52	15.77	16.02	16.28	16.55	16.83	17.11	17.41	17.72	18.04	18.37	18.72	19.07	19.44
.25	15.58	15.83	16.08	16.35	16.62	16.90	17.19	17.49	17.80	18.12	18.46	18.80	19.16	19.54	19.93
.50	15.88	16.14	16.40	16.68	16.96	17.25	17.55	17.87	18.19	18.53	18.88	19.24	19.62	20.01	20.42
.75	16.18	16.45	16.72	17.01	17.30	17.61	17.92	18.25	18.59	18.94	19.31	19.69	20.08	20.49	20.92
+15.00	16.48	16.76	17.04	17.34	17.65	17.96	18.29	18.63	18.99	19.35	19.74	20.13	20.55	20.98	21.43
.25	16.79	17.07	17.37	17.68	18.00	18.33	18.67	19.02	19.39	19.77	20.17	20.59	21.02	21.47	21.94
.50	17.09	17.39	17.69	18.01	18.34	18.68	19.04	19.41	19.79	20.19	20.61	21.04	21.50	21.97	22.46
.75	17.39	17.70	18.02	18.35	18.70	19.05	19.42	19.81	20.21	20.62	21.06	21.51	21.98	22.48	22.99
+16.00	17.70	18.02	18.35	18.69	19.05	19.42	19.80	20.20	20.62	21.05	21.51	21.98	22.47	22.99	23.53
.25	18.01	18.34	18.68	19.03	19.40	19.79	20.19	20.60	21.04	21.49	21.96	22.45	22.97	23.51	24.07
.50	18.31	18.65	19.01	19.38	19.76	20.16	20.57	21.01	21.46	21.93	22.42	22.93	23.47	24.03	24.63
.75	18.62	18.97	19.34	19.72	20.12	20.53	20.96	21.41	21.88	22.37	22.88	23.42	23.98	24.57	25.19
+17.00	18.93	19.30	19.68	20.07	20.48	20.91	21.36	21.82	22.31	22.82	**23.35**	23.91	24.50	25.11	25.76
.25	19.24	19.62	20.01	20.42	20.85	21.29	21.75	22.24	22.74	23.27	23.83	24.41	25.02	25.66	26.34
.50	19.55	19.94	20.35	20.77	21.21	21.67	22.15	22.65	23.18	23.73	24.31	24.91	25.55	26.22	26.92
.75	19.87	20.27	20.69	21.12	21.58	22.06	22.55	23.07	23.62	24.19	24.79	25.42	26.08	26.78	27.52
+18.00	20.18	20.59	21.03	21.48	21.95	22.44	22.96	23.50	24.06	24.66	25.28	25.94	26.63	27.36	28.12
.25	20.49	20.92	21.37	21.84	22.32	22.83	23.37	23.93	24.51	25.13	**25.78**	26.46	27.18	27.94	28.74
.50	20.81	21.25	21.71	22.20	22.70	23.23	23.78	24.36	24.97	25.61	26.28	26.99	27.74	28.53	29.37
.75	21.13	21.58	22.06	22.56	23.08	23.62	24.19	24.79	25.42	26.09	26.79	27.52	28.30	29.13	30.00
+19.00	21.44	21.91	22.41	22.92	23.46	24.02	24.61	25.23	25.89	26.57	27.30	28.06	28.88	29.73	30.65
.25	21.76	22.25	22.75	23.28	23.84	24.42	25.03	25.68	26.35	27.07	27.82	28.61	29.46	30.35	31.30
.50	22.08	22.58	23.10	23.65	24.22	24.82	25.46	26.12	26.82	27.56	28.34	29.17	30.05	30.98	31.97
.75	22.40	22.92	23.46	24.02	24.61	25.23	25.88	26.57	27.30	28.06	28.87	29.73	30.64	31.61	32.64
+20.00	22.73	23.26	23.81	24.39	25.00	25.64	26.32	27.03	27.78	28.57	29.41	30.30	31.25	32.26	33.33

	6	7	8	9	10	11	12	13	14	15	16	17	18	19	20
-0.25	0.25	0.25	0.25	0.25	0.25	0.25	0.25	0.25	0.25	0.25	0.25	0.25	0.25	0.25	0.25
-0.50	0.50	0.50	0.50	0.50	0.50	0.50	0.50	0.50	0.50	0.50	0.50	0.50	0.50	0.50	0.50
-0.75	0.75	0.75	0.75	0.75	0.74	0.74	0.74	0.74	0.74	0.74	0.74	0.74	0.74	0.74	0.74
-1.00	0.99	0.99	0.99	0.99	0.99	0.99	0.99	0.99	0.99	0.99	0.98	0.98	0.98	0.98	0.98
-1.25	1.24	1.24	1.24	1.24	1.23	1.23	1.23	1.23	1.23	1.23	1.23	1.22	1.22	1.22	1.22
-1.50	1.49	1.48	1.48	1.48	1.48	1.48	1.47	1.47	1.47	1.47	1.46	1.46	1.46	1.46	1.46
-1.75	1.73	1.73	1.73	1.72	1.72	1.72	1.71	1.71	1.71	1.71	1.70	1.70	1.70	1.69	1.69
-2.00	1.98	1.97	1.97	1.96	1.96	1.96	1.95	1.95	1.95	1.94	1.94	1.93	1.93	1.93	1.92
-2.25	2.22	2.22	2.21	2.21	2.20	2.20	2.19	2.19	2.18	2.18	2.17	2.17	2.16	2.16	2.15
-2.50	2.46	2.46	2.45	2.44	2.44	2.43	2.43	2.42	2.42	2.41	2.40	2.40	2.39	2.39	2.38
-2.75	2.71	2.70	2.69	2.68	2.68	2.67	2.66	2.66	2.65	2.64	2.63	2.63	2.62	2.61	2.61
-3.00	2.95	2.94	2.93	2.92	2.91	2.90	2.90	2.89	2.88	2.87	2.86	2.85	2.85	2.84	2.83
-3.25	3.19	3.18	3.17	3.16	3.15	3.14	3.13	3.12	3.11	3.10	3.09	3.08	3.07	3.06	3.05
-3.50	3.43	3.42	3.40	3.39	3.38	3.37	3.36	3.35	3.34	3.33	3.31	3.30	3.29	3.28	3.27
-3.75	3.67	3.65	3.64	3.63	3.61	3.60	3.59	3.58	3.56	3.55	3.54	3.52	3.51	3.50	3.49
-4.00	3.91	3.89	3.88	3.86	3.85	3.83	3.82	3.80	3.79	3.77	3.76	3.75	3.73	3.72	3.70
-4.25	4.14	4.13	4.11	4.09	4.08	4.06	4.04	4.03	4.01	4.00	3.98	3.96	3.95	3.93	3.92
-4.50	4.38	4.36	4.34	4.33	4.31	4.29	4.27	4.25	4.23	4.22	4.20	4.18	4.16	4.15	4.13
-4.75	4.62	4.60	4.58	4.56	4.54	4.51	4.49	4.47	4.45	4.43	4.42	4.40	4.38	4.36	4.34
-5.00	4.85	4.83	4.81	4.78	4.76	4.74	4.72	4.69	4.67	4.65	4.63	4.61	4.59	4.57	4.55
-5.25	5.09	5.06	5.04	5.01	4.99	4.96	4.94	4.91	4.89	4.87	4.84	4.82	4.80	4.77	4.75
-5.50	5.32	5.30	5.27	5.24	5.21	5.19	5.16	5.13	5.11	5.08	5.06	5.03	5.01	4.98	4.96
-5.75	5.56	5.53	5.50	5.47	5.44	5.41	5.38	5.35	5.32	5.29	5.27	5.24	5.21	5.18	5.16
-6.00	5.79	5.76	5.72	5.69	5.66	5.63	5.60	5.56	5.53	5.50	5.47	5.44	5.41	5.39	5.36
-6.25	6.02	5.99	5.95	5.92	5.88	5.85	5.81	5.78	5.75	5.71	5.68	5.65	5.62	5.59	5.56
-6.50	6.26	6.22	6.18	6.14	6.11	6.07	6.03	6.00	5.96	5.92	5.89	5.85	5.82	5.79	5.75
-6.75	6.49	6.45	6.41	6.37	6.33	6.29	6.25	6.21	6.17	6.13	6.09	6.06	6.02	5.98	5.95
-7.00	6.72	6.67	6.63	6.58	6.54	6.50	6.46	6.41	6.37	6.33	6.29	6.25	6.22	6.18	6.14
-7.25	6.94	6.90	6.85	6.81	6.76	6.72	6.67	6.63	6.58	6.54	6.50	6.46	6.41	6.37	6.33
-7.50	7.18	7.13	7.08	7.03	6.98	6.93	6.88	6.84	6.79	6.74	6.70	6.65	6.61	6.57	6.52
-7.75	7.41	7.35	7.30	7.25	7.19	7.14	7.09	7.04	6.99	6.94	6.90	6.85	6.80	6.76	6.71
-8.00	7.63	7.58	7.52	7.46	7.41	7.35	7.30	7.25	7.19	7.14	7.09	7.04	6.99	6.94	6.90
-8.25	7.86	7.80	7.74	7.68	7.62	7.56	7.51	7.45	7.40	7.34	7.29	7.24	7.18	7.13	7.08
-8.50	8.09	8.03	7.96	7.90	7.84	7.78	7.72	7.66	7.60	7.54	7.49	7.43	7.37	7.32	7.27
-8.75	8.31	8.24	8.18	8.11	8.05	7.98	7.92	7.86	7.79	7.73	7.67+	7.62	7.56	7.50	7.45
-9.00	8.54	8.47	8.40	8.33	8.26	8.19	8.12	8.06	7.99	7.93	7.87	7.81	7.75	7.69	7.63
-9.25	8.76	8.69	8.61	8.54	8.47	8.40	8.33	8.26	8.19	8.12	8.06	7.99	7.93	7.87	7.81
-9.50	8.98	8.90	8.83	8.75	8.67	8.60	8.53	8.45	8.38	8.31	8.24	8.18	8.11	8.05	7.98
-9.75	9.21	9.12	9.04	8.96	8.88	8.80	8.73	8.65	8.58	8.50	8.43	8.36	8.29	8.22	8.16
-10.00	9.43	9.35	9.26	9.17	9.09	9.01	8.93	8.85	8.77	8.70	8.62	8.55	8.47	8.40	8.33
-10.25	9.65+	9.56	9.47	9.38	9.29	9.21	9.12	9.04	8.96	8.88	8.80	8.73	8.65+	8.58	8.50
-10.50	9.88	9.78	9.69	9.59	9.50	9.41	9.32	9.24	9.15+	9.07	8.99	8.91	8.83	8.75+	8.68
-10.75	10.10	10.00	9.90	9.80	9.71	9.61	9.52	9.43	9.34	9.26	9.17	9.09	9.01	8.93	8.85
-11.00	10.32	10.21	10.11	10.01	9.91	9.81	9.72	9.62	9.53	9.44	9.35+	9.27	9.18	9.10	9.02
-11.25	10.54	10.43	10.32	10.22	10.11	10.01	9.91	9.81	9.72	9.63	9.53	9.44	9.36	9.27	9.18
-11.50	10.76	10.64	10.53	10.42	10.31	10.21	10.11	10.00	9.90	9.81	9.71	9.62	9.53	9.44	9.35
-11.75	10.98	10.86	10.74	10.63	10.51	10.40	10.30	10.19	10.09	9.99	9.89	9.79	9.70	9.61	9.51

Appendix A (contd)

Ocular refraction (D) for vertex distances (mm) of:

Spectacle refraction or spectacle lens power (BVP) (D)	6	7	8	9	10	11	12	13	14	15	16	17	18	19	20
-12.00	11.19	11.07	10.95-	10.83	10.71	10.60	10.49	10.38	10.27	10.17	10.07	9.97	9.87	9.77	9.68
.25	11.41	11.28	11.16	11.03	10.91	10.80	10.68	10.57	10.46	10.35	10.24	10.14	10.04	9.94	9.84
.50	11.63	11.49	11.36	11.24	11.11	10.99	10.87	10.75+	10.64	10.53	10.42	10.31	10.20	10.10	10.00
.75	11.84	11.71	11.57	11.44	11.31	11.18	11.06	10.94	10.82	10.70	10.59	10.48	10.37	10.26	10.16
-13.00	12.06	11.92	11.78	11.64	11.50	11.37	11.25	11.12	11.00	10.88	10.76	10.65	10.54	10.43	10.32
.25	12.27	12.13	11.98	11.84	11.70	11.56	11.43	11.30	11.18	11.05-	10.93	10.81	10.70	10.59	10.47
.50	12.49	12.34	12.18	12.04	11.89	11.76	11.62	11.49	11.35-	11.23	11.10	10.98	10.86	10.74	10.63
.75	12.70	12.54	12.39	12.24	12.09	11.94	11.80	11.66	11.53	11.40	11.27	11.14	11.02	10.90	10.78
-14.00	12.91	12.75+	12.59	12.43	12.28	12.13	11.99	11.84	11.71	11.57	11.44	11.31	11.18	11.06	10.94
.25	13.13	12.96	12.79	12.63	12.47	12.32	12.17	12.02	11.88	11.74	11.60	11.47	11.34	11.21	11.09
.50	13.34	13.16	12.99	12.83	12.66	12.50	12.35+	12.20	12.05+	11.91	11.77	11.63	11.50	11.37	11.24
.75	13.55+	13.37	13.19	13.02	12.85+	12.69	12.53	12.38	12.22	12.08	11.93	11.79	11.66	11.52	11.39
-15.00	13.76	13.57	13.39	13.22	13.04	12.87	12.71	12.55+	12.40	12.24	12.10	11.95+	11.81	11.67	11.54
.25	13.97	13.78	13.59	13.41	13.23	13.06	12.89	12.73	12.57	12.41	12.26	12.11	11.97	11.82	11.69
.50	14.18	13.98	13.79	13.60	13.42	13.24	13.07	12.90	12.74	12.58	12.42	12.27	12.12	11.97	11.83
.75	14.39	14.19	13.99	13.80	13.61	13.42	13.25	13.07	12.90	12.74	12.58	12.42	12.27	12.12	11.98
-16.00	14.60	14.39	14.18	13.99	13.79	13.61	13.42	13.25	13.07	12.90	12.74	12.58	12.42	12.27	12.12
.25	14.81	14.59	14.38	14.18	13.98	13.79	13.60	13.42	13.24	13.07	12.90	12.73	12.57	12.42	12.26
.50	15.01	14.79	14.58	14.37	14.16	13.96	13.77	13.59	13.40	13.23	13.05+	12.88	12.72	12.56	12.41
.75	15.22	14.99	14.77	14.56	14.35-	14.14	13.95	13.76	13.57	13.39	13.21	13.04	12.87	12.71	12.55
-17.00	15.43	15.19	14.97	14.74	14.53	14.32	14.12	13.92	13.73	13.55	13.37	13.19	13.02	12.85+	12.69
.25	15.63	15.39	15.16	14.93	14.71	14.50	14.29	14.09	13.89	13.70	13.52	13.34	13.16	12.99	12.83
.50	15.84	15.59	15.35+	15.12	14.89	14.68	14.46	14.26	14.06	13.86	13.67	13.49	13.31	13.13	12.96
.75	16.04	15.79	15.54	15.30	15.07	14.85+	14.63	14.42	14.22	14.02	13.82	13.64	13.45+	13.27	13.10
-18.00	16.24	15.98	15.73	15.49	15.25+	15.02	14.80	14.59	14.38	14.17	13.97	13.78	13.59	13.41	13.23
.25	16.45+	16.18	15.93	15.68	15.43	15.20	14.97	14.75+	14.54	14.33	14.13	13.93	13.74	13.55+	13.37
.50	16.65+	16.38	16.12	15.86	15.61	15.37	15.14	14.91	14.70	14.48	14.28	14.07	13.88	13.69	13.50
.75	16.85+	16.58	16.31	16.04	15.79	15.54	15.31	15.08	14.85+	14.63	14.42	14.22	14.02	13.83	13.64
-19.00	17.06	16.77	16.49	16.23	15.97	15.72	15.47	15.24	15.01	14.79	14.57	14.36	14.16	13.96	13.77
.25	17.26	16.96	16.68	16.41	16.14	15.89	15.64	15.40	15.16	14.94	14.72	14.50	14.30	14.09	13.90
.50	17.46	17.16	16.87	16.59	16.32	16.06	15.80	15.56	15.32	15.09	14.86	14.65	14.43	14.23	14.03
.75	17.66	17.35+	17.06	16.77	16.49	16.23	15.97	15.72	15.47	15.24	15.01	14.79	14.57	14.36	14.16
-20.00	17.86	17.54	17.24	16.95	16.67	16.39	16.13	15.87	15.62	15.38	15.15+	14.93	14.71	14.49	14.29
.25	18.06	17.74	17.43	17.13	16.84	16.56	16.29	16.03	15.78	15.53	15.29	15.06	14.84	14.62	14.41
.50	18.25	17.93	17.61	17.31	17.01	16.73	16.45	16.19	15.93	15.68	15.44	15.20	14.97	14.75+	14.54
.75	18.45-	18.12	17.80	17.49	17.19	16.89	16.61	16.34	16.08	15.83	15.58	15.34	15.11	14.88	14.66

	6	7	8	9	10	11	12	13	14	15	16	17	18	19	20
-21.00	18.65-	18.31	17.98	17.66	17.36	17.06	16.77	16.50	16.23	15.97	15.72	15.48	15.24	15.01	14.79
.25	18.85-	18.50	18.16	17.84	17.53	17.22	16.93	16.65	16.38	16.11	15.86	15.61	15.37	15.14	14.91
.50	19.04	18.69	18.35-	18.01	17.70	17.39	17.09	16.80	16.53	16.26	16.00	15.75-	15.50	15.26	15.04
.75	19.24	18.88	18.53	18.19	17.86	17.55+	17.25-	16.95+	16.67	16.40	16.13	15.88	15.63	15.39	15.16
-22.00	19.43	19.05+	18.71	18.36	18.03	17.71	17.40	17.11	16.82	16.54	16.27	16.01	15.76	15.51	15.28
.25	19.63	19.25-	18.89	18.54	18.20	17.88	17.56	17.26	16.97	16.68	16.41	16.14	15.89	15.64	15.40
.50	19.82	19.44	19.07	18.71	18.37	18.04	17.72	17.41	17.11	16.82	16.54	16.30	16.01	15.76	15.52
.75	20.02	19.62	19.25-	18.88	18.53	18.20	17.87	17.56	17.25	16.96	16.68	16.40	16.14	15.88	15.63
-23.00	20.21	19.81	19.43	19.05+	18.70	18.36	18.02	17.71	17.40	17.10	16.81	16.53	16.27	16.01	15.75+
.25	20.40	20.00	19.60	19.23	18.86	18.52	18.18	17.85+	17.54	17.24	16.95	16.66	16.39	16.13	15.87
.50	20.60	20.18	19.78	19.40	19.03	18.67	18.33	18.00	17.68	17.38	17.08	16.79	16.52	16.25-	15.99
.75	20.79	20.36	19.96	19.57	19.19	18.83	18.48	18.15-	17.82	17.51	17.21	16.92	16.64	16.37	16.10
-24.00	20.98	20.55-	20.13	19.74	19.35+	18.99	18.63	18.29	17.96	17.65	17.34	17.04	16.76	16.48	16.22
.25	21.17	20.73	20.31	19.90	19.52	19.14	18.78	18.44	18.10	17.78	17.47	17.17	16.88	16.60	16.33
.50	21.36	20.91	20.48	20.07	19.68	19.30	18.93	18.58	18.24	17.91	17.60	17.30	17.00	16.72	16.44
.75	21.55+	21.10	20.66	20.24	19.84	19.45+	19.08	18.73	18.38	18.05	17.73	17.42	17.12	16.83	16.56
-25.00	21.74	21.28	20.83	20.41	20.00	19.61	19.23	18.87	18.52	18.18	17.86	17.54	17.24	16.95-	16.67
.25	21.93	21.46	21.01	20.58	20.16	19.76	19.38	19.01	18.66	18.32	17.99	17.67	17.36	17.06	16.78
.50	22.12	21.64	21.18	20.74	20.32	19.91	19.52	19.15-	18.79	18.44	18.11	17.79	17.48	17.18	16.89
.75	22.31	21.82	21.35+	20.91	20.48	20.07	19.67	19.29	18.93	18.58	18.24	17.91	17.60	17.29	17.00
-26.00	22.49	22.00	21.52	21.07	20.64	20.22	19.82	19.43	19.06	18.71	18.36	18.03	17.71	17.40	17.11
.25	22.68	22.17	21.69	21.23	20.79	20.37	19.96	19.57	19.19	18.83	18.48	18.15	17.83	17.51	17.21
.50	22.86	22.35+	21.86	21.39	20.95-	20.52	20.10	19.71	19.33	18.96	18.61	18.27	17.94	17.62	17.32
.75	23.05+	22.53	22.04	21.56	21.11	20.67	20.25	19.85-	19.46	19.09	18.73	18.39	18.06	17.74	17.43
-27.00	23.23	22.71	22.20	21.72	21.26	20.82	20.39	19.98	19.59	19.22	18.85+	18.50	18.17	17.84	17.53
.25	23.42	22.88	22.37	21.88	21.41	20.96	20.53	20.12	19.72	19.34	18.98	18.62	18.28	17.95+	17.64
.50	23.61	23.06	22.54	22.05-	21.57	21.11	20.68	20.26	19.86	19.47	19.10	18.74	18.40	18.06	17.74
.75	23.79	23.23	22.71	22.20	21.72	21.26	20.82	20.39	19.98	19.59	19.22	18.85+	18.50	18.17	17.84
-28.00	23.97	23.41	22.88	22.36	21.87	21.41	20.96	20.53	20.11	19.72	19.34	18.97	18.62	18.28	17.95-
.25	24.15+	23.58	23.04	22.52	22.03	21.55+	21.10	20.66	20.24	19.84	19.46	19.08	18.73	18.38	18.05+
.50	24.34	23.76	23.21	22.68	22.18	21.70	21.24	20.79	20.37	19.96	19.57	19.20	18.84	18.49	18.15+
.75	24.52	23.93	23.38	22.84	22.33	21.84	21.38	20.93	20.50	20.09	19.69	19.31	18.95-	18.59	18.25+
-29.00	24.70	24.11	23.54	23.00	22.48	21.99	21.51	21.06	20.63	20.21	19.81	19.43	19.05+	18.70	18.36
.25	24.88	24.28	23.70	23.15	22.63	22.13	21.65	21.19	20.75	20.33	19.92	19.54	19.16	18.80	18.45+
.50	25.06	24.45-	23.87	23.31	22.78	22.27	21.79	21.32	20.88	20.45	20.04	19.65	19.27	18.90	18.55+
.75	25.25-	24.62	24.03	23.47	22.93	22.42	21.93	21.45+	21.00	20.57	20.16	19.76	19.38	19.01	18.65+
-30.00	25.42	24.79	24.19	23.62	23.08	22.56	22.06	21.58	21.13	20.69	20.27	19.87	19.48	19.11	18.75

Appendix B: Tables of radius/power considerations

Table B.I Surface power (D) for various radii and refractive index differences

Radii, r (mm)	Surface powers (D) for refractive index differences of								
	1.568–1	1.530–1	1.470–1	1.4448–1	1.430–1	1.410–1	1.376–1	1.3375–1	1.490–1.336
5.00	113.600	106.000	94.000	88.960	86.000	82.000	75.200	67.500	30.800
5.10	111.373	103.922	92.157	87.216	84.314	80.392	73.725	66.176	30.196
5.20	109.231	101.923	90.385	85.538	82.692	78.846	72.308	64.904	29.615
5.30	107.170	100.000	88.679	83.925	81.132	77.358	70.943	63.679	29.057
5.40	105.185	98.148	87.037	82.370	79.630	75.926	69.630	62.500	28.519
5.50	103.273	96.364	85.455	80.873	78.182	74.545	68.364	61.364	28.000
5.60	101.429	94.643	83.929	79.429	76.786	73.214	67.143	60.268	27.500
5.70	99.649	92.982	82.456	78.035	75.439	71.930	65.965	59.211	27.018
5.80	97.931	91.379	81.034	76.690	74.138	70.690	64.828	58.190	26.552
5.90	96.271	89.831	79.661	75.390	72.881	69.492	63.729	57.203	26.102
6.00	94.667	88.333	78.333	74.133	71.667	68.333	62.667	56.250	25.667
6.10	93.115	86.885	77.049	72.918	70.492	67.213	61.639	55.328	25.246
6.20	91.613	85.484	75.806	71.742	69.355	66.129	60.645	54.435	24.839
6.30	90.159	84.127	74.603	70.603	68.254	65.079	59.683	53.571	24.444
6.40	88.750	82.813	73.438	69.500	67.189	64.063	58.750	52.734	24.063
6.50	87.385	81.538	72.308	68.431	66.154	63.077	57.846	51.923	23.692
6.60	86.061	80.303	71.212	67.394	65.152	62.121	56.970	51.136	23.333
6.70	84.776	79.104	70.149	66.388	64.179	61.194	56.119	50.373	22.985
6.80	83.529	77.941	69.118	65.412	63.235	60.294	55.294	49.632	22.647
6.90	82.319	76.812	68.116	64.464	62.319	59.420	54.493	48.913	22.319
7.00	81.143	75.714	67.143	63.543	61.429	58.571	53.714	48.214	22.000
7.05	80.567	75.177	66.667	63.092	60.993	58.156	53.333	47.872	21.844
7.10	80.000	74.648	66.197	62.648	60.563	57.746	52.958	47.535	21.690
7.15	79.441	74.126	65.734	62.210	60.140	57.343	52.587	47.203	21.538
7.20	78.889	73.611	65.278	61.778	59.722	56.944	52.222	46.875	21.389
7.25	78.345	73.103	64.829	61.352	59.310	56.552	51.862	46.552	21.241
7.30	77.808	72.603	64.384	60.932	58.904	56.164	51.507	46.233	21.096
7.35	77.279	72.109	63.946	60.517	58.503	55.782	51.156	45.918	20.952
7.40	76.757	71.622	63.514	60.108	58.108	55.405	50.811	45.608	20.811
7.45	76.242	71.141	63.087	59.705	57.718	55.034	50.470	45.302	20.671
7.50	75.733	70.667	62.667	59.307	57.333	54.667	50.133	45.000	20.533
7.55	75.232	70.199	62.252	58.914	56.954	54.305	49.801	44.702	20.397
7.60	74.737	69.737	61.842	58.526	56.579	53.947	49.474	44.408	20.263
7.65	74.248	69.281	61.438	58.144	56.209	53.595	49.150	44.118	20.131
7.70	73.766	68.831	61.039	57.766	55.844	53.247	48.831	43.831	20.000
7.75	73.290	68.387	60.645	57.394	55.484	52.903	48.516	43.548	19.871
7.80	72.821	67.949	60.256	57.026	55.128	52.564	48.205	43.269	19.744
7.85	72.357	67.516	59.873	56.662	54.777	52.229	47.898	42.994	19.618
7.90	71.899	67.089	59.494	56.304	54.430	51.899	47.595	42.722	19.494
7.95	71.447	66.667	59.119	55.950	54.088	51.572	47.296	42.453	19.371
8.00	71.000	66.250	58.750	55.600	53.750	51.250	47.000	42.188	19.250
8.05	70.559	65.839	58.385	55.255	53.416	50.932	46.708	41.925	19.130
8.10	70.123	65.432	58.025	54.914	53.086	50.617	46.420	41.667	19.012
8.15	69.693	65.031	57.669	54.577	52.761	50.307	46.135	41.411	18.896
8.20	69.268	64.634	57.317	54.244	52.439	50.000	45.854	41.159	18.780
8.25	68.848	64.242	56.970	53.915	52.121	49.697	45.576	40.909	18.667
8.30	68.434	63.855	56.627	53.590	51.807	49.398	45.301	40.663	18.554
8.35	68.024	63.473	56.287	53.269	51.497	49.102	45.030	40.419	18.443
8.40	67.619	63.095	55.952	52.952	51.190	48.810	44.762	40.179	18.333
8.45	67.219	62.722	55.621	52.639	50.888	48.521	44.497	39.941	18.225
8.50	66.824	62.353	55.294	52.329	50.588	48.235	44.235	39.706	18.118
8.55	66.433	61.988	54.971	52.023	50.292	47.953	43.977	39.474	18.012
8.60	66.047	61.628	54.651	51.721	50.000	47.674	43.721	39.244	17.907
8.65	65.665	61.272	54.335	51.422	49.711	47.399	43.468	39.017	17.803

Table B.I (*contd*)

Radii, r (mm)	Surface powers (D) *for refractive index differences of*								
	1.568–1	*1.530–1*	*1.470–1*	*1.4448–1*	*1.430–1*	*1.410–1*	*1.376–1*	*1.3375–1*	*1.490–1.336*
8.70	65.287	60.920	54.023	51.126	49.425	47.126	43.218	38.793	17.701
8.75	64.914	60.571	53.714	50.834	49.143	46.857	42.971	38.571	17.600
8.80	64.545	60.227	53.409	50.545	48.864	46.591	42.727	38.352	17.500
8.85	64.181	59.887	53.107	50.260	48.589	46.328	42.486	38.136	17.401
8.90	63.820	59.551	52.809	49.978	48.315	46.067	42.247	37.921	17.303
8.95	63.464	59.218	52.514	49.698	48.045	45.810	42.011	37.709	17.207
9.00	63.111	58.889	52.222	49.422	47.778	45.556	41.778	37.500	17.111
9.10	62.418	58.242	51.648	48.879	47.253	45.055	41.319	37.088	16.923
9.20	61.739	57.609	51.087	48.348	46.739	44.565	40.870	36.685	16.739
9.30	61.075	56.989	50.538	47.828	46.237	44.086	40.430	36.290	16.559
9.40	60.426	56.383	50.000	47.319	45.745	43.617	40.000	35.904	16.382
9.50	59.789	55.789	49.474	46.821	45.263	43.158	39.579	35.526	16.211
9.60	59.167	55.208	48.958	46.333	44.792	42.708	39.167	35.156	16.042
9.70	58.557	54.639	48.454	45.856	44.330	42.268	38.763	34.794	15.876
9.80	57.959	54.082	47.959	45.388	43.878	41.837	38.367	34.438	15.714
9.90	57.374	53.535	47.475	44.929	43.434	41.414	37.980	34.091	15.556
10.00	56.800	53.000	47.000	44.480	43.000	41.000	37.600	33.750	15.400
10.10	56.238	52.475	46.535	44.040	42.574	40.594	37.228	33.416	15.248
10.20	55.686	51.961	46.078	43.608	42.157	40.196	36.863	33.088	15.098
10.30	55.146	51.456	45.631	43.184	41.748	39.806	36.505	32.767	14.951
10.40	54.615	50.962	45.192	42.769	41.346	39.423	36.154	32.452	14.808
10.50	54.095	50.476	44.762	42.362	40.952	39.048	35.810	32.143	14.667
10.60	53.585	50.000	44.340	41.962	40.566	38.679	35.472	31.840	14.528
10.70	53.084	49.533	43.925	41.570	40.187	38.318	35.140	31.542	14.393
10.80	52.593	49.074	43.519	41.185	39.815	37.963	34.815	31.250	14.259
10.90	52.110	48.624	43.119	40.807	39.450	37.615	34.495	30.963	14.128
11.00	51.636	48.182	42.727	40.436	39.091	37.272	34.182	30.682	14.000
11.10	51.171	47.748	42.342	40.072	38.739	36.937	33.874	30.405	13.874
11.20	50.714	47.321	41.964	39.714	38.393	36.607	33.571	30.134	13.750
11.30	50.265	46.903	41.593	39.363	38.053	36.283	33.274	29.867	13.628
11.40	49.825	46.491	41.228	39.018	37.719	35.965	32.982	29.605	13.509
11.50	49.391	46.087	40.870	38.678	37.391	35.652	32.696	29.348	13.391
11.60	48.966	45.690	40.517	38.345	37.069	35.345	32.414	29.095	13.276
11.70	48.547	45.299	40.171	38.017	36.752	35.043	32.137	28.846	13.162
11.80	48.136	44.915	39.831	37.695	36.441	34.746	31.864	28.602	13.051
11.90	47.731	44.538	39.496	37.378	36.134	34.454	31.597	28.361	12.941
12.00	47.333	44.167	39.167	37.067	35.833	34.167	31.333	28.125	12.833

For refractive index differences 1.49–1 and 1.336–1 *see Tables B.II* and *B.V* respectively.

Chapters 3, 10 and 11 give details of the refractive indices of most of the rigid and soft contact lenses materials currently produced. So many contact lens materials are available with refractive indices varying from approximately 1.38 to 1.57 that just a representative sample is covered here.

The refractive indices given pertain to the following materials:

1.568	Hyfrax
1.530	Butylstyrene polymer (e.g. Wesley–Jessen Airlens)
1.490	Polymethyl methacrylate
1.470*	Siloxy methacrylate–itaconate copolymers
1.4448	Hydrated HEMA (e.g. Hydroflex and others)
1.430	Hydrated HEMA (e.g. Weicon 38, Bausch & Lomb Soflens and others)
1.410	Hydrated HEMA copolymer (e.g. Pilkington Barnes–Hind Hydrocurve II 55 and others)
1.376	Cornea
1.3375	Most keratometers
1.336	Tears

*This is an average refractive index for this group of rigid gas permeable copolymers.

Table B.II Surface powers in air for $n = 1.49$ (PMMA), r = radius of curvature, F = surface power

r (mm)	F (D)	r (mm)	F (D)	r (mm)	F (D)	r (mm)	F (D)	r (mm)	F (D)	r (mm)	F (D)	r (mm)	F (D)
4.90	100.00	5.30	92.45	5.70	85.96	6.10	80.33	6.50	75.38	6.90	71.01	7.30	67.12
.91	99.80	.31	92.28	.71	85.81	.11	80.20	.51	75.27	.91	70.91	.31	67.03
.92	99.59	.32	92.11	.72	85.66	.12	80.07	.52	75.15	.92	70.81	.32	66.94
.93	99.39	.33	91.93	.73	85.51	.13	79.93	.53	75.04	.93	70.71	.33	66.85
.94	99.19	.34	91.76	.74	85.37	.14	79.80	.54	74.92	.94	70.60	.34	66.76
.95	98.99	.35	91.59	.75	85.22	.15	79.67	.55	74.81	.95	70.50	.35	66.67
.96	98.79	.36	91.42	.76	85.07	.16	79.55	.56	74.70	.96	70.40	.36	66.58
.97	98.59	.37	91.25	.77	84.92	.17	79.42	.57	74.58	.97	70.30	.37	66.49
.98	98.39	.38	91.08	.78	84.78	.18	79.29	.58	74.47	.98	70.20	.38	66.40
.99	98.20	.39	90.91	.79	84.63	.19	79.16	.59	74.36	.99	70.10	.39	66.31
5.00	98.00	5.40	90.74	5.80	84.48	6.20	79.03	6.60	74.24	7.00	70.00	7.40	66.22
.01	97.80	.41	90.57	.81	84.34	.21	78.90	.61	74.13	.01	69.90	.41	66.13
.02	97.61	.42	90.41	.82	84.19	.22	78.78	.62	74.02	.02	69.80	.42	66.04
.03	97.42	.43	90.24	.83	84.05	.23	78.65	.63	73.91	.03	69.70	.43	65.95
.04	97.22	.44	90.07	.84	83.90	.24	78.53	.64	73.80	.04	69.60	.44	65.86
.05	97.03	.45	89.91	.85	83.76	.25	78.40	.65	73.68	.05	69.50	.45	65.77
.06	96.84	.46	89.74	.86	83.62	.26	78.27	.66	73.57	.06	69.41	.46	65.68
.07	96.65	.47	89.58	.87	83.48	.27	78.15	.67	73.46	.07	69.31	.47	65.60
.08	96.46	.48	89.42	.88	83.33	.28	78.03	.68	73.35	.08	69.21	.48	65.51
.09	96.27	.49	89.25	.89	83.19	.29	77.90	.69	73.24	.09	69.11	.49	65.42
5.10	96.08	5.50	89.09	5.90	83.05	6.30	77.78	6.70	73.13	7.10	69.01	7.50	65.33
.11	95.89	.51	88.93	.91	82.91	.31	77.65	.71	73.03	.11	68.92	.51	65.25
.12	95.70	.52	88.77	.92	82.77	.32	77.53	.72	72.92	.12	68.82	.52	65.16
.13	95.52	.53	88.61	.93	82.63	.33	77.41	.73	72.81	.13	68.72	.53	65.07
.14	95.33	.54	88.45	.94	82.49	.34	77.29	.74	72.70	.14	68.63	.54	64.99
.15	95.15	.55	88.29	.95	82.35	.35	77.17	.75	72.59	.15	68.53	.55	64.90
.16	94.96	.56	88.13	.96	82.21	.36	77.04	.76	72.49	.16	68.44	.56	64.81
.17	94.78	.57	87.97	.97	82.08	.37	76.92	.77	72.38	.17	68.34	.57	64.73
.18	94.59	.58	87.81	.98	81.94	.38	76.80	.78	72.27	.18	68.25	.58	64.64
.19	94.41	.59	87.66	.99	81.80	.39	76.68	.79	72.16	.19	68.15	.59	64.56
5.20	94.23	5.60	87.50	6.00	81.67	6.40	76.56	6.80	72.06	7.20	68.06	7.60	64.47
.21	94.05	.61	87.34	.01	81.53	.41	76.44	.81	71.95	.21	67.96	.61	64.39
.22	93.87	.62	87.19	.02	81.40	.42	76.32	.82	71.85	.22	67.87	.62	64.30
.23	93.69	.63	87.03	.03	81.26	.43	76.21	.83	71.74	.23	67.77	.63	64.22
.24	93.51	.64	86.88	.04	81.13	.44	76.09	.84	71.64	.24	67.68	.64	64.14
.25	93.33	.65	86.73	.05	80.99	.45	75.97	.85	71.53	.25	67.59	.65	64.05
.26	93.16	.66	86.57	.06	80.86	.46	75.85	.86	71.43	.26	67.49	.66	63.97
.27	92.98	.67	86.42	.07	80.72	.47	75.73	.87	71.32	.27	67.40	.67	63.89
.28	92.80	.68	86.27	.08	80.59	.48	75.62	.88	71.22	.28	67.31	.68	63.80
.29	92.63	.69	86.12	.09	80.46	.49	75.50	.89	71.12	.29	67.22	.69	63.72

r (mm)	F (D)	r (mm)	F (D)	r (mm)	F (D)	r (mm)	F (D)	r (mm)	F (D)	r (mm)	F (D)	r (mm)	F (D)	r (mm)	F (D)
7.70	63.64	8.10	60.49	8.50	57.65	8.90	55.06	9.30	52.69	9.70	50.52	10.10	48.51		
.71	63.55	.11	60.42	.51	57.58	.91	54.99	.31	52.63	.71	50.46	.11	48.47		
.72	63.47	.12	60.34	.52	57.51	.92	54.93	.32	52.58	.72	50.41	.12	48.42		
.73	63.39	.13	60.27	.53	57.44	.93	54.87	.33	52.52	.73	50.36	.13	48.37		
.74	63.31	.14	60.20	.54	57.38	.94	54.81	.34	52.46	.74	50.31	.14	48.32		
.75	63.23	.15	60.12	.55	57.31	.95	54.75	.35	52.41	.75	50.26	.15	48.28		
.76	63.14	.16	60.05	.56	57.24	.96	54.69	.36	52.35	.76	50.20	.16	48.23		
.77	63.06	.17	59.98	.57	57.18	.97	54.63	.37	52.29	.77	50.15	.17	48.18		
.78	62.98	.18	59.90	.58	57.11	.98	54.57	.38	52.24	.78	50.10	.18	48.13		
.79	62.90	.19	59.83	.59	57.04	.99	54.51	.39	52.18	.79	50.05	.19	48.09		
7.80	62.82	8.20	59.76	8.60	56.98	9.00	54.44	9.40	52.13	9.80	50.00	10.20	48.04		
.81	62.74	.21	59.68	.61	56.91	.01	54.38	.41	52.07	.81	49.95	.21	47.99		
.82	62.66	.22	59.61	.62	56.84	.02	54.32	.42	52.02	.82	49.90	.22	47.95		
.83	62.58	.23	59.54	.63	56.78	.03	54.26	.43	51.96	.83	49.85	.23	47.90		
.84	62.50	.24	59.47	.64	56.71	.04	54.20	.44	51.91	.84	49.80	.24	47.85		
.85	62.42	.25	59.39	.65	56.65	.05	54.14	.45	51.85	.85	49.75	.25	47.81		
.86	62.34	.26	59.32	.66	56.58	.06	54.08	.46	51.80	.86	49.70	.26	47.76		
.87	62.26	.27	59.25	.67	56.52	.07	54.02	.47	51.74	.87	49.65	.27	47.71		
.88	62.18	.28	59.18	.68	56.45	.08	53.96	.48	51.69	.88	49.60	.28	47.67		
.89	62.10	.29	59.11	.69	56.39	.09	53.91	.49	51.63	.89	49.54	.29	47.62		
7.90	62.03	8.30	59.04	8.70	56.32	9.10	53.85	9.50	51.58	9.90	49.49	10.30	47.57		
.91	61.95	.31	58.97	.71	56.26	.11	53.79	.51	51.52	.91	49.45	.31	47.53		
.92	61.87	.32	58.89	.72	56.19	.12	53.73	.52	51.47	.92	49.40	.32	47.48		
.93	61.79	.33	58.82	.73	56.13	.13	53.67	.53	51.42	.93	49.35	.33	47.44		
.94	61.71	.34	58.75	.74	56.06	.14	53.61	.54	51.36	.94	49.30	.34	47.39		
.95	61.64	.35	58.68	.75	56.00	.15	53.55	.55	51.31	.95	49.25	.35	47.34		
.96	61.56	.36	58.61	.76	55.94	.16	53.49	.56	51.25	.96	49.20	.36	47.30		
.97	61.48	.37	58.54	.77	55.87	.17	53.43	.57	51.20	.97	49.15	.37	47.25		
.98	61.40	.38	58.47	.78	55.81	.18	53.38	.58	51.15	.98	49.10	.38	47.21		
.99	61.33	.39	58.40	.79	55.75	.19	53.32	.59	51.09	.99	49.05	.39	47.16		
8.00	61.25	8.40	58.33	8.80	55.68	9.20	53.26	9.60	51.04	10.00	49.00	10.40	47.12		
.01	61.17	.41	58.26	.81	55.62	.21	53.20	.61	50.99	.01	48.95	.41	47.07		
.02	61.10	.42	58.19	.82	55.56	.22	53.15	.62	50.94	.02	48.90	.42	47.03		
.03	61.02	.43	58.13	.83	55.49	.23	53.09	.63	50.88	.03	48.85	.43	46.98		
.04	60.95	.44	58.06	.84	55.43	.24	53.03	.64	50.83	.04	48.80	.44	46.94		
.05	60.87	.45	57.99	.85	55.37	.25	52.97	.65	50.78	.05	48.76	.45	46.89		
.06	60.79	.46	57.92	.86	55.30	.26	52.92	.66	50.72	.06	48.71	.46	46.85		
.07	60.72	.47	57.85	.87	55.24	.27	52.86	.67	50.67	.07	48.66	.47	46.80		
.08	60.64	.48	57.78	.88	55.18	.28	52.80	.68	50.62	.08	48.61	.48	46.76		
.09	60.57	.49	57.72	.89	55.12	.29	52.75	.69	50.57	.09	48.56	.49	46.71		

Table B.II (*contd*)

r (mm)	F (D)	r (mm)	F (D)	r (mm)	F (D)	r (mm)	F (D)	r (mm)	F (D)	r (mm)	F (D)
10.50	46.67	10.90	44.95	11.30	43.36	11.70	41.88	12.10	40.50	12.50	39.20
.51	46.62	.91	44.91	.31	43.32	.71	41.84	.11	40.46	.51	39.17
.52	46.58	.92	44.87	.32	43.29	.72	41.81	.12	40.43	.52	39.14
.53	46.53	.93	44.83	.33	43.25	.73	41.77	.13	40.40	.53	39.11
.54	46.49	.94	44.79	.34	43.21	.74	41.74	.14	40.36	.54	39.08
.55	46.45	.95	44.75	.35	43.17	.75	41.70	.15	40.33	.55	39.04
.56	46.40	.96	44.71	.36	43.13	.76	41.67	.16	40.30	.56	39.01
.57	46.36	.97	44.67	.37	43.10	.77	41.63	.17	40.26	.57	38.98
.58	46.31	.98	44.63	.38	43.06	.78	41.60	.18	40.23	.58	38.95
.59	46.27	.99	44.59	.39	43.02	.79	41.56	.19	40.20	.59	38.92
10.60	46.23	11.00	44.55	11.40	42.98	11.80	41.53	12.20	40.16	12.60	38.89
.61	46.18	.01	44.51	.41	42.95	.81	41.49	.21	40.13		
.62	46.14	.02	44.47	.42	42.91	.82	41.46	.22	40.10		
.63	46.10	.03	44.43	.43	42.87	.83	41.42	.23	40.07		
.64	46.05	.04	44.38	.44	42.83	.84	41.39	.24	40.03		
.65	46.01	.05	44.34	.45	42.80	.85	41.35	.25	40.00		
.66	45.97	.06	44.30	.46	42.76	.86	41.32	.26	39.97		
.67	45.92	.07	44.26	.47	42.72	.87	41.28	.27	39.94		
.68	45.88	.08	44.22	.48	42.68	.88	41.25	.28	39.90		
.69	45.84	.09	44.18	.49	42.65	.89	41.21	.29	39.87		
10.70	45.79	11.10	44.14	11.50	42.61	11.90	41.18	12.30	39.84		
.71	45.75	.11	44.10	.51	42.57	.91	41.14	.31	39.81		
.72	45.71	.12	44.07	.52	42.54	.92	41.11	.32	39.77		
.73	45.67	.13	44.03	.53	42.50	.93	41.07	.33	39.74		
.74	45.62	.14	43.99	.54	42.46	.94	41.04	.34	39.71		
.75	45.58	.15	43.95	.55	42.43	.95	41.00	.35	39.68		
.76	45.54	.16	43.91	.56	42.39	.96	40.97	.36	39.64		
.77	45.50	.17	43.87	.57	42.35	.97	40.94	.37	39.61		
.78	45.46	.18	43.83	.58	42.31	.98	40.90	.38	39.58		
.79	45.41	.19	43.79	.59	42.28	.99	40.87	.39	39.55		
10.80	45.37	11.20	43.75	11.60	42.24	12.00	40.83	12.40	39.52		
.81	45.33	.21	43.71	.61	42.21	.01	40.80	.41	39.48		
.82	45.29	.22	43.67	.62	42.17	.02	40.77	.42	39.45		
.83	45.25	.23	43.63	.63	42.13	.03	40.73	.43	39.42		
.84	45.20	.24	43.60	.64	42.10	.04	40.70	.44	39.39		
.85	45.16	.25	43.56	.65	42.06	.05	40.66	.45	39.36		
.86	45.12	.26	43.52	.66	42.02	.06	40.63	.46	39.33		
.87	45.08	.27	43.48	.67	41.99	.07	40.60	.47	39.29		
.88	45.04	.28	43.44	.68	41.95	.08	40.56	.48	39.26		
.89	45.00	.29	43.40	.69	41.92	.09	40.53	.49	39.23		

Table B.III Change in surface power (D) when radius (r₁) is changed to new radius (r₂), for plastics (n = 1.49) in air (see Appendix E, program index no. 1)

Change in surface power (D) at new radius, r₂ (mm) of

Initial radius, r₁ (mm)	7.0	7.1	7.2	7.3	7.4	7.5	7.6	7.7	7.8	7.9	8.0	8.1	8.2	8.3	8.4	8.5	8.6	8.7	8.8	8.9
	D																			
9.0	15.56	14.57	13.62	12.68	11.78	10.89	10.03	9.20	8.38	7.59	6.81	6.05	5.32	4.60	3.89	3.21	2.54	1.88	1.24	0.62
8.9	14.94	13.95	13.00	12.06	11.16	10.27	9.41	8.58	7.76	6.97	6.19	5.43	4.70	3.98	3.27	2.59	1.92	1.26	0.62	
8.8	14.32	13.33	12.38	11.44	10.54	9.65	8.79	7.96	7.14	6.35	5.57	4.81	4.08	3.36	2.65	1.97	1.30	0.64		
8.7	13.68	12.69	11.74	10.80	9.90	9.01	8.15	7.32	6.50	5.71	4.93	4.17	3.44	2.72	2.01	1.33	0.66			
8.6	13.02	12.03	11.08	10.14	9.24	8.35	7.49	6.66	5.84	5.05	4.27	3.51	2.78	2.06	1.35	0.67				
8.5	12.35	11.36	10.41	9.47	8.57	7.68	6.82	5.99	5.17	4.38	3.60	2.84	2.02	1.39	0.68					
8.4	11.67	10.68	9.73	8.79	7.89	7.00	6.14	5.31	4.49	3.70	2.92	2.16	1.43	0.71						
8.3	10.96	9.97	9.02	8.08	7.18	6.29	5.03	4.60	3.78	2.99	2.21	1.45	0.72							
8.2	10.24	9.25	8.30	7.36	6.46	5.57	4.71	3.88	3.06	2.27	1.49	0.73								
8.1	9.51	8.52	7.57	6.63	5.73	4.84	3.98	3.15	2.33	1.54	0.76									
8.0	8.75	7.76	6.81	5.87	4.97	4.08	3.22	2.39	1.57	0.78										
7.9	7.97	6.98	6.03	5.09	4.19	3.30	2.44	1.61	0.79											
7.8	7.18	6.19	5.24	4.30	3.40	2.51	1.65	0.82												
7.7	6.36	5.37	4.42	3.48	2.58	1.69	0.83													
7.6	5.53	4.54	3.59	2.65	1.75	0.86														
7.5	4.67	3.68	2.73	1.79	0.89															
7.4	3.78	2.79	1.84	0.90																
7.3	2.88	1.89	0.94																	
7.2	1.94	0.95																		
7.1	0.99																				

Table B.IV Change in reduced vergence due to thickness for a given initial vergence and refractive index of 1.49 (plastic in air). In each cell, the upper figure applies to divergent light, and the lower figure to convergent light.

Initial vergence (D)	.01	.02	.03	.04	.05	.06	.07	.08	.09	.10	.11	.12	.13	.14	.15	.16
									Thickness (mm)							
100.0	.07 / .07	.13 / .14	.20 / .20	.27 / .27	.34 / .34	.40 / .41	.47 / .48	.54 / .54	.60 / .61	.67 / .68	.74 / .75	.80 / .82	.86 / .88	.93 / .95	1.00 / 1.02	1.06 / 1.09
98.0	.06 / .06	.13 / .13	.19 / .20	.26 / .26	.32 / .32	.38 / .39	.45 / .46	.51 / .52	.58 / .58	.64 / .65	.70 / .72	.77 / .78	.83 / .85	.89 / .91	.96 / .98	1.02 / 1.05
96.0	.06 / .06	.12 / .12	.18 / .19	.24 / .25	.30 / .31	.37 / .37	.43 / .43	.49 / .50	.55 / .56	.61 / .62	.67 / .68	.73 / .75	.79 / .81	.85 / .87	.92 / .94	.98 / 1.00
94.0	.06 / .06	.12 / .12	.18 / .18	.24 / .24	.30 / .30	.35 / .36	.41 / .42	.47 / .48	.53 / .54	.59 / .60	.65 / .66	.71 / .72	.76 / .78	.82 / .84	.88 / .90	.94 / .96
92.0	.06 / .06	.11 / .11	.17 / .17	.22 / .23	.28 / .28	.34 / .34	.39 / .40	.45 / .46	.50 / .51	.56 / .57	.62 / .63	.67 / .69	.73 / .74	.78 / .80	.84 / .86	.90 / .92
90.0	.05 / .06	.11 / .11	.16 / .16	.22 / .22	.27 / .28	.32 / .33	.38 / .38	.43 / .44	.49 / .50	.54 / .55	.59 / .60	.65 / .66	.70 / .72	.75 / .77	.80 / .82	.86 / .88
88.0	.05 / .05	.10 / .10	.16 / .16	.21 / .21	.26 / .26	.31 / .31	.36 / .36	.42 / .42	.47 / .47	.52 / .52	.57 / .57	.62 / .63	.67 / .68	.72 / .73	.78 / .78	.83 / .84
86.0	.05 / .05	.10 / .10	.15 / .15	.20 / .20	.24 / .25	.29 / .30	.34 / .35	.39 / .40	.44 / .45	.49 / .50	.54 / .55	.59 / .60	.64 / .65	.69 / .70	.74 / .76	.78 / .81
84.0	.05 / .05	.09 / .10	.14 / .14	.19 / .19	.24 / .24	.28 / .29	.33 / .34	.38 / .38	.42 / .43	.47 / .48	.52 / .53	.56 / .58	.61 / .62	.66 / .67	.70 / .72	.75 / .77
82.0	.04 / .04	.09 / .09	.14 / .14	.18 / .18	.22 / .22	.27 / .27	.32 / .32	.36 / .36	.40 / .40	.45 / .45	.49 / .50	.54 / .54	.58 / .59	.63 / .63	.67 / .68	.71 / .73
80.0	.04 / .04	.09 / .09	.13 / .13	.17 / .17	.22 / .22	.26 / .26	.30 / .30	.34 / .34	.39 / .39	.43 / .43	.47 / .47	.51 / .52	.56 / .56	.60 / .61	.64 / .65	.68 / .69
78.0	.04 / .04	.08 / .08	.12 / .12	.16 / .16	.20 / .20	.25 / .25	.29 / .29	.33 / .33	.37 / .37	.41 / .41	.45 / .45	.49 / .49	.53 / .54	.57 / .58	.61 / .62	.65 / .66
76.0	.04 / .04	.08 / .08	.12 / .12	.16 / .16	.20 / .20	.23 / .23	.27 / .27	.31 / .31	.35 / .35	.39 / .39	.43 / .43	.47 / .47	.50 / .51	.54 / .55	.58 / .58	.62 / .62
74.0	.04 / .04	.07 / .07	.11 / .11	.15 / .15	.18 / .18	.22 / .22	.26 / .26	.30 / .30	.33 / .33	.37 / .37	.41 / .41	.44 / .44	.48 / .48	.51 / .52	.55 / .56	.59 / .59
72.0	.04 / .04	.07 / .07	.10 / .10	.14 / .14	.18 / .18	.21 / .21	.24 / .24	.28 / .28	.32 / .32	.35 / .35	.38 / .38	.42 / .42	.45 / .46	.49 / .49	.52 / .52	.55 / .56
70.0	.03 / .03	.07 / .07	.10 / .10	.13 / .13	.16 / .16	.20 / .20	.23 / .23	.26 / .26	.30 / .30	.33 / .33	.36 / .36	.39 / .40	.43 / .43	.46 / .46	.49 / .50	.52 / .51
68.0	.03 / .03	.06 / .06	.09 / .09	.12 / .12	.16 / .16	.19 / .19	.22 / .22	.25 / .25	.28 / .28	.31 / .31	.34 / .34	.37 / .37	.40 / .41	.43 / .44	.46 / .47	.50 / .50
66.0	.03 / .03	.06 / .06	.09 / .09	.12 / .12	.14 / .15	.17 / .17	.20 / .20	.23 / .23	.26 / .26	.29 / .29	.32 / .32	.35 / .35	.38 / .38	.41 / .41	.44 / .44	.46 / .47
64.0	.03 / .03	.05 / .06	.08 / .08	.11 / .11	.14 / .14	.16 / .17	.19 / .20	.22 / .22	.24 / .25	.27 / .28	.30 / .31	.33 / .33	.35 / .36	.38 / .39	.41 / .42	.44 / .44
62.0	.03 / .03	.05 / .05	.08 / .08	.10 / .10	.13 / .13	.16 / .16	.18 / .18	.21 / .21	.23 / .23	.26 / .26	.28 / .29	.31 / .31	.34 / .34	.36 / .36	.38 / .39	.41 / .42
60.0	.02 / .02	.05 / .05	.07 / .07	.10 / .10	.12 / .12	.14 / .14	.17 / .17	.19 / .19	.22 / .22	.24 / .24	.26 / .26	.29 / .29	.31 / .32	.34 / .34	.36 / .36	.38 / .39
58.0	.02 / .02	.04 / .05	.07 / .07	.09 / .09	.11 / .12	.13 / .14	.15 / .16	.18 / .18	.20 / .21	.22 / .23	.24 / .25	.27 / .28	.29 / .30	.31 / .32	.34 / .34	.36 / .37
56.0	.02 / .02	.04 / .04	.06 / .06	.08 / .08	.10 / .10	.13 / .13	.15 / .15	.17 / .17	.19 / .19	.21 / .21	.23 / .23	.25 / .25	.27 / .27	.29 / .29	.32 / .32	.34 / .34
54.0	.02 / .02	.04 / .04	.06 / .06	.08 / .08	.10 / .10	.11 / .12	.13 / .14	.15 / .16	.17 / .18	.19 / .20	.21 / .22	.23 / .24	.25 / .26	.27 / .28	.29 / .30	.31 / .31
52.0	.02 / .02	.04 / .04	.05 / .05	.07 / .07	.09 / .09	.11 / .11	.13 / .13	.14 / .14	.16 / .16	.18 / .18	.20 / .20	.22 / .22	.23 / .24	.25 / .26	.27 / .28	.29 / .29
50.0	.02 / .02	.03 / .03	.05 / .05	.07 / .07	.08 / .08	.10 / .10	.12 / .12	.14 / .14	.15 / .15	.17 / .17	.19 / .19	.20 / .20	.22 / .22	.23 / .24	.25 / .26	.27 / .27
48.0	.02 / .02	.03 / .03	.04 / .05	.06 / .06	.08 / .08	.09 / .10	.10 / .11	.12 / .13	.14 / .14	.15 / .16	.17 / .18	.18 / .19	.20 / .20	.21 / .22	.23 / .24	.25 / .25
46.0	.01 / .01	.03 / .03	.04 / .04	.06 / .06	.07 / .07	.08 / .08	.10 / .10	.11 / .11	.13 / .13	.14 / .14	.15 / .16	.17 / .17	.18 / .18	.20 / .20	.21 / .22	.22 / .23
44.0	.01 / .01	.03 / .03	.04 / .04	.05 / .05	.06 / .06	.08 / .08	.09 / .09	.10 / .10	.12 / .12	.13 / .13	.14 / .14	.16 / .16	.17 / .17	.18 / .18	.20 / .20	.21 / .21
42.0	.01 / .01	.02 / .02	.04 / .04	.05 / .05	.06 / .06	.07 / .07	.08 / .08	.10 / .10	.11 / .11	.12 / .12	.13 / .13	.14 / .14	.16 / .16	.17 / .17	.18 / .18	.19 / .19
40.0	.01 / .01	.02 / .02	.03 / .03	.04 / .04	.06 / .06	.07 / .07	.08 / .08	.09 / .09	.10 / .10	.11 / .11	.12 / .12	.13 / .13	.14 / .14	.15 / .15	.16 / .16	.17 / .18

Table B.IV (*contd*)

.17	.18	.19	.20	.21	.22	.23	.24	.25	.26	.27	.28	.29	.30	.31	.32	.33	.34
1.12 / 1.16	1.19 / 1.22	1.26 / 1.29	1.32 / 1.36	1.38 / 1.43	1.45 / 1.50	1.52 / 1.57	1.58 / 1.64	1.64 / 1.70	1.71 / 1.77	1.78 / 1.84	1.84 / 1.91	1.90 / 1.98	1.97 / 2.05	2.03 / 2.12	2.10 / 2.19	2.16 / 2.26	2.23 / 2.33
1.08 / 1.11	1.14 / 1.18	1.21 / 1.24	1.27 / 1.31	1.33 / 1.38	1.40 / 1.44	1.46 / 1.51	1.52 / 1.57	1.58 / 1.64	1.65 / 1.71	.171 / 1.77	1.77 / 1.84	1.84 / 1.90	1.90 / 1.97	1.96 / 2.04	2.02 / 2.11	2.08 / 2.17	2.14 / 2.24
1.04 / 1.06	1.10 / 1.12	1.16 / 1.19	1.22 / 1.25	1.28 / 1.31	1.34 / 1.38	1.40 / 1.44	1.46 / 1.51	1.52 / 1.57	1.58 / 1.63	1.64 / 1.70	1.70 / 1.76	1.76 / 1.83	1.82 / 1.89	1.88 / 1.96	1.94 / 2.02	2.00 / 2.08	2.06 / 2.15
1.00 / 1.02	1.05 / 1.08	1.11 / 1.14	1.17 / 1.20	1.23 / 1.26	1.29 / 1.32	1.34 / 1.38	1.40 / 1.44	1.46 / 1.50	1.52 / 1.57	1.58 / 1.63	1.63 / 1.69	1.69 / 1.75	1.75 / 1.81	1.81 / 1.87	1.86 / 1.93	1.92 / 2.00	1.97 / 2.06
.95 / .98	1.01 / 1.03	1.06 / 1.09	1.12 / 1.15	1.18 / 1.21	1.23 / 1.27	1.28 / ·1.33	1.34 / 1.39	1.40 / 1.44	1.45 / 1.50	1.50 / 1.56	1.56 / 1.62	1.62 / 1.68	1.67 / 1.74	1.72 / 1.80	1.78 / 1.86	1.84 / 1.92	1.89 / 1.98
.91 / .94	.96 / .99	1.02 / 1.04	1.07 / 1.10	1.12 / 1.16	1.18 / 1.21	1.23 / 1.27	1.28 / 1.32	1.34 / 1.38	1.39 / 1.44	1.44 / 1.49	1.49 / 1.55	1.55 / 1.60	1.60 / 1.66	1.65 / 1.72	1.70 / 1.77	1.76 / 1.83	1.81 / 1.89
.88 / .89	.91 / .94	.98 / 1.00	1.03 / 1.05	1.08 / 1.10	1.13 / 1.16	1.18 / 1.21	1.23 / 1.27	1.28 / 1.32	1.33 / 1.37	1.38 / 1.43	1.43 / 1.48	1.48 / 1.54	1.53 / 1.59	1.58 / 1.64	1.63 / 1.70	1.68 / 1.75	1.73 / 1.81
.83 / .86	.88 / .91	.93 / .96	.98 / 1.01	1.03 / 1.06	1.08 / 1.11	1.12 / 1.16	1.17 / 1.21	1.22 / 1.26	1.27 / 1.32	1.32 / 1.37	1.36 / 1.42	1.41 / 1.47	1.46 / 1.52	1.51 / 1.57	1.56 / 1.62	1.60 / 1.67	1.65 / 1.72
.80 / .82	.85 / .86	.89 / .91	.94 / .96	.99 / 1.01	1.03 / 1.06	1.08 / 1.11	1.12 / 1.16	1.17 / 1.20	1.22 / 1.25	1.26 / 1.30	1.31 / 1.35	1.35 / 1.40	1.40 / 1.45	1.44 / 1.50	1.49 / 1.55	1.54 / 1.60	1.58 / 1.65
.76 / .77	.80 / .82	.85 / .86	.89 / .91	.93 / .96	.98 / 1.00	1.02 / 1.05	1.07 / 1.10	1.11 / 1.14	1.15 / 1.19	1.20 / 1.24	1.24 / 1.29	1.29 / 1.33	1.33 / 1.38	1.37 / 1.43	1.42 / 1.47	1.46 / 1.52	1.51 / 1.57
.72 / .74	.77 / .78	.81 / .83	.85 / .87	.89 / .91	.93 / .96	.98 / 1.00	1.02 / 1.05	1.06 / 1.09	1.10 / 1.13	1.14 / 1.18	1.19 / 1.22	1.23 / 1.27	1.27 / 1.31	1.31 / 1.36	1.35 / 1.40	1.39 / 1.44	1.43 / 1.49
.69 / .70	.73 / .75	.77 / .79	.81 / .83	.85 / .87	.89 / .91	.93 / .95	.97 / .99	1.01 / 1.04	1.05 / 1.08	1.09 / 1.12	1.13 / 1.16	1.17 / 1.20	1.21 / 1.24	1.25 / 1.28	1.29 / 1.33	1.33 / 1.37	1.37 / 1.41
.66 / .66	.69 / .70	.73 / .74	.77 / .78	.81 / .82	.85 / .86	.88 / .90	.92 / .94	.96 / .98	1.00 / 1.02	1.04 / 1.06	1.07 / 1.10	1.11 / 1.14	1.15 / 1.18	1.19 / 1.22	1.22 / 1.26	1.26 / 1.30	1.30 / 1.34
.62 / .63	.66 / .67	.69 / .70	.73 / .74	.77 / .78	.80 / .82	.84 / .85	.87 / .89	.91 / .93	.95 / .97	.98 / 1.01	1.02 / 1.04	1.05 / 1.08	1.09 / 1.12	1.12 / 1.16	1.16 / 1.20	1.20 / 1.23	1.23 / 1.27
.59 / .60	.62 / .63	.66 / .66	.69 / .70	.72 / .74	.76 / .77	.79 / .81	.83 / .84	.86 / .88	.89 / .92	.93 / .95	.96 / .99	1.00 / 1.02	1.03 / 1.06	1.06 / 1.10	1.10 / 1.13	1.13 / 1.17	1.17 / 1.20
.55 / .56	.59 / .59	.62 / .63	.65 / .66	.68 / .69	.71 / .73	.75 / .76	.78 / .80	.81 / .83	.84 / .86	.87 / .90	.91 / .93	.94 / .97	.97 / 1.00	1.00 / 1.03	1.03 / 1.07	1.07 / 1.10	1.10 / 1.14
.53 / .53	.56 / .57	.59 / .60	.62 / .63	.65 / .66	.68 / .69	.71 / .72	.74 / .75	.77 / .78	.80 / .82	.83 / .85	.86 / .88	.89 / .91	.92 / .94	.95 / .97	.98 / 1.00	1.01 / 1.04	1.04 / 1.07
.49 / .50	.52 / .53	.55 / .56	.58 / .59	.61 / .62	.64 / .65	.67 / .68	.70 / .71	.72 / .74	.75 / .77	.78 / .80	.81 / .83	.84 / .86	.87 / .89	.90 / .92	.93 / .95	.95 / .98	.98 / 1.00
.47 / .47	.49 / .50	.52 / .52	.55 / .55	.58 / .58	.60 / .61	.63 / .64	.65 / .67	.68 / .70	.71 / .72	.73 / .75	.76 / .78	.78 / .81	.81 / .84	.84 / .87	.86 / .90	.89 / .92	.92 / .95
.44 / .44	.46 / .47	.48 / .49	.51 / .52	.54 / .55	.56 / .57	.58 / .60	.61 / .62	.64 / .65	.66 / .68	.68 / .70	.71 / .73	.74 / .75	.76 / .78	.79 / .81	.81 / .83	.84 / .86	.86 / .89
.41 / .42	.43 / .44	.46 / .46	.48 / .49	.50 / .51	.53 / .54	.55 / .56	.58 / .59	.60 / .61	.62 / .63	.65 / .66	.67 / .68	.70 / .71	.72 / .73	.74 / .76	.77 / .78	.79 / .80	.81 / .83
.38 / .39	.40 / .41	.43 / .44	.45 / .46	.47 / .48	.49 / .51	.52 / .53	.54 / .55	.56 / .58	.58 / .60	.60 / .62	.63 / .64	.65 / .67	.67 / .69	.69 / .71	.71 / .74	.74 / .76	.76 / .78
.36 / .36	.38 / .38	.40 / .40	.42 / .42	.44 / .44	.46 / .46	.48 / .49	.50 / .51	.52 / .53	.54 / .55	.56 / .57	.58 / .60	.60 / .62	.62 / .64	.64 / .66	.66 / .68	.68 / .70	.70 / .72
.33 / .33	.35 / .35	.37 / .37	.39 / .39	.41 / .41	.43 / .43	.45 / .45	.47 / .47	.48 / .49	.50 / .51	.52 / .53	.54 / .55	.56 / .57	.58 / .59	.60 / .61	.62 / .63	.64 / .65	.66 / .67
.31 / .31	.32 / .33	.34 / .35	.36 / .37	.38 / .39	.40 / .41	.41 / .42	.43 / .44	.45 / .46	.47 / .48	.49 / .50	.50 / .51	.52 / .53	.54 / .55	.56 / .57	.58 / .59	.59 / .61	.61 / .63
.28 / .29	.30 / .31	.31 / .32	.33 / .34	.35 / .36	.36 / .37	.38 / .39	.40 / .41	.42 / .42	.43 / .44	.45 / .46	.47 / .48	.48 / .49	.50 / .51	.52 / .53	.53 / .54	.55 / .56	.56 / .58
.26 / .26	.28 / .28	.29 / .30	.31 / .31	.32 / .33	.34 / .34	.36 / .36	.37 / .37	.38 / .39	.40 / .41	.42 / .42	.43 / .44	.44 / .45	.46 / .47	.48 / .49	.49 / .50	.50 / .52	.52 / .53
.24 / .24	.25 / .26	.27 / .28	.28 / .29	.29 / .30	.31 / .32	.32 / .33	.34 / .35	.35 / .36	.36 / .37	.38 / .39	.39 / .40	.41 / .42	.42 / .43	.43 / .44	.45 / .46	.46 / .48	.48 / .49
.22 / .22	.23 / .23	.25 / .25	.26 / .26	.27 / .27	.29 / .29	.30 / .30	.31 / .31	.32 / .32	.34 / .34	.35 / .35	.36 / .36	.38 / .38	.39 / .39	.40 / .40	.41 / .42	.43 / .43	.44 / .45
.20 / .20	.22 / .22	.23 / .23	.24 / .24	.25 / .25	.26 / .26	.27 / .28	.28 / .29	.30 / .30	.31 / .31	.32 / .32	.33 / .34	.34 / .35	.35 / .36	.36 / .37	.37 / .38	.39 / .40	.40 / .41
.18 / .19	.19 / .20	.20 / .21	.21 / .22	.22 / .23	.23 / .24	·.24 / .25	.25 / .26	.26 / .27	.28 / .28	.29 / .29	.30 / .30	.31 / .31	.32 / .32	.33 / .33	.34 / .34	.35 / .35	.36 / .36

Table B.IV (contd)

Initial vergence (D)	Thickness (mm) .35	.36	.37	.38	.39	.40	.41	.42	.43	.44	.45	.46	.47	.48	.49	.50
100.00	2.29	2.35	2.42	2.48	2.55	2.61	2.67	2.74	2.80	2.87	2.93	2.99	3.06	3.12	3.19	3.25
	2.40	2.48	2.55	2.62	2.69	2.76	2.83	2.90	2.97	3.04	3.12	3.19	3.26	3.33	3.40	3.47
98.00	2.20	2.27	2.33	2.39	2.45	2.51	2.57	2.63	2.69	2.75	2.82	2.88	2.94	3.00	3.06	3.12
	2.31	2.38	2.45	2.51	2.58	2.65	2.72	2.79	2.85	2.92	2.99	3.06	3.13	3.19	3.26	3.33
96.00	2.12	2.17	2.23	2.29	2.35	2.41	2.47	2.53	2.59	2.65	2.70	2.76	2.82	2.88	2.94	3.00
	2.22	2.28	2.34	2.41	2.48	2.54	2.61	2.67	2.74	2.80	2.87	2.94	3.00	3.07	3.13	3.20
94.0	2.03	2.09	2.14	2.20	2.25	2.31	2.37	2.42	2.48	2.53	2.59	2.65	2.70	2.76	2.81	2.87
	2.12	2.18	2.24	2.31	2.37	2.43	2.49	2.56	2.62	2.68	2.74	2.81	2.87	2.93	3.00	3.06
92.00	1.94	2.00	2.06	2.11	2.16	2.22	2.27	2.33	2.38	2.44	2.49	2.54	2.60	2.65	2.71	2.76
	2.04	2.09	2.15	2.21	2.27	2.33	2.39	2.45	2.51	2.57	2.63	2.69	2.75	2.81	2.87	2.93
90.00	1.86	1.91	1.96	2.02	2.07	2.12	2.17	2.22	2.28	2.33	2.38	2.43	2.48	2.54	2.59	2.64
	1.94	2.00	2.06	2.12	2.17	2.23	2.29	2.34	2.40	2.46	2.52	2.57	2.63	2.69	2.74	2.80
88.0	1.78	1.83	1.88	1.93	1.98	2.03	2.08	2.13	2.18	2.23	2.28	2.32	2.37	2.42	2.47	2.52
	1.86	1.91	1.97	2.02	2.08	2.13	2.18	2.24	2.30	2.35	2.40	2.46	2.52	2.57	2.62	2.68
86.0	1.70	1.75	1.80	1.84	1.89	1.94	1.99	2.03	2.08	2.13	2.18	2.22	2.27	2.32	2.36	2.41
	1.78	1.83	1.88	1.93	1.98	2.03	2.08	2.14	2.19	2.24	2.30	2.35	2.40	2.45	2.51	2.55
84.00	1.62	1.67	1.72	1.76	1.80	1.85	1.90	1.94	1.98	2.03	2.08	2.12	2.16	2.21	2.26	2.30
	1.70	1.74	1.79	1.84	1.89	1.94	1.99	2.04	2.09	2.14	2.19	2.24	2.29	2.34	2.39	2.44
82.0	1.55	1.59	1.64	1.68	1.73	1.77	1.81	1.86	1.90	1.94	1.98	2.03	2.07	2.11	2.16	2.20
	1.62	1.66	1.71	1.76	1.80	1.85	1.90	1.94	1.99	2.04	2.08	2.13	2.18	2.23	2.27	2.32
80.0	1.48	1.52	1.56	1.60	1.64	1.68	1.72	1.76	1.80	1.84	1.88	1.93	1.97	2.01	2.05	2.09
	1.54	1.58	1.62	1.67	1.72	1.76	1.80	1.85	1.90	1.94	1.98	2.03	2.08	2.12	2.16	2.21
78.0	1.40	1.44	1.48	1.52	1.56	1.60	1.64	1.68	1.72	1.76	1.80	1.83	1.87	1.91	1.95	1.99
	1.46	1.50	1.54	1.58	1.63	1.67	1.71	1.76	1.80	1.84	1.88	1.93	1.97	2.01	2.06	2.10
76.0	1.34	1.37	1.41	1.45	1.48	1.52	1.56	1.59	1.63	1.67	1.70	1.74	1.78	1.82	1.85	1.89
	1.38	1.42	1.46	1.50	1.54	1.58	1.62	1.66	1.70	1.74	1.78	1.83	1.87	1.91	1.95	1.99
74.0	1.26	1.30	1.34	1.37	1.40	1.44	1.48	1.51	1.54	1.58	1.62	1.65	1.68	1.72	1.76	1.79
	1.31	1.35	1.39	1.42	1.46	1.50	1.54	1.58	1.61	1.65	1.69	1.73	1.77	1.80	1.84	1.88
72.0	1.20	1.23	1.27	1.30	1.34	1.37	1.40	1.44	1.47	1.50	1.54	1.57	1.60	1.63	1.67	1.70
	1.24	1.28	1.31	1.35	1.38	1.42	1.46	1.49	1.53	1.56	1.60	1.64	1.67	1.71	1.74	1.78
70.0	1.13	1.16	1.19	1.23	1.26	1.29	1.32	1.35	1.39	1.42	1.45	1.48	1.51	1.55	1.58	1.61
	1.17	1.20	1.24	1.27	1.31	1.34	1.37	1.41	1.44	1.48	1.51	1.54	1.58	1.61	1.65	1.68
68.0	1.07	1.10	1.13	1.16	1.19	1.22	1.25	1.28	1.31	1.34	1.37	1.40	1.43	1.46	1.49	1.52
	1.10	1.13	1.16	1.20	1.23	1.26	1.29	1.33	1.36	1.39	1.42	1.46	1.49	1.52	1.56	1.59
66.0	1.01	1.04	1.07	1.09	1.12	1.15	1.18	1.21	1.23	1.26	1.29	1.32	1.35	1.37	1.40	1.43
	1.04	1.07	1.10	1.13	1.16	1.19	1.22	1.25	1.28	1.31	1.34	1.37	1.40	1.43	1.46	1.49
64.0	.94	.97	1.00	1.03	1.05	1.08	1.11	1.13	1.16	1.19	1.22	1.24	1.27	1.30	1.32	1.35
	.98	1.01	1.04	1.06	1.09	1.12	1.15	1.18	1.20	1.23	1.26	1.29	1.32	1.34	1.37	1.40
62.0	.89	.92	.94	.97	.99	1.02	1.04	1.07	1.09	1.12	1.14	1.16	1.19	1.21	1.24	1.26
	.92	.94	.97	1.00	1.02	1.05	1.08	1.10	1.13	1.16	1.18	1.21	1.24	1.27	1.29	1.32
60.0	.84	.86	.88	.90	.93	.95	.97	1.00	1.02	1.04	1.06	1.09	1.11	1.13	1.16	1.18
	.86	.88	.90	.93	.96	.98	1.00	1.03	1.06	1.08	1.10	1.13	1.16	1.18	1.20	1.23
58.0	.78	.80	.82	.85	.87	.89	.91	.93	.96	.98	1.00	1.02	1.04	1.07	1.09	1.11
	.80	.83	.85	.87	.90	.92	.94	.97	.99	1.01	1.04	1.06	1.08	1.10	1.13	1.15
56.0	.72	.75	.77	.79	.81	.83	.85	.87	.89	.91	.93	.95	.97	.99	1.01	1.03
	.74	.77	.79	.81	.83	.85	.87	.89	.92	.94	.96	.98	1.00	1.03	1.05	1.07
54.0	.68	.69	.71	.73	.75	.77	.79	.81	.83	.85	.86	.88	.90	.92	.94	.96
	.69	.71	.73	.75	.77	.79	.81	.83	.85	.87	.90	.92	.94	.96	.98	1.00
52.0	.63	.65	.67	.68	.70	.72	.74	.75	.77	.79	.80	.82	.84	.86	.87	.89
	.64	.66	.68	.70	.72	.74	.76	.78	.79	.81	.83	.85	.87	.88	.90	.92
50.0	.58	.60	.61	.63	.64	.66	.68	.69	.71	.73	.74	.76	.78	.80	.81	.83
	.60	.61	.63	.65	.66	.68	.70	.71	.73	.75	.76	.78	.80	.82	.83	.85
48.0	.54	.55	.56	.58	.60	.61	.62	.64	.66	.67	.68	.70	.72	.73	.74	.76
	.55	.57	.58	.60	.61	.63	.65	.66	.68	.69	.71	.73	.74	.76	.77	.79
46.0	.49	.50	.52	.53	.55	.56	.57	.59	.60	.62	.63	.64	.66	.67	.69	.70
	.50	.52	.54	.55	.56	.58	.59	.61	.62	.64	.65	.66	.68	.69	.71	.72
44.0	.45	.46	.47	.49	.50	.51	.52	.54	.55	.56	.58	.59	.60	.61	.63	.64
	.46	.47	.49	.50	.52	.53	.54	.56	.57	.58	.60	.61	.62	.63	.65	.66
42.0	.41	.42	.43	.45	.46	.47	.48	.49	.50	.51	.52	.54	.55	.56	.57	.58
	.42	.43	.44	.46	.47	.48	.49	.50	.52	.53	.54	.55	.56	.58	.59	.60
40.0	.37	.38	.39	.40	.41	.42	.43	.44	.45	.46	.48	.49	.50	.51	.52	.53
	.38	.39	.40	.41	.42	.43	.44	.45	.46	.47	.48	.50	.51	.52	.53	.54

Table B.IV (*contd*)

.51	.52	.53	.54	.55	.56	.57	.58	.59	.60	.61	.62	.63	.64	.65	.66	.67	.68
3.31 3.54	3.37 3.62	3.44 3.69	3.50 3.76	3.56 3.84	3.62 3.91	3.68 3.98	3.75 4.05	3.81 4.13	3.87 4.20	3.93 4.27	3.99 4.35	4.06 4.42	4.12 4.49	4.18 4.56	4.24 4.64	4.30 4.71	4.37 4.78
3.18 3.40	3.24 3.47	3.30 3.54	3.36 3.61	3.42 3.68	3.48 3.75	3.54 3.82	3.60 3.89	3.66 3.96	3.72 4.03	3.78 4.10	3.84 4.17	3.90 4.24	3.96 4.31	4.02 4.38	4.07 4.45	4.13 4.52	4.19 4.59
3.06 3.27	3.11 3.33	3.17 3.40	3.23 3.46	3.28 3.53	3.34 3.60	3.40 3.66	3.46 3.73	3.51 3.79	3.57 3.86	3.63 3.93	3.68 3.99	3.74 4.06	3.80 4.13	3.86 4.20	3.91 4.26	3.97 4.33	4.03 4.40
2.93 3.12	2.98 3.19	3.04 3.25	3.09 3.32	3.15 3.38	3.21 3.44	3.26 3.51	3.32 3.57	3.37 3.64	3.43 3.70	3.48 3.76	3.54 3.83	3.60 3.89	3.65 3.96	3.70 4.02	3.76 4.08	3.82 4.15	3.87 4.21
2.81 2.99	2.87 3.05	2.92 3.11	2.97 3.17	3.02 3.24	3.08 3.30	3.13 3.36	3.18 3.42	3.24 3.48	3.29 3.54	3.34 3.60	3.39 3.66	3.45 3.73	3.50 3.79	3.55 3.85	3.60 3.91	3.65 3.97	3.71 4.04
2.69 2.86	2.74 2.92	2.79 2.97	2.84 3.03	2.90 3.09	2.95 3.15	3.00 3.21	3.05 3.26	3.10 3.32	3.15 3.38	3.20 3.44	3.25 3.50	3.30 3.56	3.35 3.62	3.40 3.68	3.45 3.73	3.50 3.79	3.55 3.85
2.57 2.74	2.62 2.79	2.67 2.84	2.72 2.90	2.76 2.96	2.81 3.01	2.86 3.06	2.91 3.12	2.96 3.18	3.01 3.23	3.06 3.29	3.11 3.34	3.15 3.40	3.20 3.45	3.25 3.51	3.30 3.57	3.35 3.62	3.39 3.68
2.46 2.61	2.50 2.67	2.55 2.72	2.60 2.77	2.64 2.82	2.69 2.88	2.74 2.93	2.79 2.98	2.83 3.04	2.88 3.09	2.93 3.14	2.97 3.20	3.02 3.25	3.06 3.30	3.11 3.36	3.16 3.41	3.20 3.46	3.25 3.51
2.34 2.49	2.39 2.54	2.44 2.59	2.48 2.64	2.52 2.69	2.57 2.74	2.62 2.79	2.66 2.84	2.70 2.89	2.75 2.94	2.79 2.99	2.84 3.04	2.88 3.09	2.93 3.14	2.97 3.20	3.01 3.25	3.06 3.30	3.10 3.35
2.24 2.37	2.28 2.42	2.33 2.46	2.37 2.51	2.41 2.56	2.45 2.61	2.49 2.66	2.54 2.70	2.58 2.75	2.62 2.80	2.66 2.85	2.70 2.90	2.75 2.95	2.79 3.00	2.83 3.04	2.87 3.09	2.91 3.14	2.96 3.19
2.13 2.26	2.17 2.30	2.21 2.34	2.25 2.39	2.30 2.44	2.34 2.48	2.38 2.52	2.42 2.57	2.46 2.62	2.50 2.66	2.54 2.71	2.58 2.75	2.62 2.80	2.66 2.84	2.70 2.89	2.74 2.94	2.78 2.98	2.82 3.03
2.03 2.14	2.07 2.19	2.11 2.23	2.15 2.27	2.18 2.32	2.22 2.36	2.26 2.40	2.30 2.44	2.34 2.49	2.38 2.53	2.42 2.57	2.46 2.62	2.49 2.66	2.53 2.71	2.57 2.75	2.61 2.79	2.65 2.84	2.68 2.88
1.93 2.03	1.96 2.07	2.00 2.11	2.04 2.15	2.08 2.20	2.11 2.24	2.15 2.28	2.19 2.32	2.22 2.36	2.26 2.40	2.30 2.44	2.33 2.48	2.37 2.52	2.40 2.56	2.44 2.60	2.48 2.65	2.51 2.69	2.55 2.73
1.82 1.92	1.86 1.96	1.90 2.00	1.93 2.04	1.96 2.08	2.00 2.11	2.04 2.15	2.07 2.19	2.10 2.23	2.14 2.27	2.18 2.31	2.21 2.35	2.24 2.39	2.28 2.43	2.32 2.47	2.35 2.51	2.38 2.55	2.42 2.59
1.73 1.82	1.77 1.85	1.80 1.89	1.83 1.93	1.86 1.96	1.90 2.00	1.93 2.04	1.96 2.08	2.00 2.11	2.03 2.15	2.06 2.19	2.10 2.22	2.13 2.26	2.16 2.30	2.20 2.34	2.23 2.37	2.26 2.41	2.29 2.45
1.64 1.72	1.67 1.75	1.70 1.78	1.73 1.82	1.76 1.86	1.80 1.89	1.83 1.92	1.86 1.96	1.89 2.00	1.92 2.03	1.95 2.06	1.98 2.10	2.01 2.14	2.04 2.17	2.08 2.20	2.11 2.24	2.14 2.28	2.17 2.31
1.55 1.62	1.58 1.65	1.61 1.69	1.64 1.72	1.66 1.75	1.69 1.78	1.72 1.81	1.75 1.85	1.78 1.88	1.81 1.91	1.84 1.94	1.87 1.98	1.90 2.01	1.93 2.04	1.96 2.08	1.99 2.11	2.02 2.14	2.05 2.17
1.46 1.52	1.49 1.55	1.51 1.58	1.54 1.61	1.57 1.64	1.60 1.68	1.63 1.71	1.65 1.74	1.68 1.77	1.71 1.80	1.74 1.83	1.76 1.86	1.79 1.89	1.82 1.92	1.84 1.96	1.87 1.99	1.90 2.02	1.93 2.05
1.38 1.43	1.40 1.46	1.43 1.49	1.45 1.52	1.48 1.54	1.51 1.57	1.53 1.60	1.56 1.63	1.58 1.66	1.61 1.69	1.64 1.72	1.66 1.75	1.69 1.78	1.71 1.81	1.74 1.84	1.77 1.86	1.79 1.89	1.82 1.92
1.28 1.35	1.31 1.37	1.34 1.40	1.36 1.43	1.38 1.46	1.41 1.48	1.44 1.51	1.46 1.54	1.48 1.56	1.51 1.59	1.53 1.62	1.56 1.64	1.58 1.67	1.61 1.70	1.63 1.72	1.65 1.75	1.68 1.78	1.70 1.81
1.20 1.26	1.23 1.28	1.25 1.31	1.28 1.33	1.30 1.36	1.32 1.39	1.35 1.41	1.37 1.44	1.40 1.46	1.42 1.49	1.44 1.52	1.46 1.54	1.49 1.56	1.51 1.59	1.53 1.62	1.55 1.64	1.57 1.66	1.60 1.69
1.13 1.17	1.15 1.20	1.18 1.22	1.20 1.25	1.22 1.27	1.24 1.29	1.26 1.32	1.29 1.34	1.31 1.37	1.33 1.39	1.35 1.41	1.37 1.44	1.40 1.46	1.42 1.48	1.44 1.50	1.46 1.53	1.48 1.55	1.51 1.57
1.05 1.09	1.07 1.11	1.09 1.14	1.11 1.16	1.13 1.18	1.15 1.20	1.17 1.22	1.19 1.25	1.21 1.27	1.23 1.29	1.25 1.31	1.27 1.33	1.29 1.36	1.31 1.38	1.34 1.40	1.36 1.42	1.38 1.44	1.40 1.47
.98 1.02	1.00 1.04	1.02 1.06	1.04 1.08	1.06 1.10	1.07 1.12	1.09 1.14	1.11 1.16	1.13 1.18	1.15 1.20	1.17 1.22	1.19 1.24	1.21 1.26	1.23 1.28	1.24 1.30	1.26 1.33	1.28 1.35	1.30 1.37
.91 .94	.93 .96	.94 .98	.96 1.00	.98 1.02	1.00 1.03	1.02 1.05	1.03 1.07	1.05 1.09	1.07 1.11	1.09 1.13	1.10 1.15	1.12 1.17	1.14 1.19	1.16 1.20	1.17 1.22	1.19 1.24	1.21 1.26
.85 .87	.86 .89	.88 .90	.89 .92	.91 .94	.93 .96	.94 .98	.96 .99	.97 1.01	.99 1.03	1.01 1.05	1.02 1.06	1.04 1.08	1.05 1.10	1.07 1.12	1.09 1.13	1.10 1.15	1.12 1.17
.78 .81	.79 .82	.80 .84	.82 .85	.84 .87	.85 .89	.86 .90	.88 .92	.90 .93	.91 .95	.92 .97	.94 .98	.96 1.00	.97 1.01	.98 1.03	1.00 1.05	1.02 1.06	1.03 1.08
.71 .74	.73 .75	.74 .76	.76 .78	.77 .80	.78 .81	.80 .82	.81 .84	.83 .86	.84 .87	.85 .88	.87 .90	.88 .92	.89 .93	.90 .94	.92 .96	.93 .98	.94 .99
.65 .67	.67 .69	.68 .70	.69 .71	.70 .72	.72 .74	.73 .75	.74 .76	.76 .78	.77 .79	.78 .80	.79 .82	.81 .83	.82 .85	.83 .86	.84 .87	.85 .89	.87 .90
.59 .61	.60 .62	.62 .64	.63 .65	.64 .66	.65 .67	.66 .68	.68 .70	.69 .71	.70 .72	.71 .73	.72 .75	.73 .76	.74 .77	.76 .78	.77 .80	.78 .81	.79 .82
.54 .55	.55 .56	.56 .57	.57 .58	.58 .60	.59 .61	.60 .62	.61 .63	.62 .64	.63 .65	.64 .66	.65 .67	.66 .69	.67 .70	.68 .71	.70 .72	.71 .73	.72 .75

Table B.IV (*contd*)

Initial vergence (D)	Thickness (mm)															
	.69	.70	.71	.72	.73	.74	.75	.76	.77	.78	.79	.80	.81	.82	.83	.84
100.0	4.43 / 4.86	4.49 / 4.93	4.55 / 5.00	4.61 / 5.08	4.67 / 5.15	4.73 / 5.23	4.80 / 5.30	4.86 / 5.37	4.92 / 5.45	4.98 / 5.52	5.04 / 5.60	5.10 / 5.67	5.16 / 5.75	5.22 / 5.82	5.28 / 5.90	5.34 / 5.97
98.0	4.25 / 4.66	4.31 / 4.73	4.37 / 4.80	4.43 / 4.87	4.49 / 4.94	4.55 / 5.01	4.60 / 5.08	4.66 / 5.16	4.72 / 5.23	4.78 / 5.30	4.84 / 5.37	4.90 / 5.44	4.96 / 5.51	5.02 / 5.59	5.07 / 5.66	5.13 / 5.73
96.0	4.08 / 4.46	4.14 / 4.53	4.20 / 4.60	4.25 / 4.67	4.31 / 4.74	4.37 / 4.81	4.42 / 4.88	4.48 / 4.94	4.54 / 5.01	4.60 / 5.08	4.65 / 5.15	4.71 / 5.22	4.76 / 5.29	4.82 / 5.36	4.88 / 5.43	4.93 / 5.50
94.0	3.92 / 4.28	3.98 / 4.34	4.03 / 4.41	4.09 / 4.47	4.14 / 4.54	4.20 / 4.60	4.25 / 4.67	4.30 / 4.74	4.36 / 4.80	4.41 / 4.87	4.47 / 4.93	4.52 / 5.00	4.57 / 5.07	4.63 / 5.13	4.68 / 5.20	4.73 / 5.26
92.0	3.76 / 4.10	3.81 / 4.16	3.86 / 4.22	3.91 / 4.28	3.97 / 4.35	4.02 / 4.41	4.07 / 4.47	4.12 / 4.53	4.17 / 4.59	4.23 / 4.66	4.28 / 4.72	4.33 / 4.78	4.38 / 4.84	4.43 / 4.91	4.48 / 4.97	4.53 / 5.03
90.0	3.60 / 3.91	3.65 / 3.97	3.70 / 4.03	3.75 / 4.09	3.80 / 4.15	3.85 / 4.21	3.90 / 4.27	3.95 / 4.33	4.00 / 4.39	4.05 / 4.45	4.10 / 4.51	4.15 / 4.57	4.20 / 4.63	4.25 / 4.69	4.30 / 4.75	4.35 / 4.81
88.0	3.44 / 3.73	3.49 / 3.79	3.54 / 3.85	3.59 / 3.90	3.63 / 3.96	3.68 / 4.02	3.73 / 4.08	3.78 / 4.13	3.83 / 4.19	3.87 / 4.25	3.92 / 4.30	3.97 / 4.36	4.02 / 4.42	4.06 / 4.48	4.11 / 4.53	4.16 / 4.59
86.0	3.29 / 3.57	3.34 / 3.62	3.39 / 3.67	3.43 / 3.73	3.48 / 3.78	3.52 / 3.84	3.57 / 3.89	3.62 / 3.94	3.66 / 4.00	3.71 / 4.05	3.75 / 4.11	3.80 / 4.16	3.84 / 4.22	3.89 / 4.27	3.94 / 4.32	3.98 / 4.38
84.0	3.15 / 3.40	3.19 / 3.45	3.23 / 3.50	3.28 / 3.55	3.32 / 3.61	3.36 / 3.66	3.40 / 3.71	3.45 / 3.76	3.49 / 3.81	3.53 / 3.87	3.58 / 3.92	3.62 / 3.97	3.66 / 4.02	3.71 / 4.07	3.75 / 4.13	3.80 / 4.18
82.0	3.00 / 3.24	3.04 / 3.29	3.08 / 3.34	3.12 / 3.39	3.17 / 3.44	3.21 / 3.49	3.25 / 3.54	3.29 / 3.58	3.33 / 3.63	3.38 / 3.68	3.42 / 3.73	3.46 / 3.78	3.50 / 3.83	3.54 / 3.88	3.58 / 3.93	3.62 / 3.98
80.0	2.86 / 3.07	2.90 / 3.12	2.94 / 3.17	2.98 / 3.21	3.02 / 3.26	3.06 / 3.31	3.10 / 3.36	3.13 / 3.40	3.17 / 3.45	3.21 / 3.50	3.25 / 3.54	3.29 / 3.59	3.33 / 3.64	3.37 / 3.68	3.41 / 3.73	3.45 / 3.78
78.0	2.72 / 2.93	2.76 / 2.97	2.80 / 3.01	2.84 / 3.06	2.87 / 3.10	2.91 / 3.15	2.95 / 3.19	2.99 / 3.23	3.03 / 3.28	3.06 / 3.32	3.10 / 3.37	3.14 / 3.41	3.18 / 3.46	3.21 / 3.50	3.25 / 3.54	3.29 / 3.59
76.0	2.58 / 2.77	2.62 / 2.81	2.66 / 2.85	2.69 / 2.89	2.73 / 2.94	2.76 / 2.98	2.80 / 3.02	2.84 / 3.06	2.87 / 3.10	2.91 / 3.15	2.94 / 3.19	2.98 / 3.23	3.02 / 3.27	3.05 / 3.32	3.09 / 3.36	3.12 / 3.40
74.0	2.46 / 2.63	2.49 / 2.67	2.52 / 2.71	2.56 / 2.75	2.59 / 2.79	2.63 / 2.83	2.66 / 2.86	2.69 / 2.90	2.73 / 2.94	2.76 / 2.98	2.80 / 3.02	2.83 / 3.06	2.86 / 3.10	2.90 / 3.14	2.93 / 3.18	2.97 / 3.22
72.0	2.33 / 2.48	2.36 / 2.52	2.39 / 2.56	2.42 / 2.60	2.46 / 2.63	2.49 / 2.67	2.52 / 2.71	2.55 / 2.75	2.58 / 2.79	2.62 / 2.82	2.65 / 2.86	2.68 / 2.90	2.71 / 2.94	2.74 / 2.97	2.78 / 3.01	2.81 / 3.05
70.0	2.20 / 2.34	2.23 / 2.38	2.26 / 2.42	2.29 / 2.45	2.32 / 2.48	2.35 / 2.52	2.38 / 2.56	2.42 / 2.59	2.45 / 2.62	2.48 / 2.66	2.51 / 2.70	2.54 / 2.73	2.57 / 2.77	2.60 / 2.80	2.63 / 2.84	2.66 / 2.87
68.0	2.08 / 2.21	2.11 / 2.24	2.14 / 2.27	2.17 / 2.31	2.20 / 2.34	2.23 / 2.38	2.26 / 2.41	2.28 / 2.44	2.31 / 2.48	2.34 / 2.51	2.37 / 2.55	2.40 / 2.58	2.43 / 2.61	2.46 / 2.65	2.48 / 2.68	2.51 / 2.71
66.0	1.95 / 2.08	1.98 / 2.11	2.01 / 2.14	2.04 / 2.17	2.06 / 2.20	2.09 / 2.23	2.12 / 2.26	2.15 / 2.30	2.18 / 2.33	2.20 / 2.36	2.23 / 2.39	2.26 / 2.42	2.29 / 2.45	2.31 / 2.48	2.34 / 2.52	2.37 / 2.55
64.0	1.84 / 1.95	1.87 / 1.98	1.90 / 2.01	1.92 / 2.04	1.95 / 2.07	1.97 / 2.10	2.00 / 2.13	2.03 / 2.16	2.05 / 2.19	2.08 / 2.22	2.10 / 2.25	2.13 / 2.28	2.16 / 2.31	2.18 / 2.34	2.20 / 2.37	2.23 / 2.40
62.0	1.73 / 1.83	1.75 / 1.86	1.78 / 1.89	1.80 / 1.92	1.82 / 1.94	1.85 / 1.97	1.88 / 2.00	1.90 / 2.03	1.92 / 2.06	1.95 / 2.08	1.98 / 2.11	2.00 / 2.14	2.02 / 2.17	2.05 / 2.19	2.07 / 2.22	2.10 / 2.25
60.0	1.62 / 1.72	1.64 / 1.74	1.66 / 1.77	1.69 / 1.79	1.71 / 1.82	1.73 / 1.84	1.76 / 1.87	1.78 / 1.90	1.80 / 1.92	1.82 / 1.95	1.85 / 1.97	1.87 / 2.00	1.89 / 2.03	1.92 / 2.05	1.94 / 2.08	1.96 / 2.10
58.0	1.53 / 1.60	1.55 / 1.62	1.57 / 1.64	1.59 / 1.67	1.61 / 1.69	1.63 / 1.72	1.66 / 1.74	1.68 / 1.76	1.70 / 1.79	1.72 / 1.81	1.74 / 1.84	1.76 / 1.86	1.78 / 1.88	1.80 / 1.91	1.82 / 1.94	1.84 / 1.96
56.0	1.42 / 1.49	1.44 / 1.51	1.46 / 1.53	1.48 / 1.56	1.50 / 1.58	1.52 / 1.60	1.54 / 1.62	1.55 / 1.65	1.57 / 1.67	1.59 / 1.69	1.61 / 1.72	1.63 / 1.74	1.65 / 1.76	1.67 / 1.78	1.69 / 1.81	1.71 / 1.83
54.0	1.32 / 1.39	1.34 / 1.41	1.36 / 1.43	1.38 / 1.45	1.39 / 1.47	1.41 / 1.49	1.43 / 1.51	1.45 / 1.53	1.47 / 1.55	1.48 / 1.57	1.50 / 1.59	1.52 / 1.61	1.54 / 1.63	1.56 / 1.65	1.58 / 1.67	1.60 / 1.69
52.0	1.22 / 1.28	1.24 / 1.30	1.26 / 1.32	1.27 / 1.34	1.29 / 1.36	1.31 / 1.38	1.32 / 1.40	1.34 / 1.41	1.36 / 1.43	1.38 / 1.45	1.39 / 1.47	1.41 / 1.49	1.43 / 1.51	1.44 / 1.53	1.46 / 1.55	1.48 / 1.57
50.0	1.13 / 1.18	1.15 / 1.20	1.17 / 1.22	1.18 / 1.24	1.20 / 1.25	1.21 / 1.27	1.23 / 1.29	1.25 / 1.31	1.26 / 1.33	1.28 / 1.34	1.29 / 1.36	1.31 / 1.38	1.33 / 1.40	1.34 / 1.42	1.36 / 1.43	1.37 / 1.45
48.0	1.04 / 1.09	1.06 / 1.11	1.08 / 1.13	1.09 / 1.14	1.10 / 1.16	1.12 / 1.17	1.14 / 1.19	1.15 / 1.21	1.16 / 1.22	1.18 / 1.24	1.20 / 1.25	1.21 / 1.27	1.22 / 1.29	1.24 / 1.30	1.25 / 1.32	1.27 / 1.33
46.0	.96 / 1.00	.97 / 1.02	.98 / 1.03	1.00 / 1.05	1.01 / 1.06	1.03 / 1.08	1.04 / 1.09	1.05 / 1.10	1.07 / 1.12	1.08 / 1.13	1.10 / 1.15	1.11 / 1.16	1.12 / 1.18	1.14 / 1.19	1.15 / 1.20	1.16 / 1.22
44.0	.88 / .92	.89 / .93	.90 / .94	.92 / .96	.93 / .97	.94 / .98	.96 / 1.00	.97 / 1.01	.98 / 1.02	.99 / 1.03	1.01 / 1.05	1.02 / 1.06	1.03 / 1.07	1.04 / 1.09	1.06 / 1.10	1.07 / 1.12
42.0	.80 / .84	.81 / .85	.82 / .86	.83 / .87	.85 / .89	.86 / .90	.87 / .91	.88 / .92	.89 / .93	.91 / .95	.92 / .96	.93 / .97	.94 / .98	.95 / .99	.96 / 1.01	.97 / 1.02
40.0	.73 / .76	.74 / .77	.75 / .78	.76 / .79	.77 / .80	.78 / .81	.79 / .82	.80 / .84	.81 / .85	.82 / .86	.83 / .87	.84 / .88	.85 / .89	.86 / .90	.87 / .91	.88 / .92

Table B.IV (*contd*)

.85	.86	.87	.88	.89	.90	.91	.92	.93	.94	.95	.96	.97	.98	.99	1.00	1.01	1.02
5.40	5.46	5.52	5.58	5.64	5.70	5.76	5.82	5.88	5.94	6.00	6.05	6.11	6.17	6.23	6.29	6.35	6.41
6.05	6.13	6.20	6.28	6.35	6.43	6.51	6.58	6.66	6.73	6.81	6.89	6.96	7.04	7.11	7.19	7.27	7.35
5.19	5.25	5.31	5.36	5.42	5.48	5.54	5.59	5.65	5.71	5.76	5.82	5.88	5.94	5.99	6.05	6.11	6.16
5.80	5.88	5.95	6.02	6.10	6.17	6.24	6.32	6.39	6.46	6.54	6.61	6.68	6.75	6.83	6.90	6.97	7.05
4.98	5.04	5.10	5.15	5.20	5.26	5.32	5.37	5.42	5.48	5.54	5.59	5.64	5.70	5.76	5.81	5.86	5.92
5.56	5.63	5.70	5.77	5.84	5.91	5.98	6.05	6.12	6.19	6.26	6.33	6.40	6.47	6.54	6.61	6.68	6.75
4.78	4.84	4.89	4.94	5.00	5.05	5.10	5.16	5.21	5.26	5.32	5.37	5.42	5.47	5.53	5.58	5.63	5.68
5.33	5.40	5.46	5.53	5.59	5.66	5.73	5.79	5.86	5.93	6.00	6.06	6.13	6.20	6.26	6.33	6.40	6.47
4.58	4.64	4.69	4.74	4.79	4.84	4.89	4.94	4.99	5.04	5.10	5.15	5.20	5.25	5.30	5.35	5.40	5.45
5.10	5.16	5.22	5.28	5.35	5.41	5.47	5.54	5.60	5.67	5.73	5.79	5.86	5.92	6.00	6.05	6.12	6.18
4.40	4.44	4.49	4.54	4.59	4.64	4.69	4.74	4.79	4.84	4.88	4.93	4.98	5.03	5.08	5.13	5.18	5.23
4.87	4.93	4.99	5.05	5.11	5.17	5.23	5.29	5.36	5.42	5.48	5.54	5.60	5.67	5.73	5.79	5.85	5.91
4.20	4.25	4.30	4.35	4.39	4.44	4.49	4.53	4.58	4.63	4.68	4.72	4.77	4.82	4.86	4.91	4.96	5.00
4.65	4.71	4.77	4.82	4.88	4.94	5.00	5.06	5.11	5.17	5.23	5.29	5.35	5.40	5.46	5.52	5.58	5.64
4.02	4.07	4.12	4.16	4.20	4.25	4.29	4.34	4.38	4.43	4.47	4.51	4.56	4.60	4.65	4.69	4.73	4.78
4.44	4.49	4.54	4.60	4.66	4.71	4.77	4.82	4.88	4.93	4.99	5.05	5.10	5.16	5.21	5.27	5.33	5.38
3.84	3.88	3.93	3.97	4.02	4.06	4.10	4.14	4.19	4.23	4.27	4.31	4.35	4.40	4.44	4.48	4.52	4.56
4.23	4.28	4.33	4.39	4.44	4.49	4.54	4.60	4.65	4.70	4.76	4.81	4.86	4.91	4.97	5.02	5.07	5.13
3.66	3.71	3.75	3.79	3.83	3.87	3.91	3.95	3.99	4.03	4.08	4.12	4.16	4.20	4.24	4.28	4.32	4.36
4.02	4.07	4.12	4.17	4.22	4.27	4.32	4.37	4.42	4.47	4.52	4.58	4.63	4.68	4.73	4.78	4.83	4.88
3.49	3.53	3.57	3.61	3.65	3.69	3.73	3.77	3.81	3.85	3.88	3.92	3.96	4.00	4.04	4.08	4.12	4.16
3.82	3.87	3.92	3.97	4.01	4.06	4.11	4.16	4.20	4.25	4.30	4.35	4.40	4.44	4.49	4.54	4.59	4.64
3.32	3.36	3.40	3.44	3.47	3.51	3.55	3.58	3.62	3.66	3.69	3.73	3.77	3.81	3.84	3.88	3.92	3.95
3.64	3.68	3.72	3.77	3.82	3.86	3.90	3.95	4.00	4.04	4.08	4.13	4.18	4.22	4.26	4.31	4.36	4.40
3.16	3.20	3.23	3.27	3.30	3.34	3.38	3.41	3.44	3.48	3.52	3.55	3.58	3.62	3.66	3.69	3.72	3.76
3.44	3.49	3.53	3.57	3.62	3.66	3.70	3.74	3.79	3.83	3.87	3.91	3.95	4.00	4.04	4.08	4.12	4.17
3.00	3.03	3.07	3.10	3.14	3.17	3.20	3.24	3.27	3.30	3.34	3.37	3.40	3.43	3.47	3.50	3.53	3.57
3.26	3.30	3.34	3.38	3.42	3.46	3.50	3.54	3.58	3.62	3.66	3.71	3.75	3.79	3.83	3.87	3.91	3.95
2.84	2.87	2.90	2.94	2.97	3.00	3.03	3.06	3.10	3.13	3.16	3.19	3.22	3.26	3.29	3.32	3.35	3.38
3.08	3.12	3.16	3.20	3.23	3.27	3.30	3.35	3.39	3.43	3.46	3.50	3.54	3.58	3.62	3.66	3.70	3.74
2.69	2.72	2.75	2.78	2.81	2.84	2.87	2.90	2.93	2.96	2.99	3.02	3.05	3.08	3.11	3.14	3.17	3.20
2.91	2.95	2.98	3.02	3.05	3.09	3.13	3.16	3.20	3.23	3.27	3.31	3.34	3.38	3.41	3.45	3.49	3.52
2.54	2.57	2.60	2.62	2.65	2.68	2.71	2.74	2.77	2.80	2.82	2.85	2.88	2.91	2.94	2.97	3.00	3.03
2.74	2.78	2.81	2.84	2.88	2.91	2.94	2.98	3.01	3.05	3.08	3.11	3.15	3.18	3.22	3.25	3.28	3.32
2.40	2.42	2.45	2.48	2.50	2.53	2.56	2.58	2.61	2.64	2.66	2.69	2.72	2.75	2.77	2.80	2.83	2.85
2.58	2.61	2.64	2.68	2.71	2.74	2.77	2.80	2.84	2.87	2.90	2.93	2.96	3.00	3.03	3.06	3.09	3.12
2.26	2.28	2.30	2.33	2.36	2.38	2.41	2.43	2.46	2.48	2.51	2.54	2.56	2.59	2.61	2.64	2.66	2.69
2.42	2.45	2.48	2.51	2.54	2.57	2.60	2.63	2.66	2.69	2.72	2.75	2.78	2.81	2.84	2.87	2.90	2.93
2.12	2.14	2.17	2.19	2.22	2.24	2.26	2.29	2.31	2.34	2.36	2.38	2.41	2.43	2.46	2.48	2.50	2.53
2.28	2.30	2.33	2.36	2.38	2.41	2.44	2.47	2.49	2.52	2.55	2.58	2.61	2.63	2.66	2.69	2.72	2.75
1.98	2.01	2.03	2.05	2.08	2.10	2.12	2.14	2.17	2.19	2.21	2.23	2.25	2.28	2.30	2.32	2.34	2.36
2.13	2.16	2.18	2.21	2.23	2.26	2.29	2.31	2.34	2.36	2.39	2.42	2.44	2.47	2.49	2.52	2.55	2.57
1.86	1.89	1.91	1.93	1.95	1.97	1.99	2.01	2.03	2.05	2.08	2.10	2.12	2.14	2.16	2.18	2.20	2.22
1.98	2.01	2.04	2.06	2.08	2.11	2.13	2.16	2.18	2.21	2.23	2.25	2.28	2.30	2.33	2.35	2.37	2.40
1.73	1.75	1.77	1.79	1.81	1.83	1.85	1.87	1.89	1.91	1.93	1.95	1.97	1.99	2.01	2.03	2.05	2.07
1.85	1.87	1.89	1.92	-1.94	1.96	1.98	2.01	2.03	2.05	2.08	2.10	2.12	2.14	2.17	2.19	2.21	2.24
1.62	1.63	1.65	1.67	1.69	1.71	1.73	1.75	1.76	1.78	1.80	1.82	1.84	1.85	1.87	1.89	1.91	1.93
1.72	1.74	1.76	1.78	1.80	1.82	1.84	1.86	1.88	1.90	1.92	1.95	1.97	1.99	2.01	2.03	2.05	2.07
1.50	1.51	1.53	1.55	1.56	1.58	1.60	1.61	1.63	1.65	1.66	1.68	1.70	1.72	1.73	1.75	1.77	1.78
1.59	1.61	1.63	1.65	1.67	1.69	1.71	1.73	1.75	1.77	1.78	1.80	1.82	1.84	1.86	1.88	1.90	1.92
1.39	1.41	1.42	1.44	1.45	1.47	1.49	1.50	1.51	1.53	1.55	1.56	1.57	1.59	1.61	1.62	1.64	1.65
1.47	1.49	1.51	1.52	1.54	1.56	1.58	1.60	1.61	1.63	1.65	1.67	1.69	1.70	1.72	1.74	1.76	1.78
1.28	1.29	1.31	1.32	1.34	1.35	1.36	1.38	1.40	1.41	1.42	1.44	1.46	1.47	1.48	1.50	1.51	1.53
1.35	1.37	1.38	1.40	1.41	1.43	1.45	1.46	1.48	1.50	1.52	1.53	1.55	1.57	1.58	1.60	1.62	1.63
1.18	1.19	1.20	1.21	1.23	1.24	1.25	1.27	1.28	1.30	1.31	1.32	1.34	1.35	1.37	1.38	1.39	1.41
1.24	1.25	1.26	1.28	1.30	1.31	1.33	1.34	1.36	1.37	1.39	1.41	1.42	1.44	1.45	1.47	1.48	1.50
1.08	1.09	1.10	1.12	1.13	1.14	1.15	1.16	1.18	1.19	1.20	1.21	1.22	1.24	1.25	1.26	1.27	1.28
1.13	1.14	1.16	1.17	1.19	1.20	1.21	1.23	1.24	1.26	1.27	1.28	1.30	1.31	1.33	1.34	1.35	1.37
.98	1.00	1.01	1.02	1.03	1.04	1.05	1.06	1.07	1.08	1.10	1.11	1.12	1.13	1.14	1.15	1.16	1.17
1.03	1.04	1.05	1.07	1.08	1.09	1.10	1.12	1.13	1.14	1.16	1.17	1.18	1.19	1.21	1.22	1.23	1.24
.89	.90	.91	.92	.93	.94	.95	.96	.97	.98	1.00	1.01	1.02	1.03	1.04	1.05	1.06	1.07
.94	.95	.96	.97	.98	.99	1.00	1.01	1.02	1.03	1.04	1.06	1.07	1.08	1.09	1.10	1.11	1.12

Table B.IV (*contd*)

Initial vergence (D)	Thickness (mm)															
	1.03	1.04	1.05	1.06	1.07	1.08	1.09	1.10	1.11	1.12	1.13	1.14	1.15	1.16	1.17	1.18
100.0	6.46 / 7.42	6.52 / 7.50	6.58 / 7.58	6.64 / 7.66	6.70 / 7.74	6.75 / 7.81	6.81 / 7.89	6.87 / 7.97	6.93 / 8.05	6.99 / 8.13	7.04 / 8.21	7.10 / 8.29	7.16 / 8.36	7.22 / 8.44	7.28 / 8.52	7.33 / 8.60
98.0	6.22 / 7.12	6.27 / 7.20	6.33 / 7.27	6.39 / 7.34	6.44 / 7.42	6.50 / 7.49	6.55 / 7.57	6.61 / 7.64	6.67 / 7.72	6.72 / 7.79	6.78 / 7.87	6.83 / 7.94	6.89 / 8.02	6.95 / 8.10	7.00 / 8.17	7.06 / 8.25
96.0	5.97 / 6.82	6.03 / 6.89	6.08 / 6.96	6.13 / 7.04	6.19 / 7.11	6.24 / 7.18	6.30 / 7.25	6.35 / 7.32	6.40 / 7.39	6.46 / 7.46	6.51 / 7.54	6.57 / 7.61	6.62 / 7.68	6.67 / 7.75	6.73 / 7.82	6.78 / 7.90
94.0	5.74 / 6.53	5.79 / 6.60	5.84 / 6.67	5.89 / 6.74	5.94 / 6.81	6.00 / 6.87	6.05 / 6.94	6.10 / 7.01	6.15 / 7.08	6.20 / 7.15	6.26 / 7.22	6.31 / 7.29	6.36 / 7.36	6.41 / 7.42	6.46 / 7.49	6.52 / 7.56
92.0	5.50 / 6.24	5.55 / 6.31	5.60 / 6.38	5.65 / 6.44	5.70 / 6.50	5.75 / 6.57	5.80 / 6.64	5.85 / 6.70	5.90 / 6.77	5.95 / 6.83	6.00 / 6.90	6.05 / 6.96	6.10 / 7.03	6.15 / 7.10	6.20 / 7.16	6.25 / 7.23
90.0	5.27 / 5.98	5.32 / 6.04	5.37 / 6.10	5.42 / 6.16	5.47 / 6.22	5.51 / 6.29	5.56 / 6.35	5.61 / 6.41	5.66 / 6.47	5.70 / 6.53	5.75 / 6.60	5.80 / 6.66	5.84 / 6.72	5.89 / 6.78	5.94 / 6.84	5.99 / 6.91
88.0	5.05 / 5.70	5.09 / 5.76	5.14 / 5.82	5.19 / 5.87	5.23 / 5.93	5.28 / 5.99	5.32 / 6.05	5.37 / 6.11	5.42 / 6.17	5.46 / 6.23	5.50 / 6.29	5.55 / 6.35	5.60 / 6.41	5.64 / 6.47	5.68 / 6.53	5.73 / 6.59
86.0	4.82 / 5.44	4.87 / 5.49	4.91 / 5.55	4.95 / 5.61	5.00 / 5.66	5.04 / 5.72	5.09 / 5.77	5.13 / 5.83	5.17 / 5.89	5.22 / 5.94	5.26 / 6.00	5.31 / 6.06	5.35 / 6.12	5.39 / 6.17	5.44 / 6.23	5.48 / 6.29
84.0	4.61 / 5.18	4.65 / 5.23	4.69 / 5.28	4.73 / 5.34	4.77 / 5.39	4.82 / 5.44	4.86 / 5.50	4.90 / 5.55	4.94 / 5.60	4.98 / 5.66	5.03 / 5.72	5.07 / 5.77	5.11 / 5.82	5.15 / 5.88	5.19 / 5.94	5.24 / 5.99
82.0	4.40 / 4.93	4.44 / 4.98	4.48 / 5.03	4.52 / 5.08	4.56 / 5.13	4.60 / 5.18	4.64 / 5.23	4.68 / 5.28	4.72 / 5.33	4.76 / 5.38	4.80 / 5.44	4.84 / 5.49	4.88 / 5.54	4.92 / 5.59	4.96 / 5.64	5.00 / 5.70
80.0	4.19 / 4.68	4.23 / 4.73	4.27 / 4.78	4.31 / 4.83	4.35 / 4.88	4.38 / 4.92	4.42 / 4.97	4.46 / 5.02	4.50 / 5.07	4.54 / 5.12	4.57 / 5.17	4.61 / 5.22	4.65 / 5.26	4.69 / 5.31	4.73 / 5.36	4.76 / 5.41
78.0	3.99 / 4.45	4.03 / 4.49	4.06 / 4.54	4.10 / 4.59	4.14 / 4.63	4.18 / 4.68	4.21 / 4.72	4.25 / 4.77	4.29 / 4.82	4.32 / 4.86	4.36 / 4.91	4.39 / 4.95	4.43 / 5.00	4.47 / 5.05	4.50 / 5.09	4.54 / 5.14
76.0	3.80 / 4.21	3.83 / 4.26	3.86 / 4.30	3.90 / 4.34	3.94 / 4.39	3.97 / 4.43	4.00 / 4.48	4.04 / 4.52	4.07 / 4.56	4.11 / 4.61	4.14 / 4.65	4.18 / 4.70	4.21 / 4.74	4.24 / 4.78	4.28 / 4.83	4.31 / 4.87
74.0	3.60 / 3.99	3.63 / 4.03	3.66 / 4.08	3.70 / 4.12	3.73 / 4.16	3.76 / 4.20	3.80 / 4.24	3.83 / 4.28	3.86 / 4.32	3.90 / 4.36	3.93 / 4.40	3.96 / 4.44	4.00 / 4.48	4.03 / 4.53	4.06 / 4.57	4.09 / 4.61
72.0	3.41 / 3.77	3.44 / 3.81	3.48 / 3.85	3.51 / 3.89	3.54 / 3.93	3.57 / 3.96	3.60 / 4.00	3.63 / 4.04	3.66 / 4.08	3.69 / 4.12	3.73 / 4.16	3.76 / 4.20	3.79 / 4.24	3.82 / 4.27	3.85 / 4.31	3.89 / 4.35
70.0	3.23 / 3.56	3.26 / 3.59	3.29 / 3.63	3.32 / 3.67	3.35 / 3.70	3.38 / 3.74	3.41 / 3.77	3.44 / 3.81	3.47 / 3.85	3.50 / 3.88	3.53 / 3.92	3.56 / 3.96	3.59 / 4.00	3.62 / 4.03	3.65 / 4.07	3.68 / 4.11
68.0	3.05 / 3.35	3.08 / 3.39	3.11 / 3.42	3.14 / 3.45	3.17 / 3.49	3.19 / 3.52	3.22 / 3.56	3.25 / 3.59	3.28 / 3.62	3.31 / 3.66	3.33 / 3.70	3.36 / 3.73	3.39 / 3.76	3.42 / 3.80	3.45 / 3.84	3.47 / 3.87
66.0	2.88 / 3.16	2.91 / 3.19	2.94 / 3.22	2.96 / 3.25	2.99 / 3.28	3.02 / 3.32	3.04 / 3.35	3.07 / 3.38	3.10 / 3.41	3.12 / 3.45	3.15 / 3.48	3.17 / 3.51	3.20 / 3.54	3.23 / 3.58	3.25 / 3.61	3.28 / 3.64
64.0	2.72 / 2.96	2.74 / 2.99	2.76 / 3.02	2.79 / 3.05	2.82 / 3.08	2.84 / 3.11	2.86 / 3.14	2.89 / 3.17	2.92 / 3.20	2.94 / 3.23	2.96 / 3.26	2.99 / 3.29	3.02 / 3.32	3.04 / 3.36	3.06 / 3.39	3.09 / 3.42
62.0	2.55 / 2.77	2.57 / 2.80	2.60 / 2.83	2.62 / 2.86	2.64 / 2.89	2.66 / 2.91	2.69 / 2.94	2.71 / 2.97	2.73 / 3.00	2.76 / 3.03	2.78 / 3.06	2.81 / 3.09	2.83 / 3.12	2.85 / 3.14	2.88 / 3.17	2.90 / 3.20
60.0	2.39 / 2.60	2.41 / 2.62	2.43 / 2.65	2.45 / 2.68	2.47 / 2.70	2.50 / 2.73	2.52 / 2.75	2.54 / 2.78	2.56 / 2.81	2.59 / 2.83	2.61 / 2.86	2.63 / 2.89	2.66 / 2.92	2.68 / 2.94	2.70 / 2.97	2.72 / 3.00
58.0	2.24 / 2.42	2.26 / 2.45	2.28 / 2.47	2.31 / 2.49	2.33 / 2.52	2.35 / 2.54	2.37 / 2.57	2.39 / 2.59	2.41 / 2.62	2.43 / 2.64	2.45 / 2.66	2.47 / 2.69	2.50 / 2.72	2.52 / 2.74	2.54 / 2.76	2.56 / 2.79
56.0	2.09 / 2.26	2.11 / 2.28	2.12 / 2.30	2.14 / 2.33	2.16 / 2.35	2.18 / 2.37	2.20 / 2.40	2.22 / 2.42	2.24 / 2.44	2.26 / 2.46	2.28 / 2.49	2.30 / 2.51	2.32 / 2.53	2.34 / 2.55	2.36 / 2.57	2.38 / 2.60
54.0	1.94 / 2.09	1.96 / 2.11	1.98 / 2.14	2.00 / 2.16	2.02 / 2.18	2.03 / 2.20	2.05 / 2.22	2.07 / 2.24	2.09 / 2.26	2.11 / 2.28	2.12 / 2.31	2.14 / 2.33	2.16 / 2.35	2.18 / 2.37	2.20 / 2.39	2.21 / 2.42
52.0	1.80 / 1.94	1.82 / 1.96	1.84 / 1.98	1.85 / 2.00	1.87 / 2.02	1.89 / 2.04	1.90 / 2.06	1.92 / 2.08	1.94 / 2.10	1.95 / 2.12	1.97 / 2.14	1.99 / 2.16	2.00 / 2.18	2.02 / 2.19	2.04 / 2.21	2.06 / 2.23
50.0	1.67 / 1.79	1.68 / 1.81	1.70 / 1.83	1.72 / 1.85	1.73 / 1.87	1.75 / 1.88	1.76 / 1.90	1.78 / 1.92	1.80 / 1.94	1.81 / 1.96	1.83 / 1.97	1.84 / 1.99	1.86 / 2.01	1.88 / 2.03	1.89 / 2.05	1.91 / 2.06
48.0	1.54 / 1.65	1.56 / 1.66	1.57 / 1.68	1.58 / 1.70	1.60 / 1.71	1.61 / 1.73	1.63 / 1.74	1.64 / 1.76	1.66 / 1.78	1.67 / 1.79	1.68 / 1.81	1.70 / 1.83	1.72 / 1.84	1.73 / 1.86	1.74 / 1.88	1.76 / 1.90
46.0	1.42 / 1.52	1.43 / 1.53	1.44 / 1.54	1.46 / 1.56	1.47 / 1.58	1.48 / 1.59	1.50 / 1.60	1.51 / 1.62	1.52 / 1.64	1.54 / 1.65	1.55 / 1.66	1.56 / 1.68	1.58 / 1.70	1.59 / 1.71	1.60 / 1.72	1.61 / 1.74
44.0	1.30 / 1.38	1.31 / 1.40	1.32 / 1.41	1.33 / 1.42	1.34 / 1.44	1.36 / 1.45	1.37 / 1.47	1.38 / 1.48	1.39 / 1.49	1.41 / 1.51	1.42 / 1.52	1.43 / 1.54	1.44 / 1.55	1.46 / 1.56	1.47 / 1.58	1.48 / 1.59
42.0	1.18 / 1.26	1.19 / 1.27	1.20 / 1.28	1.22 / 1.29	1.23 / 1.30	1.24 / 1.32	1.25 / 1.33	1.26 / 1.34	1.27 / 1.35	1.28 / 1.37	1.29 / 1.38	1.30 / 1.39	1.32 / 1.40	1.33 / 1.42	1.34 / 1.43	1.35 / 1.44
40.0	1.08 / 1.14	1.09 / 1.15	1.10 / 1.16	1.11 / 1.17	1.12 / 1.18	1.13 / 1.20	1.14 / 1.21	1.15 / 1.22	1.16 / 1.23	1.17 / 1.24	1.18 / 1.25	1.19 / 1.26	1.20 / 1.28	1.21 / 1.29	1.22 / 1.30	1.23 / 1.31

Table B.IV (contd)

1.19	1.20	1.21	1.22	1.23	1.24	1.25	1.26	1.27	1.28	1.29	1.30	1.31	1.32	1.33	1.34	1.35	1.36
7.39 / 8.68	7.45 / 8.76	7.51 / 8.84	7.56 / 8.92	7.62 / 9.00	7.68 / 9.08	7.74 / 9.16	7.79 / 9.24	7.85 / 9.32	7.91 / 9.40	7.96 / 9.48	8.02 / 9.56	8.08 / 9.64	8.13 / 9.72	8.19 / 9.80	8.25 / 9.88	8.30 / 9.96	8.36 / 10.05
7.11 / 8.32	7.17 / 8.40	7.22 / 8.48	7.28 / 8.55	7.34 / 8.63	7.39 / 8.70	7.44 / 8.78	7.50 / 8.86	7.56 / 8.93	7.61 / 9.01	7.66 / 9.08	7.72 / 9.16	7.77 / 9.24	7.83 / 9.32	7.88 / 9.39	7.94 / 9.47	7.99 / 9.55	8.04 / 9.63
6.84 / 7.97	6.89 / 8.04	6.94 / 8.11	7.00 / 8.19	7.05 / 8.26	7.10 / 8.34	7.16 / 8.41	7.21 / 8.48	7.26 / 8.56	7.31 / 8.63	7.37 / 8.71	7.42 / 8.78	7.47 / 8.85	7.52 / 8.93	7.58 / 9.00	7.63 / 9.08	7.68 / 9.15	7.73 / 9.22
6.57 / 7.63	6.62 / 7.70	6.67 / 7.77	6.72 / 7.84	6.77 / 7.91	6.82 / 7.98	6.87 / 8.05	6.92 / 8.12	6.97 / 8.19	7.02 / 8.26	7.07 / 8.33	7.12 / 8.40	7.17 / 8.47	7.22 / 8.54	7.27 / 8.61	7.32 / 8.68	7.38 / 8.76	7.43 / 8.83
6.30 / 7.29	6.35 / 7.36	6.40 / 7.43	6.45 / 7.49	6.50 / 7.56	6.55 / 7.63	6.60 / 7.70	6.64 / 7.76	6.69 / 7.83	6.74 / 7.90	6.79 / 7.96	6.84 / 8.03	6.89 / 8.10	6.94 / 8.17	6.98 / 8.23	7.03 / 8.30	7.08 / 8.37	7.13 / 8.44
6.03 / 6.97	6.08 / 7.03	6.13 / 7.09	6.17 / 7.16	6.22 / 7.22	6.27 / 7.29	6.32 / 7.35	6.36 / 7.41	6.41 / 7.48	6.46 / 7.54	6.50 / 7.61	6.55 / 7.67	6.60 / 7.73	6.64 / 7.80	6.69 / 7.86	6.74 / 7.93	6.78 / 7.99	6.83 / 8.05
5.78 / 6.65	5.82 / 6.71	5.86 / 6.77	5.91 / 6.83	5.96 / 6.89	6.00 / 6.95	6.04 / 7.02	6.09 / 7.08	6.14 / 7.14	6.18 / 7.20	6.22 / 7.26	6.27 / 7.32	6.32 / 7.38	6.36 / 7.44	6.40 / 7.50	6.45 / 7.56	6.50 / 7.62	6.54 / 7.69
5.53 / 6.34	5.57 / 6.40	5.61 / 6.46	5.66 / 6.52	5.70 / 6.57	5.74 / 6.63	5.78 / 6.69	5.83 / 6.75	5.87 / 6.81	5.91 / 6.86	5.96 / 6.92	6.00 / 6.98	6.04 / 7.04	6.09 / 7.10	6.13 / 7.15	6.17 / 7.21	6.22 / 7.27	6.26 / 7.35
5.28 / 6.04	5.32 / 6.10	5.36 / 6.15	5.41 / 6.21	5.45 / 6.26	5.49 / 6.32	5.53 / 6.37	5.57 / 6.42	5.61 / 6.48	5.66 / 6.53	5.70 / 6.59	5.74 / 6.64	5.78 / 6.70	5.82 / 6.75	5.86 / 6.81	5.90 / 6.86	5.94 / 6.92	5.98 / 6.98
5.04 / 5.75	5.08 / 5.80	5.12 / 5.85	5.16 / 5.90	5.20 / 5.96	5.24 / 6.01	5.28 / 6.06	5.31 / 6.11	5.35 / 6.16	5.39 / 6.22	5.43 / 6.27	5.47 / 6.32	5.51 / 6.37	5.55 / 6.43	5.59 / 6.48	5.63 / 6.53	5.67 / 6.58	5.71 / 6.64
4.80 / 5.46	4.84 / 5.51	4.88 / 5.56	4.92 / 5.61	4.95 / 5.66	4.99 / 5.71	5.03 / 5.76	5.07 / 5.80	5.11 / 5.85	5.14 / 5.90	5.18 / 5.95	5.22 / 6.00	5.26 / 6.05	5.29 / 6.10	5.33 / 6.15	5.37 / 6.20	5.40 / 6.25	5.44 / 6.30
4.57 / 5.18	4.61 / 5.23	4.65 / 5.28	4.68 / 5.32	4.72 / 5.37	4.75 / 5.42	4.79 / 5.46	4.83 / 5.51	4.86 / 5.56	4.90 / 5.61	4.93 / 5.65	4.97 / 5.70	5.01 / 5.75	5.04 / 5.79	5.08 / 5.84	5.11 / 5.89	5.15 / 5.94	5.19 / 5.98
4.35 / 4.92	4.38 / 4.96	4.42 / 5.00	4.45 / 5.05	4.48 / 5.09	4.52 / 5.14	4.56 / 5.18	4.59 / 5.22	4.62 / 5.27	4.66 / 5.31	4.70 / 5.36	4.73 / 5.40	4.76 / 5.44	4.80 / 5.49	4.83 / 5.53	4.87 / 5.58	4.90 / 5.62	4.93 / 5.66
4.13 / 4.65	4.16 / 4.69	4.19 / 4.73	4.23 / 4.77	4.26 / 4.82	4.29 / 4.86	4.32 / 4.90	4.36 / 4.94	4.39 / 4.98	4.42 / 5.03	4.46 / 5.07	4.49 / 5.11	4.52 / 5.15	4.55 / 5.19	4.59 / 5.24	4.62 / 5.28	4.65 / 5.32	4.68 / 5.36
3.92 / 4.39	3.95 / 4.43	3.98 / 4.47	4.01 / 4.51	4.04 / 4.55	4.07 / 4.59	4.10 / 4.63	4.14 / 4.67	4.17 / 4.71	4.20 / 4.75	4.23 / 4.79	4.26 / 4.83	4.29 / 4.87	4.32 / 4.91	4.35 / 4.95	4.38 / 4.99	4.41 / 5.02	4.44 / 5.06
3.71 / 4.14	3.74 / 4.18	3.77 / 4.22	3.80 / 4.25	3.83 / 4.29	3.86 / 4.33	3.88 / 4.36	3.91 / 4.40	3.94 / 4.44	3.97 / 4.48	4.00 / 4.51	4.03 / 4.55	4.06 / 4.59	4.09 / 4.63	4.12 / 4.66	4.15 / 4.70	4.18 / 4.74	4.20 / 4.78
3.50 / 3.90	3.53 / 3.94	3.56 / 3.98	3.59 / 4.01	3.61 / 4.05	3.64 / 4.08	3.67 / 4.12	3.70 / 4.15	3.73 / 4.18	3.75 / 4.22	3.78 / 4.26	3.81 / 4.29	3.84 / 4.32	3.86 / 4.36	3.89 / 4.40	3.92 / 4.43	3.94 / 4.46	3.97 / 4.50
3.30 / 3.68	3.33 / 3.71	3.36 / 3.74	3.38 / 3.77	3.41 / 3.81	3.43 / 3.84	3.46 / 3.87	3.49 / 3.90	3.51 / 3.93	3.54 / 3.97	3.56 / 4.00	3.59 / 4.03	3.62 / 4.06	3.64 / 4.10	3.67 / 4.13	3.69 / 4.16	3.72 / 4.20	3.75 / 4.23
3.12 / 3.45	3.14 / 3.48	3.16 / 3.51	3.19 / 3.54	3.21 / 3.57	3.24 / 3.60	3.26 / 3.64	3.28 / 3.67	3.31 / 3.70	3.33 / 3.73	3.36 / 3.76	3.38 / 3.79	3.40 / 3.82	3.43 / 3.85	3.46 / 3.88	3.48 / 3.91	3.50 / 3.94	3.53 / 3.97
2.93 / 3.23	2.95 / 3.26	2.97 / 3.29	3.00 / 3.32	3.02 / 3.35	3.04 / 3.38	3.06 / 3.40	3.09 / 3.43	3.11 / 3.46	3.13 / 3.49	3.16 / 3.52	3.18 / 3.55	3.20 / 3.58	3.23 / 3.61	3.25 / 3.64	3.27 / 3.67	3.30 / 3.70	3.32 / 3.72
2.75 / 3.02	2.77 / 3.05	2.79 / 3.08	2.81 / 3.10	2.83 / 3.13	2.85 / 3.15	2.88 / 3.18	2.90 / 3.21	2.92 / 3.23	2.94 / 3.26	2.96 / 3.28	2.98 / 3.31	3.00 / 3.34	3.02 / 3.36	3.05 / 3.39	3.07 / 3.42	3.09 / 3.44	3.11 / 3.47
2.58 / 2.82	2.60 / 2.84	2.62 / 2.86	2.64 / 2.89	2.66 / 2.92	2.68 / 2.94	2.70 / 2.96	2.72 / 2.99	2.74 / 3.02	2.76 / 3.04	2.78 / 3.06	2.80 / 3.09	2.82 / 3.12	2.84 / 3.14	2.86 / 3.16	2.88 / 3.19	2.90 / 3.22	2.93 / 3.24
2.40 / 2.62	2.42 / 2.64	2.44 / 2.66	2.46 / 2.69	2.48 / 2.71	2.50 / 2.74	2.52 / 2.76	2.53 / 2.78	2.55 / 2.81	2.57 / 2.83	2.59 / 2.86	2.61 / 2.88	2.63 / 2.90	2.65 / 2.93	2.67 / 2.95	2.69 / 2.97	2.70 / 3.00	2.72 / 3.02
2.23 / 2.44	2.25 / 2.46	2.27 / 2.48	2.29 / 2.50	2.30 / 2.52	2.32 / 2.54	2.34 / 2.56	2.36 / 2.59	2.38 / 2.61	2.39 / 2.63	2.41 / 2.65	2.43 / 2.67	2.45 / 2.69	2.47 / 2.71	2.48 / 2.74	2.50 / 2.76	2.52 / 2.78	2.54 / 2.80
2.07 / 2.25	2.09 / 2.27	2.11 / 2.29	2.12 / 2.31	2.14 / 2.33	2.16 / 2.35	2.18 / 2.37	2.19 / 2.39	2.21 / 2.41	2.23 / 2.43	2.24 / 2.45	2.26 / 2.47	2.28 / 2.49	2.29 / 2.51	2.31 / 2.53	2.32 / 2.55	2.34 / 2.57	2.36 / 2.59
1.92 / 2.08	1.94 / 2.10	1.95 / 2.12	1.97 / 2.14	1.99 / 2.15	2.00 / 2.17	2.01 / 2.19	2.03 / 2.21	2.05 / 2.23	2.06 / 2.24	2.07 / 2.26	2.09 / 2.28	2.11 / 2.30	2.12 / 2.32	2.13 / 2.33	2.15 / 2.35	2.17 / 2.37	2.18 / 2.39
1.78 / 1.91	1.79 / 1.93	1.80 / 1.95	1.82 / 1.96	1.83 / 1.98	1.85 / 2.00	1.86 / 2.02	1.87 / 2.03	1.89 / 2.05	1.90 / 2.07	1.92 / 2.08	1.93 / 2.10	1.94 / 2.12	1.96 / 2.13	1.97 / 2.15	1.99 / 2.17	2.00 / 2.18	2.01 / 2.20
1.63 / 1.76	1.64 / 1.77	1.65 / 1.78	1.67 / 1.80	1.68 / 1.82	1.69 / 1.83	1.70 / 1.84	1.72 / 1.86	1.73 / 1.88	1.74 / 1.89	1.76 / 1.90	1.77 / 1.92	1.78 / 1.94	1.80 / 1.95	1.81 / 1.97	1.82 / 1.98	1.84 / 2.00	1.85 / 2.02
1.50 / 1.61	1.51 / 1.62	1.52 / 1.63	1.53 / 1.65	1.55 / 1.66	1.56 / 1.68	1.57 / 1.69	1.58 / 1.70	1.59 / 1.72	1.61 / 1.73	1.62 / 1.75	1.63 / 1.76	1.64 / 1.77	1.65 / 1.79	1.67 / 1.80	1.68 / 1.82	1.69 / 1.83	1.70 / 1.84
1.36 / 1.46	1.37 / 1.47	1.38 / 1.48	1.39 / 1.50	1.40 / 1.51	1.41 / 1.52	1.42 / 1.54	1.44 / 1.55	1.45 / 1.56	1.46 / 1.57	1.47 / 1.59	1.48 / 1.60	1.49 / 1.61	1.50 / 1.63	1.51 / 1.64	1.52 / 1.65	1.54 / 1.66	1.55 / 1.68
1.24 / 1.32	1.25 / 1.33	1.26 / 1.34	1.27 / 1.35	1.28 / 1.37	1.29 / 1.38	1.30 / 1.39	1.31 / 1.40	1.32 / 1.41	1.33 / 1.43	1.34 / 1.44	1.35 / 1.45	1.36 / 1.46	1.37 / 1.47	1.38 / 1.48	1.39 / 1.49	1.40 / 1.50	1.41 / 1.52

Table B.IV (*contd*)

Initial vergence (D)	Thickness (mm)													
	1.37	1.38	1.39	1.40	1.41	1.42	1.43	1.44	1.45	1.46	1.47	1.48	1.49	1.50
100.0	*8.42* 10.13	*8.48* 10.21	*8.53* 10.29	*8.59* 10.37	*8.65* 10.45	*8.70* 10.53	*8.76* 10.62	*8.81* 10.70	*8.87* 10.78	*8.93* 10.86	*8.98* 10.94	*9.04* 11.03	*9.09* 11.11	*9.15* 11.19
98.0	*8.10* 9.71	*8.15* 9.78	*8.21* 9.86	*8.26* 9.94	*8.31* 10.02	*8.37* 10.10	*8.42* 10.18	*8.48* 10.26	*8.53* 10.34	*8.58* 10.41	*8.64* 10.49	*8.69* 10.57	*8.75* 10.65	*8.80* 10.73
96.0	*7.78* 9.30	*7.84* 9.37	*7.89* 9.45	*7.94* 9.52	*7.99* 9.60	*8.04* 9.67	*8.10* 9.74	*8.15* 9.82	*8.20* 9.90	*8.25* 9.97	*8.30* 10.04	*8.36* 10.12	*8.41* 10.20	*8.46* 10.27
94.0	*7.48* 8.90	*7.53* 8.97	*7.58* 9.04	*7.63* 9.11	*7.68* 9.18	*7.73* 9.25	*7.78* 9.33	*7.83* 9.40	*7.88* 9.47	*7.93* 9.54	*7.98* 9.61	*8.03* 9.69	*8.08* 9.76	*8.13* 9.83
92.0	*7.18* 8.51	*7.22* 8.57	*7.27* 8.64	*7.32* 8.71	*7.37* 8.78	*7.42* 8.85	*7.46* 8.91	*7.51* 8.98	*7.56* 9.05	*7.61* 9.12	*7.66* 9.19	*7.70* 9.25	*7.75* 9.32	*7.80* 9.39
90.0	*6.88* 8.12	*6.93* 8.18	*6.97* 8.25	*7.02* 8.31	*7.07* 8.38	*7.11* 8.44	*7.16* 8.51	*7.20* 8.57	*7.25* 8.64	*7.30* 8.71	*7.34* 8.77	*7.39* 8.84	*7.43* 8.90	*7.48* 8.97
88.0	*6.58* 7.75	*6.63* 7.81	*6.68* 7.87	*6.72* 7.93	*6.76* 7.99	*6.81* 8.05	*6.85* 8.12	*6.90* 8.18	*6.94* 8.24	*6.98* 8.30	*7.03* 8.36	*7.07* 8.43	*7.12* 8.49	*7.16* 8.55
86.0	*6.30* 7.39	*6.34* 7.44	*6.39* 7.50	*6.43* 7.56	*6.47* 7.62	*6.51* 7.68	*6.56* 7.74	*6.60* 7.80	*6.64* 7.86	*6.68* 7.91	*6.72* 7.97	*6.77* 8.03	*6.81* 8.09	*6.85* 8.15
84.0	*6.02* 7.03	*6.06* 7.09	*6.10* 7.14	*6.14* 7.20	*6.18* 7.26	*6.22* 7.31	*6.26* 7.37	*6.30* 7.42	*6.34* 7.48	*6.39* 7.54	*6.43* 7.59	*6.47* 7.65	*6.51* 7.70	*6.55* 7.76
82.0	*5.75* 6.69	*5.79* 6.74	*5.83* 6.80	*5.87* 6.85	*5.91* 6.90	*5.95* 6.96	*5.98* 7.01	*6.02* 7.06	*6.06* 7.12	*6.10* 7.17	*6.14* 7.22	*6.17* 7.27	*6.21* 7.33	*6.25* 7.38
80.0	*5.48* 6.35	*5.52* 6.40	*5.55* 6.45	*5.59* 6.50	*5.63* 6.55	*5.66* 6.60	*5.70* 6.65	*5.74* 6.70	*5.78* 6.76	*5.81* 6.81	*5.85* 6.86	*5.89* 6.91	*5.92* 6.96	*5.96* 7.01
78.0	*5.22* 6.03	*5.26* 6.08	*5.29* 6.12	*5.33* 6.17	*5.36* 6.22	*5.40* 6.27	*5.43* 6.31	*5.47* 6.36	*5.50* 6.41	*5.54* 6.46	*5.57* 6.51	*5.61* 6.55	*5.64* 6.60	*5.68* 6.65
76.0	*4.97* 5.71	*5.00* 5.75	*5.04* 5.80	*5.07* 5.84	*5.10* 5.89	*5.14* 5.93	*5.17* 5.98	*5.20* 6.02	*5.24* 6.07	*5.27* 6.12	*5.30* 6.16	*5.33* 6.21	*5.37* 6.25	*5.40* 6.30
74.0	*4.71* 5.40	*4.75* 5.45	*4.78* 5.49	*4.81* 5.53	*4.84* 5.57	*4.87* 5.62	*4.91* 5.66	*4.94* 5.70	*4.97* 5.74	*5.00* 5.79	*5.03* 5.83	*5.07* 5.87	*5.10* 5.92	*5.13* 5.96
72.0	*4.47* 5.10	*4.50* 5.14	*4.53* 5.18	*4.56* 5.22	*4.59* 5.26	*4.62* 5.30	*4.65* 5.34	*4.68* 5.38	*4.72* 5.42	*4.75* 5.47	*4.78* 5.51	*4.81* 5.55	*4.84* 5.59	*4.87* 5.63
70.0	*4.23* 4.82	*4.26* 4.85	*4.29* 4.89	*4.32* 4.93	*4.35* 4.97	*4.38* 5.01	*4.41* 5.04	*4.44* 5.08	*4.46* 5.12	*4.49* 5.16	*4.52* 5.20	*4.55* 5.23	*4.58* 5.27	*4.61* 5.31
68.0	*4.00* 4.54	*4.03* 4.57	*4.05* 4.60	*4.08* 4.64	*4.11* 4.68	*4.14* 4.71	*4.16* 4.75	*4.19* 4.78	*4.22* 4.82	*4.25* 4.86	*4.28* 4.89	*4.30* 4.93	*4.33* 4.96	*4.36* 5.00
66.0	*3.77* 4.26	*3.80* 4.29	*3.82* 4.33	*3.85* 4.36	*3.88* 4.39	*3.90* 4.43	*3.93* 4.46	*3.95* 4.50	*3.98* 4.53	*4.01* 4.56	*4.03* 4.60	*4.06* 4.63	*4.08* 4.67	*4.11* 4.70
64.0	*3.56* 4.00	*3.58* 4.03	*3.60* 4.06	*3.63* 4.09	*3.65* 4.12	*3.68* 4.15	*3.70* 4.19	*3.73* 4.22	*3.75* 4.25	*3.77* 4.28	*3.80* 4.31	*3.82* 4.35	*3.85* 4.38	*3.87* 4.41
62.0	*3.34* 3.75	*3.36* 3.78	*3.39* 3.81	*3.41* 3.84	*3.43* 3.87	*3.46* 3.90	*3.48* 3.93	*3.50* 3.96	*3.52* 3.98	*3.55* 4.01	*3.57* 4.04	*3.59* 4.07	*3.62* 4.10	*3.64* 4.13
60.0	*3.13* 3.50	*3.16* 3.53	*3.18* 3.55	*3.20* 3.58	*3.22* 3.61	*3.24* 3.64	*3.27* 3.66	*3.29* 3.69	*3.31* 3.72	*3.33* 3.75	*3.35* 3.78	*3.38* 3.80	*3.40* 3.83	*3.42* 3.86
58.0	*2.95* 3.26	*2.97* 3.29	*2.99* 3.32	*3.01* 3.34	*3.03* 3.37	*3.05* 3.39	*3.07* 3.42	*3.09* 3.44	*3.11* 3.47	*3.13* 3.50	*3.15* 3.52	*3.17* 3.55	*3.19* 3.57	*3.21* 3.60
56.0	*2.74* 3.04	*2.76* 3.06	*2.78* 3.09	*2.80* 3.11	*2.82* 3.13	*2.84* 3.16	*2.86* 3.18	*2.88* 3.21	*2.90* 3.23	*2.91* 3.25	*2.93* 3.28	*2.95* 3.30	*2.97* 3.33	*2.99* 3.35
54.0	*2.56* 2.82	*2.57* 2.85	*2.59* 2.87	*2.61* 2.89	*2.63* 2.91	*2.64* 2.93	*2.66* 2.95	*2.68* 2.97	*2.70* 3.00	*2.71* 3.02	*2.73* 3.04	*2.75* 3.06	*2.76* 3.08	*2.78* 3.10
52.0	*2.37* 2.61	*2.39* 2.63	*2.40* 2.65	*2.42* 2.67	*2.44* 2.69	*2.45* 2.71	*2.47* 2.73	*2.49* 2.75	*2.50* 2.77	*2.52* 2.79	*2.54* 2.81	*2.56* 2.83	*2.57* 2.85	*2.59* 2.87
50.0	*2.19* 2.41	*2.21* 2.42	*2.23* 2.44	*2.24* 2.46	*2.26* 2.48	*2.27* 2.50	*2.29* 2.52	*2.30* 2.54	*2.32* 2.56	*2.34* 2.57	*2.35* 2.59	*2.37* 2.61	*2.38* 2.63	*2.40* 2.65
48.0	*2.03* 2.22	*2.04* 2.24	*2.06* 2.25	*2.07* 2.27	*2.08* 2.29	*2.10* 2.30	*2.11* 2.32	*2.13* 2.34	*2.14* 2.36	*2.15* 2.37	*2.17* 2.39	*2.18* 2.41	*2.20* 2.42	*2.21* 2.44
46.0	*1.86* 2.03	*1.87* 2.05	*1.89* 2.06	*1.90* 2.08	*1.91* 2.10	*1.93* 2.11	*1.94* 2.12	*1.96* 2.14	*1.97* 2.16	*1.98* 2.17	*2.00* 2.18	*2.01* 2.20	*2.03* 2.22	*2.04* 2.23
44.0	*1.71* 1.86	*1.73* 1.87	*1.74* 1.89	*1.75* 1.90	*1.76* 1.91	*1.77* 1.93	*1.79* 1.94	*1.80* 1.96	*1.81* 1.97	*1.82* 1.98	*1.83* 2.00	*1.85* 2.01	*1.86* 2.03	*1.87* 2.04
42.0	*1.56* 1.69	*1.57* 1.70	*1.58* 1.72	*1.59* 1.73	*1.60* 1.74	*1.61* 1.75	*1.62* 1.77	*1.63* 1.78	*1.64* 1.79	*1.66* 1.80	*1.67* 1.81	*1.68* 1.83	*1.69* 1.84	*1.70* 1.85
40.0	*1.42* 1.53	*1.43* 1.54	*1.44* 1.55	*1.45* 1.56	*1.46* 1.57	*1.47* 1.58	*1.48* 1.60	*1.49* 1.61	*1.50* 1.62	*1.51* 1.63	*1.52* 1.64	*1.53* 1.66	*1.54* 1.67	*1.55* 1.68

Table B.V Surface powers in air for $n = 1.336$ (Tears), r = radius of curvature, F = surface power

r (mm)	F (D)	r (mm)	F (D)	r (mm)	F (D)	r (mm)	F (D)	r (mm)	F (D)	r (mm)	F (D)	r (mm)	F (D)
4.90	68.57	5.30	63.40	5.70	58.95−	6.10	55.08	6.50	51.69	6.90	48.70	7.30	46.03
.91	68.43	.31	63.28	.71	58.84	.11	54.99	.51	51.61	.91	48.63	.31	45.96
.92	68.29	.32	63.16	.72	58.74	.12	54.90	.52	51.53	.92	48.55+	.32	45.90
.93	68.15	.33	63.04	.73	58.64	.13	54.81	.53	51.45+	.93	48.48	.33	45.84
.94	68.02	.34	62.92	.74	58.54	.14	54.72	.54	51.38	.94	48.41	.34	45.78
.95	67.88	.35	62.80	.75	58.43	.15	54.63	.55	51.30	.95	48.35−	.35	45.71
.96	67.74	.36	62.69	.76	58.33	.16	54.55−	.56	51.22	.96	48.28	.36	45.65+
.97	67.61	.37	62.57	.77	58.23	.17	54.46	.57	51.14	.97	48.21	.37	45.59
.98	67.47	.38	62.45+	.78	58.13	.18	54.37	.58	51.06	.98	48.14	.38	45.53
.99	67.33	.39	62.34	.79	58.03	.19	54.28	.59	50.99	.99	48.07	.39	45.47
5.00	67.20	5.40	62.22	5.80	57.93	6.20	54.19	6.60	50.91	7.00	48.00	7.40	45.41
.01	67.07	.41	62.11	.81	57.83	.21	54.11	.61	50.83	.01	47.93	.41	45.34
.02	66.93	.42	61.99	.82	57.73	.22	54.02	.62	50.76	.02	47.86	.42	45.28
.03	66.80	.43	61.88	.83	57.63	.23	53.93	.63	50.68	.03	47.80	.43	45.22
.04	66.67	.44	61.76	.84	57.53	.24	53.85−	.64	50.60	.04	47.73	.44	45.16
.05	66.53	.45	61.65+	.85	57.44	.25	53.76	.65	50.53	.05	47.66	.45	45.10
.06	66.40	.46	61.54	.86	57.34	.26	53.67	.66	50.45+	.06	47.59	.46	45.04
.07	66.27	.47	61.43	.87	57.24	.27	53.59	.67	50.37	.07	47.52	.47	44.98
.08	66.14	.48	61.31	.88	57.14	.28	53.50	.68	50.30	.08	47.46	.48	44.92
.09	66.01	.49	61.20	.89	57.05−	.29	53.42	.69	50.22	.09	47.39	.49	44.86
5.10	65.88	5.50	61.09	5.90	56.95−	6.30	53.33	6.70	50.15−	7.10	47.32	7.50	44.80
.11	65.75+	.51	60.98	.91	56.85+	.31	53.25−	.71	50.07	.11	47.26	.51	44.74
.12	65.62	.52	60.87	.92	56.76	.32	53.16	.72	50.00	.12	47.19	.52	44.68
.13	65.50	.53	60.76	.93	56.66	.33	53.08	.73	49.93	.13	47.12	.53	44.62
.14	65.37	.54	60.65−	.94	56.57	.34	53.00	.74	49.85+	.14	47.06	.54	44.56
.15	65.24	.55	60.54	.95	56.47	.35	52.91	.75	49.78	.15	46.99	.55	44.50
.16	65.12	.56	60.43	.96	56.38	.36	52.83	.76	49.70	.16	46.93	.56	44.44
.17	64.99	.57	60.32	.97	56.28	.37	52.75−	.77	49.63	.17	46.86	.57	44.39
.18	64.86	.58	60.22	.98	56.19	.38	52.66	.78	49.56	.18	46.80	.58	44.33
.19	64.74	.59	60.11	.99	56.09	.39	52.58	.79	49.48	.19	46.73	.59	44.27
5.20	64.62	5.60	60.00	6.00	56.00	6.40	52.50	6.80	49.41	7.20	46.67	7.60	44.21
.21	64.49	.61	59.89	.01	55.91	.41	52.42	.81	49.34	.21	46.60	.61	44.15+
.22	64.37	.62	59.79	.02	55.81	.42	52.34	.82	49.27	.22	46.54	.62	44.09
.23	64.24	.63	59.68	.03	55.72	.43	52.26	.83	49.19	.23	46.47	.63	44.04
.24	64.12	.64	59.57	.04	55.63	.44	52.17	.84	49.12	.24	46.41	.64	43.98
.25	64.00	.65	59.47	.05	55.54	.45	52.09	.85	49.05	.25	46.34	.65	43.92
.26	63.88	.66	59.36	.06	55.45−	.46	52.01	.86	48.98	.26	46.28	.66	43.86
.27	63.76	.67	59.26	.07	55.35+	.47	51.93	.87	48.91	.27	46.22	.67	43.81
.28	63.64	.68	59.15+	.08	55.26	.48	51.85+	.88	48.84	.28	46.15+	.68	43.75−
.29	63.52	.69	59.05+	.09	55.17	.49	51.77	.89	48.77	.29	46.09	.69	43.69

Table B.V *(contd)*

r (mm)	F (D)	r (mm)	F (D)	r (mm)	F (D)	r (mm)	F (D)	r (mm)	F (D)	r (mm)	F (D)	r (mm)	F (D)
7.70	43.64	8.10	41.48	8.50	39.53	8.90	37.75+	9.30	36.13	9.70	34.64	10.50	32.00
.71	43.58	.11	41.43	.51	39.48	.91	37.71	.31	36.09	.71	34.60	10.55	31.85−
.72	43.52	.12	41.38	.52	39.44	.92	37.67	.32	36.05+	.72	34.57	10.60	31.70
.73	43.47	.13	41.33	.53	39.39	.93	37.63	.33	36.01	.73	34.53	10.65	31.55−
.74	43.41	.14	41.28	.54	39.34	.94	37.58	.34	35.97	.74	34.50	10.70	31.40
.75	43.35+	.15	41.23	.55	39.30	.95	37.54	.35	35.94	.75	34.46	10.75	31.26
.76	43.30	.16	41.18	.56	39.25+	.96	37.50	.36	35.90	.76	34.43	10.80	31.11
.77	43.24	.17	41.13	.57	39.21	.97	37.46	.37	35.86	.77	34.39	10.85	30.97
.78	43.19	.18	41.08	.58	39.16	.98	37.42	.38	35.82	.78	34.36	10.90	30.83
.79	43.13	.19	41.03	.59	39.12	.99	37.37	.39	35.78	.79	34.32	10.95	30.68
7.80	43.08	8.20	40.98	8.60	39.07	9.00	37.33	9.40	35.74	9.80	34.29	11.00	30.55−
.81	43.02	.21	40.93	.61	39.02	.01	37.29	.41	35.71	.81	34.25	11.05	30.41
.82	42.97	.22	40.88	.62	38.98	.02	37.25+	.42	35.67	.82	34.22	11.10	30.27
.83	42.91	.23	40.83	.63	38.93	.03	37.21	.43	35.63	.83	34.18	11.15	30.13
.84	42.86	.24	40.78	.64	38.89	.04	37.17	.44	35.59	.84	34.15−	11.20	30.00
.85	42.80	.25	40.73	.65	38.84	.05	37.13	.45	35.56	.85	34.11	11.25	29.87
.86	42.75−	.26	40.68	.66	38.80	.06	37.09	.46	35.52	.86	34.08	11.30	29.73
.87	42.69	.27	40.63	.67	38.75+	.07	37.05−	.47	35.48	.87	34.04	11.35	29.60
.88	42.64	.28	40.58	.68	38.71	.08	37.00	.48	35.44	.88	34.01	11.40	29.47
.89	42.59	.29	40.53	.69	38.67	.09	36.96	.49	35.41	.89	33.97	11.45	29.34
7.90	42.53	8.30	40.48	8.70	38.62	9.10	36.92	9.50	35.37	9.90	33.94	11.50	29.22
.91	42.48	.31	40.43	.71	38.58	.11	36.88	.51	35.33	.91	33.91	11.55	29.09
.92	42.42	.32	40.38	.72	38.53	.12	36.84	.52	35.29	.92	33.87	11.60	28.97
.93	42.37	.33	40.34	.73	38.49	.13	36.80	.53	35.26	.93	33.84	11.65	28.84
.94	42.32	.34	40.29	.74	38.44	.14	36.76	.54	35.22	.94	33.80	11.70	28.72
.95	42.26	.35	40.24	.75	38.40	.15	36.72	.55	35.18	.95	33.77	11.75	28.60
.96	42.21	.36	40.19	.76	38.36	.16	36.68	.56	35.15−	.96	33.73	11.80	28.47
.97	42.16	.37	40.14	.77	38.31	.17	36.64	.57	35.11	.97	33.70	11.85	28.35+
.98	42.11	.38	40.10	.78	38.27	.18	36.60	.58	35.07	.98	33.67	11.90	28.24
.99	42.05+	.39	40.05−	.79	38.23	.19	36.56	.59	35.04	.99	33.63	11.95	28.12
8.00	42.00	8.40	40.00	8.80	38.18	9.20	36.52	9.60	35.00	10.00	33.60	12.00	28.00
.01	41.95−	.41	39.95+	.81	38.14	.21	36.48	.61	34.96	10.05	33.43	12.05	27.88
.02	41.90	.42	39.91	.82	38.10	.22	36.44	.62	34.93	10.10	33.27	12.10	27.77
.03	41.84	.43	39.86	.83	38.05+	.23	36.40	.63	34.89	10.15	33.10	12.15	27.65+
.04	41.79	.44	39.81	.84	38.01	.24	36.36	.64	34.85+	10.20	32.94	12.20	27.54
.05	41.74	.45	39.76	.85	37.97	.25	36.32	.65	34.82	10.25	32.78	12.25	27.43
.06	41.69	.46	39.72	.86	37.92	.26	36.28	.66	34.78	10.30	32.62	12.30	27.32
.07	41.64	.47	39.67	.87	37.88	.27	36.25−	.67	34.75−	10.35	32.46	12.35	27.21
.08	41.58	.48	39.62	.88	37.84	.28	36.21	.68	34.71	10.40	32.31	12.40	27.10
.09	41.53	.49	39.58	.89	37.80	.29	36.17	.69	34.67	10.45	32.15	12.45	26.99

Table B.VI Change in surface power (D) when radius (r_1) is changed to new radius (r_2), for liquid lens ($n = 1.336$) in air

Initial radius, r_1 (mm)	Change in surface power (D) *for new radius*, r_2 (mm)																			
	7.0	7.1	7.2	7.3	7.4	7.5	7.6	7.7	7.8	7.9	8.0	8.1	8.2	8.3	8.4	8.5	8.6	8.7	8.8	8.9
9.0	10.67	9.99	9.34	8.70	8.08	7.47	6.88	6.31	5.75	5.20	4.67	4.15	3.65	3.15	2.67	2.20	1.74	1.29	0.85	0.42
8.9	10.25	9.57	8.92	8.28	7.66	7.05	6.46	5.89	5.33	4.78	4.25	3.73	3.23	2.73	2.25	1.78	1.32	0.87	0.43	
8.8	9.82	9.14	8.49	7.85	7.23	6.62	6.03	5.46	4.90	4.35	3.82	3.30	2.80	2.30	1.82	1.35	0.89	0.44		
8.7	9.38	8.70	8.05	7.41	6.76	6.18	5.59	5.02	4.46	3.91	3.38	2.86	2.36	1.86	1.38	0.91	0.45			
8.6	8.93	8.25	7.60	6.96	6.34	5.73	5.14	4.57	4.01	3.46	2.93	2.41	1.91	1.41	0.93	0.46				
8.5	8.47	7.79	7.14	6.50	5.88	5.27	4.68	4.11	3.55	3.00	2.47	1.95	1.45	0.95	0.47					
8.4	8.00	7.32	6.67	6.03	5.41	4.80	4.21	3.64	3.08	2.53	2.00	1.48	0.98	0.48						
8.3	7.52	6.84	6.19	5.55	4.93	4.32	3.73	3.16	2.60	2.05	1.52	1.00	0.50							
8.2	7.02	6.34	5.69	5.05	4.43	3.82	3.23	2.66	2.10	1.55	1.02	0.50								
8.1	6.52	5.84	5.19	4.55	3.93	3.32	2.73	2.16	1.60	1.05	0.52									
8.0	6.00	5.32	4.67	4.03	3.41	2.80	2.21	1.64	1.08	0.53										
7.9	5.47	4.79	4.14	3.50	2.88	2.27	1.68	1.11	0.55											
7.8	4.92	4.24	3.59	2.95	2.33	1.72	1.13	0.56												
7.7	4.36	3.68	3.03	2.39	1.77	1.16	0.57													
7.6	3.79	3.11	2.46	1.82	1.20	0.59														
7.5	3.20	2.52	1.87	1.23	0.61															
7.4	2.59	1.91	1.26	0.62																
7.3	1.97	1.29	0.64																	
7.2	1.33	0.65																		
7.1	0.68																			

Table B.VII Change in reduced vergence due to thickness for a given initial vergence and refractive index of 1.336 (liquid lens in air)
Where there are two figures in one cell, the upper figure applies to divergent light and the lower figure to convergent light

Initial vergence (D)	Thickness (mm)				Initial vergence (D)	Thickness (mm)			
	0.05	0.10	0.15	0.20		0.05	0.10	0.15	0.20
20.00	.01	.03	.05	.06	42.00	.06	.13	.20	.27
21.00	.02	.03	.05	.07	43.00	.07	.14	.21	.28
22.00	.02	.04	.05	.07	44.00	.07	.15	.22	.29
23.00	.02	.04	.06	.08	45.00	.07	.15	.23	.31
24.00	.02	.04	.06	.09	46.00	.08	.16	.24	.32
25.00	.02	.05	.07	.09	47.00	.08	.17	.25	.33
26.00	.03	.05	.08	.10	48.00	.08	.17	.26	.35
27.00	.03	.05	.08	.11	49.00	.09	.18	.27	.36
28.00	.03	.06	.09	.12	50.00	.09	.19	.28	.38
29.00	.03	.06	.09	.13	51.00	.10	.20	.29	.39
30.00	.03	.07	.10	.14	52.00	.10	.20	.30	.41
31.00	.04	.07	.11	.14	53.00	.10	.21	.31	.42
32.00	.04	.08	.12	.15	54.00	.11	.22	.33	.44
33.00	.04	.08	.12	.16	55.00	.11	.23	.34	.46
34.00	.04	.09	.13	.17	56.00	.12	.24	.35	.47
35.00	.05	.09	.14	.18	57.00	.12	.24	.37	*.48* / .49
36.00	.05	.10	.15	.20	58.00	.13	.25	.38	*.50* / .51
37.00	.05	.10	.15	.21	59.00	.13	.26	.39	*.52* / .53
38.00	.05	.11	.16	.22	60.00	.14	.27	.41	*.53* / .54
39.00	.05	.11	.17	.23	61.00	.14	.28	.42	*.55* / .56
40.00	.06	.12	.18	.24	62.00	.14	.29	.43	*.57* / .58
41.00	.06	.13	.19	.25					

Table B.VIII Change in surface power (D) when radius (r_1) is changed to new radius (r_2), for liquid lens ($n = 1.336$), in contact with plastics ($n = 1.49$). Thus $n_R = 0.154$. (See Appendix E, program index no. 4)

Change in surface power (D) for new radius, r_2 (mm)

Initial radius, r_1 (mm)	7.0	7.1	7.2	7.3	7.4	7.5	7.6	7.7	7.8	7.9	8.0	8.1	8.2	8.3	8.4	8.5	8.6	8.7	8.8	8.9
9.0	4.89	4.58	4.28	3.99	3.70	3.42	3.15	2.89	2.63	2.38	2.14	1.90	1.67	1.44	1.22	1.01	0.80	0.59	0.39	0.19
8.9	4.70	4.39	4.09	3.80	3.51	3.23	2.96	2.70	2.44	2.19	1.95	1.71	1.48	1.25	1.03	0.82	0.61	0.40	0.20	
8.8	4.50	4.19	3.89	3.60	3.31	3.03	2.76	2.50	2.24	1.99	1.75	1.51	1.28	1.05	0.83	0.62	0.41	0.20		
8.7	4.30	3.99	3.69	3.40	3.11	2.83	2.56	2.30	2.04	1.79	1.55	1.31	1.08	0.85	0.63	0.42	0.21			
8.6	4.09	3.78	3.48	3.19	2.90	2.62	2.35	2.09	1.83	1.58	1.34	1.10	0.87	0.64	0.42	0.21				
8.5	3.88	3.57	3.27	2.98	2.69	2.41	2.14	1.88	1.62	1.37	1.13	0.89	0.66	0.43	0.21					
8.4	3.67	3.36	3.06	2.77	2.48	2.20	1.93	1.67	1.41	1.16	0.92	0.68	0.45	0.22						
8.3	3.45	3.14	2.84	2.55	2.26	1.98	1.71	1.45	1.19	0.94	0.70	0.46	0.23							
8.2	3.22	2.91	2.61	2.32	2.03	1.75	1.48	1.22	0.96	0.71	0.47	0.23								
8.1	2.99	2.68	2.38	2.09	1.80	1.52	1.25	0.99	0.73	0.48	0.24									
8.0	2.75	2.44	2.14	1.85	1.56	1.28	1.01	0.75	0.49	0.24										
7.9	2.51	2.20	1.90	1.61	1.32	1.04	0.77	0.51	0.25											
7.8	2.26	1.95	1.65	1.36	1.07	0.79	0.52	0.26												
7.7	2.00	1.69	1.39	1.10	0.81	0.53	0.26													
7.6	1.74	1.43	1.13	0.84	0.55	0.27														
7.5	1.47	1.16	0.86	0.57	0.28															
7.4	1.19	0.88	0.58	0.29																
7.3	0.90	0.59	0.29																	
7.2	0.61	0.30																		
7.1	0.31																			

Table B.IX Surface powers in air for plastics material of $n = 1.560$ (as used for fused bifocal contact lens segments)

r (mm)	F (D)	Difference in F for 0.01 change in r	r (mm)	F (D)	Difference in F for 0.01 change in r
5.00	112.0000		7.00	80.0000	
		0.2196			0.1127
.10	109.8039		.10	78.8732	
		0.2112			0.1095
.20	107.6923		.20	77.7778	
		0.2032			0.1066
.30	105.6604		.30	76.7123	
		0.1957			0.1037
.40	103.7037		.40	75.6757	
		0.1886			0.1009
.50	101.8182		.50	74.6667	
		0.1818			0.0982
.60	100.0000		.60	73.6842	
		0.1754			0.0957
.70	98.2456		.70	72.7273	
		0.1694			0.0932
.80	96.5517		.80	71.7949	
		0.1636			0.0909
.90	94.9153		.90	70.8861	
		0.1582			0.0886
6.00	93.3333		8.00	70.0000	
		0.1530			0.0864
.10	91.8033		.10	69.1358	
		0.1481			0.0843
.20	90.3226		.20	68.2927	
		0.1434			0.0823
.30	88.8889		.30	67.4699	
		0.1389			0.0803
.40	87.5000		.40	66.6667	
		0.1346			0.0784
.50	86.1538		.50	65.8824	
		0.1305			0.0766
.60	84.8484		.60	65.1163	
		0.1266			0.0748
.70	83.5821		.70	64.3678	
		0.2290			0.0731
.80	82.3529		.80	63.6364	
		0.1194			0.0715
.90	81.1594		.90	62.9213	
		0.1159			0.0699
7.00	80.0000		9.00	62.2223	

Table B.X Surface powers in tears ($n = 1.336$) for plastics material of $n = 1.560$ (as used for fused bifocal contact lens segments)

r (mm)	F (D)	Difference in F for 0.01 change in r	r (mm)	F (D)	Difference in F for 0.01 change in r
5.00	44.8000		7.00	32.0000	
		0.0878			0.0451
.10	43.9216		.10	31.5493	
		0.0845–			0.0438
.20	43.0769		.20	31.1111	
		0.0813			0.0426
.30	42.2642		.30	30.6849	
		0.0783			0.0415
.40	41.4815–		.40	30.2703	
		0.0754			0.0404
.50	40.7273		.50	29.8667	
		0.0727			0.0393
.60	40.0000		.60	29.4737	
		0.0702			0.0383
.70	39.2982		.70	29.0909	
		0.0678			0.0373
.80	38.6207		.80	28.7180	
		0.0655–			0.0364
.90	37.9661		.90	28.3544	
		0.0633			0.0354
6.00	37.3333		8.00	28.0000	
		0.0612			0.0346
.10	36.7213		.10	27.6543	
		0.0592			0.0337
.20	36.1290		.20	27.3171	
		0.0573			0.0329
.30	35.5556		.30	26.9880	
		0.0556			0.0321
.40	35.0000		.40	26.6667	
		0.0539			0.0314
.50	34.4615+		.50	26.3530	
		0.0522			0.0306
.60	33.9394		.60	26.0465+	
		0.0507			0.0299
.70	33.4328		.70	25.7471	
		0.0492			0.0292
.80	32.9412		.80	25.4546	
		0.0477			0.0286
.90	32.4638		.90	25.1685+	
		0.0464			0.0280
7.00	32.0000		9.00	24.8889	

Table B.XI Fused bifocal lens contact surface powers for a refractive index difference of 1.560–1.490 and change in surface power for radius, r (mm), when refractive index changes from 1.490 to 1.560 (as on the back surface of a fused bifocal, back surface segment contact lens)

r (mm)	F (D)	Difference in F for 0.01 change in r	r (mm)	F (D)	Difference in F for 0.01 change in r
5.00	14.0000		7.00	10.0000	
		0.0275			0.0141
.10	13.7255−		.10	9.8592	
		0.0264			0.0137
.20	13.4615+		.20	9.7222	
		0.0254			0.0133
.30	13.2075+		.30	9.5890	
		0.0244			0.0130
.40	12.9630		.40	9.4595−	
		0.0236			0.0126
.50	12.7273		.50	9.3333	
		0.0227			0.0123
.60	12.5000		.60	9.2105	
		0.0219			0.0120
.70	12.2807		.70	9.0909	
		0.0212			0.0116
.80	12.0690		.80	8.9744	
		0.0205			0.0114
.90	11.8644		.90	8.8608	
		0.0198			0.0111
6.00	11.6667		8.00	8.7500	
		0.0191			0.0108
.10	11.4754		.10	8.6420	
		0.0185			0.0105
.20	11.2903		.20	8.5366	
		0.0179			0.0103
.30	11.1111		.30	8.4337	
		0.0174			0.0100
.40	10.9375		.40	8.3333	
		0.0168			0.0098
.50	10.7692		.50	8.2353	
		0.0163			0.0096
.60	10.6061		.60	8.1395+	
		0.0158			0.0094
.70	10.4478		.70	8.0460	
		0.0154			0.0092
.80	10.2941		.80	7.9545+	
		0.0149			0.0089
.90	10.1449		.90	7.8652	
		0.0145			0.0087
7.00	10.0000		9.00	7.7778	

Table B.XII Contact surface radii (mm) for fused bifocal corneal lenses for refractive indices of 1.490 (main lens) and 1.560 (fused segment), for various back optic zone radii and near additions

$r_2 = BOZR$ (mm)	Radius, r_3, (mm) of contact surface required to give the near additions of						
	+1.00 D	+1.50 D	+2.00 D	+2.50 D	+3.00 D	+3.50 D	+4.00 D
6.00	5.5263	5.3164	5.1219	4.9412	4.7727	4.6154	4.4681
.10	5.6110	5.3948	5.1947	5.0088	4.8358	4.6743	4.5233
.20	5.6955+	5.4729	5.2670	5.0760	4.8984	4.7328	4.5781
.30	5.7798•	5.5507	5.3390	5.1429	4.9606	4.7909	4.6324
.40	5.8639	5.6281	5.4106	5.2093	5.0224	4.8485−	4.6862
.50	5.9477	5.7053	5.4819	5.2754	5.0838	4.9057	4.7396
.60	6.0313	5.7822	5.5529	5.3410	5.1448	4.9624	4.7925
.70	6.1147	5.8588	5.6235−	5.4063	5.2053	5.0187	4.8450
.80	6.1979	5.9352	5.6938	5.4713	5.2655−	5.0746	4.8971
.90	6.2809	6.0112	5.7637	5.5358	5.3253	5.1301	4.9488
7.00	6.3636	6.0870	5.8333	5.6000	5.3846	5.1852	5.0000
.10	6.4461	6.1624	5.9026	5.6638	5.4436	5.2398	5.0508
.20	6.5285+	6.2376	5.9716	5.7273	5.5022	5.2941	5.1012
.30	6.6106	6.3126	6.0402	5.7904	5.5604	5.3480	5.1512
.40	6.6925−	6.3872	6.1085−	5.8531	5.6182	5.4014	5.2008
.50	6.7742	6.4616	6.1765−	5.9155	5.6757	5.4546	5.2500
.60	6.8557	6.5356	6.2441	5.9775+	5.7328	5.5073	5.2988
.70	6.9369	6.6094	6.3115−	6.0392	5.7895−	5.5596	5.3472
.80	7.0180	6.6830	6.3785−	6.1005+	5.8458	5.6115−	5.3952
.90	7.0988	6.7562	6.4452	6.1615+	5.9018	5.6631	5.4429
8.00	7.1795−	6.8293	6.5116	6.2222	5.9574	5.7143	5.4902
.10	7.2599	6.9020	6.5777	6.2825	6.0127	5.7651	5.5371
.20	7.3401	6.9745−	6.6435+	6.3425	6.0676	5.8156	5.5837
.30	7.4202	7.0467	6.7090	6.4022	6.1223	5.8657	5.6299
.40	7.5000	7.1187	6.7742	6.4616	6.1765−	5.9155+	5.6757
.50	7.5796	7.1903	6.8391	6.5205+	6.2304	5.9649	5.7212
.60	7.5111	7.1287	6.7833	6.4698	6.1840	5.9224	5.7663
.70	7.7382	7.3329	6.9679	6.6376	6.3371	6.0627	5.8111
.80	7.8173	7.4039	7.0320	6.6957	6.3901	6.1111	5.8555+
.90	7.8960	7.4745−	7.0956	6.7534	6.4426	6.1592	5.8996
9.00	7.9747	7.5449	7.1591	6.8108	6.4948	6.2069	5.9434

Bifocal contact lenses ($n_1 = 1.490$; $n_2 = 1.560$) (*See Figure 5.28*)

Appendix C: Sagitta

See Appendix E, program index no. 11

Radii (mm)	Optic diameters (chords) (mm)																				
	3.0	3.2	3.4	3.6	3.8	4.0	4.2	4.4	4.6	4.8	5.0	5.2	5.4	5.6	5.8	6.0	6.2	6.4	6.6	6.8	7.0
5.00	0.230	0.263	0.298	0.335	0.375	0.417	0.462	0.510	0.560	0.614	0.670	0.729	0.792	0.858	0.927	1.000	1.077	1.158	1.244	1.334	1.429
5.25	0.219	0.250	0.283	0.318	0.356	0.396	0.438	0.483	0.531	0.581	0.633	0.689	0.748	0.809	0.874	0.942	1.013	1.088	1.167	1.250	1.337
5.50	0.209	0.238	0.269	0.303	0.339	0.377	0.417	0.459	0.504	0.551	0.601	0.653	0.708	0.766	0.827	0.890	0.957	1.027	1.100	1.177	1.257
5.75	0.199	0.227	0.257	0.289	0.323	0.359	0.397	0.438	0.480	0.525	0.572	0.621	0.673	0.728	0.785	0.845	0.907	0.973	1.041	1.113	1.188
6.00	0.191	0.217	0.246	0.276	0.309	0.343	0.380	0.418	0.458	0.501	0.546	0.593	0.642	0.693	0.747	0.804	0.863	0.925	0.989	1.056	1.127
6.25	0.183	0.209	0.236	0.265	0.296	0.329	0.364	0.400	0.439	0.479	0.522	0.566	0.613	0.662	0.714	0.767	0.823	0.881	0.942	1.006	1.072
6.50	0.175	0.200	0.226	0.254	0.284	0.315	0.349	0.384	0.421	0.459	0.500	0.543	0.587	0.634	0.683	0.724	0.787	0.842	0.900	0.960	1.023
6.75	0.169	0.193	0.218	0.245	0.273	0.303	0.335	0.369	0.404	0.441	0.480	0.521	0.564	0.608	0.655	0.703	0.754	0.807	0.862	0.919	0.978
7.00	0.163	0.185	0.210	0.235	0.263	0.292	0.322	0.355	0.389	0.424	0.462	0.501	0.542	0.584	0.629	0.675	0.724	0.774	0.827	0.881	0.938
7.10	0.160	0.183	0.207	0.232	0.259	0.289	0.318	0.349	0.383	0.418	0.455	0.493	0.533	0.575	0.619	0.665	0.713	0.762	0.814	0.867	0.923
7.20	0.158	0.180	0.204	0.229	0.255	0.283	0.313	0.344	0.377	0.412	0.448	0.486	0.525	0.567	0.610	0.655	0.702	0.750	0.801	0.853	0.908
7.30	0.156	0.178	0.201	0.225	0.252	0.279	0.309	0.339	0.372	0.406	0.441	0.479	0.518	0.558	0.601	0.645	0.691	0.739	0.788	0.840	0.894
7.40	0.154	0.175	0.198	0.222	0.248	0.275	0.304	0.335	0.367	0.400	0.435	0.472	0.510	0.550	0.592	0.635	0.681	0.728	0.777	0.827	0.880
7.50	0.152	0.173	0.195	0.219	0.245	0.272	0.300	0.330	0.361	0.394	0.429	0.465	0.503	0.542	0.583	0.626	0.671	0.717	0.765	0.815	0.867
7.60	0.150	0.170	0.193	0.216	0.241	0.268	0.296	0.325	0.356	0.389	0.423	0.459	0.496	0.535	0.575	0.617	0.661	0.707	0.754	0.803	0.854
7.70	0.148	0.168	0.190	0.213	0.238	0.264	0.292	0.321	0.352	0.384	0.417	0.452	0.489	0.527	0.567	0.608	0.652	0.696	0.743	0.791	0.841
7.80	0.146	0.166	0.188	0.211	0.235	0.261	0.288	0.317	0.347	0.378	0.411	0.446	0.482	0.520	0.559	0.600	0.642	0.687	0.732	0.780	0.829
7.90	0.144	0.164	0.185	0.208	0.232	0.257	0.284	0.313	0.342	0.373	0.406	0.440	0.476	0.513	0.552	0.592	0.634	0.677	0.722	0.769	0.818

Radii (mm)	Optic diameters (chords) (mm)																				
	7.2	7.4	7.6	7.8	8.0	8.2	8.4	8.6	8.8	9.0	9.2	9.4	9.6	9.8	10.0	10.2	10.4	10.6	10.8	11.0	11.2
5.00	1.530	1.637	1.750	1.871	2.000	2.138	2.287	2.449	2.625	2.821	3.040	3.294	3.600	4.005	5.000						
5.25	1.429	1.525	1.628	1.735	1.850	1.971	2.100	2.238	2.386	2.546	2.720	2.911	3.123	3.365	3.649	4.004	4.527				
5.50	1.342	1.431	1.524	1.622	1.725	1.834	1.949	2.071	2.200	2.338	2.485	2.643	2.815	3.002	3.209	3.441	3.708	4.030	4.456	5.500	
5.75	1.266	1.349	1.435	1.525	1.619	1.719	1.823	1.933	2.048	2.171	2.300	2.438	2.584	2.741	2.911	3.094	3.296	3.520	3.775	4.073	4.445
6.00	1.200	1.277	1.357	1.440	1.528	1.619	1.715	1.816	1.921	2.031	2.148	2.270	2.400	2.537	2.683	2.839	3.007	3.188	3.385	3.602	3.846
6.25	1.141	1.213	1.288	1.366	1.448	1.533	1.622	1.714	1.811	1.913	2.019	2.130	2.247	2.370	2.500	2.637	2.783	2.938	3.103	3.281	3.475
6.50	1.088	1.156	1.226	1.300	1.377	1.456	1.539	1.626	1.716	1.810	1.908	2.010	2.117	2.229	2.347	2.470	2.600	2.737	2.882	3.036	3.200
6.75	1.040	1.104	1.171	1.241	1.313	1.388	1.466	1.547	1.631	1.719	1.810	1.905	2.004	2.108	2.215	2.328	2.446	2.570	2.700	2.837	2.981
7.00	0.997	1.058	1.121	1.187	1.255	1.326	1.400	1.476	1.556	1.638	1.724	1.813	1.905	2.001	2.101	2.205	2.314	2.427	2.546	2.670	2.800
7.10	0.980	1.040	1.103	1.167	1.234	1.303	1.375	1.450	1.528	1.608	1.692	1.778	1.868	1.962	2.059	2.160	2.266	2.376	2.490	2.610	2.735
7.20	0.965	1.023	1.084	1.148	1.213	1.281	1.352	1.425	1.501	1.580	1.661	1.746	1.833	1.925	2.019	2.118	2.220	2.327	2.438	2.553	2.675
7.30	0.949	1.007	1.067	1.129	1.193	1.260	1.329	1.401	1.475	1.552	1.632	1.714	1.800	1.889	1.981	2.077	2.177	2.280	2.388	2.500	2.617
7.40	0.935	0.991	1.050	1.111	1.174	1.240	1.307	1.378	1.450	1.525	1.603	1.684	1.768	1.855	1.945	2.038	2.135	2.236	2.340	2.449	2.563
7.50	0.920	0.976	1.034	1.094	1.156	1.220	1.286	1.355	1.426	1.500	1.576	1.655	1.737	1.822	1.910	2.001	2.095	2.193	2.295	2.401	2.511
7.60	0.907	0.961	1.018	1.077	1.138	1.201	1.266	1.333	1.403	1.475	1.550	1.628	1.708	1.791	1.876	1.965	2.057	2.153	2.252	2.355	2.462
7.70	0.893	0.947	1.003	1.061	1.120	1.182	1.246	1.313	1.381	1.452	1.525	1.601	1.679	1.760	1.844	1.931	2.021	2.114	2.211	2.311	2.415
7.80	0.880	0.933	0.988	1.045	1.104	1.164	1.227	1.292	1.360	1.429	1.501	1.575	1.652	1.731	1.813	1.898	1.986	2.077	2.172	2.269	2.370
7.90	0.868	0.920	0.974	1.030	1.088	1.147	1.209	1.273	1.339	1.407	1.477	1.550	1.625	1.703	1.784	1.867	1.953	2.042	2.134	2.229	2.328

Radii (mm)	Optic diameters (chords) (mm)																			
	11.4	11.6	11.8	12.00	12.25	12.50	12.75	13.00	13.25	13.50	13.75	14.00	14.25	14.50	14.75	15.00	15.25	15.50	15.75	16.00
5.00																				
5.25																				
5.50																				
5.75	4.993																			
6.00	4.127	4.464	4.909	6.000																
6.25	3.686	3.921	4.188	4.500	5.006	6.250														
6.50	3.376	3.566	3.772	4.000	4.324	4.715	5.231	6.500												
6.75	3.134	3.297	3.471	3.658	3.913	4.200	4.531	4.930	5.457	6.750										
7.00	2.937	3.081	3.233	3.394	3.612	3.848	4.109	4.402	4.740	5.146	5.683	7.000								
7.10	2.867	3.005	3.150	3.304	3.509	3.731	3.974	4.243	4.547	4.898	5.327	5.913								
7.20	2.801	2.934	3.073	3.220	3.415	3.625	3.853	4.103	4.381	4.695	5.061	5.515	6.163							
7.30	2.739	2.867	3.001	3.142	3.328	3.528	3.743	3.977	4.234	4.520	4.846	5.229	5.711	6.447						
7.40	2.681	2.804	2.933	3.069	3.247	3.438	3.642	3.863	4.103	4.367	4.662	5.000	5.401	5.918	6.792					
7.50	2.626	2.745	2.870	3.000	3.172	3.354	3.549	3.759	3.984	4.231	4.503	4.807	5.158	5.580	6.136	7.500				
7.60	2.573	2.689	2.809	2.935	3.101	3.276	3.462	3.662	3.876	4.108	4.360	4.640	4.955	5.320	5.764	6.371				
7.70	2.523	2.635	2.752	2.874	3.034	3.001	3.382	3.572	3.776	3.995	4.232	4.492	4.780	5.106	5.487	5.956	5.628			
7.80	2.476	2.585	2.698	2.816	2.970	3.133	3.306	3.488	3.683	3.891	4.116	4.359	4.626	4.923	5.260	5.658	6.157	6.918		
7.90	2.430	2.536	2.646	2.761	2.911	3.068	3.234	3.410	3.598	3.795	4.008	4.238	4.498	4.762	5.068	5.418	5.834	6.397	7.272	

Radii (mm)	Optic diameters (chords) (mm)																					
	3.0	3.2	3.4	3.6	3.8	4.0	4.2	4.4	4.6	4.8	5.0	5.2	5.4	5.6	5.8	6.0	6.2	6.4	6.6	6.8	7.0	7.2
.00	0.142	0.162	0.183	0.205	0.229	0.254	0.281	0.308	0.338	0.369	0.401	0.434	0.469	0.506	0.544	0.584	0.625	0.668	0.712	0.758	0.806	0.856
.10	0.140	0.160	0.180	0.203	0.226	0.251	0.277	0.305	0.333	0.364	0.395	0.429	0.463	0.499	0.537	0.576	0.617	0.659	0.703	0.748	0.795	0.844
.20	0.138	0.158	0.178	0.200	0.223	0.248	0.274	0.301	0.329	0.359	0.390	0.423	0.457	0.493	0.530	0.568	0.609	0.650	0.693	0.738	0.784	0.833
.30	0.137	0.156	0.176	0.198	0.220	0.245	0.270	0.297	0.325	0.355	0.385	0.418	0.451	0.487	0.523	0.561	0.601	0.642	0.684	0.728	0.774	0.821
.40	0.135	0.154	0.174	0.195	0.218	0.242	0.267	0.292	0.321	0.350	0.381	0.413	0.446	0.480	0.516	0.554	0.593	0.633	0.675	0.719	0.764	0.811
.50	0.133	0.152	0.172	0.193	0.215	0.239	0.264	0.290	0.317	0.346	0.376	0.407	0.440	0.474	0.510	0.547	0.585	0.625	0.667	0.710	0.754	0.800
.60	0.132	0.150	0.170	0.191	0.213	0.236	0.260	0.286	0.313	0.342	0.371	0.402	0.435	0.469	0.504	0.540	0.578	0.618	0.658	0.701	0.744	0.790
.70	0.130	0.148	0.168	0.188	0.210	0.233	0.257	0.283	0.310	0.338	0.367	0.398	0.430	0.463	0.498	0.534	0.571	0.610	0.650	0.692	0.735	0.780
.80	0.129	0.147	0.166	0.186	0.208	0.230	0.254	0.279	0.306	0.334	0.363	0.393	0.424	0.457	0.492	0.527	0.564	0.602	0.642	0.683	0.726	0.770
.90	0.127	0.145	0.164	0.184	0.205	0.228	0.251	0.276	0.302	0.330	0.358	0.388	0.419	0.452	0.486	0.521	0.557	0.595	0.634	0.675	0.717	0.761
.00	0.126	0.143	0.162	0.182	0.203	0.225	0.248	0.273	0.299	0.326	0.354	0.384	0.415	0.447	0.480	0.515	0.551	0.588	0.627	0.667	0.708	0.751
.10	0.125	0.142	0.160	0.180	0.201	0.223	0.246	0.270	0.296	0.322	0.350	0.379	0.410	0.441	0.474	0.509	0.544	0.581	0.619	0.659	0.700	0.742
.20	0.123	0.140	0.158	0.178	0.198	0.220	0.243	0.267	0.292	0.319	0.346	0.375	0.405	0.436	0.469	0.503	0.538	0.574	0.612	0.651	0.692	0.734
.30	0.122	0.139	0.157	0.176	0.196	0.218	0.240	0.264	0.289	0.315	0.342	0.371	0.401	0.432	0.464	0.497	0.532	0.568	0.605	0.644	0.684	0.725
.40	0.121	0.137	0.155	0.174	0.194	0.215	0.238	0.261	0.286	0.312	0.339	0.367	0.396	0.427	0.459	0.492	0.526	0.561	0.598	0.636	0.676	0.717
.50	0.119	0.136	0.153	0.172	0.192	0.213	0.235	0.258	0.283	0.308	0.335	0.363	0.392	0.422	0.453	0.486	0.520	0.555	0.592	0.629	0.668	0.709
.60	0.118	0.134	0.152	0.170	0.190	0.211	0.233	0.256	0.280	0.305	0.331	0.359	0.388	0.417	0.448	0.481	0.514	0.549	0.585	0.622	0.661	0.701
.70	0.117	0.133	0.150	0.169	0.188	0.208	0.230	0.253	0.277	0.302	0.328	0.355	0.383	0.413	0.444	0.476	0.509	0.543	0.579	0.615	0.653	0.693
.80	0.116	0.132	0.149	0.167	0.186	0.206	0.228	0.250	0.274	0.298	0.324	0.351	0.379	0.409	0.439	0.470	0.503	0.537	0.572	0.609	0.646	0.685
.90	0.114	0.130	0.147	0.165	0.184	0.204	0.225	0.248	0.271	0.295	0.321	0.348	0.375	0.404	0.434	0.465	0.498	0.531	0.566	0.602	0.639	0.678

Radii (mm)	Optic diameters (chords) (mm)																					
	7.4	7.6	7.8	8.0	8.2	8.4	8.6	8.8	9.0	9.2	9.4	9.6	9.8	10.0	10.2	10.4	10.6	10.8	11.0	11.2	11.4	11.6
8.00	0.907	0.960	1.015	1.072	1.131	1.191	1.254	1.319	1.386	1.455	1.526	1.600	1.676	1.755	1.836	1.921	2.008	2.097	2.191	2.287	2.387	2.490
8.10	0.894	0.947	1.001	1.057	1.114	1.174	1.236	1.299	1.365	1.433	1.503	1.575	1.650	1.727	1.807	1.890	1.975	2.063	2.154	2.248	2.345	2.446
8.20	0.882	0.934	0.987	1.042	1.099	1.157	1.218	1.280	1.345	1.412	1.481	1.552	1.625	1.701	1.779	1.860	1.943	2.029	2.118	2.210	2.305	2.403
8.30	0.870	0.921	0.973	1.027	1.083	1.141	1.201	1.262	1.326	1.391	1.459	1.529	1.601	1.675	1.752	1.831	1.913	1.997	2.084	2.174	2.267	2.363
8.40	0.859	0.909	0.960	1.014	1.069	1.125	1.184	1.245	1.307	1.371	1.438	1.507	1.577	1.650	1.725	1.803	1.883	1.966	2.051	2.139	2.230	2.324
8.50	0.848	0.897	0.948	1.000	1.054	1.110	1.168	1.227	1.289	1.352	1.418	1.485	1.554	1.626	1.700	1.776	1.855	1.936	2.019	2.105	2.194	2.286
8.60	0.837	0.885	0.935	0.987	1.040	1.095	1.152	1.211	1.271	1.334	1.398	1.464	1.532	1.603	1.675	1.750	1.827	1.907	1.989	2.073	2.160	2.250
8.70	0.826	0.874	0.923	0.974	1.027	1.081	1.137	1.195	1.254	1.316	1.379	1.444	1.511	1.580	1.652	1.725	1.801	1.879	1.959	2.042	2.127	2.215
8.80	0.816	0.863	0.911	0.962	1.013	1.067	1.122	1.179	1.238	1.298	1.360	1.424	1.490	1.558	1.629	1.701	1.775	1.852	1.931	2.012	2.096	2.182
8.90	0.806	0.852	0.900	0.950	1.001	1.053	1.108	1.164	1.221	1.281	1.342	1.405	1.470	1.537	1.606	1.677	1.750	1.825	1.903	1.983	2.065	2.149
9.00	0.796	0.842	0.889	0.938	0.988	1.040	1.094	1.149	1.206	1.264	1.325	1.387	1.451	1.517	1.584	1.654	1.726	1.800	1.876	1.954	2.035	2.118
9.10	0.786	0.831	0.878	0.926	0.976	1.027	1.080	1.134	1.191	1.248	1.308	1.369	1.432	1.497	1.563	1.632	1.703	1.775	1.850	1.927	2.006	2.088
9.20	0.777	0.821	0.868	0.915	0.964	1.015	1.067	1.120	1.176	1.233	1.291	1.351	1.413	1.477	1.543	1.611	1.680	1.752	1.825	1.901	1.979	2.059
9.30	0.768	0.812	0.857	0.904	0.953	1.002	1.054	1.107	1.161	1.217	1.275	1.334	1.396	1.458	1.523	1.590	1.658	1.728	1.801	1.875	1.952	2.030
9.40	0.759	0.802	0.847	0.894	0.941	0.990	1.041	1.093	1.147	1.202	1.259	1.318	1.378	1.440	1.504	1.569	1.637	1.706	1.777	1.850	1.925	2.003
9.50	0.750	0.793	0.837	0.883	0.930	0.979	1.029	1.080	1.133	1.188	1.244	1.302	1.361	1.422	1.485	1.550	1.616	1.684	1.754	1.826	1.900	1.976
9.60	0.742	0.784	0.828	0.873	0.920	0.968	1.017	1.068	1.120	1.174	1.229	1.286	1.345	1.405	1.467	1.530	1.596	1.663	1.732	1.803	1.875	1.950
9.70	0.733	0.775	0.819	0.863	0.909	0.956	1.005	1.055	1.107	1.160	1.215	1.271	1.329	1.388	1.449	1.512	1.576	1.642	1.710	1.780	1.851	1.925
9.80	0.725	0.767	0.809	0.853	0.899	0.946	0.994	1.043	1.094	1.147	1.201	1.256	1.313	1.371	1.432	1.493	1.557	1.622	1.689	1.758	1.828	1.901
9.90	0.717	0.758	0.801	0.844	0.889	0.935	0.983	1.032	1.082	1.134	1.187	1.241	1.298	1.355	1.415	1.476	1.538	1.602	1.668	1.736	1.806	1.877

Radii (mm)	Optic diameters (chords) (mm)																					
	11.8	12.00	12.25	12.50	12.75	13.00	13.25	13.50	13.75	14.00	14.25	14.50	14.75	15.00	15.25	15.50	15.75	16.00	17.00	18.00	19.00	20.00
8.00	2.597	2.708	2.854	3.006	3.167	3.336	3.516	3.706	3.909	4.127	4.362	4.618	4.900	5.216	5.579	6.016	6.591	8.000				
8.10	2.550	2.658	2.800	2.948	3.103	3.267	3.440	3.623	3.817	4.024	4.247	4.488	4.750	5.041	5.367	5.745	6.204	6.831				
8.20	2.505	2.611	2.748	2.892	3.043	3.201	3.368	3.544	3.731	3.929	4.141	4.369	4.615	4.885	5.183	5.521	5.914	6.400				
8.30	2.462	2.565	2.699	2.839	2.985	3.139	3.300	3.470	3.650	3.840	4.043	4.259	4.492	4.745	5.021	5.329	5.678	6.089				
8.40	2.421	2.521	2.652	2.788	2.930	3.079	3.236	3.500	3.574	3.757	3.951	4.158	4.379	4.617	4.876	5.160	5.477	5.839				
8.50	2.381	2.479	2.606	2.739	2.878	3.023	3.175	3.334	3.502	3.678	3.865	4.063	4.274	4.500	4.744	5.018	5.301	5.628	8.500			
8.60	2.343	2.439	2.563	2.693	2.828	2.969	3.116	3.271	3.433	3.604	3.784	3.974	4.176	4.392	4.623	4.872	5.144	5.444	7.292			
8.70	2.306	2.400	2.522	2.648	2.780	2.917	3.061	3.211	3.369	3.534	3.708	3.891	4.085	4.291	4.511	4.747	5.002	5.281	6.845			
8.80	2.271	2.363	2.481	2.605	2.734	2.868	3.008	3.154	3.307	3.467	3.635	3.812	3.999	4.197	4.407	4.631	4.873	5.134	6.522			
8.90	2.237	2.327	2.443	2.564	2.690	2.821	2.957	3.099	3.248	3.404	3.567	3.738	3.918	4.108	4.310	4.524	4.753	5.000	6.262			
9.00	2.204	2.292	2.406	2.524	2.647	2.775	2.908	3.047	3.192	3.343	3.501	3.667	3.842	4.025	4.219	4.424	4.643	4.877	6.042	9.000		
9.10	2.172	2.258	2.370	2.486	2.605	2.731	2.816	2.997	3.139	3.285	3.439	3.600	3.769	3.946	4.133	4.331	4.540	4.763	5.850	7.755		
9.20	2.141	2.226	2.335	2.449	2.567	2.689	2.817	2.949	3.087	3.230	3.380	3.536	3.700	3.872	4.052	4.242	4.443	4.657	5.680	7.292		
9.30	2.111	2.194	2.302	2.413	2.529	2.649	2.773	2.903	3.037	3.177	3.323	3.475	3.634	3.801	3.976	4.159	4.353	4.558	5.526	6.957		
9.40	2.082	2.164	2.270	2.379	2.492	2.610	2.732	2.858	2.990	3.126	3.269	3.417	3.572	3.733	3.903	4.080	4.267	4.464	5.386	6.687		
9.50	2.054	2.135	2.238	2.345	2.457	2.572	2.691	2.815	2.944	3.077	3.216	3.361	3.512	3.669	3.833	4.006	4.186	4.377	5.257	6.459	9.500	
9.60	2.027	2.106	2.208	2.313	2.422	2.535	2.652	2.774	2.900	3.030	3.166	3.307	3.454	3.608	3.767	3.935	4.110	4.293	5.138	6.259	8.218	
9.70	2.001	2.078	2.178	2.282	2.389	2.500	2.615	2.734	2.857	2.985	3.118	3.256	3.399	3.549	3.704	3.867	4.037	4.215	5.027	6.082	7.740	
9.80	1.975	2.051	2.150	2.252	2.357	2.466	2.579	2.695	2.816	2.941	3.071	3.206	3.346	3.492	3.644	3.802	3.967	4.140	4.923	5.922	7.394	
9.90	1.950	2.025	2.122	2.222	2.326	2.433	2.543	2.658	2.776	2.899	3.027	3.159	3.296	3.438	3.586	3.740	3.900	4.068	4.825	5.776	7.114	

Appendix C (*contd*)
See Appendix E, program index no. 11

Radii (mm)	Optic diameters (chords) (mm)																
	5.0	5.2	5.4	5.6	5.8	6.0	6.2	6.4	6.6	6.8	7.0	7.2	7.4	7.6	7.8	8.0	8.2
10.00	0.318	0.344	0.371	0.400	0.430	0.461	0.493	0.526	0.560	0.596	0.633	0.670	0.710	0.750	0.792	0.835	0.879
10.25	0.310	0.335	0.362	0.390	0.419	0.449	0.480	0.512	0.546	0.580	0.616	0.653	0.691	0.730	0.771	0.813	0.856
10.50	0.302	0.327	0.353	0.380	0.408	0.438	0.468	0.500	0.532	0.566	0.601	0.636	0.674	0.712	0.751	0.792	0.834
10.75	0.295	0.319	0.345	0.371	0.399	0.427	0.457	0.487	0.519	0.552	0.586	0.621	0.657	0.694	0.732	0.772	0.813
11.00	0.288	0.312	0.337	0.362	0.389	0.417	0.446	0.476	0.507	0.539	0.572	0.606	0.641	0.677	0.715	0.753	0.793
11.25	0.282	0.305	0.329	0.354	0.380	0.408	0.436	0.465	0.495	0.527	0.559	0.592	0.626	0.661	0.698	0.736	0.774
11.50	0.275	0.298	0.321	0.346	0.372	0.398	0.426	0.454	0.484	0.514	0.546	0.578	0.611	0.646	0.681	0.718	0.756
11.75	0.269	0.292	0.315	0.339	0.364	0.390	0.416	0.444	0.473	0.503	0.534	0.566	0.598	0.632	0.666	0.702	0.739
12.00	0.263	0.285	0.308	0.331	0.356	0.381	0.407	0.435	0.463	0.492	0.522	0.553	0.585	0.618	0.651	0.686	0.722
12.25	0.258	0.279	0.302	0.325	0.349	0.373	0.399	0.426	0.453	0.481	0.511	0.541	0.573	0.605	0.638	0.672	0.707
12.50	0.253	0.273	0.295	0.318	0.341	0.365	0.390	0.417	0.443	0.471	0.500	0.530	0.560	0.592	0.624	0.657	0.692
12.75	0.248	0.268	0.289	0.312	0.335	0.358	0.383	0.408	0.435	0.462	0.490	0.519	0.549	0.580	0.612	0.644	0.677
13.00	0.243	0.263	0.283	0.305	0.328	0.351	0.375	0.400	0.426	0.452	0.480	0.508	0.538	0.568	0.599	0.631	0.663
13.25	0.238	0.258	0.278	0.299	0.322	0.344	0.368	0.393	0.418	0.444	0.471	0.498	0.527	0.557	0.587	0.619	0.651
13.50	0.234	0.253	0.273	0.294	0.315	0.338	0.361	0.385	0.410	0.435	0.462	0.489	0.517	0.546	0.576	0.606	0.638
13.75	0.229	0.248	0.268	0.288	0.309	0.332	0.354	0.378	0.402	0.427	0.453	0.480	0.507	0.536	0.565	0.595	0.626
14.00	0.225	0.244	0.263	0.283	0.304	0.325	0.348	0.371	0.394	0.419	0.445	0.471	0.498	0.526	0.554	0.584	0.614
14.25	0.221	0.239	0.258	0.278	0.298	0.320	0.342	0.364	0.388	0.412	0.437	0.463	0.489	0.516	0.544	0.573	0.603
14.50	0.217	0.235	0.254	0.273	0.293	0.314	0.335	0.358	0.381	0.404	0.429	0.454	0.480	0.507	0.534	0.563	0.592
14.75	0.214	0.231	0.249	0.268	0.288	0.308	0.330	0.352	0.374	0.398	0.422	0.447	0.472	0.498	0.525	0.553	0.581
5.00	0.210	0.227	0.245	0.264	0.283	0.303	0.324	0.345	0.368	0.390	0.414	0.438	0.463	0.489	0.516	0.543	0.571
5.25	0.207	0.224	0.241	0.259	0.278	0.298	0.318	0.340	0.362	0.384	0.407	0.431	0.456	0.481	0.507	0.534	0.562
5.50	0.203	0.220	0.237	0.255	0.274	0.293	0.313	0.334	0.355	0.378	0.400	0.424	0.448	0.473	0.499	0.525	0.552
15.75	0.200	0.216	0.233	0.251	0.269	0.288	0.308	0.329	0.350	0.372	0.394	0.417	0.441	0.466	0.491	0.517	0.543
16.00	0.197	0.213	0.229	0.247	0.265	0.284	0.303	0.323	0.344	0.365	0.388	0.410	0.434	0.458	0.483	0.508	0.534
17.00	0.185	0.200	0.216	0.232	0.249	0.267	0.285	0.304	0.323	0.343	0.364	0.386	0.408	0.430	0.453	0.477	0.502

Radii (mm)	Optic diameters (chords) (mm)																
	8.4	8.6	8.8	9.0	9.2	9.4	9.6	9.8	10.0	10.2	10.4	10.6	10.8	11.0	11.2	11.4	11.6
10.00	0.925	0.972	1.020	1.070	1.121	1.173	1.227	1.283	1.340	1.398	1.458	1.520	1.583	1.648	1.715	1.784	1.854
10.25	0.900	0.946	0.992	1.041	1.090	1.141	1.193	1.247	1.302	1.359	1.417	1.477	1.538	1.601	1.665	1.731	1.799
10.50	0.877	0.921	0.966	1.013	1.061	1.111	1.161	1.213	1.267	1.322	1.378	1.436	1.495	1.556	1.618	1.682	1.747
10.75	0.854	0.897	0.942	0.987	1.034	1.082	1.131	1.182	1.234	1.287	1.341	1.397	1.455	1.514	1.574	1.636	1.699
11.00	0.833	0.875	0.918	0.963	1.008	1.055	1.103	1.152	1.202	1.254	1.307	1.361	1.417	1.474	1.532	1.592	1.653
11.25	0.814	0.854	0.896	0.940	0.984	1.029	1.076	1.124	1.172	1.223	1.274	1.327	1.381	1.436	1.493	1.551	1.611
11.50	0.794	0.834	0.875	0.917	0.960	1.004	1.050	1.096	1.144	1.193	1.243	1.294	1.347	1.400	1.456	1.512	1.570
11.75	0.777	0.815	0.855	0.896	0.938	0.981	1.025	1.071	1.117	1.165	1.214	1.263	1.315	1.367	1.420	1.475	1.532
12.00	0.759	0.797	0.836	0.876	0.917	0.959	1.002	1.046	1.091	1.138	1.185	1.234	1.284	1.335	1.387	1.440	1.495
12.25	0.743	0.780	0.818	0.857	0.897	0.938	0.980	1.023	1.067	1.112	1.159	1.206	1.255	1.304	1.355	1.407	1.460
12.50	0.727	0.763	0.800	0.838	0.877	0.917	0.958	1.000	1.044	1.088	1.133	1.179	1.227	1.275	1.325	1.375	1.427
12.75	0.712	0.747	0.784	0.821	0.859	0.897	0.938	0.979	1.022	1.065	1.109	1.154	1.200	1.248	1.296	1.345	1.396
13.00	0.697	0.732	0.767	0.804	0.841	0.879	0.919	0.959	1.000	1.042	1.085	1.129	1.175	1.221	1.268	1.316	1.366
13.25	0.684	0.717	0.752	0.788	0.824	0.862	0.900	0.940	0.980	1.021	1.063	1.107	1.151	1.195	1.242	1.289	1.337
13.50	0.670	0.703	0.737	0.772	0.808	0.845	0.882	0.921	0.960	1.000	1.042	1.084	1.127	1.171	1.216	1.262	1.309
13.75	0.658	0.690	0.723	0.757	0.792	0.828	0.865	0.903	0.942	0.981	1.021	1.063	1.105	1.148	1.192	1.237	1.283
14.00	0.645	0.677	0.709	0.743	0.777	0.813	0.849	0.886	0.923	0.962	1.002	1.042	1.083	1.126	1.169	1.213	1.258
14.25	0.633	0.665	0.697	0.729	0.763	0.797	0.833	0.869	0.906	0.944	0.983	1.022	1.063	1.104	1.147	1.190	1.234
14.50	0.622	0.652	0.684	0.716	0.749	0.783	0.818	0.853	0.889	0.926	0.964	1.003	1.043	1.084	1.125	1.167	1.211
14.75	0.611	0.641	0.672	0.704	0.736	0.769	0.803	0.838	0.873	0.910	0.947	0.986	1.024	1.064	1.104	1.146	1.189
15.00	0.600	0.630	0.660	0.691	0.723	0.755	0.789	0.823	0.858	0.894	0.930	0.968	1.006	1.045	1.085	1.125	1.167
15.25	0.590	0.619	0.649	0.679	0.711	0.743	0.775	0.809	0.843	0.878	0.914	0.951	0.989	1.027	1.066	1.105	1.146
15.50	0.580	0.608	0.638	0.668	0.698	0.730	0.762	0.795	0.829	0.863	0.898	0.934	0.971	1.009	1.047	1.086	1.126
15.75	0.570	0.598	0.627	0.657	0.687	0.718	0.750	0.782	0.815	0.849	0.883	0.919	0.955	0.992	1.030	1.068	1.107
16.00	0.561	0.589	0.617	0.646	0.676	0.706	0.737	0.769	0.801	0.835	0.869	0.903	0.939	0.975	1.012	1.050	1.088
17.00	0.527	0.553	0.579	0.606	0.634	0.663	0.692	0.721	0.752	0.783	0.815	0.847	0.880	0.914	0.949	0.984	1.020

Radii (mm)	11.8	12.00	12.25	12.50	12.75	13.00	13.25	13.50	13.75	14.00	14.25	14.50	14.75	15.00	15.25	15.50	15.75

Optic diameters (chords) (mm)

Radii (mm)	11.8	12.00	12.25	12.50	12.75	13.00	13.25	13.50	13.75	14.00	14.25	14.50	14.75	15.00	15.25	15.50	15.75
10.00	1.926	2.000	2.095	2.194	2.295	2.401	2.509	2.622	2.738	2.859	2.983	3.113	3.247	3.386	3.530	3.680	3.837
10.25	1.868	1.940	2.031	2.126	2.224	2.325	2.429	2.536	2.648	2.763	2.881	3.004	3.132	3.263	3.400	3.542	3.689
10.50	1.814	1.883	1.972	2.063	2.157	2.254	2.354	2.457	2.564	2.674	2.787	2.905	3.026	3.152	3.281	3.416	3.555
10.75	1.764	1.830	1.916	2.004	2.094	2.188	2.284	2.383	2.486	2.591	2.700	2.813	2.929	3.049	3.172	3.300	3.432
11.00	1.716	1.780	1.863	1.948	2.036	2.126	2.219	2.315	2.413	2.515	2.619	2.727	2.839	2.953	3.072	3.194	3.320
11.25	1.672	1.734	1.814	1.896	1.981	2.068	2.158	2.250	2.345	2.443	2.544	2.648	2.755	2.865	2.978	3.095	3.216
11.50	1.629	1.689	1.767	1.847	1.929	2.013	2.100	2.189	2.281	2.376	2.473	2.573	2.676	2.782	2.891	3.004	3.119
11.75	1.589	1.648	1.723	1.800	1.880	1.962	2.046	2.132	2.221	2.313	2.407	2.503	2.603	2.705	2.810	2.918	3.030
12.00	1.551	1.608	1.681	1.756	1.833	1.913	1.995	2.078	2.165	2.253	2.344	2.438	2.534	2.633	2.734	2.838	2.945
12.25	1.515	1.570	1.641	1.715	1.790	1.867	1.946	2.028	2.111	2.197	2.285	2.376	2.469	2.564	2.662	2.763	2.867
12.50	1.480	1.534	1.603	1.675	1.748	1.823	1.900	1.979	2.060	2.144	2.229	2.317	2.407	2.500	2.595	2.693	2.793
12.75	1.448	1.500	1.568	1.637	1.708	1.781	1.856	1.933	2.012	2.093	2.177	2.262	2.349	2.439	2.531	2.626	2.723
13.00	1.416	1.467	1.533	1.601	1.670	1.742	1.815	1.890	1.967	2.046	2.126	2.209	2.294	2.382	2.471	2.563	2.657
13.25	1.386	1.436	1.501	1.567	1.634	1.704	1.775	1.848	1.923	2.000	2.079	2.159	2.242	2.327	2.414	2.503	2.599
13.50	1.358	1.407	1.469	1.534	1.600	1.668	1.737	1.809	1.882	1.957	2.033	2.112	2.193	2.275	2.360	2.446	2.535
13.75	1.331	1.379	1.440	1.503	1.567	1.633	1.701	1.771	1.842	1.915	1.990	2.067	2.145	2.226	2.308	2.392	2.478
14.00	1.304	1.351	1.411	1.473	1.536	1.600	1.667	1.735	1.804	1.876	1.949	2.023	2.100	2.178	2.259	2.341	2.425
14.25	1.279	1.325	1.383	1.444	1.506	1.569	1.634	1.700	1.768	1.838	1.909	1.982	2.057	2.133	2.212	2.292	2.374
14.50	1.255	1.300	1.357	1.416	1.478	1.539	1.602	1.667	1.733	1.802	1.871	1.943	2.016	2.090	2.167	2.245	2.325
14.75	1.232	1.276	1.332	1.390	1.449	1.509	1.572	1.635	1.700	1.767	1.835	1.905	1.976	2.049	2.124	2.200	2.278
15.00	1.209	1.252	1.308	1.364	1.422	1.482	1.542	1.605	1.668	1.734	1.800	1.868	1.938	2.010	2.083	2.157	2.233
15.25	1.188	1.230	1.284	1.340	1.396	1.455	1.514	1.575	1.638	1.701	1.767	1.834	1.902	1.972	2.043	2.116	2.191
15.50	1.167	1.208	1.262	1.316	1.372	1.429	1.487	1.547	1.608	1.671	1.735	1.800	1.867	1.935	2.005	2.077	2.150
15.75	1.147	1.188	1.240	1.294	1.348	1.404	1.461	1.520	1.580	1.641	1.704	1.768	1.833	1.900	1.969	2.039	2.110
16.00	1.128	1.168	1.219	1.271	1.325	1.380	1.436	1.494	1.552	1.613	1.674	1.737	1.801	1.867	1.934	2.002	2.072
17.00	1.057	1.094	1.142	1.191	1.241	1.292	1.344	1.398	1.452	1.508	1.565	1.623	1.683	1.744	1.806	1.869	1.934

Radii (mm)	16.0	17.0	18.0	19.0	20.0	21.0	22.0	23.0	24.0	25.0	26.0	27.0	28.0	29.0	30.0
10.00	4.000	4.638	5.641	6.878	10.000										
10.25	3.842	4.522	5.345	6.401	8.000										
10.50	3.699	4.336	5.092	6.028	7.298	10.500									
10.75	3.569	4.169	4.871	5.719	6.805	8.445									
11.00	3.450	4.018	4.675	5.455	6.417	7.721	11.000								
11.25	3.340	3.880	4.500	5.224	6.096	7.211	8.892								
11.50	3.239	3.754	4.341	5.019	5.821	6.810	8.221	11.500							
11.75	3.144	3.638	4.196	4.835	5.581	6.476	7.619	9.339							
12.00	3.056	3.529	4.063	4.669	5.367	6.191	7.204	8.572	12.000						
12.25	2.973	3.429	3.940	4.516	5.175	5.940	6.859	8.030	9.788						
12.50	2.895	3.335	3.825	4.376	5.000	5.718	6.563	7.601	9.000	12.500					
12.75	2.822	3.247	3.719	4.246	4.840	5.517	6.303	7.244	8.442	10.238					
13.00	2.753	3.164	3.619	4.126	4.693	5.335	6.072	6.938	8.000	9.429	13.000				
13.25	2.688	3.086	3.526	4.014	4.557	5.168	5.863	6.669	7.632	8.855	10.688				
13.50	2.626	3.012	3.438	3.908	4.431	5.015	5.674	6.429	7.315	8.401	9.860	13.500			
13.75	2.567	2.942	3.355	3.810	4.313	4.872	5.500	6.213	6.937	8.022	9.271	11.140			
14.00	2.511	2.876	3.276	3.717	4.202	4.740	5.340	6.016	6.789	7.695	8.804	10.292	14.000		
14.25	2.458	2.813	3.202	3.629	4.095	4.616	5.191	5.835	6.565	7.408	8.414	9.688	11.592		
14.50	2.407	2.753	3.131	3.546	4.000	4.500	5.053	5.668	6.361	7.152	8.077	9.208	10.725	14.500	
14.75	2.358	2.695	3.064	3.467	3.907	4.391	4.923	5.514	6.173	6.920	7.781	8.808	10.106	12.046	
15.00	2.311	2.641	3.000	3.392	3.820	4.288	4.802	5.369	6.000	6.708	7.517	8.462	9.615	11.159	15.000
15.25	2.267	2.589	2.939	3.321	3.736	4.191	4.688	5.234	5.839	6.514	7.277	8.157	9.203	10.526	12.500
15.50	2.224	2.539	2.881	3.253	3.657	4.098	4.580	5.108	5.689	6.335	7.059	7.884	8.848	10.023	11.595
15.75	2.183	2.491	2.825	3.189	3.582	4.011	4.478	4.988	5.549	6.168	6.858	7.638	8.535	9.601	10.948
16.00	2.144	2.445	2.771	3.126	3.510	3.927	4.381	4.876	5.417	6.013	6.673	7.412	8.254	9.236	10.432
17.00	2.000	2.278	2.578	2.920	3.252	3.630	4.039	4.480	4.958	5.478	6.046	6.668	7.356	8.126	9.000

Optic diameters (chords) (mm)

Appendix D: Back and front vertex powers for various centre thicknesses and back optic zone radii, calculated on the basis of a refractive index of 1.49

Table D.I Centre thickness 0.08 mm

Back vertex powers (D)	Front vertex powers (D) for back optic zone radii							
	5.0 mm	6.0 mm	7.0 mm	7.5 mm	8.0 mm	8.5 mm	9.0 mm	10.0 mm
+ 20	19.77	19.81	19.83	19.84	19.85	19.86	19.86	19.87
19	18.78	18.82	18.84	18.85	18.86	18.86	18.87	18.88
18	17.80	17.83	17.85	17.86	17.87	17.87	17.88	17.89
17	16.81	16.84	16.86	16.87	16.87	16.88	16.89	16.90
16	15.82	15.85	15.87	15.88	15.88	15.89	15.89	15.90
15	14.83	14.86	14.88	14.88	14.89	14.90	14.90	14.91
14	13.84	13.87	13.89	13.89	13.90	13.90	13.91	13.92
13	12.86	12.88	12.89	12.90	12.91	12.91	12.92	12.92
12	11.87	11.89	11.90	11.91	11.91	11.92	11.92	11.93
11	10.88	10.90	10.91	10.92	10.92	10.93	10.93	10.94
10	9.89	9.91	9.92	9.93	9.93	9.93	9.94	9.94
9	8.90	8.92	8.93	8.93	8.94	8.94	8.94	8.95
8	7.91	7.93	7.94	7.94	7.94	7.95	7.95	7.96
7	6.92	6.94	6.95	6.95	6.95	6.95	6.96	6.96
6	5.94	5.95	5.95	5.96	5.96	5.96	5.96	5.97
5	4.95	4.96	4.96	4.96	4.97	4.97	4.97	4.97
4	3.96	3.96	3.97	3.97	3.97	3.98	3.98	3.98
3	2.97	2.97	2.98	2.98	2.98	2.98	2.98	2.98
2	1.98	1.98	1.99	1.99	1.99	1.99	1.99	1.99
1	0.99	0.99	0.99	0.99	0.99	0.99	0.99	1.00
0	0.00	0.00	0.00	0.00	0.00	0.00	0.00	0.00
− 1	0.99	0.99	0.99	0.99	0.99	0.99	0.99	1.00
2	1.98	1.98	1.99	1.99	1.99	1.99	1.99	1.99
3	2.97	2.97	2.98	2.98	2.98	2.98	2.98	2.99
4	3.96	3.97	3.97	3.97	3.98	3.98	3.98	3.98
5	4.95	4.96	4.96	4.97	4.97	4.97	4.97	4.98
6	5.94	5.95	5.96	5.96	5.96	5.97	5.97	5.97
7	6.93	6.94	6.95	6.95	6.96	6.96	6.96	6.97
8	7.92	7.93	7.94	7.95	7.95	7.95	7.96	7.96
9	8.91	8.93	8.94	8.94	8.95	8.95	8.95	8.96
10	9.90	9.92	9.93	9.94	9.94	9.94	9.95	9.95
11	10.89	10.91	10.92	10.93	10.93	10.94	10.94	10.95
12	11.88	11.90	11.92	11.92	11.93	11.93	11.94	11.95
13	12.87	12.90	12.91	12.92	12.92	12.93	12.93	12.94
14	13.86	13.89	13.91	13.91	13.92	13.92	13.93	13.94
15	14.86	14.88	14.90	14.91	14.91	14.92	14.93	14.93
16	15.85	15.87	15.89	15.90	15.91	15.92	15.92	15.93
17	16.84	16.87	16.88	16.90	16.90	16.91	16.92	16.93
18	17.83	17.86	17.88	17.89	17.90	17.91	17.91	17.92
19	18.82	18.85	18.88	18.89	18.90	18.90	18.91	18.92
20	19.81	19.85	19.87	19.88	19.89	19.90	19.91	19.92
21	20.80	20.84	20.87	20.88	20.89	20.89	20.90	20.91
22	21.80	21.83	21.86	21.87	21.88	21.89	21.90	21.91
23	22.79	22.83	22.86	22.87	22.88	22.89	22.89	22.91
24	23.78	23.82	23.85	23.86	23.87	23.88	23.89	23.91
25	24.77	24.82	24.85	24.86	24.87	24.88	24.89	24.90
26	25.76	25.81	25.84	25.86	25.87	25.88	25.89	25.90
27	26.76	26.80	26.84	26.85	26.86	26.87	26.88	26.90
28	27.75	27.80	27.83	27.85	27.86	27.87	27.88	27.90
29	28.74	28.79	28.83	28.84	28.86	28.87	28.88	28.89
30	29.73	29.79	29.82	29.84	29.85	29.86	29.87	29.89

Table D.II Centre thickness 0.10 mm

Back vertex powers (D)	Front vertex powers (D) for back optic zone radii							
	5.0 mm	6.0 mm	7.0 mm	7.5 mm	8.0 mm	8.5 mm	9.0 mm	10.0 mm
+ 20	19.71	19.76	19.79	19.80	19.81	19.82	19.83	19.84
19	18.73	18.77	18.80	18.81	18.82	18.83	18.84	18.85
18	17.74	17.78	17.81	17.82	17.83	17.84	17.85	17.86
17	16.76	16.80	16.82	16.83	16.84	16.85	16.86	16.87
16	15.78	15.81	15.83	15.84	15.85	15.86	15.87	15.88
15	14.79	14.82	14.85	14.85	14.86	14.87	14.88	14.89
14	13.81	13.84	13.86	13.87	13.87	13.88	13.89	13.90
13	12.82	12.85	12.87	12.88	12.88	12.89	12.89	12.90
12	11.83	11.86	11.88	11.89	11.89	11.90	11.90	11.91
11	10.85	10.87	10.89	10.90	10.90	10.91	10.91	10.92
10	9.86	9.89	9.90	9.91	9.91	9.92	9.92	9.93
9	8.88	8.90	8.91	8.92	8.92	8.93	8.93	8.94
8	7.89	7.91	7.92	7.93	7.93	7.93	7.94	7.94
7	6.91	6.92	6.93	6.94	6.94	6.94	6.95	6.95
6	5.92	5.93	5.94	5.95	5.95	5.95	5.95	5.96
5	4.93	4.94	4.95	4.96	4.96	4.96	4.96	4.97
4	3.95	3.96	3.96	3.96	3.97	3.97	3.97	3.97
3	2.96	2.97	2.97	2.97	2.98	2.98	2.98	2.98
2	1.97	1.98	1.98	1.98	1.98	1.98	1.99	1.99
1	0.99	0.99	0.99	0.99	0.99	0.99	0.99	0.99
0	0.00	0.00	0.00	0.00	0.00	0.00	0.00	0.00
− 1	0.99	0.99	0.99	0.99	0.99	0.99	0.99	0.99
2	1.97	1.98	1.98	1.98	1.98	1.99	1.99	1.99
3	2.96	2.97	2.97	2.97	2.98	2.98	2.98	2.98
4	3.95	3.96	3.96	3.97	3.97	3.97	3.97	3.98
5	4.94	4.95	4.96	4.96	4.96	4.96	4.97	4.97
6	5.92	5.94	5.95	5.95	5.95	5.96	5.96	5.96
7	6.91	6.93	6.94	6.94	6.95	6.95	6.95	6.96
8	7.90	7.92	7.93	7.94	7.94	7.94	7.95	7.95
9	8.89	8.91	8.92	8.93	8.93	8.94	8.94	8.95
10	9.88	9.90	9.91	9.92	9.93	9.93	9.93	9.94
11	10.87	10.89	10.91	10.91	10.92	10.92	10.93	10.94
12	11.85	11.88	11.90	11.91	11.91	11.92	11.92	11.93
13	12.84	12.87	12.89	12.90	12.91	12.91	12.92	12.93
14	13.83	13.86	13.88	13.89	13.90	13.91	13.91	13.92
15	14.82	14.85	14.88	14.88	14.89	14.90	14.91	14.92
16	15.81	15.84	15.87	15.88	15.89	15.89	15.90	15.91
17	16.80	16.83	16.86	16.87	16.88	16.89	16.90	16.91
18	17.79	17.83	17.85	17.87	17.87	17.88	17.89	17.90
19	18.78	18.82	18.85	18.86	18.87	18.88	18.89	18.90
20	19.77	19.81	19.84	19.85	19.86	19.87	19.88	19.90
21	20.76	20.80	20.83	20.85	20.86	20.87	20.88	20.89
22	21.75	21.79	21.83	21.84	21.85	21.86	21.87	21.89
23	22.74	22.79	22.82	22.84	22.85	22.86	22.87	22.89
24	23.73	23.78	23.81	23.83	23.84	23.85	23.86	23.88
25	24.72	24.77	24.81	24.82	24.84	24.85	24.86	24.88
26	25.71	25.76	25.80	25.82	25.83	25.85	25.86	25.88
27	26.70	26.76	26.80	26.81	26.83	26.84	26.85	26.87
28	27.69	27.75	27.79	27.81	27.82	27.84	27.85	27.87
29	28.68	28.74	28.79	28.80	28.82	28.83	28.85	28.87
30	29.67	29.73	29.78	29.80	29.82	29.83	29.84	29.86

Table D.III Centre thickness 0.12 mm

Back vertex powers (D)	Front vertex powers (D) for back optic zone radii							
	5.0 mm	6.0 mm	7.0 mm	7.5 mm	8.0 mm	8.5 mm	9.0 mm	10.0 mm
+ 20	19.66	19.71	19.75	19.76	19.77	19.78	19.79	19.81
19	18.68	18.72	18.76	18.77	18.79	18.80	18.81	18.82
18	17.69	17.74	17.77	17.79	17.80	17.81	17.82	17.83
17	16.71	16.76	16.79	16.80	16.81	16.82	16.83	16.84
16	15.73	15.77	15.80	15.81	15.82	15.83	15.84	15.85
15	14.75	14.79	14.81	14.83	14.84	14.84	14.85	14.86
14	13.77	13.80	13.83	13.84	13.85	13.86	13.86	13.88
13	12.78	12.82	12.84	12.85	12.86	12.87	12.87	12.89
12	11.80	11.83	11.85	11.86	11.87	11.88	11.88	11.89
11	10.82	10.85	10.87	10.88	10.88	10.89	10.90	10.90
10	9.84	9.86	9.88	9.89	9.89	9.90	9.91	9.91
9	8.85	8.88	8.89	8.90	8.91	8.91	8.92	8.92
8	7.87	7.89	7.91	7.91	7.92	7.92	7.93	7.93
7	6.89	6.91	6.92	6.92	6.93	6.93	6.94	6.94
6	5.90	5.92	5.93	5.94	5.94	5.94	5.95	5.95
5	4.92	4.93	4.94	4.95	4.95	4.95	4.95	4.96
4	3.94	3.95	3.95	3.96	3.96	3.96	3.96	3.97
3	2.95	2.96	2.97	2.97	2.97	2.97	2.97	2.98
2	1.97	1.97	1.98	1.98	1.98	1.98	1.98	1.98
1	0.98	0.99	0.99	0.99	0.99	0.99	0.99	0.99
0	0.00	0.00	0.00	0.00	0.00	0.00	0.00	0.00
− 1	0.98	0.99	0.99	0.99	0.99	0.99	0.99	0.99
2	1.97	1.97	1.98	1.98	1.98	1.98	1.98	1.99
3	2.95	2.96	2.97	2.97	2.97	2.97	2.98	2.98
4	3.94	3.95	3.96	3.96	3.96	3.96	3.97	3.97
5	4.92	4.94	4.95	4.95	4.95	4.96	4.96	4.96
6	5.91	5.93	5.94	5.94	5.94	5.95	5.95	5.96
7	6.90	6.91	6.93	6.93	6.94	6.94	6.94	6.95
8	7.88	7.90	7.92	7.92	7.93	7.93	7.94	7.94
9	8.87	8.89	8.91	8.91	8.92	8.92	8.93	8.94
10	9.85	9.88	9.90	9.90	9.91	9.92	9.92	9.93
11	10.84	10.87	10.89	10.90	10.90	10.91	10.91	10.92
12	11.82	11.86	11.88	11.89	11.89	11.90	11.91	11.92
13	12.81	12.84	12.87	12.88	12.89	12.89	12.90	12.91
14	13.80	13.83	13.86	13.87	13.88	13.89	13.89	13.91
15	14.78	14.82	14.85	14.86	14.87	14.88	14.89	14.90
16	15.77	15.81	15.84	15.85	15.86	15.87	15.88	15.90
17	16.76	16.80	16.83	16.85	16.86	16.87	16.88	16.89
18	17.75	17.79	17.82	17.84	17.85	17.86	17.87	17.89
19	18.73	18.78	18.82	18.83	18.84	18.85	18.86	18.88
20	19.72	19.77	19.81	19.82	19.84	19.85	19.86	19.88
21	20.71	20.76	20.80	20.82	20.83	20.84	20.85	20.87
22	21.70	21.75	21.79	21.81	21.82	21.84	21.85	21.87
23	22.68	22.74	22.79	22.80	22.82	22.83	22.84	22.86
24	23.67	23.73	23.78	23.80	23.81	23.83	23.84	23.86
25	24.66	24.72	24.77	24.79	24.81	24.82	24.83	24.85
26	25.65	25.72	25.76	25.78	25.80	25.81	25.83	25.85
27	26.64	26.71	26.76	26.78	26.79	26.81	26.82	26.85
28	27.63	27.70	27.75	27.77	27.79	27.80	27.82	27.84
29	28.61	28.69	28.74	28.76	28.78	28.80	28.81	28.84
30	29.60	29.68	29.74	29.76	29.78	29.80	29.81	29.84

Table D.IV Centre thickness 0.14 mm

Back vertex powers (D)	Front vertex powers (D) for back optic zone radii							
	5.0 mm	6.0 mm	7.0 mm	7.5 mm	8.0 mm	8.5 mm	9.0 mm	10.0 mm
+ 20	19.60	19.66	19.70	19.72	19.74	19.75	19.76	19.78
19	18.62	18.68	18.72	18.74	18.75	18.76	18.77	18.79
18	17.64	17.70	17.74	17.75	17.77	17.78	17.79	17.81
17	16.67	16.72	16.75	16.77	16.78	16.79	16.80	16.82
16	15.69	15.73	15.77	15.78	15.79	15.80	15.81	15.83
15	14.71	14.75	14.78	14.80	14.81	14.82	14.83	14.84
14	13.73	13.77	13.80	13.81	13.82	13.83	13.84	13.85
13	12.75	12.79	12.82	12.83	12.84	12.85	12.85	12.87
12	11.77	11.81	11.83	11.84	11.85	11.86	11.87	11.88
11	10.79	10.82	10.85	10.86	10.86	10.87	10.88	10.89
10	9.81	9.84	9.86	9.87	9.88	9.88	9.89	9.90
9	8.83	8.86	8.88	8.88	8.89	8.90	8.90	8.91
8	7.85	7.87	7.89	7.90	7.90	7.91	7.91	7.92
7	6.87	6.89	6.90	6.91	6.92	6.92	6.92	6.93
6	5.89	5.91	5.92	5.92	5.93	5.93	5.94	5.94
5	4.91	4.92	4.93	4.94	4.94	4.94	4.95	4.95
4	3.93	3.94	3.95	3.95	3.95	3.96	3.96	3.96
3	2.95	2.95	2.96	2.96	2.97	2.97	2.97	2.97
2	1.96	1.97	1.97	1.98	1.98	1.98	1.98	1.98
1	0.98	0.99	0.99	0.99	0.99	0.99	0.99	0.99
0	0.00	0.00	0.00	0.00	0.00	0.00	0.00	0.00
− 1	0.98	0.99	0.99	0.99	0.99	0.99	0.99	0.99
2	1.96	1.97	1.97	1.98	1.98	1.98	1.98	1.98
3	2.95	2.96	2.96	2.96	2.97	2.97	2.97	2.97
4	3.93	3.94	3.95	3.95	3.96	3.96	3.96	3.97
5	4.91	4.93	4.94	4.94	4.95	4.95	4.95	4.96
6	5.89	5.91	5.93	5.93	5.94	5.94	5.94	5.95
7	6.88	6.90	6.91	6.92	6.93	6.93	6.93	6.94
8	7.86	7.89	7.90	7.91	7.92	7.92	7.93	7.93
9	8.84	8.87	8.89	8.90	8.91	8.91	8.92	8.93
10	9.83	9.86	9.88	9.89	9.90	9.90	9.91	9.92
11	10.81	10.84	10.87	10.88	10.89	10.89	10.90	10.91
12	11.80	11.83	11.86	11.87	11.88	11.88	11.89	11.90
13	12.78	12.82	12.85	12.86	12.87	12.88	12.88	12.90
14	13.76	13.81	13.84	13.85	13.86	13.87	13.88	13.89
15	14.75	14.79	14.83	14.84	14.85	14.86	14.87	14.88
16	15.73	15.78	15.82	15.83	15.84	15.85	15.86	15.88
17	16.72	16.77	16.81	16.82	16.83	16.84	16.85	16.87
18	17.70	17.76	17.80	17.81	17.83	17.84	17.85	17.87
19	18.69	18.75	18.79	18.80	18.82	18.83	18.84	18.86
20	19.67	19.73	19.78	19.79	19.81	19.82	19.83	19.85
21	20.66	20.72	20.77	20.79	20.80	20.82	20.83	20.85
22	21.65	21.71	21.76	21.78	21.79	21.81	21.82	21.84
23	22.63	22.70	22.75	22.77	22.79	22.80	22.82	22.84
24	23.62	23.69	23.74	23.76	23.78	23.80	23.81	23.83
25	24.60	24.68	24.73	24.75	24.77	24.79	24.80	24.83
26	25.59	25.67	25.72	25.75	25.77	25.78	25.80	25.83
27	26.58	26.66	26.72	26.74	26.76	26.78	26.79	26.82
28	27.56	27.65	27.71	27.73	27.75	27.77	27.79	27.82
29	28.55	28.64	28.70	28.73	28.75	28.77	28.78	28.81
30	29.54	29.63	29.69	29.72	29.74	29.76	29.78	29.81

Table D.V Centre thickness 0.16 mm

Back vertex powers (D)	Front vertex powers (D) for back optic zone radii							
	5.0 mm	6.0 mm	7.0 mm	7.5 mm	8.0 mm	8.5 mm	9.0 mm	10.0 mm
+ 20	19.54	19.61	19.66	19.68	19.70	19.71	19.73	19.75
19	18.57	18.63	18.68	18.70	18.72	18.73	18.74	18.76
18	17.59	17.66	17.70	17.72	17.73	17.75	17.76	17.78
17	16.62	16.68	16.72	16.73	16.75	16.76	16.77	16.79
16	15.64	15.70	15.74	15.75	15.77	15.78	15.79	15.81
15	14.67	14.72	14.75	14.77	14.78	14.79	14.80	14.82
14	13.69	13.74	13.77	13.79	13.80	13.81	13.82	13.83
13	12.71	12.76	12.79	12.80	12.81	12.82	12.83	12.85
12	11.74	11.78	11.81	11.82	11.83	11.84	11.85	11.86
11	10.76	10.80	10.82	10.84	10.84	10.85	10.86	10.87
10	9.78	9.82	9.84	9.85	9.86	9.87	9.87	9.89
9	8.81	8.84	8.86	8.87	8.87	8.88	8.89	8.90
8	7.83	7.86	7.87	7.88	7.89	7.90	7.90	7.91
7	6.85	6.87	6.89	6.90	6.90	6.91	6.91	6.92
6	5.87	5.89	5.91	5.91	5.92	5.92	5.93	5.93
5	4.89	4.91	4.92	4.93	4.93	4.94	4.94	4.95
4	3.92	3.93	3.94	3.94	3.95	3.95	3.95	3.96
3	2.94	2.95	2.95	2.96	2.96	2.96	2.96	2.97
2	1.96	1.97	1.97	1.97	1.97	1.98	1.98	1.98
1	0.98	0.98	0.99	0.99	0.99	0.99	0.99	0.99
0	0.00	0.00	0.00	0.00	0.00	0.00	0.00	0.00
− 1	0.98	0.98	0.99	0.99	0.99	0.99	0.99	0.99
2	1.96	1.97	1.97	1.97	1.97	1.98	1.98	1.98
3	2.94	2.95	2.96	2.96	2.96	2.96	2.97	2.97
4	3.92	3.93	3.94	3.95	3.95	3.95	3.96	3.96
5	4.90	4.92	4.93	4.93	4.94	4.94	4.95	4.95
6	5.88	5.90	5.92	5.92	5.93	5.93	5.93	5.94
7	6.86	6.88	6.90	6.91	6.91	6.92	6.92	6.93
8	7.84	7.87	7.89	7.90	7.90	7.91	7.91	7.92
9	8.82	8.85	8.88	8.88	8.89	8.90	8.90	8.92
10	9.80	9.84	9.86	9.87	9.88	9.89	9.90	9.91
11	10.79	10.82	10.85	10.86	10.87	10.88	10.89	10.90
12	11.77	11.81	11.84	11.85	11.86	11.87	11.88	11.89
13	12.75	12.79	12.83	12.84	12.85	12.86	12.87	12.88
14	13.73	13.78	13.81	13.83	13.84	13.85	13.86	13.88
15	14.71	14.76	14.80	14.82	14.83	14.84	14.85	14.87
16	15.70	15.75	15.79	15.81	15.82	15.83	15.84	15.86
17	16.68	16.74	16.78	16.79	16.81	16.82	16.83	16.85
18	17.66	17.72	17.77	17.78	17.80	17.81	17.83	17.85
19	18.64	18.71	18.76	18.77	18.79	18.81	18.82	18.84
20	19.63	19.70	19.75	19.76	19.78	19.80	19.81	19.83
21	20.61	20.68	20.73	20.76	20.77	20.79	20.80	20.83
22	21.60	21.67	21.72	21.75	21.77	21.78	21.80	21.82
23	22.58	22.66	22.71	22.74	22.76	22.77	22.79	22.82
24	23.56	23.65	23.70	23.73	23.75	23.77	23.78	23.81
25	24.55	24.63	24.69	24.72	24.74	24.76	24.78	24.81
26	25.53	25.62	25.69	25.71	25.73	25.75	25.77	25.80
27	26.52	26.61	26.68	26.70	26.73	26.75	26.76	26.80
28	27.50	27.60	27.67	27.69	27.72	27.74	27.76	27.79
29	28.49	28.59	28.66	28.69	28.71	28.73	28.75	28.79
30	29.47	29.58	29.65	29.68	29.70	29.73	29.75	29.78

Table D.VI Centre thickness 0.18 mm

Back vertex powers (D)	Front vertex powers (D) *for back optic zone radii*							
	5.0 mm	6.0 mm	7.0 mm	7.5 mm	8.0 mm	8.5 mm	9.0 mm	10.0 mm
+ 20	19.49	19.56	19.62	19.64	19.66	19.68	19.69	19.72
19	18.52	18.59	18.64	18.66	18.68	18.70	18.71	18.73
18	17.54	17.61	17.66	17.68	17.70	17.71	17.73	17.75
17	16.57	16.64	16.68	16.70	16.72	16.73	16.74	16.77
16	15.60	15.66	15.70	15.72	15.74	15.75	15.76	15.78
15	14.63	14.68	14.72	14.74	14.75	14.77	14.78	14.80
14	13.65	13.71	13.74	13.76	13.77	13.78	13.79	13.81
13	12.68	12.73	12.76	12.78	12.79	12.80	12.81	12.83
12	11.70	11.75	11.78	11.80	11.81	11.82	11.83	11.84
11	10.73	10.77	10.80	10.81	10.83	10.83	10.84	10.86
10	9.76	9.79	9.82	9.83	9.84	9.85	9.86	9.87
9	8.78	8.82	8.84	8.85	8.86	8.87	8.87	8.89
8	7.81	7.84	7.86	7.87	7.88	7.88	7.89	7.90
7	6.83	6.86	6.88	6.89	6.89	6.90	6.90	6.91
6	5.86	5.88	5.90	5.90	5.91	5.91	5.92	5.93
5	4.88	4.90	4.91	4.92	4.92	4.93	4.93	4.94
4	3.91	3.92	3.93	3.94	3.94	3.94	3.95	3.95
3	2.93	2.94	2.95	2.95	2.96	2.96	2.96	2.96
2	1.95	1.96	1.97	1.97	1.97	1.97	1.97	1.98
1	0.98	0.98	0.98	0.98	0.99	0.99	0.99	0.99
0	0.00	0.00	0.00	0.00	0.00	0.00	0.00	0.00
− 1	0.98	0.98	0.98	0.99	0.99	0.99	0.99	0.99
2	1.95	1.96	1.97	1.97	1.97	1.97	1.97	1.98
3	2.93	2.94	2.95	2.95	2.96	2.96	2.96	2.97
4	3.91	3.92	3.94	3.94	3.94	3.95	3.95	3.96
5	4.89	4.91	4.92	4.93	4.93	4.93	4.94	4.94
6	5.87	5.89	5.90	5.91	5.92	5.92	5.93	5.93
7	6.84	6.87	6.89	6.90	6.90	6.91	6.92	6.92
8	7.82	7.85	7.87	7.88	7.89	7.90	7.90	7.91
9	8.80	8.84	8.86	8.87	8.88	8.89	8.89	8.90
10	9.78	9.82	9.85	9.86	9.87	9.87	9.88	9.90
11	10.76	10.80	10.83	10.84	10.85	10.86	10.87	10.89
12	11.74	11.78	11.82	11.83	11.84	11.85	11.86	11.88
13	12.72	12.77	12.80	12.82	12.83	12.84	12.85	12.87
14	13.70	13.75	13.79	13.81	13.82	13.83	13.84	13.86
15	14.68	14.74	14.78	14.79	14.81	14.82	14.83	14.85
16	15.66	15.72	15.76	15.78	15.80	15.81	15.82	15.84
17	16.64	16.70	16.75	16.77	16.79	16.80	16.81	16.84
18	17.62	17.69	17.74	17.76	17.78	17.79	17.80	17.83
19	18.60	18.67	18.73	18.75	18.77	18.78	18.80	18.82
20	19.58	19.66	19.71	19.74	19.76	19.77	19.79	19.81
21	20.56	20.64	20.70	20.73	20.75	20.76	20.78	20.81
22	21.55	21.63	21.69	21.71	21.74	21.75	21.77	21.80
23	22.53	22.62	22.68	22.70	22.73	22.75	22.76	22.79
24	23.51	23.60	23.67	23.69	23.72	23.74	23.76	23.79
25	24.49	24.59	24.66	24.68	24.71	24.73	24.75	24.78
26	25.47	25.57	25.65	25.67	25.70	25.72	25.74	25.78
27	26.46	26.56	26.64	26.67	26.69	26.71	26.74	26.77
28	27.44	27.55	27.63	27.66	27.68	27.71	27.73	27.77
29	28.42	28.54	28.62	28.65	28.68	28.70	28.72	28.76
30	29.41	29.52	29.61	29.64	29.67	29.69	29.72	29.76

Table D.VII Centre thickness 0.20 mm

Back vertex powers (D)	Front vertex powers (D) for back optic zone radii							
	5.0 mm	6.0 mm	7.0 mm	7.5 mm	8.0 mm	8.5 mm	9.0 mm	10.0 mm
+ 20	19.43	19.52	19.58	19.60	19.62	19.64	19.66	19.69
19	18.46	18.54	18.60	18.62	18.64	18.66	18.68	18.71
18	17.49	17.57	17.62	17.65	17.67	17.68	17.70	17.72
17	16.52	16.60	16.65	16.67	16.69	16.70	16.72	16.74
16	15.55	15.62	15.67	15.69	15.71	15.72	15.74	15.76
15	14.58	14.65	14.69	14.71	14.73	14.74	14.75	14.78
14	13.61	13.67	13.72	13.73	13.75	13.76	13.77	13.79
13	12.64	12.70	12.74	12.75	12.77	12.78	12.79	12.81
12	11.67	11.71	11.76	11.77	11.79	11.80	11.81	11.83
11	10.70	10.75	10.78	10.79	10.81	10.82	10.83	10.84
10	9.73	9.77	9.80	9.81	9.82	9.83	9.84	9.86
9	8.76	8.80	8.82	8.83	8.84	8.85	8.86	8.87
8	7.79	7.82	7.84	7.85	7.86	7.87	7.88	7.89
7	6.81	6.84	6.86	6.87	6.88	6.89	6.89	6.90
6	5.84	5.87	5.88	5.89	5.90	5.90	5.91	5.92
5	4.89	4.89	4.90	4.91	4.92	4.92	4.92	4.93
4	3.90	3.91	3.92	3.93	3.93	3.94	3.94	3.95
3	2.92	2.93	2.94	2.95	2.95	2.95	2.96	2.96
2	1.95	1.96	1.96	1.97	1.97	1.97	1.97	1.97
1	0.97	0.98	0.98	0.98	0.98	0.99	0.99	0.99
0	0.00	0.00	0.00	0.00	0.00	0.00	0.00	0.00
− 1	0.97	0.98	0.98	0.98	0.98	0.99	0.99	0.99
2	1.95	1.96	1.96	1.97	1.97	1.97	1.97	1.97
3	2.92	2.94	2.95	2.95	2.95	2.96	2.96	2.96
4	3.90	3.92	3.93	3.93	3.94	3.94	3.94	3.95
5	4.87	4.90	4.91	4.92	4.92	4.93	4.93	4.94
6	5.85	5.88	5.89	5.90	5.91	5.91	5.92	5.93
7	6.83	6.86	6.88	6.89	6.89	6.90	6.91	6.92
8	7.80	7.84	7.86	7.87	7.88	7.89	7.89	7.90
9	8.78	8.82	8.84	8.86	8.86	8.87	8.88	8.89
10	9.76	9.80	9.83	9.84	9.85	9.86	9.87	9.88
11	10.73	10.78	10.81	10.83	10.84	10.85	10.86	10.89
12	11.71	11.76	11.80	11.81	11.82	11.84	11.85	11.86
13	12.69	12.74	12.78	12.80	12.81	12.82	12.83	12.85
14	13.66	13.72	13.77	13.78	13.80	13.81	13.82	13.84
15	14.64	14.71	14.75	14.77	14.79	14.80	14.81	14.83
16	15.62	15.69	15.74	15.76	15.77	15.79	15.80	15.83
17	16.60	16.67	16.72	16.74	16.76	16.78	16.79	16.82
18	17.58	17.65	17.71	17.73	17.75	17.77	17.78	17.81
19	18.56	18.64	18.70	18.72	18.74	18.76	18.77	18.80
20	19.54	19.62	19.68	19.71	19.73	19.75	19.76	19.79
21	20.52	20.61	20.67	20.69	20.72	20.74	20.75	20.79
22	21.50	21.59	21.66	21.68	21.71	21.73	21.75	21.78
23	22.48	22.57	22.64	22.67	22.70	22.72	22.74	22.77
24	23.46	23.56	23.63	23.66	23.69	23.71	23.73	23.76
25	24.44	24.54	24.62	24.65	24.68	24.70	24.72	24.76
26	25.42	25.53	25.61	25.64	25.67	25.69	25.71	25.75
27	26.40	26.51	26.60	26.63	26.66	26.68	26.71	26.75
28	27.38	27.50	27.58	27.62	27.65	27.68	27.70	27.74
29	28.36	28.48	28.57	28.61	28.64	28.67	28.69	28.73
30	29.34	29.47	29.56	29.60	29.63	29.66	29.69	29.73

Table D.VIII Centre thickness 0.22 mm

Back vertex powers (D)	Front vertex powers (D) for back optic zone radii							
	5.0 mm	6.0 mm	7.0 mm	7.5 mm	8.0 mm	8.5 mm	9.0 mm	10.0 mm
+ 20	19.38	19.47	19.54	19.56	19.59	19.61	19.63	19.66
19	18.41	18.50	18.56	18.59	18.61	18.63	18.65	18.68
18	17.44	17.53	17.59	17.61	17.63	17.65	17.67	17.70
17	16.48	16.56	16.61	16.64	16.66	16.67	16.69	16.72
16	15.51	15.59	15.64	15.66	15.68	15.69	15.71	15.73
15	14.54	14.61	14.66	14.68	14.70	14.72	14.73	14.75
14	13.58	13.64	13.69	13.71	13.72	13.74	13.75	13.77
13	12.61	12.67	12.71	12.73	12.74	12.76	12.77	12.79
12	11.64	11.70	11.74	11.75	11.77	11.78	11.79	11.81
11	10.67	10.72	10.76	10.77	10.79	10.80	10.81	10.83
10	9.70	9.75	9.78	9.80	9.81	9.82	9.83	9.84
9	8.73	8.78	8.81	8.82	8.83	8.84	8.85	8.86
8	7.76	7.80	7.83	7.84	7.85	7.86	7.86	7.88
7	6.80	6.83	6.85	6.86	6.87	6.88	6.88	6.89
6	5.83	5.85	5.87	5.88	5.89	5.89	5.90	5.91
5	4.86	4.88	4.90	4.90	4.91	4.91	4.92	4.93
4	3.88	3.90	3.92	3.92	3.93	3.93	3.93	3.94
3	2.91	2.93	2.94	2.94	2.95	2.95	2.95	2.96
2	1.94	1.95	1.96	1.96	1.96	1.97	1.97	1.97
1	0.97	0.98	0.98	0.98	0.98	0.98	0.98	0.99
0	0.00	0.00	0.00	0.00	0.00	0.00	0.00	0.00
− 1	0.97	0.98	0.98	0.98	0.98	0.98	0.98	0.99
2	1.94	1.95	1.96	1.96	1.97	1.97	1.97	1.97
3	2.92	2.93	2.94	2.94	2.95	2.95	2.95	2.96
4	3.89	3.91	3.92	3.93	3.93	3.94	3.94	3.95
5	4.86	4.89	4.90	4.91	4.91	4.92	4.92	4.93
6	5.84	5.86	5.88	5.89	5.90	5.90	5.91	5.92
7	6.81	6.84	6.87	6.87	6.88	6.89	6.90	6.91
8	7.78	7.82	7.85	7.86	7.87	7.88	7.88	7.90
9	8.76	8.80	8.83	8.84	8.85	8.86	8.87	8.88
10	9.73	9.78	9.81	9.82	9.84	9.85	9.86	9.87
11	10.71	10.76	10.79	10.81	10.82	10.83	10.84	10.86
12	11.68	11.74	11.78	11.79	11.81	11.82	11.83	11.85
13	12.66	12.72	12.76	12.78	12.79	12.81	12.82	12.84
14	13.63	13.70	13.74	13.76	13.78	13.79	13.81	13.83
15	14.61	14.68	14.73	14.75	14.77	14.78	14.79	14.82
16	15.58	15.66	15.71	15.73	15.75	15.77	15.78	15.81
17	16.56	16.64	16.70	16.72	16.74	16.76	16.77	16.80
18	17.54	17.62	17.68	17.70	17.73	17.74	17.76	17.79
19	18.51	18.60	18.67	18.69	18.71	18.73	18.75	18.78
20	19.49	19.58	19.65	19.68	19.70	19.72	19.74	19.77
21	20.47	20.57	20.64	20.66	20.69	20.71	20.73	20.76
22	21.45	21.55	21.62	21.65	21.68	21.70	21.72	21.76
23	22.42	22.53	22.61	22.64	22.67	22.69	22.71	22.75
24	23.40	23.51	23.59	23.63	23.66	23.68	23.70	23.74
25	24.38	24.50	24.58	24.62	24.64	24.67	24.69	24.73
26	25.36	25.48	25.57	25.60	25.63	25.66	25.69	25.73
27	26.34	26.47	26.56	26.59	26.62	26.65	26.68	26.72
28	27.32	27.45	27.54	27.58	27.61	27.64	27.67	27.71
29	28.30	28.43	28.53	28.57	28.60	28.63	28.66	28.71
30	29.28	29.42	29.52	29.56	29.60	29.63	29.65	29.70

Table D.IX Centre thickness 0.24 mm

Back vertex powers (D)	Front vertex powers (D) for back optic zone radii							
	5.0 mm	6.0 mm	7.0 mm	7.5 mm	8.0 mm	8.5 mm	9.0 mm	10.0 mm
+ 20	19.32	19.42	19.49	19.52	19.55	19.57	19.59	19.63
19	18.36	18.45	18.52	18.55	18.57	18.60	18.62	18.65
18	17.40	17.49	17.55	17.58	17.60	17.62	17.64	17.67
17	16.43	16.52	16.58	16.60	16.62	16.64	16.66	16.69
16	15.47	15.55	15.61	15.63	15.65	15.67	15.68	15.71
15	14.50	14.58	14.63	14.65	14.67	14.69	14.71	14.73
14	13.54	13.61	13.66	13.68	13.70	13.71	13.73	13.75
13	12.57	12.64	12.69	12.70	12.72	12.74	12.75	12.77
12	11.61	11.67	11.71	11.73	11.74	11.76	11.77	11.79
11	10.64	10.70	10.74	10.75	10.77	10.78	10.79	10.81
10	9.68	9.73	9.76	9.78	9.79	9.80	9.81	9.83
9	8.71	8.76	8.79	8.80	8.81	8.82	8.83	8.85
8	7.74	7.78	7.81	7.82	7.83	7.84	7.85	7.87
7	6.78	6.81	6.84	6.85	6.86	6.86	6.87	6.88
6	5.81	5.84	5.86	5.87	5.88	5.88	5.89	5.90
5	4.84	4.87	4.89	4.89	4.90	4.91	4.91	4.92
4	3.87	3.89	3.91	3.92	3.92	3.92	3.93	3.94
3	2.91	2.92	2.93	2.94	2.94	2.94	2.95	2.95
2	1.94	1.95	1.96	1.96	1.96	1.96	1.97	1.97
1	0.97	0.97	0.98	0.98	0.98	0.98	0.98	0.98
0	0.00	0.00	0.00	0.00	0.00	0.00	0.00	0.00
− 1	0.97	0.97	0.98	0.98	0.98	0.98	0.98	0.99
2	1.94	1.95	1.96	1.96	1.96	1.96	1.97	1.97
3	2.91	2.92	2.94	2.94	2.94	2.95	2.95	2.96
4	3.88	3.90	3.91	3.92	3.93	3.93	3.93	3.94
5	4.85	4.88	4.89	4.90	4.91	4.91	4.92	4.93
6	5.82	5.85	5.87	5.88	5.89	5.90	5.90	5.91
7	6.79	6.83	6.85	6.86	6.87	6.88	6.89	6.90
8	7.76	7.80	7.83	7.84	7.85	7.86	7.87	7.89
9	8.74	8.78	8.81	8.83	8.84	8.85	8.86	8.87
10	9.71	9.76	9.79	9.81	9.82	9.83	9.84	9.86
11	10.68	10.74	10.78	10.79	10.81	10.82	10.83	10.85
12	11.65	11.71	11.76	11.77	11.79	11.80	11.82	11.84
13	12.63	12.69	12.74	12.76	12.77	12.79	12.80	12.82
14	13.60	13.67	13.72	13.74	13.76	13.77	13.79	13.81
15	14.57	14.65	14.70	14.72	14.74	14.76	14.78	14.80
16	15.55	15.63	15.69	15.71	15.73	15.75	15.76	15.79
17	16.52	16.61	16.67	16.69	16.72	16.73	16.75	16.78
18	17.50	17.59	17.65	17.68	17.70	17.72	17.74	17.77
19	18.47	18.57	18.64	18.66	18.69	18.71	18.73	18.76
20	19.45	19.55	19.62	19.65	19.67	19.70	19.72	19.75
21	20.42	20.53	20.60	20.63	20.66	20.69	20.71	20.74
22	21.40	21.51	21.59	21.62	21.65	21.67	21.70	21.73
23	22.37	22.49	22.57	22.61	22.64	22.66	22.69	22.73
24	23.35	23.47	23.56	23.59	23.62	23.65	23.68	23.72
25	24.33	24.45	24.54	24.58	24.61	24.64	24.67	24.71
26	25.30	25.43	25.53	25.57	25.60	25.63	25.66	25.70
27	26.28	26.42	26.52	26.56	26.59	26.62	26.65	26.69
28	27.26	27.40	27.50	27.54	27.58	27.61	27.64	27.69
29	28.24	28.38	28.49	28.53	28.57	28.60	28.63	28.68
30	29.21	29.37	29.48	29.52	29.56	29.59	29.62	29.67

Table D.X Centre thickness 0.26 mm

Back vertex powers (D)	Front vertex powers (D) *for back optic zone radii*									
	5.0 mm	5.5 mm	6.0 mm	6.5 mm	7.0 mm	7.5 mm	8.0 mm	8.5 mm	9.0 mm	10.0 mm
+ 20	19.27	19.33	19.38	19.42	19.45	19.48	19.51	19.54	19.56	19.60
19	18.31	18.36	18.41	18.45	18.48	18.51	18.54	18.56	18.58	18.62
18	17.35	17.40	17.44	17.48	17.51	17.54	17.57	17.59	17.61	17.64
17	16.39	16.44	16.48	16.51	16.54	16.57	16.59	16.61	16.63	16.66
16	15.42	15.47	15.51	15.54	15.57	15.60	15.62	15.64	15.66	15.69
15	14.46	14.51	14.54	14.58	14.60	14.63	14.65	14.67	14.68	14.71
14	13.50	13.54	13.58	13.61	13.63	13.65	13.67	13.69	13.71	13.73
13	12.54	12.58	12.61	12.64	12.66	12.68	12.70	12.71	12.73	12.75
12	11.58	11.61	11.64	11.67	11.69	11.71	11.72	11.74	11.75	11.77
11	10.61	10.65	10.67	10.70	10.72	10.73	10.75	10.76	10.77	10.79
10	9.65	9.68	9.70	9.73	9.74	9.76	9.77	9.79	9.80	9.81
9	8.69	8.71	8.74	8.75	8.77	8.79	8.80	8.81	8.82	8.83
8	7.72	7.75	7.77	7.78	7.80	7.81	7.82	7.83	7.84	7.85
7	6.76	6.78	6.80	6.81	6.82	6.84	6.84	6.85	6.86	6.87
6	5.79	5.81	5.83	5.84	5.85	5.86	5.87	5.88	5.88	5.89
5	4.83	4.84	4.86	4.87	4.88	4.88	4.89	4.90	4.90	4.91
4	3.86	3.88	3.89	3.89	3.90	3.91	3.91	3.92	3.92	3.93
3	2.90	2.91	2.92	2.92	2.93	2.93	2.94	2.94	2.94	2.95
2	1.93	1.94	1.94	1.95	1.95	1.95	1.96	1.96	1.96	1.97
1	0.97	0.97	0.97	0.97	0.98	0.98	0.98	0.98	0.98	0.98
0	0.00	0.00	0.00	0.00	0.00	0.00	0.00	0.00	0.00	0.00
− 1	0.97	0.97	0.97	0.97	0.98	0.98	0.98	0.98	0.98	0.98
2	1.93	1.94	1.95	1.95	1.95	1.96	1.96	1.96	1.96	1.97
3	2.90	2.91	2.92	2.92	2.93	2.93	2.94	2.94	2.95	2.95
4	3.87	3.88	3.89	3.90	3.91	3.91	3.92	3.92	3.93	3.94
5	4.84	4.85	4.87	4.88	4.88	4.89	4.90	4.91	4.91	4.92
6	5.81	5.82	5.84	5.85	5.86	5.87	5.88	5.89	5.89	5.91
7	6.76	6.80	6.81	6.83	6.84	6.85	6.86	6.87	6.88	6.89
8	7.74	7.77	7.79	7.80	7.82	7.83	7.84	7.85	7.86	7.88
9	8.71	8.74	8.76	8.78	8.80	8.81	8.82	8.84	8.85	8.86
10	9.68	9.71	9.74	9.76	9.78	9.79	9.81	9.82	9.83	9.85
11	10.65	10.69	10.71	10.74	10.76	10.77	10.79	10.80	10.81	10.84
12	11.62	11.66	11.69	11.71	11.74	11.76	11.77	11.79	11.80	11.82
13	12.60	12.63	12.67	12.69	12.72	12.74	12.76	12.77	12.79	12.81
14	13.57	13.61	13.64	13.67	13.70	13.72	13.74	13.76	13.77	13.80
15	14.54	14.58	14.62	14.66	14.68	14.70	14.72	14.74	14.76	14.79
16	15.51	15.56	15.60	15.63	15.66	15.69	15.71	15.73	15.74	15.77
17	16.48	16.53	16.57	16.61	16.64	16.67	16.69	16.71	16.73	16.76
18	17.45	17.51	17.55	17.59	17.62	17.65	17.68	17.70	17.72	17.75
19	18.43	18.48	18.53	18.57	18.61	18.64	18.66	18.69	18.71	18.74
20	19.40	19.46	19.51	19.55	19.59	19.62	19.65	19.67	19.69	19.73
21	20.37	20.44	20.49	20.53	20.57	20.60	20.63	20.66	20.68	20.72
22	21.35	21.41	21.47	21.51	21.55	21.59	21.62	21.65	21.67	21.71
23	22.32	22.39	22.45	22.50	22.54	22.57	22.61	22.63	22.66	22.70
24	23.30	23.37	23.43	23.48	23.52	23.56	23.59	23.62	23.65	23.69
25	24.27	24.34	24.41	24.46	24.51	24.55	24.58	24.61	24.64	24.69
26	25.25	25.32	25.39	25.44	25.49	25.53	25.57	25.60	25.63	25.68
27	26.22	26.30	26.37	26.43	26.48	26.52	26.56	26.59	26.62	26.67
28	27.20	27.28	27.35	27.41	27.46	27.51	27.54	27.58	27.61	27.66
29	28.17	28.26	28.33	28.39	28.45	28.49	28.53	28.57	28.60	28.65
30	29.15	29.24	29.31	29.38	29.43	29.48	29.52	29.56	29.59	29.65

Table D.XI Centre thickness 0.28 mm

Back vertex powers (D)	Front vertex powers (D) for back optic zone radii									
	5.0 mm	5.5 mm	6.0 mm	6.5 mm	7.0 mm	7.5 mm	8.0 mm	8.5 mm	9.0 mm	10.0 mm
+ 20	19.21	19.28	19.33	19.37	19.41	19.45	19.48	19.50	19.52	19.56
19	18.26	18.32	18.37	18.41	18.45	18.48	18.51	18.53	18.55	18.59
18	17.30	17.35	17.40	17.42	17.48	17.51	17.53	17.56	17.58	17.61
17	16.34	16.39	16.44	16.48	16.51	16.54	16.56	16.59	16.61	16.64
16	15.38	15.43	15.47	15.51	15.54	15.57	15.59	15.61	15.63	15.66
15	14.42	14.47	14.51	14.54	14.57	14.60	14.62	14.64	14.66	14.69
14	13.46	13.51	13.55	13.58	13.60	13.63	13.65	13.67	13.68	13.71
13	12.50	12.55	12.58	12.61	12.63	12.66	12.68	12.69	12.71	12.73
12	11.54	11.58	11.61	11.64	11.66	11.69	11.70	11.72	11.73	11.76
11	10.58	10.62	10.65	10.67	10.69	10.71	10.73	10.74	10.76	10.78
10	9.62	9.96	9.68	9.70	9.72	9.74	9.76	9.77	9.78	9.80
9	8.66	8.69	8.72	8.74	8.75	8.77	8.78	8.79	8.80	8.82
8	7.70	7.73	7.75	7.77	7.78	7.80	7.81	7.82	7.83	7.84
7	6.74	6.76	6.78	6.80	6.81	6.82	6.83	6.84	6.85	6.86
6	5.78	5.80	5.81	5.83	5.84	5.85	5.86	5.87	5.87	5.88
5	4.82	4.89	4.85	4.86	4.87	4.88	4.88	4.89	4.90	4.91
4	3.85	3.87	3.88	3.89	3.89	3.90	3.91	3.91	3.92	3.92
3	2.89	2.90	2.91	2.92	2.92	2.93	2.93	2.93	2.94	2.94
2	1.93	1.93	1.94	1.94	1.95	1.95	1.95	1.96	1.96	1.96
1	0.96	0.97	0.97	0.97	0.97	0.98	0.98	0.98	0.98	0.98
0	0.00	0.00	0.00	0.00	0.00	0.00	0.00	0.00	0.00	0.00
− 1	0.96	0.97	0.97	0.97	0.97	0.98	0.98	0.98	0.98	0.98
2	1.93	1.94	1.94	1.95	1.95	1.95	1.96	1.96	1.96	1.96
3	2.89	2.90	2.91	2.92	2.92	2.93	2.93	2.94	2.94	2.95
4	3.86	3.87	3.88	3.89	3.90	3.91	3.91	3.92	3.92	3.93
5	4.83	4.84	4.85	4.87	4.88	4.88	4.89	4.90	4.90	4.91
6	5.79	5.81	5.83	5.84	5.85	5.86	5.87	5.88	5.89	5.90
7	6.76	6.78	6.80	6.82	6.83	6.84	6.85	6.86	6.87	6.88
8	7.73	7.75	7.77	7.79	7.81	7.82	7.83	7.84	7.85	7.87
9	8.69	8.72	8.75	8.77	8.78	8.80	8.81	8.82	8.83	8.85
10	9.66	9.69	9.72	9.74	9.76	9.78	9.79	9.81	9.82	9.84
11	10.63	10.66	10.69	10.72	10.74	10.76	10.77	10.79	10.80	10.82
12	11.60	11.63	11.67	11.69	11.72	11.74	11.76	11.77	11.78	11.81
13	12.56	12.61	12.64	12.67	12.70	12.72	12.74	12.75	12.77	12.80
14	13.53	13.58	13.62	13.65	13.67	13.70	13.72	13.74	13.75	13.78
15	14.50	14.55	14.59	14.62	14.65	14.70	14.70	14.72	14.74	14.77
16	15.47	15.52	15.57	15.60	15.63	15.66	15.69	15.71	15.72	15.76
17	16.44	16.50	16.54	16.58	16.61	16.64	16.67	16.69	16.71	16.74
18	17.41	17.47	17.52	17.56	17.59	17.63	17.65	17.68	17.70	17.73
19	18.38	18.44	18.50	18.54	18.58	18.61	18.64	18.66	18.68	18.72
20	19.36	19.42	19.47	19.52	19.56	19.59	19.62	19.65	19.67	19.71
21	20.33	20.39	20.45	20.50	20.54	20.57	20.61	20.63	20.66	20.70
22	21.30	21.37	21.43	21.48	21.52	21.56	21.59	21.62	21.65	21.69
23	22.27	22.34	22.41	22.46	22.50	22.54	22.58	22.61	22.63	22.68
24	23.24	23.32	23.38	23.44	23.49	23.53	23.56	23.59	23.62	23.67
25	24.22	24.30	24.36	24.42	24.47	24.51	24.55	24.58	24.61	24.66
26	25.19	25.27	25.34	25.40	25.45	25.50	25.54	25.57	25.60	25.65
27	26.16	26.25	26.32	26.38	26.44	26.48	26.52	26.56	26.59	26.64
28	27.14	27.23	27.30	27.37	27.42	27.47	27.51	27.55	27.58	27.64
29	28.11	28.20	28.28	28.35	28.41	28.45	29.50	28.54	28.57	28.63
30	29.09	29.18	29.26	29.33	29.39	29.44	29.49	29.53	29.56	29.62

Table D.XII Centre thickness 0.30 mm

Back vertex powers (D)	Front vertex powers (D) for back optic zone radii									
	5.0 mm	5.5 mm	6.0 mm	6.5 mm	7.0 mm	7.5 mm	8.0 mm	8.5 mm	9.0 mm	10.0 mm
+ 20	19.16	19.23	19.28	19.33	19.37	19.41	19.44	19.47	19.49	19.53
19	18.20	18.27	18.32	18.37	18.41	18.44	18.47	18.50	18.52	18.56
18	17.25	17.31	17.36	17.40	17.44	17.47	17.50	17.53	17.55	17.59
17	16.29	16.35	16.40	16.44	16.48	16.51	16.53	16.56	16.58	16.61
16	15.34	15.39	15.44	15.48	15.51	15.54	15.56	15.59	15.61	15.64
15	14.38	14.43	14.48	14.51	14.54	14.57	14.59	14.61	14.63	14.66
14	13.43	13.47	13.51	13.55	13.58	13.60	13.62	13.64	13.66	13.69
13	12.47	12.51	12.55	12.58	12.61	12.63	12.65	12.67	12.69	12.71
12	11.51	11.55	11.59	11.62	11.64	11.66	11.68	11.70	11.71	11.74
11	10.56	10.59	10.62	10.65	10.67	10.69	10.71	10.73	10.74	10.76
10	9.60	9.63	9.66	9.68	9.71	9.72	9.74	9.75	9.77	9.79
9	8.64	8.67	8.70	8.72	8.74	8.75	8.77	8.78	8.79	8.81
8	7.68	7.71	7.73	7.75	7.77	7.78	7.79	7.81	7.82	7.83
7	6.72	6.75	6.77	6.78	6.80	6.81	6.82	6.83	6.84	6.85
6	5.76	5.78	5.80	5.82	5.83	5.84	5.85	5.86	5.86	5.88
5	4.80	4.82	4.84	4.85	4.86	4.87	4.87	4.88	4.89	4.90
4	3.84	3.86	3.87	3.88	3.89	3.89	3.90	3.91	3.91	3.92
3	2.88	2.89	2.90	2.91	2.92	2.92	2.93	2.93	2.93	2.94
2	1.92	1.93	1.94	1.94	1.94	1.95	1.95	1.95	1.96	1.96
1	0.96	0.96	0.97	0.97	0.97	0.97	0.98	0.98	0.98	0.98
0	0.00	0.00	0.00	0.00	0.00	0.00	0.00	0.00	0.00	0.00
− 1	0.96	0.97	0.97	0.97	0.97	0.97	0.98	0.98	0.98	0.98
2	1.92	1.93	1.94	1.94	1.95	1.95	1.95	1.96	1.96	1.96
3	2.89	2.90	2.91	2.91	2.92	2.92	2.93	2.93	2.94	2.94
4	3.85	3.86	3.88	3.88	3.89	3.90	3.91	3.91	3.92	3.93
5	4.81	4.83	4.84	4.86	4.87	4.88	4.88	4.89	4.90	4.91
6	5.78	5.80	5.81	5.83	5.84	5.85	5.86	5.87	5.88	5.89
7	6.74	6.76	6.79	6.80	6.82	6.83	6.84	6.85	6.86	6.87
8	7.71	7.73	7.76	7.77	7.79	7.81	7.82	7.83	7.84	7.86
9	8.67	8.70	8.73	8.75	8.77	8.78	8.80	8.81	8.82	8.84
10	9.64	9.67	9.70	9.72	9.74	9.76	9.78	9.79	9.80	9.83
11	10.60	10.64	10.67	10.70	10.72	10.74	10.76	10.77	10.79	10.81
12	11.57	11.61	11.64	11.67	11.70	11.72	11.74	11.75	11.77	11.80
13	12.53	12.58	12.62	12.65	12.67	12.70	12.72	12.74	12.75	12.78
14	13.50	13.55	13.59	13.62	13.65	13.68	13.70	13.72	13.74	13.77
15	14.47	14.52	14.56	14.60	14.63	14.66	14.68	14.70	14.72	14.75
16	15.44	15.49	15.54	15.57	15.61	15.64	15.66	15.69	15.71	15.74
17	16.40	16.46	16.51	16.55	16.59	16.62	16.65	16.67	16.69	16.73
18	17.37	17.43	17.49	17.53	17.57	17.60	17.63	17.65	17.68	17.71
19	18.34	18.41	18.46	18.51	18.55	18.58	18.61	18.64	18.66	18.70
20	19.31	19.38	19.44	19.48	19.53	19.56	19.59	19.62	19.65	19.69
21	20.28	20.35	20.41	20.46	20.51	20.54	20.58	20.61	20.63	20.68
22	21.25	21.32	21.39	21.44	21.49	21.53	21.56	21.59	21.62	21.67
23	22.22	22.30	22.36	22.42	22.47	22.51	22.55	22.58	22.61	22.66
24	23.19	23.27	23.34	23.40	23.45	23.49	23.53	23.57	23.60	23.65
25	24.16	24.25	24.32	24.38	24.43	24.48	24.52	24.55	24.58	24.64
26	25.13	25.22	25.30	25.36	25.41	25.46	25.50	25.54	25.57	25.63
27	26.10	26.20	26.27	26.34	26.40	26.45	26.49	26.53	26.56	26.62
28	27.08	27.17	27.25	27.32	27.38	27.43	27.48	27.51	27.55	27.61
29	28.05	28.15	28.23	28.30	28.36	28.42	28.46	28.50	28.54	28.60
30	29.02	29.12	29.21	29.28	29.35	29.40	29.45	29.49	29.53	29.59

Table D.XIII Centre thickness 0.32 mm

Back vertex powers (D)	Front vertex powers (D) for back optic zone radii									
	5.0 mm	5.5 mm	6.0 mm	6.5 mm	7.0 mm	7.5 mm	8.0 mm	8.5 mm	9.0 mm	10.0 mm
+ 20	19.10	19.18	19.24	19.29	19.33	19.37	19.40	19.43	19.46	19.50
19	18.15	18.22	18.28	18.33	18.37	18.40	18.44	18.46	18.49	18.53
18	17.20	17.27	17.32	17.36	17.40	17.44	17.47	17.50	17.52	17.56
17	16.25	16.31	16.36	16.40	16.44	16.47	16.50	16.53	16.55	16.59
16	15.30	15.35	15.40	15.44	15.48	15.51	15.54	15.56	15.58	15.62
15	14.34	14.40	14.44	14.48	14.51	14.54	14.57	14.59	14.61	14.64
14	13.39	13.44	13.48	13.52	13.55	13.58	13.60	13.62	13.64	13.67
13	12.44	12.48	12.52	12.55	12.58	12.61	12.63	12.65	12.67	12.70
12	11.48	11.52	11.56	11.59	11.62	11.64	11.66	11.68	11.69	11.72
11	10.53	10.57	10.60	10.63	10.65	10.67	10.69	10.71	10.72	10.75
10	9.57	9.61	9.64	9.66	9.69	9.71	9.72	9.74	9.75	9.77
9	8.62	8.65	8.68	8.70	8.72	8.74	8.75	8.76	8.78	8.80
8	7.66	7.69	7.71	7.73	7.75	7.77	7.78	7.79	7.80	7.82
7	6.71	6.73	6.75	6.77	6.78	6.80	6.81	6.82	6.83	6.85
6	5.75	5.77	5.79	5.80	5.82	5.83	5.84	5.85	5.86	5.87
5	4.79	4.81	4.82	4.84	4.85	4.86	4.87	4.87	4.88	4.89
4	3.83	3.85	3.86	3.87	3.88	3.89	3.89	3.90	3.91	3.91
3	2.88	2.89	2.90	2.90	2.91	2.92	2.92	2.93	2.93	2.94
2	1.92	1.92	1.93	1.94	1.94	1.94	1.95	1.95	1.95	1.96
1	0.96	0.96	0.97	0.97	0.97	0.97	0.97	0.98	0.98	0.98
0	0.00	0.00	0.00	0.00	0.00	0.00	0.00	0.00	0.00	0.00
− 1	0.96	0.96	0.97	0.97	0.97	0.97	0.97	0.98	0.98	0.98
2	1.92	1.93	1.93	1.94	1.94	1.95	1.95	1.95	1.96	1.96
3	2.88	2.89	2.90	2.91	2.91	2.92	2.92	2.93	2.93	2.94
4	3.84	3.85	3.87	3.88	3.89	3.89	3.90	3.91	3.91	3.92
5	4.80	4.82	4.83	4.85	4.86	4.87	4.88	4.88	4.89	4.90
6	5.76	5.78	5.80	5.82	5.83	5.84	5.85	5.86	5.87	5.88
7	6.72	6.75	6.77	6.79	6.80	6.82	6.83	6.84	6.85	6.87
8	7.69	7.72	7.74	7.76	7.78	7.79	7.81	7.82	7.83	7.85
9	8.65	8.68	8.71	8.73	8.75	8.77	8.79	8.80	8.81	8.83
10	9.61	9.65	9.68	9.70	9.73	9.75	9.76	9.78	9.79	9.81
11	10.58	10.62	10.65	10.68	10.70	10.72	10.74	10.76	10.77	10.80
12	11.54	11.58	11.62	11.65	11.68	11.70	11.72	11.74	11.75	11.78
13	12.50	12.55	12.59	12.62	12.65	12.68	12.70	12.72	12.74	12.77
14	13.47	13.52	13.56	13.60	13.63	13.66	13.68	13.70	13.72	13.75
15	14.43	14.49	14.53	14.57	14.61	14.63	14.66	14.68	14.70	14.74
16	15.40	15.46	15.51	15.55	15.58	15.61	15.64	15.66	15.69	15.72
17	16.37	16.43	16.48	16.52	16.56	16.59	16.62	16.65	16.67	16.71
18	17.33	17.40	17.45	17.50	17.54	17.57	17.60	17.63	17.65	17.70
19	18.30	18.37	18.43	18.47	18.52	18.55	18.59	18.61	18.64	18.68
20	19.27	19.34	19.40	19.45	19.49	19.53	19.57	19.60	19.62	19.67
21	20.23	20.31	20.37	20.43	20.47	20.51	20.55	20.58	20.61	20.66
22	21.20	21.28	21.35	21.40	21.45	21.50	21.53	21.57	21.60	21.65
23	22.17	22.25	22.32	22.38	22.43	22.48	22.52	22.55	22.58	22.63
24	23.14	23.22	23.30	23.36	23.41	23.46	23.50	23.54	23.57	23.62
25	24.11	24.20	24.27	24.34	24.39	24.44	24.49	24.52	24.56	24.61
26	25.08	25.17	25.25	25.32	25.38	25.43	25.47	25.51	25.54	25.60
27	26.05	26.14	26.23	26.30	26.36	26.41	26.46	26.50	26.53	26.59
28	27.02	27.12	27.20	27.28	27.34	27.39	27.44	27.48	27.52	27.58
29	27.99	28.09	28.18	28.26	28.32	28.38	28.43	28.47	28.51	28.58
30	28.96	29.07	29.16	29.24	29.30	29.36	29.41	29.46	29.50	29.57

Table D.XIV Centre thickness 0.34 mm

Back vertex powers (D)	Front vertex powers (D) for back optic zone radii									
	5.0 mm	5.5 mm	6.0 mm	6.5 mm	7.0 mm	7.5 mm	8.0 mm	8.5 mm	9.0 mm	10.0 mm
+ 20	19.05	19.13	19.19	19.24	19.29	19.33	19.37	19.40	19.43	19.47
19	18.10	18.17	18.23	18.28	18.33	18.37	18.40	18.43	18.46	18.50
18	17.15	17.22	17.28	17.33	17.37	17.41	17.44	17.47	17.49	17.53
17	16.20	16.27	16.32	16.37	16.41	16.44	16.47	16.50	16.52	16.56
16	15.25	15.31	15.37	15.41	15.45	15.48	15.51	15.53	15.55	15.59
15	14.30	14.36	14.41	14.45	14.48	14.51	14.54	14.56	14.59	14.62
14	13.35	13.41	13.45	13.49	13.52	13.55	13.57	13.60	13.62	13.65
13	12.40	12.45	12.49	12.53	12.56	12.58	12.61	12.63	12.65	12.68
12	11.45	11.50	11.53	11.57	11.59	11.62	11.64	11.66	11.68	11.70
11	10.50	10.54	10.58	10.60	10.63	10.65	10.67	10.69	10.71	10.73
10	9.55	9.58	9.62	9.64	9.67	9.69	9.70	9.72	9.73	9.76
9	8.59	8.63	8.66	8.68	8.70	8.72	8.74	8.75	8.76	8.78
8	7.64	7.67	7.70	7.72	7.74	7.75	7.77	7.78	7.79	7.81
7	6.69	6.71	6.74	6.75	6.77	6.79	6.80	6.81	6.82	6.84
6	5.73	5.76	5.78	5.79	5.81	5.82	5.83	5.84	5.85	5.86
5	4.78	4.80	4.81	4.83	4.84	4.85	4.86	4.87	4.87	4.89
4	3.82	3.84	3.85	3.86	3.87	3.88	3.89	3.89	3.90	3.91
3	2.87	2.88	2.89	2.90	2.90	2.91	2.92	2.92	2.93	2.93
2	1.91	1.92	1.93	1.93	1.94	1.94	1.94	1.95	1.95	1.96
1	0.96	0.96	0.96	0.97	0.97	0.97	0.97	0.97	0.98	0.98
0	0.00	0.00	0.00	0.00	0.00	0.00	0.00	0.00	0.00	0.00
− 1	0.96	0.96	0.96	0.97	0.97	0.97	0.97	0.97	0.98	0.98
2	1.91	1.92	1.93	1.93	1.94	1.94	1.95	1.95	1.95	1.96
3	2.87	2.88	2.89	2.90	2.91	2.91	2.92	2.93	2.93	2.94
4	3.83	3.85	3.86	3.87	3.88	3.89	3.89	3.90	3.91	3.92
5	4.79	4.81	4.82	4.84	4.85	4.86	4.87	4.88	4.88	4.90
6	5.75	5.77	5.79	5.81	5.82	5.83	5.84	5.85	5.86	5.88
7	6.71	6.73	6.76	6.78	6.79	6.81	6.82	6.83	6.84	6.86
8	7.67	7.70	7.72	7.75	7.76	7.78	7.80	7.81	7.82	7.84
9	8.63	8.66	8.69	8.72	8.74	8.76	8.77	8.79	8.80	8.82
10	9.59	9.63	9.66	9.69	9.71	9.73	9.75	9.76	9.78	9.80
11	10.55	10.59	10.63	10.66	10.68	10.71	10.73	10.74	10.76	10.79
12	11.51	11.56	11.60	11.63	11.66	11.68	11.70	11.72	11.74	11.77
13	12.47	12.52	12.57	12.60	12.63	12.66	12.68	12.70	12.72	12.75
14	13.44	13.49	13.54	13.57	13.61	13.64	13.66	13.68	13.70	13.74
15	14.40	14.46	14.51	14.55	14.58	14.61	14.64	14.66	14.68	14.72
16	15.36	15.42	15.48	15.52	15.56	15.59	15.62	15.64	15.67	15.71
17	16.33	16.39	16.45	16.49	16.53	16.57	16.60	16.63	16.65	16.69
18	17.29	17.36	17.42	17.47	17.51	17.55	17.58	17.61	17.63	17.68
19	18.26	18.33	18.39	18.44	18.49	18.53	18.56	18.59	18.62	18.66
20	19.22	19.30	19.36	19.42	19.46	19.50	19.54	19.57	19.60	19.65
21	20.19	20.27	20.33	20.39	20.44	20.48	20.52	20.56	20.59	20.64
22	21.15	21.24	21.31	21.37	21.42	21.47	21.50	21.54	21.57	21.62
23	22.12	22.21	22.28	22.34	22.40	22.45	22.49	22.52	22.56	22.61
24	23.09	23.18	23.26	23.32	23.38	23.43	23.47	23.51	23.54	23.60
25	24.05	24.15	24.23	24.30	24.36	24.41	24.45	24.49	24.53	24.59
26	25.02	25.12	25.20	25.28	25.34	25.39	25.44	25.48	25.52	25.58
27	25.99	26.09	26.18	26.25	26.32	26.37	26.42	26.46	26.50	26.57
28	26.96	27.06	27.16	27.23	27.30	27.36	27.41	27.45	27.49	27.56
29	27.93	28.04	28.13	28.21	28.28	28.34	28.39	28.44	28.48	28.55
30	28.90	29.01	29.11	29.19	29.26	29.32	29.38	29.43	29.47	29.54

Table D.XV Centre thickness 0.36 mm

Back vertex powers (D)	Front vertex powers (D) for back optic zone radii									
	5.0 mm	5.5 mm	6.0 mm	6.5 mm	7.0 mm	7.5 mm	8.0 mm	8.5 mm	9.0 mm	10.0 mm
+ 20	19.00	19.08	19.14	19.20	19.25	19.29	19.33	19.36	19.39	19.44
19	18.05	18.13	18.19	18.24	18.29	18.33	18.37	18.40	18.43	18.47
18	17.10	17.18	17.24	17.29	17.33	17.37	17.40	17.43	17.46	17.51
17	16.16	16.23	16.28	16.33	16.37	16.41	16.44	16.47	16.50	16.54
16	15.21	15.27	15.33	15.37	15.41	15.45	15.48	15.50	15.53	15.57
15	14.26	14.32	14.37	14.42	14.45	14.49	14.51	14.54	14.56	14.60
14	13.32	13.37	13.42	13.46	13.49	13.52	13.55	13.57	13.59	13.63
13	12.37	12.42	12.46	12.50	12.53	12.56	12.59	12.61	12.63	12.66
12	11.42	11.47	11.51	11.54	11.57	11.60	11.62	11.64	11.66	11.69
11	10.47	10.51	10.55	10.58	10.61	10.63	10.65	10.67	10.69	10.72
10	9.52	9.56	9.59	9.62	9.65	9.67	9.69	9.70	9.72	9.74
9	8.57	8.61	8.64	8.66	8.69	8.70	8.72	8.74	8.75	8.77
8	7.62	7.65	7.68	7.70	7.72	7.74	7.75	7.77	7.78	7.80
7	6.67	6.70	6.72	6.74	6.76	6.77	6.79	6.80	6.81	6.83
6	5.72	5.74	5.76	5.78	5.79	5.81	5.82	5.83	5.84	5.85
5	4.77	4.79	4.80	4.82	4.83	4.84	4.85	4.86	4.87	4.88
4	3.81	3.83	3.84	3.85	3.86	3.87	3.88	3.89	3.89	3.90
3	2.86	2.87	2.88	2.89	2.90	2.91	2.91	2.92	2.92	2.93
2	1.91	1.92	1.92	1.93	1.93	1.94	1.94	1.95	1.95	1.95
1	0.95	0.96	0.96	0.96	0.97	0.97	0.97	0.97	0.97	0.98
0	0.00	0.00	0.00	0.00	0.00	0.00	0.00	0.00	0.00	0.00
− 1	0.95	0.96	0.96	0.96	0.97	0.97	0.97	0.97	0.97	0.98
2	1.91	1.92	1.92	1.93	1.94	1.94	1.94	1.95	1.95	1.95
3	2.87	2.88	2.89	2.90	2.90	2.91	2.92	2.92	2.93	2.93
4	3.82	3.84	3.85	3.86	3.87	3.88	3.89	3.90	3.90	3.91
5	4.78	4.80	4.81	4.83	4.84	4.85	4.86	4.87	4.88	4.89
6	5.73	5.76	5.78	5.80	5.81	5.82	5.84	5.85	5.85	5.87
7	6.69	6.72	6.74	6.76	6.78	6.80	6.81	6.82	6.83	6.85
8	7.65	7.68	7.71	7.73	7.75	7.77	7.78	7.80	7.81	7.83
9	8.61	8.64	8.67	8.70	8.72	8.74	8.76	8.77	8.79	8.81
10	9.57	9.61	9.64	9.67	9.69	9.72	9.73	9.75	9.77	9.79
11	10.52	10.57	10.61	10.64	10.67	10.69	10.71	10.73	10.74	10.77
12	11.48	11.53	11.57	11.61	11.64	11.66	11.69	11.71	11.72	11.76
13	12.44	12.50	12.54	12.58	12.61	12.64	12.66	12.69	12.70	12.74
14	13.40	13.46	13.51	13.55	13.58	13.61	13.64	13.66	13.69	13.72
15	14.37	14.43	14.48	14.52	14.56	14.59	14.62	14.64	14.67	14.70
16	15.33	15.39	15.45	15.49	15.53	15.57	15.60	15.62	15.65	15.69
17	16.29	16.36	16.42	16.46	16.51	16.54	16.58	16.60	16.63	16.67
18	17.25	17.32	17.38	17.44	17.48	17.52	17.55	17.58	17.61	17.66
19	18.21	18.29	18.35	18.41	18.46	18.50	18.53	18.57	18.59	18.64
20	19.18	19.26	19.33	19.38	19.43	19.48	19.51	19.55	19.58	19.63
21	20.14	20.22	20.30	20.36	20.41	20.46	20.49	20.53	20.56	20.62
22	21.10	21.19	21.27	21.33	21.39	21.43	21.48	21.51	21.55	21.60
23	22.07	22.16	22.24	22.31	22.36	22.41	22.46	22.50	22.53	22.59
24	23.03	23.13	23.21	23.28	23.34	23.39	23.44	23.48	23.52	23.58
25	24.00	24.10	24.19	24.26	24.32	24.37	24.42	24.46	24.50	24.57
26	24.96	25.07	25.16	25.23	25.30	25.36	25.40	25.45	25.49	25.55
27	25.93	26.04	26.13	26.21	26.28	26.34	26.39	26.43	26.47	26.54
28	26.90	27.01	27.11	27.19	27.26	27.32	27.37	27.42	27.46	27.53
29	27.87	27.98	28.08	28.17	28.24	28.30	28.36	28.41	28.45	28.52
30	28.83	28.95	29.06	29.14	29.22	29.28	29.34	29.39	29.44	29.51

Table D.XVI Centre thickness 0.38 mm

Back vertex powers (D)	Front vertex powers (D) for back optic zone radii									
	5.0 mm	5.5 mm	6.0 mm	6.5 mm	7.0 mm	7.5 mm	8.0 mm	8.5 mm	9.0 mm	10.0 mm
+ 20	18.94	19.03	19.10	19.16	19.21	19.25	19.29	19.33	19.36	19.41
19	18.00	18.08	18.15	18.20	18.25	18.30	18.33	18.37	18.40	18.45
18	17.06	17.13	17.20	17.25	17.30	17.34	17.37	17.40	17.43	17.48
17	16.11	16.18	16.24	16.30	16.34	16.38	16.41	16.44	16.47	16.51
16	15.17	15.24	15.29	15.34	15.38	15.42	15.45	15.48	15.50	15.55
15	14.22	14.29	14.34	14.39	14.42	14.46	14.49	14.51	14.54	14.58
14	13.28	13.34	13.39	13.43	13.47	13.50	13.53	13.55	13.57	13.61
13	12.33	12.39	12.44	12.47	12.51	12.54	12.56	12.59	12.61	12.64
12	11.39	11.44	11.48	11.52	11.55	11.58	11.60	11.62	11.64	11.67
11	10.44	10.49	10.53	10.56	10.59	10.61	10.64	10.65	10.67	10.70
10	9.50	9.54	9.57	9.60	9.63	9.65	9.67	9.69	9.70	9.73
9	8.55	8.59	8.62	8.64	8.67	8.69	8.71	8.72	8.74	8.76
8	7.60	7.63	7.66	7.69	7.71	7.72	7.74	7.75	7.77	7.79
7	6.65	6.68	6.71	6.73	6.75	6.76	6.77	6.79	6.80	6.82
6	5.70	5.73	5.75	5.77	5.78	5.80	5.81	5.82	5.83	5.84
5	4.75	4.77	4.79	4.81	4.82	4.83	4.84	4.85	4.86	4.87
4	3.80	3.82	3.84	3.85	3.86	3.87	3.87	3.88	3.89	3.90
3	2.85	2.87	2.88	2.89	2.89	2.90	2.91	2.91	2.92	2.92
2	1.90	1.91	1.92	1.92	1.93	1.93	1.94	1.94	1.95	1.95
1	0.95	0.96	0.96	0.96	0.97	0.97	0.97	0.97	0.97	0.98
0	0.00	0.00	0.00	0.00	0.00	0.00	0.00	0.00	0.00	0.00
− 1	0.95	0.96	0.96	0.96	0.97	0.97	0.97	0.97	0.97	0.98
2	1.91	1.91	1.92	1.93	1.93	1.94	1.94	1.94	1.95	1.95
3	2.86	2.87	2.88	2.89	2.90	2.91	2.91	2.92	2.92	2.93
4	3.81	3.83	3.84	3.85	3.87	3.87	3.88	3.89	3.90	3.91
5	4.77	4.79	4.80	4.82	4.83	4.84	4.85	4.86	4.87	4.88
6	5.72	5.75	5.77	5.78	5.80	5.81	5.83	5.84	5.85	5.86
7	6.67	6.70	6.73	6.75	6.77	6.78	6.80	6.81	6.82	6.84
8	7.63	7.66	7.69	7.72	7.74	7.76	7.77	7.79	7.80	7.82
9	8.59	8.62	8.66	8.68	8.71	8.73	8.75	8.76	8.78	8.80
10	9.54	9.58	9.62	9.65	9.68	9.70	9.72	9.74	9.75	9.78
11	10.50	10.55	10.59	10.62	10.65	10.67	10.69	10.71	10.73	10.76
12	11.46	11.51	11.55	11.59	11.62	11.65	11.67	11.69	11.71	11.74
13	12.41	12.47	12.52	12.56	12.59	12.62	12.64	12.67	12.69	12.72
14	13.37	13.43	13.48	13.52	13.56	13.59	13.62	13.65	13.67	13.71
15	14.33	14.39	14.45	14.49	14.53	14.57	14.60	14.62	14.65	14.69
16	15.29	15.36	15.42	15.46	15.51	15.54	15.57	15.60	15.63	15.67
17	16.25	16.32	16.38	16.43	16.48	16.52	16.55	16.58	16.61	16.65
18	17.21	17.29	17.35	17.41	17.45	17.49	17.53	17.56	17.59	17.64
19	18.17	18.25	18.32	18.38	18.43	18.47	18.51	18.54	18.57	18.62
20	19.13	19.22	19.29	19.35	19.40	19.45	19.49	19.52	19.55	19.61
21	20.09	20.18	20.26	20.32	20.38	20.43	20.47	20.50	20.54	20.59
22	21.06	21.15	21.23	21.30	21.35	21.40	21.45	21.49	21.52	21.58
23	22.02	22.12	22.20	22.27	22.33	22.38	22.43	22.47	22.51	22.57
24	22.98	23.08	23.17	23.25	23.31	23.36	23.41	23.45	23.49	23.55
25	23.95	24.05	24.14	24.22	24.28	24.34	24.39	24.43	24.47	24.54
26	24.91	25.02	25.11	25.19	25.26	25.32	25.37	25.42	25.46	25.53
27	25.87	25.94	26.09	26.17	26.24	26.30	26.36	26.40	26.45	26.52
28	26.84	26.96	27.06	27.14	27.22	27.28	27.34	27.39	27.43	27.51
29	27.80	27.93	28.03	28.12	28.20	28.26	28.32	28.37	28.42	28.50
30	28.77	28.90	29.01	29.10	29.18	29.25	29.31	29.36	29.41	29.49

Table D.XVII Centre thickness 0.40 mm

Back vertex powers (D)	Front vertex powers (D) for back optic zone radii									
	5.0 mm	5.5 mm	6.0 mm	6.5 mm	7.0 mm	7.5 mm	8.0 mm	8.5 mm	9.0 mm	10.0 mm
+ 20	18.89	18.98	19.05	19.11	19.17	19.22	19.26	19.29	19.33	19.38
19	17.95	18.03	18.10	18.16	18.21	18.26	18.30	18.33	18.36	18.42
18	17.01	17.09	17.16	17.21	17.26	17.30	17.34	17.37	17.40	17.45
17	16.07	16.14	16.21	16.26	16.31	16.35	16.38	16.41	16.44	16.49
16	15.13	15.20	15.26	15.31	15.35	15.39	15.42	15.45	15.48	15.52
15	14.19	14.25	14.31	14.35	14.40	14.43	14.46	14.49	14.51	14.56
14	13.24	13.30	13.36	13.40	13.44	13.47	13.50	13.53	13.55	13.59
13	12.30	12.36	12.41	12.45	12.48	12.51	12.54	12.56	12.59	12.62
12	11.36	11.41	11.46	11.49	11.53	11.55	11.58	11.60	11.62	11.65
11	10.41	10.46	10.50	10.54	10.57	10.59	10.62	10.64	10.65	10.69
10	9.47	9.51	9.55	9.58	9.61	9.63	9.65	9.67	9.69	9.72
9	8.52	8.56	8.60	8.63	8.65	8.67	8.69	8.71	8.72	8.75
8	7.58	7.61	7.64	7.67	7.69	7.71	7.73	7.74	7.76	7.78
7	6.63	6.64	6.69	6.71	6.73	6.75	6.76	6.78	6.79	6.81
6	5.69	5.71	5.74	5.76	5.77	5.79	5.80	5.81	5.82	5.84
5	4.74	4.76	4.78	4.80	4.81	4.82	4.83	4.84	4.85	4.87
4	3.79	3.81	3.83	3.84	3.85	3.86	3.87	3.88	3.88	3.89
3	2.85	2.86	2.87	2.88	2.89	2.90	2.90	2.91	2.91	2.92
2	1.90	1.91	1.91	1.92	1.93	1.93	1.94	1.94	1.94	1.95
1	0.95	0.95	0.96	0.96	0.96	0.97	0.97	0.97	0.97	0.97
0	0.00	0.00	0.00	0.00	0.00	0.00	0.00	0.00	0.00	0.00
− 1	0.95	0.95	0.96	0.96	0.96	0.97	0.97	0.97	0.97	0.97
2	1.90	1.91	1.92	1.92	1.93	1.93	1.94	1.94	1.94	1.95
3	2.85	2.86	2.88	2.88	2.89	2.90	2.91	2.91	2.92	2.93
4	3.80	3.82	3.83	3.85	3.86	3.87	3.88	3.88	3.89	3.90
5	4.75	4.78	4.79	4.81	4.82	4.84	4.85	4.86	4.86	4.88
6	5.71	5.73	5.75	5.77	5.79	5.80	5.82	5.83	5.84	5.86
7	6.66	6.69	6.72	6.74	6.76	6.77	6.79	6.80	6.81	6.83
8	7.61	7.65	7.68	7.70	7.72	7.74	7.76	7.77	7.79	7.81
9	8.57	8.60	8.64	8.67	8.69	8.71	8.73	8.75	8.76	8.79
10	9.52	9.56	9.60	9.63	9.66	9.68	9.71	9.72	9.74	9.77
11	10.47	10.52	10.56	10.60	10.63	10.66	10.68	10.70	10.72	10.75
12	11.43	11.48	11.53	11.57	11.60	11.63	11.65	11.67	11.69	11.73
13	12.38	12.44	12.49	12.53	12.57	12.60	12.63	12.65	12.67	12.71
14	13.34	13.40	13.46	13.50	13.54	13.57	13.60	13.63	13.65	13.69
15	14.30	14.36	14.42	14.47	14.51	14.55	14.58	14.60	14.63	14.67
16	15.25	15.33	15.39	15.44	15.48	15.52	15.55	15.58	15.61	15.65
17	16.21	16.29	16.35	16.41	16.45	16.49	16.53	16.56	16.59	16.64
18	17.17	17.25	17.32	17.38	17.43	17.47	17.51	17.54	17.57	17.62
19	18.13	18.21	18.29	18.35	18.40	18.44	18.48	18.52	18.55	18.60
20	19.09	19.18	19.25	19.32	19.37	19.42	19.46	19.50	19.53	19.59
21	20.05	20.14	20.22	20.29	20.35	20.40	20.44	20.48	20.51	20.57
22	21.01	21.11	21.19	21.26	21.32	21.37	21.42	21.46	21.49	21.56
23	21.97	22.07	22.16	22.23	22.29	22.35	22.40	22.44	22.48	22.54
24	22.93	23.04	23.13	23.20	23.27	23.33	23.38	23.42	23.46	23.53
25	23.89	24.00	24.10	24.18	24.25	24.31	24.36	24.41	24.45	24.52
26	24.85	24.97	25.07	25.15	25.22	25.29	25.34	25.39	25.43	25.51
27	25.82	25.94	26.04	26.13	26.20	26.26	26.32	26.37	26.42	26.49
28	26.78	26.90	27.01	27.10	27.18	27.24	27.30	27.36	27.40	27.48
29	27.74	27.87	27.98	28.08	28.16	28.23	28.29	28.34	28.39	28.47
30	28.71	28.84	28.96	29.05	29.13	29.21	29.27	29.33	29.38	29.46

Table D.XVIII Centre thickness 0.50 mm

Back vertex powers (D)	Front vertex powers (D) for back optic zone radii										
	5.0 mm	5.5 mm	6.0 mm	6.5 mm	7.0 mm	7.5 mm	8.0 mm	8.5 mm	9.0 mm	9.5 mm	10.0 mm
+ 20	18.63	18.73	18.82	18.90	18.97	19.03	19.08	19.12	19.16	19.20	19.23
19	17.70	17.80	17.89	17.96	18.03	18.08	18.13	18.17	18.21	18.24	18.28
18	16.77	16.87	16.95	17.02	17.08	17.14	17.18	17.22	17.26	17.29	17.32
17	15.85	15.94	16.02	16.08	16.14	16.19	16.23	16.27	16.30	16.34	16.36
16	14.92	15.01	15.08	15.14	15.19	15.24	15.28	15.32	15.35	15.38	15.41
15	13.99	14.07	14.14	14.20	14.25	14.29	14.33	14.37	14.40	14.43	14.45
14	13.06	13.14	13.20	13.26	13.30	13.34	13.38	13.41	13.44	13.47	13.49
13	12.13	12.20	12.26	12.31	12.36	12.40	12.43	12.46	12.48	12.51	12.53
12	11.20	11.27	11.32	11.37	11.41	11.45	11.48	11.50	11.53	11.55	11.57
11	10.27	10.33	10.38	10.43	10.46	10.50	10.52	10.55	10.57	10.59	10.61
10	9.34	9.40	9.44	9.48	9.52	9.54	9.57	9.59	9.61	9.63	9.65
9	8.41	8.46	8.50	8.54	8.57	8.59	8.62	8.64	8.65	8.67	8.69
8	7.48	7.52	7.56	7.59	7.62	7.64	7.66	7.68	7.70	7.71	7.72
7	6.55	6.58	6.62	6.64	6.67	6.69	6.71	6.72	6.74	6.75	6.76
6	5.61	5.65	5.67	5.70	5.72	5.73	5.75	5.76	5.78	5.79	5.80
5	4.68	4.71	4.73	4.75	4.77	4.78	4.79	4.80	4.81	4.82	4.83
4	3.74	3.77	3.79	3.80	3.81	3.83	3.84	3.85	3.85	3.86	3.87
3	2.81	2.83	2.84	2.85	2.86	2.87	2.88	2.88	2.89	2.90	2.90
2	1.87	1.88	1.89	1.90	1.91	1.91	1.92	1.92	1.93	1.93	1.94
1	0.94	0.94	0.95	0.95	0.95	0.96	0.96	0.96	0.96	0.97	0.97
0	0.00	0.00	0.00	0.00	0.00	0.00	0.00	0.00	0.00	0.00	0.00
− 1	0.94	0.94	0.95	0.95	0.96	0.96	0.96	0.96	0.97	0.97	0.97
2	1.88	1.89	1.90	1.90	1.91	1.92	1.92	1.93	1.93	1.93	1.94
3	2.82	2.83	2.85	2.86	2.87	2.88	2.88	2.89	2.90	2.90	2.91
4	3.75	3.78	3.79	3.81	3.82	3.84	3.85	3.86	3.86	3.87	3.88
5	4.69	4.72	4.75	4.76	4.78	4.80	4.81	4.82	4.83	4.84	4.85
6	5.64	5.67	5.70	5.72	5.74	5.76	5.77	5.79	5.80	5.81	5.82
7	6.58	6.61	6.65	6.67	6.70	6.72	6.74	6.75	6.77	6.78	6.79
8	7.52	7.56	7.60	7.63	7.66	7.68	7.70	7.72	7.74	7.75	7.76
9	8.46	8.51	8.55	8.59	8.62	8.64	8.67	8.69	8.71	8.72	8.74
10	9.40	9.46	9.51	9.54	9.58	9.61	9.63	9.66	9.68	9.69	9.71
11	10.35	10.41	10.46	10.50	10.54	10.57	10.60	10.63	10.65	10.67	10.69
12	11.29	11.36	11.41	11.46	11.50	11.54	11.57	11.60	11.62	11.64	11.66
13	12.24	12.31	12.37	12.42	12.46	12.50	12.54	12.57	12.59	12.62	12.64
14	13.18	13.26	13.32	13.38	13.43	13.47	13.50	13.54	13.57	13.59	13.62
15	14.13	14.21	14.28	14.34	14.39	14.43	14.47	14.51	14.54	14.57	14.59
16	15.08	15.16	15.24	15.30	15.36	15.40	15.44	15.48	15.51	15.54	15.57
17	16.02	16.12	16.20	16.26	16.32	16.37	16.41	16.45	16.49	16.52	16.55
18	16.97	17.07	17.15	17.22	17.29	17.34	17.39	17.43	17.46	17.50	17.53
19	17.92	18.02	18.11	18.19	18.25	18.31	18.36	18.40	18.44	18.47	18.51
20	18.87	18.98	19.07	19.15	19.22	19.28	19.33	19.38	19.42	19.45	19.49
21	19.82	19.93	20.03	20.12	20.19	20.25	20.30	20.35	20.39	20.43	20.47
22	20.77	20.89	20.99	21.08	21.15	21.22	21.28	21.33	21.37	21.41	21.45
23	21.72	21.85	21.95	22.05	22.12	22.19	22.25	22.30	22.35	22.39	22.43
24	22.67	22.81	22.92	23.01	23.09	23.16	23.23	23.28	23.33	23.38	23.42
25	23.63	23.76	23.88	23.98	24.06	24.14	24.20	24.26	24.31	24.36	24.40
26	24.58	24.72	24.84	24.95	25.03	25.11	25.18	25.24	25.29	25.34	25.38
27	25.53	25.68	25.81	25.91	26.01	26.09	26.16	26.22	26.27	26.32	26.37
28	26.49	26.64	26.77	26.88	26.98	27.06	27.13	27.20	27.26	27.31	27.35
29	27.44	27.60	27.74	27.85	27.95	28.04	28.11	28.18	28.24	28.29	28.34
30	28.40	28.56	28.70	28.82	28.92	29.01	29.09	29.16	29.22	29.28	29.33

Table D.XIX Centre thickness 0.60 mm

Back vertex powers (D)	Front vertex powers (D) for back optic zone radii										
	5.0 mm	5.5 mm	6.0 mm	6.5 mm	7.0 mm	7.5 mm	8.0 mm	8.5 mm	9.0 mm	9.5 mm	10.0 mm
+ 20	18.27	18.49	18.60	18.69	18.77	18.84	18.90	18.95	19.00	19.04	19.08
19	17.46	17.57	17.68	17.77	17.84	17.91	17.96	18.01	18.06	18.10	18.14
18	16.54	16.66	16.75	16.84	16.91	16.97	17.02	17.07	17.12	17.15	17.19
17	15.63	15.74	15.83	15.91	15.97	16.03	16.08	16.13	16.17	16.21	16.24
16	14.72	14.82	14.90	14.98	15.04	15.10	15.14	15.19	15.23	15.26	15.29
15	13.80	13.90	13.98	14.05	14.11	14.16	14.20	14.24	14.28	14.31	14.34
14	12.89	12.98	13.05	13.12	13.17	13.22	13.26	13.30	13.33	13.36	13.39
13	11.97	12.05	12.12	12.18	12.24	12.28	12.32	12.35	12.39	12.41	12.44
12	11.06	11.13	11.20	11.25	11.30	11.34	11.38	11.41	11.44	11.46	11.49
11	10.14	10.21	10.27	10.32	10.36	10.40	10.43	10.46	10.49	10.51	10.53
10	9.22	9.28	9.34	9.38	9.42	9.46	9.49	9.51	9.54	9.56	9.58
9	8.30	8.36	8.41	8.45	8.48	8.51	8.54	8.57	8.59	8.61	8.62
8	7.38	7.43	7.48	7.51	7.54	7.57	7.60	7.62	7.64	7.65	7.67
7	6.46	6.51	6.54	6.58	6.60	6.63	6.65	6.67	6.68	6.70	6.71
6	5.54	5.58	5.61	5.64	5.66	5.68	5.70	5.72	5.73	5.74	5.76
5	4.62	4.65	4.68	4.70	4.72	4.74	4.75	4.77	4.78	4.79	4.80
4	3.70	3.72	3.75	3.76	3.78	3.79	3.80	3.82	3.82	3.83	3.84
3	2.77	2.79	2.81	2.82	2.83	2.85	2.85	2.86	2.87	2.88	2.88
2	1.85	1.86	1.87	1.88	1.89	1.90	1.90	1.91	1.91	1.92	1.92
1	0.93	0.93	0.94	0.94	0.95	0.95	0.95	0.96	0.96	0.96	0.96
0	0.00	0.00	0.00	0.00	0.00	0.00	0.00	0.00	0.00	0.00	0.00
− 1	0.93	0.93	0.94	0.94	0.95	0.95	0.95	0.96	0.96	0.96	0.96
2	1.85	1.87	1.88	1.89	1.89	1.90	1.91	1.91	1.92	1.92	1.93
3	2.78	2.80	2.82	2.83	2.84	2.85	2.86	2.87	2.88	2.88	2.89
4	3.71	3.73	3.76	3.77	3.79	3.80	3.82	3.83	3.84	3.85	3.85
5	4.64	4.67	4.70	4.72	4.74	4.76	4.77	4.79	4.80	4.81	4.82
6	5.57	5.60	5.64	5.67	5.69	5.71	5.73	5.74	5.76	5.77	5.78
7	6.50	6.54	6.58	6.61	6.64	6.66	6.69	6.70	6.72	6.74	6.75
8	7.43	7.48	7.52	7.56	7.59	7.62	7.64	7.67	7.69	7.70	7.72
9	8.36	8.42	8.47	8.51	8.54	8.58	8.60	8.63	8.65	8.67	8.69
10	9.29	9.36	9.41	9.46	9.50	9.53	9.56	9.59	9.61	9.64	9.66
11	10.22	10.30	10.36	10.41	10.45	10.49	10.52	10.55	10.58	10.60	10.63
12	11.16	11.24	11.30	11.36	11.41	11.45	11.48	11.52	11.55	11.57	11.60
13	12.09	12.18	12.25	12.31	12.36	12.41	12.45	12.48	12.51	12.54	12.57
14	13.03	13.12	13.20	13.26	13.32	13.37	13.41	13.45	13.48	13.51	13.54
15	13.96	14.06	14.14	14.21	14.27	14.33	14.37	14.41	14.45	14.48	14.51
16	14.90	15.00	15.09	15.17	15.23	15.29	15.34	15.38	15.42	15.45	15.49
17	15.84	15.95	16.04	16.12	16.19	16.25	16.30	16.35	16.39	16.43	16.46
18	16.78	16.89	16.99	17.07	17.15	17.21	17.27	17.32	17.36	17.40	17.43
19	17.72	17.84	17.94	18.03	18.11	18.17	18.23	18.28	18.33	18.37	18.41
20	18.66	18.78	18.89	18.99	19.07	19.14	19.20	19.25	19.30	19.35	19.39
21	19.60	19.73	19.85	19.94	20.03	20.10	20.17	20.23	20.28	20.32	20.36
22	20.54	20.68	20.80	20.90	20.99	21.07	21.14	21.20	21.25	21.30	21.34
23	21.48	21.63	21.75	21.86	21.95	22.04	22.11	22.17	22.23	22.28	22.32
24	22.42	22.58	22.71	22.82	22.92	23.00	23.08	23.14	23.20	23.25	23.30
25	23.36	23.53	23.66	23.78	23.88	23.97	24.05	24.12	24.18	24.23	24.28
26	24.31	24.48	24.62	24.74	24.85	24.94	25.02	25.09	25.15	25.21	25.26
27	25.25	25.43	25.58	25.70	25.81	25.91	25.99	26.07	26.13	26.19	26.25
28	26.20	26.38	26.54	26.67	26.78	26.88	26.97	27.04	27.11	27.17	27.23
29	27.15	27.33	27.49	27.63	27.75	27.85	27.94	28.02	28.09	28.15	28.21
30	28.09	28.29	28.45	28.59	28.72	28.82	28.91	28.90	29.07	29.14	29.20

Table D.XX Centre thickness 0.70 mm

Back vertex powers (D)	Front vertex powers (D) for back optic zone radii										
	5.0 mm	5.5 mm	6.0 mm	6.5 mm	7.0 mm	7.5 mm	8.0 mm	8.5 mm	9.0 mm	9.5 mm	10.0 mm
+ 20	18.12	18.26	18.38	18.49	18.58	18.66	18.73	18.79	18.84	18.89	18.94
19	17.22	17.36	17.47	17.57	17.66	17.73	17.80	17.86	17.91	17.96	18.00
18	16.32	16.45	16.56	16.65	16.74	16.81	16.87	16.92	16.97	17.02	17.06
17	15.42	15.54	15.65	15.74	15.81	15.88	15.94	15.99	16.04	16.08	16.12
16	14.52	14.63	14.73	14.82	14.89	14.95	15.01	15.06	15.10	15.14	15.18
15	13.62	13.73	13.82	13.90	13.97	14.02	14.08	14.12	14.16	14.20	14.23
14	12.72	12.82	12.90	12.98	13.04	13.10	13.14	13.19	13.23	13.26	13.29
13	11.81	11.91	11.99	12.05	12.11	12.17	12.21	12.25	12.29	12.33	12.35
12	10.91	11.00	11.07	11.13	11.19	11.23	11.28	11.31	11.35	11.38	11.40
11	10.00	10.08	10.15	10.21	10.26	10.30	10.34	10.38	10.41	10.43	10.46
10	9.10	9.17	9.23	9.29	9.33	9.37	9.41	9.44	9.46	9.49	9.51
9	8.19	8.25	8.31	8.36	8.40	8.44	8.47	8.50	8.52	8.54	8.56
8	7.29	7.34	7.39	7.44	7.47	7.50	7.53	7.56	7.58	7.60	7.62
7	6.38	6.43	6.47	6.51	6.54	6.57	6.59	6.62	6.63	6.65	6.67
6	5.47	5.51	5.55	5.58	5.61	5.63	5.65	5.67	5.69	5.70	5.72
5	4.56	4.60	4.63	4.65	4.68	4.70	4.71	4.73	4.74	4.76	4.77
4	3.65	3.68	3.70	3.72	3.74	3.76	3.77	3.79	3.80	3.81	3.82
3	2.74	2.76	2.78	2.79	2.81	2.82	2.83	2.84	2.85	2.86	2.86
2	1.83	1.84	1.85	1.86	1.87	1.88	1.89	1.89	1.90	1.91	1.91
1	0.91	0.92	0.93	0.93	0.94	0.94	0.94	0.95	0.95	0.95	0.96
0	0.00	0.00	0.00	0.00	0.00	0.00	0.00	0.00	0.00	0.00	0.00
− 1	0.91	0.92	0.93	0.93	0.94	0.94	0.95	0.95	0.95	0.95	0.96
2	1.83	1.84	1.86	1.87	1.88	1.88	1.89	1.90	1.90	1.91	1.91
3	2.75	2.77	2.79	2.80	2.82	2.83	2.84	2.85	2.86	2.86	2.87
4	3.66	3.69	3.72	3.74	3.76	3.77	3.79	3.80	3.81	3.82	3.83
5	4.58	4.62	4.65	4.67	4.70	4.72	4.74	4.75	4.77	4.78	4.79
6	5.50	5.54	5.58	5.61	5.64	5.66	5.69	5.70	5.72	5.74	5.75
7	6.42	6.47	6.51	6.55	6.58	6.61	6.64	6.66	6.68	6.69	6.71
8	7.34	7.40	7.45	7.49	7.53	7.56	7.59	7.61	7.63	7.65	7.67
9	8.26	8.33	8.38	8.43	8.47	8.51	8.54	8.57	8.59	8.61	8.64
10	9.18	9.25	9.32	9.37	9.42	9.46	9.49	9.52	9.55	9.58	9.60
11	10.10	10.18	10.25	10.31	10.36	10.41	10.45	10.48	10.51	10.54	10.56
12	11.03	11.12	11.19	11.25	11.31	11.36	11.40	11.44	11.47	11.50	11.53
13	11.95	12.05	12.13	12.20	12.26	12.31	12.36	12.40	12.43	12.47	12.50
14	12.88	12.98	13.07	13.14	13.21	13.26	13.31	13.36	13.40	13.43	13.46
15	13.80	13.91	14.01	14.09	14.16	14.22	14.27	14.32	14.36	14.40	14.43
16	14.73	14.85	14.95	15.03	15.11	15.17	15.23	15.28	15.32	15.36	15.40
17	15.66	15.78	15.89	15.98	16.06	16.13	16.19	16.24	16.29	16.33	16.37
18	16.58	16.72	16.83	16.93	17.01	17.08	17.15	17.21	17.26	17.30	17.34
19	17.51	17.66	17.78	17.88	17.97	18.04	18.11	18.17	18.22	18.27	18.31
20	18.44	18.59	18.72	18.83	18.92	19.00	19.07	19.13	19.19	19.24	19.29
21	19.38	19.53	19.66	19.78	19.87	19.96	20.03	20.10	20.16	20.21	20.26
22	20.31	20.47	20.61	20.73	20.83	20.92	21.00	21.07	21.13	21.19	21.24
23	21.24	21.41	21.56	21.68	21.79	21.88	21.96	22.04	22.10	22.16	22.21
24	22.17	22.35	22.50	22.63	22.74	22.84	22.93	23.00	23.07	23.13	23.19
25	23.11	23.29	23.45	23.59	23.70	23.80	23.89	23.97	24.04	24.11	24.17
26	24.04	24.24	24.40	24.54	24.66	24.77	24.86	24.94	25.02	25.08	25.14
27	24.98	25.18	25.35	25.50	25.62	25.73	25.83	25.92	25.99	26.06	26.12
28	25.92	26.12	26.30	26.45	26.58	26.70	26.80	26.89	26.97	27.04	27.10
29	26.85	27.07	27.25	27.41	27.55	27.66	27.77	27.86	27.94	28.02	28.08
30	27.79	28.02	28.21	28.37	28.51	28.63	28.74	28.83	28.92	29.00	29.07

Table D.XXI Centre thickness 0.80 mm

Back vertex powers (D)	Front vertex powers (D) for back optic zone radii										
	5.0 mm	5.5 mm	6.0 mm	6.5 mm	7.0 mm	7.5 mm	8.0 mm	8.5 mm	9.0 mm	9.5 mm	10.0 mm
+ 20	17.87	18.03	18.17	18.29	18.39	18.48	18.55	18.62	18.69	18.74	18.79
19	16.98	17.14	17.27	17.38	17.48	17.56	17.64	17.70	17.76	17.81	17.86
18	16.10	16.24	16.37	16.47	16.57	16.65	16.72	16.78	16.83	16.88	16.93
17	15.21	15.35	15.47	15.57	15.65	15.73	15.80	15.85	15.91	15.95	16.00
16	14.32	14.46	14.56	14.66	14.74	14.81	14.87	14.93	14.98	15.02	15.06
15	13.44	13.56	13.66	13.75	13.83	13.89	13.95	14.00	14.05	14.09	14.13
14	12.55	12.66	12.76	12.84	12.91	12.97	13.03	13.08	13.12	13.16	13.20
13	11.66	11.76	11.85	11.93	12.00	12.05	12.10	12.15	12.19	12.23	12.26
12	10.76	10.86	10.95	11.02	11.08	11.13	11.18	11.22	11.26	11.29	11.32
11	9.87	9.96	10.04	10.10	10.16	10.21	10.25	10.29	10.33	10.36	10.38
10	8.98	9.06	9.13	9.19	9.24	9.29	9.33	9.36	9.39	9.42	9.44
9	8.09	8.16	8.22	8.28	8.32	8.36	8.40	8.43	8.46	8.48	8.50
8	7.19	7.26	7.31	7.36	7.40	7.44	7.47	7.50	7.52	7.54	7.56
7	6.30	6.35	6.40	6.44	6.48	6.51	6.54	6.56	6.58	6.60	6.62
6	5.40	5.45	5.49	5.53	5.56	5.58	5.61	5.63	5.65	5.66	5.68
5	4.50	4.54	4.58	4.61	4.63	4.66	4.68	4.69	4.71	4.72	4.74
4	3.60	3.64	3.66	3.69	3.71	3.73	3.74	3.76	3.77	3.78	3.79
3	2.70	2.73	2.75	2.77	2.78	2.80	2.81	2.82	2.83	2.84	2.84
2	1.80	1.82	1.83	1.85	1.86	1.87	1.87	1.88	1.89	1.89	1.90
1	0.90	0.91	0.92	0.92	0.93	0.93	0.94	0.94	0.94	0.95	0.95
0	0.00	0.00	0.00	0.00	0.00	0.00	0.00	0.00	0.00	0.00	0.00
− 1	0.90	0.91	0.92	0.92	0.93	0.93	0.94	0.94	0.94	0.95	0.95
2	1.81	1.82	1.84	1.85	1.86	1.87	1.88	1.88	1.89	1.90	1.90
3	2.71	2.74	2.76	2.78	2.79	2.80	2.82	2.83	2.84	2.85	2.85
4	3.62	3.65	3.68	3.70	3.72	3.74	3.76	3.77	3.78	3.80	3.81
5	4.52	4.57	4.60	4.63	4.66	4.68	4.70	4.72	4.73	4.75	4.76
6	5.43	5.48	5.52	5.56	5.59	5.62	5.64	5.66	5.68	5.70	5.71
7	6.34	6.40	6.45	6.49	6.53	6.56	6.59	6.61	6.63	6.65	6.67
8	7.25	7.32	7.37	7.42	7.46	7.50	7.53	7.56	7.58	7.61	7.63
9	8.16	8.23	8.30	8.35	8.40	8.44	8.48	8.51	8.54	8.56	8.59
10	9.07	9.15	9.23	9.29	9.34	9.38	9.42	9.46	9.49	9.52	9.54
11	9.98	10.08	10.15	10.22	10.28	10.33	10.37	10.41	10.44	10.48	10.50
12	10.90	11.00	11.08	11.15	11.22	11.27	11.32	11.36	11.40	11.43	11.47
13	11.81	11.92	12.01	12.09	12.16	12.22	12.27	12.32	12.36	12.39	12.43
14	12.73	12.84	12.94	13.03	13.10	13.16	13.22	13.27	13.31	13.35	13.39
15	13.64	13.77	13.87	13.96	14.04	14.11	14.17	14.22	14.27	14.31	14.35
16	14.56	14.69	14.81	14.90	14.99	15.06	15.12	15.18	15.23	15.28	15.32
17	15.48	15.62	15.74	15.84	15.93	16.01	16.08	16.14	16.19	16.24	16.28
18	16.40	16.55	16.67	16.78	16.88	16.96	17.03	17.10	17.15	17.20	17.25
19	17.32	17.47	17.61	17.72	17.82	17.91	17.99	18.06	18.12	18.17	18.22
20	18.24	18.40	18.55	18.67	18.77	18.86	18.94	19.02	19.08	19.14	19.19
21	19.20	19.33	19.48	19.61	19.72	19.82	19.90	19.98	20.04	20.10	20.16
22	20.08	20.27	20.42	20.55	20.67	20.77	20.86	20.94	21.01	21.07	21.13
23	21.00	21.20	21.36	21.50	21.62	21.73	21.82	21.90	21.98	22.04	22.10
24	21.93	22.13	22.30	22.45	22.57	22.68	22.78	22.87	22.94	23.01	23.08
25	22.86	23.06	23.24	23.39	23.53	23.64	23.74	23.83	23.91	23.98	24.05
26	23.78	24.00	24.19	24.34	24.48	24.60	24.71	24.80	24.88	24.96	25.02
27	24.71	24.94	25.13	25.29	25.44	25.56	25.67	25.77	25.85	25.93	26.00
28	25.64	25.87	26.07	26.24	26.39	26.52	26.63	26.73	26.82	26.90	26.98
29	26.57	26.81	27.02	27.19	27.35	27.48	27.60	27.70	27.80	27.88	27.96
30	27.50	27.75	27.96	28.15	28.31	28.44	28.57	28.67	28.77	28.86	28.94

Table D.XXII Centre thickness 0.90 mm

Back vertex powers (D)	Front vertex powers (D) for back optic zone radii										
	5.0 mm	5.5 mm	6.0 mm	6.5 mm	7.0 mm	7.5 mm	8.0 mm	8.5 mm	9.0 mm	9.5 mm	10.0 mm
+ 20	17.63	17.81	17.96	18.09	18.20	18.30	18.38	18.46	18.53	18.59	18.65
19	16.75	16.92	17.07	17.19	17.30	17.39	17.48	17.55	17.61	17.67	17.73
18	15.88	16.04	16.18	16.30	16.40	16.49	16.57	16.63	16.70	16.75	16.80
17	15.01	15.16	15.29	15.40	15.50	15.58	15.65	15.72	15.78	15.83	15.88
16	14.13	14.28	14.40	14.50	14.59	14.67	14.74	14.80	14.86	14.91	14.95
15	13.26	13.39	13.51	13.60	13.69	13.76	13.83	13.89	13.94	13.98	14.03
14	12.38	12.51	12.61	12.70	12.78	12.85	12.91	12.97	13.02	13.06	13.10
13	11.50	11.62	11.72	11.80	11.88	11.94	12.00	12.05	12.09	12.13	12.17
12	10.62	10.73	10.82	10.90	10.97	11.03	11.08	11.13	11.17	11.21	11.24
11	9.74	9.84	9.93	10.00	10.06	10.12	10.16	10.21	10.25	10.28	10.31
10	8.86	8.95	9.03	9.10	9.15	9.20	9.25	9.28	9.32	9.35	9.38
9	7.98	8.06	8.13	8.19	8.24	8.29	8.33	8.36	8.39	8.42	8.45
8	7.10	7.17	7.23	7.28	7.33	7.37	7.41	7.44	7.46	7.49	7.51
7	6.22	6.28	6.33	6.38	6.42	6.45	6.48	6.51	6.54	6.56	6.58
6	5.33	5.38	5.43	5.47	5.50	5.53	5.56	5.58	5.60	5.62	5.64
5	4.44	4.49	4.53	4.56	4.59	4.61	4.64	4.66	4.67	4.69	4.70
4	3.56	3.59	3.62	3.65	3.67	3.69	3.71	3.73	3.74	3.75	3.76
3	2.67	2.70	2.72	2.74	2.76	2.77	2.79	2.80	2.81	2.82	2.83
2	1.78	1.80	1.81	1.83	1.84	1.85	1.86	1.87	1.87	1.88	1.88
1	0.89	0.90	0.91	0.91	0.92	0.93	0.93	0.93	0.94	0.94	0.94
0	0.00	0.00	0.00	0.00	0.00	0.00	0.00	0.00	0.00	0.00	0.00
− 1	0.89	0.90	0.91	0.92	0.92	0.93	0.93	0.93	0.94	0.94	0.94
2	1.79	1.80	1.82	1.83	1.84	1.85	1.86	1.87	1.88	1.88	1.89
3	2.68	2.71	2.73	2.75	2.77	2.78	2.80	2.81	2.82	2.83	2.84
4	3.57	3.61	3.64	3.67	3.69	3.71	3.73	3.74	3.76	3.77	3.78
5	4.47	4.52	4.55	4.59	4.62	4.64	4.66	4.68	4.70	4.72	4.73
6	5.37	5.42	5.47	5.51	5.54	5.57	5.60	5.62	5.64	5.66	5.68
7	6.26	6.33	6.38	6.43	6.47	6.51	6.54	6.56	6.59	6.61	6.63
8	7.16	7.24	7.30	7.35	7.40	7.44	7.47	7.51	7.53	7.56	7.58
9	8.06	8.15	8.22	8.28	8.33	8.37	8.41	8.45	8.48	8.51	8.54
10	8.97	9.06	9.13	9.20	9.26	9.31	9.35	9.39	9.43	9.46	9.49
11	9.87	9.97	10.05	10.13	10.19	10.25	10.30	10.34	10.38	10.41	10.44
12	10.77	10.88	10.97	11.05	11.12	11.18	11.24	11.29	11.33	11.37	11.40
13	11.67	11.79	11.90	11.98	12.06	12.12	12.18	12.23	12.28	12.32	12.36
14	12.58	12.71	12.82	12.91	12.99	13.06	13.12	13.18	13.23	13.28	13.32
15	13.49	13.62	13.74	13.84	13.93	14.01	14.07	14.13	14.18	14.23	14.28
16	14.39	14.54	14.67	14.77	14.87	14.95	15.02	15.08	15.14	15.19	15.24
17	15.30	15.46	15.59	15.71	15.80	15.89	15.97	16.03	16.10	16.15	16.20
18	16.21	16.38	16.52	16.64	16.74	16.84	16.92	16.99	17.05	17.11	17.16
19	17.12	17.30	17.45	17.57	17.68	17.78	17.87	17.94	18.01	18.07	18.13
20	18.03	18.22	18.38	18.51	18.63	18.73	18.82	18.90	18.97	19.03	19.09
21	18.95	19.14	19.31	19.45	19.57	19.68	19.77	19.85	19.93	20.00	20.06
22	19.86	20.06	20.24	20.38	20.51	20.63	20.72	20.81	20.89	20.96	21.03
23	20.77	20.99	21.17	21.32	21.46	21.58	21.68	21.77	21.85	21.93	21.99
24	21.69	21.91	22.10	22.26	22.40	22.53	22.63	22.73	22.82	22.89	22.96
25	22.61	22.84	23.04	23.20	23.35	23.48	23.59	23.69	23.78	23.86	23.93
26	23.52	23.77	23.97	24.15	24.30	24.43	24.55	24.65	24.75	24.83	24.91
27	24.44	24.69	24.91	25.09	25.25	25.39	25.51	25.62	25.71	25.80	25.88
28	25.36	25.62	25.85	26.04	26.20	26.34	26.47	26.58	26.68	26.77	26.85
29	26.28	26.55	26.79	26.98	27.15	27.30	27.43	27.55	27.65	27.75	27.83
30	27.21	27.49	27.72	27.93	28.10	28.26	28.39	28.51	28.62	28.72	28.81

Table D.XXIII Centre thickness 1.00 mm

Back vertex powers (D)	Front vertex powers (D) for back optic zone radii										
	5.0 mm	5.5 mm	6.0 mm	6.5 mm	7.0 mm	7.5 mm	8.0 mm	8.5 mm	9.0 mm	9.5 mm	10.0 mm
+ 20	17.39	17.58	17.75	17.89	18.01	18.12	18.22	18.30	18.38	18.45	18.51
19	16.53	16.72	16.87	17.01	17.13	17.23	17.32	17.40	17.47	17.53	17.59
18	15.67	15.85	16.00	16.12	16.23	16.33	16.42	16.49	16.56	16.62	16.68
17	14.81	14.97	15.12	15.24	15.34	15.43	15.51	15.59	15.65	15.71	15.76
16	13.95	14.10	14.24	14.35	14.45	14.54	14.61	14.68	14.74	14.79	14.84
15	13.08	13.23	13.35	13.46	13.55	13.64	13.71	13.77	13.83	13.88	13.92
14	12.22	12.36	12.47	12.57	12.66	12.73	12.80	12.86	12.91	12.96	13.00
13	11.35	11.48	11.59	11.68	11.76	11.83	11.89	11.95	12.00	12.04	12.08
12	10.49	10.60	10.70	10.79	10.86	10.93	10.99	11.04	11.08	11.12	11.16
11	9.62	9.73	9.82	9.90	9.97	10.02	10.08	10.12	10.17	10.20	10.24
10	8.75	8.85	8.93	9.00	9.07	9.12	9.17	9.21	9.25	9.28	9.31
9	7.88	7.97	8.04	8.11	8.16	8.21	8.26	8.29	8.33	8.36	8.39
8	7.01	7.09	7.15	7.21	7.26	7.30	7.34	7.38	7.41	7.44	7.46
7	6.14	6.20	6.26	6.31	6.36	6.40	6.43	6.46	6.49	6.51	6.53
6	5.26	5.32	5.37	5.42	5.45	5.49	5.51	5.54	5.56	5.58	5.60
5	4.39	4.44	4.48	4.52	4.55	4.57	4.60	4.62	4.64	4.66	4.67
4	3.51	3.55	3.59	3.61	3.64	3.66	3.68	3.70	3.71	3.73	3.74
3	2.64	2.67	2.69	2.71	2.73	2.75	2.76	2.78	2.79	2.80	2.81
2	1.76	1.78	1.80	1.81	1.82	1.83	1.84	1.85	1.86	1.87	1.87
1	0.88	0.89	0.90	0.91	0.91	0.92	0.92	0.93	0.93	0.93	0.94
0	0.00	0.00	0.00	0.00	0.00	0.00	0.00	0.00	0.00	0.00	0.00
− 1	0.88	0.89	0.90	0.91	0.91	0.92	0.92	0.93	0.93	0.93	0.94
2	1.76	1.78	1.80	1.81	1.83	1.84	1.85	1.86	1.86	1.87	1.88
3	2.65	2.68	2.70	2.72	2.74	2.76	2.77	2.79	2.80	2.81	2.82
4	3.53	3.57	3.60	3.63	3.66	3.68	3.70	3.72	3.73	3.75	3.76
5	4.42	4.47	4.51	4.54	4.58	4.60	4.63	4.65	4.67	4.69	4.70
6	5.30	5.36	5.41	5.46	5.50	5.53	5.56	5.58	5.61	5.63	5.65
7	6.19	6.26	6.32	6.37	6.42	6.45	6.49	6.52	6.55	6.57	6.59
8	7.08	7.16	7.23	7.29	7.34	7.38	7.42	7.45	7.49	7.51	7.54
9	7.97	8.06	8.14	8.20	8.26	8.31	8.35	8.39	8.43	8.46	8.49
10	8.86	8.96	9.05	9.12	9.18	9.24	9.29	9.33	9.37	9.40	9.44
11	9.75	9.86	9.96	10.04	10.11	10.17	10.22	10.27	10.31	10.35	10.39
12	10.65	10.77	10.87	10.96	11.03	11.10	11.16	11.21	11.26	11.30	11.34
13	11.54	11.67	11.78	11.88	11.96	12.03	12.10	12.15	12.20	12.25	12.29
14	12.44	12.58	12.70	12.80	12.89	12.97	13.03	13.10	13.15	13.20	13.24
15	13.33	13.48	13.61	13.72	13.82	13.90	13.97	14.04	14.10	14.15	14.20
16	14.23	14.39	14.53	14.65	14.75	14.84	14.92	14.99	15.05	15.10	15.16
17	15.13	15.30	15.45	15.57	15.68	15.77	15.86	15.93	16.00	16.06	16.11
18	16.03	16.21	16.37	16.50	16.61	16.71	16.80	16.88	16.95	17.01	17.07
19	16.93	17.12	17.29	17.43	17.55	17.65	17.75	17.83	17.90	17.97	18.03
20	17.83	18.03	18.21	18.35	18.48	18.59	18.69	18.78	18.86	18.93	18.99
21	18.74	18.95	19.13	19.28	19.42	19.54	19.64	19.73	19.82	19.89	19.96
22	19.64	19.86	20.05	20.22	20.36	20.48	20.59	20.69	20.77	20.85	20.92
23	20.55	20.78	20.98	21.15	21.30	21.43	21.54	21.64	21.73	21.81	21.89
24	21.45	21.70	21.91	22.08	22.24	22.37	22.49	22.60	22.69	22.78	22.85
25	22.36	22.61	22.83	23.02	23.18	23.32	23.44	23.55	23.65	23.74	23.82
26	23.27	23.54	23.76	23.96	24.12	24.27	24.40	24.51	24.61	24.71	24.79
27	24.18	24.46	24.69	24.89	25.07	25.22	25.35	25.47	25.58	25.67	25.76
28	25.09	25.38	25.62	25.83	26.01	26.17	26.31	26.43	26.54	26.64	26.73
29	26.01	26.30	26.55	26.77	26.96	27.12	27.27	27.39	27.51	27.61	27.71
30	26.92	27.23	27.49	27.71	27.91	28.07	28.22	28.36	28.48	28.58	28.68

Table D.XXIV Centre thickness 1.10 mm

Back vertex powers (D)	Front vertex powers (D) for back optic zone radii										
	5.0 mm	5.5 mm	6.0 mm	6.5 mm	7.0 mm	7.5 mm	8.0 mm	8.5 mm	9.0 mm	9.5 mm	10.0 mm
+ 20	17.16	17.37	17.55	17.70	17.83	17.95	18.05	18.14	18.23	18.30	18.37
19	16.31	16.51	16.68	16.83	16.95	17.06	17.16	17.25	17.33	17.40	17.46
18	15.46	15.65	15.81	15.95	16.07	16.18	16.27	16.35	16.43	16.49	16.55
17	14.61	14.79	14.95	15.08	15.19	15.29	15.38	15.45	15.52	15.59	15.64
16	13.76	13.93	14.08	14.20	14.31	14.40	14.48	14.56	14.62	14.68	14.73
15	12.91	13.07	13.21	13.32	13.42	13.51	13.59	13.66	13.72	13.77	13.82
14	12.06	12.21	12.33	12.44	12.54	12.62	12.69	12.75	12.81	12.86	12.91
13	11.21	11.34	11.46	11.56	11.65	11.72	11.79	11.85	11.91	11.95	12.00
12	10.35	10.48	10.59	10.68	10.76	10.83	10.89	10.95	11.00	11.04	11.08
11	9.49	9.61	9.71	9.80	9.87	9.93	9.99	10.04	10.09	10.13	10.17
10	8.64	8.74	8.83	8.91	8.98	9.04	9.09	9.14	9.18	9.21	9.25
9	7.78	7.87	7.96	8.03	8.09	8.14	8.19	8.23	8.27	8.30	8.33
8	6.92	7.00	7.08	7.14	7.19	7.24	7.28	7.32	7.35	7.38	7.41
7	6.06	6.13	6.20	6.25	6.30	6.34	6.38	6.41	6.44	6.46	6.49
6	5.20	5.26	5.32	5.36	5.40	5.44	5.47	5.50	5.52	5.54	5.57
5	4.33	4.39	4.43	4.47	4.51	4.53	4.56	4.58	4.61	4.62	4.64
4	3.47	3.51	3.55	3.58	3.61	3.63	3.65	3.67	3.69	3.70	3.72
3	2.60	2.64	2.66	2.69	2.71	2.73	2.74	2.75	2.77	2.78	2.79
2	1.74	1.76	1.78	1.79	1.81	1.82	1.83	1.84	1.85	1.85	1.86
1	0.87	0.88	0.89	0.90	0.90	0.91	0.92	0.92	0.92	0.93	0.93
0	0.00	0.00	0.00	0.00	0.00	0.00	0.00	0.00	0.00	0.00	0.00
− 1	0.87	0.88	0.89	0.90	0.91	0.91	0.92	0.92	0.93	0.93	0.93
2	1.74	1.76	1.78	1.80	1.81	1.82	1.83	1.84	1.85	1.86	1.87
3	2.61	2.65	2.67	2.70	2.72	2.74	2.75	2.77	2.78	2.79	2.80
4	3.49	3.53	3.57	3.60	3.63	3.65	3.67	3.69	3.71	3.72	3.74
5	4.36	4.42	4.46	4.50	4.54	4.57	4.59	4.62	4.64	4.66	4.67
6	5.24	5.30	5.36	5.41	5.45	5.48	5.52	5.54	5.57	5.59	5.61
7	6.12	6.19	6.26	6.31	6.36	6.40	6.44	6.47	6.50	6.53	6.55
8	7.00	7.08	7.16	7.22	7.27	7.32	7.36	7.40	7.44	7.47	7.49
9	7.88	7.97	8.06	8.13	8.19	8.24	8.29	8.33	8.37	8.41	8.44
10	8.76	8.87	8.96	9.04	9.11	9.17	9.22	9.27	9.31	9.35	9.38
11	9.64	9.76	9.86	9.95	10.02	10.09	10.15	10.20	10.25	10.29	10.33
12	10.52	10.65	10.76	10.86	10.94	11.01	11.08	11.14	11.19	11.23	11.27
13	11.41	11.55	11.67	11.77	11.86	11.94	12.01	12.07	12.13	12.18	12.22
14	12.29	12.45	12.58	12.69	12.78	12.87	12.94	13.01	13.07	13.12	13.17
15	13.18	13.34	13.48	13.60	13.71	13.80	13.88	13.95	14.01	14.07	14.12
16	14.07	14.24	14.39	14.52	14.63	14.73	14.81	14.89	14.96	15.02	15.07
17	14.96	15.14	15.30	15.44	15.56	15.66	15.75	15.83	15.90	15.97	16.03
18	15.85	16.05	16.21	16.36	16.48	16.59	16.69	16.77	16.85	16.92	16.98
19	16.74	16.95	17.13	17.28	17.41	17.53	17.63	17.72	17.80	17.87	17.94
20	17.64	17.85	18.04	18.20	18.34	18.46	18.57	18.67	18.75	18.83	18.90
21	18.53	18.76	18.96	19.12	19.27	19.40	19.51	19.61	19.70	19.78	19.86
22	19.43	19.67	19.87	20.05	20.20	20.34	20.46	20.56	20.66	20.74	20.82
23	20.32	20.58	20.79	20.98	21.14	21.28	21.40	21.51	21.61	21.70	21.78
24	21.22	21.49	21.71	21.90	22.07	22.22	22.35	22.46	22.57	22.66	22.74
25	22.12	22.40	22.63	22.83	23.01	23.16	23.30	23.42	23.52	23.62	23.71
26	23.02	23.31	23.55	23.76	23.95	24.10	24.24	24.37	24.48	24.58	24.67
27	23.92	24.22	24.48	24.69	24.88	25.05	25.20	25.33	25.44	25.55	25.64
28	24.83	25.14	25.40	25.63	25.82	26.00	26.15	26.28	26.40	26.51	26.61
29	25.73	26.05	26.33	26.56	26.77	26.94	27.10	27.24	27.37	27.48	27.58
30	26.64	26.97	27.26	27.50	27.71	27.89	28.06	28.20	28.33	28.45	28.55

Table D.XXV Centre thickness 1.20 mm

Back vertex powers (D)	Front vertex powers (D) for back optic zone radii										
	5.0 mm	5.5 mm	6.0 mm	6.5 mm	7.0 mm	7.5 mm	8.0 mm	8.5 mm	9.0 mm	9.5 mm	10.0 mm
+ 20	16.93	17.15	17.35	17.51	17.65	17.78	17.89	17.99	18.08	18.16	18.23
19	16.09	16.31	16.49	16.65	16.78	16.90	17.01	17.10	17.19	17.26	17.33
18	15.26	16.46	15.63	15.78	15.91	16.03	16.13	16.21	16.29	16.37	16.43
17	14.42	14.61	14.78	14.92	15.04	15.15	15.24	15.32	15.40	15.47	15.53
16	13.58	13.76	13.92	14.05	14.17	14.27	14.36	14.43	14.51	14.57	14.63
15	12.74	12.91	13.06	13.18	13.29	13.38	13.47	13.54	13.61	13.67	13.72
14	11.90	12.06	12.20	12.31	12.41	12.50	12.58	12.65	12.71	12.77	12.82
13	11.06	11.21	11.33	11.44	11.54	11.62	11.69	11.75	11.81	11.86	11.91
12	10.22	10.35	10.47	10.57	10.66	10.73	10.80	10.86	10.91	10.96	11.00
11	9.37	9.50	9.60	9.70	9.78	9.85	9.91	9.96	10.01	10.05	10.10
10	8.53	8.64	8.74	8.82	8.89	8.96	9.01	9.06	9.11	9.15	9.18
9	7.68	7.78	7.87	7.95	8.01	8.07	8.12	8.16	8.20	8.24	8.27
8	6.83	6.92	7.00	7.07	7.13	7.18	7.22	7.26	7.30	7.33	7.36
7	5.98	6.06	6.13	6.19	6.24	6.28	6.32	6.36	6.39	6.42	6.44
6	5.13	5.20	5.26	5.31	5.35	5.39	5.42	5.45	5.48	5.51	5.53
5	4.28	4.34	4.39	4.43	4.46	4.50	4.52	4.55	4.57	4.59	4.61
4	3.43	3.47	3.51	3.54	3.57	3.60	3.62	3.64	3.66	3.68	3.69
3	2.57	2.61	2.64	2.66	2.68	2.70	2.72	2.73	2.75	2.76	2.77
2	1.72	1.74	1.76	1.78	1.79	1.80	1.81	1.82	1.83	1.84	1.85
1	0.86	0.87	0.88	0.89	0.90	0.90	0.91	0.91	0.92	0.92	0.93
0	0.00	0.00	0.00	0.00	0.00	0.00	0.00	0.00	0.00	0.00	0.00
− 1	0.86	0.87	0.88	0.89	0.90	0.90	0.91	0.91	0.92	0.92	0.93
2	1.72	1.74	1.76	1.78	1.80	1.81	1.82	1.83	1.84	1.85	1.85
3	2.58	2.62	2.65	2.67	2.70	2.71	2.73	2.75	2.76	2.77	2.78
4	3.45	3.49	3.53	3.57	3.60	3.62	3.64	3.66	3.68	3.70	3.71
5	4.31	4.37	4.42	4.46	4.50	4.53	4.56	4.58	4.61	4.63	4.65
6	5.18	5.25	5.31	5.36	5.40	5.44	5.47	5.51	5.53	5.56	5.58
7	6.05	6.13	6.20	6.26	6.31	6.35	6.39	6.43	6.46	6.49	6.51
8	6.91	7.01	7.09	7.15	7.21	7.27	7.31	7.35	7.39	7.42	7.45
9	7.78	7.89	7.98	8.05	8.12	8.18	8.23	8.28	8.32	8.35	8.39
10	8.66	8.77	8.87	8.96	9.03	9.10	9.15	9.20	9.25	9.29	9.33
11	9.53	9.66	9.76	9.86	9.94	10.01	10.08	10.13	10.18	10.23	10.27
12	10.40	10.54	10.66	10.76	10.85	10.93	11.00	11.06	11.12	11.17	11.21
13	11.28	11.43	11.56	11.67	11.77	11.85	11.93	11.99	12.05	12.11	12.15
14	12.15	12.32	12.46	12.58	12.68	12.77	12.85	12.93	12.99	13.05	13.10
15	13.03	13.21	13.36	13.49	13.60	13.70	13.78	13.86	13.93	13.99	14.05
16	13.91	14.10	14.26	14.40	14.52	14.62	14.71	14.79	14.87	14.93	14.99
17	14.79	14.99	15.16	15.31	15.43	15.55	15.64	15.73	15.81	15.88	15.94
18	15.67	15.89	16.07	16.22	16.35	16.47	16.58	16.67	16.75	16.83	16.90
19	16.56	16.78	16.97	17.13	17.28	17.40	17.51	17.61	17.70	17.78	17.85
20	17.44	17.68	17.88	18.05	18.20	18.33	18.45	18.55	18.64	18.73	18.80
21	18.33	18.57	18.79	18.97	19.13	19.26	19.38	19.49	19.59	19.68	19.76
22	19.22	19.47	19.70	19.89	20.05	20.20	20.32	20.44	20.54	20.63	20.71
23	20.10	20.38	20.61	20.81	20.98	21.13	21.26	21.38	21.49	21.59	21.67
24	20.99	21.28	21.52	21.73	21.91	22.07	22.21	22.33	22.44	22.54	22.63
25	21.89	22.18	22.43	22.65	22.84	23.00	23.15	23.28	23.40	23.50	23.60
26	22.78	23.09	23.35	23.57	23.77	23.94	24.09	24.23	24.35	24.46	24.56
27	23.67	23.99	24.27	24.50	24.70	24.88	25.04	25.18	25.31	25.42	25.52
28	24.57	24.90	25.18	25.43	25.64	25.82	25.99	26.13	26.26	26.38	26.49
29	25.46	25.81	26.10	26.36	26.58	26.77	26.94	27.09	27.22	27.35	27.46
30	26.36	26.72	27.02	27.28	27.51	27.71	27.89	28.05	28.19	28.31	28.43

Table D.XXVI Centre thickness 1.30 mm

Back vertex powers (D)	Front vertex powers (D) for back optic zone radii										
	5.0 mm	5.5 mm	6.0 mm	6.5 mm	7.0 mm	7.5 mm	8.0 mm	8.5 mm	9.0 mm	9.5 mm	10.0 mm
+ 20	16.71	16.94	17.15	17.32	17.48	17.61	17.73	17.83	17.93	18.01	18.09
19	15.88	16.11	16.30	16.47	16.62	16.74	16.86	16.96	17.05	17.13	17.20
18	15.06	15.27	15.46	15.62	15.75	15.88	15.98	16.08	16.16	16.24	16.31
17	14.23	14.44	14.61	14.76	14.89	15.01	15.11	15.20	15.28	15.35	15.42
16	13.41	13.60	13.76	13.90	14.03	14.13	14.23	14.31	14.39	14.46	14.52
15	12.58	12.76	12.91	13.05	13.16	13.26	13.35	13.43	13.50	13.57	13.62
14	11.75	11.92	12.06	12.19	12.29	12.39	12.47	12.55	12.61	12.67	12.73
13	10.92	11.08	11.21	11.32	11.42	11.51	11.59	11.66	11.72	11.78	11.83
12	10.09	10.23	10.36	10.46	10.55	10.64	10.71	10.77	10.83	10.88	10.93
11	9.25	9.39	9.50	9.60	9.68	9.76	9.82	9.88	9.93	9.98	10.02
10	8.42	8.54	8.64	8.73	8.81	8.88	8.94	8.99	9.04	9.08	9.12
9	7.58	7.69	7.79	7.87	7.94	8.00	8.05	8.10	8.14	8.18	8.22
8	6.75	6.84	6.93	7.00	7.06	7.11	7.16	7.20	7.24	7.28	7.31
7	5.91	5.99	6.07	6.13	6.18	6.23	6.27	6.31	6.34	6.37	6.40
6	5.07	5.14	5.20	5.26	5.30	5.34	5.38	5.41	5.44	5.47	5.49
5	4.23	4.29	4.34	4.38	4.42	4.46	4.49	4.51	4.54	4.56	4.58
4	3.38	3.43	3.47	3.51	3.54	3.57	3.59	3.61	3.63	3.65	3.67
3	2.54	2.58	2.61	2.64	2.66	2.68	2.70	2.71	2.73	2.74	2.75
2	1.70	1.72	1.74	1.76	1.77	1.79	1.80	1.81	1.82	1.83	1.84
1	0.85	0.86	0.87	0.88	0.89	0.89	0.90	0.91	0.91	0.92	0.92
0	0.00	0.00	0.00	0.00	0.00	0.00	0.00	0.00	0.00	0.00	0.00
− 1	0.85	0.86	0.87	0.88	0.89	0.90	0.90	0.91	0.91	0.92	0.92
2	1.70	1.72	1.75	1.76	1.78	1.79	1.81	1.82	1.83	1.83	1.84
3	2.55	2.59	2.62	2.65	2.67	2.69	2.71	2.73	2.74	2.75	2.77
4	3.41	3.46	3.50	3.53	3.57	3.59	3.62	3.64	3.66	3.68	3.69
5	4.26	4.32	4.38	4.42	4.46	4.49	4.52	4.55	4.58	4.60	4.62
6	5.12	5.19	5.25	5.31	5.36	5.40	5.43	5.47	5.50	5.52	5.55
7	5.97	6.06	6.14	6.20	6.25	6.30	6.35	6.38	6.42	6.45	6.49
8	6.83	6.93	7.02	7.09	7.15	7.21	7.26	7.30	7.34	7.38	7.41
9	7.69	7.81	7.90	7.98	8.05	8.12	8.17	8.22	8.26	8.30	8.34
10	8.56	8.68	8.79	8.88	8.96	9.03	9.09	9.14	9.19	9.23	9.27
11	9.42	9.56	9.67	9.77	9.86	9.94	10.00	10.06	10.12	10.17	10.21
12	10.28	10.43	10.56	10.67	10.77	10.85	10.92	10.99	11.05	11.10	11.15
13	11.15	11.31	11.45	11.57	11.67	11.76	11.84	11.91	11.98	12.04	12.09
14	12.02	12.19	12.34	12.47	12.58	12.68	12.76	12.84	12.91	12.97	13.03
15	12.89	13.07	13.23	13.37	13.49	13.59	13.69	13.77	13.84	13.91	13.97
16	13.76	13.96	14.13	14.27	14.40	14.51	14.61	14.70	14.78	14.85	14.92
17	14.63	14.84	15.02	15.18	15.31	15.43	15.54	15.63	15.72	15.79	15.86
18	15.50	15.73	15.92	16.08	16.23	16.35	16.47	16.57	16.65	16.73	16.81
19	16.38	16.61	16.82	16.99	17.14	17.28	17.40	17.50	17.59	17.68	17.76
20	17.25	17.50	17.72	17.90	18.06	18.20	18.33	18.44	18.54	18.63	18.71
21	18.13	18.39	18.62	18.81	18.98	19.13	19.26	19.38	19.48	19.57	19.66
22	19.01	19.28	19.52	19.72	19.90	20.06	20.19	20.32	20.42	20.52	20.61
23	19.89	20.18	20.43	20.64	20.82	20.99	21.13	21.26	21.37	21.47	21.57
24	20.77	21.07	21.33	21.55	21.75	21.92	22.07	22.20	22.32	22.43	22.53
25	21.65	21.97	22.24	22.47	22.67	22.85	23.00	23.14	23.27	23.38	23.48
26	22.54	22.87	23.15	23.39	23.60	23.78	23.95	24.09	24.22	24.34	24.44
27	23.42	23.76	24.06	24.31	24.53	24.72	24.89	25.04	25.17	25.29	25.41
28	24.31	24.66	24.97	25.23	25.46	25.65	25.83	25.99	26.13	26.25	26.37
29	25.20	25.57	25.88	26.15	26.39	26.59	26.78	26.94	27.08	27.22	27.33
30	26.09	26.47	26.80	27.08	27.32	27.53	27.72	27.89	28.04	28.18	28.30

Table D.XXVII Centre thickness 1.40 mm

Back vertex powers (D)	Front vertex powers (D) for back optic zone radii										
	5.0 mm	5.5 mm	6.0 mm	6.5 mm	7.0 mm	7.5 mm	8.0 mm	8.5 mm	9.0 mm	9.5 mm	10.0 mm
+ 20	16.49	16.74	16.96	17.14	17.30	17.45	17.57	17.68	17.78	17.87	17.96
19	15.68	15.92	16.12	16.30	16.45	16.59	16.71	16.81	16.91	16.99	17.07
18	14.86	15.09	15.29	15.45	15.60	15.73	15.84	15.94	16.03	16.11	16.19
17	14.05	14.26	14.45	14.61	14.75	14.87	14.97	15.07	15.16	15.23	15.30
16	13.23	13.44	13.61	13.76	13.89	14.00	14.11	14.20	14.28	14.35	14.42
15	12.42	12.61	12.77	12.91	13.03	13.14	13.24	13.32	13.40	13.46	13.53
14	11.60	11.78	11.93	12.06	12.18	12.28	12.36	12.44	12.51	12.58	12.64
13	10.78	10.95	11.09	11.21	11.32	11.41	11.49	11.56	11.63	11.69	11.74
12	9.96	10.11	10.24	10.36	10.45	10.54	10.62	10.68	10.75	10.80	10.85
11	9.14	9.28	9.40	9.50	9.59	9.67	9.74	9.80	9.86	9.91	9.96
10	8.31	8.44	8.55	8.64	8.73	8.80	8.86	8.92	8.97	9.02	9.06
9	7.49	7.60	7.70	7.79	7.86	7.93	7.98	8.03	8.08	8.12	8.16
8	6.66	6.77	6.85	6.93	6.99	7.05	7.10	7.15	7.19	7.23	7.26
7	5.83	5.92	6.00	6.07	6.13	6.18	6.22	6.26	6.30	6.33	6.36
6	5.01	5.08	5.15	5.21	5.26	5.30	5.34	5.37	5.40	5.43	5.45
5	4.17	4.24	4.29	4.34	4.38	4.42	4.45	4.48	4.51	4.53	4.55
4	3.34	3.39	3.44	3.48	3.51	3.54	3.56	3.59	3.61	3.63	3.64
3	2.51	2.55	2.58	2.61	2.63	2.66	2.68	2.69	2.71	2.72	2.73
2	1.67	1.70	1.72	1.74	1.76	1.77	1.79	1.80	1.81	1.82	1.83
1	0.84	0.85	0.86	0.87	0.88	0.89	0.89	0.90	0.90	0.91	0.91
0	0.00	0.00	0.00	0.00	0.00	0.00	0.00	0.00	0.00	0.00	0.00
− 1	0.84	0.85	0.86	0.87	0.88	0.89	0.90	0.90	0.91	0.91	0.92
2	1.68	1.71	1.73	1.75	1.76	1.78	1.79	1.80	1.81	1.82	1.83
3	2.52	2.56	2.59	2.62	2.65	2.67	2.69	2.71	2.72	2.74	2.75
4	3.37	3.42	3.46	3.50	3.53	3.56	3.59	3.61	3.63	3.65	3.67
5	4.21	4.28	4.33	4.38	4.42	4.46	4.49	4.52	4.55	4.57	4.59
6	5.06	5.14	5.20	5.26	5.31	5.35	5.39	5.43	5.46	5.49	5.51
7	5.91	6.00	6.08	6.14	6.20	6.25	6.30	6.34	6.38	6.41	6.44
8	6.75	6.86	6.95	7.03	7.09	7.15	7.20	7.25	7.29	7.33	7.36
9	7.61	7.72	7.82	7.91	7.99	8.05	8.11	8.16	8.21	8.25	8.29
10	8.46	8.59	8.70	8.80	8.88	8.96	9.02	9.08	9.13	9.18	9.22
11	9.31	9.46	9.58	9.69	9.78	9.86	9.93	10.00	10.05	10.11	10.15
12	10.17	10.33	10.46	10.58	10.68	10.77	10.85	10.92	10.98	11.04	11.09
13	11.02	11.20	11.34	11.47	11.58	11.67	11.76	11.84	11.90	11.97	12.02
14	11.88	12.07	12.23	12.36	12.48	12.58	12.68	12.76	12.83	12.90	12.96
15	12.74	12.94	13.11	13.26	13.38	13.49	13.59	13.68	13.76	13.83	13.90
16	13.60	13.82	14.00	14.15	14.29	14.41	14.51	14.61	14.69	14.77	14.84
17	14.47	14.69	14.88	15.05	15.19	15.32	15.43	15.53	15.62	15.70	15.78
18	15.33	15.57	15.77	15.95	16.10	16.24	16.36	16.46	16.56	16.64	16.72
19	16.20	16.45	16.67	16.85	17.01	17.15	17.28	17.39	17.49	17.58	17.67
20	17.06	17.33	17.56	17.75	17.92	18.07	18.21	18.32	18.43	18.53	18.61
21	17.93	18.21	18.45	18.66	18.84	18.99	19.13	19.26	19.37	19.47	19.56
22	18.80	19.10	19.35	19.56	19.75	19.92	20.06	20.19	20.31	20.42	20.51
23	19.67	19.98	20.25	20.47	20.67	20.84	20.99	21.13	21.25	21.36	21.46
24	20.55	20.87	21.14	21.38	21.59	21.77	21.93	22.07	22.20	22.31	22.42
25	21.42	21.76	22.05	22.29	22.51	22.69	22.86	23.01	23.14	23.26	23.37
26	22.30	22.65	22.95	23.20	23.43	23.62	23.80	23.95	24.09	24.22	24.33
27	23.18	23.54	23.85	24.12	24.35	24.55	24.74	24.90	25.04	25.17	25.29
28	24.06	24.43	24.76	25.03	25.28	25.49	25.67	25.84	25.99	26.13	26.25
29	24.94	25.33	25.66	25.95	26.20	26.42	26.62	26.79	26.95	27.08	27.21
30	25.82	26.23	26.57	26.87	27.13	27.36	27.56	27.74	27.90	28.04	28.18

Table D.XXVIII Centre thickness 1.50 mm

Back vertex powers (D)	Front vertex powers (D) for back optic zone radii										
	5.0 mm	5.5 mm	6.0 mm	6.5 mm	7.0 mm	7.5 mm	8.0 mm	8.5 mm	9.0 mm	9.5 mm	10.0 mm
+ 20	16.27	16.54	16.77	16.96	17.13	17.28	17.41	17.53	17.64	17.73	17.82
19	15.47	15.72	15.94	16.03	16.29	16.43	16.56	16.67	16.77	16.86	16.95
18	14.67	14.91	15.12	15.29	15.45	15.58	15.70	15.81	15.91	15.99	16.07
17	13.87	14.10	14.29	14.46	14.60	14.73	14.84	14.94	15.04	15.12	15.19
16	13.06	13.28	13.46	13.62	13.76	13.88	13.98	14.08	14.16	14.24	14.31
15	12.26	12.46	12.63	12.78	12.91	13.02	13.12	13.21	13.29	13.36	13.43
14	11.45	11.64	11.80	11.94	12.06	12.16	12.26	12.34	12.42	12.48	12.55
13	10.64	10.82	10.97	11.10	11.21	11.31	11.39	11.47	11.54	11.60	11.66
12	9.83	9.99	10.13	10.25	10.36	10.45	10.53	10.60	10.66	10.72	10.77
11	9.02	9.17	9.30	9.41	9.50	9.59	9.66	9.73	9.78	9.84	9.89
10	8.21	8.34	8.46	8.56	8.65	8.72	8.79	8.85	8.90	8.95	9.00
9	7.40	7.52	7.62	7.71	7.79	7.86	7.92	7.97	8.02	8.06	8.10
8	6.58	6.69	6.78	6.86	6.93	6.99	7.04	7.09	7.14	7.17	7.21
7	5.76	5.81	5.94	6.01	6.07	6.12	6.17	6.21	6.25	6.28	6.32
6	4.94	5.03	5.10	5.15	5.21	5.25	5.29	5.33	5.36	5.39	5.42
5	4.12	4.19	4.25	4.30	4.34	4.38	4.42	4.45	4.47	4.50	4.52
4	3.30	3.36	3.40	3.44	3.48	3.51	3.54	3.56	3.58	3.60	3.62
3	2.48	2.52	2.55	2.58	2.61	2.63	2.65	2.67	2.69	2.70	2.72
2	1.65	1.68	1.70	1.72	1.74	1.76	1.77	1.78	1.79	1.80	1.81
1	0.83	0.84	0.85	0.86	0.87	0.88	0.89	0.89	0.90	0.90	0.91
0	0.00	0.00	0.00	0.00	0.00	0.00	0.00	0.00	0.00	0.00	0.00
− 1	0.83	0.84	0.86	0.87	0.87	0.88	0.89	0.89	0.90	0.91	0.91
2	1.66	1.69	1.71	1.73	1.75	1.76	1.78	1.79	1.80	1.81	1.82
3	2.49	2.53	2.57	2.60	2.63	2.65	2.67	2.69	2.70	2.72	2.73
4	3.33	3.38	3.43	3.47	3.50	3.54	3.56	3.59	3.61	3.63	3.65
5	4.16	4.23	4.29	4.34	4.38	4.42	4.46	4.49	4.52	4.54	4.56
6	5.00	5.08	5.15	5.21	5.27	5.31	5.35	5.39	5.42	5.45	5.48
7	5.84	5.93	6.02	6.09	6.15	6.20	6.25	6.30	6.33	6.37	6.40
8	6.68	6.79	6.88	6.96	7.03	7.10	7.15	7.20	7.25	7.29	7.32
9	7.52	7.64	7.75	7.84	7.92	7.99	8.05	8.11	8.16	8.20	8.25
10	8.36	8.50	8.62	8.72	8.81	8.89	8.96	9.02	9.07	9.12	9.17
11	9.21	9.36	9.49	9.60	9.70	9.79	9.86	9.93	9.99	10.05	10.10
12	10.05	10.22	10.36	10.48	10.59	10.69	10.77	10.84	10.91	10.97	11.03
13	10.90	11.08	11.24	11.37	11.49	11.59	11.68	11.76	11.83	11.90	11.96
14	11.75	11.94	12.11	12.26	12.38	12.49	12.59	12.68	12.75	12.82	12.89
15	12.60	12.81	12.99	13.14	13.28	13.40	13.50	13.59	13.68	13.75	13.82
16	13.45	13.68	13.87	14.03	14.18	14.30	14.41	14.51	14.60	14.68	14.76
17	14.31	14.54	14.75	14.92	15.08	15.21	15.33	15.44	15.53	15.62	15.70
18	15.16	15.41	15.63	15.82	15.98	16.12	16.25	16.36	16.46	16.55	16.64
19	16.02	16.29	16.52	16.71	16.88	17.03	17.17	17.29	17.39	17.49	17.58
20	16.88	17.16	17.40	17.61	17.79	17.95	18.09	18.21	18.33	18.43	18.52
21	17.74	18.03	18.29	18.51	18.70	18.86	19.01	19.14	19.26	19.37	19.46
22	18.60	18.91	19.18	19.40	19.60	19.78	19.94	20.07	20.20	20.31	20.41
23	19.47	19.79	20.07	20.31	20.52	20.70	20.86	21.01	21.14	21.25	21.36
24	20.33	20.67	20.96	21.21	21.43	21.62	21.79	21.94	22.08	22.20	22.31
25	21.20	21.50	21.85	22.11	22.34	22.54	22.72	22.88	23.02	23.15	23.26
26	22.07	22.43	22.75	23.02	23.26	23.47	23.65	23.82	23.96	24.10	24.22
27	22.94	23.32	23.65	23.93	24.18	24.39	24.58	24.76	24.91	25.05	25.17
28	23.81	24.21	24.55	24.84	25.10	25.32	25.52	25.70	25.86	26.00	26.13
29	24.68	25.09	25.45	25.76	26.02	26.25	26.46	26.64	26.81	26.96	27.09
30	25.56	25.98	26.35	26.66	26.94	27.18	27.40	27.59	27.76	27.91	28.05

Table D.XXIX Centre thickness 1.60 mm

Back vertex powers (D)	Front vertex powers (D) for back optic zone radii										
	5.0 mm	5.5 mm	6.0 mm	6.5 mm	7.0 mm	7.5 mm	8.0 mm	8.5 mm	9.0 mm	9.5 mm	10.0 mm
+ 20	16.06	16.34	16.58	16.78	16.96	17.12	17.26	17.39	17.50	17.60	17.69
19	15.27	15.54	15.76	15.96	16.13	16.28	16.41	16.53	16.64	16.73	16.82
18	14.48	14.73	14.95	15.13	15.30	15.44	15.57	15.68	15.78	15.87	15.95
17	13.69	13.93	14.13	14.31	14.46	14.60	14.71	14.82	14.92	15.00	15.08
16	12.90	13.12	13.31	13.48	13.62	13.75	13.86	13.96	14.05	14.13	14.21
15	12.10	12.31	12.49	12.65	12.78	12.90	13.01	13.10	13.19	13.26	13.33
14	11.31	11.50	11.67	11.82	11.94	12.06	12.15	12.24	12.32	12.39	12.46
13	10.51	10.69	10.85	10.98	11.10	11.21	11.30	11.38	11.45	11.52	11.58
12	9.71	9.88	10.02	10.15	10.26	10.35	10.44	10.51	10.58	10.64	10.70
11	8.91	9.06	9.20	9.31	9.41	9.50	9.58	9.65	9.71	9.77	9.82
10	8.11	8.25	8.37	8.47	8.57	8.65	8.72	8.78	8.84	8.89	8.93
9	7.30	7.43	7.54	7.63	7.72	7.79	7.85	7.91	7.96	8.01	8.05
8	6.50	6.61	6.71	6.79	6.87	6.93	6.99	7.04	7.08	7.12	7.16
7	5.69	5.79	5.88	5.95	6.01	6.07	6.12	6.16	6.20	6.24	6.27
6	4.88	4.97	5.04	5.10	5.16	5.21	5.25	5.29	5.32	5.35	5.38
5	4.07	4.14	4.21	4.26	4.30	4.34	4.38	4.41	4.44	4.47	4.49
4	3.26	3.32	3.37	3.41	3.45	3.48	3.51	3.53	3.56	3.58	3.60
3	2.45	2.49	2.53	2.56	2.59	2.61	2.63	2.65	2.67	2.69	2.70
2	1.63	1.66	1.69	1.71	1.73	1.74	1.76	1.77	1.78	1.79	1.80
1	0.82	0.83	0.84	0.86	0.86	0.87	0.88	0.89	0.89	0.90	0.90
0	0.00	0.00	0.00	0.00	0.00	0.00	0.00	0.00	0.00	0.00	0.00
− 1	0.82	0.83	0.85	0.86	0.87	0.87	0.88	0.89	0.89	0.90	0.90
2	1.64	1.67	1.69	1.72	1.73	1.75	1.76	1.78	1.79	1.80	1.81
3	2.46	2.51	2.54	2.58	2.60	2.63	2.65	2.67	2.69	2.70	2.72
4	3.29	3.35	3.39	3.44	3.47	3.51	3.54	3.56	3.59	3.61	3.63
5	4.11	4.19	4.25	4.30	4.35	4.39	4.42	4.46	4.49	4.51	4.54
6	4.94	5.03	5.10	5.17	5.22	5.27	5.31	5.35	5.39	5.42	5.45
7	5.77	5.87	5.96	6.03	6.10	6.16	6.21	6.25	6.29	6.33	6.36
8	6.60	6.72	6.82	6.90	6.98	7.04	7.10	7.15	7.20	7.24	7.28
9	7.43	7.56	7.68	7.77	7.86	7.93	8.00	8.06	8.11	8.16	8.20
10	8.27	8.41	8.54	8.64	8.74	8.82	8.89	8.96	9.02	9.07	9.12
11	9.10	9.26	9.40	9.52	9.62	9.71	9.79	9.87	9.93	9.99	10.04
12	9.94	10.11	10.27	10.39	10.51	10.61	10.69	10.77	10.84	10.91	10.97
13	10.78	10.97	11.13	11.27	11.39	11.50	11.60	11.68	11.76	11.83	11.89
14	11.62	11.82	12.00	12.15	12.28	12.40	12.50	12.59	12.68	12.75	12.82
15	12.46	12.68	12.87	13.03	13.17	13.30	13.41	13.51	13.60	13.68	13.75
16	13.31	13.54	13.74	13.91	14.07	14.20	14.32	14.42	14.52	14.60	14.68
17	14.15	14.40	14.62	14.80	14.96	15.10	15.23	15.34	15.44	15.53	15.61
18	15.00	15.26	15.49	15.68	15.86	16.01	16.14	16.26	16.37	16.46	16.55
19	15.85	16.13	16.37	16.57	16.75	16.91	17.05	17.18	17.29	17.39	17.49
20	16.70	16.99	17.25	17.46	17.65	17.82	17.97	18.10	18.22	18.33	18.43
21	17.55	17.86	18.13	18.36	18.56	18.73	18.89	19.03	19.15	19.27	19.37
22	18.40	18.73	19.01	19.25	19.46	19.64	19.81	19.95	20.09	20.20	20.31
23	19.26	19.60	19.89	20.14	20.36	20.56	20.73	20.88	21.02	21.14	21.26
24	20.12	20.47	20.78	21.04	21.27	21.47	21.65	21.81	21.96	22.09	22.20
25	20.98	21.35	21.67	21.94	22.18	22.39	22.58	22.75	22.90	23.03	23.15
26	21.84	22.22	22.56	22.84	23.09	23.31	23.51	23.68	23.84	23.98	24.11
27	22.70	23.10	23.45	23.74	24.00	24.23	24.44	24.62	24.78	24.93	25.06
28	23.56	23.98	24.34	24.65	24.92	25.16	25.37	25.55	25.72	25.88	26.01
29	24.43	24.86	25.24	25.55	25.84	26.08	26.30	26.49	26.67	26.83	26.97
30	25.30	25.75	26.13	26.46	26.75	27.01	27.24	27.44	27.62	27.78	27.93

Appendix E: Visual optics and contact lens calculations, computer programs

The following programs were written on an Amstrad PC1640 HD20 which is said to be compatible with the IBM PC so they should run on similar computers. The language used is BASIC 2. The programs enable many calculations to be completed easily and rapidly, and they obviate the need for numerous tables.

To use the programs it is, of course, necessary to enter them into your computer. This is a bit tedious but should only need to be done once as, once entered, they can be recorded onto a floppy disk. The programs have been written so that each of them will run on its own in case one does not wish to use (or enter) all of them. A MENU or INDEX is provided (lines 100 to 450) which facilitates the work and speeds up the process, especially if a number of programs have to be used in the calculation.

Whether you use the entire listing or just one or two programs, the computer will request the information it needs to complete the calculation as and when it is required. It will also give an example of the order and the form in which data should be presented where appropriate. The Amstrad computer treats all numbers as positive values unless they are preceded by a minus sign so there is no need to use the plus sign when entering positive lens powers.

The following notes, which apply to the Amstrad computer, may be helpful to those who are not accustomed to entering computer programs. Users of other makes of computer should consult their users' manual.

Programs are entered into the BASIC 2 APP file, access to which is via GEM Desktop. Having opened the BASIC2 application, press the key F10 to select 'EDIT' mode and expand the EDIT window to full screen size by clicking the mouse arrow on the diamond in the top right corner of the EDIT window. This makes it much easier to read the program as it is being entered and the length of the program lines will correspond more closely to those on the printed page. All that is required now is to type the program lines *exactly* as printed. The following points should be noted.

1. Lines beginning with REM are not essential to the running of the program and may be omitted.
2. A program line may occupy more than one line on the printed page or on the screen.
3. Each program line begins with a line number.
4. The '£' symbol appears frequently in the programs. This is due to a peculiarity of the author's printer and the hash symbol '#' should be entered whenever the '£' symbol is printed.
5. When you reach the end of a program line press the carriage return key before typing the number of the next line.
6. It is absolutely essential that every detail of the program is entered precisely as printed including punctuation marks and spaces. For example, the following version of program line 280 would fail and stop the running of the program because it requires a comma (not a semicolon) between the third and fourth numbers after the word BOX. The line would also fail if there was not a space between the word BOX and the figure 5.

```
280  PRINT AT(1;1)    "To CANCEL & begin again;  press Ctrl & C  together;
release both; then press F9": BOX 5;4765,8530;270 COLOUR 4
```

Similarly, the following version of line 290 would fail because it must have a semicolon (not a comma) between the third and fourth numbers after the word LINE.

```
290  PRINT AT(28;20)"Then press RETURN":  LINE  4965;368,5165,368,5165;600
START 1
```

Fortunately the computer is very helpful and, if an attempt is made to run a program in which there is a syntax error, the program will stop automatically, switch itself to EDIT mode and display the relevant section of the program with the cursor indicating the offending line.

7. Having entered the program you must record it. Put the mouse arrow onto the word File at the top left corner of the screen, then click on the word Save. Before clicking on OK the program must be given a name so that it can be found on the disk later. The filename can have up to eight letters, then a full stop, followed by a three letter filetype. A suitable name would be OPTICALC.BAS. Using BAS as the filetype causes the program to run automatically each time it is loaded, otherwise pressing the key F9 will start the program running. Type your chosen name and filetype, then click on OK or press the carriage return key.

Ocular *RX* (effectivity) program, lines 460–680 (index no. 8)

Given the vertex distance and spectacle *Rx* this program will calculate the ocular *Rx* taking account of astigmatic refraction.

Corneal astigmatism program, lines 690–830 (index no. 5)

Given the K readings this program will calculate the corneal astigmatism.

Induced cyl, and back surface cyl, in air program, lines 840–970 (index nos 4 and 1)

Given the back optic zone radii this program will calculate either the power of the cyl produced by the back surface in air or the power of the cyl induced when the lens is worn.

The same mathematics are used in both of these programs but, because the presentation of the results is different, the computer needs a marker to tell it which result you require. This is done automatically if the full program (including the MENU) is used but if the program is entered without the MENU it will be necessary to type m1=1 into the Dialogue window, then press the carriage return key, before running the program if the back surface cyl in air is required or m1=4 if you want the induced cyl (on the eye).

Sag and edge lift program, lines 980–1910 (index nos 11, 12 and 2)

Given the surface specifications this program will calculate either the sag of a single spherical surface, the primary sag or the axial and radial edge lift of a multicurve spherical lens.

The same mathematics are used in both of these programs but, because the presentation of the results is different, the computer needs a marker to tell it which result you require. This is done automatically if the full program (including the MENU) is used but if the program is entered without the MENU it will be necessary to type m1=2:f=0:GOTO 1040 into the Dialogue window, then press the carriage return key, before running the program if the edge lift is required, m1=11 if the sag of a single spherical surface is needed or m1=12:f=1:GOTO 1040 if the primary sag of a multicurve spherical lens is required.

Obliquely crossed cyl program, lines 1920–2440 (index no. 7)

This program will calculate the *Rx* resulting from the combination of any two sphero/cyl or plano/cyl lenses. Lens powers may be entered in either + or − cyl transposition, or in any combination of transpositions. 0 should be entered for plano.

The effective power of the second lens, in the plane of the first lens is given if vertex distance is significant, then the resultant lens in both + and − cyl transpositions is given with the powers rounded to 0.01 D. Finally the resultant lens is shown with the powers rounded to the nearest 0.25 D. In all cases the cyl axis is rounded to the nearest half degree.

It may be noticed that occasionally, in the 0.25 D version, there is a discrepancy of 0.25 D between the + and − cyl transpositions. This is not an error. The accurate values are used for the internal calculations and the results shown are within 0.25 D of the accurate figure. The discrepancy occurs in cases where simply to transpose the first *Rx* would double the rounded margin of error and render the result outside the required tolerance.

The program can eliminate vertex distance problems with highly ametropic patients if over refraction is carried out with the patient wearing their own glasses and, because it takes account of vertex distance it can be used to combine over refraction and contact lens power.

Power changes due to the flexure of rigid lenses, lines 2450–3150 (index no. 9)

Given the original BOZR, BOZD, FOZD, BVP, t_c, TD, and refractive index, and K readings of the front surface of the lens, the program will calculate the power change in air and the effective power change *in situ*, taking account of the cyls produced by flexure at both surfaces of the lens and at the front surface of the tear lens.

Front optic zone radius program, lines 3160–3290 (index no. 3)

Given the BOZR, BVP, t_c, and refractive index the program calculates the FOZR.

Multicurve spherical lens design program, lines 3300–4090 (index no. 6)

This program will design the back surface of C2, C3, or C4 spherical lenses. It offers you a number of choices. It can design a 'standard' lens having 9.50 mm TD, or a 'one off' lens, the dimensions of which you are free to choose. You may stipulate the total edge lift the lens should have or the edge lift to be provided by each peripheral zone individually. You may also stipulate the accuracy to which the calculated peripheral zone radii should be rounded.

The quit program, lines 4100–4130 (index no. 10)

This short program simply restores the graphic screen to normal so that the BASIC 2 facility can be used for other calculations.

Computer programs

```
        REM collected programmes for visual optics & contact lens calculations.
Feb. 1989.  Line 100 sets up the graphics screen.
100 WINDOW £2 CLOSE: CLOSE WINDOW 3: CLOSE WINDOW 4: WINDOW £1 FULL ON: CLS
110 PRINT AT(16;3)"VISUAL OPTICS AND CONTACT LENS CALCULATIONS."
120 LINE 1655;4291,6409;4291: PRINT AT(34;4)"Feb.1989.": OPTION TRAP ON
130    REM this menu allows the selection of any desired program section.
140 PRINT AT(15;5)"Index No.                        Category."
150 LINE 1545;3823,2428;3823: LINE 5184;3823,6088;3823
160 PRINT AT(19;6)"1                        Back surface Cyl. in air."
170 PRINT AT(19;7)"2                        Edge lift of known lens."
180 PRINT AT(19;8)"3                        Front optic zone radius."
190 PRINT AT(19;9)"4                        Induced Cyl."
200 PRINT AT(19;10)"5                        K.Astigmatism."
210 PRINT AT(19;11)"6                        Multicurve spherical lens design."
220 PRINT AT(19;12)"7                        Obliquely crossed Cyls."
230 PRINT AT(19;13)"8                        Ocular Rx.(Effectivity)"
240 PRINT AT(19;14)"9                        Power change due to flexure."
250 PRINT AT(18;15)"10                       QUIT."
260 PRINT AT(18;16)"11                       Sag of spherical surface."
270 PRINT AT(18;17)"12                       Sag of multicurve spherical lens."
280 PRINT AT(1;1)    "To CANCEL & begin again; press Ctrl & C together; release
both; then press F9": BOX 5;4765,8530,270 COLOUR 4
290 PRINT AT(28;20)"Then press RETURN": LINE 4965;368,5165;368,5165;600 START 1
300 INPUT AT(19;19)"Please type your chosen index number;",m1
310 IF (m1<1)OR(m1>12) THEN GOTO 430
320 IF (m1=1)OR(m1=4) THEN GOTO 850
330 IF m1 = 2 THEN f = 0: GOTO 1040
340 IF m1 = 3 THEN GOTO 3170
350 IF m1 = 5 THEN GOTO 700
360 IF m1 = 6 THEN GOTO 3310
370 IF m1 = 7 THEN GOTO 1930
380 IF m1 = 8 THEN GOTO 470
390 IF m1 = 9 THEN GOTO 2450
400 IF m1 = 10 THEN GOTO 4100
410 IF m1 = 11 THEN GOTO 990
420 IF m1 = 12 THEN f = 1: GOTO 1040
430 PRINT AT(4;2)CHR$(7);CHR$(7);CHR$(96)m1"´is an invalid index number; please
choose another number(1 to 12)"
440 LINE 6178;650,6778;650 WIDTH 5 COLOUR 2 START 1
450 BOX 235;4510,7856,290 WIDTH 3 COLOUR 2: GOTO 300

              REM ***Start of effectivity program.***
460 CLS: WINDOW £1 FULL ON: WINDOW £2 CLOSE: CLOSE WINDOW 3: CLOSE WINDOW 4
470 CLS: OPTION TRAP ON: PRINT AT(29;11)"y = yes / n = no": c = 0: GOSUB 660
480 PRINT AT(30;15)"Type ";CHR$(96)"y´ or ";CHR$(96)"n´";
490 INPUT AT(21;7)"Does the spectacle Rx.have a Cyl.";q$:CLS:GOSUB 660:GOSUB 680
500 PRINT AT(12;6)"Please type spectacle Rx. and vertex distance(in mm.)"
510 PRINT AT(9;7)"using commas to separate each item. ";
520 IF q$="y" THEN PRINT "eg. 12.75, -4.25, 165, 11":  LINE 7640;1740,7640;3370
COLOUR 2 END 1 ELSE PRINT "eg. 8.75, 11":LINE 6210;1740,6210;3370 COLOUR 2 END 1
530 IF q$="y" THEN INPUT AT(49;9)"",specsph,speccyl,ax,vd ELSE INPUT AT(49;9)"",
specsph,vd
540 IF q$ = "n" THEN speccyl = 0
550 IF (specsph=0)OR((specsph+speccyl)=0) THEN specsph = specsph + .001
560 IF vd => 0 THEN bvd = (0 - vd)/1000 ELSE bvd = vd/1000
570 CLS:orf = 1/(1/specsph+bvd):ors = 1/(1/(specsph+speccyl)+bvd):oastig=ors-orf
580 PRINT AT(16;8)"Spectacle Rx. "ROUND(specsph,2)"Sph.";
590 IF speccyl <> 0 THEN PRINT"/";speccyl"Cyl.Ax.";ax
600 PRINT AT(25;10)"At bvd";vd"mm. becomes:-"
610 PRINT AT(19;12)"Ocular Rx. "ROUND(orf,2)"Sph.";
620 IF speccyl <> 0 THEN PRINT"/"ROUND(oastig,2)"Cyl.Ax.";ax
630 PRINT AT(30;17)"Type ";CHR$(96)"y´ or ";CHR$(96)"n´": GOSUB 660
```

Effectivity program (*contd*)

```
640 INPUT AT(25;15)"Again.? y = yes / n = no",q$
650 IF q$ = "y" THEN GOTO 470 ELSE RUN
660 PRINT AT(28;20)"Then press RETURN": LINE 4965;368,5165;368,5165;600 START 1
670 PRINT AT(1;1)    "To CANCEL & begin again; press Ctrl & C together; release
both; then press F9": BOX 5;4765,8530,270 COLOUR 4: RETURN
680 BOX 432;1470,7612,270 COLOUR 2:  PRINT AT(6;15)"Please note that a comma is
NOT required after the last data entry.": RETURN

          REM ***Start of K. astigmatism program.***
690 CLS: WINDOW £1 FULL ON: WINDOW £2 CLOSE: CLOSE WINDOW 3: CLOSE WINDOW 4
700 CLS: OPTION TRAP ON:  PRINT AT(14;6)"Please type K. readings(in mm.),  flat
meridian first,";
710 PRINT AT(14;7)"and axes,  using commas to separate each item.": GOSUB 810
720 PRINT AT(29;9)"eg. 8.27,180, 7.94,90":LINE 5430;1740,5430;2903COLOUR 2 END 1
730 GOSUB 830: INPUT AT(33;11)"",kf,afl,ks,ast
740 BOX 432;1470,7612,270 COLOUR 0: LINE 5430;1740,5430;2903 COLOUR 0 END 1
750 PRINT AT(6;15)"
          " :ff = 337.5/kf: fs = 337.5/ks: kastig = ff - fs
760 PRINT AT(20;16)"Power of cornea is ";ROUND(ff,2)"D. along";afl
770 PRINT AT(20;17)" ''    ''    ''    '' ";ROUND(fs,2)"D. along";ast
780 LINE 4303;1015, 4854;1015: BOX 1645;768,4900,280 COLOUR 2
790 PRINT AT(17;18)"Corneal astigmatism is ";ROUND((ff-fs),2)"D.Cyl.Ax.";afl
800 INPUT AT(25;20)"Again.? y = yes / n = no",q$:IF q$="y"THEN GOTO 700 ELSE RUN
810 PRINT AT(28;20)"Then press RETURN": LINE 4965;368,5165;368,5165;600 START 1
820 PRINT AT(1;1)    "To CANCEL & begin again; press Ctrl & C together; release
both; then press F9": BOX 5;4765,8530,270 COLOUR 4: RETURN
830 BOX 432;1470,7612,270 COLOUR 2:  PRINT AT(6;15)"Please note that a comma is
NOT required after the last data entry.": RETURN

          REM ***Start of air & induced cyl. programs.***
840 CLS: WINDOW £1 FULL ON: WINDOW £2 CLOSE: CLOSE WINDOW 3: CLOSE WINDOW 4
850 CLS: OPTION TRAP ON: PRINT AT(11;6)"Please type back optic zone radii,(flat
meridian first)"
860 PRINT AT(11;7)"and refractive index,  using commas to separate each item."
870 PRINT AT(30;9)"eg.  8.25, 7.75, 1.49":LINE 5540;1740,5540;2903COLOUR 2 END 1
880 BOX 432;1470,7612,270 COLOUR 2:  PRINT AT(6;15)"Please note that a comma is
NOT required after the last data entry.": GOSUB 960
890 INPUT AT(35;11)"",bozrf,bozrs,u: ua = (u-1)*1000: ub = (u - 1.336)*1000
900 indcyl = ub/bozrf - ub/bozrs: bacyl = ua/bozrf - ua/bozrs: CLS:GOSUB 970
910 PRINT AT(12;11)"For toric surface"bozrf"/"bozrs"of refractive index"u
920 IF m1=1 THEN PRINT AT(1;15)"The back surface Cyl.in air is ";ROUND(bacyl,2)"
D. axis along the flat(";bozrf")meridian.";ELSE PRINT AT(7;15)"The induced Cyl.
is ";ROUND(indcyl,2)"D. axis along the flat(";bozrf")meridian."
930 IF m1=1 THEN BOX 10;1470,8496,270COLOUR 2 ELSE BOX 502;1470,7332,270COLOUR 2
940 PRINT AT(30;19)"Type ";CHR$(96)"y´ or ";CHR$(96)"n´": GOSUB 960
950 INPUT AT(25;17)"Again.? y = yes / n = no",q$:IF q$="y"THEN GOTO 850 ELSE RUN
960 PRINT AT(28;20)"Then press RETURN": LINE 4965;368,5165;368,5165;600 START 1
970      PRINT AT(1;1)"To CANCEL & begin again; press Ctrl & C together; release
both; then press F9": BOX 5;4765,8530,270 COLOUR 4: RETURN

          REM *** Start of edge lift & sag program.***
980 CLS: WINDOW £1 FULL ON: WINDOW £2 CLOSE: CLOSE WINDOW 3: CLOSE WINDOW 4
990 CLS:  OPTION TRAP ON:  PRINT AT(14;7)      "Please type Radius and Diameter,
separated by a comma";
1000 PRINT AT(31;9)"eg.       7.95, 9.5": LINE 5210;1740,5210;2903 COLOUR 2 END 1:
 GOSUB 1850: GOSUB 1870
1010 INPUT AT(39;10)"",ro,bozd: s = ro - SQR(ro^2-(bozd/2)^2): CLS: GOSUB 1850
1020 PRINT AT(3;8)"The sag of radius"ro"mm., over a diameter of"bozd"mm.,rounded
 to 0.0001": PRINT AT(30;10)"is  "ROUND(s,4): BOX 3520;2640,1103,270 COLOUR 2
1030 GOSUB 1880: IF q$ = "y" THEN GOTO 990 ELSE RUN
1040 CLS: PRINT AT(13;8)"Please type the number of zones there are on the back";
1050 GOSUB 1850: INPUT AT(13;9)"surface of the lens, including the BOZR.",q1
```

Sag and edge lift program (*contd*)

```
1060 IF q1 > 5 THEN GOTO 1830
1070 IF q1 < 2 THEN GOTO 1840
1080 CLS:PRINT AT(7;6)"Please type the specification of the back surface of the
lens ": PRINT AT(7;8)"using commas to separate each item.": GOSUB 1850
1090 GOSUB 1870: IF q1 = 3 THEN GOTO 1230
1100 IF q1 = 4 THEN GOTO 1370
1110 IF q1 = 5 THEN GOTO 1510
1120 PRINT AT(11;7)"in the following sequence;  BOZR,BOZD,  BPR1,TD"
1130 PRINT AT(22;10)"eg.  7.85,7.5,  10.5,8.6  (for a C2 lens)"
1140 LINE 4990;1740,4990;2669 COLOUR 2 END 1
1150 INPUT AT(27;12)"",ro,bozd,bpr1,bpd1: GOSUB 1540
1160 PRINT AT(21;9)USING"The C2 lens  £.££:£.££/ £.££:£.££"ro;bozd;bpr1;bpd1
1170 IF f = 1 THEN PRINT AT(19;7)"The primary sag,(rounded to 0.0001),of":PRINT
AT(30;10)"is  "ROUND((s1+s2-s3),4): GOSUB 1900: GOSUB 1880: GOTO 1220
1180 PRINT AT(19;10)"will provide the following edge lift:-"
1190 PRINT AT(28;12)"AXIAL        RADIAL"
1200 LINE 2979;2184,3531;2184: LINE 4303;2184,4965;2184
1210 PRINT AT(27;13)USING"£.££££"ROUND(ael1,4):       PRINT AT(34;13)USING"mm.
£.££££"ROUND(rel1,4):PRINT AT(47;13)"mm.": GOSUB 1880
1220 IF q$ = "y" THEN GOTO 1040 ELSE RUN
1230 PRINT AT(7;7)"in the following sequence;  BOZR,BOZD, BPR1,BPD1,  BPR2,TD"
1240 PRINT AT(16;10)"eg.  7.9,7,  9.15,7.8,  11.2,8.6  (for a C3 lens)"
1250 LINE 5210;1740,5210;2669 COLOUR 2 END 1
1260 INPUT AT(21;12)"",ro,bozd,bpr1,bpd1,bpr2,bpd2: GOSUB 1540
1270 PRINT AT(17;8)USING"  The C3 lens  £.££:£.££/ £.££:£.££/ £.££:£.££"ro;bozd
bpr1;bpd1;bpr2;bpd2
1280 IF f = 1 THEN PRINT AT(19;6)"The primary sag,(rounded to 0.0001),of":PRINT
AT(30;10)"is  "ROUND((s1+s2-s3+s4-s5),4): GOSUB 1900: GOSUB 1880: GOTO 1360
1290 PRINT AT(2;9)"will provide the following edge lift:-";
1300 PRINT AT(14;11)"AXIAL          RADIAL"
1310 LINE 1434;2418,1986;2418: LINE 3088;2418,3750;2418
1320 PRINT AT(13;12)USING"£.££££"ROUND(ael1,4):  PRINT AT(19;12)USING" mm.
£.££££"ROUND(rel1,4):PRINT AT(36;12)"mm. From the 1st. back peripheral zone ";
1330 PRINT AT(13;13)USING"£.££££"ROUND(ael2,4):  PRINT AT(19;13)USING" mm.
£.££££"ROUND(rel2,4):PRINT AT(36;13)"mm.  '  ''  2nd. '' '  '' ''";
LINE 1434;1950,2096;1950: LINE 3088;1950,3750;1950
1340 PRINT AT(7;14)USING"Total £.££££"ROUND((ael1+ael2),4): PRINT AT(36;14)"mm.'
1350 PRINT AT(20;14)USING"mm.      £.££££"ROUND((rel1+rel2),4): GOSUB 1880
1360 IF q$ = "y" THEN GOTO 1040 ELSE RUN
1370 PRINT AT(5;7)" in the following sequence; BOZR,BOZD, BPR1,BPD1, BPR2,BPD2,
BPR3,TD": LINE 5541;1740,5541;2669 COLOUR 2 END 1
1380 PRINT AT(9;10)"eg. 8.1,7,  8.95,7.8,  10.1,8.6,  11.3,9.2  (for a C4 lens)'
1390 INPUT AT(13;12)"",ro,bozd,bpr1,bpd1,bpr2,bpd2,bpr3,bpd3: GOSUB 1540
1400 PRINT AT(9;7)USING"The C4 lens  £.££:£.££/ £.££:£.££/ £.££:£.££/ £.££:£.££'
ro;bozd;bpr1;bpd1;bpr2;bpd2;bpr3;bpd3;
1410 IF f = 1 THEN PRINT AT(19;5)"The primary sag,(rounded to 0.0001),of":PRINT
AT(30;10)"is  "ROUND((s1+s2-s3+s4-s5+s6-s7),4):GOSUB 1900:GOSUB 1880:GOTO 1500
1420 PRINT"  will provide the following edge lift:-"
1430 PRINT AT(14;10)"AXIAL          RADIAL"
1440 LINE 1434;2652,1986;2652: LINE 3088;2652,3750;2652
1450 PRINT AT(13;11)USING"£.££££"ROUND(ael1,4):  PRINT AT(19;11)USING" mm.
£.££££"ROUND(rel1,4): PRINT AT(36;11)"mm. From the 1st. back peripheral zone ";
1460 PRINT AT(13;12)USING"£.££££"ROUND(ael2,4):  PRINT AT(19;12)USING" mm.
£.££££"ROUND(rel2,4): PRINT AT(36;12)"mm.  '  ''  2nd. '' '  '' ''";
1470 PRINT AT(13;13)USING"£.££££"ROUND(ael3,4):  PRINT AT(19;13)USING" mm.
£.££££"ROUND(rel3,4): PRINT AT(36;13)"mm.  '  ''  3rd. '' '  '' ''";
1480 LINE 1324;1950,1986;1950: LINE 3088;1950,3750;1950
1490 PRINT AT(7;14)USING"Total £.££££"ROUND((ael1+ael2+ael3),4): PRINT AT(20;14'
USING"mm.      £.££££"ROUND((rel1+rel2+rel3),4): PRINT AT(36;14)"mm.":GOSUB 188(
1500 IF q$ = "y" THEN GOTO 1040 ELSE RUN
1510 PRINT AT(6;7)"in this sequence;BOZR,BOZD, BPR1,BPD1, BPR2,BPD2, BPR3,BPD3,
BPR4,TD"
```

Sag and edge lift program (*contd*)

```
1520 PRINT AT(2;10)"  eg.  7.9,7.5,  9.05,8.2,  10.2,9,  11.45,9.5,  12.85,9.9
(for a C5 lens)": LINE 6535;1740,6535;2669 COLOUR 2 END 1
1530 INPUT AT(9;12)"",ro,bozd,bpr1,bpd1,bpr2,bpd2,bpr3,bpd3,bpr4,bpd4
1540 CLS: GOSUB 1850
1550 yo = bozd/2: y1 = bpd1/2: s1a = ro-SQR(ro^2-y1^2): s1 = ro-SQR(ro^2-yo^2)
1560 s2 = bpr1-SQR(bpr1^2-y1^2): s3 = bpr1-SQR(bpr1^2-yo^2)
1570 ael1 = (s1a-s1)-(s2-s3): rel1 = SQR((ro-(s1+s2-s3))^2+y1^2)-ro
1580 IF q1 = 2 THEN RETURN
1590 y2 = bpd2/2: s1b = ro-SQR(ro^2-y2^2): s4 = bpr2-SQR(bpr2^2-y2^2)
1600 s5 = bpr2-SQR(bpr2^2-y1^2): ael2 = (s1b-s1a)-(s4-s5)
1610 rel2t = SQR((ro-(s1+s2-s3+s4-s5))^2+y2^2)-ro: rel2 = rel2t - rel1
1620 IF q1 = 3 THEN RETURN
1630 y3 = bpd3/2: s1c = ro-SQR(ro^2-y3^2): s6 = bpr3-SQR(bpr3^2-y3^2)
1640 s7 = bpr3-SQR(bpr3^2-y2^2): ael3 = (s1c-s1b)-(s6-s7)
1650 rel3t = SQR((ro-(s1+s2-s3+s4-s5+s6-s7))^2+y3^2)-ro: rel3 = rel3t - rel2t
1660 IF q1 = 4 THEN RETURN
1670 y4 = bpd4/2: s1d = ro-SQR(ro^2-y4^2): s8 = bpr4-SQR(bpr4^2-y4^2)
1680 s9 = bpr4-SQR(bpr4^2-y3^2): ael4 = (s1d-s1c)-(s8-s9)
1690 rel4t = SQR((ro-(s1+s2-s3+s4-s5+s6-s7+s8-s9))^2+y4^2)-ro:rel4 = rel4t-rel3t
1700 PRINT AT(4;5)USING"The C5 lens £.££:£.££/ £.££:£.££/ £.££:£.££/ £.££:£.££/
£.££:£.££"ro;bozd;bpr1;bpd1;bpr2;bpd2;bpr3;bpd3;bpr4;bpd4
1710 IF f = 1 THEN PRINT AT(19;3)"The primary sag,(rounded to 0.0001),of":PRINT
AT(30;10)"is  "ROUND((s1+s2-s3+s4-s5+s6-s7+s8-s9),4)
1720 IF f = 1 THEN GOSUB 1900 :GOSUB 1880:GOTO 1820
1730 PRINT"  will provide the following edge lift:-"
1740 PRINT AT(14;8)"AXIAL          RADIAL"
1750 LINE 1434;3120,1986;3120: LINE 3088;3120,3750;3120
1760 PRINT AT(13;9)USING"£.££££"ROUND(ael1,4):   PRINT AT(19;9)USING" mm.
£.££££"ROUND(rel1,4): PRINT AT(36;9)"mm.  From the 1st. back peripheral zone ";
1770 PRINT AT(13;10)USING"£.££££"ROUND(ael2,4):  PRINT AT(19;10)USING" mm.
£.££££"ROUND(rel2,4): PRINT AT(36;10)"mm.  ´´ ´´   2nd. ´´ ´´   ´´ ´´   ´´´";
1780 PRINT AT(13;11)USING"£.££££"ROUND(ael3,4):  PRINT AT(19;11)USING" mm.
£.££££"ROUND(rel3,4): PRINT AT(36;11)"mm.  ´´ ´´   3rd. ´´ ´´   ´´ ´´   ´´´";
1790 PRINT AT(13;12)USING"£.££££"ROUND(ael4,4):  PRINT AT(19;12)USING" mm.
£.££££"ROUND(rel4,4): PRINT AT(36;12)"mm.  ´´ ´´   4th.";
1800 LINE 1434;2184,2096;2184: LINE 3088;2184,3750;2184
1810 PRINT AT(4;13)USING"  Total £.££££"ROUND((ael1+ael2+ael3+ael4),4):PRINT AT
(20;13)USING"mm.      £.££££"ROUND((rel1+rel2+rel3+rel4),4):PRINT AT(36;13)"mm."
1820 GOSUB 1880: IF q$ = "y" THEN GOTO 1040 ELSE RUN
1830 PRINT AT(4;3)CHR$(7)CHR$(7)"Sorry! the programme does not extend to lenses
with more than 5 curves.": BOX 212;4281, 8020,260 COLOUR 2
1840 PRINT AT(14;15)CHR$(7)"Please choose another number, 2, 3, 4, or 5.":  BOX
1314;1470,5077,270 COLOUR 2: LINE 3240;1740,3240;2890 COLOUR 2 END 1: GOTO 1050
1850 PRINT AT(28;20)"Then press RETURN": LINE 4965;368,5165;368,5165;600 START 1
1860    PRINT AT(1;1)"To CANCEL & begin again; press Ctrl & C together; release
both; then press F9": BOX 5;4765,8530,270 COLOUR 4: RETURN
1870 BOX 432;1470,7612,270 COLOUR 2: PRINT AT(6;15)"Please note that a comma is
NOT required after the last data entry.": RETURN
1880 PRINT AT(30;19)"Type ";CHR$(96)"y´ or  ";CHR$(96)"n´"": GOSUB 1850
1890 INPUT AT(26;17)"Again? y = yes / n = no",q$: RETURN
1900 BOX 3520;2640,1103,270 COLOUR 2: BOX 652;1704,6950,520 STYLE 5 COLOUR 3
1910 PRINT AT(8;14)"Axial edge thickness(tea) = total sag - sag of front surface
":PRINT AT(12;13)"NOTE:- Total sag = primary sag + centre thickness(tc)":RETURN

     REM ***Start of obliquely crossed cyls. program.***
1920 CLS: WINDOW £1 FULL ON: WINDOW £2 CLOSE: CLOSE WINDOW 3: CLOSE WINDOW 4
1930 CLS:  OPTION TRAP ON: c=0: PRINT AT(6;4)"This programme will calculate the
Rx. resulting from the combination": OPTION DEGREES: GOSUB 2410
1940 PRINT AT(4;5)"of any two sphero/cyl. or plano/cyl. lenses."
1950 PRINT AT(5;7)" Lens powers may be entered in + or - Cyl. transposition, or
in any": PRINT AT(4;8)"combination of transpositions.         Enter 0 for plano."
1960 PRINT AT(2;10)"    The computer treats all numbers as ";CHR$(96)"+´ unless
```

Obliquely crossed cyl program (*contd*)

```
they are preceeded": PRINT AT(4;11)"by a ";CHR$(96)"-´ sign."
1970 PRINT AT(6;14)"To start the programme, type the Rx.of the first lens using
commas": PRINT AT(4;15)"to separate Sph,Cyl,and Ax      eg. 4.25,-1.75,165":
LINE 6210;1015,6210;1514 COLOUR 2 END 1: GOSUB 2440
1980 INPUT AT(43;16)"",s1,c1,a1: CLS: GOSUB 2410
1990 PRINT AT(3;7)"Now please enter the second lens, in the following sequence;
Sph, Cyl, Ax": PRINT AT(3;8)"using commas to separate each item.":GOSUB 2440
2000 PRINT AT(22;10)"eg.    12.75, -4.25, 12.5";
2010 LINE 4990;1035,4990;2669COLOUR 2 END 1
2020 INPUT AT(28;11)"",s2,c2,a2: CLS: GOSUB 2410
2030 PRINT AT(1;5)"   Now type the vertex distance of the second lens,from the
first lens,in mm";
2040 PRINT AT(6;14)"Enter O if first and second lenses are in the same plane,or
if vertex": INPUT AT(6;15)"distance doesn´t matter.",vd: CLS: GOSUB 2410
2050 BOX 1645;4280,5030,470 STYLE 3 COLOUR 4: IF vd > 0 THEN vd = 0-vd
        REM the next 5 lines set the position of the"degree"symbol in the printou
2060 IF ABS(s1)>9.999 THEN c=c+1
2070 IF ABS(c1)>9.999 THEN c=c+1
2080 IF a1>9.6 THEN c=c+1
2090 IF a1>99.6 THEN c=c+1
2100 IF FRAC(a1)<>0 THEN c=c+2 ELSE GOTO 2120
2110 PRINT AT(17;2)"First lens : ";USING"-£.££ Sph./-£.££ Cyl.Ax £.£";s1,c1,a1
PRINT AT((55+c);2)CHR$(248): GOTO 2140
2120 PRINT AT(17;2)"First lens : ";USING"-£.££ Sph./-£.££ Cyl.Ax £";s1,c1,a1
2130 PRINT AT((55+c);2)CHR$(248): PRINT AT(63;5)"1st. lens";
2140 PRINT AT(17;3)"Second lens: ";s2"Sph./";c2"Cyl.Ax.";a2;CHR$(248)
2150 IF vd<>0 THEN se2 = 1/(1/s2+(vd/1000)): se2r = ROUND(se2,2) ELSE GOTO 2190
2160 fe2 = 1/(1/(s2+c2)+(vd/1000)): ce2 = fe2-se2: ce2r = ROUND(ce2,2)
2170 PRINT AT(6;5)"The effective power of the 2nd. lens,in the plane of the";
2180 PRINT AT(9;6)"(at vd.";vd"mm., and with the power rounded to 0.01D.) is:-"
s2 = se2: c2 = ce2: PRINT AT(23;7)se2r"Sph./";ce2r"Cyl.Ax.";a2;CHR$(248)
2190 x1 = c1*COS(2*a1): x2 = c2*COS(2*a2): y1 = c1*SIN(2*a1): y2 = c2*SIN(2*a2)
2200 xr= x1+x2:yr= y1+y2:cr= SQR(xr^2+yr^2): crr= ROUND(cr,2): ar= .5*ATN(yr/xr
2210 IF ar <= 0 THEN ar = ar+180
2220 IF ar > 180 THEN ar = ar-180
2230 IF xr+yr < 0 THEN GOSUB 2430
2240 arr = INT(ar*2+.5)/2: sr = s2+s1+(c2+c1-cr)/2: srr = ROUND(sr,2)
2250 PRINT AT(29;9)"The resultant lens"
2260 IF (srr<>0)AND(crr<>0) THEN PRINT AT(12;10)"Power rounded to 0.01D."
2270 IF crr<>0THEN PRINT AT(36;10)"and axis rounded to 0.5";CHR$(248)"is:-"ELSE
PRINT AT(32;10)"is:-"
2280 PRINT AT(23;12)srr"Sph./";: IF crr<>0 THEN PRINT crr"Cyl.Ax.";arr;CHR$(248
2290 srrt = srr+crr: crrt = 0-crr: IF arr<=90 THEN arrt=arr+90 ELSE arrt=arr-90
2300 IF crr<>0THEN PRINT AT(20;13)"or ";srrt"Sph./";crrt"Cyl.Ax.";arrt;CHR$(248
2310 srr2 = INT(sr*4+.5)/4: crr2 = INT(cr*4+.5)/4
2320 IF(srr2=srr)AND(crr2=crr)THEN GOTO 2390
2330 PRINT AT(20;15)"Rounded to 0.25D:-"
2340 IF (srr2<>srr) OR (crr2<>0) THEN PRINT AT(23;16)srr2"Sph./";
2350 IF crr2<>0THEN PRINT crr2"Cyl.Ax.";arr;CHR$(248)ELSE IF srr2<>srr THEN BOX
1930;1230,2320,520 COLOUR 2
2360 srrt2 = INT(srrt*4+.5)/4: crrt2 = INT(crrt*4+.5)/4
2370 IF crrt2<>0 THEN PRINT AT(20;17)    "or ";srrt2"Sph./";crrt2"Cyl.Ax.";arrt;
CHR$ (248): BOX 1930;1000,4050,750 WIDTH 3 COLOUR 2
2380 PRINT AT(18;20)"Type ";CHR$(96)"y´ or ";CHR$(96)"n´": GOSUB 2410
2390 CLOSE WINDOW 4: INPUT AT(25;19)"Again.? y = yes / n = no",q$
2400 IF q$ = "y" THEN GOTO 1930 ELSE RUN
2410 PRINT AT(36;20)"Then press RETURN": LINE 5845;368,6045;368,6045;600 START 1
2420    PRINT AT(1;1)"To CANCEL & begin again; press Ctrl & C together; release
both; then press F9": BOX 5;4765,8530,270 COLOUR 4: RETURN
2430 IF ar <= 90 THEN ar = ar + 90: RETURN ELSE ar = ar - 90: RETURN
2440 BOX 432;765,7612,270 COLOUR 2:  PRINT AT(6;18)"Please note that a comma is
NOT required after the last data entry.": RETURN
```

```
      REM***Start of program for power changes due to flexure of rigid lenses***
2450 CLS: WINDOW £1 FULL ON: WINDOW £2 CLOSE: CLOSE WINDOW 3: CLOSE WINDOW 4
2460 OPTION TRAP ON: LINE 1324;4056,7060;4056
2470 PRINT AT(13;4)"POWER CHANGES DUE TO FLEXURE OF RIGID CONTACT LENSES."
2480     PRINT AT(1;1)"To CANCEL & begin again; press Ctrl & C together; release
both; then press F9": BOX 5;4765,8530,270 COLOUR 4:
2490 PRINT AT(2;8)        "Please type the lens details, including front surface K
readings,KL(f)&KL(s)";
2500 PRINT " in the following sequence, using commas to separate each item.";
2510 PRINT AT(28;20)"Then press RETURN": LINE 4965;368,5165;368,5165;600 START 1
2520 PRINT AT(10;11)"BOZR,BOZD,BVP,Tc,TD,FOZD,Refractive Index,KL(f),KL(s)";
2530 PRINT AT(20;13)"eg.   8.1,7.5,-6.25,.16,9.5,9.5,1.47,9.065,9.01";
2540 PRINT AT(6;16)"Enter TD for FOZD if the front surface is not lenticulated."
2550 BOX 432;1236,6775,270 COLOUR 3: LINE 5407;1506,5407;1960 COLOUR 3 END 1
2560 BOX 432;765,7612,270 COLOUR 2:   PRINT AT(6;18)"Please note that a comma is
NOT required after the last data entry.":LINE 7402;1035,7402;1963 COLOUR 2 END 1
2570 INPUT AT(27;14)"",bozr,bozd,fv,tc,td,fozd,u,fozraf,fozras: CLS: tcr=tc/u:
ua=(u-1)*1000: fozr=ua/(ua/bozr+fv)+(u-1)*tcr: IF fozd=td THEN fozd=bozd
2580 PRINT AT(25;2)"Calculated lens parameters.":LINE 2648;4525,5628;4525
2590     PRINT AT(1;1)"To CANCEL & begin again; press Ctrl & C together; release
both; then press F9":BOX 5;4765,8530,270 COLOUR 4:IF bozd>fozd THEN bozd = fozd
2600 y = fozd/2: fozr=SQR(fozr^2-y^2): vfr = PI*(3*fozr-sfr)*sfr^2/3
2610 sb = bozr-SQR(bozr^2-y^2): vb = PI*(3*bozr-sb)*sb^2/3: te = sb+tc-sfr
2620 vc = PI*y^2*te: vl = vfr+vc-vb
2630 rf = 1: ya = y-rf: GOSUB 2660
2640 WHILE ROUND((vl-vla),4)<0: ya = ya-rf: GOSUB 2660
2650 WEND: ya=ya+rf: rf=rf/10:
2660 sfra=fozraf-SQR(fozraf^2-ya^2): sba=sfra+te-tc: bozra=(ya^2+sba^2)/(2*sba)
2670 vfra = PI*(3*fozraf-sfra)*sfra^2/3: vba = PI*(3*bozra-sba)*sba^2/3
2680 vca = PI*ya^2*te
2690 vla = vfra+vca-vba: IF ROUND((vl-vla),4)<>0 THEN GOTO 2640
2700 IF fozraf <> fozras THEN fozraff = fozraf ELSE fozrafs = fozraf
2710 dif = fozraf - fozr: IF fozraf <> fozras THEN GOSUB 2920 ELSE GOSUB 2940
2720 IF fozraf<>fozras THEN PRINT AT(8;3) "fozr =";ROUND(fozr,4)", Flexed KL(f)
=";fozraf", which is";ROUND(ABS(dif),4)
2730 IF fozraf=fozras THEN PRINT AT(8;4)   "fozr =";ROUND(fozr,4)", Flexed KL(s)
=";fozraf", which is";ROUND(ABS(dif),4): LINE 4083;4057,4634;4057
2740 IF fozraf=fozras THEN PRINT AT(31;5)"Diff =";ROUND((fozraff-fozrafs),3)
2750 IF fozraf <> fozras THEN bozraf = bozra ELSE bozras = bozra
2760 dif = bozra - bozr: IF fozraf <> fozras THEN GOSUB 2960 ELSE GOSUB 2980
2770 IF fozraf<>fozras THEN PRINT AT(8;6)      "BOZR =";bozr", Flexed BOZR(f) =";
ROUND(bozra,4)", which is";ROUND(ABS(dif),4)
2780 IF fozraf=fozras THEN PRINT AT(8;7)      "BOZR =";bozr", Flexed BOZR(s) =";
ROUND(bozra,4)", which is";ROUND(ABS(dif),4): LINE 4082;3354,4744;3354
2790 fvf=1000/(1000/(ua/fozraf)-tcr)+(ua/(0-bozra)): IF fozraf<>fozras THEN axf=
ROUND(bozra,3) ELSE PRINT AT(31;8)"Diff =";ROUND((bozraf-bozras),4)
2800 IF fozraf <> fozras THEN fvff = fvf ELSE fvfs = fvf
2810 dif = fv - fvf: IF fozraf <> fozras THEN GOSUB 3000 ELSE GOSUB 3050
2820 IF fozraf <> fozras THEN PRINT AT(8;9)      "BVP =";fv", Flexed BVP(f)  =";
ROUND(fvf,4)", which is";ROUND(ABS(dif),4)
2830 IF fozraf = fozras THEN PRINT AT(8;10)      "BVP =";fv", Flexed BVP(s)  =";
ROUND(fvf,4)", which is";ROUND(ABS(dif),4)
2840 IF fozraf = fozras THEN GOTO 3140
2850 IF fozraf = fozras THEN LINE 3862;2652,4524;2652
2860 IF fozraf = fozras THEN PRINT AT(29;11)"Diff =";ROUND((fvff-fvfs),4)
2870 IF fozraf <> fozras THEN GOTO 3100 ELSE BOX 1866;768,4593,280: GOSUB 3110
2880 PRINT AT(20;20)"Type ";CHR$(96)"y´ or ";CHR$(96)"n´"
2890 PRINT AT(38;20)"Then press RETURN": LINE 6065;368,6265;368,6265;600 START 1
2900 INPUT AT(19;18)"Have you another lens to calculate, y/n";q$
2910 IF q$ = "y" THEN CLS: GOTO 2480 ELSE RUN
2920 IF dif>0 THEN PRINT AT(63;3)"flatter.";ELSE PRINT AT(63;3)"steeper.";
```

Power changes due to the flexure of rigid lenses (*contd*)

```
2930 RETURN
2940 IF dif>0 THEN PRINT AT(63;4)"flatter.";ELSE PRINT AT(63;4)"steeper.";
2950 RETURN
2960 IF dif>0 THEN PRINT AT(65;6)"flatter.";ELSE PRINT AT(65;6)"steeper.";
2970 RETURN
2980 IF dif>0 THEN PRINT AT(65;7)"flatter.";ELSE PRINT AT(65;7)"steeper.";
2990 RETURN
3000 IF fv >0 THEN GOTO 3010 ELSE GOTO 3030
3010 IF fvf < fv THEN PRINT AT(64;9)"less +ve.";ELSE PRINT AT(64;9)"more +ve.";
3020 RETURN
3030 IF fvf > fv THEN PRINT AT(64;9)"less -ve.";ELSE PRINT AT(64;9)"more -ve.";
3040 RETURN
3050 IF fv > 0 THEN GOTO 3060 ELSE GOTO 3080
3060 IF fvf<fv THEN PRINT AT(64;10)"less +ve.";ELSE PRINT AT(64;10)"more +ve.";
3070 RETURN
3080 IF fvf>fv THEN PRINT AT(64;10)"less -ve.";ELSE PRINT AT(64;10)"more -ve.";
3090 RETURN
3100 fozraf = fozras: GOTO 2630:
3110 PRINT AT(1;12)               "BVP of flexed lens in air = "ROUND(fvff,4)"/
ROUND((fvfs-fvff),4)"Cyl.Ax.along flat("axf")radius"
3120 cif = 134/bozraf-134/bozras:PRINT AT(4;14)"Induced cyl. due to flexure is
ROUND(cif,4)"Cyl.Ax.along flat("axf")radius.": cetot = cif+fvfs-fvff
3130 PRINT AT(1;16)               "Effective Rx(flexed lens) = "ROUND(fvff,4)"/
ROUND(cetot,4)"Cyl.Ax.along flat("axf")radius": RETURN
3140 IF (fvfs < 0) OR (fvfs > 9.99) THEN LINE 4082;2652,4744;2652 ELSE GOTO 285(
3150 PRINT AT(31;11)"Diff ="ROUND((fvff-fvfs),4): GOTO 2870

               REM***Front optic zone radius program.***
3160 CLS: WINDOW £1 FULL ON: WINDOW £2 CLOSE: CLOSE WINDOW 3: CLOSE WINDOW 4
3170 CLS:   OPTION TRAP ON:  PRINT AT(6;6) "Please type the lens details, in the
following sequence":LINE 7180;1015,7180;2943 COLOUR 2 END 1: GOSUB 3290
3180 PRINT AT(6;8)"BOZR,BVP,Centre thickness,Refractive index": GOSUB 3270
3190 PRINT AT(6;9)"using commas to separate each item.   eg. 7.95,6.75,.39,1.49'
3200 INPUT AT(48;10)"",bozr,fv,tc,u: CLS: tcr = tc/u: ua = (u-1)*1000
3210 PRINT AT(9;6) "The FRONT OPTIC ZONE RADIUS of a lens having BVP"fv"
3220 PRINT AT(9;7)  "BOZR"bozr" tc"tc"and "CHR$(230)u:   BOX 1866;768,4593,280:
PRINT AT(62;6)",": PRINT AT(18;7)",": fozr = ua/(ua/bozr+fv)+(u-1)*tcr
3230 PRINT AT(30;10)"is:-  "ROUND(fozr,3): BOX 3742;2640,993,270 COLOUR 2
3240 PRINT AT(18;20)"Type ";CHR$(96)"y´ or ";CHR$(96)"n´": GOSUB 3270
3250 INPUT AT(19;18)"Have you another lens to calculate, y/n";q$
3260 IF q$ = "y" THEN GOTO 3170 ELSE RUN
3270 PRINT AT(36;20)"Then press RETURN": LINE 5845;368,6045;368,6045;600 START
3280    PRINT AT(1;1)"To CANCEL & begin again; press Ctrl & C together; release
both; then press F9": BOX 5;4765,8530,270 COLOUR 4: RETURN
3290 BOX 432;765,7612,270 COLOUR 2:  PRINT AT(6;18)"Please note that a comma is
NOT required after the last data entry.": RETURN

               REM***Start of multicurve spherical lens design program***
3300 CLS: WINDOW £1 FULL ON: WINDOW £2 CLOSE: CLOSE WINDOW 3: CLOSE WINDOW 4
3310 OPTION TRAP ON:CLS:PRINT AT(18;4)"MULTICURVE SPHERICAL LENS DESIGN PROGRAM.
3320 PRINT AT(11;9)"This program will design the back surface of multicurve"
3330 PRINT AT(11;10)"spherical lenses,(C2, C3, or C4).":LINE 1876;4057,6289;4057
3340 PRINT AT(17;13)"Please type the number of zones you wish the": GOSUB 4080
3350 INPUT AT(17;14)"back surface to have, including the BOZD.",c:CLS:GOSUB 408(
3360 PRINT AT(6;4)"Given the BOZR, the computer can design a"CHR$(96)"standard´
lens having 9.50 mm.";
3370 PRINT AT(2;5)"total diameter,or a"CHR$(96)"one off´lens,the specifications
for which you will be";
3380 PRINT AT(2;6)"asked to provide, as and when the program requires them.";
3390 PRINT AT(6;9)" Do you wish the computer to design a"CHR$(96)"standard´lens
or will you supply": PRINT AT(2;10)"the data for a"CHR$(96)"non-standard´lens?";
3400 PRINT AT(18;13)"For "CHR$(96)"standard´, please type the letter  s";
```

Multicurve spherical lens design program (*contd*)

```
3410 PRINT AT(29;15)CHR$(96)"non-standard´ = ns"
3420 INPUT AT(23;19)"Please type your design chioce;",q$
          REM Conditional branching for standard lens design.
3430 IF q$ = "s" THEN GOTO 3990 ELSE CLS: GOSUB 4080
          REM conditional branching for rounding to a stipulated accuracy.
3440 PRINT AT(10;8)"Do you wish the calculated peripheral radii to be rounded";
3450 PRINT AT(27;12)"y = yes          n = no";
3460 PRINT AT(30;19)"Type "CHR$(96)"y´ or "CHR$(96)"n´"
3470 INPUT AT(10;9)"to a stipulated accuracy";q$: CLS: GOSUB 4080
3480 IF q$ = "n" THEN sa = .01: GOTO 3510
          REM "sa" stands for stipulated accuracy.
3490 PRINT AT(3;8)"Please type the value to which the peripheral radii should be
 rounded.": PRINT AT(23;12)"eg.  .05, .02, .01, or .001, etc. etc.";
3500 INPUT AT(23;19)"Please type your design chioce;",sa: CLS: GOSUB 4080
          REM Collects data for non-standard lens.
3510 PRINT AT(2;6)"Please type the BOZR and Diameters required on the back surfa
ce of the lens,";
3520 IF c = 2 THEN GOTO 3630
3530 IF c = 3 THEN GOTO 3700
3540 PRINT AT(11;7)"in the following sequence;   BOZR,BOZD,  BPD1,  BPD2,  TD";
3550 PRINT AT(20;8)"using commas to separate each item.": GOSUB 4070
3560 PRINT AT(13;10)"eg.  8.1,7,  7.8,  8.6,  9.2       (for a C4 lens)";
3570 LINE 4440;1740,4440;2669 COLOUR 2 END 1
3580 INPUT AT(18;12)"",ro,bozd,bpd1,bpd2,bpd3: CLS: GOSUB 4080
3590 PRINT AT(6;6) "Please type the amount of AEL required from each peripheral
zone,": PRINT AT(6;7)"in the following sequence;  BPZ1, BPZ2, BPZ3";
3600 PRINT AT(23;10)"eg.  .033,   .081,   .076"
3610 LINE 5320;1740,5320;2669 COLOUR 2 END 1: GOSUB 4070
3620 INPUT AT(29;12)"",ael1,ael2,ael3: CLS: GOSUB 4080: GOTO 3790
3630 PRINT AT(19;7)"in the following sequence;  BOZR, BOZD, TD";
3640 PRINT AT(20;8)"using commas to separate each item.": GOSUB 4070
3650 PRINT AT(19;10)"eg.  8.1, 7, 8.8       (for a C2 lens)";
3660 LINE 3780;1740,3780;2669 COLOUR 2 END 1
3670 INPUT AT(24;12)"",ro,bozd,bpd1: CLS: GOSUB 4090
3680 PRINT AT(4;8)      "Please type the amount of axial edge lift the lens should
have(in mm.).": LINE 4965;368,5165;368,5165;600 START 1
3690 INPUT AT(28;20)"Then press RETURN",ael: ael1 = ael: CLS: GOTO 3790
3700 PRINT AT(14;7)"in the following sequence;  BOZR,BOZD,  BPD1,   TD";
3710 PRINT AT(20;8)"using commas to separate each item.": GOSUB 4070
3720 PRINT AT(19;10)"eg.  8.1,7,  8,  9.2       (for a C3 lens)";
3730 LINE 4220;1740,4220;2669 COLOUR 2 END 1
3740 INPUT AT(24;12)"",ro,bozd,bpd1,bpd2: CLS: GOSUB 4080
3750 PRINT AT(6;6) "Please type the amount of AEL required from each peripheral
zone,": PRINT AT(8;7)"in the following sequence;  BPZ1, BPZ2,";
3760 PRINT AT(23;10)"eg.  .045,   .105"
3770 LINE 4440;1740,4440;2669 COLOUR 2 END 1: GOSUB 4070
3780 INPUT AT(29;12)"",ael1,ael2: CLS: ael = ael1+ael2: GOSUB 4080
          REM Calculates value of x for first peripheral zone.
3790 x1=(ro-SQR(ro^2-(bpd1/2)^2))-(ro-SQR(ro^2-(bozd/2)^2))-ael1
          REM Calculates BPR1.
3800 bpr1=SQR(((((bpd1/2)^2-(bozd/2)^2-x1^2)/(2*x1))^2+(bpd1/2)^2)
          REM Rounds BPR1 to stipulated accuracy (bpr1r)
3810 bpr1r=INT(bpr1*(1/sa)+.5)/(1/sa): IF c = 2 THEN GOTO 3900
          REM Same for BPR2 & BPR3 as for BPR1 above.
3820 x2=(ro-SQR(ro^2-(bpd2/2)^2))-(ro-SQR(ro^2-(bpd1/2)^2))-ael2
3830 bpr2=SQR(((((bpd2/2)^2-(bpd1/2)^2-x2^2)/(2*x2))^2+(bpd2/2)^2)
3840 bpr2r=INT(bpr2*(1/sa)+.5)/(1/sa): IF c = 3 THEN GOTO 3910
3850 x3=(ro-SQR(ro^2-(bpd3/2)^2))-(ro-SQR(ro^2-(bpd2/2)^2))-ael3
3860 bpr3=SQR(((((bpd3/2)^2-(bpd2/2)^2-x3^2)/(2*x2))^2+(bpd3/2)^2)
3870 bpr3r=INT(bpr3*(1/sa)+.5)/(1/sa): ael=ael1+ael2+ael3
3880 PRINT AT(16;8)USING"£.££:£.££/ £.££:£.££/ £.££:£.££/ £.££:£.££"    ro;bozd;
bpr1r;bpd1;bpr2r;bpd2;bpr3r;bpd3: BOX 1535;3108,5075,270 COLOUR 2: GOTO 3920
```

Multicurve spherical lens design program (*contd*)

```
3890 PRINT AT(8;10)"The peripheral radius has been rounded to the nearest"sa"mm
3900 PRINT AT(28;8)USING"£.££:£.££/ £.££:£.££"ro;bozd;bpr1r;bpd1: BOX 2859;3108
2427,270 COLOUR 2: GOTO 3930
3910 PRINT AT(22;8)USING"£.££:£.££/ £.££:£.££/ £.££:£.££"    ro;bozd;bpr1r;bpd1
bpr2r;bpd2: BOX 2179;3108,3751,270 COLOUR 2
3920 PRINT AT(8;10)"The peripheral radii have been rounded to the nearest"sa"mm
3930 PRINT AT(20;6)"The required lens, in C"c" format is:-";
3940 PRINT AT(25;11)"The chosen AEL is"ael"mm.";
3950 BOX 1425;767,5517,770 STYLE 3 COLOUR 7 ROUNDED
3960 PRINT AT(23;18)"Type "CHR$(96)"y´ for yes / "CHR$(96)"n´ for no.";
3970 INPUT AT(15;16)"Do you wish to do another lens of the same type";q$
        REM Conditional branching to design another lens.
3980 IF q$ = "y" THEN CLS: GOTO 3340 ELSE RUN
        REM Sets program to round peripheral radii to 0.05 mm.
3990 sa = .05: CLS
        REM Collects data for ´standard´ lens.
4000 GOSUB 4080: INPUT AT(24;8)"Plese type the BOZR (in mm.)",ro: CLS:GOSUB 409
4010 LINE 4965;368,5165;368,5165;600 START 1:  PRINT AT(7;8)    "Please type the
total amount of axial edge lift the lens should have(in mm.).";
4020 INPUT AT(28;20)"Then press RETURN",ael: bozd = 7.5: CLS
        REM Sets parameters for ´standard´ lens & apportions AEL.
4030 IF c = 2 THEN bpd1 = 9.5: aell = ael: GOSUB 4080: GOTO 3790
4040 IF c = 3 THEN bpd1 = 8.5:bpd2 = 9.5:aell = ael*.3:ael2 = ael*.7:GOSUB 4080
GOTO 3790
4050 IF c = 4 THEN bpd1 = 8.2: bpd2 = 9: bpd3 = 9.5
4060 aell = ael*.174: ael2 = ael*.426: ael3 = ael*.4: GOSUB 4080: GOTO 3790
4070 BOX 432;1470,7612,270 COLOUR 2: PRINT AT(6;15)"Please note that a comma is
NOT required after the last data entry.": RETURN
4080 PRINT AT(28;20)"Then press RETURN": LINE 4965;368,5165;368,5165;600 START
4090 PRINT AT(1;1)"To CANCEL & begin again; press Ctrl & C together; release bo
h; then press F9": BOX 5;4765,8530,270 COLOUR 4: RETURN
END
4100 CLS
4110 WINDOW £1 FULL OFF
4120 WINDOW £2 OPEN
4130 END
```

Appendix F: Appropriate drugs and solutions for use with contact lenses

Table F.I Solutions and drops for use with hard and rigid gas permeable lenses

Most soft lens solutions may also be used for hard lenses (*see Table F.II*). However, for lens materials other than polymethyl methacrylate the manufacturer's instructions regarding solutions should be followed, as lenses containing silicone and cellulose acetate butyrate, for example, may not be compatible with all preservatives.

Name of solutions and sizes available	Manufacturer	Preservatives with percentage concentration	Remarks
Soaking solutions (which may also be used for cleaning)			
Contique Cleaning and Soaking, 120 ml	Alcon	B Cl 0.02; EDTA 0.1	
Clean-N-Soak, 120 ml	Allergan	PMN 0.004	Dual purpose cleaner
Wet-N-Soak, 120 ml	Allergan	B Cl 0.004	Dual purpose wetting
Duracare, 120 ml*	Allergan	B Cl 0.004	Dual purpose wetting
Soquette, 10 ml, 120 ml	Barnes–Hind	B Cl 0.01; EDTA 0.2	Available UK only
Boots Soaking Solution, 120 ml	Boots	B Cl 0.004; CHX 0.006; EDTA 0.128	
Contactasoak, 7 ml, 120 ml	CIBA Vision	B Cl 0.004; CHX 0.006; EDTA 0.1	
Duo-Flow Cleaning and Soaking, 120 ml	CIBA Vision	B Cl 0.013; EDTA 0.25	Italy and USA only
Kelsoak, 10 ml, 120 ml	CIBA Vision	B Cl 0.01; EDTA 0.1	Germany only
Hoya Hard Daily Soaking/ Cleaning, 120 ml	Hoya	EDTA 0.1; CHX 0.005	
Hydron Formula H*	Hydron Europe (Allergan)	B Cl 0.01; EDTA 0.2	
ICN Unicare (red), 25 ml, 100 ml	ICN Pharmaceuticals	EDTA ?; THI 0.0015	Combined clean and storage
ICN Unihard, 25 ml, 100 ml	ICN Pharmaceuticals	EDTA ?; THI 0.0015	Recommended in combination with Uniclean
Steri-Soak, 110 ml	Sauflon Pharmaceuticals	B Cl 0.002; CHB 0.4; EDTA 0.1	
Transoak, 120 ml	Smith & Nephew	B Cl 0.01; EDTA 0.2	
Wetting solutions (which may also be used for re-wetting on the eye)			
Adapt, 2 ml, 15 ml	Alcon	EDTA 0.05; THI 0.002	
Dualwet, 60 ml	Alcon	B Cl 0.01; EDTA 0.05	
Liquifilm Wetting, 20 ml, 60 ml	Allergan	B Cl 0.004; EDTA 0.1	
Boots Wetting, 60 ml	Boots	B Cl 0.004; CHX 0.006; EDTA 0.128	
Barnes–Hind Wetting, 35 ml, 60 ml	Barnes–Hind	B Cl 0.004; EDTA 0.02	
Contactasol, 10 ml, 60 ml	CIBA Vision	B Cl 0.004; CHX 0.006; EDTA 0.1	
Hy-Flow, 60 ml	CIBA Vision	B Cl 0.01; EDTA 0.025	Italy and USA only
Kelvinol, 10 ml, 58 ml	CIBA Vision	B Cl 0.005; EDTA 0.1	Germany only
Hydron Formula H Wetting*	Hydron Europe (Allergan)	B Cl 0.005; EDTA 0.02	
Steri-Clens, 60 ml	Sauflon Pharmaceuticals	EDTA 0.1; THI 0.004	Suitable for cleaning
Transol, 50 ml	Smith & Nephew	B Cl 0.004; EDTA 0.02	
Combined soaking and wetting solutions (which may also be used for cleaning)			
Soaclens, 120 ml	Alcon	EDTA 0.1; THI 0.004	
Total, 60 ml, 120 ml	Allergan	B Cl 0.004; EDTA?	
One Solution, 90 ml	Barnes–Hind	B Cl 0.01; EDTA 0.02	USA only
Barnes–Hind Wetting and Soaking, 120 ml	Barnes–Hind	B Cl 0.005; EDTA 0.1	
GP Wetting and Soaking, 120 ml*	Barnes–Hind	CHX 0.003; EDTA 0.02; PS 0.13	

* Formulated specifically for RGP lenses.

Table F.I (*contd*)

Name of solutions and sizes available	Manufacturer	Preservatives with percentage concentration	Remarks
Conditioning Solution (Wetting and Soaking Solution)*, 120 ml	Bausch & Lomb	CHX 0.06; EDTA 0.05	In UK, called wetting and soaking solution for rigid gas permeable lenses
Boston Conditioning Solution* 120 ml	Polymer Technology	CHX 0.06; EDTA 0.05	
Complete Care*, 120 ml	CIBA Vision	B Cl 0.01; EDTA 0.05	
Cleaning solutions (see also Soft lens cleaning solutions, Table F. II)			
Clens, 60 ml	Alcon	B Cl 0.02; EDTA 0.1	
Contique Hard Cleaning, 30 ml	Alcon	B Cl 0.02	
Polyclens (Opticlean), 12 ml, 24 ml	Alcon	EDTA 0.1; THI 0.004	Contains polymeric beads
Polyclens II (Opticlean II), 12 ml, 24 ml	Alcon	EDTA 0.1; Polyquad 0.001	Contains polymeric beads
Duraclean Daily Cleaner, 30 ml	Allergan	Self-preserving	
LC 65, 15 ml, 30 ml, 60 ml	Allergan	EDTA 0.01; THI 0.001	
Oxyclean Daily Cleaner, 15 ml	Allergan	Self-preserving	
Titan, 30 ml	Barnes–Hind	B Cl 0.02; EDTA 0.2	
Gel Clean, 30 g tube	Barnes–Hind	THI 0.004	
GP Daily Cleaner, 30 ml*	Barnes–Hind	EDTA 2.0; PS 0.13	
Concentrated Cleaner, 30 ml*	Bausch & Lomb	Self-preserving	Contains sodium tridecylether sulphate 10%. In UK, called cleaner for rigid gas permeable lenses
Boots Cleaning, 35 ml	Boots	B Cl 0.004; CHX 0.006; EDTA 0.128	
Contactaclean, 35 ml	CIBA Vision	B Cl 0.004; CHX 0.006; EDTA 0.1	
D-Film, 25 ml	CIBA Vision	B Cl 0.013; EDTA 0.1	
Hoya Hard Cleaner, 60 ml	Hoya	EDTA 0.1; CHX 0.005	
Hydron Formula H Cleaning*	Hydron Europe (Allergan)	B Cl 0.01; EDTA 0.1	
ICN Uniclean, 5 ml, 60 ml	ICN Pharmaceuticals	EDTA ?; THI 0.0015	Universal cleanser of hard, soft and RGP lenses
Boston cleaner*, 60 ml	Polymer Technology	Self-preserving	Contains sodium tridecylether sulphate 10%
Transclean, 10 ml	Smith & Nephew	B Cl 0.01; EDTA 0.1	
Re-wetting solutions (see also Soft lens re-wetting solutions, Table F.II)			
Adapettes, 15 ml	Alcon	EDTA 0.1; THI 0.004	
Blink-N-Clean, 15 ml	Allergan	CHB 0.5	Poloxyl 40 stearate and polyethylene glycol 300 as surfactants
Comfort Drops, 15 ml	Barnes–Hind	B Cl 0.005; EDTA 0.02	
Lens Lubricant	Barnes–Hind	EDTA 0.1; THI 0.004	For hard and soft
Aqua-Flow, 25 ml	CIBA Vision	B Cl 0.005; EDTA 0.025	Italy only
Boston Reconditioning Drops	Polymer Technology	CHX 0.006; EDTA 0.05	
Transdrop, 10 ml	Smith & Nephew	B Cl 0.004; EDTA 0.02	

* Formulated specifically for RGP lenses.

Table F.I (*contd*)

Name of solutions and sizes available	Manufacturer	Preservatives with percentage concentration	Remarks
Artificial tears drops (which may be used for re-wetting hard lenses)			
Adsorbotear, 15 ml	Alcon	EDTA 0.05; THI 0.002	Pharmacy Medicine
Tears Naturale, 15 ml	Alcon	B Cl 0.01; EDTA 0.05	Pharmacy Medicine
Isopto Plain (Isopto Tears), 15 ml	Alcon	B Cl 0.01	Pharmacy Medicine
Isopto Alkaline, 15 ml	Alcon	B Cl 0.01	Pharmacy Medicine
Liquifilm Tears, 15 ml	Allergan	CHB 0.5	Pharmacy Medicine
Liquifilm Forte, 15 ml	Allergan	EDTA 0.01; THI 0.002	Polyvinyl alcohol 3.0%
Tears Plus, 15 ml	Allergan	CHB 0.5	Polyvinyl alcohol 1.4%, povidone 0.6%
Neoteers, 15 ml	Barnes–Hind	EDTA 0.02; THI 0.004	Pharmacy Medicine Awaiting a product licence
Snotears, 10 ml	Smith & Nephew	B Cl 0.004; EDTA 0.02	Pharmacy Medicine
Vit-A-Drops, 15 ml	Vision Pharmaceuticals	Preservative-free	Contains 500 IU vitamin A and Polysorbate 80
Conjunctival decongestants (see also Table F. III) (these are all Pharmacy Medicines)			
Isoptofrin, 15 ml	Alcon	B Cl 0.01	Contains PHE 0.12%
Zincfrin, 15 ml	Alcon	B Cl 0.01	PHE 0.12%; Z S 0.25%
Naphcon	Alcon	B Cl 0.01; NAPH 0.012	
Naphcon A	Alcon	B Cl 0.01; NAPH 0.025; pheniramine maleate 0.3	
Prefrin, 15 ml	Allergan	B Cl 0.004; EDTA 0.001	PHE 0.12%, PVA 1.4%
Prefrin-Z, 15 ml	Allergan	THI 0.005	PHE 0.12%, zinc sulphate 0.25%, PVA 1.4%
Albalon, 15 ml	Allergan	EDTA 0.01; B Cl 0.004	NAPH-HCL 0.1%, PVA 1.4%
Albalon-A, 15 ml	Allergan	EDTA 0.01; B Cl 0.004	NAPH 0.05%, antazoline phosphate 0.5%, PVA 1.4%
Miscellaneous solutions			
O₂ Care, 100 ml	Toyo	EDTA 0.02; bromonitroprophylene glycol 0.001	For Menicon RGP lenses
Eyesoothe, 120 ml with eyebath	CIBA Vision	B Cl 0.004	Eye lotion contains PHE 0.01%
O₂ Solution, 110 ml	Sauflon Pharmaceuticals	BCl 0.005; EDTA 0.128	For all GP lenses including surface treated

* Formulated specifically for RGP lenses.

B Cl, benzalkonium chloride; CHB, chlorbutol; CHX, chlorhexidine gluconate; EDTA ethylenediamine tetraacetic acid; NAPH, naphazoline; PHE, phenylephrine hydrochloride; PVA, polyvinyl alcohol; PMN, phenylmercuric nitrate; PS, potassium sorbate; THI, thimerosal; Z S, zinc sulphate; ?, concentration not available.

Note that not all products or volume sizes are available in all countries, and the proprietary names often differ slightly from one country to another.

Table F.II Solutions and drops for use with soft lenses

Most soft lens solutions may also be used for hard lenses (*see Table F.I*). However, for lens materials other than polymethyl methacrylate the manufacturer's instructions regarding solutions should be followed, as lenses containing silicone and cellulose acetate butyrate, for example, may not be compatible with all preservatives. The same caution should be observed with any soft lens made of a new material, as preservatives may bind to the material, and cleaning solutions and systems might alter the lens parameters.

Name of solutions and sizes available	Manufacturer	Preservatives with percentage concentration	Remarks
Disinfecting and storage (soaking) solutions (these are basically saline, except where indicated)			
Hydrophilic lenses			
Aosept, 237 ml, 250 ml	CIBA Vision	Self-preserving	3% hydrogen peroxide Sodium stannate + sodium nitrate as stabilizers Isotonic, buffered
Ami-10, 40 ml, 200 ml	Abatron	CHX 0.005; EDTA 0.01; THI 0.001	
Flexsol, 120 ml, 175 ml	Alcon	CHX 0.005; EDTA 0.1; THI 0.001	
Flexcare, 250 ml, 355 ml	Alcon	CHX 0.005; EDTA 0.1; THI 0.001	
Contigel, 120 ml	Alcon	CHX 0.005; EDTA 0.02; THI 0.0005	
Pliacide, 7.5 ml*	Alcon	IOD 0.1	Not for use with lenses of greater than 53% water content
used with			
Nutraflow, 110 ml	Alcon	EDTA 0.1; S A 0.1	
Opti-Free, 120 ml, 240 ml	Alcon	EDTA 0.1; Polyquad 0.001	
Opti-Soft, 120 ml, 240 ml	Alcon	EDTA 0.1; Polyquad 0.001	Not to be used with lenses over 45% water content
Softab (Opti-tabs) 32 tabs	Alcon	Sodium dichloro-isocyanurate 0.065 mg	Chlorine release To be used with unpreserved saline only
Hydrocare Soaking and Cleaning, 120 ml, 240 ml, 360 ml	Allergan	ATAC 0.03; THI 0.002	Contains surfactant for daily cleaning
Oxysept 1, 235 ml, 360 ml	Allergan		Hydrogen peroxide 3% used for a minimum of 20 minutes followed by neutralization in Oxysept 2
Hexidin (Soft Mate Disinfecting Solution), 120 ml, 240 ml	Barnes–Hind	CHX 0.005; EDTA 0.02; THI 0.001	
Soft Mate Consept 1	Barnes–Hind		Hydrogen peroxide 3% with surfactant
HP 1 (Quick Sept 1), 120 ml, 240 ml	Bausch & Lomb		Hydrogen peroxide 3%
Sensitive Eyes Soaking Solution (Disinfecting Solution), 120 ml, 240 ml, 335 ml	Bausch & Lomb	Dymed 0.00005	
Boots Soft Lens Soaking, 120 ml	Boots	CHX 0.0025; EDTA 0.128; THI 0.0025	
Contactasol 10·10, 120 ml, 250 ml	CIBA Vision	H_2O_2 3.0	
Lensan A	CIBA Vision	H_2O_2 3.0	
In A Wink, 240 ml	CIBA Vision	H_2O_2 3.0	
Titmus H_2O_2 Solution 1	CIBA Vision	H_2O_2 0.6	

* Contains sodium hexametaphosphate (chelating agent) for prevention and removal of calcium ions.

Table F.II (*contd*)

Name of solutions and sizes available	Manufacturer	Preservatives with percentage concentration	Remarks
Lensept, 240 ml (Septicon system)	CIBA Vision		Hydrogen peroxide 3% solution used for 20 min followed by soak in Lensrins with platinum disc to neutralize residual hydrogen peroxide or Lensept Neutralising Solution
used with			
Lensrins	CIBA Vision	THI 0.001; EDTA 0.1	
Lensrins NT	CIBA Vision	EDTA 0.1; SA 0.1	
Hydrosoak, 10 ml, 120 ml	CIBA Vision	CHX 0.0025; EDTA 0.128; THI 0.0025	
Medisoak, 35 ml, 120 ml	CIBA Vision	CHX 0.0025; EDTA 0.128; THI 0.0025	Belgium and Germany only
Mirasept 1, 120 ml, 250 ml	CIBA Vision		Hydrogen peroxide 3%
Hydron Soft Lens Soaking, 120 ml	Hydron Europe	CHX 0.0025; EDTA 0.128; THI 0.0025	
ICN Unicare (blue), 25 ml, 240 ml	ICN Pharmaceuticals	EDTA ?; THI 0.0015	Combined cleaning and storage
ICN Unisept, 240 ml	ICN Pharmaceuticals	EDTA ?; H_2O_2 3.0; cleansing agent 0.0025	Recommended in combination with ICN Unirins
ICN Unirins, 240 ml	ICN Pharmaceuticals	EDTA ?; THI 0.001; catalytic enzyme 0.3%	In combination with ICN Unisept
ICN Unisoft, 25 ml, 240 ml	ICN Pharmaceuticals	EDTA ?; THI 0.0015	In combination with ICN Uniclean
Murine Puresept, 237 ml	Ross Labs	H_2O_2 3.0	
Steri-Sal, 110 ml	Sauflon Pharmaceuticals	CHX 0.001; EDTA 0.1; THI 0.002	
Steri-Sal 2, 110 ml	Sauflon Pharmaceuticals	CHX 0.002; EDTA 0.1; THI 0.002	
Steri-Soft Soaking Solution, 110 ml, 250 ml	Sauflon Pharmaceuticals	EDTA 0.1; NIPA 0.02	Not available in UK
Aerotab (32/pack)	Sauflon Pharmaceuticals	HAL 0.16 mg	Effervescent tablets (8 ppm available chlorine)
Prymesoak, 120 ml	Smith & Nephew	CHX 0.002	
Silicone lenses			
Silicolens, 120 ml	Alcon	EDTA 0.1; THI 0.004	
Consil Wetting and Storage, 90 ml	Barnes–Hind	CHX 0.005; EDTA 0.1; THI 0.001	Europe only

Name of solutions and sizes available	Manufacturer	Preservatives with percentage concentration	Suitable for boiling
Preserved saline solution (which is used for rinsing)			
(Most of the disinfecting and storage solutions are basically preserved physiological saline solutions, also suitable for rinsing)			
Alcon Preserved Saline	Alcon	SA 0.1; EDTA 0.1	Yes
Boil-N-Soak, 240 ml	Alcon	EDTA 0.1; THI 0.001	Yes
Normol, 175 ml, 250 ml	Alcon	CHX 0.005; EDTA 0.1; THI 0.001	No
Thermosal, 250 ml	Alcon	EDTA 0.1; THI 0.001	Yes
Nutraflow, 110 ml	Alcon	EDTA 0.1; S A 0.1	Yes
Sorbisal Saline Solution, 240 ml*	Allergan	S A 0.1	Yes

* Contains sodium hexametaphosphate (chelating agent) for prevention and removal of calcium ions.

Table F.II (*contd*)

Name of solutions and sizes available	Manufacturer	Preservatives with percentage concentration	Suitable for boiling
Oxysept 2, 235 ml	Allergan	EDTA 0.1; THI 0.001‡	No
Hydrocare Preserved Saline 240 ml*	Allergan	EDTA 0.01; THI 0.001	Yes
Oxysept 2 Unit Dose, 25 × 15 ml	Allergan	‡	Preservative-free neutralizer Buffered
Consept 2, Aerosol, 240 ml	Barnes–Hind	†	Unpreserved
Soft-Therm, 240 ml†	Barnes–Hind	EDTA 0.1; THI 0.001	Yes (UK only)
Soft Mate PS Saline, 240 ml	Barnes–Hind	EDTA 0.025; PS 0.13	Yes (not available in UK)
Soft Mate Consept 2 360 ml	Barnes–Hind	CHX 0.001; †	
HP 2 (Quik Sept 2), 120 ml, 240 ml†	Bausch & Lomb	Dymed 0.00004	No
Sensitive Eyes Saline, 120 ml, 240 ml, 355 ml	Bausch & Lomb	EDTA 0.1; THI 0.001	Yes
Contactasol 10.10 Rinsing and Neutralising Solution, 15 ml unit dose	CIBA Vision		Preservative-free neutralizer containing 0.5% sodium pyruvate
Lensept Neutraliser, 120 ml, 240 ml	CIBA Vision	EDTA, 0.2; SA 0.1‡	No
Lensan B, 130 ml	CIBA Vision	THI 0.001‡	
In A Wink Neutralising Rinse, 240 ml	CIBA Vision	EDTA 0.2; SA 0.1‡	No
Titmus H_2O_2 Solution 2, 10 ml unit dose	CIBA Vision	‡	Preservative-free neutralizer
Mirasol, 120 ml, 250 ml	CIBA Vision	EDTA 0.1; S A 0.1; THI 0.001	No
ICN Eyefresh, 240 ml	ICN Pharmaceuticals	EDTA ?; THI 0.001	No
Murine Preserved All-Purpose Saline, 237 ml, 355 ml	Ross Labs	EDTA 0.1; SA 0.1	Yes, buffered

Name of solutions and sizes available	Manufacturer	Preservatives with percentage concentration	Remarks
Sterile unpreserved saline solution (for rinsing and heat disinfection)			
Amidose, 30 ml	Abatron	–	Screw-capped tubes
Polyrinse, 15 ml	Alcon (France, Germany)		Unit dose
Alcon Aerosol Saline (Opti-pure), 240 ml	Alcon		Aerosol can
Isosol Saline, 20 × 20 ml	Allergan		Unit dose (buffered)
Isosol Plus Saline, 20 × 10 ml	Allergan		Unit dose (buffered)
Lens Plus, 90 ml, 360 ml	Allergan		Aerosol (buffered)
Soft Mate Unpreserved 30 × 15 ml	Barnes–Hind		Unit dose (buffered)
Soft Mate Saline Spray, 90 ml, 360 ml	Barnes–Hind	–	Aerosol (buffered)
B & L Aerosol Saline, 90ml, 240 ml, 360 ml	Bausch & Lomb	–	
B & L Saline plus, 500 ml	Bausch & Lomb	EDTA 0.11	Buffered

* Contains sodium hexametaphosphate (chelating agent) for prevention and removal of calcium ions.
† Contains 0.5% sodium thiosulphate as neutralizer for hydrogen peroxide.
‡ Contains catalase as neutralizer for hydrogen peroxide

Table F.II (*contd*)

Name of solutions and sizes available	Manufacturer	Preservatives with percentage concentration	Remarks
Solar Saline, 275 ml, 115 ml	CIBA Vision		Aerosol (buffered)
Hydron non-preserved Sterile Saline, 250 ml	Hydron Europe (Allergan)	–	Aerosol can (unbuffered)
Hydron Stabilised Saline, 250 ml	Hydron Europe (Allergan)		Aerosol can (buffered)
Sauflon Saline Solution, 300 ml	Sauflon Pharmaceuticals	–	Aerosol can (buffered)
Salettes, 10 ml	Sauflon Pharmaceuticals	–	Sachets
Sauflon Saline Solution, 10 ml	Sauflon Pharmaceuticals	–	Sachets

Daily cleaning solutions (for use on removal of the lenses from the eyes)
(These solutions may also be used with hard and RGP lenses, subject to the provisions stated in Table F.I)

Hydrophilic lenses

Name of solutions and sizes available	Manufacturer	Preservatives with percentage concentration	Remarks
Amiclean gel, 15 ml	Abatron	PMN 0.002	Screw-capped tube
Amiclean solution, 10 ml, 60 ml	Abatron	CHX 0.005; EDTA 0.01; THI 0.01	
Preflex, 10 ml, 45 ml	Alcon	EDTA 0.2; THI 0.004	
Pliagel, 25 ml	Alcon	EDTA 0.5; SA 0.1	
Polyclens (Opti-Clean), 12 ml, 24 ml	Alcon	EDTA 0.1; THI 0.004	Contains polymeric beads
Polyclens II (Opti-Clean II), 12 ml, 24 ml	Alcon	EDTA 0.1; Polyquad 0.001	Contains polymeric beads
LC 65, 15 ml, 30 ml, 60 ml	Allergan	EDTA 0.01; THI 0.001	
Oxyclean Daily Cleaner, 15 ml	Allergan	Self-preserving	
SorbiClean Daily Cleaner, 30 ml	Allergan	EDTA 0.2; SA 0.1	
Cleaner No.4 (Softmate), 35 ml	Barnes–Hind	EDTA 0.2; THI 0.004	UK only
Soft Mate PS Daily Cleaner, 35 ml	Barnes–Hind	PS 0.13	
Daily Cleaner, 30 ml	Bausch & Lomb	EDTA 0.2; SA 2.5	
Boots Soft Lens Cleaner, 35 ml	Boots	CHX 0.0025; EDTA 0.128; THI 0.0025	
Hydroclean, 35 ml	CIBA Vision	CHX 0.0025; EDTA 0.1; THI 0.0025	
Miraflow, 10 ml, 15 ml, 25 ml, 35 ml	CIBA Vision	Self-preserving	Contains 20% isopropyl alcohol
Mediclean, 20 ml, 35 ml	CIBA Vision	CHX 0.0025; EDTA 0.1; THI 0.0025	Belgium and Germany only
Hoya Soft Cleaner, 60 ml	Hoya	EDTA 0.1; SA 0.1	
Hydron Soft Lens Cleaning, 20 ml	Hydron Europe (Allergan)	CHX 0.0025; EDTA 0.128; THI 0.0025	
ICN Uniclean, 5 ml, 60 ml	ICN Pharmaceuticals	EDTA ?; THI 0.0015	Universal cleanser of hard, soft and RGP lenses
Sterisoft Cleaning, 20/60 ml	Sauflon Pharmaceuticals	EDTA 0.1; NIPA 0.02	Not available in UK
Sauflon Soft Lens Daily Cleaner, 20 ml	Sauflon Pharmaceuticals	EDTA 0.1; THI 0.004	
Steri-Solv, 60 ml	Sauflon Pharmaceuticals	EDTA 0.1; THI 0.004	
Prymeclean, 10 ml	Smith & Nephew	CHX 0.002	Active ingredient poloxamer 0.5%

Table F.II (*contd*)

Name of solutions and sizes available	Manufacturer	Preservatives with percentage concentration	Remarks
Silicone lenses			
Silclens, 45 ml	Alcon	EDTA 0.2; THI 0.004	
Consil Clean, 35 ml	Barnes–Hind	THI 0.001	UK only
Occasional cleaners (those which do not involve heating are also suitable for hard lenses)			
Amiclair tablets used with Amiclair-O, 200 ml, sterile purified water	Abatron	EDTA 0.074	Contains the chelating agent EDTA, and three enzymes; a lipase, and two proteases, one being pronase for removal of lipids, mucin and protein
Polyzym (Opti-Zyme)	Alcon	Pancreatin	Triphasic, acts against protein, lipids, mucin
Clean-O-Gel, powder in pouches	Alcon		Contains a lipase and surfactant
Liprofin, powder in sachets	Alcon		Oxidizing agent used hot or cold Unsuitable for Menicon soft lenses. For practitioner use only
Hydrocare Protein (Enzyme) Remover Tablets	Allergan		Contains papain, a proteolytic enzyme Also marketed as Bausch & Lomb protein removal tablets
Ultrazyme Protein Remover Tablets	Allergan		Active ingredient subtilisin A Suitable for dissolving in hydrogen peroxide
Soft Mate Weekly Cleaner (Intensive Cleaner)	Barnes–Hind	EDTA 0.1; THI 0.001	Surfactant combination
Soft Mate Protein Remover, 8 × 8 ml, 12 × 8 ml	Barnes–Hind	–	Surfactant combination unpreserved
Sensitive Eyes Effervescent Cleaning Tablets (Renu Effervescent)	Bausch & Lomb		Subtilisin B 25 mg/tab
Sensitive Eyes Thermal Cleaning Tablets (Renu Thermal)	Bausch & Lomb		Subtilisin B 25 mg/tab
Sauflon Enzyme Tablets	Sauflon Pharmaceuticals		Contains EDTA (chelating), lipase (esterase), mucolytic enzyme (glycosidase), protease (pancreatin)
Monoclens powder in sachets	Sauflon Pharmaceuticals	EDTA; S P	Oxidizing system using heat for practitioner use only
Prymecare protein remover tablets, 8, 16	Smith & Nephew		Contain papain for protein removal
Re-wetting solutions (these may be used for hard and RGP lenses)			
Amilis Wetting, 20 ml	Abatron	PMN 0.003	
Adapettes, 2 ml, 15 ml	Alcon	EDTA 0.1; THI 0.004	
Opti-Tears, 15 ml	Alcon	Dextran; EDTA 0.1; Polyquad 0.001	Known as Opti-Free Comfort Drops in Australia

Table F.II (*contd*)

Name of solutions and sizes available	Manufacturer	Preservatives with percentage concentration	Remarks
Soft Mate PS Comfort Drops, 15 ml	Barnes–Hind	EDTA 0.1; PS 0.13	Not available in UK
Soft Lens Comfort Drops, 15 ml	Barnes–Hind	EDTA 0.1; THI 0.004	Available UK only
Lens Lubricant	Barnes–Hind	EDTA 0.1; THI 0.004	
Bausch & Lomb Lubricant, 15 ml	Bausch & Lomb	S A 2.5	
Boots Comfort Drops, 10 ml	Boots	CHX 0.0025; EDTA 0.128; THI 0.0025	
Hydrosol, 20 ml	CIBA Vision	CHX 0.0025; EDTA 0.1; THI 0.0025	Intended to be rubbed into lens surfaces prior to wear
Clerz, 15 ml, 25 ml	CIBA Vision	EDTA 0.1; S A 0.1	Available as single dose units
Hydron Soft Lens Comfort, 20 ml	Hydron Europe (Allergan)	CHX 0.0025; EDTA 0.128; THI 0.0025	
Sterifresh, 10 ml	Sauflon Pharmaceuticals	CHX 0.001; EDTA 0.1; THI 0.002	
Vit-A-Drops, 15 ml	Vision Pharmaceuticals	Preservative-free	Contains 5000 IU vitamin A and Polysorbate 80

ATAC, alkyl triethanol ammonium chloride; B A, benzoic acid; CHB, chlorbutol; CHX, chlorhexidine gluconate; EDTA, ethylenediamine tetraacetic acid; IOD, iodine; NIPA, Nipastat; PMN, phenylmercuric nitrate; POV, povidone; PS, potassium sorbate; S A, sorbic acid; SP, sodium perborate; THI, thimerosal.

Table F.III Drugs used in contact lens practice

Drug	Concentrations used (%)	Legal category	Use by UK Optometrists	Available in single dose units
Topical anaesthetics				
Amethocaine hydrochloride	0.5, 1.0	POM	U	Yes
Proxymetacaine hydrochloride	0.5	POM	U	No
Oxybuprocaine hydrochloride	0.5	POM	U	Yes
Lignocaine hydrochloride	4.0	POM	U	Only combined with 0.25% fluorescein
Conjunctival decongestants (vasoconstrictors) (see also Table F.I)				
Adrenaline acid tartrate	0.1	P	U/S	No
Naphazoline hydrochloride	0.1	POM	U/S	No
Xylometazoline hydrochloride	0.05			
with antazoline sulphate	0.5	P	U/S	No
Diagnostic staining agents				
Fluorescein sodium	1.0, 2.0	P	U/S	Yes, and as paper strips
Rose bengal	1.0	P	U/S	Yes
Chemotherapeutic (antimicrobial) agents				
Drops				
Framycetin sulphate	0.5	POM	U	No
Mafenide propionate	5.0	POM	U/S	No
Sulphacetamide sodium	10.0, 15.0, 20.0, 30.0	POM	U/S	Only in 10% strength
Sulphacetamide sodium	5.0			
with zinc sulphate	0.1	POM	U/S	No
and cetrimide	0.01			
Propamide isethionate	0.1	P	U/S	No
Ointments				
Framycetin sulphate	0.5	POM	U	No
Sulphacetamide sodium	2.5, 6.0, 10.0	POM	U/S	No
Dibromopropamidine isethionate	0.15	P	U/S	No
Miscellaneous agents				
Hypertonic saline solution				
Sodium chloride	2.0, 5.0	POM	U	No

P, Pharmacy medicine; POM, Prescription Only Medicine; U, use only; U/S, use and supply for prophylaxis only. More details of the following ophthalmic preparations mentioned in Chapter 4 are obtainable from *Mims*, published monthly by Haymarket Publishing Limited, Medical Division, 76 Dean Street, London W1A 1BU, and the *Data Sheet Compendium* published yearly by the Association of the British Pharmaceutical Industry (Pharmind Publications). These publications give brand names and names of the various manufacturing drug houses, as well as strengths, dosages, legal categories, contra-indications, side effects etc.

Index